Clinical Cardiogenetics

Hubert F. Baars
Pieter A. F. M. Doevendans
Arjan C. Houweling • J. Peter van Tintelen
Editors

Clinical Cardiogenetics

Third Edition

Springer

Editors
Hubert F. Baars
Director of the DNA Clinic
Bosch en Duin
The Netherlands

Consultant Cardiologist at the Outpatient
Clinic for Cardiogenetics
The Hague
The Netherlands

Consultant Cardiologist at the
OLVG Hospital
Amsterdam
The Netherlands

Arjan C. Houweling
Amsterdam University Medical Center
Amsterdam
The Netherlands

Pieter A. F. M. Doevendans
Utrecht University
Utrecht
The Netherlands

J. Peter van Tintelen
University Medical Center Utrecht
Utrecht
The Netherlands

ISBN 978-3-030-45459-3 ISBN 978-3-030-45457-9 (eBook)
https://doi.org/10.1007/978-3-030-45457-9

This Springer imprint is published by the registered company Springer Nature Switzerland AG
The registered company address is: Gewerbestrasse 11, 6330 Cham, Switzerland

Preface

Dear colleagues,

Four years after the release of the second edition of Clinical Cardiogenetics we are proud to present this updated third edition. The majority of the chapters have been extensively revised and updated in accordance with recent developments, insights, and guidelines. In addition, separate chapters on metabolic cardiomyopathies, cardiac amyloidosis, preimplantation genetic diagnostics, and a chapter on induced pluripotent stem cells have been added. These chapters emphasize the expanding horizon of clinical cardiogenetics.

In addition, we have also attempted to create a more uniform chapter layout throughout this edition of Clinical Cardiogenetics. With contributions of worldwide leading experts in their fields, we believe this textbook will provide an up-to-date and useful reference for those interested in the field of cardiogenetics. We expect this third edition will provide the reader guidance to cope with challenges in their day-to-day work.

The Hague, The Netherlands	Hubert F. Baars
Utrecht, The Netherlands	Pieter A. F. M. Doevendans
Amsterdam, The Netherlands	Arjan C. Houweling
Utrecht, The Netherlands	J. Peter van Tintelen

Contents

Contributors

Y. Arens Department of Clinical Genetics, Maastricht University Medical Center, Maastricht, Netherlands

Annette F. Baas Department of Clinical Genetics, University Medical Center Utrecht, Utrecht, The Netherlands

Geerthe Margriet Balk Department of Cardiology, Division Heart and Lungs, University Medical Center Utrecht, Utrecht, Netherlands

Elijah R. Behr Cardiovascular Medicine, Cardiology Clinical Academic Group, St. George's, University of London, London, UK

St. George's University Hospitals NHS Foundation Trust, London, UK

Andreas C. Blank Division Pediatrics, Wilhelmina Children's Hospital, University Medical Center Utrecht, Utrecht, The Netherlands

Lennart J. Blom Department of Cardiology, University Medical Center Utrecht, Utrecht, The Netherlands

G. Bonne Center of Research in Myology, Sorbonne Université, INSERM UMRS 974, Paris, France, Institut de Myologie, Paris, France

R.L. Braam Gelre Hospitals, ApeldoornThe Netherlands

Johannes M.P.J. Breur Division Pediatrics, Wilhelmina Children's Hospital, University Medical Center Utrecht, Utrecht, The Netherlands

Josep Brugada Centro de Investigación Biomédica en Red de Enfermedades Cardiovasculares (CIBERCV), Madrid, Spain

Arrhythmia Unit, Hospital Sant Joan de Déu, University of Barcelona, Barcelona, Spain

Arrhythmia Section, Cardiovascular Institute, Hospital Clinic, University of Barcelona, Barcelona, Catalonia, Spain

Ramon Brugada Cardiovascular Genetics Centre, University of Girona-IDIBGI, Girona, Spain

Medical Science Department, School of Medicine, University of Girona, Girona, Spain

Centro de Investigación Biomédica en Red de Enfermedades Cardiovasculares (CIBERCV), Madrid, Spain

Familial Cardiomyopathies Unit, Hospital Josep Trueta de Girona, Girona, Spain

Jan Willem Buikema Department of Cardiology, Division Heart and Lungs, University Medical Center Utrecht, Utrecht, Netherlands

Julia Cadrin-Tourigny Cardiovascular Genetics Center, Montreal Heart Institute, Montréal, Canada, Department of Medicine, Université de Montréal, Montréal, Canada

Oscar Campuzano Cardiovascular Genetics Centre, University of Girona-IDIBGI, Girona, Spain

Medical Science Department, School of Medicine, University of Girona, Girona, Spain

Centro de Investigación Biomédica en Red de Enfermedades Cardiovasculares (CIBERCV), Madrid, Spain

Imke Christiaans Department of Clinical Genetics, University Medical Centre Groningen, Groningen, The Netherlands

Jason R. Cowan Dorothy M. Davis Heart and Lung Research Institute, The Ohio State University College of Medicine, Columbus, OH, USA

Divisions of Human Genetics, The Ohio State University College of Medicine, Columbus, OH, USA

Moniek G.P.J. Cox Department of Cardiology, University Medical Center Utrecht, Utrecht, The Netherlands

Netherlands Heart Institute, Utrecht, The Netherlands

A.J. Cupido Department of Vascular Medicine, Academic Medical Center, University of Amsterdam, Amsterdam, The Netherlands

Julie De Backer Department of Cardiology and Center for Medical Genetics, Ghent University Hospital, Ghent, Belgium

Isabelle Denjoy AP-HP, Hôpital Bichat, Département de Cardiologie et Centre de Référence des Maladies Cardiaques Héréditaires, Université Paris Diderot, Sorbonne Paris Cité, Paris, France

Pieter A. F. M. Doevendans Department of Cardiology, Division Heart and Lungs, University Medical Center Utrecht, Utrecht, Netherlands

Netherlands Heart Institute, Utrecht, Netherlands

Perry M. Elliott Institute for Cardiovascular Science, University College London, London, UK

Jeanette Erdmann Institute for Cardiogenetics, University of Lübeck, Lübeck, Germany

Sabine A. Fuchs Division Pediatrics, Wilhelmina Children's Hospital (Part of UMC Utrecht), Utrecht, The Netherlands

Tjeerd Germans Department of Cardiology, Northwest Clinics Alkmaar, Amsterdam University Medical Centres, Amsterdam, The Netherlands

Michael H. Gollob Inherited Arrhythmia and Cardiomyopathy Program, Peter Munk Cardiac Centre, Division of Cardiology, Toronto General Hospital, University of Toronto, Toronto, ON, Canada

Rutger J. Hassink Department of Cardiology, University Medical Center Utrecht, Utrecht, The Netherlands

Richard N.W. Hauer Department of Cardiology, University Medical Center Utrecht, Utrecht, The Netherlands

Netherlands Heart Institute, Utrecht, The Netherlands

Ray E. Hershberger Dorothy M. Davis Heart and Lung Research Institute, The Ohio State University College of Medicine, Columbus, OH, USA

Divisions of Human Genetics, The Ohio State University College of Medicine, Columbus, OH, USA

Cardiovascular Medicine, Department of Internal Medicine, The Ohio State University College of Medicine, Columbus, OH, USA

Masayasu Hiraoka Tokyo Medical and Dental University, Bunkyo-ku, Tokyo, Japan

Yvonne M. Hoedemaekers Department of Clinical Genetics, Radboudumc, Radboud University Nijmegen, Nijmegen, The Netherlands

Jodie Ingles Agnes Ginges Centre for Molecular Cardiology, Centenary Institute, Sydney, NSW, Australia

Sydney Medical School, University of Sydney, Sydney, NSW, Australia

Department of Cardiology, Royal Prince Alfred Hospital, Sydney, NSW, Australia

Jan D.H. Jongbloed Department of Genetics, University Medical Center Groningen, University of Groningen, Groningen, The Netherlands

Daniel P. Judge Charleston, SC, USA

J.J.P. Kastelein Department of Vascular Medicine, Amsterdam University Medical Centers - location AMC, University of Amsterdam, Amsterdam, The Netherlands

Klaas Koop Division Pediatrics, Wilhelmina Children's Hospital, University Medical Center Utrecht, Utrecht, The Netherlands

Antoine Leenhardt Cardiology Department, APHP, Hopital Bichat, Refering Centre for Cardiac Hereditary Diseases, Paris Sorbonne University, Paris, France

Ronald H. Lekanne Deprez Department of Clinical Genetics, Academic Medical Center, University of Amsterdam, Amsterdam, The Netherlands

Krystien V. Lieve Department of Clinical and Experimental Cardiology, Amsterdam Cardiovascular Sciences, Amsterdam UMC, University of Amsterdam, Heart Centre, Amsterdam, The Netherlands

Aleš Linhart First Faculty of Medicine, Charles University, General University Hospital, Prague, Czech Republic

Bart Loeys Center of Medical Genetics, Faculty of Medicine and Health Sciences, University of Antwerp and Antwerp University Hospital, Antwerp, Belgium

Department of Human Genetics, Radboud University Nijmegen Medical Center, Nijmegen, The Netherlands

Alice Maltret M3C-Necker, Hôpital Universitaire Necker Enfants Malades, Université Paris Descartes, Paris, France

Michelle Michels Department of Cardiology, Erasmus Medical Centre, Rotterdam, The Netherlands

Barbara J.M. Mulder Department of Cardiology, Academic Medical Centre, Amsterdam, The Netherlands

E.A. Nannenberg Department of Clinical Genetics, Amsterdam UMC, University of Amsterdam, AZ, Amsterdam, Netherlands

Klaus Neef Department of Cardiology, Division Heart and Lungs, University Medical Center Utrecht, Utrecht, Netherlands

Toon Oomen Antonius Hospital Sneek, Sneek, Netherlands

Ana J. Pérez Matos Antonius Hospital Sneek, Sneek, Netherlands

J.G. Post Gelre Hospitals, ApeldoornThe Netherlands, University Medical Center Utrecht, Utrecht, The Netherlands

Jason D. Roberts Arrhythmia Service, Division of Cardiology, University of Western Ontario, London, ON, Canada

Jolien Roos-Hesselink Department of Cardiology, Erasmus Medical Centre, Rotterdam, The Netherlands

Georgia Sarquella-Brugada Arrhythmia Unit, Hospital Sant Joan de Déu, University of Barcelona, Barcelona, Spain

Tetsuo Sasano Department of Cardiovascular Medicine, Tokyo Medical and Dental University, Bunkyo-ku, Tokyo, Japan

Eric Schulze-Bahr Klinikum Ludwigsburg, Department of Medicine – Cardiology, Ludwigsburg, Germany

Institut für Genetik von Herzerkrankungen (IfGH), Universitätsklinikum Münster (UKM), Münster, Germany

Heribert Schunkert Deutsches Herzzentrum München, Klinik für Herz- und Kreislauferkrankungen, Technische Universität München, Munich, Germany

Joost P.G. Sluijter Department of Cardiology, Division Heart and Lungs, University Medical Center Utrecht, Utrecht, Netherlands

R.M. Stoekenbroek Department of Vascular Medicine, Amsterdam University Medical Centers - location AMC, University of Amsterdam, Amsterdam, The Netherlands

Rafik Tadros Cardiovascular Genetics Center, Montreal Heart Institute, Montréal, Canada

Department of Medicine, Université de Montréal, Montréal, Canada

Department of Experimental and Clinical Cardiology, Academic Medical Center, Amsterdam, Netherlands

Anneline S.J.M. te Riele Department of Cardiology, University Medical Center Utrecht, Utrecht, The Netherlands, Netherlands Heart Institute, Utrecht, The Netherlands

Ingrid M.B.H. van de Laar Department of Clinical Genetics, Erasmus Medical Center, Rotterdam, The Netherlands

Maarten P. van den Berg Departments of Genetics (P.A.v.d.Z.) and Cardiology (M.P.v.d.B.), University Medical Center Groningen, University of Groningen, Groningen, The Netherlands

A.J. van der Kooi Amsterdam UMC, Academic Medical Center (AMC), Neuroscience Institute, University of Amsterdam, Amsterdam, The Netherlands

J.J. van der Smagt University Medical Centre Utrecht, Utrecht, The Netherlands

Christian van der Werf Department of Clinical and Experimental Cardiology, Amsterdam Cardiovascular Sciences, Amsterdam UMC, University of Amsterdam, Heart Centre, Amsterdam, The Netherlands

Paul A. van der Zwaag Departments of Genetics (P.A.v.d.Z.) and Cardiology (M.P.v.d.B.), University Medical Center Groningen, University of Groningen, Groningen, The Netherlands

Alain van Mil Department of Cardiology, Division Heart and Lungs, University Medical Center Utrecht, Utrecht, Netherlands

Karin Y. van Spaendonck-Zwarts Department of Clinical Genetics, Amsterdam University Medical Centre, Amsterdam, The Netherlands

Genetic Health Queensland, Royal Brisbane and Women's Hospital, Herston, QLD, Australia

J. Peter van Tintelen University Medical Center Utrecht, Department of Genetics, Sneek, The Netherlands

S.M. Schade van Westrum Amsterdam UMC, Academic Medical Center (AMC), Neuroscience Institute, University of Amsterdam, Amsterdam, The Netherlands

Matteo Vatta Invitae Corporation, San Francisco, CA, USA

Department of Medical and Molecular Genetics, Indiana University School of Medicine, Indianapolis, IN, USA

Department of Medicine, Indiana University School of Medicine, Indianapolis, IN, USA

Aline Verstraeten Center of Medical Genetics, Faculty of Medicine and Health Sciences, University of Antwerp and Antwerp University Hospital, Antwerp, Belgium

Aryan Vink Department of Pathology, University Medical Center Utrecht, Utrecht, The Netherlands

K. Wahbi APHP, Cochin Hospital, Cardiology Department, FILNEMUS, Paris-Descartes, Sorbonne Paris Cité University, Paris, France

Yanushi D. Wijeyeratne Cardiovascular Medicine, Cardiology Clinical Academic Group, St. George's, University of London, London, UK

St. George's University Hospitals NHS Foundation Trust, LondonUK

Christian Wolpert Klinikum Ludwigsburg, Department of Medicine – Cardiology, Ludwigsburg, Germany

Institut für Genetik von Herzerkrankungen (IfGH), Universitätsklinikum Münster (UKM), Münster, Germany

Liza S.M. Wong Amsterdam, The Netherlands

Part I

Genetics

Introduction to Molecular Genetics

1

Jan D. H. Jongbloed, Ronald H. Lekanne Deprez, and Matteo Vatta

Introduction

In recent years, comprehensive developments in genetics vastly improved our knowledge of inherited human diseases, including genetic cardiac disorders. While previously only one to several candidate genes could be studied to search for putative disease-causing mutations, currently whole-exome sequencing (WES) and whole-genome sequencing (WGS) enable the analysis of all variants within a personal genome, including those predisposing to disease. Important in this respect is the fact that the sequencing of a full genome can now be performed in reasonable time and at a relatively low cost, as the $1000 genome is nowadays within reach. Moreover, this and other genotyping techniques provide the possibility to identify variants, modifiers, which have an effect on disease development by either leading to more severe symptoms or protecting carriers of pathogenic mutations from getting seriously ill. Interestingly, these developments also confronted the clinical genetics community with the challenges of handling "big data" and building bioinformatics tools and methods to extract the truly relevant ones from the wealth of variants identified using these techniques. The identification of disease-associated genes in unsolved families no longer requires linkage (-like) techniques. Moreover, with the rapidly growing numbers of reported disease-associated genes and gene variants, we are challenged to distinguish the definitely disease-causing ones from (relatively) innocent variants. The latter demands intelligent genomic *in silico* solutions, as well as "old-fashioned" wet but preferably high-throughput laboratory experimental setups to functionally study the effect of identified variants. Gene and variant curation remains one of the important goals for the near future. Logically, in the field of inherited cardiac disorders, to perform this properly, close collaboration between cardiologists (and other clinical specialists involved), clinical geneticists/genetic counselors, and laboratory specialists is essential. In the following paragraphs, the abovementioned topics and challenges will be addressed.

J. D. H. Jongbloed (✉)
Department of Genetics, University Medical Center Groningen, University of Groningen, Groningen, The Netherlands
e-mail: j.d.h.jongbloed@umcg.nl

R. H. Lekanne Deprez
Department of Clinical Genetics, Academic Medical Center, University of Amsterdam, Amsterdam, The Netherlands
e-mail: r.h.lekanne@amc.uva.nl

M. Vatta
Invitae Corporation, San Francisco, CA, USA

Department of Medical and Molecular Genetics, Indiana University School of Medicine, Indianapolis, IN, USA

Department of Medicine, Indiana University School of Medicine, Indianapolis, IN, USA
e-mail: mvatta@iu.edu

DNA, RNA, and Proteins

All information necessary to "build" a human is secured within genomic and mitochondrial DNA (deoxyribonucleic acid) and the variation on that theme therefore too. The simple concept, however, of parts of the DNA (the genes) being transcribed into RNA molecules that provide the prescriptions to produce proteins that then form the building blocks of this complex organism is no longer valid. In reality, the situation is much more complex. Both other genetic factors, like regulatory RNAs (ribonucleic acids) and imprinting processes, and nongenetic factors like metabolites and other environmental influences have important effects on the final outcome of the information captured in genes. In this paragraph, the basic principles of the molecular factors involved will be described and their interplay discussed.

DNA molecules are composed of four nucleotides, which all consist of a deoxyribose and a phosphate group, together forming the sugar-phosphate backbone of the molecule, and vary in the base side chains adenine (A), guanine (G), cytosine (C), or thymine (T) (see Fig. 1.1). These nucleotides are connected via phosphodiester linkages, and the resulting nucleic acid strands entwine each other in an antiparallel

H. F. Baars et al. (eds.), *Clinical Cardiogenetics*, https://doi.org/10.1007/978-3-030-45457-9_1

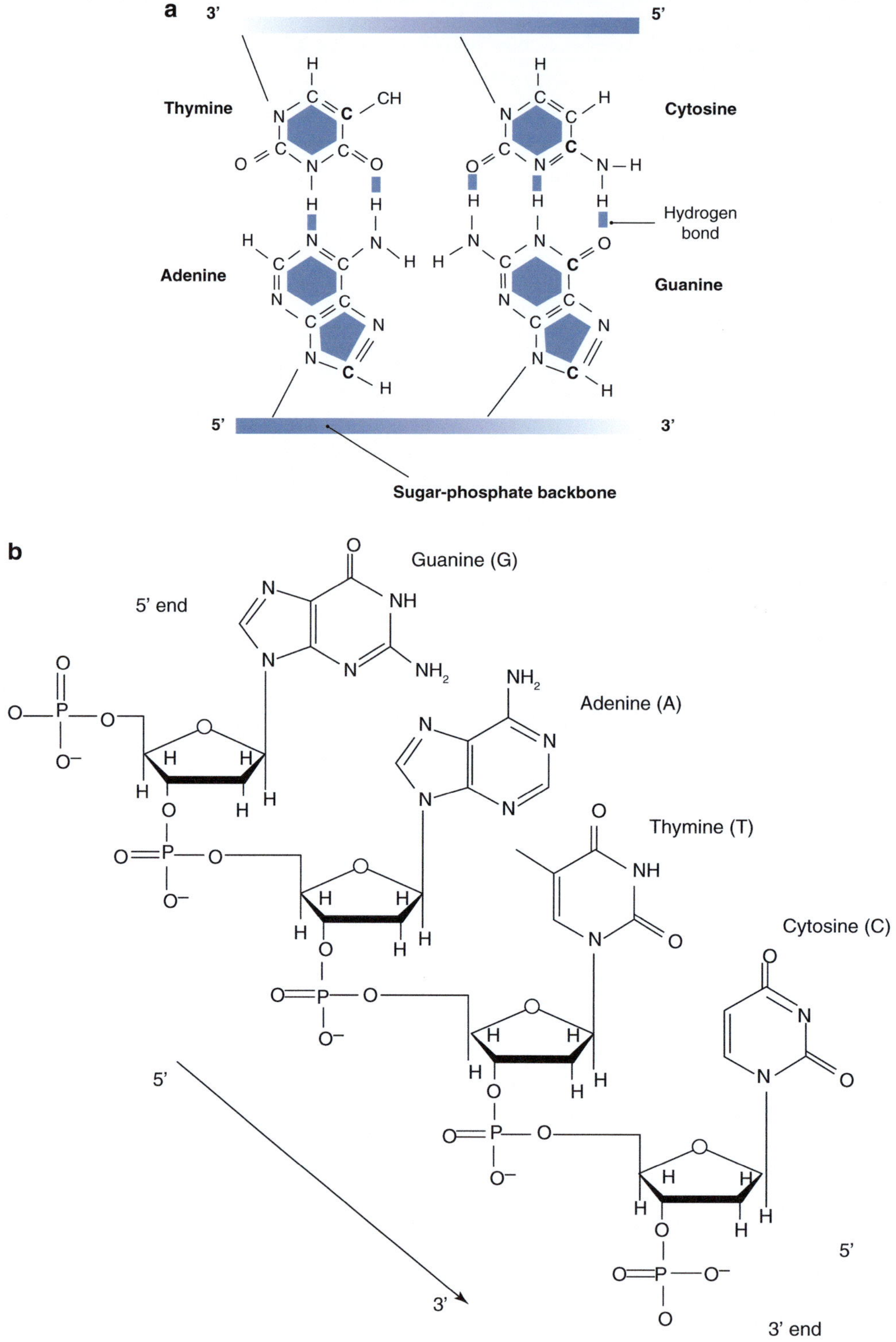

Fig. 1.1 Structure of DNA. A base (C, T, A, or G) combined with a deoxyribose and a phosphate group is called a nucleotide. These nucleotides are polymerized through phosphodiester linkage. DNA is read from the 5′ to the 3′ end. (**a**) The four bases that make up the actual DNA code. Alanine always pairs with thymine with two hydrogen bonds, and cytosine always pairs with guanine using three hydrogen bonds. (**b**) Chemical structure of DNA, showing the sugar backbone and the polymerization through phosphodiester linkage; as DNA is read in 5′–3′ direction, the code of this stretch of DNA would read GATC. (**c**) DNA double-helix structure; the base pairs in the middle are aligned around the helical axis. The major and minor grooves are the result of imperfect winding of the helix. Adapted from Clinical Cardiogenetics edition 2011

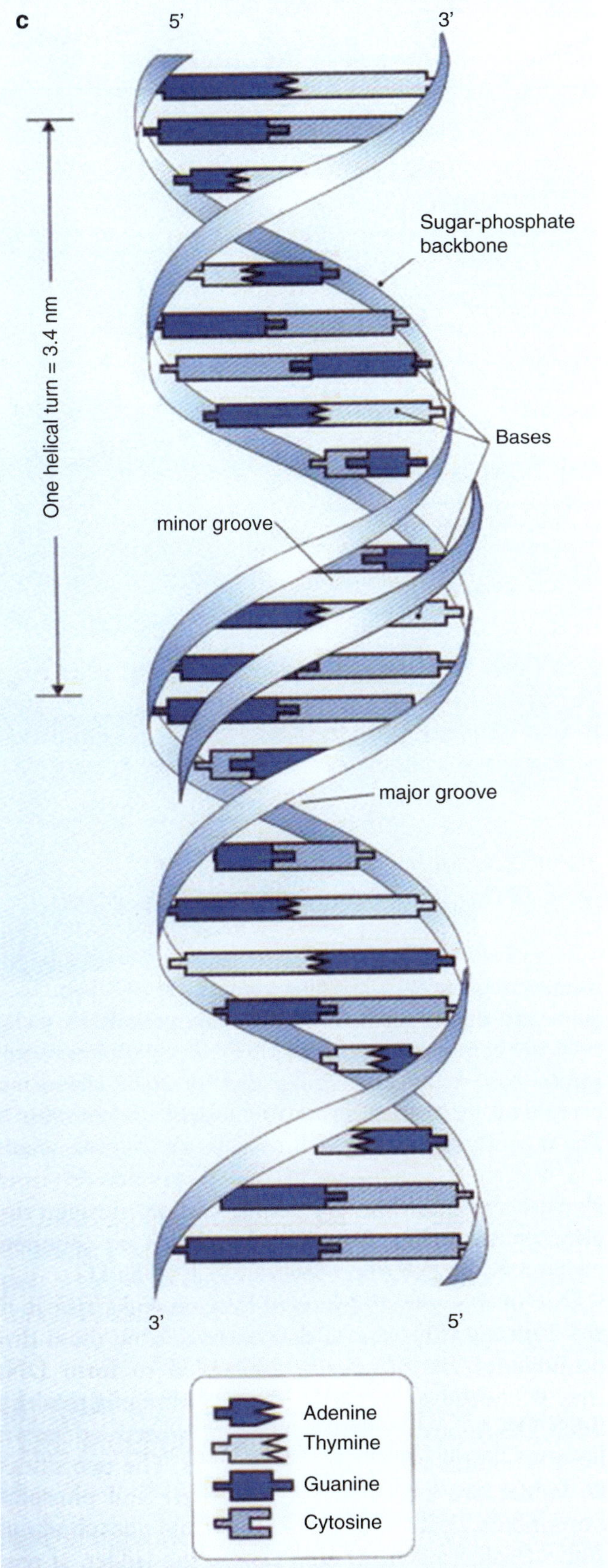

Fig. 1.1 (continued)

fashion, leading to the very stable double-helix structure first described by Watson and Crick in 1953. The antiparallel pairing, meaning that these strands run in opposite directions (5′–3′ vs. 3′–5′), of the nucleotide strands is mediated via hydrogen bonds between adenine and thymine or guanine and cytosine bases. As AT pairs are formed by two hydrogen bonds and CG pairs by three, the latter bonds are stronger. When the total DNA of a human cell would be placed in a row, it would form a thin stretch that measures between 2 and 3 m. This long DNA fiber has to fit in the nucleus of the cell, which in humans has an average diameter of 6 μm and therefore has to be very condensed. This condensation is realized within chromosomes in which the antiparallel DNA molecules are tightly packed with the help of histone molecules. Each human cell contains two pairs (diploid) of 23 different chromosomes (homologues) that vary in size, chromosome 1 being the largest and chromosomes 21 and 22 being the smallest. Of these, 22 chromosome pairs, the autosomes, are present in both male and female cells, while the sex chromosomal (the 23rd chromosome) content differs: male cells carry one X and one Y chromosome (XY), while female cells contain an X chromosome pair (XX). In general, the full genetic content is maintained in every cell, and to accomplish this, the DNA has to be duplicated before every cell division. A complex of proteins is involved in unpacking chromosomes, unwinding the helical DNA structure to make the antiparallel strands accessible for this process and subsequent replication of the DNA molecules, resulting in two copies of the original strand. During this replication process, mistakes occur, and in spite of the presence of DNA repair mechanisms correcting such mistakes, on average 1 in 10^9 mismatches remain, potentially resulting in mutations. During cell division within the human organism, these mutations (somatic mutations) generally only affect the specific tissue in which they arise, however, sometimes causing serious nonhereditary diseases, for example, cancer. When occurring during sexual reproduction, such mutation (germline mutations) may be transmitted to the next generation and form the origin of a hereditary disease in the offspring. Moreover, while chromosomes stay diploid (two copies per cell) during somatic cell division, they become haploid (one copy per cell) during gametogenesis (the production of sperm or egg cells), and in the course of that process, recombination occurs. This is the exchange of genetic material between homologous chromosomes. This process is an important driving force for evolutionary diversity however may also result in mutations at the chromosomal level. For more information on the variety of mutations underlying human diseases, see the section "Genetic Mutations."

It is important to note that only ~2% of the human genome encodes proteins and this part of the genetic information is contained within the coding exons of genes. The genome consists of up to 30,000 different genes. These genes generally

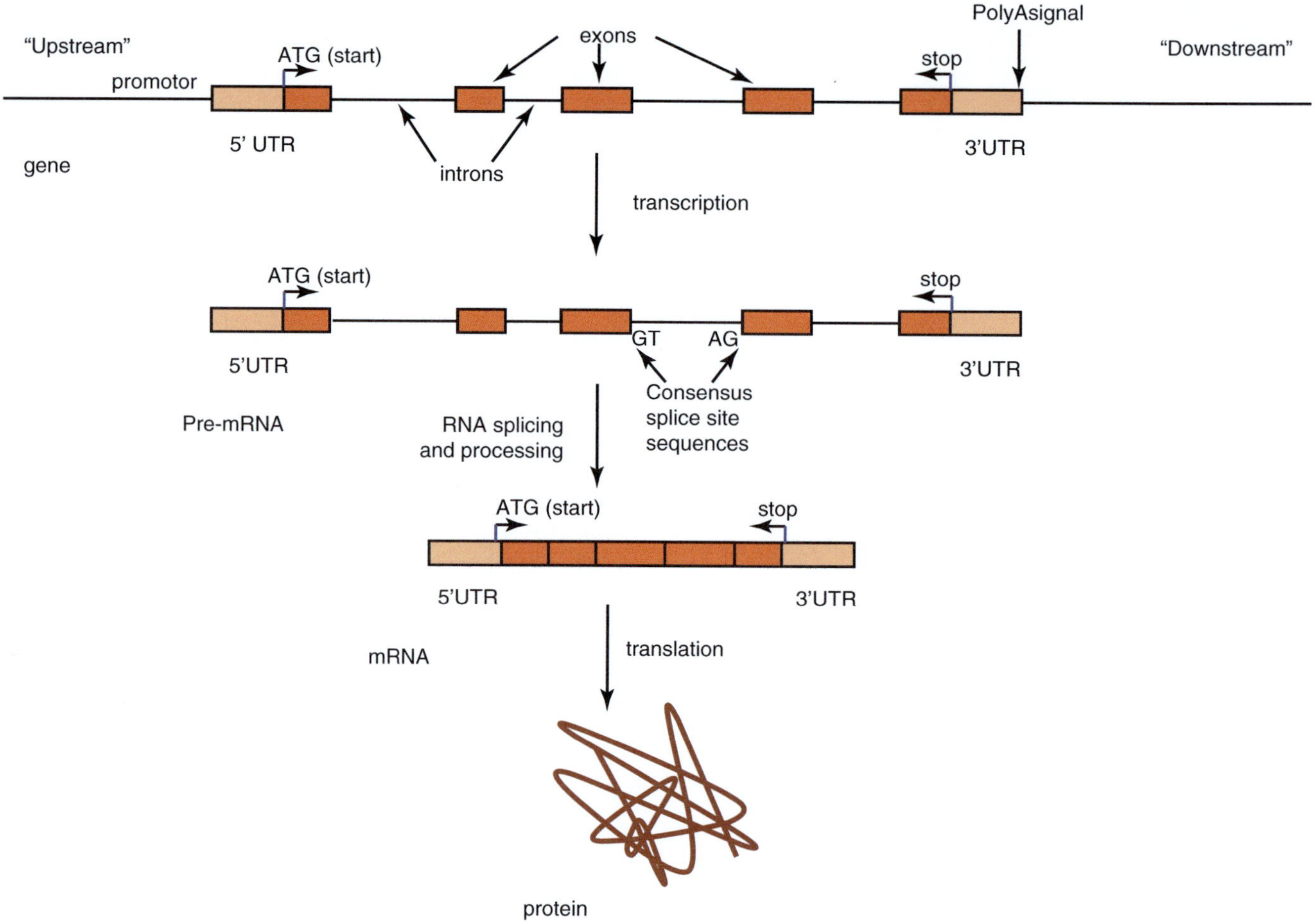

Fig. 1.2 Organization of a human gene and its processing via pre-mRNA and mRNA into protein. For explanation of the different features and aspects shown, see the main text

consist of "upstream" 5′ promoter sequences, regulatory and/or stabilizing 5′ UTR (untranslated region)-containing exons, alternating coding exons and noncoding introns, regulatory/stabilizing 3′UTR exons, and "downstream" 3′ sequences (Fig. 1.2). Notably, the 5′UTR and 3′UTR sequences lie within the first and last exon or exons, respectively, and also exons containing only UTR sequences without protein-encoding parts can be present. The promoter region contains sequences that are recognized by the transcription machinery and transcription-modulating factors that, in collaboration with RNA polymerase, are responsible for the transcription of genes. During transcription, which starts at the transcription start site lying within the first nucleotides of the 5′ UTR, the full sequence between the transcription start site and the polyadenylation signal at the end of the 3′ UTR is being transcribed into pre-mRNA (see also Fig. 1.2). For this purpose, the part of the DNA molecule on which a particular gene is located is unwinded, making it accessible for the previously mentioned transcription machinery. The resulting pre-mRNA molecule is the antiparallel copy of a gene (so the complementary sequence), a situation comparable to DNA being duplicated during replication. Therefore, pre-mRNA molecules are composed comparable to DNA molecules, except for the base thymine being replaced for uracil and ribose being used for the sugar backbone instead of deoxyribose. The pre-mRNA molecule still contains intronic sequences, and these are spliced out and the mRNA is further processed by another complex machinery, the mRNA-processing complex, within the nucleus (see also Fig. 1.2). The resulting mature mRNA, now only consisting of regulatory 5′ and 3′ UTR sequences and exonic sequences encoding the amino acid sequence of the respective protein, is then transported to the cytosol. In the cytosol, ribosomes, complexes of proteins and ribosomal RNAs (rRNAs), are responsible for translating the amino acid-encoding part of the mRNA molecule into protein. Proteins contain 20 different amino acids, and each of these is encoded by nucleotide triplets (codons). In total, 64 different codons encode these 20 amino acids, meaning that most amino acids are encoded by more than one triplet (see Table 1.1). The exceptions are phenylalanine (F), trypto-

Table 1.1 The genetic code

	T		C		A		G	
T	TTT	Phc (F)	CTT	Leu (L)	ATT	Ile (I)	GTT	Val (V)
	TTC	Leu (L)	CTC	Leu(L)	ATC	Ile (I)	GTC	Val (V)
	TTA	Ser (S)	CTA	Leu (L)	ATA	Ile (I)	GTA	Val (V)
	TTG	Leu (L)	CTG	Leu (L)	ATG	Met (M)	GTG	Val (V)
C	TCT	Ser (S)	CCT	Phe (F)	ACT	Thr (T)	GCT	Ala (A)
	TCG	Ser (S)	CCG	Phe (F)	ATT	Thr (T)	GCC	Ala (A)
	TCA	Ser (S)	CCA	Phe (F)	ATA	Thr (T)	GCA	Ala (A)
	TCG	Ser (S)	CCG	Phe (F)	ACG	Thr (T)	GCG	Ala (A)
A	TAT	Tyr (Y)	CAT	His (H)	AAT	Asn (N)	GAT	Asp (D)
	TAC	Tyr (Y)	CAC	His (H)	AAC	Asn (N)	GAC	Asp (D)
	TAA	Stop (X)	CAA	Gln (Q)	AAA	Lys (K)	GAA	Glu (H)
	TAG	Stop (X)	CAG	Gln (Q)	AAG	Lys (K)	GAG	Glu (E)
G	TGT	Cys (C)	CGT	Arg (R)	ACT	Ser (S)	GGT	Gly (G)
	TGC	Cys (C)	CGC	Arg (R)	AGC	Ser (S)	GGC	Gly (G)
	TGA	Stop (X)	CGA	Arg (R)	AGA	Arg (R)	GGA	Gly (G)
	TGG	Trp (W)	CGG	Arg (R)	AGG	Arg (R)	GGG	Gly (G)

The 64 genetic triplets and the respective amino acids. In the upper row, the first nucleotide of each codon is depicted (at the DNA level; in RNA. the thymine (T) would be a uracil (U)). In the most left column, the second nucleotide of each codon is depicted. Amino acids are indicated with both their three letter and single letter codes: *Ala* alanine, *Arg* arginine, *Asn* asparagines, *Asp* aspartic acid, *Cys* cysteine, *Gln* glutamine, *Glu* glutamic acid, *Gly* glycine. *His* histidine, *Ile* isoleucine, *Leu* leucine, *Lys* lysine, *Met* methionine, *Phe* phenylalanine, *Ser* serine, *Stop* codon, *Thr* threonine, *Trp* tryptophan, *Tyr* tyrosine, *Val* Valine

phan (W), and methionine (M), which are encoded by one triplet only. Importantly, the codon of the latter is also recognized as start codon at which translation of the protein is initiated. Moreover, three codons encode so-called stop codons indicating the end of an amino acid sequence. During protein translation, tRNA molecules operate as amino acid carriers and recognize the respective triplets encoding these amino acids. By binding to specific codons on the mRNA within a ribosome, the respective amino acid can be linked to the previous amino acid of a growing peptide. By repeating this and thus linking subsequent amino acids to each other, a complete protein is being produced. During or after completion of this process, the protein will fold into its final conformation, unless it first has to be transported to other cellular organelles, like the endoplasmic reticulum (ER), mitochondria, etc. Notably, often also posttranslational modifications of proteins occur, like glycosylation of proteins in the ER and the Golgi complex. As mentioned earlier, only a small part (2%) of DNA is actually encoding proteins. In contrast, about 25% of the DNA codes for introns, the sequences separating subsequent exon sequences, which generally are longer than exons. The remainder of the genome may have different functions: sequences can have regulatory roles (i.e., promoter and enhancer sequences), can be involved in stabilizing and/or maintaining the DNA (e.g., binding modules for histones), or play a role in replication and recombination processes. Part of the DNA may also simply be the remains of ancient evolutionary events and have no function anymore. For example, a considerable number of so-called pseudogenes are known that resemble parts of genes or sometimes full genes that are, however, not being processed into functional proteins, even though these pseudogenes sometimes only differ from the functional gene for only a limited number of nucleotides. It is also increasingly recognized that the genome encodes a wide range of noncoding RNAs that, however, do play functional roles. Among these are tRNAs and rRNAs, but also many more recently identified catalytic and regulatory RNAs, like small nuclear RNAs (snRNAs), small nucleolar RNAs (snoRNAs), microRNAs (miRNAs), transcription initiation RNAs (tiRNAs), splicing RNAs (spliRNAs), and long noncoding RNAs (lncRNAs) [1]. miRNAs were shown to recognize specific nucleotide sequences within 3′ UTRs and by doing so modulate protein synthesis, while lncRNAs are believed to be involved in the regulation of differentiation and development. For many of these functional RNAs, their precise roles still have to be elucidated. Moreover, yet unknown new functions of DNA sequences may still be revealed in the near future. Finally, it is very likely that also variations in the different noncoding but functional sequences do contribute to the spectrum of disease-causing mutations.

Genetic Mutations

As mentioned previously, during DNA replication and recombination processes, errors occur and, in spite of the existence of repair mechanisms, these errors can form the basis of somatic or germline mutations. Moreover, mutations can also occur as the result of chemical modification due to the effects of sunlight (UV), smoking, air pollution, radioactivity, and/or simply the chemical instability of DNA. While somatic mutations may lead to disease in individuals (like the development of cancer), germline mutations (those that did arise during gametogenesis) may be the basis of inherited disease, like those in cardiogenetics. Mutations differ in size, varying from only one nucleotide being changed up to the deletion or duplication of a complete chromosome (like that of chromosome 21 leading to the well-known Down syndrome, including cardiac abnormalities). Different types of mutations are described in the following sections. In the section "Molecular Genetic Techniques," techniques used to identify these mutations will be addressed. Mutations affecting only one nucleotide can have different outcomes. This of course depends on the nucleotide change itself, but also whether the affected base is located within regulatory, coding, or intronic sequences. When considering mutations in coding sequences, these can sort different effects at the amino acid level. The substitution of one nucleotide can result in an amino acid change, a missense mutation that impairs the function of the protein either because the activity of the protein is affected, but with the production of an intact molecule (gain or loss of function mutations), or because it leads to misfolding or unfolding and thus instability of the protein. In the latter case, this most likely leads to an approximately 50% reduction in the production of that protein. Notably, the other half of produced protein is the result of the transcription of the intact ("wild type") gene copy on the other chromosome and subsequent translation of its mRNA product. However, when this amount is insufficient for proper functioning of the protein, this can have immediate or long-term deleterious effects. This phenomenon is known as haploinsufficiency. The same basically accounts to single-nucleotide substitutions leading to an amino acid-encoding triplet being changed into a stop codon-encoding triplet, which at the protein level result in a nonsense mutation (see below for other examples leading to haploinsufficiency). This introduction of a premature stop codon (also called truncating mutation) was for years by definition considered pathogenic. However, the large-scale sequencing efforts of the last decennium have shown that every human genome actually contains several dozens of truncating mutations without being disease causing. And in relation to that, it has been shown that such mutations exert no or only mild effects in a significant number of disease genes, while, in contrast, missense mutations in the same gene may have significant effects. When truncating mutations are tolerated, this is most likely related to the availability of an intact gene copy on the other chromosome still resulting in the production of sufficient protein. Of course in cases where both gene copies are mutated, the situation is different and this is almost always deleterious. Although most nucleotide substitutions in intronic or regulatory sequences are most likely benign, it is rather difficult to predict the pathogenic nature of such mutations, except for those close to the exon-intron boundaries within consensus sequences that are being recognized by the RNA-splicing machinery. The latter mutations are frequently deleterious as these often lead to the skipping of exons, resulting in either the deletion of a significant part of the protein or a reading frameshift often leading to haploinsufficiency. Finally, with respect to the previously mentioned alterations, some intronic/regulatory mutations or (silent or missense) coding mutations that seem nondeleterious at the protein level may introduce an alternative (cryptic) splice site also resulting in aberrant RNA splicing. In addition to single-nucleotide substitutions, the deletion or insertion (indels) of one or more nucleotides occurs also quite regularly. When this affects nucleotide triplets within reading frames, it will delete or add the encoding amino acids. This may have effects similar to that of missense mutations, leading to stable but dysfunctional proteins or instable and therefore degraded proteins. However, when the number of deleted/inserted nucleotides does not equal 3 or a multitude of that, it will lead to a disruption of the normal reading frame and thus a frameshift mutation. At the protein level, this will result in a completely different protein sequence (and structure, in the unlikely case that this would lead to a stable product) from that position or more frequently to the loss of protein. The latter is because the frameshift frequently leads to the introduction of a premature termination codon, thus resulting in haploinsufficiency. The presence of a premature stop codon (as a result of a frameshift or nonsense mutations) is often already recognized during the process of (pre-) mRNA processing, and the respective RNA molecule is degraded. This process is known as "nonsense-mediated decay" (NMD), and a large complex of proteins is involved. Important to note is that premature stop codons that are positioned at the 3′ end of coding sequences do escape this NMD pathway, leading to the production of a truncated protein (however with a limited number of amino acids being truncated; this applies to both nonsense and frameshift mutations) or an extended protein of which the C-terminal amino acid sequence is divergent from the normal sequence, starting from the position of the respective mutation (in this case only applying to frameshift mutations). As a general "rule of thumb," this applies to premature stop codon introducing mutations in the last coding exon and in the 3′ 50–55 nucleotides of the second to last exon. Important to realize is that with both Sanger sequencing and nowadays routinely used next-generation sequencing (NGS) applications, the possibility to accurately identify larger indels (>10–15 nucleotides, depending on the technique used) is limited. Standardized methods to identify deletions or insertions that are larger than 10–15 nucleotides and those that encompass one to several exons, as described below, are currently limited. In addition to single-nucleotide mutations and small indels, larger insertions, duplications, or deletions may cause disease. First of all and already mentioned earlier, this may concern the deletion or duplication of one to several exons within a gene. Generally, this will also result in haploinsufficiency, as the affected gene will not be (properly) expressed. For example, the deletion of only exon 3 of the *RYR2* gene was shown to cause cardiomyopathy, dilated (DCM), or left ventricular noncompaction (LVNC) and catecholaminergic polymorphic ventricular tachycardia (CPVT) [2]. Moreover, the deletion of several coding exons of the *PKP2* gene was shown to be involved in the development of arrhythmogenic right ventricular cardiomyopathy (ARVC) [3]. These types of mutations are often detected by using the multiple ligation probe amplification (MLPA) technique and very recently by using CNV detection with NGS reads ("Molecular Genetic Techniques"). Deletions or duplications, however, often include one or more genes, so-called microdeletions or duplications. The pathogenicity of microdeletions is well established (e.g., the deletion of the region including the *TAB2* gene leading to dominantly inherited congenital heart defects: [4]), whereas that of duplications is more debated. As long as the insertion of DNA sequences that are duplicated does not affect the functionality of the gene duplicated or that of a gene or region in which it is inserted, duplications can be harmless. Identifying such mutations is generally done by array-comparative genomic hybridization (CGH) or single-nucleotide polymorphism (SNP)-array technologies and/or by performing copy number variation (CNV) analysis of NGS-derived data ("Molecular Genetic Techniques"). Finally, deletions/duplications of a large part of a chromosome or full chromosomes can also underlie cardiac diseases, however, often as part of a broad spectrum including other clinical features. The already mentioned Down syndrome (trisomy of chromosome 21) is a well-known example. Moreover, translocation of parts of chromosomes during gametogenesis results in the deletions and concomitant duplications of parts of chromosomes that may lead to an imbalanced situation in the resulting oocytes or spermatozoids resulting in a child with a severe clinical phenotype, including cardiac abnormalities (often congenital heart defects (CHDs)). These aberrations can be identified using "old-fashioned" karyotyping and fluorescence in situ hybridization (FISH) methods, QF-PCR (quantitative fluorescent polymerase chain reaction), or CNV analyses of NGS-derived data, including analysis of sequences that were affected by the translocation event.

Genes in Families and Populations

In the previous paragraph, different kinds of mutations, from those only affecting one specific nucleotide up to full chromosome duplications or deletions, have been described. When such mutations arise during sexual reproduction, these can be transmitted to following generations and, thus, form the basis of inherited diseases. In general, this does not apply to very large deletions/duplications, as these often have rather drastic effects, often already resulting in a spontaneous abortion. In the following sections, different aspects related to the inheritance of mutations (or variations; in particular when concerning multifactorial diseases) are described.

Modes of Inheritance

Depending on which chromosome or gene is affected by mutations and how, different ways of inheritance are recognized. Most well-established genetic diseases are Mendelian-inherited diseases, those caused by mutations on autosomal or sex chromosomal genes. These mutations can be inherited in a dominant or recessive manner. Important in this respect is that the terms dominant and recessive describe the inheritance of genetic disease and not the genes or mutations themselves. When dominantly inherited, carrying the mutation on one allele (one chromosome) is sufficient to cause disease, and as a result, children of mutation carriers have a 50% chance of inheriting the same mutation. When such mutation causes disease mainly after the reproductive age, it can be transmitted through pedigrees for numerous generations. In contrast, recessively inherited mutations result in disease development only when both alleles are affected. In general, this implicates that patients having both alleles mutated, inheriting a mutation from both parents (each carrying one copy of the mutated allele) without being affected. Such mutations are often also transmitted through numerous generations and through populations and only causing disease in the rare situation where two mutations come together in one individual. This is seen relatively frequently in situations where consanguinity is involved: the parents of an affected child being closely or more distantly (sometimes some generations ago) related. In this case, it most likely concerns homozygous mutations: the same mutation on both alleles. In more rare situations, compound heterozygous mutations may be encountered: different, deleterious mutations on the two alleles (i.e., two chromosomes) but in the same gene. In addition to the situation of parents not being affected in case of recessively inherited diseases, this also applies to cases were mutations are actually "*de novo*." This means that these did arise early in the development of the embryo or in the reproductive cells of the father or the mother and were transmitted to the affected child. Of course, when the disease course is not too severe, this can be the start of a dominantly inherited disease in following generations. In the situations described above, mutations are generally located on the autosomes and not on the sex chromosomes (X or Y). Mutations can, however, also be present on the X or Y chromosomes. Y-chromosome inheritance is quite uncommon and has until now never been described for heart-related diseases. X-linked cardiac diseases are often recognized by the fact that female carriers do not exhibit disease, or only mildly, while their sons are severely affected. Logically, this mode of inheritance is often recognized in pedigrees because of affected male family members being connected via mildly or unaffected females. If consanguinity is present in these families, a homozygous, X-linked mutation may cause severe disease in females too. Notably, the exception to this is the situation in which male carriership is actually lethal, while female carriers of one X-linked mutation are being affected (comparable to the above-described dominant inheritance on autosomes). As mitochondria also contain a genome that is duplicated independently from the nuclear genome and transmitted to new mitochondria, mutations in mitochondrial DNA can also be transmitted to next generations, and mitochondrial inheritance is being recognized too. Important to note is that mitochondrial diseases also show a maternal segregation pattern (like X-linked diseases), and recognizing this inheritance patterns is being complicated by the fact that mitochondria contain multiple genome copies that are not necessarily all mutated. Actually, mitochondrial inherited diseases are non-Mendelian diseases, as are multifactorial (polygenic) diseases. The latter will be discussed in more detail in the section "Multifactorial Inheritance."

Penetrance and Disease Expressivity

It is important to realize that carrying a mutation does not necessarily mean that disease will develop. In particular in dominantly inherited diseases, the phenomenon of reduced penetrance is often present. When the respective disease is 90% penetrant, this means that 90% of carriers develop disease. Often penetrance is age dependent, that is, symptoms of disease develop during the course of life. Moreover, disease expressivity can differ considerably. For example, the founder mutation c.40_42delAGA; p.(Arg14del) in the *PLN* gene predisposes to ACM and/or DCM [5, 6]. In a cohort of over 400 people in the Netherlands carrying this deletion, the phenotype ranges from severe outcomes as sudden cardiac death (SCD) or heart transplantation in young adults to fully healthy elderly individuals in their 70s even though they are performing quite extensive sport activities. Moreover, the same mutation can have different outcomes. For example, families have been described in which a mutation in a cardiomyopathy gene resulted in dilated, hypertrophic, or noncompaction cardiomyopathy in different family members. Both reduced penetrance and differences in disease expressivity may be explained by either nongenetic, environmental factors or genetic factors, that is, secondary mutations and/or modifiers. Although the effect size of such genetic factors is still difficult to establish or predict, current genome-wide association studies (GWAS) and, in particular, NGS approaches now enable the search for these genetic variations.

Genetic Heterogeneity

With the increasing possibilities to detect underlying genetic mutations in inherited diseases, we have seen an exponential growth in the number of identified disease genes, also within the field of cardiogenetics. As a result, it has become evident that a disease or disease type is rarely explained by a single underlying gene. Often several genes can be involved. For example, currently, more than 50 genes have been identified that are associated with dilated cardiomyopathy (DCM). In combination with the fact that mutations in the yet known genes only explain half of the patients suffering from the inherited form of this disease, this underscores that many DCM genes are still to be uncovered. Moreover, it is also increasingly recognized that mutations in the same gene can result in different phenotypes (which is different from the same mutation being differently expressed, as discussed earlier). Again within the cardiomyopathies, significant "genetic overlap" is observed, as mutations in one gene can underlie different cardiomyopathy subtypes, some even being associated with every subtype known. Furthermore, genes can even be involved in several cardiac diseases. For example, mutations in the *SCN5A* gene are known to cause cardiomyopathy, but also channelopathies like Brugada syndrome or long QT syndrome or conduction disease. Likewise, in addition to leading to cardiomyopathies, mutations in the *LMNA* or *DES* genes can also underlie generalized muscular diseases (i.e., limb girdle, desminopathy) or, in the case of *LMNA*, noncardiac disorders like lipodystrophy (caused by specific heterozygous mutations) or Hutchinson-Gilford progeria syndrome (in which a specific heterozygous *LMNA* mutation is the cause). Finally, several syndromes, like Noonan or Danon syndrome, may include cardiac manifestations, sometimes dependent on the underlying gene defect and/or mutation.

Multifactorial Inheritance

So far we only described monogenetic diseases. However, in a significant number of cases, the disease is not purely monogenic and considering multigenic or multifactorial inheritance is more appropriate. This can vary from digenic inheritance in which two genes together underlie disease up to polygenic diseases in which many variants, individually giving rise to very small effect sizes, together increase the chances of developing disease or multifactorial disease where a combination of genetic variants and environmental factors underlie disease expressivity. Of course, it is rather difficult, if at all possible, to identify all components of such multigenic diseases, even with all the novel genetic technologies and concomitant bioinformatics tools that have recently become available. Moreover, even when all could be identified, estimating both the individual and the total effect is almost impossible. In addition, variations that actually have protective effects (and quantifying those) and that thus modify the negative effects of the putatively disease-associated ones exist. Likewise, it is also increasingly recognized that monogenetic diseases are actually not really monogenetic and that several other genetic factors may modify disease (both negatively and positively), although with the major disease gene mutation being the one asserting the strongest effect. Despite the difficulties described earlier with interpreting these results, numerous studies to identify causal variants involved in polygenic diseases, as well as modifying factors in more Mendelian-inherited disease, have been performed in the last decades. In this respect, also within the field of cardiogenetics, many GWAS have been performed to find SNPs that are associated with cardiological traits. For this purpose, large groups of individuals suffering from the same disease, at least several hundreds, have to be analyzed using arrays containing a large amount of SNPs in order to identify variants that show a statistically relevant association with the respective trait. In addition, when detected, such association is often only valued after being confirmed in an independent large cohort (preferably from another ethnic origin). As discussed earlier, the relevance of such findings for the individual patient is debatable; however, the results may help in understanding and further elucidating underlying molecular pathways and mechanisms, and the identified genes linked with these variants could serve as potential drug targets. As these types of analyses are limited to the SNPs captured on these arrays, this approach may only identify variants in the direct genetic neighborhood of the affected gene that is linked to the phenotype studied, but not the actual variant. Therefore, with all the new NGS-based technologies available, the sequencing of thousands of exomes and genomes now enables the identification of many more of such variants. However, the wealth of data that have already become available indicates that every individual is carrying many private variants (even truncating mutations that are not always clinically relevant), and distinguishing the irrelevant ones from the relevant ones in polygenic disease will be a tremendous challenge. On the other hand, all ongoing whole-exome and whole-genome sequencing activities will help in separating relevant from irrelevant genetic information in the future.

Molecular Genetic Techniques from Past to Future

The last 20 years have seen unprecedented advances in technology and the development of innovative techniques in molecular genetics for the discovery of genes related to human diseases as well as the application of such knowledge to molecular genetic diagnostics as a powerful tool in patient care. The year 2016 marked the 20th anniversary from the publication of the first comprehensive genetic map of the human genome based on 5264 microsatellites [7]. Although a "report of the DNA committee and catalogues of cloned and mapped genes, markers formatted for PCR and DNA polymorphisms," was previously published in 1991 [8], the 1996 map represented the most powerful tool in the hand to human geneticists for employment of PCR-based polymorphic dinucleotide and tetranucleotide microsatellite markers for pursuing gene mapping via linkage analysis. In addition, it provided the possibility to study structural chromosomal alterations such as loss of heterozygosity (LOH) as what commonly occurs in cancer, in which one copy of a tumor suppressor gene is deleted due to various rearrangements [9]. Furthermore, these highly polymorphic markers provided the possibility to detect copy-neutral LOH, uniparental disomy (UPD) [10], as well as microsatellite instability (MSI) resulting from abnormal DNA mismatch repair (MMR) [11]. Molecular genetics and cytogenetics have since witnessed an exciting 20 years of technical and technological progress, which will be discussed in the following paragraphs.

Cytogenetics

Cytogenetics is the branch of genetics that studies the number, structure, and function of the chromosomes, which contain the highly organized and packed nuclear DNA of the cell. The first observation of chromosomes occurred in 1842 in plant cells by Carl Wilhelm von Nägeli. Later, in 1882, Walther Flemming discovered the somatic cell division (mitosis) in eukaryotic cells, in which the nucleus vanished and a highly organized and packed nuclear DNA of the cell appeared and was named chromatin. In 1888, a German anatomist, Heinrich von Waldeyer, coined the term chromosome to indicate the chromatin at its most compacted structure. Thanks also to the discovery and development of proper solution for the preparation of metaphase and interphase cells, further studies on the structure and function of chromosomes could take place. In the early twentieth century, the development and the application of the Giemsa banding (G-banding) staining technique of metaphase chromosomes allowed the description of the first human karyotype by Hans von Winiwarter in 1912, reporting 47 chromosomes in sperm cells and 48 in egg cells, inferring the mechanism of sex determination. The employment of the karyotyping technique allows researchers to define the structure of the normal complete chromosome set and identify alterations linked to biological abnormalities. In particular, the application to human genetics and clinical practice led to the discovery of defects in chromosome number (aneuploidy) in a cell leading to human diseases such as trisomy 21 (Down syndrome), trisomy 13 (Patau syndrome), and trisomy 18 (Edwards syndrome). Furthermore, karyotype analysis by Mary F. Lyon of somatic cells led to uncovering the process of X-chromosome inactivation (Xi) in female mouse [12] and in 1962 in female human subjects [13]. This pivotal observation paved the way for future investigations in the field of epigenetic regulation. In addition to aneuploidy, the use of karyotype analysis using the G-banding technique permitted the identification of even more subtle aberration, such as the constriction at the subtelomeric position of chromosome X with which Herbert Lubs [14] in 1969 discovered the cytogenetic basis of the fragile X syndrome, the most common inherited cause of intellectual disability in males. The investigation of the subtle changes in banding pattern was instrumental in determining not only the loss of the genetic material but also its exchange between chromosomes with a mechanism called balanced translocation. The study of the karyotypes from patients with various diseases allowed the identification of syndromes caused by the transfer of a piece of a chromosome detaching from its original location and translocating to another chromosome through the exchange of genetic materials. In some cases, depending on the genes involved, this mechanism could lead to the constitutive activation of fusion (chimeric) gene product leading to novel aberrant function. Many forms of leukemia may stem from this very mechanism. An example of such mechanism is represented by the Philadelphia chromosome, which results from the translocation of genetic material between chromosomes 9 and 22, defined with the cytogenetic nomenclature as t(9;22)(q34;q11) and associated with the development of most cases with chronic myeloid leukemia (CML) in which the fusion of part of the breakpoint cluster region (BCR) protein gene from chromosome 22 with part the Abelson murine leukemia viral oncogene homolog 1 (*ABL1*) gene from chromosome 9 leads to a constitutively active tyrosine kinase. The molecular mechanism prompted by the Philadelphia chromosome has allowed researchers in pharmaceutical industry to design a monoclonal antibody to act as tyrosine kinase function inhibitor. Tyrosine kinase inhibitors such as imatinib and sunitinib have been shown to be effective in CML subjects.

All the abovementioned examples underscore the profound impact in clinical diagnosis and management derived from the application of the karyotype analysis, also defined as traditional cytogenetics. However, despite much advances in the DNA molecule stretching and in the banding technique, karyotyping suffers from a lack of resolution, which prevents it from the detection of submicroscopic chromosomal aberration, in particular deletions and duplications of genetic material. Although normally utilized by cytogenetic laboratories, the answer to the need in increasing the resolution came from molecular genetic approaches, such as fluorescent in situ hybridization (FISH), comparative genomic hybridization (CGH), and single-nucleotide polymorphism (SNP) arrays. In a significant number of cases, the use of CGH or SNP array technologies allowed the identification of submicroscopic genomic rearrangements leading to genomic architecture aberrations associated with the occurrence of genetic diseases. Such genomic architecture aberrations could be the result of mispairing of highly homologous repetitive sequences called low-copy repeats (LCR), which are segmental duplications of DNA blocks ranging from 1 to 400 kb, leading to recurrent chromosomal rearrangement [15]. The plasticity of the human genome does not only depend on the LCRs, but other mechanisms can lead to interstitial or subtelomeric deletion/duplication causing copy number variation (CNV), which represents a much greater source of structural diversity of the human genome than previously expected [16–18]. However, in most cases, when a firm clinical diagnosis is achieved and a specific defect, such as a microscopic deletion or duplication is a known mechanism of the disease, a more targeted approach such as Fluorescence in situ hybridization (FISH), which does not include a genome-wide analysis such as conventional karyotyping, CGH or SNP array, can be employed. The development of fluorescent molecular probes pairing to a specific genomic region, exploiting the high complementarity to a given DNA sequence, is the basis of FISH and allows the detection or lack thereof of a specific signal in an interphase or metaphase chromosome preparation. Probably, the first (in 1993) and best-known cardiovascular disease in which FISH was used and is still currently widely employed in clinical practice is the 22q11 deletion syndrome, previously known as DiGeorge syndrome and velocardiofacial syndrome, among others [19]. The most commonly used genome-wide cytogenetic approaches are still array-based due to the their resolution capable of detecting relatively small genomic aberrations such as sub-chromosomal deletions and gain of genetic material. For that characteristics, CGH or SNP arrays are mostly used to identify variants associated with CHDs or syndromes involving cardiovascular abnormalities. However, genome-wide arrays bear intrinsic limitations in the detection of genomic rearrangements such as balanced chromosomal rearrangements like translocations or inversions.

Molecular DNA Techniques

Among the technical advances in molecular biology, which have been widely utilized in genetic research and in clinical molecular diagnostics, two represent absolute milestones: Sanger sequencing, developed in 1977 by Frederick Sanger [20], which won the Nobel Prize in Chemistry in 1980 along with Walter Gilbert, and the polymerase chain reaction (PCR) developed in 1983 by Kary Mullis [21], also awarded with the Nobel Prize in Chemistry in 1993 with Michael Smith. PCR is a process used to exponentially amplify a specific DNA sequence, through sequential repetitive cycles, at several orders of magnitude starting even from a single DNA molecule and leading to thousands to millions of copies of the desired DNA target. PCR found immediate applications in biological research and molecular diagnostics including DNA cloning for sequencing, forensic genetic fingerprinting, and diagnosis in infectious diseases, evolutionary biology, and quantitative gene expression analysis, among others [22–24]. A natural application of PCR was the ability to provide the rapid availability of sufficient DNA target for sequencing, compared to previous laborious DNA isolation techniques. In addition, the exploitation of the exponential phase of the PCR along with the employment of fluorescently labeled primers, probes or dyes, led to the development of a real-time quantitative PCR (qPCR) method for the accurate and sensitive detection and quantification of nucleic acids [25]. Among the various applications in clinical practice, an important role was played by qPCR in the detection of infective agents load in endomyocardial specimen from patients with myocarditis [26] or in post heart and lung transplant subjects at risk of rejection [27]. The latest development of such technology led to digital PCR (dPCR), which can be used to provide the direct absolute quantification of the initial nucleic acid sample amount by partitioning the specimen into a large number of separated micro wells or emulsion reactions, allowing for a large data point collection and more sensitive measurement of the target nucleic acid amount [28] including small deletions and duplications, as well as copy number variants, in a manner independent on the number of amplification cycles [29].

Another frequently used molecular technique, namely, multiplex ligation-dependent probe amplification (MLPA), is extensively employed in clinical diagnostics for the detection of copy number variation and exon-based small and large deletion/duplication analysis [30]. MLPA represents a derivative of multiplex PCR that allows multiple targets to be amplified simultaneously using various pairs of forward and reverse oligonucleotide primer probes recognizing adjacent target sites on the DNA. Only, when both probes perfectly anneal to their respective targets, they can be ligated into a complete probe and amplified into a fluorescently labeled PCR product of unique length and can then be separated and identified by capillary electrophoresis [30]. The comparison of the detected fluorescent peak patterns between the test sample and a reference sample can provide a quantitative ratio of each amplicon stemming from the relative amount of the target sequence along with the relative quantity of each obtained product [30].

In addition to the numerous applications of PCR and all its derivatives, PCR has become the perfect mate of the Sanger technique, which is the chain-termination method for sequencing DNA molecules. Sanger sequencing exploits the inability of dideoxynucleotides to allow another DNA base to be added to the newly synthesized DNA strand. Its extraordinariness is represented by the ability to determine rapidly and accurately the sequence composition of long stretches of DNA such as the 16,569 base pairs of the human mitochondrial genomic DNA [31], the 48,502 base pairs of the bacteriophage λ [32], and the complete and accurate sequence of the 3 billion DNA base pairs that compose the human genome [33, 34].

NGS

For several decades, Sanger sequencing has been the gold standard for the determination of variants in nucleic acid molecules in both biological research and clinical molecular diagnostics. However, the pace of gene discoveries along with unveiling the increasing genetic heterogeneity in most diseases, and especially in primary cardiomyopathies and arrhythmias syndrome, overcame the ability to target all most relevant genes to increase the detection rate and improve molecular diagnostics. Since the announcement of the completion of the first draft of the Human Genome Project in 2003, it became apparent that the throughput employed until then was insufficient to compete with the upcoming challenges in genetics and genomic research and clinical practice. In particular, the high demand of cost-efficient methods for large-scale sequencing projects pushed toward the development of high-throughput sequencing or next-generation sequencing (NGS) technologies that provide massive parallel sequencing, producing thousands or millions of sequences simultaneously. The technique was initially applied to determine gene expression levels by counting the number of individual messenger RNA (mRNA) molecules produced by each gene. The NGS technology evolved between the end of the 1990s and the beginning of the twenty-first century with the advent of the 454-pyrosequencing machine for DNA sequencing, which could drastically reduce the cost of sequencing compared to Sanger and produce 20 million bases (20 Mbp) worth of data [35]. In the following years, the throughput increased almost exponentially. Almost simultaneously, another platform, the Genome Analyzer (GA), entered the market based on the sequencing by synthesis (SBS) technology using reversible dye-terminator chemistry generating up to 50 billion bases (50 Bbp) of usable data per run [36]. Another platform based on the SBS technology is the single-molecule real-time (SMRT) sequencing in which the DNA is synthesized in zero-mode waveguides (ZMWs), a nanophotonic confinement structure consisting of a hole in an aluminum shell film deposited on a clear silica substrate in which a single DNA polymerase enzyme is attached to the bottom of a ZMW with a single molecule of DNA as a template where fluorescently labeled nucleotides are added to the growing DNA molecule allowing reads of up to 60,000 nucleotides or more, with average read lengths of 5000 bases [37]. In addition to the aforementioned technologies, various companies developed a vast selection of machines able to yield up to 600 G bases of data with increasing read length and coverage depth with the capacity to sequence a human genome in about 24 h, 20 exomes in a day, or 30 transcriptomes (RNA sequencing) samples in as little as 5 h. Other technologies are also developed such as sequencing by oligo ligation detection, employed by the SOLiD platform, and the semiconductor technology used by the Ion Torrent sequencer, which is based on the detection of hydrogen ions that are released during the polymerization of DNA. Of great interest are methods recently commercialized such as nanopore sequencing, which relies on the retrieval of electrical signals from nucleotides passing through nanopores changing conformation of the pore and the ion flow going through it according to the shape, size, and length of the DNA sequence. Nanopore sequencing benefits from generally long reads (10–30 Kbp) and is capable to achieve ultra-long reads (50–882 Kbp) with great sequence data mappability [38]. Very long reads capacity may allow the detection of expansion variants and discriminate between the intended target and homologous, paralogous, and pseudogene sequences. In addition, there are new methods recently developed to improve the base accuracy of the nanopore technology, such as circularizing cDNA molecules followed by rolling circle amplification [39]. However, despite great promises, a major limitation for large-scale application of nanopore sequencing remains the single base reading accuracy, which prevents its use in clinical diagnostics. The use of NGS has allowed an increasing amount of DNA to be targeted for sequencing. Depending on the desired application, NGS can be applied to target a panel of candidate genes, known to be associated with a specific disease or spectrum of disorders, or can be used to capture the entire 35Mbp of the coding sequence collection, namely, whole-exome sequence (WES), or even the 3Gbp of the whole-genome sequence (WGS), thus providing with an extraordinary level of flexibility. Besides, there are important parameters to consider in NGS experiments such as the read modality, which means obtaining a sequence read from one end of a DNA fragment (single-end read) or from both (pair-end read). The single-end read usually is faster, cheaper, and usually enough for applications such as RNAseq (gene expression profile) or ChIPseq (chromatin immunoprecipitation paired with massively parallel DNA sequencing to identify the binding sites of DNA-associated proteins). Pair-end read sequencing however provides more accurate mapping of the DNA fragment to the reference genome, making it an excellent approach for clinical diagnostics and allowing the resolution of structural rearrangements such as deletions, insertions, and inversions. The application of NGS in either research or clinical diagnostics, although offering the flexibility to determine the extent of nucleic acid sequence to cover (panels, WES, WGS, RNAseq, ChiPSeq, methylome, etc.), also presents with technical limitations, which are intrinsic to the modality utilized for the test. In all applications but WGS, after fragmenting the nucleic acid molecules, specific probes to target or capture the desired sequences should be employed. There are mainly two capture modalities currently used in NGS: amplicon-based, which use oligonucleotide probes as PCR primers for amplicons, and the hybridization-based which allows the nucleic acid fragments to be used for further enrichment and clonal amplification [40]. Each capturing modality provides various levels of sequence complexity and uniformity, along with difference in depth of coverage. Constitutional genetic disorders such as cardiovascular diseases can be effectively detected using a minimum of 100× average coverage (approximately 100 reads from both directions), being derived mostly from constitutional variants. However, for somatic cancer genetics applications, much higher depth of coverage is usually required due to the genetic heterogeneity in tumor samples along with normal tissue. Further, the choice of the sequencing platform also has an important impact on the ability to detect different types of variants, and each platform comes with unique advantages as well as technical limitations in variant detection, which can be partially resolved by the use of appropriate software for alignment and variant calling that normalizes for these errors [40]. Recently, investigators have compared amplicon-based with hybridization capture-based methods, and apparently, hybridization capture-based methods resulted in better sequencing complexity and uniformity and lower false-positive and false-negative rates for single-nucleotide variants (SNVs), although the latter issue can be corrected by modifying the parameters, such as minimum variant frequency or minimum read coverage, necessary for a base call [40]. In the case of clinical molecular diagnostic re-sequencing, the raw data obtained from the various sequencing machines needs to be processed bioinformatically and assembled into contigs reconstructing the entire DNA fragment clonally amplified during the sequencing process. In addition, once the sequence fragments have been aligned in contigs, they have to be also mapped against a reference genome sequence, called assembly. An important bioinformatics issue is the filtering of repetitive sequence, segmental duplications, and pseudogenes which can be spreading all over the genome. In many cases, if a sequence cannot be uniquely assigned to a specific genomic location, it is filtered out loosing part of the information. Following this, the next steps in the procedure involve the detection of each variant compared to the reference sequence and its placement with respect to the coding, splicing, or intronic sequence, a process called variant annotation. It is only after all variants' annotation has been completed that a laborious and complex process of variant interpretation begins (see that paragraph).

The extraordinary application of NGS in cardiovascular genetics stemmed from the notion that for many decades, primary cardiac diseases such as cardiomyopathies or channelopathies have been regarded as purely monogenic Mendelian disorders characterized by high locus and allelic heterogeneity, incomplete penetrance, and clinical variability. However, recent findings challenged this view, and a significant fraction of cardiovascular patients with suspected genetic origin analyzed for large gene panels, WES or WGS, presented with the detection of multiple pathogenic variants suggesting the occurrence of a more complex genetic interaction, leading to a challenging interpretation of the clinically relevant role of each identified variant [41]. Recently the American College of Medical Genetics and Genomics (ACMG) has published the standard guidelines for the interpretation of sequence variants [42], weighing strong genetic data, such as linkage analysis and cosegregation of the variants in large pedigrees, or solid and comprehensive functional characterization of the variants along with the frequency in large controls databases, amino acid conservation analysis, *in silico* damage prediction, association studies data, and other "indirect" suggestive parameters [42]. More details on this are being provided in paragraph "analysis and interpretation".

In the last several years, NGS has allowed the gathering of data from a large set of genes, the whole sets of coding exons (exome) or the entire genome, which has also prompted the development of bioinformatics methods for the detection of CNV [43–45]. Currently, NGS is widely used in clinical diagnostic laboratories, which are employing NGS also for the detection of CNV as well as other genomic rearrangements including balanced translocations and inversions [46]. It has been recently shown that there is a significant prevalence of genomic rearrangements in Mendelian diseases and, although pathogenic CNVs for cardiovascular disorders were detected overall in 4.7% of cases, comparatively lower than other clinical areas [47], familial hypercholesterolemia showed a positive detection in almost 11% of subjects [47], while in aortopathies pathogenic CNVs were detected in up to 8.1% of cases [48].

Despite all the existing limitations and technical challenges, the increasing utilization of massive parallel sequencing technologies will continue to allow the unveiling of an increasing level of complexity in genetic causes of human diseases along with an impressive amount of data, which will permit, in a non-distant future, the hasty interpretation of genetic variants.

Analysis and Interpretation

Variant Classification

Before we will discuss the aspects involved in variant classification, we will explain why it is recommended to use the term (genomic) variant and not mutation or polymorphism when we discuss a DNA alteration. The terms "mutation" and "polymorphism" lead to confusion due to incorrect assumptions of pathogenic and benign effects, respectively. A mutation is defined as a permanent change in the nucleotide sequence, while a polymorphism is defined as a variant with a frequency above 1%. Therefore, these terms do not say anything about the biological significance (benign vs. pathogenic) of the DNA alteration [42].

In the past few years, sequencing technology has changed rapidly with the development of high-throughput sequencing methods, which are collectively referred to as NGS. In the past, Sanger sequencing has been the gold standard in molecular diagnostics. Because this test is relatively labor-intensive and rather expensive, it was not suitable for diseases that show extensive genetic heterogeneity. It was therefore either applied to diseases in which (pathogenic) genetic variants in a small number of genes could explain the phenotype or in cases of genetic heterogeneous diseases to analyze only the most prevalent disease genes. The recent technological developments in high-throughput sequencing and computing have resulted in accurate sequencing at much lower costs, which enabled testing for targeted gene panels of over 100 disease genes, as well as exomes and even genomes ("Next-Generation Sequencing"). The limiting factor in deciding on the content of the test is no longer the size of the gene or its relative contribution but more on its relevance for the disease. Inaccurate variant-disease associations represent a challenge for clinical variant interpretation, and because the amount of information about genes and genetic variants is growing daily, there is a continuous need for the reassessment of previously classified genetic variants. In daily practice, however, this is virtually impossible. Instead, it is recommended to reassess the variant if it is identified in another index patient or when the patient or family in which the variant was originally found revisits the cardiogenetic clinic or as a result of discussion on classification of a variant between different laboratories where the variant was found. When this reassessment results in another classification that affects medical care, all previously identified gene carriers should be informed about this. Molecular genetic testing is highly relevant. Finding a pathogenic variant may be of help to identify family members at risk or those that do not need cardiological surveillance any more. In addition, knowing the underlying gene variant may guide clinical treatment in some cases. Therefore, accurate variant assessment is very important but not easily accomplished as relevant information is not always available or accessible at the time of interpretation. Moreover, no standard, comprehensive, and efficient variant classification method is available that is approved and shared by the community. However, variant interpretation should be as uniform as possible, and therefore, medical genetic laboratories have developed guidelines for interpretation, including those from American (ACMG), Dutch (VKGL), and British (ACGS) Clinical Molecular Genetics Societies [42, 49–51]. Important to note is that this classification is only relevant for the interpretation of variants that cause a (suspected) inherited Mendelian disease and not intended to be used for the interpretation of pharmacogenomics, somatic or multigenic non-Mendelian diseases. In addition, care must be taken in interpreting variants in candidate disease genes (GUS, genes of uncertain significance) which will be detected when exomes and genomes are studied or when these GUS are added to a targeted panel.

It is of great importance that diagnostic laboratories use a consistent method to report variants. Therefore, the diagnostic genetic community has decided to use the guidelines available from the Human Genome Variation Society (HGVS: http://varnomen.hgvs.org). Clinical reports should include sequence reference(s) (or genome build when genomic coordinates are used) to ensure unambiguous naming of the variant at the DNA and protein level ("c." for coding DNA sequence, "p." for coding protein, and "g." for genomic sequence). There is a general agreement on using a classification system based on five variant classes. These are class 1, certainly not pathogenic or benign (diagnosis not confirmed molecularly and therefore not reported); class 2, unlikely pathogenic variants or likely benign (diagnosis not confirmed molecularly and often not reported); class 3, unknown or uncertain pathogenicity or significance (does not confirm or exclude diagnosis); class 4, likely pathogenic (consistent with the diagnosis); and class 5, (certainly) pathogenic (result confirms the diagnosis). Some laboratories subdivide class 3 variants, also known as variants of uncertain significance (VUS), even further into VUS (favors benign), VUS (unknown), and VUS (favors pathogenic). Often this is done for internal use and not reported to the referring physician. The term "likely" is used when the professional believes that the variant is about 90% benign (class 2) or pathogenic (class 4). To obtain an appropriate classification, the following major aspects are taken into account: frequency and number of alleles in patient and control populations, degree of segregation with disease, functional evidence, predicted protein effect, and comparison with the established spectrum of pathogenic variation in a gene. Basically, variant interpretation consists of two parts. In the first part, variant-specific features are calculated and scored based on *in silico* (computational) predictive programs, many of them being available on the Internet (see [42, 49, 52]) and frequency data from "control" databases, for example, from the Genome Aggregation Database (gnomAD; http://gnomad.broadinstitute.org/). The second part is using already available information from the literature or online databases or can be obtained by performing additional studies of a particular variant. Examples of this are as follows: how often has this variant been found before related to this disease, does the variant cosegregate with the disease, has it functionally been analyzed, and did the variant occur de novo (not present in both biological parents)? Many genome diagnostic labs use Alamut (http://www.interactivebiosoftware.com/alamut.html), a commercially licensed software package that allows a user-friendly environment for variant review, visualization, and interpretation combining several protein effect prediction programs and "control" and disease databases. In addition, it can be used as a database for the analyzed samples in the laboratory. Many other commercial applications for the annotation and data interpretation are available as well (see Oliver GR et al. [53]).

In Silico Predictive Programs In general, the algorithms can be divided into tools that predict whether a missense change could result in a change or loss of protein function (e.g., PolyPhen-2, SIFT, MutationTaster, Grantham score) or those that predict whether there is an effect on splicing (e.g., Human Splice Finder, NetGene2). In general, most programs for missense variant prediction are about 70% accurate when examining known disease variants [54, 55]. Although many prediction tools are based on different algorithms, they have similarities in their underlying methodology. All tools depend on criteria such as biochemical consequences of the amino acid substitution and evolutionary conservation. The predicted classification must not be considered definitive but should be considered as one aspect of a more extensive investigation (i.e., moderate evidence). Splice prediction tools in general have a greater sensitivity (about 90%; fraction or percentage of splice-site variants successfully identified) than specificity (about 70%; fraction or percentage of neutral variants successfully identified) and should only be used as a first indication [56, 57]. If possible, RNA studies should be performed to prove that the variant indeed interferes with splicing. This should be performed in an appropriate and validated tissue or cell type. Only nucleotide changes that disrupt the (essential) dinucleotide consensus splice sites (located in the intron at the intron/exon boundary, that is, positions ±1 and ±2) can be considered to disrupt the splicing without functional RNA analysis when most splice prediction tools predict the loss of splicing. However, whether this variant will be considered (truly) pathogenic depends on aspects like the role of the gene in disease and whether these types of variants have been reported before as pathogenic in this specific disease. Therefore, it is recommended to test these types of splice-site variants in RNA as well to investigate whether the alternatively spliced RNA will result in an in-frame or frameshift variation. Both types of variants often have different impact on function. A frameshift variant often results in loss of function, whereas an in-frame variant could function in a dominant-negative way.

Frequency Data from "Control" Databases Determining the frequency of a variant in the general (or control) population is useful in judging its potential pathogenicity, preferably by using ethnically matched controls. For this, several publicly available population databases as well as other resources (in house, publications) are being used. The already mentioned gnomAD database is at present the largest with frequency data from over 123,000 exomes and 15,000 whole genomes. An allele frequency higher than expected for the disease is in general considered as strong support for a benign interpretation. Several exceptions to this rule are, however, known in the literature like the common South Asian c.3628-41_3628-17del variant in *MYBPC3* that is associated with cardiomyopathies and occurs with a frequency of 3.1% in South Asian (gnomAD) and even up to 8% in certain Indian populations [58]. The absence of a variant in a large general control population indicates only a moderate piece of evidence for pathogenicity of a variant, because also many benign ones are "private" (i.e., unique to an individual or family).

Occurrence of the Variant in Disease Databases Data sharing of variants has shown to be of great value for classifying VUSs. For this reason, diagnostic labs make use of mutation/disease databases, like HGMD or Human Gene Mutation Database (http://www.hgmd.org), ClinVar (http://www.ncbi.nlm.nih.gov/clinvar), and Locus-Specific Databases (LOVD; http://www.lovd.nl) [59–61], and published literature. However, these data should be used with caution. When using these databases, it is important to know the quality of the data (e.g., Sanger-validated vs. low-quality next-generation sequencing), how often the database is updated, and the source reliability and independence of the data. Notably, dated literature may contain older nomenclature and classification. Many previously published disease-associated variants turned out to be present in population-based exome data and made the pathogenicity of these variants dubious [62, 63]. A variant is statistically more likely pathogenic if it occurs in affected individuals more frequently than expected by chance. For this, the likelihood of random occurrence (e.g., through case-control studies using Fisher's exact or chi-square test) or odds ratios (ORs, http://www.hutchon.net/confidor.htm, http://www.easycalculation.com/statistics/odds-ratio) is being calculated. In general, variants with a modest Mendelian effect size will have an OR of 3 or greater, while highly penetrant variants will have very high ORs (up to 13). When interpreting ORs, it is important to take the confidence interval (CI) around the OR into account. For instance, if the CI includes 1.0 (e.g., OR = 2.5; CI = 0.9–7.4), there is little confidence in the assertion of association [42]. Because NGS results in exponential growth of the number of variants, data sharing has become even more important. Therefore, clinical laboratories should submit variants to existing databases or should create their own sharing databases. These databases should offer the possibility to record each unique detection of the same variant to keep track of the prevalence of the disease in the general population. At present, sharing of data is unfortunately still in its infancy due to issues like insufficiently automated submissions, curation of data, patient privacy issues, and the traceability of the origin of submission. For organizational reasons, as well as to record population and/or geographic-specific information, Weiss et al. [50] recommended that diagnostic labs should start with national data-sharing initiatives that should merge into an international database. In the Netherlands, the genome diagnostic laboratories share their variant classifications with each other and with international databases like LOVD, CafeVariome, and ClinVar. Not only sharing of the variant is important but also sharing of accurate and detailed phenotypic data. This is far from optimal at present and requires good collaboration between clinic and laboratory- and software-supported approaches.

Cosegregation with the Disease Significant cosegregation of a variant with the disease in families is a strong indication for pathogenicity. However, it should be realized that the presence of partial (age-related) penetrance, phenocopies (affected family members with the disease due to a nongenetic or different genetic cause), and nonpaternity can result in erroneous interpretation. Accurate clinical evaluation and communication of this to the laboratory is of crucial importance for a reliable interpretation. In addition, the segregation of a particular variant with a phenotype in a family is evidence for linkage of the locus to the disorder but not necessarily evidence of pathogenicity of the variant itself, that is, any variant in linkage disequilibrium with the causative variant will segregate with the disease. Cosegregation in multiple distantly related family members and multiple families from diverse ethnic background and sequencing of the complete gene provide stronger proof that another variant is not involved. Linkage analysis methods have been published [64, 65] and recently a more simplified method for segregation analysis (SISA, [66]). As a rule of thumb, ten informative segregations can provide a significant LOD score (>3.0), providing significant evidence for linkage between a genetic locus and the disease. In general, extended families with cardiogenetic diseases are rare, and therefore, significant LOD scores are difficult to obtain, although LOD scores of multiple independent families carrying the same variant, but not genealogically linked, can be added together. Notably, fewer informative segregation may be sufficient in combination with other supporting data. In addition, lack of segregation of a variant with a phenotype provides strong evidence against pathogenicity.

Functional Studies A reliable functional test is regarded as an important piece of evidence to confirm pathogenicity. However, such assays are rarely available as part of routine diagnostic services. In addition, it is important to assess the validity of a functional test with respect to how closely it reflects the biological situation. Other factors to consider are, for example, validation (robustness, reproducibility) of the assay and specimen integrity including storage and transport. In general, direct analysis on patient material provides the strongest functional evidence. *In vitro* studies can be useful (e.g., patch-clamp studies for ion channels) but may not represent the biological situation completely and therefore do not always provide direct proof for causality but are only moderate evidence.

De Novo Variants A *de novo* observation in an exome or genome as such is no longer considered unequivocal evidence for pathogenicity because all individuals are expected to have approximately 1 *de novo* variant in their exome or 100 in their genome. A *de novo* variant (not present in both biological parents) is considered strong support for pathogenicity when the phenotype of the patient is in line with the gene's disease association and the family history of disease is consistent with *de novo* inheritance. This means unaffected parents for a dominant disorder, but more than one sibling can be affected if one of the parents is a germline mosaic.

Other Aspects to Consider Genes may have multiple transcripts, some of which can be tissue specific and associated with different phenotypes. When multiple variants are identified in a single gene, the phase (i.e., in cis on the same chromosome or in trans on homologous chromosomes) of the variant is of importance, in particular for recessive disorders. Variant spectrum (i.e., which type of variant gives rise to which disease) is important to take into account as well. For some genes, truncating variants (e.g., resulting in loss of function) are the primary type of pathogenic variants, as is the case for *MYBPC3* variants in HCM, whereas in other genes, missense (e.g., resulting in a dominant-negative effect) variants are the primary type of pathogenic variants, as is the case for *MYH7* variants in HCM. In addition, index patients could have multiple variants that can contribute to more severe disease [67]. These aspects need to be considered and further complicate variant interpretation.

Data Quality Issues and NGS

NGS methods (gene panels, exomes, in the future genomes) are being used by genome diagnostics laboratories worldwide because of their fast, efficient, and relatively cheap analysis of diseases that show genetic heterogeneity. Some diagnostic labs are able to use NGS data to detect copy number variants (CNVs) as well. This makes NGS even more attractive as a diagnostic tool [68]. In the past, CNV detection required the use of microarrays (for detecting large CNVs) or multiplex ligation-dependent probe amplification (MLPA) for gene/exon-sized CNVs (see also the section "Molecular Genetic Techniques"). Bioinformatics analysis applied to next-generation sequencing (NGS) data by making use of, for instance, normalized depth of coverage per region (exon) per sample and comparing this with the average coverage per region (exon) of previously analyzed samples makes CNV detection of NGS data visible. Vertical coverage per region and reproducibility of normalized coverage data determine the resolution and visibility of CNV detection with NGS.

Many NGS platforms are available and are being adjusted and improved constantly presenting their users with new challenges, at the technical, data management, interpretation (see the section "Variant Classification"), and counseling level. With the handling of NGS data, a skilled and dedicated bioinformatician as part of the analysis team in any diagnostic laboratory is mandatory. Before NGS can be used in diagnostics, all methods and equipment should be validated. Previously discussed guidelines (e.g., [50, 69, 70]) are being used to allow more standardization and agreement about quality issues and number of genes that needs to be analyzed for a particular disease. Analyzing more genes for a disease does not necessarily mean a higher yield but can instead result in more uncertainty (e.g., identification of more VUSs or obtaining unsolicited findings) for the patient [71]. A condense summary of these guidelines will be given below. Before doing that we will discuss the major components of a NGS analytical pipeline [53]. It all starts by deciding what should be analyzed. One can choose for a targeted panel, which consists of the DNA from only the proven candidate genes for a disease and is obtained by an amplicon-based strategy (PCR-based enrichment of target region) or sequence capture (hybridization based) [72, 73]. WES is also an option. For this, DNA from all coding exons using a sequence capture is isolated. Finally, the whole genome can be sequenced (WGS, starting to be introduced in diagnostics). For this, no DNA enrichment is involved. WES and WGS can be analyzed in different ways using different analysis models, for example, trio analysis (e.g., parents and affected child), for detecting *de novo* variants or specific approaches for autosomal dominant or recessive inheritance. In addition, filtering of a specific gene panel (virtual analysis) can be used. Each approach has its own quality issues that should be considered, and none of these pretend to give a "complete" analysis, although in the mind of patients who have their "genome" analyzed, this may be suggested. It is the task of the referring clinician to clearly explain the shortcomings of the test to the patient (as a part of the pretest counseling). The conditions for including a gene into a panel or what type of analysis is preferred for a certain disease should ideally be dealt with at the community level in a multidisciplinary way and is not common practice yet. Initiatives for this has been started recently by the Clinical Genome Resource (ClinGen), supported by the National Institutes of Health (NIH), to develop expertly curated and freely accessible resources defining the clinical relevance of genes and variants for use in precision medicine and research [74]. To guarantee uniform and transparent molecular testing between clinical genetic laboratories, it is recommended that a "core disease gene" list and/or "diagnostic routing" for genetic diseases will be defined and maintained [50, 69]. Variant analysis in these "core disease genes" should warrant a sequencing quality that matches current practice (i.e., high sensitivity and specificity). Sometimes this could mean that gaps ("low-coverage regions") should be sequenced with another sequencing method (e.g., Sanger sequencing). The (enriched) DNA is subsequently used for NGS. Three parts can be distinguished in the process from DNA sequencing to interpretation of NGS data. The first part is the sequencing on the sequencing instrument (e.g., MiSeq, Ion Torrent). Most instruments are also able to convert the raw signals generated by the sequencing instrument into nucleotide bases with associated quality scores in a so-called FASTQ file. The second part involves several methods that operate together to detect genomic aberrations from quality-scored sequence data and consists of several stages from which alignment of reads to the human reference genome, flagging or filtering duplicate reads (probably PCR artifacts), and variant calling are the most important. Alignment problems due to repetitive genomic regions and pseudogenes can result in the loss of sequence data as a result of relatively short read lengths generated by most NGS technologies [75]. The final output is often a VCF (variant call format) file. This file is used in the final stage, which consists of result interpretation by annotating (classifying) the variants to determine their biological significance by trained clinical laboratory geneticists using homemade pipelines or commercial programs like Alissa and Alamut (see also the section "Variant Classification"). In order to deliver high-quality diagnostics, it is important to realize the limitations of the different NGS platforms and enrichment methods (if any) used to isolate the DNA to be sequenced. Not only for the laboratory but also for the referring clinician, it is important to know which quality issues need to be considered. In general, the sensitivity of NGS depends largely on the horizontal and vertical coverage of the genomic regions of interest (Table 1.2). In this respect, one should distinguish between raw coverage and informative coverage (Table 1.2): the first is the actual number of times a certain position, that is, nucleotide, has been observed (including low-quality calls), whereas the latter reflects the true informative value of all positions within a gene target (only high-quality calls are included). This informative coverage can be calculated on the basis of a predefined set of filtering criteria: uniqueness of mapping, mapping quality of the read, position of the base within the read, and the number of individual start sites represented by the reads (independent samplings from the pool). The informative coverage is per definition at best equal to, but generally lower than, the raw coverage. By only using these informative reads, variant calling efficiency and accuracy have enhanced tremendously, thereby reducing the minimal coverage needed per nucleotide. The minimal vertical informative coverage is dependent on the platform and the strategy used. In general, the Dutch laboratories recommend at least 20–30× coverage; read depths that range from 15 to 20 are left to the expert interpretation of the laboratory specialist. In addition, the laboratory must be able to guarantee that reported variants are associated with the analyzed patient by using a SNP control test or confirmation on a second (independent) DNA sample to rule out sample swaps. Other aspects that influence data quality are the way in which target enrichment is performed. Amplicon-based strategies can result in losing important sequence information because of allelic dropout (due to rare polymorphisms), whereas an important drawback of hybridization-based enrichment strategies is reduced coverage in GC-rich regions [72, 73]. To make this issue more transparent, a rating system (A, B, or C) for NGS diagnostics has been proposed [69]. With a type-A test reserved for genes or gene panels analyzed with the highest possible quality, no sequence gaps in the target region are allowed. In a type-B test, the lab describes exactly which regions are sequenced with the highest possible quality and which are not (only for some regions sequence gaps are filled with another sequencing method). The type-C test solely relies on the quality of NGS sequencing (no additional Sanger (or other) sequencing is offered) as is the case for exomes. If a test is based on exome of genome sequencing, then it should be realized that with the current possibilities, quality issues related to insufficient sequence depth of many regions should be accepted. Rehm [76] stated this in the following way: "although exome and genome sequencing are often referred to as 'whole' exome or genome sequencing, these services might better be called 'hole' exome and genome sequencing." Nevertheless in cases of extreme locus heterogeneity (e.g., in pediatric cardiac diseases), WES can be the best choice because the reduced sensitivity per gene compared with conventional sequencing may be compensated by the large number of genes that can be included in this test, resulting in a higher diagnostic yield (i.e., the number of patients that receive a molecular confir-

Table 1.2 Definitions and used terminologies (see also [50])

Target	Selected template region that needs to be investigated
Raw coverage	Percentage of reads that map to reference genome
Horizontal coverage	Percentage of target mapped reads that are on or near the target
Vertical coverage	Read depth, uniquely mapped reads at a specific locus
Informative coverage	Uniquely mapped (high-quality) reads, excluding duplicate reads
Core disease gene list	Disease genes that are considered essential to establish a molecular diagnosis (i.e., genes containing proven pathogenic variants that explain the disease)
Diagnostic routing	Flowchart, indicating the routing of genetic tests within the laboratory for a specific disease, can be a combination of different techniques

mation of a given clinical diagnosis). In addition, the quality of exomes have improved in the years because of better capture strategies.

Reporting of Results

The writing of diagnostic reports is challenging, as they should be as concise as possible but contain the essential information in understandable wording and according to international diagnostic standards ISO15189, ACMG [77–80], CMGS [81], or RCPA [82]. In this section, the most important issues will be discussed. Further details about this subject can be found in the diagnostic standards referred above and other guidelines [42, 49, 50]. In summary, a report should contain all of the essential elements of the test performed, an interpretation, relevant references, methodology, proposed follow-up tests if appropriate, and disclaimers. The variants should be described using HGVS nomenclature (see also the section "Classification of Variants"). It is important that test characteristics (e.g., the minimal vertical coverage, the average vertical coverage (per gene), the complete gene list and analyzed gene parts, the data analysis pipeline and version, and the diagnostic routing) are included or provided in an alternative manner. In Fig. 1.3, an example letter from a diagnostic laboratory is shown including all relevant test characteristics in the Appendix. It is strongly recommended to use the five class system for reporting variants (see the section "Classification of Variants"). Class 1 and 2 variants are generally not reported as this could lead to misinterpretation outside of the laboratory. In general, class 4 and 5 variants are always reported. Reporting of class 3 variants depends on the DNA test performed. Class 3 variants are reported when targeted panels containing proven candidate genes are analyzed but often not reported when a class 3 variant is detected in a gene of uncertain significance (GUS) [50]. Class 3 variants have the potential to cause confusion and should therefore be communicated to adequately trained clinicians. Most of the time, this would be a clinical geneticist or genetic counselor. As indicated above, not all variants will be reported to the referring clinician, but all variants are recorded within the laboratory. In addition, it is not essential to document all lines of evidence obtained in a report because this can be confusing to the clinician, but complete records must be stored in the laboratory.

Finding New Disease Genes

As exemplified in the coming chapters, many genes associated with various cardiovascular diseases have been identified in the past decennia. Nevertheless, all these genes still do not explain all known genetic cardiac disorders, and more genes still have to be uncovered. Up to the current NGS era, in general new genes were discovered by studying large families in which many affected family members were available to be genetically analyzed. In order to identify the most likely disease-associated region within a family of polymorphic markers, often dinucleotide repeats (and in some cases repeats of three or more nucleotides) that differ in length between individuals covering the full genome were being used. By mapping these markers in all affected family members and comparing with nonaffected family members, so-called linkage analysis (or also known as haplotype-sharing analysis), it was possible to identify a set of linked markers shared by all affected, most likely harboring the causal mutation in this family. Often this region still contained many possible candidate genes in which each had to be analyzed by Sanger sequencing to get to the true disease gene. Of course, genes known to be related to the heart or for which expression in cardiac tissue was shown were the ones prioritized for this. In case of suspected recessive-inherited disease, mostly because of known consanguinity in the respective family, polymorphic markers were also mapped but limited to the affected child (and often also the parents). In such analysis, the underlying genetic cause was supposed to be identical on both alleles (homozygous), and thus, (a) region(s) with a large number of subsequent identical markers were analyzed for mutations. This so-called homozygosity mapping has, however, been successful in only a limited part of all inherited cardiac disorders. When high-density SNP arrays became available, linkage-like analyses and homozygosity mapping were adapted to using such arrays as these had higher resolution, thereby in most cases reducing the size of the linked/homozygous region and limiting the amount of candidate genes to be Sanger sequenced. Another way to identify new disease genes was by comparing the deleted (or occasionally duplicated) regions on the same chromosomal region in a number of patients with the same phenotype and deducing the minimal deleted region shared. By including as many of such patients as possible, the regions could be considerably minimized to one containing only several genes. By subsequently sequencing these putative candidate genes in another group of patients with the same or a very comparable phenotype, but in which no deletion of the respective region could be found, the identification of causal point mutations in one of these genes would pinpoint to the actual disease gene in the deleted region of the initial patient cohort. Nowadays, NGS is generally being employed to find new disease genes. Comparably to the situation in previously described linkage/haplotype sharing analyses, now several affected family members are being analyzed by WES of GWS after which the identified exome- or genome-wide variation is being compared. In order to perform a proper comparison, first all variants that are rather frequent in the general population (>1%) are removed from the analysis. Only then the list of remaining variants will be short enough to enable the detection of the shared, potentially pathogenic variant. However, this is still not an easy task, and predictions on pathogenicity of the different shared candidate variants are required to identify the truly pathogenic variant.

To: Consultant Clinical Geneticist
Date:
Letter ID:
Our reference: FFxxxxx,

Dear colleague,

Enclosed the results of the DNA-analysis you requested:
Name: A. Patient
Date of birth: ....
Gender: ....
Date application: ....
Indication(s): Confirmation of clinical diagnosis of Dilated Cardiomyopathy
Performed diagnostics: Next-generation sequence analysis of the cardiomyopathy panel (56 genes)
Diagnosed materials: 18Dxxxx (DNA from EDTA blood)

Performed diagnostics and result
Sequence analysis of the gene panel for cardiomyopathy by NGS (18D6763):
1. PLN (Chr6: NM_002667.4) c.40_42del p.(Arg14del) (class 5): heterozygous

CNV analysis of the gene panel for cardiomyopathy by NGS (18D6763):
2. No (possibly) pathogenic variant detected

Variant classification: 5 = Pathogenic; 4 = Likely pathogenic; 3 = Uncertain significance; 2 = Likely benign; 1 = Benign;
RF = Risk factor; DR = Drug response

Conclusion
Patient is heterozygous for the pathogeni cvariant c.40_42del; p.(Arg14del) in the PLN gene (class 5 variant, pathogenic). This result confirms the clinical diagnosis of dilated cardiomyopathy in the patient.
Genetic testing of at risk family members is possible.

Explanation
The nucleotide change c.40_42del results in a deletion of three nucleotides predicting a deletion of amino acid Aginine at position 14 (p.(Arg14del) in the PLN protein. The deleted amino acid (Arg14) is strongly conserved. In literature this variant has been described before in DCM families (de Witt MM et al., J Am Coll Cardiol 2006;48:1396-1398; Haghighi K et al., Proc Natl Acad Sci 2006;103:1388-93). Introduction of this mutated gene in transgenic mice results in a similar phenotype and co-transfection in HEK-293 cells shows strong inhibition of the sarcoplasmic reticulum Ca2+-ATPase (de Witt MM et al., J Am Coll Cardiol 2006;48:1396-1398). This variant is a well-known founder variant in the Netherlands (van der Zwaag PA et al., EurJ Heart Fail. 2012;14(11):1199-207).

Method and quality
All coding exons of the 56 genes (45 "Dutch core genes" for cardiomyopathy plus ALPK3, CDH2, FHL2, FKRP, FLNC, HCN4, MYLK3, PPA2, PRDM16, TNNI3K and TTN), including the 20 flanking intron nucleotides have been analyzed. The presence of larger deletions or insertions, or mutations located outside the analyzed fragments can not be excluded.
The "core disease genes" in a diagnostic test represent the genes which are considered as essential for establishing a reliable and accurate molecular diagnosis (see Weiss MM et al, 2013, Human Mutat, 34:1313-1321).

Machine: MiSeq
MiSeq experiment nr: ....
Chemistry: MiSeq Reagent Kit v2, 2 x 150 bp
Analysis programs: BWA-MEM(0.7.12-r1039), picard-tools 1.95, GATK3.8 HaplotypeCaller, Cartagenia v5.0.4.
Enrichment of the target regions: Nimblegen SeqCap easy choice (OID.....) version CMv18.
Minimal coverage (minimal MAPQ20 and BaseQ20): 30 reads.
Average vertical coverage (minimal MAPQ20 and BaseQ20): 787 (±372)
Sanger sequencing for regions with a coverage < 30 reads.
Sample swaps ruled out with a SNP control test.
We do not report variants occurring in > 0,3% of control alleles (NHLBI Exome Sequencing Project), silent variants without a clear effect on splicing (as predicted by the programs in AlaMut), class 1 (certainly not pathogenic) and class 2 (unlikely pathogenic) variants.
Based on our validation experiments we determined that the sensitivity of our combined test (NextGen and Sanger sequencing) for nucleotide substitutions and deletions, insertions and duplications up to 68 nucleotides is >99%.
CNV detection: Calculation of Depth of Coverage (DoC) per exon after performing the BWA-MEM-GATK pipeline. DoC per exon per sample are normalized to the average normalized coverage per sample and compared to the average coverage per exon of previously analyzed samples. The differences in normalized coverage are used to calculate Z-scores (see http://amcpipeline.readthedocs.io/nl/latest/seqcappipeline.html).
CNV analysis was possible for 98.6% of the nucleotides (specific data are available on request).

Genes with reference sequences:
1. ACTC1 (NM_005159.4), 2. ACTN2 (NM_001103.2, NM_001278343.1, NM_001278344.1), 3. ALPK3 (NM_020778.4), 4. ANKRD1 (NM_014391. 2), 5. BAG3 (NM_004281.3), 6. CALR3 (NM_145046.3), 7. CAV3 (NM_033337.2), 8. CDH2 (NM_001792.4, NM_001308176.1), 9. CRYAB (NM_001885.2), 10. CSRP3 (NM_003476.4), 11. CTNNA3 (NM_013266.3, NM_001291133.1), 12. DES (NM_001927.3), 13. DSC2 (NM_024422.4, NM_004949.4), 14. DSG2(NM_001943.4), 15. DSP (NM_004415.3), 16. EMD (STA) (NM_000117.2), 17. FHL1 (NM_001159702.2, NM_001159701.1, NM_001159699.1), 18. FHL2 (NM_201555.1), 19.FKRP (NM_024301.4), 20.FLNC (NM_001458.4), 21.GLA (NM_000169.2), 22. HCN4 (NM_005477.2), 23. JPH2 (NM_020433.4, NM_175913.3), 24. JUP (NM_021991.2), 25. LAMA4 (NM_001105206.2, NM_001105208.2), 26.LAMP2 (NM_002294.2, NM_013995.2, NM_001122606.1), 27. LDB3 (NM_007078.2, NM_001080116.1), 28. LMNA (NM_170707.3, NM_001257374.2, NM_005572.3; NM_001282624.1), 29. MIB1 (NM_020774.2), 30. MYBPC3 (NM_000256.3), 31. MYH6 (NM_002471.3), 32. MYH7 (NM_000257.3), 33. MYL2 (NM_000432.3), 34. MYLK3 (NM_182493.2), 35. MYL3 (NM_000258.2), 36. MYOZ2 (NM_016599.4), 37. MYPN (NM_032578.2, NM_001256268.1), 38. NEXN (NM_144573.3), 39. PKP2 (NM_004572.3), 40. PLN (NM_002667.3), 41. PPA2 (NM_176869.2), 42. PRDM16 (NM_022114.3), 43. PRKAG2 (NM_016203.3, NM_001304527.1), 44. RBM20 (NM_001134363.1), 45. SCN5A (NM_198056.2), 46. TAZ (NM_000116.3, NM_001303465.1), 47. TCAP (NM_003673.3), 48. TMEM43 (NM_024334.2), 49. TNNC1 (NM_003280.2), 50. TNNI3 (NM_000363.4), 51. TNNI3K (NM_015978.2), 52. TNNT2 (NM_000364.2,

Fig. 1.3 Example letter including quality issues sent to a referring clinical geneticist that request targeted NGS analysis for dilated cardiomyopathy

NM_001001430.2), 53. TPM1 (NM_000366.5, NM_001018005.1, NM_001018020.1, NM_001301289.1), 54. TTN (N2-B (NM_003319.4; all coding exons), N2A (NM_133378.4; all coding exons), Novex-3 (NM_133379.3; all coding exons), Novex-1 (NM_133432.3; all coding exons), Novex-2 (NM_133437.3; all coding exons), transcript variant IC (NM_001267550.1; 335 of the 362 coding exons were analyzed)), 55. TTR (NM_000371.3), 56. VCL (NM_014000.2).

Yours sincerely,

laboratory specialist in clinical genetics laboratory specialist in clinical genetics

This report is signed electronically

The Genome Diagnostics laboratory … is EN-ISO15189:2012 accredited (…. Accreditation Council, M<accreditation number>); Nomenclature according to http://www.hgvs.org/mutnomen/. Our conclusions are based on the assumption that the tubes were correctly labelled and that the information provided in the pedigree is correct. We accept no responsibility for errors involving incorrect interpretation and/or translation of our letters.

Fig. 1.3 (continued)

Combining this with an additional linkage-like approach will facilitate the search for the causal mutation, as the variation in the shared region or regions identified by the linkage method can then be prioritized. The same of course accounts to homozygosity mapping in combination with NGS and subsequent hunting for deleterious mutations in the homozygous region of patients supposedly affected with a recessive-inherited disease. Moreover, performing NGS in a cohort of patients with the same phenotype, but no deletion/duplication detected via array-based approaches, and then zooming in on regions that have been shown to be deleted in a comparable patient cohort could also result in identifying nucleotide mutations in such patients. Of course, the above-described methods can also be exploited to identify causal genes in patients that show the same phenotype and come from the same geographic region, but are not known to be related, with the underlying idea that they might share a founder mutation (and thus in the end are related). This could be done by using NGS data only but will probably be more successful in combination with a haplotype-sharing approach. Finally, in case of very rare diseases, the comparison of NGS data of several certainly not related patients (often even originating from different ethnic backgrounds) is being used to find new disease genes, however in that case with the assumption that these patients do not share the same mutation, but different drastic mutations, in the same gene. It is important to realize with respect to this type of analyses that not all patients included in such efforts necessarily share only one disease gene, and extensive computational work is needed to get to the once that do.

Clinical Genetic Diagnostics

In the last decades, clinical genetic testing has become increasingly incorporated in the clinical care for patients and their families with inherited cardiac diseases, and genetic analyses often considerably contribute to the diagnostic workup for these patients. With the recent developments in WGS possibilities, clinical genetic diagnostics may even develop toward "genotype-first" approaches, meaning that patients suspected of having a genetic cardiac disease will first undergo genetic screening, preferably by performing WGS, to identify putative pathogenic mutations in cardiac-related genes, before other diagnostic testing will be performed. It can be expected that WGS will be performed rapidly enough in the near future that waiting for the result to guide further diagnostics and prevent unnecessary examinations, treatments, and interventions may become general practice. In this respect, rapid WGS was already used to reach genetic diagnoses within several days, including that of long QT syndrome ([83], Priest et al. [84]). Moreover, with the continuing aggregation of large amounts of exome and genome sequencing data and concomitant developments in interpreting the data, personalized genetic medicine will become a reality soon as well. However, these methods are not yet within reach for every individual and will thus only be applied in particular cases, and more targeted approaches are currently daily practice and will therefore be discussed in more detail below. In the past, when only individual genes were screened sequentially, genetic screening was mostly terminated as soon as a likely pathogenic or pathogenic mutation was identified, precluding the identification of a second mutation of which it is known that these may explain the clinical phenotype in ~5–10% of cases. The early application of targeted NGS approaches within the field of cardiogenetics relates to the fact that many candidate genes were already known to be involved in different cardiac diseases but were certainly also endorsed because of the extensive genetic heterogeneity within as well as the genetic overlap between these disorders. Although the latter would support the screening of all known cardiac-related genes within one experiment in every cardiac patient, most laboratories started with developing gene-panel approaches targeting genes involved in a specific disease or disease type and which gene panel used was guided by the clinical diagnosis/suspicion. This had to do with the labs being unfamiliar with both the technique and the putative outcome of genes irregularly screened. The costs involved in using larger panels would increase because of more materials and equipment being used but also due to more (bioinformatical) processing time required. Currently, genome diagnostic labs do offer targeted NGS analyses for most diseases, among which cardiac diseases. The number of genes targeted may differ from one gene (e.g., the screening of largest known human gene TTN, in which truncating mutations explain that between 15% and 25% of inherited DCM cases is being offered as a standalone NGS test in a number of laboratories) up to several hundreds. Unfortunately, the exact content of these gene panels differs between labs. It is therefore of major importance that specialists worldwide continuously interact and reach a consensus on which genes would be mandatory to be included in disease-specific panels. Of note, the exact content may of course be influenced by regional differences. In this respect, all Dutch genome diagnostic laboratories proposed that labs should agree on and use a list of "core disease genes" for every genetic disease that should be included in a diagnostic test to establish a reliable and molecular diagnosis [50]. Therefore, the five labs in the Netherlands that provide cardiogenetic NGS tests decided on a core list of 45 cardiomyopathy genes that are included in their gene panels, despite differences in the remainder of the content of their gene panels. It is important to realize, however, that some labs may offer NGS applications targeting only a relatively small subset of genes associated with a specific disease type, while these may be included in larger panels in other genetic testing facilities. On the other hand, often also the possibility is offered to sequence a larger gene panel but subsequently filter bioinformatically for a subpanel that is related to the specific disorder. The advantage of this approach is that this provides the possibility to again analyze the data using other or no filtering when the disease-specific filter failed to identify causal mutations. Importantly, in addition to proposing the use of core disease gene lists, the Dutch genome diagnostic labs in the same manuscript published general best practice guidelines for the use of NGS applications in clinical settings to ensure high-quality diagnostics. Likewise, this was, for example, done by the ACMG [79] and EuroGentest and the European Society of Human Genetics [69]. The reason to initially offer NGS application in which disease-associated genes were specifically enriched and, subsequently, sequenced was due to insufficient sequencing quality and coverage in WES data. However, due to significant improvements in both vertical and horizontal coverage of, in particular, disease-associated genes in recently introduced WES applications, a substantial number of clinical genetic testing laboratories are now moving toward diagnostic WES with subsequent *in silico* filtering for disease-specific genes. Comparable to the possibility mentioned above to analyze subpanels within enriched larger gene panels and subsequently apply other filtering or "open" the gene panel, the same can be done with WES data, without being limited to the enriched genes. Moreover, this also enables "opening the exome," including the sequences of genes not (yet) related to the disease and by allowing the hunt for new disease genes. In spite of the already mentioned improvements in WES, WGS would still be the most preferred method, as this will provide more evenly distributed coverage and shorter sequencing time. Since this approach is becoming cheaper, WGS will most likely be the most preferred option for the near future, and several studies have proven its added value in clinical practice [83–85]. One of the advantages of the more evenly distributed sequencing data coming from WGS is that it is well suitable for quantitative analyses, in order to identify deletions and duplications [85, 86], as the normalization of data to enable the identification of aberrations in coverage indicating such deletions/duplications is easier than with WES or disease panel-specific enrichment approaches. Nevertheless, computational methods to perform this in the latter NGS data have been developed and have found their way into clinical diagnostics recently as well [87, 88]. Although these methods do not yet assure detection of all deletions/duplications, it may provide more information than previously used tests like MLPA and Q-PCR or array-based approaches, as they either focus on a limited set of genes only or have limitations in detecting smaller deletions, respectively. Nevertheless, currently, these techniques are often still used in addition to NGS applications, certainly when these types of mutations in specific genes can be expected, for example, using the respective MLPA when deletions in the *LMNA* gene are to be suspected in patients with cardiomyopathy and conduction disease. In addition to the use of these methods in parallel with NGS, other "old- fashioned" techniques are still being used in clinical genetic diagnostics. Sanger sequencing is still the preferred method to perform predictive testing in family members at risk after NGS has identified the disease-causing mutation in the respective index patient. Moreover, in numerous cases, it is still more cost-effective to first perform Sanger sequencing of the most prevalent gene or sometimes the only gene yet known to be involved in that disease before using a gene panel, WES or WGS. However, as the logistics of near-future genome diagnostic labs will almost fully be focused on NGS applications, one may anticipate that even those rare cases will all be screened by NGS first followed by targeting the respective gene(s) *in silico*. As long as WGS is not routinely introduced, in addition to applying the current NGS methodologies, several cytogenetic techniques, like karyotyping, FISH analyses, and array-CGH, are still widely used within the field of CHDs, syndromal cardiac diseases, or multiple congenital anomalies/mental retardation (MCA/MR) syndromes including cardiac abnormalities. Finally, the introduction of other techniques or approaches like the TLA technology to detect disease-causing mutations outside coding of near-coding sequences or the use of RNA sequencing instead of DNA sequencing will be implemented in diagnostics in the near future as well.

References

1. Morris KV, Mattick JS. The rise of regulatory RNA. Nat Rev Genet. 2014;15:423–37.
2. Bhuiyan ZA, van den Berg MP, van Tintelen JP, Bink-Boelkens MT, Wiesfeld AC, Alders M, Postma AV, van Langen I, Mannens MM, Wilde AA. Expanding spectrum of human RYR2 -related disease: new electrocardiographic, structural, and genetic features. Circulation. 2007;116:1569–76.
3. Roberts JD, Herkert JC, Rutberg J, Nikkel SM, Wiesfeld AC, Dooijes D, Gow RM, van Tintelen JP, Gollob MH. Detection of genomic deletions of PKP2 in arrhythmogenic right ventricular cardiomyopathy. Clin Genet. 2013;83:452–6.
4. Weiss K, Applegate C, Wang T, Batista DA. Familial TAB2 microdeletion and congenital heart defects including unusual valve dysplasia and tetralogy of fallot. Am J Med Genet A. 2015;167A:2702–6.
5. van der Zwaag PA, van Rijsingen IA, Asimaki A, Jongbloed JD, van Veldhuisen DJ, Wiesfeld AC, Cox MG, van Lochem LT, de Boer RA, Hofstra RM, Christiaans I, van Spaendonck-Zwarts KY, Lekanne dit Deprez RH, Judge DP, Calkins H, Suurmeijer AJ, Hauer RN, Saffitz JE, Wilde AA, van den Berg MP, van Tintelen JP. Phospholamban R14del mutation in patients diagnosed with dilated cardiomyopathy or arrhythmogenic right ventricular cardiomyopathy: evidence supporting the concept of arrhythmogenic cardiomyopathy. Eur J Heart Fail. 2012;14:1199–207.
6. van Rijsingen IA, van der Zwaag PA, Groeneweg JA, Nannenberg EA, Jongbloed JD, Zwinderman AH, Pinto YM, Lekanne dit Deprez RH, Post JG, Tan HL, de Boer RA, Hauer RN, Christiaans I, van den Berg MP, van Tintelen JP, Wilde AA. Outcome in phospholamban R14del carriers: results of a large multicentre cohort study. Circ Cardiovasc Genet. 2014;7:455–65.
7. Dib C, Fauré S, Fizames C, Samson D, Drouot N, Vignal A, Millasseau P, Marc S, Hazan J, Seboun E, Lathrop M, Gyapay G, Morissette J, Weissenbach J. A comprehensive genetic map of the human genome based on 5,264 microsatellites. Nature. 1996;380:152–4.
8. Williamson R, Bowcock A, Kidd K, Pearson P, Schmidtke J, Ceverha P, Chipperfield M, Cooper DN, Coutelle C, Hewitt J, Klinger K, Langley K, Beckmann J, Tolley M, Maidak B, Hewett D, Linch C, Maslen G. Report of the DNA committee and catalogues of cloned and mapped genes, markers formatted for PCR and DNA polymorphisms. Cytogenet Cell Genet. 1990;55:457–778.
9. Futreal PA, Söderkvist P, Marks JR, Iglehart JD, Cochran C, Barrett JC, Wiseman RW. Detection of frequent allelic loss on proximal chromosome 17q in sporadic breast carcinoma using microsatellite length polymorphisms. Cancer Res. 1992;52:2624–7.
10. Lindor NM, Karnes PS, Michels VV, Dewald GW, Goerss J, Jalal S, Jenkins RB, Vockley G, Thibodeau SN. Uniparental disomy in congenital disorders: a prospective study. Am J Med Genet. 1995;58:143–6.
11. Vilar E, Mork ME, Cuddy A, Borras E, Bannon SA, Taggart MW, Ying J, Broaddus RR, Luthra R, Rodriguez-Bigas MA, Lynch PM, You YQ. Role of microsatellite instability-low as a diagnostic biomarker of Lynch syndrome in colorectal cancer. Cancer Gene Ther. 2014;207:495–502.
12. Lyon MF. Gene action in the X-chromosome of the mouse (*Mus musculus* L.). Nature. 1961;190:372–3.
13. Lyon MF. Sex chromatin and gene action in the mammalian X-chromosome. Am J Hum Genet. 1962;14:135–48.
14. Lubs HA. A marker X chromosome. Am J Hum Genet. 1969;21:231–44.
15. Sharp AJ, Locke DP, McGrath SD, Cheng Z, Bailey JA, Vallente RU, Pertz LM, Clark RA, Schwartz S, Segraves R, Oseroff VV, Albertson DG, Pinkel D, Eichler EE. Segmental duplications and copy-number variation in the human genome. Am J Hum Genet. 2005;77:78–88.
16. Goidts V, Cooper DN, Armengol L, Schempp W, Conroy J, Estivill X, Nowak N, Hameister H, Kehrer-Sawatzki H. Complex patterns of copy number variation at sites of segmental duplications: an important category of structural variation in the human genome. Hum Genet. 2006;120:270–84.
17. Komura D, Shen F, Ishikawa S, Fitch KR, Chen W, Zhang J, Liu G, Ihara S, Nakamura H, Hurles ME, Lee C, Scherer SW, Jones KW, Shapero MH, Huang J, Aburatani H. Genome-wide detection of human copy number variations using high-density DNA oligonucleotide arrays. Genome Res. 2006;16:1575–84.
18. Redon R, Ishikawa S, Fitch KR, Feuk L, Perry GH, Andrews TD, Fiegler H, Shapero MH, Carson AR, Chen W, Cho EK, Dallaire S, Freeman JL, González JR, Gratacòs M, Huang J, Kalaitzopoulos D, Komura D, MacDonald JR, Marshall CR, Mei R, Montgomery L, Nishimura K, Okamura K, Shen F, Somerville MJ, Tchinda J, Valsesia A, Woodwark C, Yang F, Zhang J, Zerjal T, Zhang J, Armengol L, Conrad DF, Estivill X, Tyler-Smith C, Carter NP, Aburatani H, Lee C, Jones KW, Scherer SW, Hurles ME. Global variation in copy number in the human genome. Nature. 2006;444:444–54.
19. Driscoll DA, Salvin J, Sellinger B, Budarf ML, McDonald-McGinn DM, Zackai EH, Emanuel BS. Prevalence of 22q11 microdeletions in DiGeorge and velocardiofacial syndromes: implications for genetic counselling and prenatal diagnosis. J Med Genet. 1993;30:813–7.
20. Sanger F, Nicklen S, Coulson AR. DNA sequencing with chain terminating inhibitors. Proc Natl Acad Sci U S A. 1977;74:5463–7.
21. Mullis K, Faloona F, Scharf S, Saiki R, Horn G, Erlich H. Specific enzymatic amplification of DNA in vitro: the polymerase chain reaction. Cold Spring Harb Symp Quant Biol. 1986;51(Pt 1):263–73.
22. Jovanovich S, Bogdan G, Belcinski R, Buscaino J, Burgi D, Butts EL, Chear K, Ciopyk B, Eberhart D, El-Sissi O, Franklin H, Gangano S, Gass J, Harris D, Hennessy L, Kindwall A, King D, Klevenberg J, Li Y, Mehendale N, McIntosh R, Nielsen B, Park C, Pearson F, Schueren R, Stainton N, Troup C, Pm V, Vangbo M, Woudenberg T, Wyrick D, Williams S. Developmental validation of a fully integrated sample-to-profile rapid human identification system for processing single-source reference buccal samples. Forensic Sci Int Genet. 2015;16:181–94.
23. Klein D. Quantification using real-time PCR technology: applications and limitations. Trends Mol Med. 2002;8:257–60.
24. Ross RS, Chien KR. The polymerase chain reaction (PCR) and cardiovascular diagnosis. Trends Cardiovasc Med. 1991;1:1–5.
25. Heid CA, Stevens J, Livak KJ, Williams PM. Real time quantitative PCR. Genome Res. 1996;6:986–94.
26. Calabrese F, Thiene G. Myocarditis and inflammatory cardiomyopathy: microbiological and molecular biological aspects. Cardiovasc Res. 2003;60:11–25.
27. Guiver M, Fox AJ, Mutton K, Mogulkoc N, Egan J. Evaluation of CMV viral load using TaqMan CMV quantitative PCR and comparison with CMV antigenemia in heart and lung transplant recipients. Transplantation. 2001;71:1609–15.
28. Sykes PJ, Neoh SH, Brisco MJ, Hughes E, Condon J, Morley AA. Quantitation of targets for PCR by use of limiting dilution. BioTechniques. 1992;13:444–9.
29. Pinheiro LB, Coleman VA, Hindson CM, Herrmann J, Hindson BJ, Bhat S, Emslie KR. Evaluation of a droplet digital polymerase chain reaction format for DNA copy number quantification. Anal Chem. 2012;84:1003–11.
30. Schouten JP, McElgunn CJ, Waaijer R, Zwijnenburg D, Diepvens F, Pals G. Relative quantification of 40 nucleic acid sequences by multiplex ligation-dependent probe amplification. Nucleic Acids Res. 2002;30:e57.
31. Anderson S, Bankier AT, Barrell BG, de Bruijn MH, Coulson AR, Drouin J, Eperon IC, Nierlich DP, Roe BA, Sanger F, Schreier PH,

Smith AJ, Staden R, Young IG. Sequence and organization of the human mitochondrial genome. Nature. 1981;290:457–65.
32. Sanger F, Coulson AR, Hong GF, Hill DF, Petersen GB. Nucleotide sequence of bacteriophage lambda DNA. J Mol Biol. 1982;162:729–73.
33. International Human Genome Sequencing Consortium. Finishing the euchromatic sequence of the human genome. Nature. 2004;431:931–45.
34. Istrail S, Sutton GG, Florea L, Halpern AL, Mobarry CM, Lippert R, Walenz B, Shatkay H, Dew I, Miller JR, Flanigan MJ, Edwards NJ, Bolanos R, Fasulo D, Halldorsson BV, Hannenhalli S, Turner R, Yooseph S, Lu F, Nusskern DR, Shue BC, Zheng XH, Zhong F, Delcher AL, Huson DH, Kravitz SA, Mouchard L, Reinert K, Remington KA, Clark AG, Waterman MS, Eichler EE, Adams MD, Hunkapiller MW, Myers EW, Venter JC. Whole-genome shotgun assembly and comparison of human genome assemblies. Proc Natl Acad Sci U S A. 2004;101:1916–21.
35. Ronaghi M, Karamohamed S, Pettersson B, Uhlén M, Nyrén P. Real-time DNA sequencing using detection of pyrophosphate release. Anal Biochem. 1996;242:84–9.
36. Mardis ER. Next-generation sequencing platforms. Annu Rev Anal Chem. 2013;6:287–303.
37. Levene MJ, Korlach J, Turner SW, Foquet M, Craighead HG, Webb WW. Zero-mode waveguides for single-molecule analysis at high concentrations. Science. 2003;299:682–6.
38. Jain M, Koren S, Miga KH, Quick J, Rand AC, Sasani TA, Tyson JR, Beggs AD, Dilthey AT, Fiddes IT, Malla S, Marriott H, Nieto T, O'Grady J, Olsen HE, Pedersen BS, Rhie A, Richardson H, Quinlan AR, Snutch TP, Tee L, Paten B, Phillippy AM, Simpson JT, Loman NJ, Loose M. Nanopore sequencing and assembly of a human genome with ultra-long reads. Nat Biotechnol. 2018 Apr;36(4):338–45. https://doi.org/10.1038/nbt.4060.
39. Volden R, Palmer T, Byrne A, Cole C, Schmitz RJ, Green RE, Vollmers C. Improving nanopore read accuracy with the R2C2 method enables the sequencing of highly multiplexed full-length single-cell cDNA. Proc Natl Acad Sci U S A. 2018 Sep 10;115:9726–31. https://doi.org/10.1073/pnas.1806447115.
40. Samorodnitsky E, Jewell BM, Hagopian R, Miya J, Wing MR, Lyon E, Damodaran S, Bhatt D, Reeser JW, Datta J, Roychowdhury S. Evaluation of hybridization capture versus amplicon-based methods for whole-exome sequencing. Hum Mutat. 2015;36:903–14.
41. Vatta M, Spoonamore KG. Use of genetic testing to identify sudden cardiac death syndromes. Trends Cardiovasc Med. 2015;25:738–48.
42. Richards S, Aziz N, Bale S, Bick D, Das S, Gastier-Foster J. Standards and guidelines for the interpretation of sequence variants: a joint consensus recommendation of the American college of medical genetics and genomics and the association for molecular pathology. Genet Med. 2015;17:405–24.
43. He D, Furlotte N, Eskin E. Detection and reconstruction of tandemly organized de novo copy number variations. BMC Bioinformatics. 2010 Dec 14;11(Suppl 11):S12. https://doi.org/10.1186/1471-2105-11-S11-S12.
44. Teo SM, Pawitan Y, Ku CS, Chia KS, Salim A. Statistical challenges associated with detecting copy number variations with next-generation sequencing. Bioinformatics. 2012 Nov 1;28(21):2711–8. https://doi.org/10.1093/bioinformatics/bts535.
45. Cui H, Dhroso A, Johnson N, Korkin D. The variation game: cracking complex genetic disorders with NGS and omics data. Methods. 2015 Jun;79–80:18–31. https://doi.org/10.1016/j.ymeth.2015.04.018.
46. Hehir-Kwa JY, Tops BBJ, Kemmeren P. The clinical implementation of copy number detection in the age of next generation sequencing. Expert Rev Mol Diagn. 2018 Sep 15;18(10):907–15. https://doi.org/10.1080/14737159.2018.1523723.
47. Truty R, Paul J, Kennemer M, Lincoln SE, Olivares E, Nussbaum RL, Aradhya S. Prevalence and properties of intragenic copy-number variation in Mendelian disease genes. Genet Med. 2018 Jun 12;21(1):114–23. https://doi.org/10.1038/s41436-018-0033-5.
48. Overwater E, Marsili L, Baars MJH, Baas AF, van de Beek I, Dulfer E, van Hagen JM, Hilhorst-Hofstee Y, Kempers M, Krapels IP, Menke LA, Verhagen JMA, Yeung KK, Zwijnenburg PJG, Groenink M, van Rijn P, Weiss MM, Voorhoeve E, van Tintelen JP, Houweling AC, Maugeri A. Results of next-generation sequencing gene panel diagnostics including copy-number variation analysis in 810 patients suspected of heritable thoracic aortic disorders. Hum Mutat. 2018 Sep;39(9):1173–92. https://doi.org/10.1002/humu.23565.
49. Wallis Y, Payne S, McAnulty C, Bodmer D, Sistermans E, Robertson K, Moore D, Abbs S, Deans Z, Devereau A. 2013. Practice guidelines for the evaluation of pathogenicity and the reporting of sequence variants in clinical molecular genetics. http://www.acgs.uk.com/media/774853/evaluation_and_reporting_of_sequence_variants_bpgs_june_2013_-finalpdf.pdf
50. Weiss MM, Van der Zwaag B, Jongbloed JD, Vogel MJ, Brüggenwirth HT, Lekanne Deprez RH, Mook O, Ruivenkamp CA, van Slegtenhorst MA, van den Wijngaard A, Waisfisz Q, Nelen MR, van der Stoep N. Best practice guidelines for the use of next generation sequencing applications in genome diagnostics: a national collaborative study of Dutch genome diagnostic laboratories. Hum Mutat. 2013;34:1313–21.
51. Nykamp K, Anderson M, Powers M, Garcia J, Herrera B, Ho YY, Kobayashi Y, Patil N, Thusberg J, Westbrook M, Topper S. Sherloc: a comprehensive refinement of the ACMG–AMP variant classification criteria. Genet Med. 2017 Oct;19(10):1105–17. https://doi.org/10.1038/gim.2017.37.
52. Li Q, Wang K. InterVar: clinical interpretation of genetic variants by the 2015 ACMG-AMP guidelines. Am J Hum Genet. 2017 Feb 2;100(2):267–80. https://doi.org/10.1016/j.ajhg.2017.01.004.
53. Oliver GR, Hart SN, Klee EW. Bioinformatics for clinical next generation sequencing. Clin Chem. 2015;61:124–35.
54. Riera C, Lois S, Dom C, Fernandez-Cadenas I, Montaner J, Rodrıguez-Sureda V, de la Cruz X. Molecular damage in Fabry disease: characterization and prediction of alpha-galactosidase a pathological mutations. Proteins. 2015;83:91–104.
55. Thusberg J, Olatubosun A, Vihinen M. Performance of mutation pathogenicity prediction methods on missense variants. Hum Mutat. 2011;32:358–68.
56. Houdayer C, Caux-Montcoutier V, Krieger S, Barrois M, Bonnet F, Bourdon V, Bronner M, Buisson M, Coulet F, Gaildrat P, Lefol C, Léone M, Mazoyer S, Muller D, Remenieras A, Révillion F, Rouleau E, Sokolowska J, Jp V, Lidereau R, Soubrier F, Sobol H, Sevenet N, Bressac-de Paillerets B, Hardouin A, Tosi M, Om S, Stoppa-Lyonnet D. Guidelines for splicing analysis in molecular diagnosis derived from a set of 327 combined in silico/in vitro studies on BRCA1 and BRCA2 variants. Hum Mutat. 2012;33:1228–38.
57. Vreeswijk MP, Kraan JN, van der Klift HM, Vink GR, Cornelisse CJ, Wijnen JT, Bakker E, van Asperen CJ, Devilee P. Intronic variants in BRCA1 and BRCA2 that affect RNA splicing can be reliably selected by splice-site prediction programs. Hum Mutat. 2009;30:107–14.
58. Dhandapany PS, Sadayappan S, Xue Y, Powell GT, Rani DS, Nallari P, Rai TS, Khullar M, Soares P, Bahl A, Tharkan JM, Vaideeswar P, Rathinavel A, Narasimhan C, Ayapati DR, Ayub Q, Mehdi SQ, Oppenheimer S, Richards MB, Price AL, Patterson N, Reich D, Singh L, Tyler-Smith C, Thangaraj K. A common MYBPC3 (cardiac myosin binding protein C) variant associated with cardiomyopathies in South Asia. Nat Genet. 2009;41:187–91.
59. Fokkema IF, Taschner PE, Schaafsma GC, Celli J, Laros JF, den Dunnen JT. LOVD v.2.0: the next generation in gene variant databases. Hum Mutat. 2011;32:557–63.

60. Landrum MJ, Lee JM, Benson M, Brown G, Chao C, Chitipiralla S, Gu B, Hart J, Hoffman D, Hoover J, Jang W, Katz K, Ovetsky M, Riley G, Sethi A, Tully R, Villamarin-Salomon R, Rubinstein W, Maglott DR. ClinVar: public archive of interpretations of clinically relevant variants. Nucleic Acids Res. 2016;44:D862–8.
61. Stenson PD, Mort M, Ball EV, Shaw K, Phillips A, Cooper DN. The human gene mutation database: building a comprehensive mutation repository for clinical and molecular genetics, diagnostic testing and personalized genomic medicine. Hum Genet. 2014;133:1–9.
62. Andreasen C, Nielsen JB, Refsgaard L, Holst AG, Christensen AH, Andreasen L, Sajadieh A, Haunsø S, Svendsen JH, Olesen MS. New population-based exome data are questioning the pathogenicity of previously cardiomyopathy-associated genetic variants. Eur J Hum Genet. 2013;21:918–28.
63. Risgaard B, Jabbari R, Refsgaard L, Holst AG, Haunsø S, Sadjadieh A, Winkel BG, Olesen MS, Tfelt-Hansen J. High prevalence of genetic variants previously associated with Brugada syndrome in new exome data. Clin Genet. 2013;84:489–95.
64. Bayrak-Toydemir P, McDonald J, Mao R, Phansalkar A, Gedge F, Robles J, Goldgar D, Lyon E. Likelihood ratios to assess genetic evidence for clinical significance of uncertain variants: hereditary hemorrhagic telangiectasia as a model. Exp Mol Pathol. 2008;85:45–9.
65. Thompson D, Easton DF, Goldgar DE. A full-likelihood method for the evaluation of causality of sequence variants from family data. Am J Hum Genet. 2003;73:652–5.
66. Møller P, Clark N, Mæhle L. A simplified method for segregation analysis (SISA) to determine penetrance and expression of a genetic variant in a family. Hum Mutat. 2011;32:568–71.
67. Lekanne Deprez RH, Muurling-Vlietman JJ, Hruda J, Baars MJ, Wijnaendts LC, Stolte-Dijkstra I, Alders M, van Hagen JM. Two cases of severe neonatal hypertrophic cardiomyopathy caused by compound heterozygous mutations in the MYBPC3 gene. J Med Genet. 2006;43:829–32.
68. Fortier N, Rudy G, Scherer A. Detection of CNVs in NGS data using VS-CNV. Methods Mol Biol. 2018;1833:115–27. https://doi.org/10.1007/978-1-4939-8666-8_9.
69. Matthijs G, Souche E, Alders M, Corveleyn A, Eck S, Feenstra I, Race V, Sistermans E, Sturm M, Weiss M, Yntema H, Bakker B, Scheffer H, Bauer P. Guidelines for diagnostic next-generation sequencing. Eur J Hum Genet. 2016;24:2–5.
70. Roy S, Coldren C, Karunamurthy A, Kip NS, Klee EW, Lincoln SE, Leon A, Pullambhatla M, Temple-Smolkin RL, Voelkerding KV, Wang C, Carter AB. Standards and guidelines for validating next-generation sequencing bioinformatics pipelines: a joint recommendation of the association for molecular pathology and the college of American pathologists. J Mol Diagn. 2018 Jan;20(1):4–27. https://doi.org/10.1016/j.jmoldx.2017.11.003.
71. Pugh TJ, Kelly MA, Gowrisankar S, Hynes E, Seidman MA, Baxter SM, Bowser M, Harrison B, Aaron D, Mahanta LM, Lakdawala NK, McDermott G, White ET, Rehm HL, Lebo M, Funke BH. The landscape of genetic variation in dilated cardiomyopathy as surveyed by clinical DNA sequencing. Genet Med. 2014;16:601–8.
72. Mamanova L, Coffey AJ, Scott CE, Kozarewa I, Turner EH, Kumar A, Howard E, Shendure J, Turner DJ. Target-enrichment strategies for next-generation sequencing. Nat Methods. 2010;7:111–8.
73. Rossetti S, Hopp K, Sikkink RA, Sundsbak JL, Lee YK, Kubly V, Eckloff BW, Ward CJ, Winearls CG, Torres VE, Harris PC. Identification of gene mutations in autosomal dominant polycystic kidney disease through targeted resequencing. J Am Soc Nephrol. 2012;23:915–33.
74. Milko LV, Funke BH, Hershberger RE, Azzariti DR, Lee K, Riggs ER, Rivera-Munoz EA, Weaver MA, Niehaus A, Currey EL, Craigen WJ, Mao R, Offit K, Steiner RD, Martin CL, Rehm HL, Watson MS, Ramos EM, Plon SE, Berg JS. Development of clinical domain working groups for the clinical genome resource (ClinGen): lessons learned and plans for the future. Genet Med. 2018 Sep 5;21(4):987–93. https://doi.org/10.1038/s41436-018-0267-2.
75. Treangen TJ, Salzberg SL. Repetitive DNA and next generation sequencing: computational challenges and solutions. Nat Rev Genet. 2012;13:36–46.
76. Rehm HL. Disease-targeted sequencing: a cornerstone in the clinic. Nat Rev Genet. 2013;14:295–300.
77. Lubin IM, Caggana M, Constantin C, Gross SJ, Lyon E, Pagon RA, Trotter TL, Wilson JA, McGovern MM. Ordering molecular genetic tests and reporting results: practices in laboratory and clinical settings. J Mol Diagn. 2008;10:459–68.
78. Lubin IM, McGovern MM, Gibson Z, Gross SJ, Lyon E, Pagon RA, Pratt VM, Rashid J, Shaw C, Stoddard L, Trotter TL, Williams MS, Amos Wilson J, Pass K. Clinician perspectives about molecular genetic testing for heritable conditions and development of a clinician- friendly laboratory report. J Mol Diagn. 2009;11:162–71.
79. Rehm HL, Bale SJ, Bayrak-Toydemir P, Berg JS, Brown KK, Deignan JL, Friez MJ, Funke BH, Hegde MR, Working Group of the American College of Medical Genetics and Genomics Laboratory Quality Assurance Committee. ACMG clinical laboratory standards for next-generation sequencing. Genet Med. 2013;15:733–47.
80. Scheuner MT, Hilborne L, Brown J, Lubin IM. A report template for molecular genetic tests designed to improve communication between the clinician and laboratory. Genet Test Mol Biomarkers. 2012;16:761–9.
81. Treacy RJL, Robinson DO. Draft best practice guidelines for reporting molecular genetics results. 2013. http://www.cmgs.org/BPGs/Best_Practice_Guidelines.htm.
82. Suthers G. Guidelines for reporting molecular genetic tests to medical practitioners. 2009. http://www.rcpa.edu.au//Home.htm
83. Saunders CJ, Miller NA, Soden SE, Dinwiddie DL, Noll A, Alnadi NA, Andraws N, Patterson ML, Krivohlavek LA, Fellis J, Humphray S, Saffrey P, Kingsbury Z, Weir JC, Betley J, Grocock RJ, Margulies EH, Farrow EG, Artman M, Safina NP, Petrikin JE, Hall KP, Kingsmore SF. Rapid whole-genome sequencing for genetic disease diagnosis in neonatal intensive care units. Sci Transl Med. 2012;4:154ra135.
84. Priest JR, Ceresnak SR, Dewey FE, Malloy-Walton LE, Dunn K, Grove ME, Perez MV, Maeda K, Dubin AM, Ashley EA. Molecular diagnosis of long QT syndrome at 10 days of life by rapid whole genome sequencing. Heart Rhythm. 2014;11:1707–13.
85. Gilissen C, Hehir-Kwa JY, Thung DT, van de Vorst M, van Bon BW, Willemsen MH, Kwint M, Janssen IM, Hoischen A, Schenck A, Leach R, Klein R, Tearle R, Bo T, Pfundt R, Yntema HG, de Vries BB, Kleefstra T, Brunner HG, Vissers LE, Veltman JA. Genome sequencing identifies major causes of severe intellectual disability. Nature. 2014;511:344–7.
86. Zhao M, Wang QQ, Jia P, Zhao Z. Computational tools for copy number variation (CNV) detection using next-generation sequencing data: features and perspectives. BMC Biochem. 2013;14(Suppl 11):S1.
87. Johansson LF, van Dijk F, de Boer EN, van Dijk-Bos KK, Jongbloed JD, van der Hout AH, Westers H, Sinke RJ, Swertz MA, Sijmons RH, Sikkema-Raddatz B. CoNVaDING: single exon variation detection in targeted NGS data. Hum Mutat. 2016;37:457–64.
88. Tan R, Wang Y, Kleinstein SE, Liu Y, Zhu X, Guo H, Jiang Q, Allen AS, Zhu M. An evaluation of copy number variation detection tools from whole exome sequencing data. Hum Mutat. 2013;35:899–907.

Clinical Genetics

2

J. J. van der Smagt and Jodie Ingles

Introduction

With the rapid advances in genetic knowledge, more specifically genetic knowledge of human disease, many physicians will not find the time to keep up with the pace. Even though new generations of doctors are much better trained, both in genetics and in quickly acquiring adequate information from (Internet) databases, cooperation between "organ specialists" and "genetic specialists" seems to be the best option for the near future. Importantly, many genetic diseases are relatively rare, so that individual specialists will only encounter patients with a specific genetic disease on an occasional basis. This makes it difficult for them to obtain sufficient experience in providing adequate genetic information, in addressing the genetic questions of both patients and their families, and eventually in interpreting the often complex genetic test results.

Genetics has become increasingly important to the field of cardiology [1, 2]. There is increasing awareness that some cardiac disorders occur in families and that important genetic factors play a role in disease causation. This holds true not only for monogenic disorders such as hypertrophic cardiomyopathy, congenital long QT syndromes, and catecholaminergic polymorphic ventricular tachycardia but also for more common complex disorders such as coronary artery disease, hypertension, and diabetes. In the latter group of disorders, many different additive genetic and environmental contributions, each of relatively small effect size, are hypothesized to be disease-causing. Important progress has been made in understanding the molecular background predisposing to different types of cardiac disease.

Meanwhile, in clinical genetic practice, focus has shifted from primarily reproductive issues (parents wanting to know the risk of recurrence after the birth of a child with a mental handicap or serious congenital abnormality, e.g., a congenital heart defect) to include the assessment of risk of genetic disease, occurring later in life, in individuals with a positive family history. This started in neurology with individuals at risk for mostly untreatable neurodegenerative disease, like Huntington's chorea, wanting to know their genetic status in order to make future plans. Subsequently genetic diagnosis entered the field of oncology, where it has become an increasingly important tool in identifying individuals at high risk of getting cancer. Of course, in the field of oncology, genetic testing has important medical implications, as individuals at risk may opt for increased cancer surveillance and preventive treatment strategies—may be devised, based on genetic information.

Cardiology is another discipline of medicine where large-scale so-called presymptomatic testing of healthy at-risk individuals has become available for some of the primary electrical heart diseases and cardiomyopathies. In particular, following the sudden cardiac death of a young person, post-mortem genetic testing (i.e., extraction of DNA from post-mortem frozen blood or tissue sections for genetic analysis) can play an important role in clarifying the cause of death and risk to family members. Although for most disease entities, family studies have not yet actually been proven to be beneficial, identifying those individuals at risk seems a logical first step in the development of preventive strategies. However, genetics of cardiac disease is complicated, for example, by *genetic heterogeneity* (many different genetic causes result in clinically identical disease) and the fact that test results may be difficult to interpret. Cooperation between cardiologists and clinical geneticists is, therefore, of great importance.

J. J. van der Smagt (✉)
University Medical Centre Utrecht, Utrecht, The Netherlands
e-mail: j.j.vandersmagt@umcutrecht.nl

J. Ingles
Agnes Ginges Centre for Molecular Cardiology, Centenary Institute, Sydney, NSW, Australia

Sydney Medical School, University of Sydney, Sydney, NSW, Australia

Department of Cardiology, Royal Prince Alfred Hospital, Sydney, NSW, Australia

H. F. Baars et al. (eds.), *Clinical Cardiogenetics*, https://doi.org/10.1007/978-3-030-45457-9_2

In this chapter, basic concepts in genetics and important issues that have to be considered in case of genetic testing are discussed.

The Clinical Genetic Intake

For those cardiologists involved in caring for families with cardiogenetic disorders, it is important to gain some experience in constructing pedigrees and recording family histories.

Family History

History taking will be more time-consuming than usual as, besides the regular cardiac anamnesis, detailed information on several family members has to be obtained [3]. Usually, information on three (sometimes four) generations is considered sufficient. Whenever possible, information should be collected on first-degree relatives (parents, siblings, and children), second-degree relatives (grandparents, uncles/aunts, and nephews/nieces), and third-degree relatives (first cousins). On average, they share 50%, 25%, and 12.5% of their DNA with the index patient. Information on past generations may be sparse or even misleading as many conditions could not be correctly diagnosed in the past, whereas in contrast, younger generations will be less informative as they may not have lived long enough yet for disease symptoms to become manifest. Therefore, information on more distant relatives, like first cousins, from the same generation as the index patient may prove essential.

The reliability of the information obtained through family history taking will vary from case to case. In general, accuracy decreases with the decreasing degree of relationship. As a general rule, it is wise to confirm important information by checking medical records, whenever possible. If this involves family members, their written consent to retrieve these records will be required.

While taking a family history, it is important to be as specific as possible. People may leave out vital information when they do not think that it is important. Possible cardiac events should be specifically asked for, and approximate ages at which they occurred should be recorded. Of course, also the circumstances in which the event took place have to be noted. Depending on the nature of the condition under investigation, it may be necessary to ask for specific events, like diving or swimming accidents in case of suspected long QT syndrome type 1. It is useful to keep in mind that syncope resulting from arrhythmias may in the past have been diagnosed as seizures or epilepsy and that sudden death of an infant could have been documented as a sudden infant death syndrome (SIDS). General questions about the entire family can be asked to elicit any additional information, such as "are there any other family members who have the same heart condition as yourself?" and "are there any individuals who have died suddenly or at a young age?"

If family members are under cardiac surveillance elsewhere, it is prudent to record this, and if individuals are deceased as a result of a possible cardiac event, always inquire whether autopsy has been performed. Information on consanguinity is often not readily volunteered and should be specifically asked for. Depending on the nature of the disorder under investigation, it may also be important to inquire about medical conditions not specifically involving the heart. For example, when investigating a family with possible autosomal dominant dilated cardiomyopathy, it would be prudent to also ask for signs of skeletal muscle disease in family members.

Pedigree Construction

Drawing a *pedigree* is a helpful tool in assessing any familial disorder. Presenting family history information in a pedigree allows to quickly visualize family structure and assess the possible inheritance patterns [4, 5]. In addition, a drawn pedigree will make it more easy to see which, and how many, family members are at risk for cardiac disease and who should be contacted. The symbols commonly used for pedigree construction are represented in Fig. 2.1.

Nowadays, different software packages exist for pedigree construction. These packages have the advantage that it is easier to update pedigrees and that pedigrees can be more easily added to other digital medical files. Frequently, the software also offers options that are valuable for genetic research.

However, the great advantage of pen and paper is that the pedigree can be constructed while taking the family history, thus ensuring that no important family members are overlooked.

A few tips and tricks (see Fig. 2.2):

- Start drawing your pedigree on a separate sheet of paper. Start with your index patient in the middle of the paper and go from there.
- Add a date to your pedigree.
- Numbering: by convention, generations are denoted by a Roman numeral, whereas individuals within a generation are identified by an Arabic numeral. In this way each individual can be identified unambiguously by combining the two numbers (II-3, III-1, etc.). Additional information on a specific individual can be added in a footnote referring to this identification number.
- The most important clinical information can be directly added to the pedigree (see Fig. 2.2).
- Record approximate dates (e.g., birth year or 5-year interval), not ages. Add age at time of death.

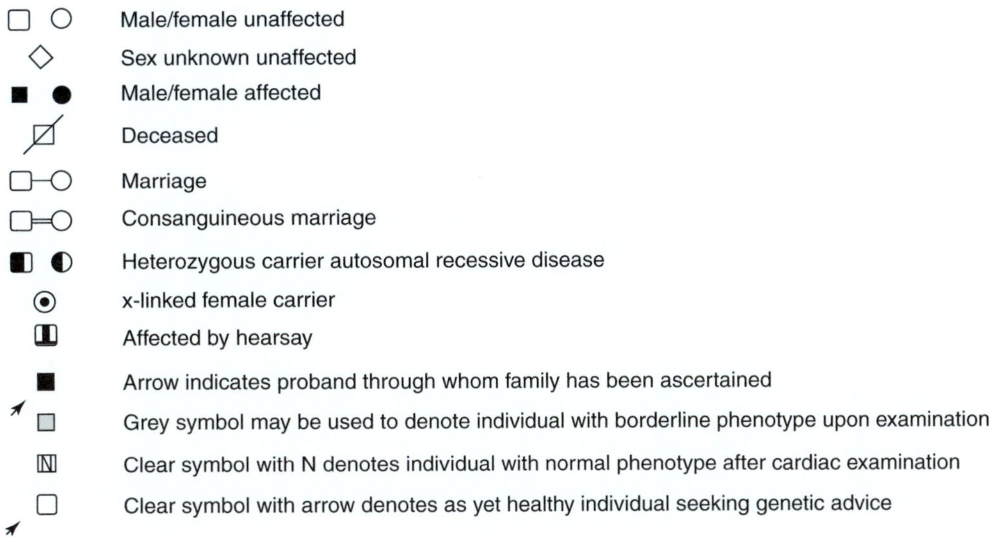

Fig. 2.1 Symbols used to denote individuals in a pedigree

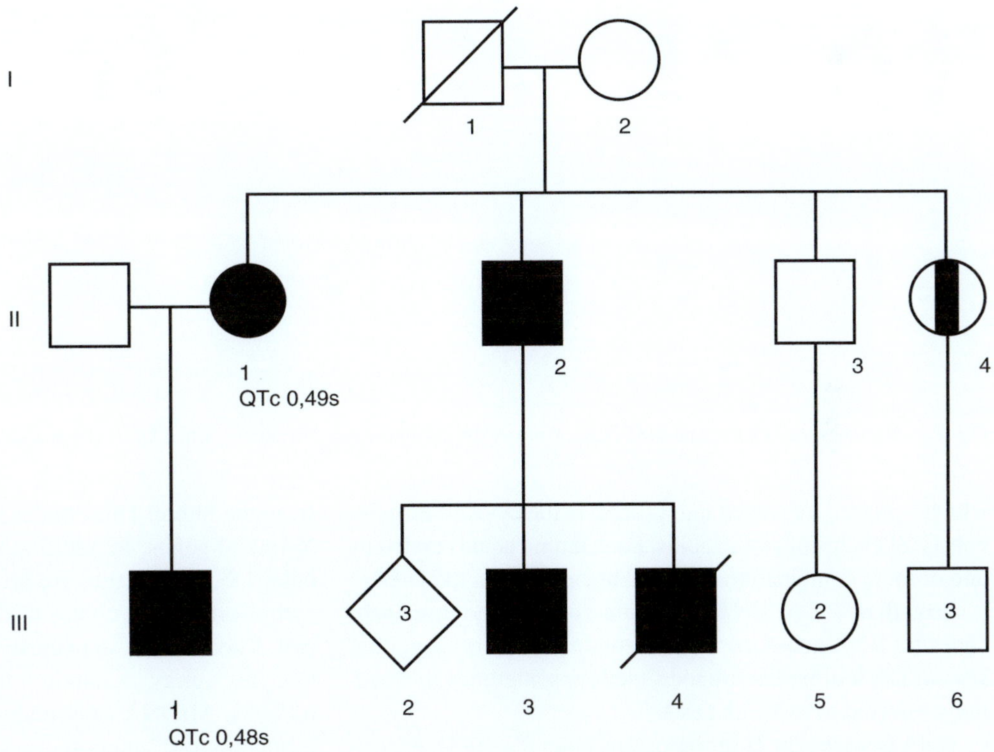

Fig. 2.2 Example of a small pedigree like one could draw up while taking a family history, during consultation of a family suspected of long QT syndrome type 1. Footnotes with this pedigree could be the following: III-1 index patient (October 27, 2000), syncope while playing soccer, spontaneous recovery, QTc 0.48 s, repolarization pattern compatible with LQT type I; I-1, no medical information, died in unilateral car accident at age 32; II-1 (March 02, 1975), no symptoms, QTc 0.49 s; II-2 (May 10, 1977), known with seizures as a child; II-4 (June 13, 1979), said to have fainted during exercise on more than one occasion. III-4, sudden death while swimming at age 12 years. No other persons known with seizures, syncope, or sudden death in the family

- Especially in case of a suspected autosomal recessive disorder, names and places of birth of all grandparents of the index patient should be recorded (usually in a footnote). Consanguinity is unlikely when paternal and maternal grandparents come from very different areas and may be more common in certain ethnic groups. If birthdates are also available, this could facilitate genealogical studies in search of consanguinity.
- Levels of evidence: for individuals that are probably affected based on heteroanamnestic information, but whose medical records have not yet been checked, the symbol "affected by hearsay" (see Fig. 2.1) can be used.
- For counseling reasons, add information on both sides of the family. Unexpected additional pathology may be of importance to your patient and his or her offspring.

Basic Concepts in Inherited Disease

A single copy of the human genome contains over 3 billion base pairs and is estimated to contain 20,000–25,000 protein coding genes [4]. Genes are transcribed into messenger RNA in the nucleus. Subsequently, the noncoding parts of genes (introns) are spliced out to form the mature messenger RNA,

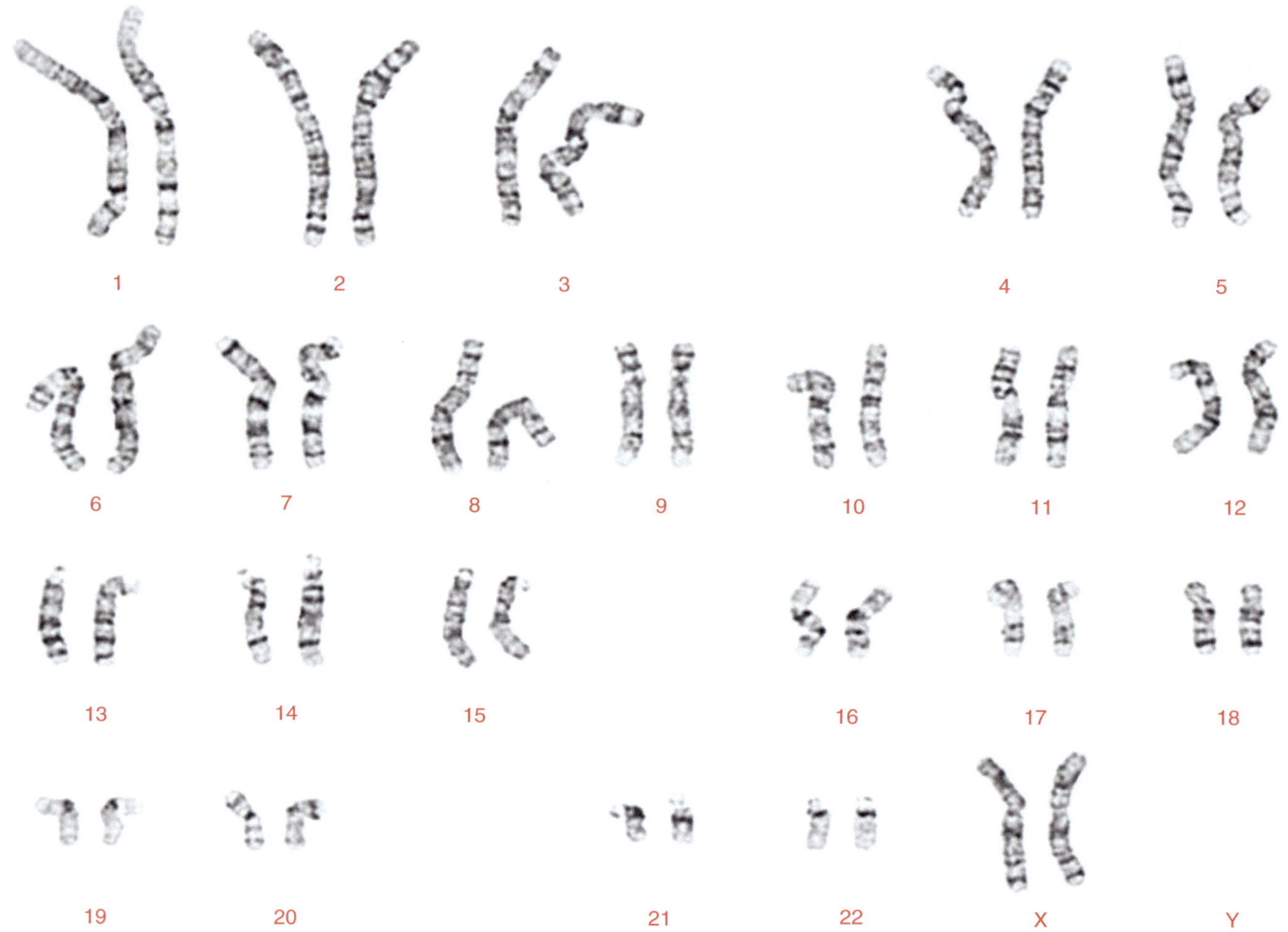

Fig. 2.3 Normal female karyogram (46, XX): the way the chromosomes are shown, when DNA is visualized through a light microscope

which is in turn translated into protein in the cytosol. Proteins consist of chains of amino acids. Each amino acid is coded by one or more combinations of three nucleotides in the DNA.

Less than 3% of DNA is protein coding. The remainder codes for RNA genes, contains regulatory sequences, or consists of DNA of undetermined function, sometimes misleadingly referred to as "junk DNA."

DNA is stored on 23 chromosome pairs (Fig. 2.3), present in the nucleus of each cell: 22 pairs of autosomes and 1 pair of sex chromosomes. During gametogenesis (the production of oocytes and sperm cells), meiosis takes place ensuring that only one copy of each pair is transmitted to the offspring. Since chromosomes are present in pairs, humans are diploid organisms. They have two complete copies of DNA, in which one copy is contributed by the father and one by the mother. Therefore, each gene at each locus is present in two copies. These are usually referred to as the two alleles of that specific gene.

The exception to this rule are the sex chromosomes, as males have only one X-chromosome and one Y-chromosome, the first being inherited from the mother while the latter from the father. Thus, males have only a single copy of most X-linked genes. In addition to the nuclear DNA, small circular DNA molecules are present in the mitochondria in the cytoplasm. Many copies of this mtDNA will be present per cell. The mtDNA is exclusively inherited from the mother. Oocytes may contain up to 100,000 copies of mtDNA. MtDNA only codes for 37 genes, all involved in mitochondrial function.

Mitosis and Meiosis

Two types of cell divisions exist: mitosis and meiosis. Mitosis ensures the equal distribution of the 46 chromosomes over both daughter cells. In order to accomplish this, first the DNA on each chromosome has to be replicated. At cell division, each chromosome consists of two identical DNA chromatids (sister chromatids), held together at a single spot: the centromere. To ensure orderly division, the DNA in the chromosome has to be neatly packaged (a process called condensation). This is when chromosomes actually become visible through a microscope. Prior to cell division, a bipolar mitotic spindle develops, the completely condensed chromosomes move to the equator of the cell, the nuclear membrane dissolves, and microtubular structures develop reaching from both poles of the spindle to the centromere of each chromosome. Subsequently, the centromeres divide, and the sister chromatids are pulled to opposite poles of the dividing cell. Cell division results in 2 daughter cells, each with 46 unreplicated chromosomes and exactly the same nuclear genetic information as the original cell (Fig. 2.4).

Meiosis is a specialized cell division that is necessary to finish the process of gametogenesis. The goal is to produce gametes that contain only 23 unreplicated chromosomes. The vital steps of meiosis are outlined in Fig. 2.5. One of the hallmarks of meiosis is that both replicated chromosomes of each pair come in close apposition to each other and actually exchange genetic material before meiosis takes place. This more or less random process is called homologous *recombination*. Recombination ensures that each individual is able to produce an infinite number of genetically different offspring. Apart from ensuring genetic diversity, recombination is also necessary for proper segregation of the homologous chromosomes during meiosis 1. During male meiosis, the X and Y are able to function as a chromosome pair, thus ensuring proper segregation of sex chromosomes. They can recombine at the tip of their short arms.

Chromosomal Abnormalities

Mutations may affect single genes, but also the genomic architecture at a larger scale can be affected. Such aberrations, when visible through a microscope, are called chromosomal abnormalities. Humans have 22 pairs of autosomes and 1 pair of sex chromosomes. Abnormalities can be divided in numerical (any deviation from 46 chromosomes) and structural

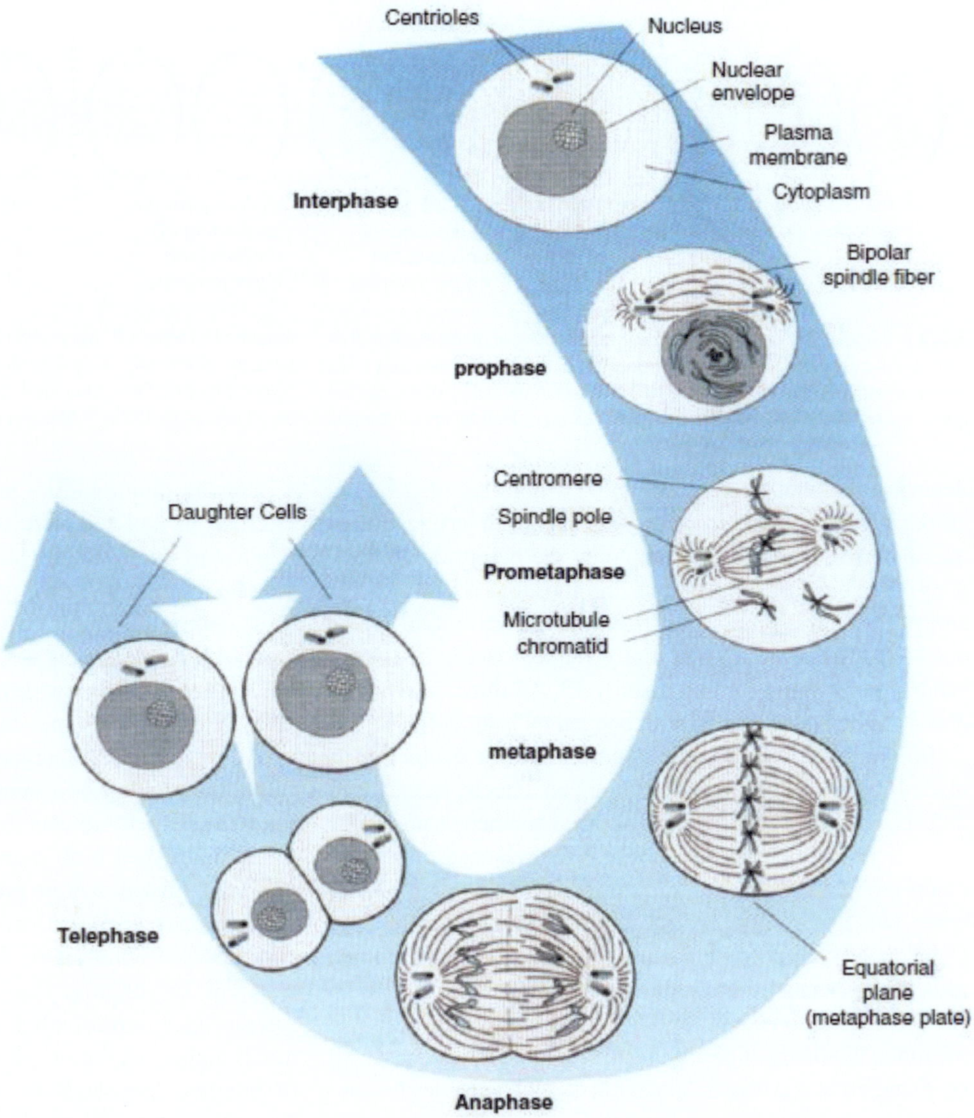

Fig. 2.4 Different stages of mitosis, leading to two daughter cells with exactly the same nuclear DNA content. (Reprinted with permission Jorde, Carey, Bamshad, White, Medical Genetics third edition, Mosby Elsevier 2006)

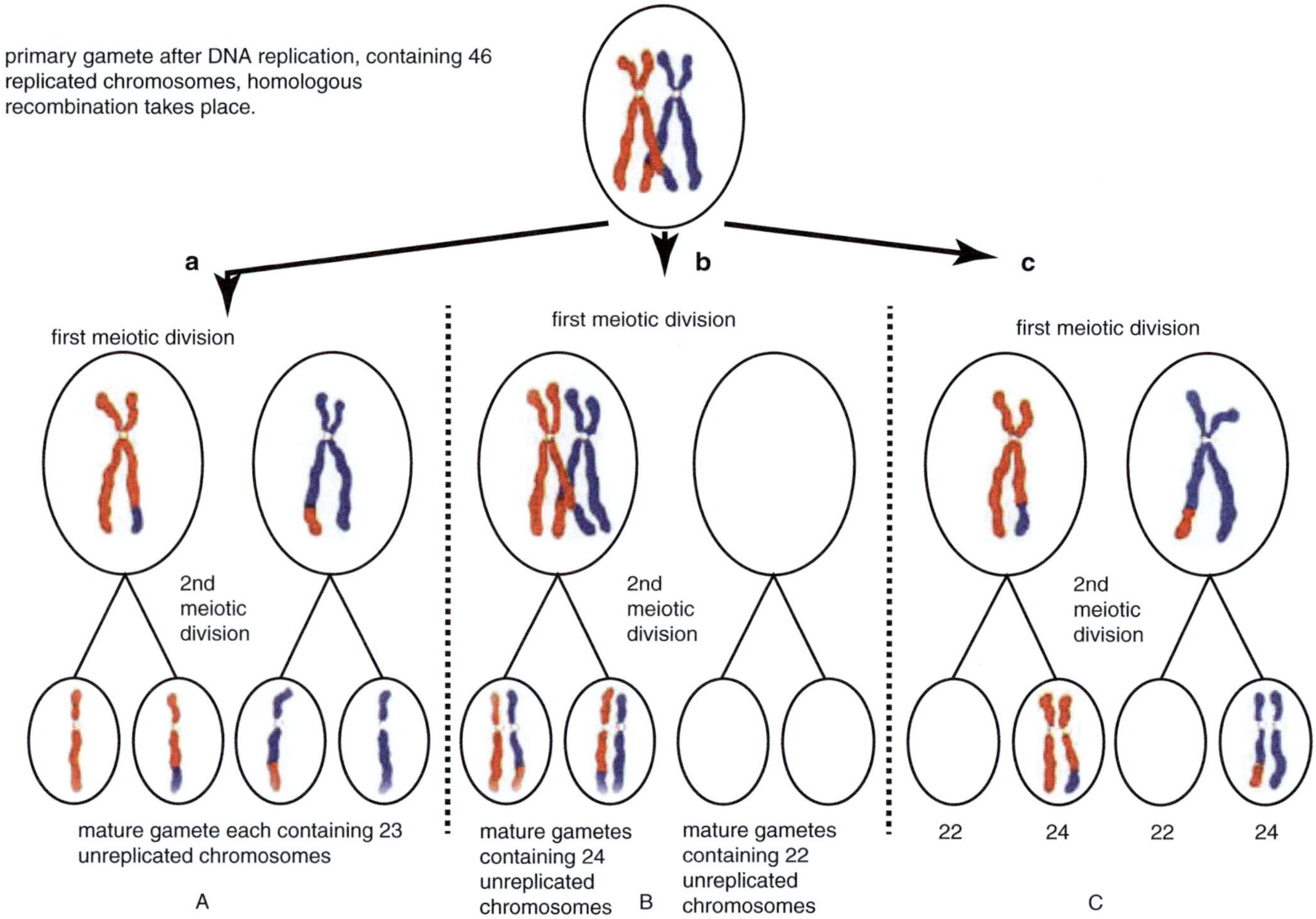

Fig. 2.5 Meiosis: (**a**) demonstrates the normal stages of meiosis (after division, 1 cell contains 23 replicated chromosomes—22 autosomes and 1 sex chromosome). (**b**) Demonstrates nondisjunction in meiosis 1 (the most frequent cause of, for instance, Down syndrome). (**c**) Demonstrates nondisjunction in meiosis 2. Appreciate the effect of recombination in the mature gamete; in this way each grandparent contributes to both copies of each autosome of his/her grandchild (**b**). (Adapted from Langman Inleiding tot de embryologie Bohn Scheltema & Holkema 9e herziene druk 1982)

defects (abnormal chromosomes). A whole set of 23 extra chromosomes is called triploidy. It results from fertilization or meiotic error. Children with triploidy die before or immediately after birth. A single extra chromosome is called a trisomy. They most often result from meiotic error. Only three autosomal trisomies are potentially viable: trisomy 21 (Down syndrome), trisomy 18, and trisomy 13. All three have a high chance of being associated with congenital heart defects.

In structural chromosome abnormalities, a distinction is made between balanced and unbalanced defects. In balanced defects, chromosome parts are displaced but there is no visible extra or missing chromosome material. Balanced rearrangements are most often not associated with an abnormal phenotype, but they may predispose to unbalanced offspring. Unbalanced chromosome abnormalities have a very high risk of being associated with mental retardation and birth defects. As heart development is a very complex process, probably involving hundreds of genes, chances are that this process will be disturbed in one way or another in case of a visible chromosomal abnormality. Indeed, heart defects are very frequent in children with structural chromosomal abnormalities.

Smaller abnormalities are not readily visible through the microscope and will be missed unless specific techniques are applied to detect them. Still, so-called microdeletions may contain a large number of genes and are often associated with heart defects. Examples of microdeletion syndromes associated with heart defects are the 22q11.2 (velo–cardio–facial/DiGeorge) deletion syndrome, Williams–Beuren syndrome, 1p36 deletion syndrome, and Wolf–Hirschhorn syndrome.

As a general rule, regardless whether a visible chromosome abnormality or a microdeletion is involved, the resulting heart defect will usually not occur as an isolated feature. Often associated birth defects, developmental delay, and/or abnormal growth will be present. Therefore, it is in this category of heart defect patients with additional anomalies that a chromosome abnormality has to be considered. Nowadays classical karyotyping (looking at chromosomes through a microscope) is most often replaced by SNP arrays (with a much higher resolution) that are able to detect copy number of hundred thousands of single SNPs across the genome. Therefore, microdeletions and microduplications will be easily detected, without ordering any specific test to detect them.

In contrast to mutation analysis, chromosome analysis by classical karyotyping requires dividing cells for the chromosomes to become visible through a microscope. Usually, white blood cells or cultured fibroblasts are used for chromosome analysis.

Inheritance Patterns

A genetic component plays a role in many diseases. Usually the genetic contribution to disease is appreciated when either a clear pattern of inheritance or significant familial clustering of a disease is noted [5].

Classical genetic disease follows a recognizable Mendelian inheritance pattern. These disorders are called monogenic disorders as a mutation at a single locus conveys a very strong risk of getting the disease. Sometimes, indeed everybody with a specific mutation develops the disease (this is called complete *penetrance*). In that case, the influence of environmental factors or contributions at other genetic loci seems negligible. In practice, however, most monogenic diseases display considerable variation in disease manifestation, severity, and age at onset (clinical variability), even within a single family (where every affected person has the same mutation). Especially in autosomal dominant disease, the chance of developing clinical manifestations of disease when a specific pathogenic mutation is present is often far less than 100% (*incomplete or reduced penetrance*). However, such clinically unaffected mutation carriers may foster severely affected children when they transmit the mutation to their offspring. So, even in so-called monogenic diseases, many other genetic and nongenetic factors can usually modify clinical outcome.

Whereas monogenic diseases are often relatively rare, there is a clear genetic contribution to many common disorders such as coronary artery disease, hypertension, and hypercholesterolemia. In the vast majority of patients, these diseases are explained by the combined additive effect of unfavorable genetic variants at multiple different loci and environmental factors (anything nongenetic), eventually causing disease. Polygenic disease, multifactorial disease, and *complex genetic disease* are all terms used to denote this category of diseases. When looking at pedigrees, apparently nonrandom clustering within the family can often be noted, however, without a clear Mendelian inheritance pattern. Very common complex disorders may mimic autosomal dominant disease, whereas in less common disorders like congenital heart defects, a genetic contribution is very likely although the majority of cases will present as sporadic cases without a positive family history. Importantly, frequent complex genetic diseases may have less common monogenic subtypes like FH (familial hypercholesterolemia) as a result of mutations in the LDL receptor or MODY (maturity-onset diabetes in the young) that are examples of monogenic subtypes of diseases that most often have a complex etiology.

Single-Gene Disorders: Mendelian Inheritance

In *single-gene disorders*, inheritance patterns can be explained in terms of Mendelian inheritance. Of importance in the first place is whether the causative gene is on one of the autosomes or on one of the sex chromosomes, more specifically on the X-chromosome (the Y-chromosome contains very few disease-related genes and will not be discussed further).

The second distinction to be made is whether mutations in the gene follow a *dominant* or *recessive* mode of inheritance.

Autosomal Dominant Inheritance

Autosomal dominant disease is caused by dominant mutations on one of the autosomes. Dominant mutations already cause disease when only one of both alleles is mutated. Most individuals with dominant disease are *heterozygous* for the mutation (they have one mutated and one normal allele). Heterozygous carriers of such a mutation have a high risk of clinically expressing disease symptoms. It is the most common form of inheritance in monogenic cardiac disease. It is characterized by (see Fig. 2.6):

- Equal chance of males and females being affected.
- Individuals in more than one generation are usually affected (unless a new mutation has occurred).
- Father-to-son transmission can occur.
- On average 50% of offspring will be affected (assuming complete penetrance).

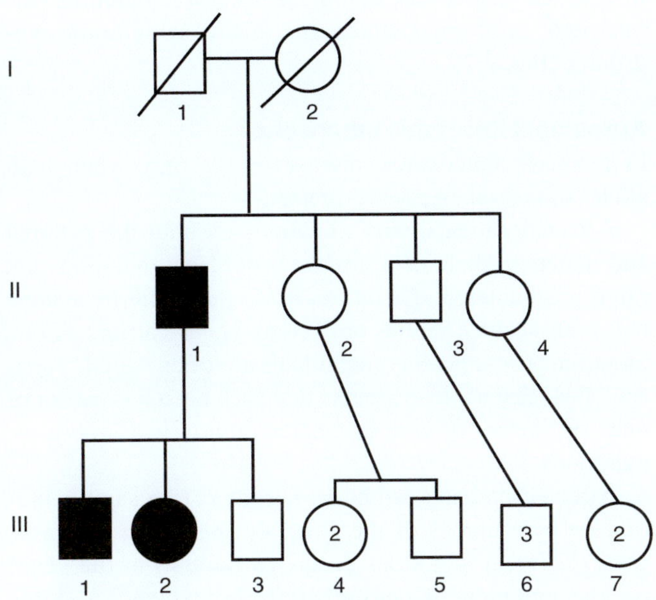

Fig. 2.6 Example of a small autosomal dominant pedigree; the observed male-to-male transmission (II-1 > III-1) excludes X-linked dominant inheritance. If we assume this disorder has full penetrance, a de novo mutation must have occurred in II-1

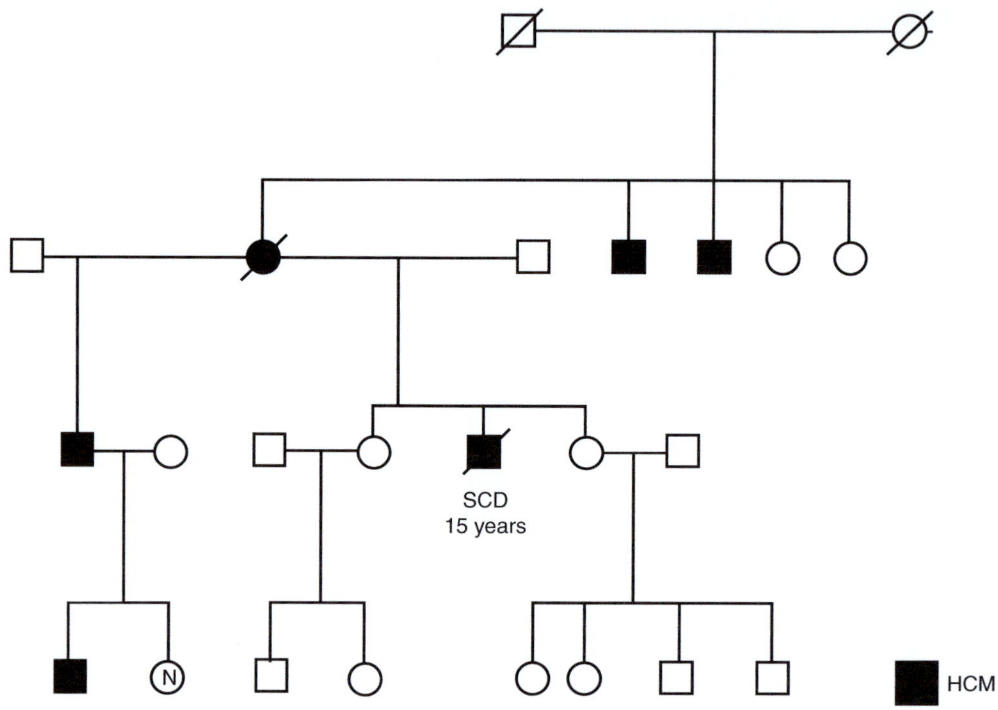

Fig. 2.7 Example of a hypertrophic cardiomyopathy (HCM) pedigree showing autosomal dominant inheritance. The proband was a 15-year-old boy who suffered a sudden cardiac death (SCD); as a result, other family members were identified on family screening

Although this inheritance pattern is rather straightforward, in practice precise predictions are often complicated by issues of penetrance and *variable expression* (see paragraph *on penetrance and variable expressivity*).

An example in cardiogenetics is hypertrophic cardiomyopathy, and a typical pedigree demonstrating autosomal dominant inheritance is shown below. The vast majority of monogenic–cardiogenetic diseases are inherited in an autosomal dominant fashion, including the inherited cardiomyopathies and many arrhythmia syndromes (Fig. 2.7).

Autosomal Recessive Inheritance

In recessive inheritance, disease occurs only when both alleles of the same gene are affected.

Affected patients carry mutations on both the paternal and maternal allele of a disease gene. New mutations are rarely encountered. Therefore, it is reasonable to assume that both healthy parents are heterozygous carriers of one mutation. These healthy individuals are often called "carriers." It is reasonable to assume that each person is carrier of one or more disease-associated *autosomal recessive* mutations.

Affected patients can be *homozygous* (the same mutation on both alleles of the gene) or *compound heterozygous* (different mutations on the two alleles of the gene) for the mutation. If *consanguinity* is involved, a single mutation that was present in the common ancestor is transmitted to the patient by both parents, leading to the homozygous state.

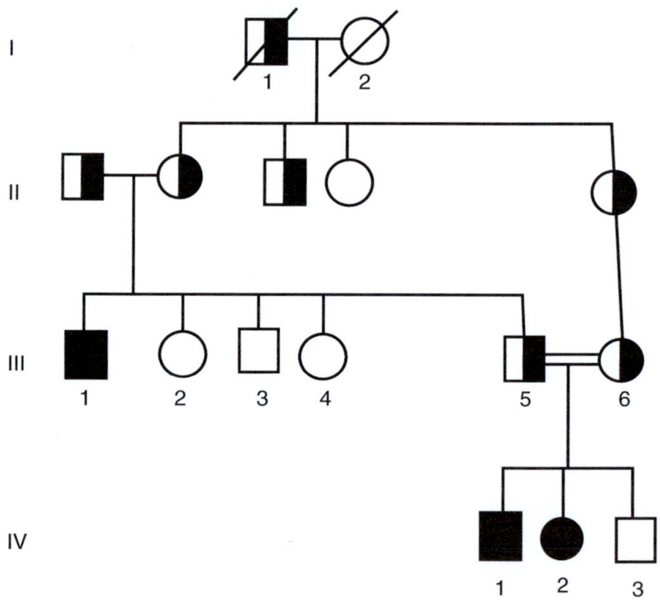

Fig. 2.8 Example of an autosomal recessive pedigree, illustrating the role of consanguinity in AR disease. III-5 and III-6 are first cousins. IV-1 and IV-2 inherited both their mutated alleles from a single heterozygous grandparent (in this case, I-1). In this pedigree, heterozygous carriers are indicated; usually heterozygous carriers for AR disorders can only be unambiguously identified by DNA analysis

In most cases, but not always, autosomal recessive conditions are limited to a single sibship (see Fig. 2.8). If vertical transmission of an autosomal recessive disease occurs, this is called "pseudodominance." Pseudodominance can be encountered in case of consanguinity in multiple generations or in case of a very high population frequency of healthy heterozygous carriers. Autosomal recessive inheritance is characterized by:

- Equal chance of males and females to be affected.
- Parents of patients are usually healthy carriers.
- The chance that the next child (a sib) will be affected is 25%.
- Affected individuals are usually limited to a single sibship.
- The presence of consanguinity in the parents favors, but does not prove, the autosomal recessive inheritance mode.

While autosomal recessive inheritance is rare among cardiogenetic diseases, there are reports including this family shown below (Fig. 2.9).

X-Linked Recessive Inheritance

X-linked disorders are caused by mutations on the X-chromosome. The X-chromosome does not contain “female-specific” genes. As females have two X-chromosomes and males only one, in X-linked disorders, usually, a difference in disease expression will be noted between males and females.

In X-linked recessive inheritance (see Fig. 2.10):

- No male-to-male transmission occurs.
- Heterozygous females are usually healthy.
- All daughters of affected males will be usually healthy carriers.
- Sons of carrier women have a 50% chance of being affected.
- Daughters of carrier women have a 50% chance of being a healthy carrier.

It should be noted that in female somatic cells, only one X-chromosome is active. The other X-chromosome is inactivated. This process of *X-inactivation* (called *Lyonization*) is random, occurs early in embryogenesis, and remains fixed, so that daughter cells will have the same X-chromosome inactivated as the cell they were derived from. Usually, in a given female tissue, approximately half of the cells will express the paternal X-chromosome and the other half of the cells, the maternal X-chromosome. However, for a variety of reasons, significant deviations of this equal distribution of active X-chromosomes may occur (called *skewing of X-inactivation*). Naturally, this may influence disease expression in case of X-linked disease. For example, if the X-chromosome containing an X-linked recessive mutation is expressed in over 90% of cells in a given tissue, disease may develop in a female like it does in males.

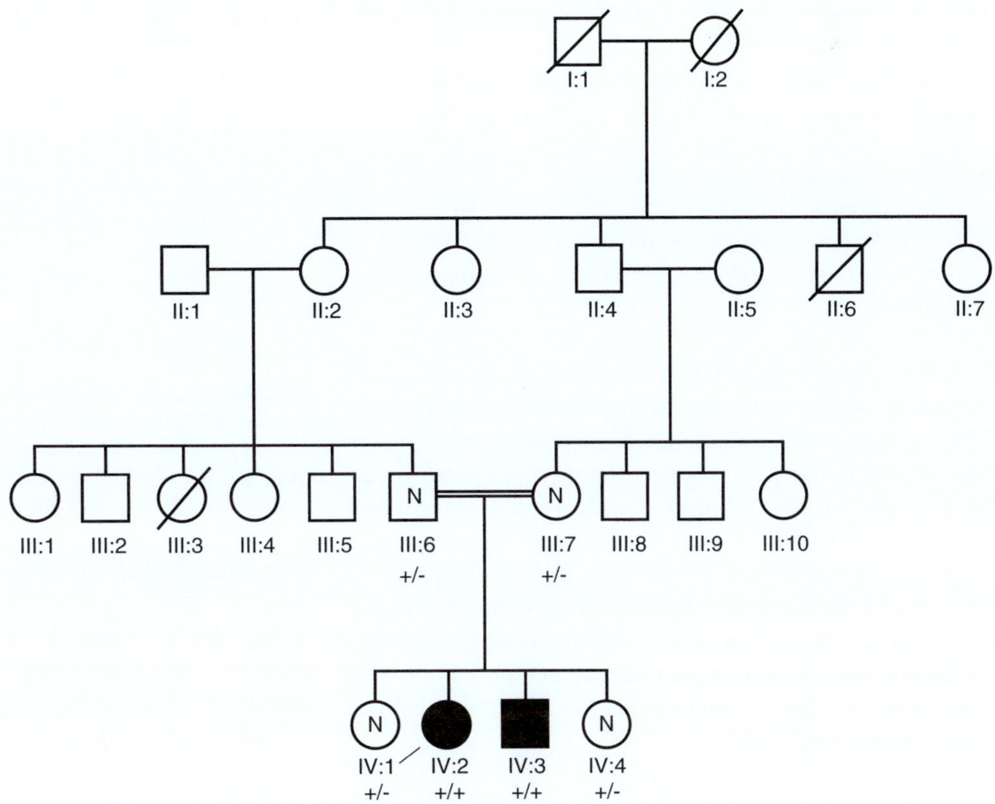

Fig. 2.9 Example of a recessively inherited form of hypertrophic cardiomyopathy (TNNI3 Arg162Trp). This family presented after the symptomatic presentation of IV:2 who subsequently required cardiac transplantation due to a severe restrictive phenotype. Her brother (IV:3) suffered a resuscitated cardiac arrest while awaiting cardiac investigation. Both parents and siblings were heterozygous carriers and showed no clinical evidence of disease + denotes presence of the p.Arg162Trp variant and - denotes absence of this variant [6]

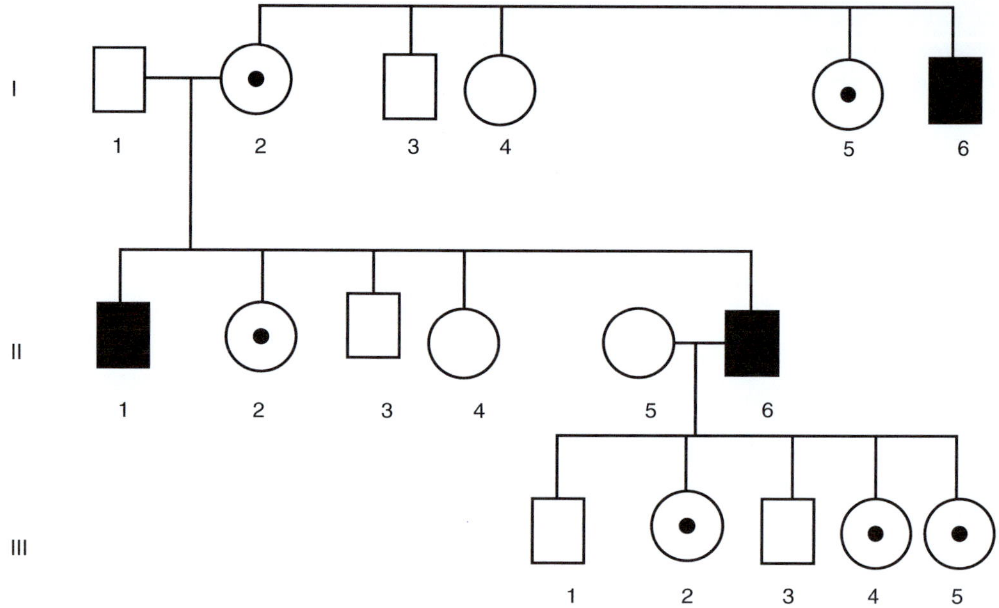

Fig. 2.10 Example of an X-linked recessive disorder; the disease is transmitted via apparently healthy heterozygous females; only hemizygous males manifest the disease. All daughters of an affected male will be carriers. Carrier females are indicated with dots within circles, and usually DNA analysis will be required to unambiguously identify carrier females

X-Linked Dominant Inheritance

In X-linked dominant disorders, heterozygous females are most likely to be affected. However, on average these heterozygous females are often less severely affected than hemizygous males. Exceptions, however, do exist.

Some X-linked dominant disorders may be lethal in hemizygous males like the oculo–facio–cardio–dental syndrome that is associated with congenital heart defects. Hemizygous males will miscarry, leading to a reduced chance of male offspring in affected females.

The characteristics of X-linked dominant inheritance are (see Fig. 2.11):

- No male-to-male transmission occurs.
- Heterozygous females are affected.
- All daughters of an affected male will also be affected.
- Affected females have a 50% chance of having affected children.

Especially in X-linked disorders, the distinction between dominant and recessive disease may be blurred, with some heterozygous females not being affected at all, while others are affected to the same degree as hemizygous men. In cardiogenetics, several X-linked disorders are known where heterozygous females may be asymptomatic but also run a high risk of significant disease, like in Fabry disease. In Duchenne muscular dystrophy, considered to be an X-linked recessive disorder, females only very rarely develop severe skeletal muscle weakness, but they are at considerable risk for dilatation of the left ventricle and should be monitored by a cardiologist (Fig. 2.12).

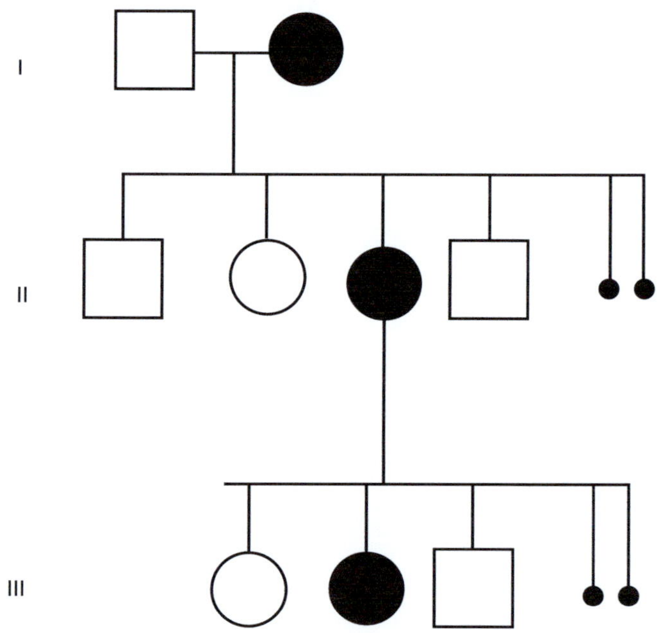

Fig. 2.11 Example pedigree of an X-linked dominant disorder with early lethality in males. Affected males that are conceived will miscarry (leading to skewed sex ratios in offspring). The black dots in the pedigree represent miscarriages. Based on such a limited pedigree, definite distinction from autosomal dominant inheritance would be impossible

Non-Mendelian Inheritance

In fact, any deviation from the classical rules of Mendel could be categorized under the heading of non-Mendelian inheritance. Such deviations can, for example, result from genome disorders (de novo deletions or duplications of larger

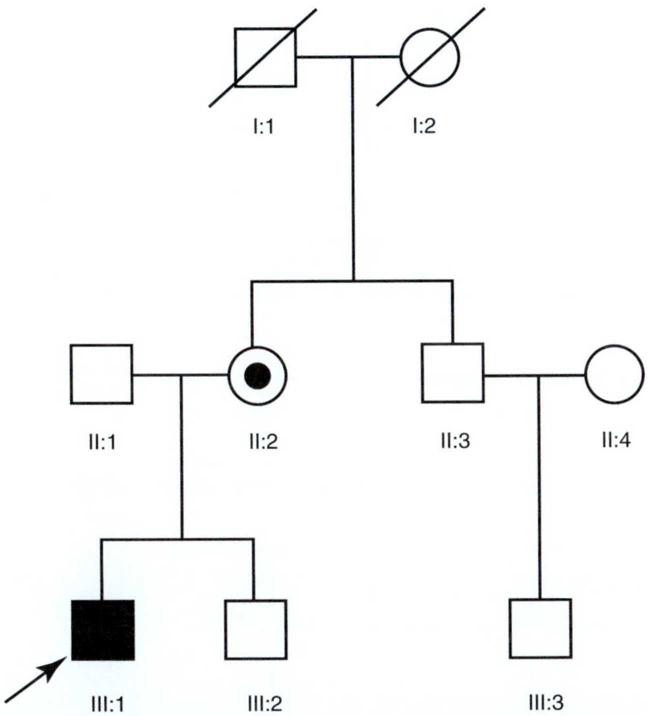

Fig. 2.12 Example of an X-linked dominantly inherited condition, Danon disease. This is a rare disease caused by mutations in the *LAMP2* gene and is a known HCM phenocopy (i.e., causing clinical characteristics similar to HCM). In this family, the proband (III:1) presented with severe concentric left ventricular hypertrophy aged 12 years. His mother (II:2) was found to be a carrier of the causative loss of function variant in *LAMP2* though had no clinical evidence of disease herself. Other family members have not been assessed. Female carriers of *LAMP2* mutations can be affected, though often less severely than males

stretches of DNA or even whole chromosomes), epigenetic factors (these are factors not changing the actual DNA code but change the way in which specific genes are expressed), and unstable mutations (trinucleotide repeat mutations such as in myotonic dystrophy that may expand over generations and lead to a more severe phenotype in subsequent generations). However, for sake of brevity, only multifactorial inheritance and maternal (mitochondrial) inheritance will be briefly discussed.

Multifactorial Inheritance

Although genetic factors very often contribute to disease, most of the time this will not be in a monogenic fashion. The majority of disorders are caused by a complex interplay of multiple unfavorable genetic variants at different loci in combination with environmental (nongenetic) factors. The genetic variants involved may each by themselves have a limited effect. It is the additive effect of multiple factors that eventually will lead to disease, hence the name *multifactorial inheritance*. In this paragraph, no distinction is made between multifactorial inheritance and polygenic inheritance (no important environmental contribution). In general practice, such a distinction is most often of no importance unless specific environmental factors can be identified that can be influenced. Hereditability is a measure used to indicate the contribution of inherited factors to a multifactorial phenotype. In animal studies, heritability can be calculated, as both environment and genetic composition of the animals can be controlled. In man, hereditability can only be estimated indirectly.

In multifactorial inheritance, sometimes clustering of a condition within a family may be observed that cannot be easily explained by chance. Especially in common diseases like diabetes or hypertension (when the underlying genetic variants occur at high frequency in the population), this clustering may mimic Mendelian inheritance. However, in more rare disorders like in congenital heart disease, an identified patient may well be the only affected one in the family. Still, family members may be at increased risk of a congenital heart defect.

Many continuous traits, for example, blood pressure, can be explained in terms of the additive effect of multiple deleterious or protective genetic and environmental factors. In case of hypertension, the sum of all these factors would be defined as disease liability, which is distributed as a Gaussian curve in the population. At the right side of the curve (highest liability), those with hypertension are found. Their close relatives who will share many of the predisposing genetic (and possibly also environmental) factors with the hypertensive patient will usually have a higher than average disease liability; however, they may not meet with the clinical criteria for hypertension. For discontinuous traits like congenital heart defects, a threshold model has been proposed (Fig. 2.13). If disease susceptibility exceeds the threshold level, disease will arise. Again, the liability of close relatives of a patient with a heart defect will be, on average, closer to the disease threshold than that of unrelated individuals, but most of them will not exceed the threshold and therefore will have anatomically normal hearts.

It is important to realize that some disorders are more multifactorial than others. Sometimes mutations at a single locus will not be sufficient to cause disease but have a strong effect. If a mutation in such a *major gene* is present, little else has to go wrong for disease to occur. Therefore, strict separation between Mendelian and multifactorial disease is artificial. Indeed, genes that are involved in rare monogenetic variants of a disease may also play a role in the more common multifactorial forms of the disease.

The following characteristics can be applied to multifactorial inheritance:

- Familial clustering may occur, but usually no Mendelian inheritance pattern can be identified.
- Recurrence risks for family members are in general lower than in monogenic disease.
- Risk of disease rapidly falls with decreasing degree of relationship to the index patient.

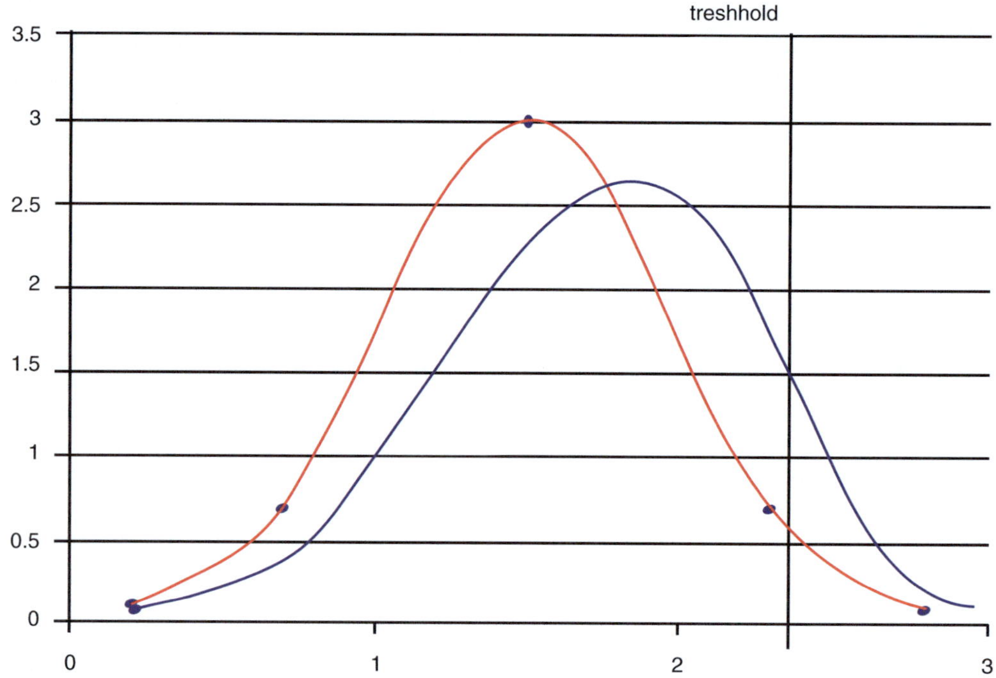

Fig. 2.13 Example of a liability distribution of a discontinuous multifactorial trait (a congenital heart defect) in a given population. The red curve is for the general population. The area under the red curve to the right of the threshold represents the proportion of individuals with CHD in the general population. The blue curve is for first-degree relatives of a patient with CHD. Since CHD is a discontinuous trait (it is either present or absent), a threshold is introduced. Everybody with a liability exceeding the threshold will have CHD. Liability for CHD will be determined by the additive effect of unfavorable genetic and environmental factors. As a result of shared unfavorable factors, the liability curve for first-degree relatives has shifted to the right explaining the fact that a larger proportion of first-degree relatives will be affected with CHD in comparison with the general population, whereas the majority of relatives has no CHD, as their liability does not exceed the threshold

- Risk may be higher for relatives of severely affected patients.
- Risk estimations are usually based on empirical (observational) data.
- These risks are not fixed risks, like in Mendelian disease. New disease cases in a family may indicate a higher genetic load and therefore a higher risk for relatives.

At this point in time, the use of cascade genetic testing in multifactorial disease is limited, as usually only a small part of morbidity can be explained by the genetics variants that have thus far been identified for these disorders. As these variants have by themselves only a small effect, the odds of getting the disease, once an unfavorable variant has been identified, are small. Still, commercial genetic tests, supplying risk profiles for many common conditions, based on genetic profiles, are readily available via the Internet. Such risk predictions may be imprecise and differ substantially between different test providers.

Although exceptions may exist, predictive genetic testing in multifactorial disease is not likely to play a role of importance in genetic counseling in the near future. In contrast, genetic tests for common disorders may play a role in clinical practice in the near future, for example, in risk stratification and in identifying groups that are eligible for specific treatments.

Maternal (Mitochondrial) Inheritance

Mitochondria are present in most cells in different numbers and are the principal providers of energy by means of the respiratory chain. Mitochondria contain small circular DNA molecules of their own (*mtDNA*). These molecules are only 16,569 base pairs in length and code for only 37 genes. Thirteen polypeptides of the respiratory chain are encoded by the mitochondrial DNA, whereas the remainder (the majority) are encoded by the nuclear DNA. The rest of the mitochondrial genes play a role in mitochondrial translation (transfer RNAs and ribosomal RNAs).

Somatic cells typically contain 1000–10,000 mtDNA molecules (2–10 molecules per mitochondrion). Mitochondrial DNA replication is under nuclear control and suited to meet with the energy requirement of the cell. It is not associated with cell division like the nuclear DNA. When a cell divides, mitochondria randomly segregate to daughter cells within the cytoplasm. Oocytes may contain up to 100,000 copies of mtDNA, whereas sperm cells usually contain only a few hundreds. Moreover, these paternal copies do not enter the oocyte at fertilization. Therefore, the paternal contribution to the mtDNA is negligible, and mtDNA is inherited exclusively via the mother, hence the concept of *maternal inheritance*.

Whereas nuclear genes are present in two copies per cell, mitochondrial genes are present in thousands of copies. In maternally inherited disease, in a specific tissue, a significant part of the mtDNA copies may carry a similar mtDNA mutation, whereas the remainder of the copies is normal (wild type). This phenomenon is called *heteroplasmy*. Here, again, a threshold is important that is determined by the specific energy requirement of the tissue. If the percentage of mutated mtDNA becomes so high that the energy requirement cannot be fulfilled, this may result in mitochondrial disease. If a mutation is present in all mtDNA molecules in a specific tissue, this is called *homoplasmy*. The mechanism that leads to homoplasmy of certain mtDNA mutations is not yet fully understood.

Mitochondrial DNA differs in many aspects from nuclear DNA. In contrast to nuclear DNA, most of the mtDNA codes for genes. Therefore, any random mutation in the mtDNA is much more likely to disrupt an actual gene than is the case in the nuclear genome. DNA repair mechanisms to repair acquired DNA damage, as are present in the nucleus, are lacking, leading to accumulation of mtDNA mutations, for example, in aging. On the other hand, since mtDNA genes are present in hundreds to thousands of copies per cell, acquired mutations rarely lead to recognizable mitochondrial disease. Only a minute fraction of mtDNA mutations will become "fixed" and will subsequently be transmitted to offspring.

It is important to realize that maternal inheritance is not equivalent to mitochondrial disease. As most of the proteins active in the mitochondrion are encoded by nuclear genes, mitochondrial diseases may be inherited in other fashions, most often in an autosomal recessive manner.

Mitochondrial disease affects many tissues, although tissues with the highest energy requirements (muscle, brain) are most often involved. Cardiac muscle may be involved in different mitochondrial conditions. Sometimes, a cardiomyopathy may be the first or most prominent manifestation of a mutation in the mtDNA.

The following characteristics apply to maternal inheritance:

- Men and women are affected with similar frequencies; however, only females transmit the disease to offspring.
- Phenotypes may be extremely variable (and unpredictable) as a result of different levels of heteroplasmy in different tissues.
- The percentage of mutated mtDNA in one specific tissue may not accurately predict the level of heteroplasmy in other tissues. This is a major problem, for example, in prenatal diagnosis.
- Affected females are likely to transmit mutated mtDNA to all of their offspring, but non-penetrance will result if the threshold for disease expression is not reached.

New (De Novo) Mutations

Mutations can occur at any time during both gametogenesis and regular cell division. If a detected mutation is present in neither of the parents (i.e., if it is absent in the blood of both parents), the mutation is called "de novo." De novo mutations may have arisen in the sperm or egg cell or may even have occurred after conception. Mutation rates in genes (the number of mutations per gene per generation) are on average very low, in the order of 10^{-5}–10^{-7}. Therefore, if in an isolated patient a de novo mutation in a candidate gene for the disorder is being found, it is usually regarded as a pathogenic mutation.

It should be realized that most new mutations will go unnoticed. When they are situated in noncoding DNA or in recessive genes, they will have no immediate effect, whereas new mutations in important dominant genes may be lethal and may therefore not be ascertained.

Mosaicism

When mutations (or chromosomal abnormalities) arise shortly after conception, *mosaicism* may result. Mosaicism is defined as the presence of genetically different cell populations (usually an abnormal and a normal cell line) within a single individual. The importance of mosaicism in relation to cardiac disease is that (at least in theory) mutations that are not detected in the blood of the affected individual may be present in the heart. Preliminary observations suggest that this may be important in some types of congenital heart disease.

Germline mosaicism is a special type of mosaicism, where a population of precursor spermatocytes or oocytes carries a specific mutation that is not detected in other tissues. As a result of germline mosaicism, a healthy (apparently noncarrier) parent may unexpectedly transmit the same disease mutation to several offspring. The classic observation of germline mosaicism is in Duchenne muscular dystrophy, where apparently noncarrier females may give birth to more than one affected son with exactly the same dystrophin mutation. However, germline mosaicism may occur in any disorder including cardiac disorders, and, therefore, it should be considered a possibility in any apparently de novo mutational event.

On Penetrance and Variable Expressivity

The *penetrance* of a specific mutation refers to its ability to cause a disease phenotype. In monogenic disease, mutations may show 100% penetrance. For instance, most pathogenic dystrophin mutations will cause Duchenne muscular dystrophy in all hemizygous males. However, especially in autosomal dominant disease, penetrance is often reduced; not everybody with the mutation actually becomes ill. Whether or not disease symptoms develop may be dependent on a constellation of other genetic (genetic background) or environmental factors, such as lifestyle. Disease penetrance is not necessarily identical to having actual clinical complaints. Especially in cardiogenetics, many clinically asymptomatic individuals with, for example, a hypertrophic cardiomyopathy or long QT syndrome may have easily noticeable abnormalities on ECG or echocardiography. Such individuals may not realize their genetic status, but they cannot be regarded as true non-penetrants. Usually, they should be under cardiac surveillance and often preventive treatment will be indicated. Penetrance, in this way, is to some extent dependent on how well individuals have been examined for disease symptoms. If true non-penetrance occurs, genetic diagnosis may be the only means to identify individuals that may transmit the disease to their offspring. For decisions with respect to patient care, it is more useful to look at penetrance of specific phenotypic traits, for example, the chance of a ventricular arrhythmia in case of a *KCNQ1* mutation in long QT syndrome type 1.

In congenital heart disease, penetrance is fixed, as the disease is either present or not. In diseases that manifest themselves later in life, this is not true. For instance, in an autosomal dominant inherited cardiomyopathy, penetrance at the age of 10 may be low, whereas at the age of 60, most individuals with the genetic defect will have developed disease manifestations. In this case, there is *age-dependent penetrance*. Of course, this will influence risk estimations based on clinical observation. At the age of 10, a child of a cardiomyopathy patient from this family may still have an almost 50% chance of having inherited the familial mutation despite a normal cardiac evaluation, while at the age of 60, a normal cardiac evaluation severely reduces the chance of the mutation being present. If sound scientific data are available on penetrance, these can be used in genetic counseling and decision-making. However, unfortunately this is often not the case.

Variable expression is used to indicate the presence of variation in disease symptoms and severity in individuals with a similar mutation. For example, in desmin myopathy, some individuals may mainly suffer from skeletal myopathy, whereas in others from the same family, cardiac manifestations may be the principal determinant of the disease.

Genotype–Phenotype Correlations

This term refers to the extent to which it is possible to predict a phenotype (i.e., clinical disease manifestation) given a specific genotype and vice versa. In an era where presymptomatic genetic testing becomes more and more customary, this is an issue of great importance. If it were possible to predict phenotype based on genotype with great accuracy, this would lend additional legitimacy to predictive genetic testing, especially if early intervention would change disease course. Indeed, there have been claims that, for example, hypertrophic cardiomyopathy caused by mutations in the gene encoding cardiac Troponin T (*TNNT2*) has a higher potential for malignant arrhythmias than cardiomyopathy caused by mutations in some other genes [7, 8]. Also within a given gene, some mutations may have a stronger pathogenic effect than others.

Without doubt significant genotype–phenotype correlations do exist, but it is prudent to regard such claims with caution, as some of them may also be the result of ascertainment and *publication bias*. From a clinical point of view, it is obvious that, if intrafamilial (where every affected individual has the same mutation) variation in disease severity and penetrance is considerable, little can be expected of phenotype predictions based on the presence of this family-specific mutation alone. As a result of the difficulty in establishing straightforward genotype–phenotype correlations, the role of genetic information in cardiac risk stratification protocols has been limited thus far. There nowadays are a few exceptions in genetic cases of DCM, where specific classes of mutations in LMNA and PLN seem to be associated with adverse outcome. In these selected cases, precise genetic diagnosis may influence clinical decision-making, for example, with regard to ICD therapy [9, 10].

The reverse situation needs also to be considered. Clinical history and clinical data such as T-wave morphology in patients suspected of having a form of long QT syndrome are very helpful in selecting the genes that should be analyzed first [11]. In the long QT syndromes, genotype–phenotype correlations can be used in practice: clinical parameters suggest a specific genotype, and subsequently, genotype-specific therapy can be instituted. Accurate clinical information may improve the yield of genetic testing and may decrease costs and time needed for these analyses.

Basic Concepts in Population Genetics

Population genetics studies genetic variation and genetic disease in the context of populations. Here, a population is defined as the group of individuals that are likely to get offspring together and the genetic diversity that is contained within this group. Populations are delimited not only by geographical boundaries such as borders, rivers, mountains, and islands but also by religious, ethnic, and cultural differences.

Some insights from population genetics are important to the field of clinical genetics and necessary for understanding genetic phenomena that are relevant to clinical practice, for instance, *founder effects*. Two important population genetic "laws" predict the distribution of neutral genetic variation (i.e., the Hardy–Weinberg equilibrium) and the frequency of disease mutations (mutation-selection equilibrium), respectively.

Hardy–Weinberg Equilibrium

The *Hardy–Weinberg equilibrium* predicts that the relative frequency of different genotypes at a locus within a population remains the same over generations. For an autosomal gene G with two alleles A and a with an allele frequency of p and q, respectively, the possible genotypes AA, Aa, and aa will occur with a frequency of p^2, $2pq$, and q^2. As there are only two alleles for G, $p + q = 1$.

However, for the Hardy–Weinberg equilibrium to be true, many assumptions have to be made. The population has to be infinitely large, there has to be random mating with respect to G, there has to be no selection against any of the G genotypes, no new mutations occur in G, and there is no migration introducing G alleles into or removing G alleles from the population. Clearly no situation in real life will ever satisfy all these criteria.

The Hardy–Weinberg equilibrium is a neutral equilibrium. Small deviations from the expected genotype frequencies occur by chance (genetic drift), and over multiple generations a significant difference in genotype frequency (when compared to the original equilibrium) may become apparent. There is no driving force correcting such chance deviations. As a matter of fact, a new Hardy–Weinberg equilibrium is established with each generation.

In real life, new mutations do occur and often selection does exist against disease-associated alleles, causing them to disappear from the gene pool. However, mutation rates for recessive disorders are extremely small and selection pressure is low, as selection works only against the homozygous affected. Therefore, in autosomal recessive disorders, the Hardy–Weinberg equilibrium can be used to calculate carrier frequencies for recessive disorders if the frequency of the disorder in the population (q^2) is known. Because of the limitations mentioned above, such calculations have to be regarded as estimates and interpreted with caution.

Mutation–Selection Equilibrium

To understand the dynamics of disease-causing (not neutral) alleles, another equilibrium is of importance: the *mutation–selection equilibrium*. New disease alleles will arise with a given frequency as a result of new mutations, but when diseased individuals are less likely to reproduce, they also disappear again from the gene pool. Therefore, the equilibrium that predicts the frequency of disease alleles is a function of the mutation rate, the reproductive fitness, and the mode of inheritance of the disease.

The easiest example is a severe congenital heart defect as a result of a new autosomal dominant mutation. If this heart defect is lethal, reproductive fitness is nil, and the population frequency of the mutated autosomal dominant gene would be identical to the mutation frequency. In, for example, long QT syndrome type 1, most mutation carriers, however, will reproduce, but reproductive fitness is somewhat reduced as a result of some affected individuals dying from arrhythmias at a young age [12]. Here, the actual frequency of the disease allele is much larger than the mutation frequency, as most disease alleles will be inherited. Still, if no new mutations would occur, the disease would eventually die out as a result of reduced fitness.

Mutation–selection equilibrium is more stable than the Hardy–Weinberg equilibrium. If for some reason more new mutations arise than expected, selective pressure increases as well since there are more affected individuals to target, moving the equilibrium again in the direction of the original state. However, if reproductive fitness increases significantly as a result of improved therapies, eventually a new equilibrium with a higher population frequency of the mutated allele will be established.

Founder Mutations

If a population descends from a relatively limited number of ancestors, the genetic variation is largely dependent on the variation that was present in this small group of ancestors. If by chance a rare disease allele was present in one of these "founders," this disease allele may achieve an unusual high frequency in this founder population, which is not found in other populations. This is especially true if selection against the mutation is small, so that the mutation is not easily eliminated from the gene pool.

For example, in the Netherlands, over 20% of hypertrophic cardiomyopathy is caused by a single c.2373_2374insG mutation in the MYBPC3 gene [13]. In order to prove that this is indeed a founder mutation and not a mutation that has occurred de novo more than once, it was established that the mutation in each patient lies on an identical genetic marker background (haplotype), which must have been present in the founder. If the mutation had occurred many times de novo, it would have been expected to be associated with different haplotypes.

Founder effects, like the one described above, can help explain why certain diseases are more frequent in some populations than others. Moreover, it is important to be aware of these mechanisms as they can aid in devising efficient strategies for molecular diagnosis in specific populations.

Genetic Isolates

Genetic isolates are small, closed communities within a larger population where people tend to marry among each other. Consanguinity is more likely and even if this is not the case, genetic variation within an isolate is much more limited, because of the absence of new genes contributing to the gene pool. As a result some genetic diseases may have a much higher frequency within an isolate than in the population as whole, while in contrast other genetic diseases may be virtually absent. Therefore, it may be important to realize whether or not a specific patient comes from a genetic isolate.

Consanguinity

Consanguineous marriages are very common in some cultures and unusual in others [14]. Marriages between first cousins are most frequent. They share 12.5% of their DNA, derived from their common ancestor. In some cultures uncles are allowed to marry their nieces. Such second-degree relatives share 25% of their DNA. This situation, from a genetic point of view, is no different from double first cousins that have all four grandparents in common and, therefore, also share 25% of their DNA.

Consanguinity may have significant social and economic advantages, especially in low-income societies. However, the genetic risks cannot be ignored, but they are highly dependent on the degree of relationship. The problem with consanguinity arises from the reduction to homozygosity in offspring of consanguineous parents. If both parents carry the same recessive mutation in their shared DNA, there is a 25% risk of the mutation being homozygous in each child. Therefore, consanguinity mainly increases the likelihood of autosomal recessive disease. The chance that a recessive disorder is caused by consanguinity increases with decreasing frequency of the disorder. In other words, the relative risk increase as a result of consanguinity is highest for the rarest recessive disorders. For example, thus far a rare form of catecholaminergic polymorphic ventricular tachycardia (CPVT) as a result of an autosomal recessive mutation in the CASQ2 gene has only been found in consanguineous families [15]. In addition, one also has to be aware of the fact that autosomal dominantly inherited disease may also run in consanguineous families. If offspring has inherited both affected alleles, the clinical picture is often severe and lethal at an early age. Examples include long QT syndrome and hypertrophic cardiomyopathy [16, 17].

If consanguinity occurs frequently within a population, the population becomes inbred. In such a population, for any genetic locus, the frequency of heterozygotes will be lower than expected under Hardy–Weinberg equilibrium (because of reduced random mating). This will lead to overestimation of carrier frequencies.

In multifactorial disease, consanguinity may play a role as well, although less conspicuous than in autosomal recessive disease. Shared predisposing genetic variants, present in heterozygous form in the parents, have a 25% chance of being present in homozygous form in the offspring, thus increasing the likelihood for multifactorial disorders.

Information on consanguinity is not always volunteered and should be specifically asked for. Sometimes consanguinity is present, but not known to the family. Most individuals have little information on relatives dating further than three generations back. If ancestors from both parents are from the same small isolated community, consanguinity may still be suspected. When of importance, genealogical studies or SNP array analysis may be used to substantiate this.

Genetic Testing

Any test to identify a genetic disease can be considered a genetic test. Genetic testing using DNA analysis is available for an increasing number of cardiac diseases and conditions that are associated with cardiovascular disease in a wider context. Two important differences between genetic DNA tests, when compared to other diagnostic tests, need mentioning. First, DNA tests usually have health implications that last a lifetime, while the genetic defect in itself is not amenable to treatment. Second, the implications of genetic test results often are not limited to the patient in front of you but also are of concern to family members including future offspring. The family and not the individual patient could be regarded as the "diagnostic unit" in genetic disease. As a result of these notions, DNA testing is and should only be offered as part of a genetic counseling procedure in order to assure that patients fully understand the scope of the tests that are being performed. This is especially true for monogenic disease and tests for very high-risk genes.

Genetic Counseling

Genetic counseling is a two-way communication process aiming at helping patients with genetic disease or at (perceived) increased risk of genetic disease, and their relatives, to understand the genetic risk and decide on a suitable course of action [18]. Genetic counseling is offered by trained medical or paramedical professionals. Its goals are:

- To help patients and their family members comprehend medical facts (diagnosis, symptoms, complications, course, variation, and management)
- To help patients and their family members understand the basic facts of the genetic contribution to their disorder, where this is relevant for communicating risks to specific family members and recurrence risks in (future) children
- To make them understand the options available to deal with risks and recurrence risks (preventive treatments, lifestyle adjustments, reproductive options, prenatal diagnosis)
- To help individuals choose a suitable course of action in view of their individual risk of disease, goals, personal and cultural values, and religious beliefs and to facilitate this course of action
- To support individuals and their families in making the best possible adjustment to their disease condition or to their increased risk of genetic disease

Most common counseling situations for cardiac disorders can be grouped into one of the three categories mentioned below. All three have their own dynamics and major issues:

- Parents who have a child with a congenital heart defect or a syndrome that has important cardiovascular implications or other pediatric cardiac disease. They may want to be informed about prognosis, recurrence risk in future children, and sometimes the possibility of prenatal diagnosis.
- Patients that have a cardiac defect or cardiac disease themselves and have questions about genetic aspects and prognosis. They may also be concerned about risk to family members, most often (future) children and/or sibs.
- Those who have been referred because of a positive family history for cardiac disease or suspicion thereof or have a family history for sudden cardiac death at a young age. They come for information on their personal risk and questions about the usefulness of presymptomatic cardiac evaluation, and, if possible, they may opt for presymptomatic genetic testing.

Some basic principles of genetic counseling:

- Nondirectiveness. Historically, nondirectiveness is an important hallmark of genetic counseling. The counselor provides adequate information and support. The counselee decides. This notion stems from time that genetic counseling was mainly concerned with reproductive issues. Naturally, counselors should have no say in the reproductive decisions made by their clients. Also, in presymptomatic testing of late-onset neurodegenerative disease, where medical interventions to change disease course are virtually absent, maximum nondirectiveness should be applied in counseling.
- However, with a changing focus in medical genetics to disorders that are, at least to some extent, amenable to early intervention or preventive treatment, the applicability of nondirective genetic counseling becomes less obvious. For example, in long QT syndrome type 1, where β-blocker therapy has been proven to be effective in symptomatic patients, nondirective counseling seems less indicated [19]. In practice, in cardiogenetics, a balance that both respects patient autonomy and assures that the appropriate medical decisions are made should be sought for.
- Informed consent. Informed consent is not unique to clinical genetics or genetic counseling. However, some institutions will require written informed consent prior to DNA testing, especially if presymptomatic testing of apparently healthy individuals is concerned. This is no rule of thumb and may vary based on individual insights and local differences in the medicolegal situation.
- Privacy issues. These are also not unique to genetic medicine but may be more urgent in this discipline. Genetic information may have a huge impact on insurability and career options. The extent to which this is true is largely dependent on legislation dealing with genetic discrimination, which varies between countries. However, a danger of discrimination on genetic grounds always exists. Therefore, maximum confidentiality of genetic information should be assured. Providing genetic information to third parties, without written permission from the individual involved, would be defendable only in case of a medical emergency. In contrast, genetic information is much harder to keep confidential because DNA is shared by relatives that are likely to benefit significantly from this information. When appropriate, permission to use genetic information for the benefit of relatives should be actively acquired by the genetic counselor. Especially in families that communicate insufficiently, clinical geneticists may encounter problems with confidentiality and find themselves confronted with conflicting duties.

Cardiac Genetic Counseling

The most notable feature of cardiogenetic diseases is the risk of sudden cardiac death. Every aspect of this devastating event defines the unique role of cardiac genetic counselors [20].These include involvement in prevention strategies, such as helping patients to make lifestyle modifications and coordinating clinical screening of at-risk relatives. Furthermore, the cardiac genetic counselor may be involved in key treatment strategies such as implantable cardioverter defibrillator therapy, thorough investigation of the family history, and in many cases dealing with a grieving family who have unexpectedly lost a loved one. Given the importance of clinical screening of first-degree relatives as a primary prevention strategy, cardiac genetic counselors frequently provide assistance in coordinating clinical surveillance of at-risk family members. Being the first point of call for many families, it is also important for cardiac genetic counselors to educate patients about how frequently clinical screening should occur and often to dispel misinformation regarding family members who have been told in the past that they never need to return for clinical assessment. A diagnosis of many of these diseases will also impose exercise restrictions, particularly relating to competitive sports, and this can be devastating to many patients making adjustment to their disease much more difficult. This is particularly relevant in the younger population where disqualification from sports participation can often lead to major psychosocial consequences. Similarly, patients deemed at increased risk of sudden death who are advised to undergo implantation of an implantable cardioverter defibrillator experience a range of emotions, and the role of the cardiac genetic counselor to provide information and emotional support can be significant. Many of the families seen in the specialized cardiac genetic clinics will have direct experience with sudden cardiac death, often having lost a close relative. In such cases, the grief of the family will be in the forefront and make the provision of information and adjustment to new diagnoses far more difficult.

Cardiac Genetic Testing

Next-generation sequencing technologies have paved the way for testing of a vast number of genes, with a typical cardiac gene panel now comprising 50–200 genes. Many of the genes included in these panels have only minimal evidence of disease association or causation, i.e., accounting for less than 5% of disease. Use of such panels has significantly increased the yield of genetic diagnosis in cardiomyopathy families. However, as could be expected, it has also resulted in an enormous expansion of the detection of VUS (variant of unknown significance) [21]. Despite databases filled with sequence data of over 120,000 controls from different populations (http://exac.broadinstitute.org/, http://gnomad.broadinstitute.org/) and the availability of different in silico prediction algorithms, many of these vusses at this moment cannot yet be satisfactorily resolved. Exome (sequencing of the entire coding region of the genome) and genome sequencing (sequencing of the entire genome) are powerful tools for research and gene discovery and becoming increasingly common in the commercial setting. Coupled with rapidly decreasing costs, and wider access and uptake, the complexity of the results generated when a cardiogenetic gene test is now ordered goes beyond the basic expertise and scope of current practices.

Genetic testing is an important component of cardiogenetic disease management. Commercial genetic tests are available for most, and increasing uptake among patients has contributed to a vastly improved knowledge of the genetic basis of these diseases. The incredible advances in genetic technologies have translated to more rapid, comprehensive, and less expensive genetic tests, completely changing the landscape of genetic testing in recent years. While there are enormous challenges, mostly relating to interpretation of variants, the value of a genetic diagnosis should not be underestimated. In almost all cases, the single greatest utility is for the predictive genetic testing of family members.

With the increasing number of uncertain variants identified after cardiac genetic testing, determining methods to ensure the highest yield of causative variants is important. One key consideration is defining the clinical phenotype both in the individual patient and the family. A complete cardiogenetic evaluation is required, which includes being certain of the clinical diagnosis in the proband. The highest yields from genetic testing are often based on patient cohorts with confirmed disease. A word of caution with respect to pathogenicity seems justified: a variant is not causative because it has been published as such. Many publications do provide neither adequate information on segregation (does the variant cosegregate with disease in the family?) nor functional data supporting pathogenicity. The fact that a variant has been reported in a series of 50 cardiomyopathy patients and was absent in 400 ethnically matched controls cannot now be regarded as sufficient evidence for pathogenicity. Indeed, large-scale population sequencing efforts demonstrate that some mutations in the past believed to be causal occur at a far too high population frequency to be actual monogenic causal pathogenic mutations [22].

The outcomes of cardiac genetic testing are summarized in Table 2.1.

Pre- and Posttest Genetic Counseling

Cardiac genetic counseling is a key component of the multidisciplinary approach to care for families with cardiogenetic diseases, and this is not more evident than in the setting of cardiac genetic testing. With increasing complexity of cardiac genetic results, ensuring individuals are well informed prior to testing is a challenging but critical task.

Table 2.1 Outcomes of cardiac genetic testing (table modified from Ingles et al. Heart Rhythm. 2014 PMID: 24632221)

Possible outcome	Consequences for the proband	Consequences for the family
No variants of potential clinical importance identified	An indeterminate gene result does not exclude a cardiac genetic disease, but reassessment of the phenotype should be considered	Predictive genetic testing cannot be offered to the family. At-risk relatives are advised to be clinically assessed according to current guidelines
Variant of uncertain significance (VUS) identified	Efforts to delineate pathogenicity of the variant are required, including cosegregation studies involving phenotyped family members	While pathogenicity of a variant is under question, it cannot be used to inform clinical management of family members. Predictive genetic testing cannot be offered. At-risk relatives are advised to be clinically assessed according to guidelines
Pathogenic mutation identified (pathogenic or likely pathogenic)	Confirm clinical diagnosis, limited therapeutic and prognostic application except in familial long QT syndrome	Predictive genetic testing of asymptomatic family members is available following genetic counseling
Multiple pathogenic mutations identified	Confirm clinical diagnosis and potentially explain a more severe clinical phenotype	Complex inheritance risk to first-degree relatives must be discussed. Predictive genetic testing of asymptomatic family members is available following genetic counseling
Incidental or secondary pathogenic mutation identified	Action regarding incidental or secondary findings must be discussed with the proband pretest	Genetic counseling to determine clinical and genetic impact to family members is available

Genetic test results should not be considered a binary (yes/no) outcome, but rather a carefully considered result along a continuum from benign to VUS, likely pathogenic, and pathogenic. The genetic test result is therefore a *probabilistic* one, in which the weight of evidence for pathogenicity determines the probability of the specific variant being disease-causing. Conveying this result to the family can be a challenge, but the basic principles of pretest counseling essentially remain unchanged with the ultimate goal of ensuring a full understanding of the process and consequences of genetic testing. There is often inherent uncertainty of the genetic test result, and therefore discussion with a health professional who can effectively explain what this means to the family is preferable [23]. There should be an understanding that the identification of a VUS may require initiation of further family investigation to clarify pathogenicity, and indeed a detailed family history at this point will give information about whether this is even possible. Furthermore, it should be highlighted clearly that there is a small chance new information will become available in the future that may change lead to reclassification of the result. Trained genetic counselors are skilled in delivering complex information in a sensitive manner and should play a key role in the testing process.

Interpreting Genetic Test Results

Interpretation of genetic results is not always straightforward. Without going into great depths, it may be appropriate to spend a few lines on this subject. Mutations can basically have effects in three different ways. They can cause decreased amounts of protein or loss of normal protein function. This is called haploinsufficiency. They can cause gain or change of normal protein function, or they can alter protein features making the protein to become toxic, if normal protein metabolism is disturbed. For example, loss of function mutations in the SCN5a gene cause Brugada syndrome and progressive conduction disease, whereas gain of function mutations in the same gene underlie long QT syndrome type 3. Loss of function (haploinsufficiency) is the most common disease-causing mechanism.

If *nonsense mutations* (leading to a stop codon) or frameshift *mutations* (leading to disruption of the reading frame, which usually causes a premature stop) occur, one can be confident that this will lead to haploinsufficiency, unless the truncation is very close to the C-terminus of the gene. As a result of a process called nonsense-mediated messenger RNA decay, only very little truncated protein will be produced. Most splice mutations (especially those disturbing the reading frame) and larger rearrangements of genes will also lead to haploinsufficiency. In certain genes where haploinsufficiency is known to be the disease-causing mechanism, these types of mutations will almost certainly be considered pathogenic. In cardiogenetic diseases, this can include MYBPC3 mutations in HCM, in PKP2 in ARVC/D, and truncating TTN mutations in familial DCM. Truncating mutations in MYH7 are an example of changes not expected to impact the protein function much, since loss of function is not thought to be the disease-causing mechanism for this gene.

Missense mutations (mutations changing only one amino acid in the protein) may lead to both loss of protein function and gain/change of function. Especially in case of structural proteins, where different protein molecules act together to form a structure, missense mutations may be more deleterious than truncating mutations, as these mutated proteins are incorporated into the structure and disrupt it. This will lead to a dominant negative effect.

However, many of the missense mutations detected will actually be rare variants without significant effect on protein function. Therefore, if a new missense mutation in a candidate gene for a specific disorder is identified, it will often be difficult to predict whether or not it is the actual causative mutation, i.e., VUS (Table 2.1). There has been almost universal adoption of variant classification criteria proposed by the American College of Medical Genetics and Genomics and the Association of Medical Pathologists (ACMG/AMP) in 2015 [24]. Since then, gene-specific modifications have been made, including a recent publication outlining classification of variants in sarcomere genes [25]. In brief, many of the principles of variant classification are shown in Table 2.2. Where there is not enough evidence for causation, a variant will remain uncertain. Unfortunately, in clinical practice VUS occur rather frequently and cannot always be satisfactorily resolved. Assumptions made regarding the pathogenic potential of missense mutations are therefore often provisional. It is important to realize this when using genetic information in clinical practice. Overinterpreting missense variants for pathogenic mutations is harmful in several ways, as on the one hand some individuals without a genetic predisposition to the disease will be stigmatized and unnecessarily kept under surveillance, while on the other hand, the actual causative

Table 2.2 Key criteria used in determining pathogenicity of variants

Key criteria	Description	Tools/approach
Absence of rarity in general population	The variant has not been reported in general population databases. In 2016, the Exome Aggregation Consortium reports >60,000 exomes giving allele frequencies by ethnicity. Absence of the variant in a large number of healthy controls is compatible with pathogenicity but merely confirms that the variant is indeed rare	ExAC and gnomAD databases *ExAC.broadinstitute.org* *gnomAD.broadinstiture.org*
Variant previously reported in disease population	Many classification criteria will require the variant to have been previously reported in >3 unrelated probands with the same phenotype. Public access databases such a NCBI ClinVar encourage laboratories and research groups to upload their details and experience of certain variants. Other disease-specific databases exist	ClinVar website *clinvar.com* ARVD/C genetic variant database *arvcdatabase.info*
De novo event	If the variant has arisen spontaneously at conception, (i.e., de novo) this can be regarded as very strong evidence in favor of pathogenicity. As mutation frequencies are exceedingly low, the chance that a new mutation would occur in the studied candidate gene just by coincidence is negligible	Genetic and clinical testing of both parents is necessary. Where there is question over paternity, this should be confirmed by haplotype analysis following discussion with the family. In recent times, due to occurrence of egg donor in vitro fertilization options, it may also be necessary to confirm maternity with a family. Paternity/maternity issues are sensitive discussion topics and should be carefully approached
Segregation with multiple affected family members	Proving that a variant cosegregates with the disease phenotype in a family can provide definite evidence for pathogenicity, but only if the family is large enough (about ten informative meiosis would be required). This is often not the case. In families where even two or more affected relatives can be shown to carry the variant, this will provide lower-level supportive evidence for pathogenicity and should be pursued where possible Absence of the variant in an affected family member is, of course, strong evidence against pathogenicity	Clinical and genetic testing of relatives is needed to gather segregation data. In general, we collect DNA samples from affected relatives only since unaffected relatives are not informative (i.e., we know there is incomplete penetrance among cardiogenetic diseases). When segregating an uncertain variant in a family, the individual should understand that the importance of the variant is unknown. Often the approach is to request the DNA as a research sample, where there is no expectation to get a result. If pathogenicity can be adequately confirmed, then the family members will be invited to the clinical service to undergo predictive genetic testing
Variant causes loss of function of a gene known to result in a phenotype by this mechanism	As described above, loss of function in a handful of genes can be very strong evidence of pathogenicity	This rule does not apply to all genes
In silico tools and conservation scores supportive of a deleterious role	There are a multitude of in silico prediction software and conservation scores, no weight should be placed on a single score, and in general whether a number of these are in support of a deleterious impact can be used as low-level evidence to support pathogenicity	Polyphen2 *genetics.bwh.harvard.edu/pph2* Polyphen HCM *genetics.bwh.harvard.edu/hcm* SIFT (sorting intolerant from tolerant) *sift.jcvi.org* CADD (combined annotation-dependent depletion) score *cadd.gs.washington.edu*

mutation may go unnoticed and individuals may be released from surveillance, based on incorrect genetic information. The fact that a specific missense mutation has been published as a pathogenic mutation in the literature cannot always be regarded as sufficient evidence (one has to go back to the original publications and weigh the evidence).

Controls

In the past, absence of a potentially pathogenic mutation from 100 or 200 controls matched for ethnicity was regarded as sufficient evidence for causality. Nowadays we know this has led to significant overinterpretation of rare variants with respect to causality; therefore, older papers claiming that a mutation is causal for a specific cardiac disease should be regarded with caution [26]. Luckily we now have online access to whole-exome data (ExAC and gnomAD) of more than 120,000 unrelated individuals across different populations that were not specifically ascertained for cardiac disease and that can therefore serve as useful controls. Causal highly penetrant autosomal dominant mutations should be present at very low frequencies in such population-based databases. On the other hand, even complete absence from these databases cannot be regarded as definite proof of pathogenicity. ExAC also provides data on evolutionary constraint for different classes of mutations; they calculated whether or not there were more certain loss of function mutations than expected, based on the size of the gene, and represent that as pLI ranging from 0.00 to 1. The closer the pLI is to 1, the stronger the evolutionary constraint is for loss of function mutations. However, even for known cardiac loss of function genes like MYBPC3 and PKP2, the pLI is actually 0.00 indicating that even individuals with definite loss of function mutations in these cardiomyopathy genes have a near-normal reproductive fitness, so they will usually reproduce before they get seriously ill. In comparison, the pLI for LAMP2 and PRKAG2 are 0.94 and 0.98 respectively, indicating very significant evolutionary constraint for loss of function mutations in these genes; and indeed loss of function mutations in those genes may lead to very severe phenotypes at a young age. Similarly for missense variants, they calculated a Z-score that may actually be negative if more missense variants were seen than expected. The higher the Z-score, the less tolerant the gene is for missense mutations.

Predictive Testing and the Dynamics of Family Studies

Predictive, *presymptomatic*, or *cascade genetic testing* is performed on family members with no apparent evidence of clinical disease to find out whether or not they have inherited a pathogenic gene variant. Often predictive testing takes place in the context of family studies. In family studies, specific individuals are targeted for evaluation based on a positive family history for genetic disease. Both predictive testing and family studies are unique features of clinical genetics practice.

Predictive DNA Testing

Predictive DNA testing is usually performed for monogenic disorders with important health risks. Demonstrating that an individual has not inherited the family-specific mutation usually reduces risks to population level, and also risks for offspring will be normalized. However, if the mutation is indeed identified, this does not automatically mean that the individual will get the disease. In many cardiac disorders, penetrance is significantly reduced. In general, presence of the familial mutation will not allow for predictions on severity of the disease or age of onset.

Most genetic cardiac disorders show significant locus heterogeneity, that is, many different genes are associated with a similar phenotype. Besides, molecular heterogeneity (the number of different mutations in a gene) is immense. Therefore, as a paradigm, predictive genetic testing in a family is only possible if a causative family-specific mutation has been identified in the index patient.

It is important to emphasize that predictive testing does not necessarily involve DNA testing. A cardiologist performing echocardiography in a symptom-free sib of a hypertrophic cardiomyopathy patient is involved in both a family study and predictive testing. The detection of, even a very mild, hypertrophy of the interventricular septum, that as yet does not need treatment, will have serious consequences for this person. The adverse consequences (see next paragraph) of predictive testing based on concealed cardiac symptoms are no different from those associated with predictive DNA testing. Therefore, in a case like this, the same standards of genetic counseling should be applied prior to echocardiography.

In families where DNA studies have been unsuccessful, family studies will have to rely solely on phenotype and therefore on cardiac evaluation. An important difference between family studies based on phenotype and those based on genotype arises when non-penetrance or age-dependent penetrance occurs. In that case, of course, a genetic test will be more sensitive to demonstrate the predisposition especially in young individuals. In conditions with age-dependent penetrance, it may be prudent to reevaluate individuals with a 50% prior chance of having inherited the genetic defect after a couple of years.

Adverse Consequences of Predictive Testing

Predictive testing may offer important medical and psychosocial benefits to the individuals tested. However, it should be realized that, in contrast to this, predictive testing can also have negative psychological and socioeconomic repercussions [27]. Individuals may perceive themselves as less healthy, even when no disease symptoms can yet be demonstrated. Coming to terms with knowledge about one's own genetic predisposition, feelings of guilt toward children that are now also at increased risk, forced lifestyle changes, and difficulty with choices regarding, for example, reproductive issues may cause a lot of distress and anxiety. Importantly, knowing that one has the predisposition for a serious late-onset disorder is likely to complicate qualifying for, for example, life or health insurance or might interfere with career options. Last but not least, predictive testing can complicate family relationships, especially if some family members want to be tested while others decline testing. Test results of one person may also yield risk information with regard to other family members that may not want to know this. Therefore, predictive testing should not be embarked on without giving these issues serious thought. Opting for predictive testing should be a well-considered and autonomous decision of the individual involved. Pressure on individuals to undergo testing, for instance, by insurance companies or employers would be absolutely unethical.

Predictive Testing in Minors

Minors cannot make their own well-informed decisions with regard to predictive testing. It is a paradigm in clinical genetics not to perform predictive genetic testing in minors if there is no direct and important medical benefit [28, 29]. Late-onset disorders, or disorders that are not amenable to preventive treatment, are not to be tested in healthy children [28]. In some countries, predictive genetic testing in minors is subject to specific restrictive legislation.

However, in many cardiac disorders like long QT syndromes, preventive therapy should be instituted at an early age. In such cases, postponing testing until children can make their own autonomous decisions is often not a realistic option. Thus, predictive genetic testing of minors can certainly be indicated. In the Netherlands, for example, predictive genetic testing of minors for cardiac disorders is performed in centers for cardiogenetics, according to a protocol that also involves participation of a psychologist or specialized social worker. It should be noted that parents who have their children tested for heritable arrhythmia syndromes are likely to experience major distress and anxiety [30]. This may influence the handling of their children, and moreover parental anxiety is likely to lead to anxiety in children.

As a rule of thumb, predictive testing in children is only performed if treatment or surveillance at a pediatric age is possible and necessary; there may be exceptions to this rule that have to be judged on a case-by-case basis. The bottom line is that predictive testing always has to be in the interest of the child. For example, should a child from a hypertrophic cardiomyopathy family be talented enough to seriously pursue a professional career in sports, it would be unfair to postpone testing, thereby depriving the child from the possibility to choose another career at an earlier stage.

Conducting Family Studies

The way individuals are selected for evaluation in a family study primarily depends on the mode of inheritance of the disease. Cardiogenetic family studies most often involve autosomal dominant conditions, in which affected individuals are likely to occur in several generations and both males and females may be affected. Family studies are conducted using the "cascade method." As soon as a new disease carrier has been identified, his or her first-degree relatives become the next targets for study. Historically information about the possibility of genetic testing was always distributed within the family by coached patients themselves [31]. This was designed in this way in order to circumvent issues of patient confidentiality and in order to retain the nondirective character of genetic testing. Nowadays alternative methods for distributing genetic information within families are being investigated as the old routine is considered to put too much burden and responsibility on the shoulders of patients that are themselves already struggling with genetic disease. At least some way of professional supervision of the information distribution process seems justified. When parents of a disease carrier are deceased, it will often be difficult to determine whether the condition has been inherited from the mother or from the father. The possibility also remains that the disease predisposition was inherited from neither parents but resulted from a de novo mutational event. A decision will have to be made whether to stop here or to pursue the family study further to aunts, uncles, and often first cousins at both sides. This decision depends in part on the medical information available on the parents and more distant relatives. Moreover, the magnitude of the risk for severe events that is associated with the familial disease, knowledge on the frequency of the familial character of the disease, and the availability of therapies that influence this risk are important issues when deciding how far family studies should be pursued.

The major justification for family studies is to unambiguously identify those individuals that run an increased risk of disease, in order to institute preventive therapies or closely monitor these individuals and enroll them in risk stratification protocols.

However, sometimes the targeted family members themselves may not be at high risk for serious disease anymore.

Contacting them may still be justified if there is a considerable chance that the predisposition to a treatable disease has been transmitted to their children. This may, for example, be the case in elderly individuals from long QT syndrome families that never experienced arrhythmias themselves. Demonstrating the predisposition in them will not necessarily lead to treatment, but exclusion of the predisposition will render further testing unnecessary for all of his or her children. The medical benefits for elderly tested individuals may be limited, but also the socioeconomic dangers of predictive testing may be less urgent in older individuals, as they will usually already have insurance and careers.

In case of a disorder that is not amenable to treatment, only reproductive counseling can be offered to family members that turn out to have the genetic predisposition. For personal reasons, family members may opt for predictive testing. Uncertainty regarding genetic status may by itself be a major cause of distress and anxiety. However, if no clear medical benefits are to be expected, family studies should only be initiated on specific demand of the relatives themselves.

Prenatal Diagnosis

Prenatal diagnosis can be requested for a number of different reasons. Termination of pregnancy may be the ultimate consequence once it has been established that the fetus has a very serious debilitating genetic disorder. However, the goal of prenatal diagnosis may also be to aid in planning peripartum medical interventions or help parents to emotionally prepare for the birth of a child with a birth defect. Parents with a previous child with a congenital heart defect will qualify for specialized ultrasound in subsequent pregnancies. Depending on the severity and type of heart defect that is detected at ultrasound, parents may decide to terminate the pregnancy or to deliver in a center where appropriate neonatal intensive care is available. On rare occasions, even fetal therapy can be applied; for instance, some fetal tachyarrhythmias can be treated by putting the mother on medication.

Prenatal diagnosis can be divided in invasive prenatal diagnosis and noninvasive imaging studies, mainly prenatal ultrasound. Invasive prenatal diagnosis involves obtaining chorionic villi (placental cells), amniocytes (fetal cells present in amniotic fluid), or rarely cord blood, for genetic and, sometimes, protein or metabolite studies. The invasive procedures are associated with a small albeit significant risk of pregnancy loss. Therefore, these should be undertaken only if the prenatal diagnosis will have medical consequences. Like in predictive genetic testing, prenatal DNA diagnosis for cardiac disorders will only be possible if the family-specific mutation has been identified beforehand.

Except for ultrasound diagnosis in pregnancies of couples to whom an earlier child with a congenital heart defect has been born, requests for prenatal diagnosis are infrequent in cardiogenetic practice. However, requests for prenatal diagnosis should always be taken seriously and the reasons should be explored. Frequently, other issues like feelings of guilt, fear of disapproval from friends or relatives, uncertainty about postnatal follow-up, and so on may be found to underlie such requests.

Preimplantation genetic diagnosis (PGD) is a technique in which in vitro fertilization (IVF) is combined with genetic diagnosis prior to implantation of the embryo into the womb. As genetic diagnosis has to be performed on one or two embryonal cells instead of millions of white blood cells, PGD is technically much more demanding. PGD may be an alternative to couples that are opposed to pregnancy termination, but would not be able to reproduce knowing that their child is at high risk of serious genetic disease. Success rates of PGD are limited by the limitations of the IVF procedure and the fact that after genetic testing, fewer viable embryos may be left for implantation. PGD has been performed for a limited number of disorders that may have major cardiac consequences like Marfan syndrome or myotonic dystrophy [32, 33].

Besides prenatal diagnosis, which is performed in selected cases because of increased risk of genetic disease, also prenatal screening programs exist. In principle, all pregnant women are eligible for prenatal screening programs that may be differently set up in different countries. In most western countries nowadays, prenatal ultrasound screening is offered to pregnant women at around 20 weeks of gestation. As congenital heart defects occur at high frequency in the general population, many more heart defects will be found by chance during ultrasound screening than by using other methods of prenatal diagnosis, even if the sensitivity of ultrasound screening may be relatively poor.

The Cardiogenetics Outclinic

Since the care for individuals with genetic cardiac disease and their relatives requires both cardiologic and genetic expertise, the multidisciplinary outpatient clinics for cardiogenetics are advocated as the ideal model of care. In these outpatient clinics that are operating within the university hospitals, cardiologists, pediatric cardiologists, clinical geneticists, molecular geneticists, genetic nurses, psychologists, and social workers cooperate to provide integrated healthcare for this specific patient group. This is of benefit to patients because the number of hospital visits can usually be reduced and also to healthcare providers because of easier communication. Besides, from a data collection and research point of view, centralization of patients with inherited cardiac disease also has obvious advantages. It will be immediately clear that most of the regular care for this patient group will have to remain with cardiologists working in regional or local hospitals. With an estimated prevalence of 1 in 500 for hypertrophic cardiomyopathy, it would not only be unnecessary to follow all these patients in outclinics for cardiogenetics but also impossible. This implicates that a general awareness among cardiologists of the genetic aspects of cardiac disease is needed.

References

1. Hofman N, van Langen I, Wilde AM. Genetic testing in cardiovascular diseases. Curr Opin Cardiol. 2010;25:243–8.
2. Cowan J, Morales A, Dagua J, Hershberger RE. Genetic testing and henetic counseling in cardiovascular genetic medicine: overview and preliminary recommendations. Congest Heart Fail. 2008;14:97–105.
3. Morales A, Cowan J, Dagua J, Hershberger RE. Family history: an essential tool for cardiovascular genetic medicine. Congest Heart Fail. 2008;14:37–45.
4. Kingston HM. Genetic assessment and pedigree analysis. In: Rimoin DL, Connor JM, Pyeritz RE, Korf BR, editors. Emery and Rimoin's principles and practice of medical genetics. 4th ed. London: Churchill Livingstone; 2002.
5. Turnpenny P, Ellard S. Emery's elements of medical genetics. 13th ed. London: Churchill Livingstone; 2008.
6. Gray B, Yeates L, Medi C, et al. Homozygous mutation in the cardiac troponin I gene: clinical heterogeneity in hypertrophic cardiomyopathy. Int J Cardiol. 2013 Sep 30;168(2):1530–1.
7. McKenna WJ, Thierfelder L, Suk HJ, Anan R, O'Donoghue A, et al. Mutations in the genes for cardiac troponin T and alpha-tropomyosin in hypertrophic cardiomyopathy. N Engl J Med. 1995;332:1058–64.
8. Gimeno JR, Monserrat L, Pérez-Sánchez I, et al. Hypertrophic cardiomyopathy. A study of the troponin-T gene in 127 Spanish families. Rev Esp Cardiol. 2009;62:1473–7.
9. van Rijsingen IA, Arbustini E, Elliott PM, et al. Risk factors for malignant ventricular arrhythmias in lamin a/c mutation carriers a European cohort study. Am Coll Cardiol. 2012 Jan 31;59(5):493–500.
10. van Rijsingen IA, van der Zwaag PA, Groeneweg JA. Outcome in phospholamban R14del carriers: results of a large multicentre cohort study. Circ Cardiovasc Genet. 2014 Aug;7(4):455–65.
11. Van Langen IM, Birnie E, Alders M, et al. The use of genotype-phenotype correlations in mutation analysis for the long QT syndrome. J Med Genet. 2003;40:141–5.
12. Schwartz PJ, Priori SG, Spazzolini C, et al. Genotype-phenotype correlation in the long-QT syndrome: gene-specific triggers for life-threatening arrhythmias. Circulation. 2001;103:89–95.
13. Alders M, Jongbloed R, Deelen W, Van den Wijngaard A, Doevendans P, Cate FT, Regitz-Zagrosek V, Vosberg HP, Langen IV, Wilde A, Dooijes D, Mannens M. The 2373insG Mutation in the MYBPC3 Gene Is a Founder Mutation, Which Accounts for Nearly One-Fourth of the HCM Cases in the Netherlands. Eur Heart J. 2003;24(20):1848–53. PMID: 14563344. https://doi.org/10.1016/s0195-668x(03)00466-4.
14. Othman H, Saadat M. Prevalence of consanguineous marriages in Syria. J Biosoc Sci. 2009;41:685–92.
15. Lahat H, Pras E, Olender T, et al. A missense mutation in a highly conserved region of CASQ2 is associated with autosomal recessive catecholamine-induced polymorphic ventricular tachycardia in Bedouin families from Israel. Am J Hum Genet. 2001;69:1378–84.
16. Hoorntje T, Alders M, van Tintelen P, et al. Homozygous premature truncation of the HERG protein: the human HERG knockout. Circulation. 1999;100:1264–7.
17. Zahka K, Kalidas K, Simpson MA, et al. Homozygous mutation of MYBPC3 associated with severe infantile hypertrophic cardiomyopathy at high frequency among the Amish. Heart. 2008;94:1326–30.
18. Resta R, Biesecker BB, Bennett RL, et al. A new definition of genetic counseling: national society of genetic counselors' task force report. J Genet Couns. 2006;15:77–83.
19. Vincent GM, Schwartz PJ, Denjoy I, et al. High efficacy of beta-blockers in long-QT syndrome type 1: contribution of noncompliance and QT-prolonging drugs to the occurrence of beta-blocker treatment "failures". Circulation. 2009;119:215–21.
20. Ingles J, Yeates L, Semsarian C. The emerging role of the cardiac genetic counselor. Heart Rhythm. 2011 Dec;8(12):1958–62.
21. Pugh TJ, Kelly MA, Gowrisankar S, et al. The landscape of genetic variation in dilated cardiomyopathy as surveyed by clinical DNA sequencing. Genet Med. 2014 Aug;16(8):601–8.
22. Andreasen C, Nielsen JB, Refsgaard L, et al. New population-based exome data are questioning the pathogenicity of previously cardiomyopathy-associated genetic variants. Eur J Hum Genet. 2013 Sep;21(9):918–28.
23. Ingles J, Semsarian C. Conveying a probabilistic genetic test result to families with an inherited heart disease. Heart Rhythm. 2014 Jun;11(6):1073–8.
24. Richards S, Aziz N, Bale S, et al. Standards and guidelines for the interpretation of sequence variants: a joint consensus recommendation of the American College of Medical Genetics and Genomics and the Association for Molecular Pathology. Genet Med. 2015 May;17(5):405–24.
25. Kelly MA, Caleshu C, Morales A, Buchan J, et al. Adaptation and validation of the ACMG/AMP variant classification framework for MYH7-associated inherited cardiomyopathies: recommendations by ClinGen's inherited cardiomyopathy expert panel. Genet Med. 2018 Mar;20(3):351–9.
26. Walsh R, Thomson KL, Ware JS, et al. Reassessment of Mendelian gene pathogenicity using 7,855 cardiomyopathy cases and 60,706 reference samples. Genet Med. 2017 Feb;19(2):192–203.
27. Hendriks KS, Hendriks MM, Birnie E, et al. Familial disease with a risk of sudden death: a longitudinal study of the psychological consequences of predictive testing for long QT syndrome. Heart Rhythm. 2008;5:719–24.
28. European Society of Human Genetics. Genetic testing in asymptomatic minors: recommendations of the European Society of Human Genetics. Eur J Hum Genet. 2009;17:720–1.
29. Borry P, Evers-Kiebooms G, Cornel MC, et al. Genetic testing in asymptomatic minors: background considerations towards ESHG Recommendations. Eur J Hum Genet. 2009 Jun;17(6):711–9.
30. Hendriks KS, Grosfeld FJ, Wilde AA, et al. High distress in parents whose children undergo predictive testing for long QT syndrome. Community Genet. 2005;8:103–13.
31. van der Roest WP, Pennings JM, Bakker M, van den Berg MP, van Tintelen JP. Family letters are an effective way to inform relatives about inherited cardiac disease. Am J Med Genet A. 2009;149A:357–63.
32. Piyamongkol W, Harper JC, Sherlock JK, et al. A successful strategy for preimplantation genetic diagnosis of myotonic dystrophy using multiplex fluorescent PCR. Prenat Diagn. 2001;21:223–32.
33. Spits C, De Rycke M, Verpoest W, et al. Preimplantation genetic diagnosis for Marfan syndrome. Fertil Steril. 2006;86:310–20.

Part II

Cardiomyopathies

Introduction to Hereditary Cardiomyopathies

3

Paul A. van der Zwaag and Maarten P. van den Berg

Cardiomyopathies are defined by the European Society of Cardiology (ESC) Working Group on Myocardial and Pericardial Diseases as myocardial disorders in which the heart muscle is structurally and functionally abnormal in the absence of coronary artery disease, hypertension, valvular heart disease, and congenital heart disease sufficient to explain the observed myocardial abnormality [1]. In other words, a cardiomyopathy is disease of the heart muscle "itself," but the requirement "sufficient" is crucial since minor structural disease is acceptable. For instance, the finding of mild concomitant coronary artery disease does not preclude the diagnosis of DCM, and by the same token, mild hypertension does not necessarily preclude the diagnosis of HCM. Conversely, patients with a genetic predisposition to a cardiomyopathy can more easily display myocardial disease caused by environmental factors such as hypertension, medication or intoxication, excessive exertion, etc. illustrating that a mutation is in essence merely a risk factor but by itself often insufficient to cause the disease. Cardiomyopathy can be part of a systemic disease (e.g., amyloidosis), syndrome (e.g., Noonan syndrome), muscular disease (e.g., limb girdle muscular dystrophy), or an isolated cardiac disorder.

Like the definition of cardiomyopathy, the classification of subtypes of cardiomyopathy has always been a matter of hot debates, reflecting the complexity of the topic and the plethora of clinical pictures and entities as well the ever-increasing knowledge on the underlying mechanisms of disease, including new insights acquired by molecular genetics. Indeed, the number of PubMed-indexed papers on "cardiomyopathy" and "genetics" has greatly increased over the years (Fig. 3.1). Of note, the classification of cardiomyopathies by ESC differs substantially from the American Heart Association (AHA) classification. The AHA focuses more on the underlying mechanism and first distinguishes "genetic" and "acquired" forms of cardiomyopathies, and by the same token, the Americans, for instance, also consider ion channel disorders to be forms of (genetic) cardiomyopathy [2]. In contrast, the vantage point of ESC Working Group on Myocardial and Pericardial Diseases is the clinical phenotype as presented to the attending physician, in particular the findings as obtained with echocardiography. Putting it simply: is there a phenotype of left ventricular hypertrophy vs. dilatation and systolic dysfunction vs. restriction vs. arrhythmias and right ventricular involvement? In this chapter, we largely adhere to the European classification, and we thus discuss five different subtypes of cardiomyopathy: hypertrophic cardiomyopathy (HCM), dilated cardiomyopathy (DCM), arrhythmogenic cardiomyopathy (ACM), restrictive cardiomyopathy (RCM), and non-compaction cardiomyopathy (NCCM). Over the years however, we have learned that there is substantial overlap between these cardiomyopathies, both clinically and genetically. For example, severe hypertrophic cardiomyopathy can progress to systolic dysfunction with dilatation of the left ventricle [3]. If not diagnosed before the dilatation started, this could therefore be misdiagnosed as DCM and not as HCM. Likewise, DCM is often accompanied by a certain measure of hypertrophy, and in particular in the setting of limited dilatation of the left ventricle and/or limited systolic dysfunction, the distinction with HCM can be arbitrary. Also, the term arrhythmogenic cardiomyopathy was coined to account for the fact arrhythmogenic right ventricular cardiomyopathy is often accompanied by some degree of left ventricular dilatation and/or dysfunction [4]. In fact, left-dominant forms have been reported with features otherwise typical for arrhythmogenic right ventricular cardiomyopathy, including fibro-fatty replacement [5]. The next step in the European classification is the distinction between hereditary and nonhereditary forms of cardiomyopathy. For instance, cardiomyopathy with phenotype of hypertrophy ("hypertrophic cardiomyopathy") can also be due to obesity or AL amyloidosis. Likewise, cardiomyopathy with phenotype of dilatation and systolic dysfunction ("dilated cardiomyopathy") can also be due to

P. A. van der Zwaag (✉) · M. P. van den Berg
Departments of Genetics (P.A.v.d.Z.) and Cardiology (M.P.v.d.B.), University Medical Center Groningen, University of Groningen, Groningen, The Netherlands
e-mail: p.a.van.der.zwaag@umcg.nl; m.p.van.den.berg@umcg.nl

H. F. Baars et al. (eds.), *Clinical Cardiogenetics*, https://doi.org/10.1007/978-3-030-45457-9_3

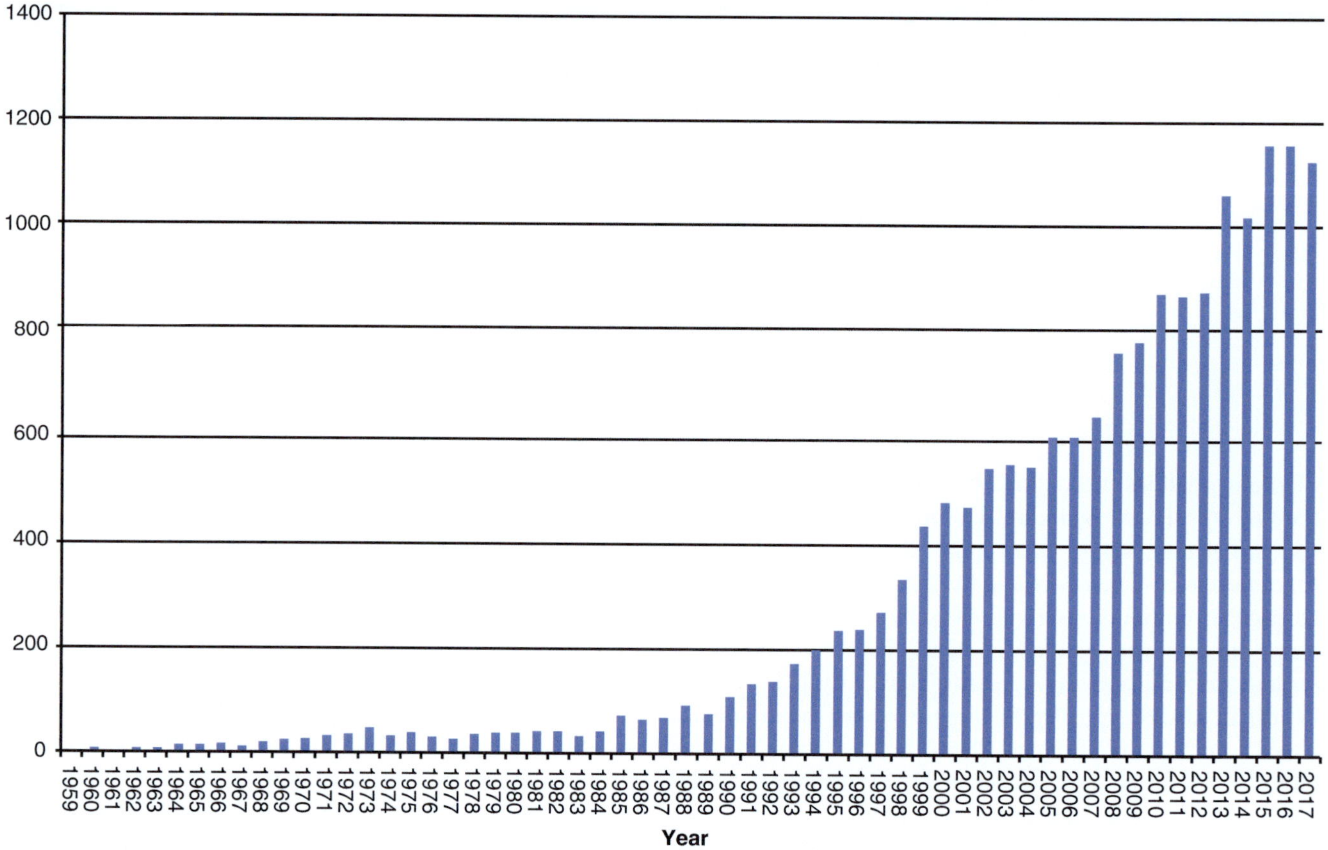

Fig. 3.1 The number of PubMed-indexed papers on "cardiomyopathy" and "genetics," on the y-axis, is shown per year, on the x-axis

myocarditis, anthracycline cardiotoxicity, etc. However, for the purpose of this chapter, these forms of nonhereditary cardiomyopathy will not be discussed further. All hereditary cardiomyopathies are characterized by incomplete and age-related penetrance. The proportion of individuals carrying a pathogenic mutation with associated clinical symptoms increases with age but virtually never reaches 100%. This incomplete penetrance implies that some mutation carriers will remain unaffected during their entire life. The onset of symptoms is usually after adolescence or in early adulthood, but children with severe forms of cardiomyopathy have been described. Some of these cases have been associated with multiple mutations [6, 7]. The type and severity of the disease and sometimes even cardiomyopathy subtype can vary widely, even within families, a concept that is called variable expression.

Hereditary cardiomyopathies are not only clinically variable, but the genetic background is also heterogeneous. For each cardiomyopathy, multiple disease genes have been identified, and mutations in several genes can cause different cardiomyopathy subtypes (Fig. 3.2). However, despite this large overlap and numerous important exceptions, some broad distinctions can be made. HCM is usually caused by mutations in genes encoding constituents of the sarcomere, and the same holds true for NCCM, whereas ACM is usually due to mutations in genes encoding constituents of the desmosome. In contrast, DCM is indeed genetically highly heterogeneous (Fig. 3.3) [8]. The number of genes associated with cardiomyopathies continues to increase and will continue to do so given the many genetically unsolved cases, including familial ones (Fig. 3.4).

Hypertrophic Cardiomyopathy

HCM is the most prevalent cardiomyopathy, affecting an estimated 1 in 500 individuals worldwide. Thereby it does not fulfill the criterion for a rare disease, which is defined as prevalence below 1:2000. HCM is the most common cause of sudden cardiac death below the age of 35 years. Familial HCM has long been recognized, mostly with an autosomal dominant pattern of inheritance, and the first mutation was identified in 1990 by the group of Seidman et al. in the gene encoding the sarcomeric protein β-myosin heavy chain (*MYH7*) [9, 10]. Soon afterward, mutations in several other sarcomere genes were identified in HCM families, resulting in the concept of genetic HCM as a disease of the sarcomere.

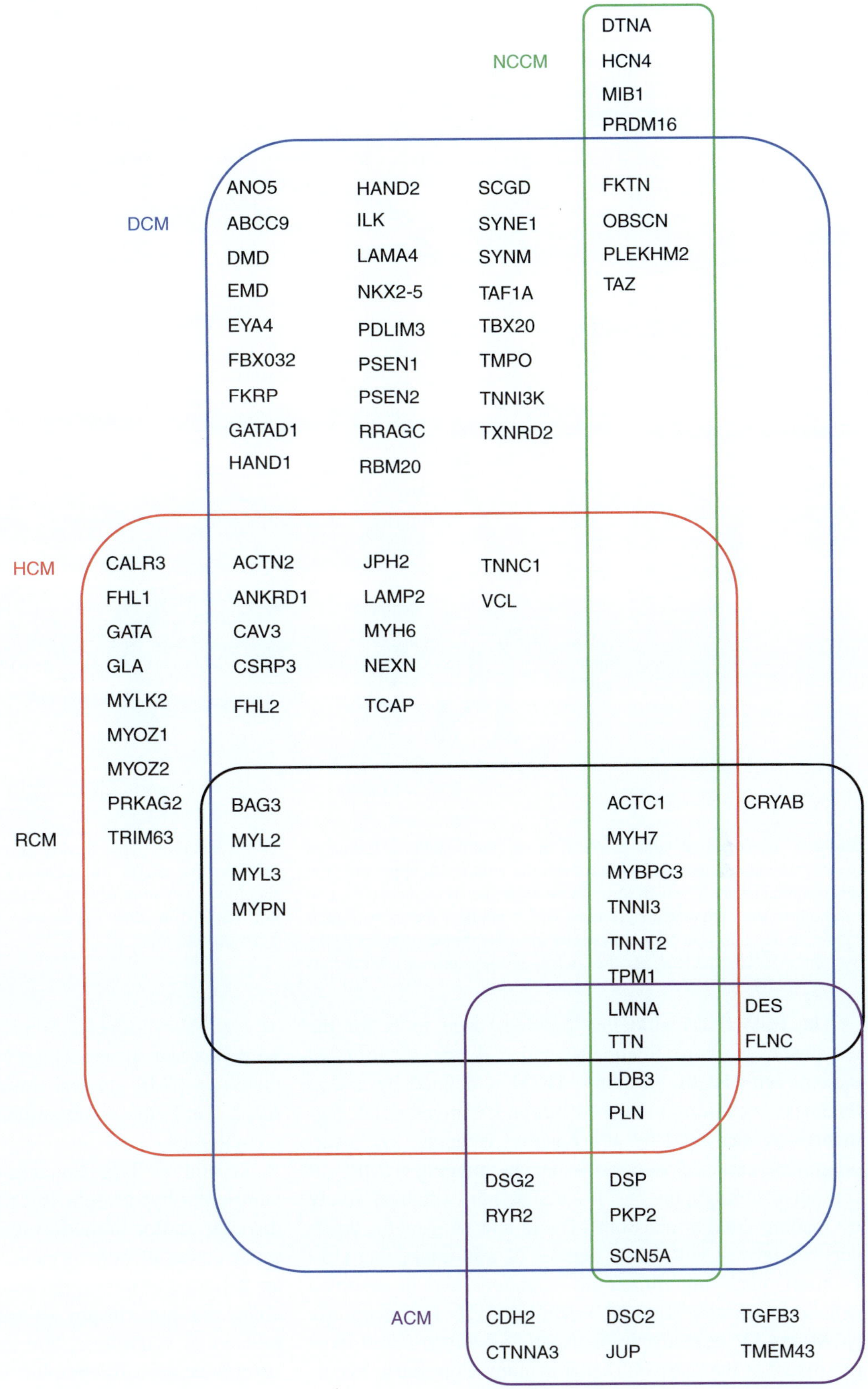

Fig. 3.2 Genetic heterogeneity and overlap in genes causing cardiomyopathies. This figure shows the genes underlying hypertrophic cardiomyopathy (HCM), dilated cardiomyopathy (DCM), arrhythmogenic cardiomyopathy (ACM), restrictive cardiomyopathy (RCM), and non-compaction cardiomyopathy (NCCM). Modified from Van der Zwaag PA. Genetic and clinical characterisation of arrhythmogenic cardiomyopathy. Doctoral Thesis, 2012 [http://irs.ub.rug.nl/ppn/352159146]

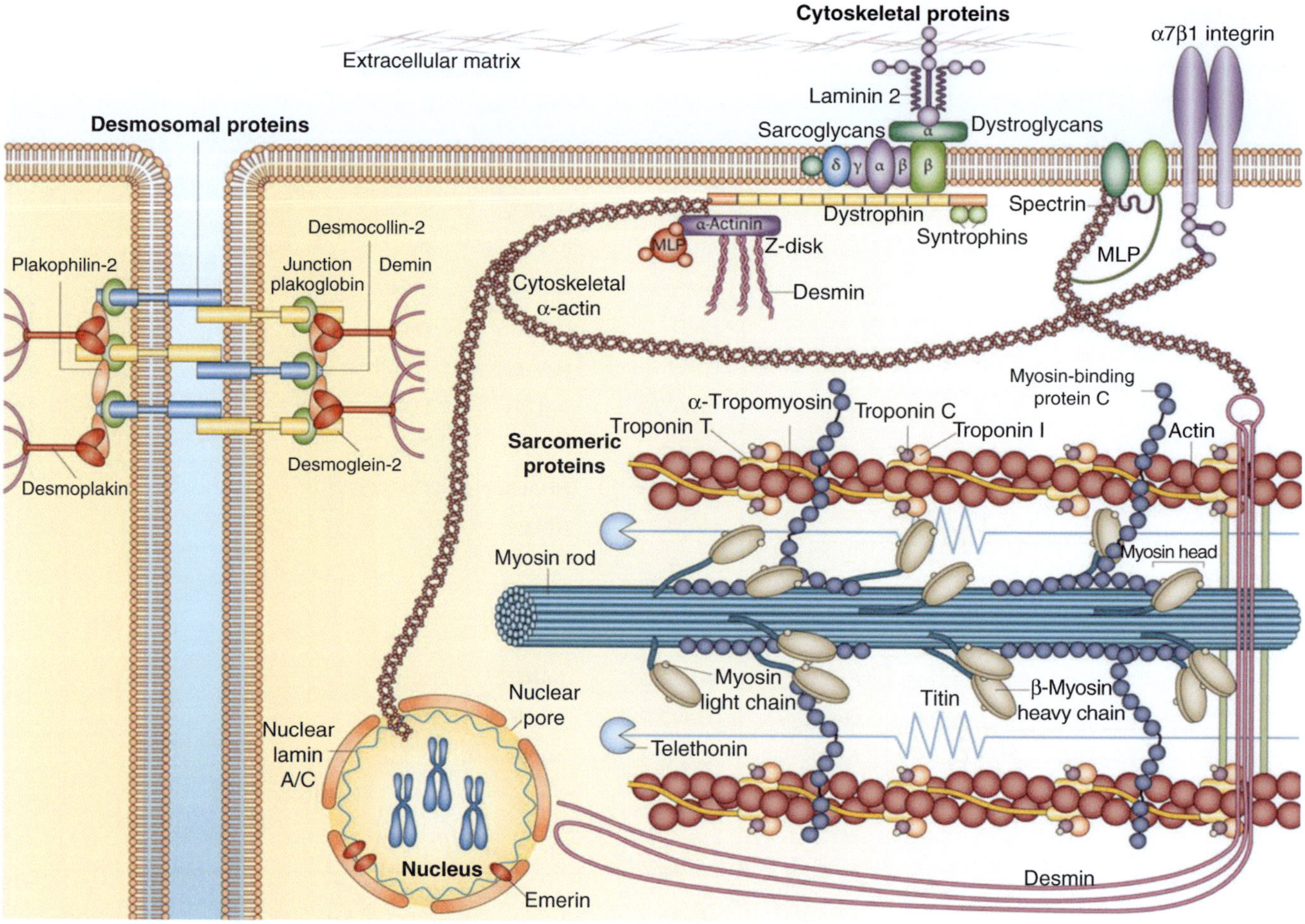

Fig. 3.3 The main proteins involved in cardiomyopathies. Indicated are the sarcomeric proteins, which form the contractile apparatus; the desmosomal proteins, which form the desmosome and connect one cell to another; the cytoskeletal proteins, which connect the extracellular matrix to the cells and connect various transmembrane proteins to the sarcomere and the nucleus; and the nuclear envelope proteins. Mutations in the encoding genes lead to aberrant function of the respective proteins and to one of the cardiomyopathy subtypes. The sarcoplasmic reticulum, where phospholamban controls SERCA2a, a Ca^{2+} pump, is not shown in this figure [8]. [Obtained with permission from SpringerNature]

The ESC HCM guideline provides clear tools for the diagnostic workup, treatment, and risk stratification of patients with HCM. In adults, HCM is defined by a wall thickness ≥15 mm in one or more LV myocardial segments—as measured by any imaging technique (echocardiography, cardiac magnetic resonance imaging (CMR), or computed tomography (CT))—that is not explained solely by loading conditions. Both genetic and nongenetic disorders can present with lesser degrees of wall thickening (13–14 mm), justifying further investigations and in assumed genetic cases also familial screening [11]. In sarcomeric HCM, the LV hypertrophy is usually asymmetric and most prominent at the interventricular septum. Concentric hypertrophy is more frequent in metabolic disorders and also suggestive of hypertension. In its workup, several causes should be excluded before considering HCM to be sarcomeric. Pathology studies show that typical myocardial disarray distinguishes sarcomeric HCM from secondary LV hypertrophy or, e.g., Fabry's disease, where myocardial cells are expanded with vacuolar spaces. The myocardial fibrosis can be appreciated on CMR studies, showing late gadolinium enhancement, and these abnormalities form a substrate for arrhythmias.

Several red flags should raise awareness that the observed ventricular hypertrophy in a patient may not be a sarcomeric disorder and/or limited to the heart [12]. Childhood onset, involvement of other organs, a family history suggestive of an X-linked or autosomal recessive inheritance pattern, and concentric hypertrophy all warrant further investigation into metabolic, syndromic, and systemic diseases. In addition, several electrocardiographic abnormalities may suggest specific diagnoses other than sarcomeric HCM, for instance, a short PR interval, AV block, low voltages or very high voltages, and extreme LVH. Metabolic causes include Pompe's disease, Danon disease, and Fabry's disease [13]. Noonan syndrome and LEOPARD syndrome are both RASopathies

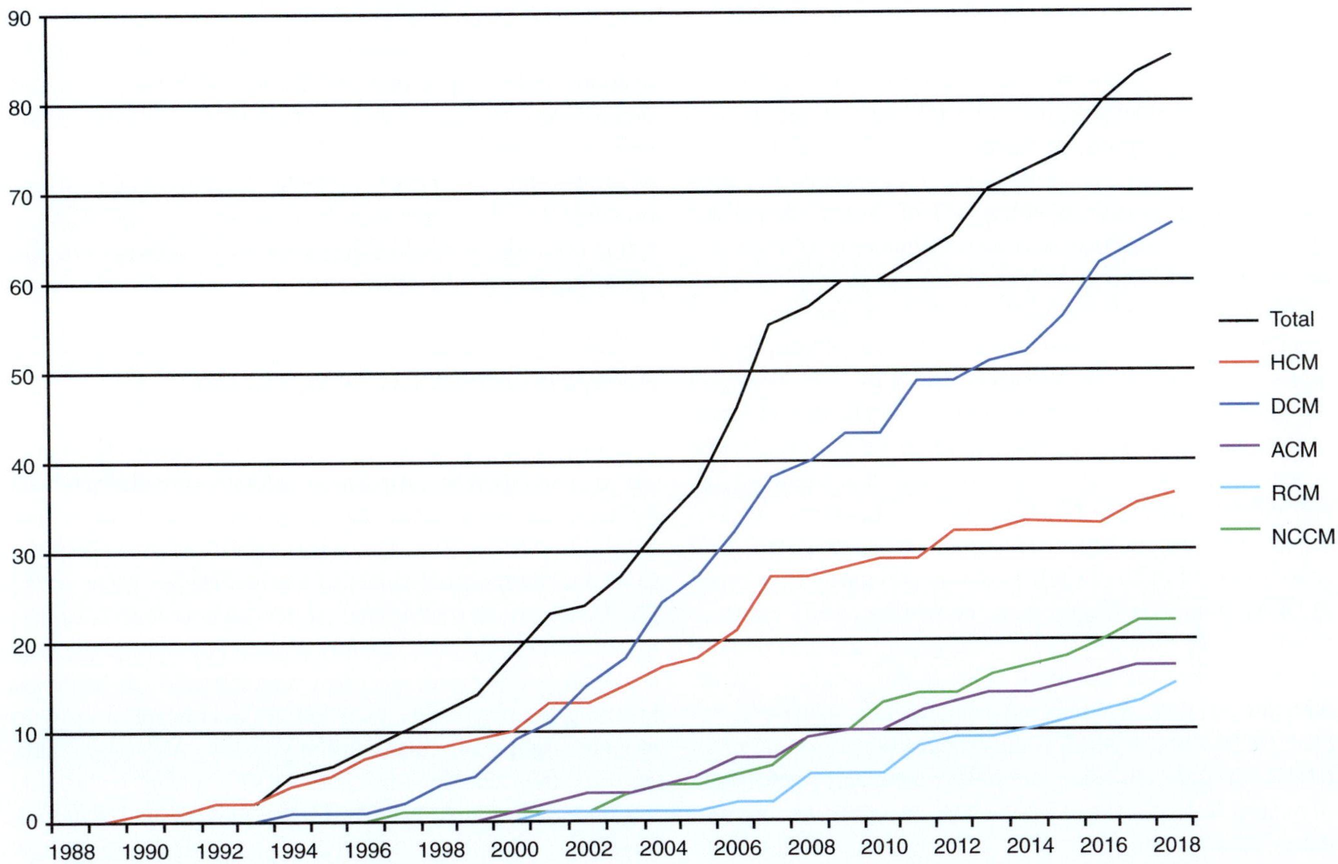

Fig. 3.4 Total number of genes associated with one or more cardiomyopathy subtype reported since 1990. The total number of associated cardiomyopathy genes is shown by the black line. Per cardiomyopathy subtype, the novel associated genes are listed since the first publication in 1990 of a mutation in the *MYH7* gene in HCM by Geisterfer-Lowrance et al. [10]. Since many genes have been associated with multiple cardiomyopathy subtypes, the line of the total number of associated genes is not the sum of all lines of the cardiomyopathy subtypes. Since the previous edition of this book, 2 years ago, nine novel genes have been implicated to cause at least one subtype of inherited cardiomyopathy

that can display HCM. RASopathies are a group of syndromes caused by mutations in genes that encode components or regulators of the Ras/mitogen-activated protein kinase (MAPK) pathway [14]. A systemic condition that can mimic sarcomeric HCM is cardiac amyloidosis, which by itself can be inherited as well due to mutations in the transthyretin (*TTR*) gene [15].

The ESC HCM guidelines recommend that patients undergo a standardized clinical evaluation to estimate the 5-year risk of sudden cardiac death (SCD) using the HCM Risk-SCD model. This model takes into account several variables, such as age, echocardiographic and Holter abnormalities, and family history, to determine risk categories for recommending ICD implantation. This online calculator can be found at http://doc2do.com/hcm/webHCM.html.

Of all cardiomyopathies, the yield of genetic testing is the highest in HCM. In a study by the Mayo Clinic, multivariate analysis identified a number of positive predictors for a positive genetic test in a cohort of >1000 unrelated HCM patients, tested for nine genes. Illustrative of the role of environmental factors is the fact that the presence of hypertension was identified as a negative predictor. A history of hypertension lowered the chance of a positive genetic test from 14% without any positive or negative predictors to 6%. The overall genetic yield in this cohort was 34% [16].

Dilated Cardiomyopathy

The criteria provided by Mestroni et al. are often used for the diagnosis of DCM in cardiogenetics [17]. DCM is thus characterized by systolic LV dysfunction (ejection fraction <45% or fractional shortening <25%) in combination with LV dilatation (LV end-diastolic volume/dimension >117% (2SD + 5%) of the predicted value corrected for age and BSA). In 2016, the ESC Working Group on Myocardial and Pericardial Diseases proposed an updated description of DCM, consisting of a preclinical or early phase and a clinical phase. The latter is further divided into "true" DCM and hypokinetic non-dilated cardiomyopathy, defined as LV or biventricular global systolic dysfunction without dilatation (defined as LVEF <45%), not explained by abnormal loading conditions or coronary artery disease [18]. As alluded to earlier, in case a patient presents with DCM, underlying (nongenetic) diseases should be excluded first. By and large, in about 50% of cases, such underlying disease/etiology can be identified [19]. In the remaining 50% of cases ("idiopathic" DCM), about one-third is likely attributable to a genetic defect, i.e., a mutation in one of the genes implicated in DCM. Dilated cardiomyopathy (DCM) is genetically the most heterogeneous of all cardiomyopathies; at least 50 different genes have been implicated in DCM. The first were the same sarcomeric genes as identified in HCM, and it was shown that DCM-causing mutations had different molecular properties when compared to mutations that cause HCM, e.g., calcium handling. The yield per gene has been low until the identification of titin (*TTN*) mutations as most prevalent cause of DCM in 2012 [20]. Titin was previously implicated in DCM, but as the largest gene, consisting of 363 exons, it was for a long time technically challenging and too costly to screen the gene for mutations. Like in the setting of HCM, there are red flags that may suggest a specific genetic defect [12]. DCM with AV block is thus suggestive of a mutation in *LMNA* (the gene encoding lamin A/C, the major constituents of nuclear lamina) or in *DES* (the gene encoding the intermediate filament desmin) [21, 22], whereas DCM with extremely low voltage is a hallmark of the Dutch *PLN* p.Arg14del founder mutation [23]. In addition, the clinician should be aware of and look for extracardiac features like learning difficulties and deafness which may point to mitochondrial disease or muscle weakness which is among others suggestive of a mutation in *LMNA* or *DES*. Of note, a recent study showed that the yield of pathogenic variants is similarly high in DCM patients and patients with hypokinetic non-dilated cardiomyopathy [24].

As a general rule, therapeutic management of patients with DCM should be performed according to the ESC guidelines for heart failure, including device therapy (CRT, ICD) [25]. However, in selected cases, knowledge of the underlying genetic defect should be taken into consideration in terms of therapeutic choices, in particular timing of ICD implantation. Whereas ICD implantation should generally be considered in cases of left ventricular ejection fraction <35%, patients with DCM due to a *LMNA* mutation have a high risk for malignant arrhythmias even in the setting of relatively preserved left ventricular ejection fraction, and they should receive an ICD when ejection fraction drops below 45% when an additional risk factor is present, i.e., non-missense mutation, male sex, and the presence of non-sustained VTs [26]. The same holds true for patients with arrhythmogenic cardiomyopathy due to the Dutch *PLN* p.Arg14del founder mutation: a left ventricular ejection fraction <45% portends a poor prognosis regarding malignant arrhythmias and cardiac arrest/sudden death, and these patients should also be considered for ICD implantation [27]. On the other hand, the available data suggest that DCM due to *TTN* mutations may behave more benign, in terms of both malignant arrhythmias and progression to advanced heart failure [28, 29]. These examples show that genetics may have a considerable impact on clinical management in individual patients with DCM, in terms not only of establishing a specific diagnosis but also regarding therapeutic choices.

Arrhythmogenic Cardiomyopathy

ACM was first described in 1982 as "right ventricular dysplasia" by Marcus et al. [30]. These patients were characterized by life-threatening ventricular arrhythmias, originating from the right ventricle (RV). The cause of the disease was believed to be a developmental defect of the myocardial tissue of the RV. However, the finding that the RV myocardium is subject to cell death and is subsequently replaced by fibrous and fatty tissue, interfering with electrical conduction of the heart and resulting in arrhythmias, later led to the concept of arrhythmogenic right ventricular cardiomyopathy (ARVC). In addition to this classic form of ARVC, biventricular and left-dominant forms have been recognized, and therefore nowadays, the term "arrhythmogenic cardiomyopathy" (ACM) is increasingly used [31, 32]. The estimated prevalence in the general population ranges from 1 in 1000 to 1 in 5000, and men are more frequently affected than women [33].

The current diagnostic criteria were published in 2010 as the modification of the original task force criteria in 1994, comprising six different categories, including structural and histological findings, depolarization and repolarization abnormalities, arrhythmias, and family history [34, 35]. ACM is considered a disease of the cardiac desmosome (Fig. 3.3) following the identification of mutations in two genes encoding desmosomal proteins, plakoglobin (*JUP*) and desmoplakin (*DSP*), in syndromic forms of ACM called Naxos disease and Carvajal disease, respectively [36, 37]. Plakophilin 2 (PKP2) is the most prevalent mutated gene in ACM. Mutations in several non-desmosomal genes however have also been identified, including PLN, TMEM43, and SCN5A [23, 38, 39]. ACM is a nice example of the added value of genetics in terms of providing insight into the pathophysiology.

In 2015, an international task force published a consensus statement on the treatment and management of ACM. These recommendations deal with electrophysiological studies, lifestyle changes such as restriction from competitive sports, pharmacotherapy, catheter ablation, and ICD implantation. These recommendations are useful for all healthcare professionals dealing with ACM, especially those who are not very familiar with this rare disease [40].

Restrictive Cardiomyopathy

RCM is characterized by impaired filling of the ventricles in the presence of normal wall thickness and normal systolic function. RCM can be part of systemic, inflammatory, or storage diseases, but it also occurs in isolated form and is often associated with sarcomeric mutations (Fig. 3.2) [41]. RCM is the least common cardiomyopathy subtype and can be observed in a variety of cardiac or multi-organ diseases such as Löffler's endocarditis, amyloidosis, sarcoidosis, hemochromatosis, and Fabry's disease [42]. Furthermore, RCM is found in patients who have undergone radiotherapy, for instance, for Hodgkin's disease [43].

As for other sarcomeric cardiomyopathies, different cardiomyopathy subtypes have been observed within families and for RCM mostly in combination with HCM [44]. There is no consensus regarding diagnostic criteria for RCM, but in a case of heart failure with abnormal diastolic function but preserved contractility, and no signs of other cardiomyopathy subtypes such as dilatation or hypertrophy, the diagnosis should be considered. Of the cardiomyopathies, RCM has the worst prognosis, especially in children, as a cardiac transplant is often necessitated within only a few years after diagnosis.

The relatively common scenario of a severely affected child with RCM of apparent healthy parents is usually attributable to the fact that the sarcomeric mutation occurred de novo. Mutations in the gene encoding the sarcomeric contractile protein troponin I (*TNNI3*) appear to be the most frequent [45, 46]. As in DCM, the presence of a conduction defect, especially AV block, in patients with RCM could unmask a *DES* mutation [47].

Non-compaction Cardiomyopathy

NCCM, also referred to as left ventricular non-compaction (LVNC), is an enigmatic disorder. Although it is a rare form of cardiomyopathy, it is relatively often diagnosed as a chance finding, in particular during echocardiography, performed for another reason. The wall of the left ventricle is thus found to be "non-compacted," i.e., in addition to the normal compacted wall (outer layer), there is an inner layer of meshy myocardium with trabeculations and recesses. According to the Jenni criteria, the ratio of the thickness of the non-compacted layer and the compacted layer should exceed 2 (end-systolic) at parasternal short-axis view on echocardiography for NCCM to be diagnosed [48]. However, this echocardiographic definition is highly arbitrary since there is no gold standard for NCCM, which is also exemplified by the fact that other criteria are used when CMR is performed. In terms of the etiology, there also is much controversy. NCCM can be part of a syndrome (e.g., Barth syndrome) or a congenital heart defect (e.g., Ebstein's anomaly), or it can present as an isolated hereditary cardiomyopathy. But even in the latter case, the picture is not always clear and there is often overlap with DCM and HCM. Moreover, in families with, for instance, HCM, some individuals may present with NCCM. This close association is supported by the fact that the most commonly implicated genes in HCM and NCCM are the same, i.e., *MYH7* and *MYBPC3* [49]. Another important observation is that individual patients may progress from one form of cardiomyopathy to another, in particular from NCCM to DCM. NCCM is thus a striking example of the clinical and genetic heterogeneity of cardiomyopathies, and taking all this into consideration, some investigators even question whether NCCM should be considered a separate entity. However, for the clinician taking care of patients with alleged NCCM, some points should be kept in mind. Due to the recesses, there is chance for thrombus formation and embolic events, and anticoagulation therapy should be considered, in particular in case of concomitant left ventricular dysfunction. In addition, some patients with NCCM may develop heart failure, and there is also a propensity for malignant arrhythmias, and as a general rule, the guidelines for heart failure (including device therapy) should be applied. As such, NCCM is not always a benign chance finding, and it may have serious consequences for the patient, and it gives reason for family screening.

Given the complexity of cardiomyopathies in terms of the phenotype, extracardiac (organ) involvement, genetics, and etiology, a group of experts have proposed a new classification, the MOGE(S) classification [50]. They identified five attributes:

- (M) The "morphofunctional" notation provides a descriptive diagnosis of the phenotype, for instance, DCM (M_D), HCM (M_H), etc.
- (O) "Organ involvement" is notated as heart only (O_H) or involvement of other organs, for instance, kidney (O_K), skeletal muscle (O_M), etc.
- (G) "Genetics" provides information on the mode of inheritance, for instance, autosomal dominant (G_{AD}), X-linked (G_{XL}), etc.
- (E) "Etiology" adds to the description of the underlying cause, including the gene/mutation, for instance, in case of HCM ($E_{G,\ MYH7}$) or DCM due to myocarditis secondary to Ebstein-Barr virus infection ($E_{V,EBV}$)
- (S) "Heart failure stage" pertains to AHA/ACC stage of heart failure (A–D) and the NHYA functional class (I–IV), for instance, S_{A-I}.

In the article, the authors provide numerous examples of how this classification works. Just to name one: in a male with Fabry's disease with a phenotype of "HCM," with involvement of the kidney, due to a mutation in GLA, the gene encoding galactosidase-α, the MOGE(S) annotation would be M_H O_k G_{X-L} $E_{G\text{-}GLA+}$. For further details, the reader is referred to this very interesting paper. The practical implications of the MOGES classification have already been shown in several subsequent papers, including a study by Hazebroek et al. [51]. These authors have applied the MOGE(S) classification in a group of patients with DCM, and using the classification, they convincingly showed the importance of gene-environment interaction in terms of clinical outcome.

Studies on induced pluripotent stem cells (iPSCs) from cardiomyopathy patients have given great insights to further elucidate the pathophysiology of cardiomyopathies. Such approaches also enable large-scale studies on possible pharmacological interventions, including precision medicine initiatives. These and other revolutionizing approaches are outlined in Chap. 26 on gene therapy and induced pluripotent stem cells. These are big steps forward in unraveling the many intricacies of cardiomyopathies, but much work is still to be done.

Take-Home Message

The five main cardiomyopathy subtypes, hypertrophic cardiomyopathy, dilated cardiomyopathy, arrhythmogenic cardiomyopathy, restrictive cardiomyopathy, and non-compaction cardiomyopathy, show substantial overlap, both clinically and genetically. For each cardiomyopathy subtype, multiple disease genes have been identified, and mutations in several genes can cause different subtypes.

All hereditary cardiomyopathies are characterized by incomplete penetrance, meaning that some mutation carriers will remain unaffected during their entire life, and variable expression, i.e., the type and severity of the disease can vary widely, even within families. The availability of diagnostic and management guidelines for different cardiomyopathies should improve the outcome of these patients and aid the clinician to identify the many rare presentations of cardiomyopathies that all can be part of a wider spectrum of multiorgan, systemic, or syndromic diseases.

References

1. Elliott P, Andersson B, Arbustini E, Bilinska Z, Cecchi F, Charron P, et al. Classification of the cardiomyopathies: a position statement from the European society of cardiology working group on myocardial and pericardial diseases. Eur Heart J. 2008;29:270–6.
2. Maron BJ, Towbin JA, Thiene G, Antzelevitch C, Corrado D, Arnett D, et al. Contemporary definitions and classification of the cardiomyopathies: an American heart association scientific statement from the council on clinical cardiology, heart failure and transplantation committee; quality of care and outcomes research and functional genomics and translational biology interdisciplinary working groups; and council on epidemiology and prevention. Circulation. 2006;113:1807–16.
3. ten Cate FJ, Roelandt J. Progression to left ventricular dilatation in patients with hypertrophic obstructive cardiomyopathy. Am Heart J. 1979;97:762–5.
4. Sen-Chowdhry S, Morgan RD, Chambers JC, McKenna WJ. Arrhythmogenic cardiomyopathy: etiology, diagnosis, and treatment. Annu Rev Med. 2010;61:233–53.
5. Sen-Chowdhry S, Syrris P, Prasad SK, Hughes SE, Merrifield R, Ward D, et al. Left-dominant arrhythmogenic cardiomyopathy an under-recognized clinical entity. J Am Coll Cardiol. 2008;52:2175–87.
6. Jeschke B, Uhl K, Weist B, Schroder D, Meitinger T, Dohlemann C, et al. A high risk phenotype of hypertrophic cardiomyopathy associated with a compound genotype of two mutated beta-myosin heavy chain genes. Hum Genet. 1998;102:299–304.
7. Lekanne Deprez RH, Muurling-Vlietman JJ, Hruda J, Baars MJ, Wijnaendts LC, Stolte-Dijkstra I, et al. Two cases of severe neonatal hypertrophic cardiomyopathy caused by compound heterozygous mutations in the MYBPC3 gene. J Med Genet. 2006;43:829–32.
8. Wilde AA, Behr ER. Genetic testing for inherited cardiac disease. Nat Rev Cardiol. 2013;10:571–83.
9. Jarcho JA, McKenna W, Pare JA, Solomon SD, Holcombe RF, Dickie S, et al. Mapping a gene for familial hypertrophic cardiomyopathy to chromosome 14q1. N Engl J Med. 1989;321:1372–8.
10. Geisterfer-Lowrance AA, Kass S, Tanigawa G, Vosberg HP, McKenna W, Seidman CE, et al. A molecular basis for familial hypertrophic cardiomyopathy: a beta cardiac myosin heavy chain gene missense mutation. Cell. 1990;62:999–1006.
11. Elliott PM, Anastasakis A, Borger MA, Borggrefe M, Cecchi F, et al. ESC guidelines on diagnosis and management of hypertrophic cardiomyopathy: the task force for the diagnosis and management of hypertrophic cardiomyopathy of the European Society of Cardiology (ESC). Eur Heart J. 2014;35:2733–79.
12. Rapezzi C, Arbustini E, Caforio AL, Charron P, Gimeno-Blanes J, Helio T, et al. Diagnostic work-up in cardiomyopathies: bridging the gap between clinical phenotypes and final diagnosis. A position statement from the ESC working group on myocardial and pericardial diseases. Eur Heart J. 2013;34:1448–58.
13. Wicks EC, Elliott PM. Genetics and metabolic cardiomyopathies. Herz. 2012;37:598–610.
14. Gelb BD, Roberts AE, Tartaglia M. Cardiomyopathies in Noonan syndrome and the other RASopathies. Prog Pediatr Cardiol. 2015;39:13–9.
15. Ruberg FL, Berk JL. Transthyretin (TTR) cardiac amyloidosis. Circulation. 2012;126:1286–300.
16. Bos JM, Will ML, Gersh BJ, Kruisselbrink TM, Ommen SR, Ackerman MJ. Characterization of a phenotype-based genetic test prediction score for unrelated patients with hypertrophic cardiomyopathy. Mayo Clin Proc. 2014;89:727–37.
17. Mestroni L, Rocco C, Gregori D, Sinagra G, Di Lenarda A, Miocic S, et al. Familial dilated cardiomyopathy: evidence for genetic and phenotypic heterogeneity. Heart muscle disease study group. J Am Coll Cardiol. 1999;34:181–90.
18. Pinto YM, Elliott PM, Arbustini E, Adler Y, Anastasakis A, Bohm M, et al. Proposal for a revised definition of dilated cardiomyopathy, hypokinetic non-dilated cardiomyopathy, and its implications for clinical practice: a position statement of the ESC working group on myocardial and pericardial diseases. Eur Heart J. 2016;37:1850–8.
19. Felker GM, Thompson RE, Hare JM, Hruban RH, Clemetson DE, Howard DL, et al. Underlying causes and long-term survival in patients with initially unexplained cardiomyopathy. N Engl J Med. 2000;342:1077–84.
20. Herman DS, Lam L, Taylor MR, Wang L, Teekakirikul P, Christodoulou D, et al. Truncations of titin causing dilated cardiomyopathy. N Engl J Med. 2012;366:619–28.

21. Arbustini E, Pilotto A, Repetto A, Grasso M, Negri A, Diegoli M, et al. Autosomal dominant dilated cardiomyopathy with atrioventricular block: a Lamin A/C defect-related disease. J Am Coll Cardiol. 2002;39:981–90.
22. Taylor MR, Slavov D, Ku L, Di Lenarda A, Sinagra G, Carniel E, et al. Prevalence of desmin mutations in dilated cardiomyopathy. Circulation. 2007;115:1244–51.
23. van der Zwaag PA, van Rijsingen IA, Asimaki A, Jongbloed JD, van Veldhuisen DJ, Wiesfeld AC, et al. Phospholamban R14del mutation in patients diagnosed with dilated cardiomyopathy or arrhythmogenic right ventricular cardiomyopathy: evidence supporting the concept of arrhythmogenic cardiomyopathy. Eur J Heart Fail. 2012;14:1199–207.
24. Hazebroek MR, Krapels I, Verdonschot J, van den Wijngaard A, Vanhoutte E, Hoos M, et al. Prevalence of pathogenic gene mutations and prognosis do not differ in isolated left ventricular dysfunction compared with dilated cardiomyopathy. Circ Heart Fail. 2018;11:e004682.
25. McMurray JJ, Adamopoulos S, Anker SD, Auricchio A, Bohm M, Dickstein K, et al. ESC guidelines for the diagnosis and treatment of acute and chronic heart failure 2012: the task force for the diagnosis and treatment of acute and chronic heart failure 2012 of the European Society of Cardiology. Developed in collaboration with the heart failure association (HFA) of the ESC. Eur Heart J. 2012;33:1787–847.
26. Van Rijsingen IA, Arbustini E, Elliott PM, Mogensen J, Hermans-van Ast JF, van der Kooi AJ, et al. Risk factors for malignant ventricular arrhythmias in Lamin a/c mutation carriers a European cohort study. J Am Coll Cardiol. 2012;59:493–500.
27. van Rijsingen IA, van der Zwaag PA, Groeneweg JA, Nannenberg EA, Jongbloed JD, Zwinderman AH, et al. Outcome in phospholamban R14del carriers: results of a large multicentre cohort study. Circ Cardiovasc Genet. 2014;7:455–65.
28. Jansweijer JA, Nieuwhof K, Russo F, Hoorntje ET, Jongbloed JD, Lekanne Deprez RH, et al. Truncating titin mutations are associated with a mild and treatable form of dilated cardiomyopathy. Eur J Heart Fail. 2017;19:512–21.
29. Tayal U, Newsome S, Buchan R, Whiffin N, Halliday B, Lota A, et al. Phenotype and clinical outcomes of titin cardiomyopathy. J Am Coll Cardiol. 2017;70:2264–74.
30. Marcus FI, Fontaine GH, Guiraudon G, Frank R, Laurenceau JL, Malergue C, et al. Right ventricular dysplasia: a report of 24 adult cases. Circulation. 1982;65:384–98.
31. Corrado D, Basso C, Thiene G, McKenna WJ, Davies MJ, Fontaliran F, et al. Spectrum of clinicopathologic manifestations of arrhythmogenic right ventricular cardiomyopathy/dysplasia: a multicenter study. J Am Coll Cardiol. 1997;30:1512–20.
32. Sen-Chowdhry S, Syrris P, Ward D, Asimaki A, Sevdalis E, McKenna WJ. Clinical and genetic characterization of families with arrhythmogenic right ventricular dysplasia/cardiomyopathy provides novel insights into patterns of disease expression. Circulation. 2007;115:1710–20.
33. Basso C, Corrado D, Marcus FI, Nava A, Thiene G. Arrhythmogenic right ventricular cardiomyopathy. Lancet. 2009;373:1289–300.
34. McKenna WJ, Thiene G, Nava A, Fontaliran F, Blomstrom-Lundqvist C, Fontaine G, et al. Diagnosis of arrhythmogenic right ventricular dysplasia/cardiomyopathy. Task Force of the working group myocardial and pericardial disease of the European Society of Cardiology and of the scientific council on cardiomyopathies of the international society and federation of cardiology. Br Heart J. 1994;71:215–8.
35. Marcus FI, McKenna WJ, Sherrill D, Basso C, Bauce B, Bluemke DA, et al. Diagnosis of arrhythmogenic right ventricular cardiomyopathy/dysplasia: proposed modification of the task force criteria. Eur Heart J. 2010;31:806–14.
36. McKoy G, Protonotarios N, Crosby A, Tsatsopoulou A, Anastasakis A, Coonar A, et al. Identification of a deletion in plakoglobin in arrhythmogenic right ventricular cardiomyopathy with palmoplantar keratoderma and woolly hair (Naxos disease). Lancet. 2000;355:2119–24.
37. Norgett EE, Hatsell SJ, Carvajal-Huerta L, Cabezas JC, Common J, Purkis PE, et al. Recessive mutation in desmoplakin disrupts desmoplakin-intermediate filament interactions and causes dilated cardiomyopathy, woolly hair and keratoderma. Hum Mol Genet. 2000;9:2761–6.
38. Merner ND, Hodgkinson KA, Haywood AF, Connors S, French VM, Drenckhahn JD, et al. Arrhythmogenic right ventricular cardiomyopathy type 5 is a fully penetrant, lethal arrhythmic disorder caused by a missense mutation in the TMEM43 gene. Am J Hum Genet. 2008;82:809–21.
39. Te Riele AS, Agullo-Pascual E, James CA, Leo-Macias A, Cerrone M, Zhang M, et al. Multilevel analyses of SCN5A mutations in arrhythmogenic right ventricular dysplasia/cardiomyopathy suggest non-canonical mechanisms for disease pathogenesis. Cardiovasc Res. 2017;113:102–11.
40. Corrado D, Wichter T, Link MS, Hauer R, Marchlinski F, Anastasakis A, et al. Treatment of arrhythmogenic right ventricular cardiomyopathy/dysplasia: an international task force consensus statement. Eur Heart J. 2015;36:3227–37.
41. Mogensen J, Arbustini E. Restrictive cardiomyopathy. Curr Opin Cardiol. 2009;24:214–20.
42. Kushwaha SS, Fallon JT, Fuster V. Restrictive cardiomyopathy. N Engl J Med. 1997;336:267–76.
43. Adams MJ, Lipsitz SR, Colan SD, Tarbell NJ, Treves ST, Diller L, et al. Cardiovascular status in long-term survivors of Hodgkin's disease treated with chest radiotherapy. J Clin Oncol. 2004;22:3139–48.
44. Mogensen J, Kubo T, Duque M, Uribe W, Shaw A, Murphy R, et al. Idiopathic restrictive cardiomyopathy is part of the clinical expression of cardiac troponin I mutations. J Clin Invest. 2003;111:209–16.
45. Kaski JP, Syrris P, Burch M, Tome-Esteban MT, Fenton M, Christiansen M, et al. Idiopathic restrictive cardiomyopathy in children is caused by mutations in cardiac sarcomere protein genes. Heart. 2008;94:1478–84.
46. Mogensen J, Hey T, Lambrecht S. A systematic review of phenotypic features associated with cardiac troponin I mutations in hereditary cardiomyopathies. Can J Cardiol. 2015;31:1377–85.
47. Arbustini E, Pasotti M, Pilotto A, Pellegrini C, Grasso M, Previtali S, et al. Desmin accumulation restrictive cardiomyopathy and atrioventricular block associated with desmin gene defects. Eur J Heart Fail. 2006;8:477–83.
48. Jenni R, Oechslin E, Schneider J, Attenhofer Jost C, Kaufmann PA. Echocardiographic and pathoanatomical characteristics of isolated left ventricular non-compaction: a step towards classification as a distinct cardiomyopathy. Heart. 2001;86:666–71.
49. Hoedemaekers YM, Caliskan K, Michels M, Frohn-Mulder I, van der Smagt JJ, Phefferkorn JE, et al. The importance of genetic counseling, DNA diagnostics, and cardiologic family screening in left ventricular noncompaction cardiomyopathy. Circ Cardiovasc Genet. 2010;3:232–9.
50. Arbustini E, Narula N, Dec GW, Reddy KS, Greenberg B, Kushwaha S, et al. The MOGE(S) classification for a phenotype-genotype nomenclature of cardiomyopathy: endorsed by the world heart federation. J Am Coll Cardiol. 2013;62:2046–72.
51. Hazebroek MR, Moors S, Dennert R, van den Wijngaard A, Krapels I, Hoos M, et al. Prognostic relevance of gene-environment interactions in patients with dilated cardiomyopathy: applying the MOGE(S) classification. J Am Coll Cardiol. 2015;66:1313–23.

Hypertrophic Cardiomyopathy

4

Imke Christiaans, Perry M. Elliott, and Michelle Michels

Introduction

The British pathologist Robert Donald Teare is assumed to be the first to describe hypertrophic cardiomyopathy (HCM) in 1958 [1], although bulky hearts and hypertrophy in sudden cardiac death (SCD) victims have been described centuries earlier [2]. Nowadays, HCM is the most common monogenic heart disease affecting at least 1 in 500 persons worldwide and a known cause of SCD in the young [3–5].

This chapter discusses not only the epidemiology, diagnosis, pathophysiology, and therapy of HCM but also deals with topics specific for cardiogenetic diseases like the genetic background, risk stratification for SCD, and the screening strategies in HCM families. It is intended to be of help for all involved in the care for HCM patients and their families.

Etiology/Pathophysiology

Teare was the first to describe left ventricular hypertrophy (LVH), the hallmark of HCM and its familial nature [1]. The most common location for LVH in HCM is the anterior part of the interventricular septum, giving rise to asymmetrical LVH. Other forms of LVH, for example, concentric and apical LVH, can also be found in HCM (Fig. 4.1). The apical form seems to occur more frequently in East Asian patients [6]. Teare also described a disordered arrangement of muscle fibers at microscopic examination, now known as myocyte disarray (Fig. 4.2) [1]. With electron microscopy, one can also notice a disordered arrangement of the myofilaments. Myocardial disarray is not confined to the thickened parts of the left ventricle (LV); LV regions with normal thickness can also be disorganized [7]. Fibrosis is another feature of HCM visualized by microscopy. Both fibrosis and myocyte disarray are thought to be related to ventricular arrhythmias [8]. Besides hypertrophy, fibrosis, and disarray, abnormalities in the intramyocardial small vessels are another pathological finding in HCM. Vessels may show a thickening of the vessel wall and a decrease in luminal size [9]. The anatomic changes in HCM can be a substrate for arrhythmias, which may lead to palpitations, syncope, and SCD.

In up to 60% of HCM patients, the disease is an autosomal dominant trait caused by pathogenic variants in sarcomere protein genes. In these patients, the early pathogenesis in HCM starts in this functional unit of contraction within the cardiomyocytes. The sarcomere is a protein complex divided into thick and thin myofilaments and proteins involved in the cytoarchitecture of the sarcomeres, like proteins in the Z-disc connecting the thin myofilaments of the sarcomere (Fig. 4.3). It is hypothesized that the genetic defect in a gene encoding a sarcomeric protein disrupts normal contraction and relaxation of the sarcomere and calcium accumulates within the sarcomere. Myocytes in mice with HCM display an inefficient use of ATP. This in combination with the increased calcium sensitivity triggers a remodeling process moderated by several transcription factors resulting in hypertrophy of cardiomyocytes. The increased mass of cardiomyocytes and inefficient use of ATP lead to an increased energy demand. When this energy demand cannot be met, ischemia can result in premature myocyte death and replacement fibrosis [10].

In 5–10% of adult cases, other genetic disorders, including inherited metabolic and neuromuscular diseases, chromosome abnormalities, and genetic syndromes, cause HCM [4]. Metabolic disorders can cause hypertrophy by accumulation of metabolites in the heart. A relatively common metabolic disease is Anderson-Fabry disease, which is X-linked, and cardiac hypertrophy can be its sole disease symptom,

I. Christiaans
Department of Clinical Genetics, University Medical Centre Groningen, Groningen, The Netherlands

P. M. Elliott
Institute for Cardiovascular Science, University College London, London, UK

M. Michels (✉)
Department of Cardiology, Erasmus Medical Centre, Rotterdam, The Netherlands
e-mail: m.michels@erasmusmc.nl

H. F. Baars et al. (eds.), *Clinical Cardiogenetics*, https://doi.org/10.1007/978-3-030-45457-9_4

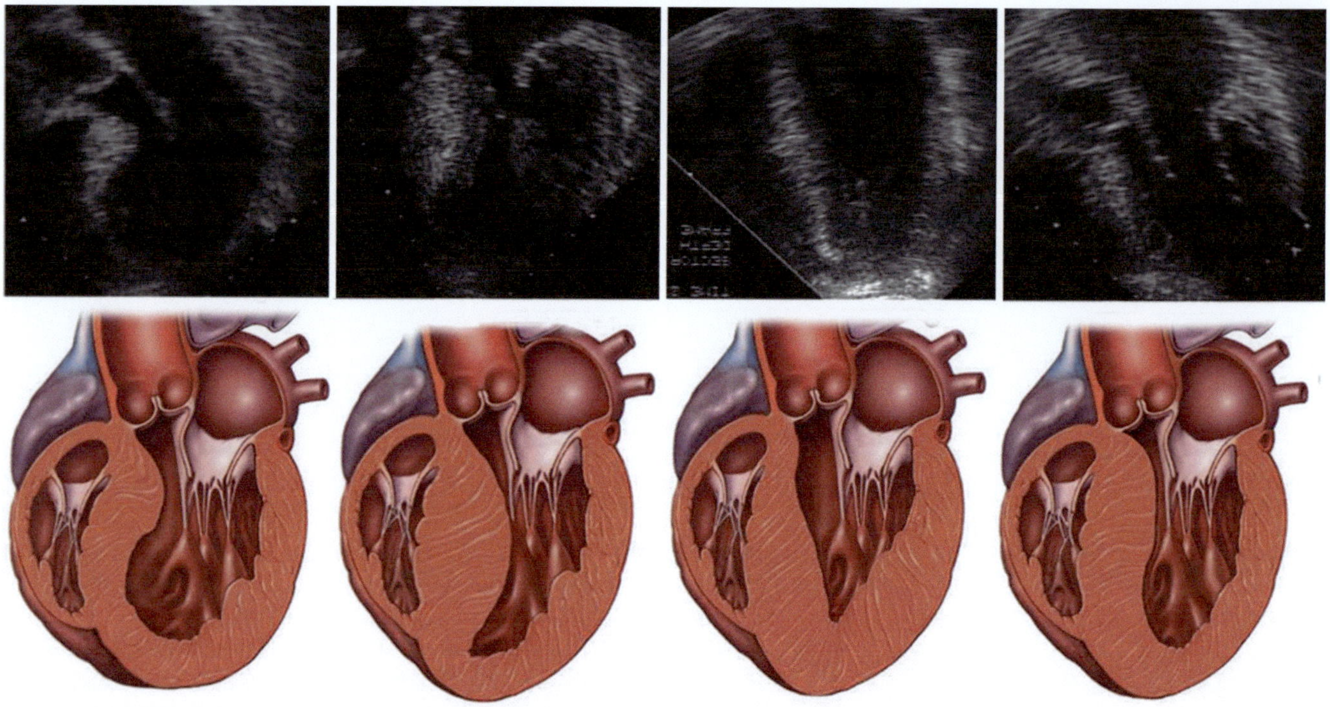

Fig. 4.1 Hypertrophic cardiomyopathy septal morphological subtypes based on standard echocardiography long-axis views taken at end diastole (top). From left to right, sigmoid, reverse curve, apical, and neutral subtypes. Figure adapted from: Echocardiography-guided genetic testing in hypertrophic cardiomyopathy: septal morphological features predict the presence of myofilament mutations. J. Binder, S.R. Ommen, B.J. Gersh, S.L. Van Driest, A.J. Tajik, R.A. Nishimura and M.J. Ackerman, *Mayo Clin. Proc.* **81** (2006), 459–467

especially in women [11]. Mitochondrial disorders can also give rise to cardiac hypertrophy among other symptoms. Disease severity, affected organs, and age of onset can vary considerably in mitochondrial disorders [12]. Cardiac hypertrophy can also be part of a genetic syndrome with multiple congenital abnormalities. The most frequent one is Noonan syndrome, which can also be very mild and may present in adulthood [13]. Infiltrative diseases like amyloidosis—both genetic and nongenetic forms—can cause cardiac hypertrophy. In some populations, founder variants in the TTR gene are present giving rise to a late-onset cardiac hypertrophy without neurological symptoms [14].

Clinical Presentation

Not only can HCM present at any age, but the clinical course is also variable, ranging from asymptomatic with a normal lifespan to premature SCD or development of end-stage heart failure. HCM in asymptomatic patients is detected by coincidence because of a heart murmur or an abnormal ECG made for screening purposes or during family screening in family members from HCM families.

Symptomatic HCM patients often complain of exertional dyspnea, chest pain, palpitations, or syncope. Embolic stroke can be the first presentation. In small infants, tachypnea, poor feeding, sweeting, and failure to thrive can be presenting symptoms.

Symptoms in HCM are caused by the typical morphological changes in HCM. The thickening of the basal septum and the systolic anterior motion (SAM) of the mitral valve cause a dynamic LV outflow tract (LVOT) obstruction in 20–30% of patients at rest, increasing with provocation measures like Valsalva and exercise ([15], Fig. 4.4). LVOT obstruction can cause exertional dyspnea and (pre) syncope at exercise. Besides LVOT obstruction, symptoms are often related to diastolic dysfunction with impaired filling of the LV due to abnormal relaxation and increased stiffness of the thickened myocardial wall, leading in turn to elevated left atrial and LV end-diastolic pressures and pulmonary congestion [16]. Systolic function is often spared but can decline in patients with the so-called "end-stage" form of HCM.

Palpitations caused by atrial fibrillation or ventricular tachycardia are frequent symptoms in HCM. About 20% of HCM patients will experience atrial fibrillation; it is associated with advanced age, congestive symptoms, and an increased left atrial size. HCM patients with atrial fibrillation have an increased risk of heart failure-related death, besides the risk of cerebrovascular accidents [17].

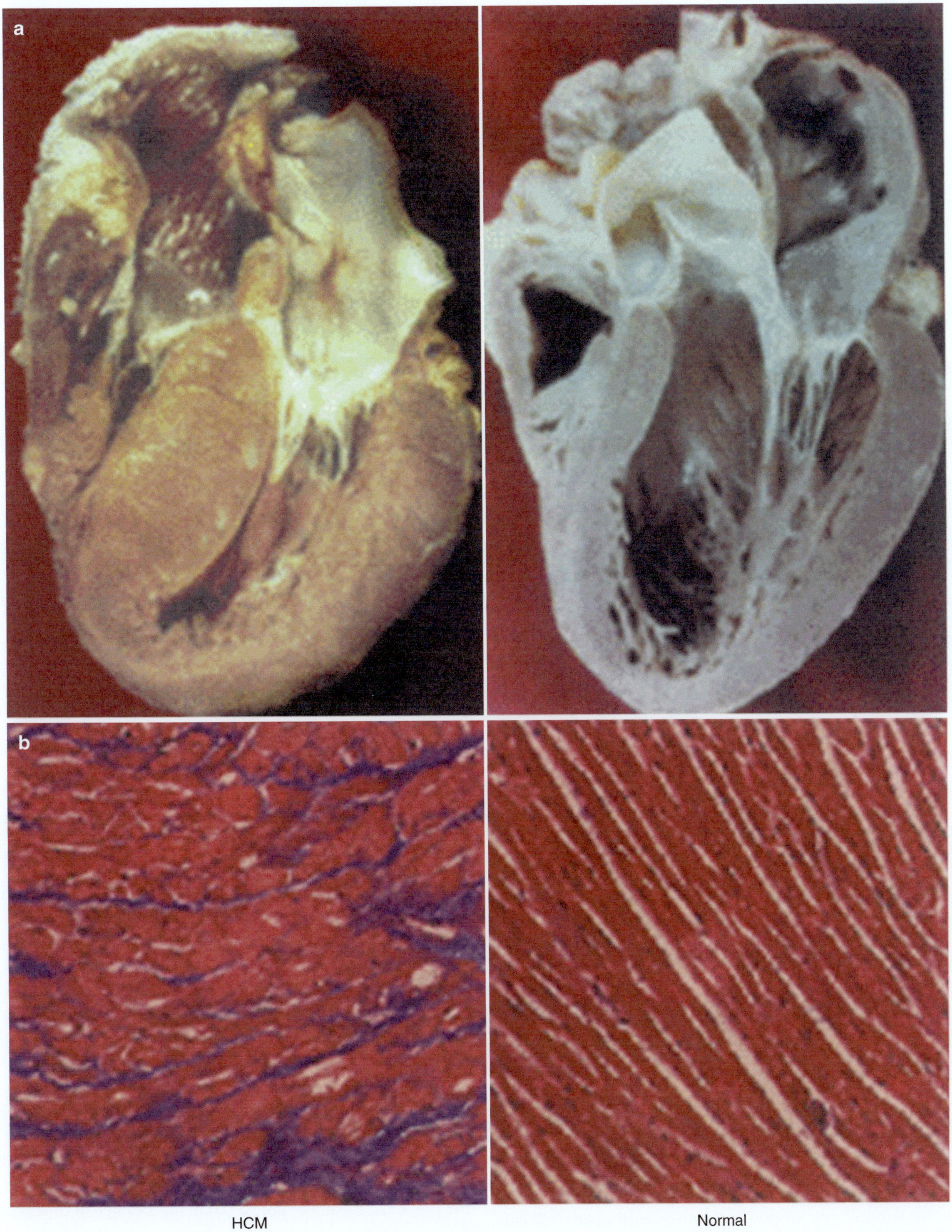

Fig. 4.2 (**a**) Normal heart and heart with hypertrophic cardiomyopathy. (**b**) Heart muscle on microscopy with structured fiber pattern in the normal heart and myocardial disarray in the heart with hypertrophic cardiomyopathy. Figure derived from: Hypertrophic cardiomyopathy: from gene defect to clinical disease. Chung, MW, Tsoutsman, T, Semsarian, C. Cell Research (2003) 13, 9–20

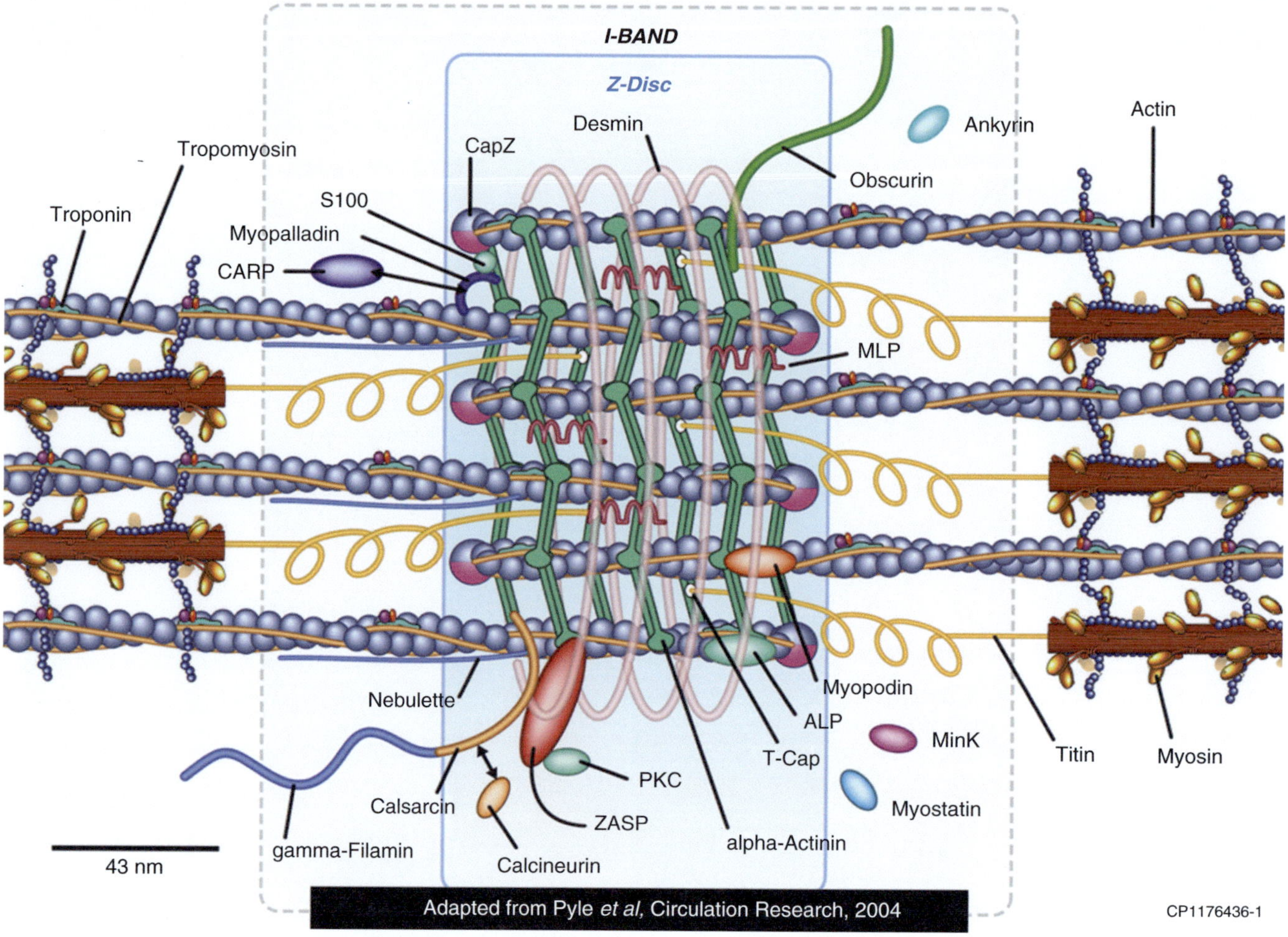

Fig. 4.3 Main sarcomeric proteins. Figure derived from: Familial hypertrophic cardiomyopathy:basic concepts and future molecular diagnostics. Rodrigues JE, McCudden CR, Willis MS. Clin Biochem 2009;42:755–765

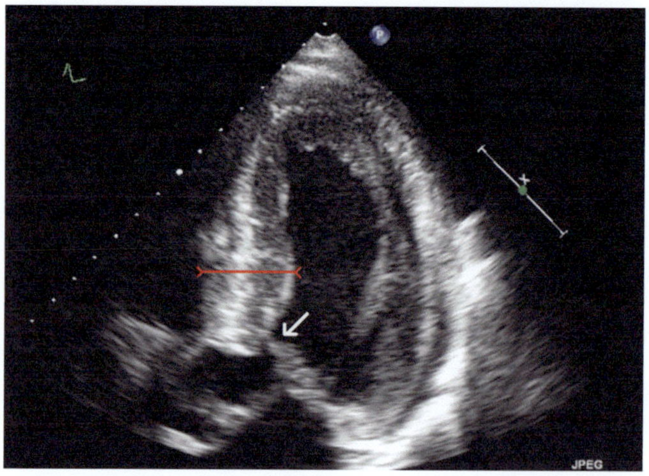

Fig. 4.4 Apical four chamber echocardiography in a HCM patient. Red arrow indicates the hypertrophic interventricular septum (>25 mm), and the white arrow indicates systolic anterior motion of a mitral valve leaflet in the left ventricular outflow tract

Genotype Specific

Cardiac hypertrophy can also be caused by non-sarcomeric genetic and nongenetic disorders (Table 4.1). In most of these disorders, the heart is not the only affected organ, and patients complain of other symptoms or have other signs of organ involvement. It is important to be aware of any so-called red flags during evaluation of a HCM patient (Table 4.2).

Clinical Diagnosis

The clinical diagnosis of HCM is made when the maximal wall thickness of the LV is ≥ 15 mm (in children >2 SD than the predicted mean (z-score > 2)) in the absence of other cardiac or systemic diseases that may cause cardiac hypertrophy, such as aortic valve stenosis and arterial hypertension

[4]. In first-degree relatives of HCM patients, the diagnosis can be made if LV wall thickness ≥13 mm is present [4]. Many other abnormalities in a relative of a HCM patient like diastolic dysfunction and incomplete SAM of the mitral valve can be interpreted as pre-phenotypic expression of the disease. Especially, patients with mild hypertrophy and the presence of possible other factors that can cause hypertrophy diagnosis can be challenging. Common diagnostic dilemmas are hypertrophy in a patient with hypertension, hypertrophy in an athlete, and isolated basal septal hypertrophy in an elderly person. Isolated basal hypertrophy is more common in elderly persons, especially females, and can be differentiated from HCM by the absence of familial disease and the sigmoid form of the septum.

Table 4.1 Non-sarcomeric causes of HCM

Categories	Examples
Metabolic disorders	Anderson-Fabry disease, Danon disease, PRKAG2 gene mutation-related HCM, Pompe disease, carnitine disorders
Mitochondrial disorders	MELAS, MERFF
Neuromuscular diseases	Friedreich's ataxia, FHL1 gene mutation-related HCM, DES gene mutation-related HCM
Malformation syndromes	Noonan syndrome, LEOPARD syndrome, Costello syndrome, CFC syndrome
Infiltrative/inflammatory diseases	Amyloidosis
Endocrine diseases	Pheochromocytoma, acromegaly, maternal diabetes
Other	Chronic use of certain drugs (anabolic steroids, tacrolimus, hydroxychloroquine)

Differential Diagnosis

The etiology of HCM is diverse and the underlying cause should be systematically searched [4].

Age is an important factor to take into account, for example, TTR-related amyloidosis is a disease of mostly men over the age of 65 years, and inherited metabolic disorders as a cause of hypertrophy are much more common in neonates and infants. A family pedigree can give insights in the mode of inheritance, which is autosomal dominant in sarcomeric HCM but X-linked in, for example, Anderson-Fabry disease. Noncardiac symptoms and typical ECG and echocardiography findings can also point to specific etiologies (Table 4.2).

Table 4.2 Differential diagnosis in hypertrophic cardiomyopathy

	Sarcomeric HCM	Mitochondrial diseases	Noonan syndrome	Anderson-Fabry	Amyloidosis	Danon disease
Clinical evaluation						
Learning difficulties	–	+	+	–	–	+
Deafness	–	+	–	+	–	–
Visual impairment	–	+	–	–	+	+
Paresthesia	–	–	–	+	+	–
Carpal tunnel syndrome	–	–	–	–	+	–
Angiokeratoma	–	–	–	+	–	–
Electrocardiogram						
Short PR interval	–	–	–	+	–	–
Preexcitation	–	–	–	–	–	+
AV block	–	+	–	+	+	–
Low QRS voltage	–	–	–	–	+	–
Echocardiography						
Increased interatrial septum thickness	–	–	–	–	+	–
Increased AV valve thickness	–	–	–	+	+	–
Increased RV thickness	–	–	+	+	+	–
Pericardial effusion	–	–	–	–	+	–
Concentric LVH	–	–	–	+	–	+
Extreme concentric LVH	–	–	–	–	–	+
RV outflow tract obstruction	–	–	+	–	–	–

Molecular Diagnosis

Sarcomeric HCM is inherited as an autosomal dominant trait. Currently, in more than half of the HCM patients, the disease-causing variant can be identified [18]. Variants can be located in many genes but are most often found in the genes encoding sarcomeric proteins (Table 4.3, Fig. 4.3). Sarcomeric genes can be divided in genes encoding for myofilament proteins and genes encoding for Z-disc proteins.

Most HCM patients are heterozygous for the variant, but in 3–5% of cases, patients carry two variants in the same gene (different alleles—compound heterozygous or homozygous) or in different genes (digenic). This is generally associated with a more severe phenotype with younger age of onset (often <10 years) and more adverse events suggesting a gene-dosage effect [19, 20]. The two most frequently mutated genes are *MYBPC3* and *MYH7*, encoding the sarcomeric proteins cardiac myosin-binding protein C and beta-myosin heavy chain, respectively (Table 4.1) [21]. Both proteins are major components of the sarcomeric thick filament. In contrast to *MYH7* and most of the other genes associated with HCM, 70% of *MYBPC3* pathogenic variants are nonsense or frameshift and are predicted to result in truncated proteins [22], causing haploinsufficiency. In the other genes, missense variants are most frequent which create a mutant protein that interferes with normal function (dominant negative effect).

Since the discovery of the first genes for HCM, many papers on genotype-phenotype correlations have been written. At first specific variants, mainly in the *MYH7* gene, were

Table 4.3 Genes associated with HCM and their detection rate

Gene	Name	Detection rate
Sarcomeric		
Myofilament		
MYBPC3	Myosin-binding protein C	13–32%
MYH7	Beta-myosin heavy chain	4–25%
TNNT2	Troponin T2	0.5–7%
TNNI3	Cardiac troponin I	<5%
MYL2	Myosin light chain 2	<5%
MYL3	Myosin light chain 3	<1%
TPM1	Alpha-tropomyosin	<1%
ACTC	Alpha-actin	<1%
TNNC1	Troponin C	<1%
Z-disc		
ACTN2	Alpha-2 actinin	4–5%
CSRP3	Cysteine- and glycine-rich protein 3	
LBD3 (or ZASP)	Lim domain-binding 3	
TCAP	Titin-cap (Telethonin)	
VCL	Vinculin	
TTN	Titin	
MYOZ2	Myozenin 2	<1%
Non-sarcomeric[a]		**Phenotype**
PRKAG2	AMP-activated protein kinase gamma 2	LVH/preexcitation (Wolf-Parkinson-White syndrome)/ conduction disturbances
LAMP2	Lysosome-associated membrane protein 2	Danon disease
GLA	Alpha-galactosidase	Anderson-Fabry disease
PTPN11	Protein-tyrosine phosphatase non-receptor type 11	Noonan, LEOPARD, CFC syndrome
KRAS2	Kirsten rat sarcoma viral oncogene homolog	Noonan, LEOPARD, CFC syndrome
SOS1	Son of sevenless homolog 1	Noonan syndrome
BRAF1	V-RAF murine sarcoma viral oncogene homolog B1	CFC syndrome
MAP2K1	Mitogen-activated protein kinase kinase 1	CFC syndrome
MAP2K2	Mitogen-activated protein kinase kinase 2	CFC syndrome
HRAS	Harvey rat sarcoma viral oncogene homolog	Costello syndrome
GAA	Glucosidase alpha acid	Pompe disease
GDE	Glycogen debranching enzyme	Glycogen storage disorder III
FXN	Frataxin	Friedreich's ataxia
TTR	Transthyretin	Amyloidosis I
Mitochondrial DNA		LVH "plus"

[a]Because of specific phenotype mutation detection rate is not provided

described that were associated with a "malignant" phenotype (decreased survival) [23]. So-called "benign" variants were reported in families with normal longevity, as well [24]. These suggested "malignant" and "benign" variants have been contradicted in many subsequent studies. Nowadays it is believed that, possibly apart from rare exceptions, there are no clear genotype-phenotype relations with respect to magnitude of LVH and incidence of SCD [25]. Moreover, genetic studies have revealed that not all carriers of a pathogenic variant are clinically affected. This suggests the existence of modifier genes, which modulate the phenotypic expression of the disease.

Non-sarcomeric genes have been associated with specific phenotypes which include besides HCM almost always a distinct noncardiac syndromic phenotype, like the PTPN11 gene in Noonan syndrome and the LAMP2 gene in Danon disease. However, variants in the GLA gene, associated with Fabry disease, can give rise to HCM without further symptoms of Fabry disease, especially in women [26]. PRKAG2 is the other non-sarcomeric gene which presents with an exclusively cardiac phenotype. The cardiac phenotype is distinct and includes electrical preexcitation in addition to HCM (Table 4.1) [27].

De novo variants and germline mosaicism occur very rarely in HCM [28, 29]. Because most mutations are private, many of the identified mutations are novel. In certain countries/populations, however, founder variants have been identified, in which haplotype analysis suggests a common ancestor. These founder variants often comprise a large part (10–25%) of the detected pathogenic variants in these countries. Founder variants have been found in the Netherlands [30], South Africa [31], Finland [32], Italy [33], Japan, India, [34], and in the Amish population of the United States [35].

Like in other genetic diseases, identified variants in HCM patients can be pathogenic (disease causing), silent polymorphisms, or unclassified variants of which the pathogenic effect is still unclear, also called variants of unknown significance (VUS). According to guidelines of the Association for Clinical Genomic Science, variants can be classified into five subtypes: class 1, clearly not pathogenic; class 2, unlikely to be pathogenic; class 3, unknown significance; class 4, likely to be pathogenic; and class 5, clearly pathogenic. Because pathogenicity is not completely clear for classes 3 and 4, the laboratory should state in their report that follow-up studies, like segregation analysis in the family, are needed to clarify the significance of a variant. Nonsense or frameshift variants are most often pathogenic because they are predicted to result in a C-terminal truncated protein that is likely to be nonfunctional. Moreover, due to the presence of two quality controls, the nonsense-mediated mRNA decay-degrading nonsense (truncated) mRNAs [36] and the ubiquitin-proteasome-degrading aberrant proteins, [37] truncating variants most often do not result in the formation of protein at all and therefore lead to haploinsufficiency of the protein encoded by the mutated allele in the cells. Missense variants create a mutant protein that either interferes with normal function (dominant negative effect) or assumes a new function. Often however it remains unclear if a missense variant results in a protein with no or abnormal function.

The amino acid substitution in missense variants can give some indications for pathogenicity. Missense variants at codons conserved between species and isoforms are more likely to be pathogenic than variants at poorly conserved regions. Different in silico methods have been developed to assess not only conservation but also the frequency of the variant in the control databases, changes in protein structure, and chemical and biophysical characteristics and interactions. These in silico methods to define pathogenicity have to be validated by comparison to a gold standard. Gold standards can be functional assays, frequently found variants (e.g., founder variants), or segregation with the phenotype. All of these potential standards, however, have their own strengths and weaknesses [38–40]. Unclassified variants and even polymorphisms in HCM-associated genes and other genes may exhibit phenotype-modifying effects. In most countries, functional analysis of uncertain variants and modifiers in HCM patients is currently performed in research setting only and not used in clinical decision-making [38].

The main reason for genetic testing in HCM is to enable genetic cascade testing in relatives which is a more cost-efficient way of detecting relatives at risk of HCM and associated HCM compared to clinical testing [41]. Because clear genotype-phenotype relations cannot be made on an individual basis, often the genetic test result in an affected patient does not influence clinical evaluation, therapy, and prognosis of the HCM patient. Exceptions can be made for double mutations and non-sarcomeric genetic causes like Anderson-Fabry disease.

Genetic testing in HCM has shifted from testing of a few genes in order of frequency toward testing of large panels of cardiomyopathy-associated genes, often including common non-sarcomeric genetic causes like the GLA gene for Anderson-Fabry disease. The latter is a form of next-generation sequencing and has a higher yield of pathogenic variants and a short turnaround time. On the other hand, because more genes are evaluated including non-HCM genes and genes of which little is known yet, the chance of VUS is large. A lower number of tested genes make interpretation of test results easier, with less VUS but also with a lower yield of pathogenic variants. A high number of tested genes make test interpretation more difficult and give rise to more VUS, but the probability of detecting a pathogenic variant increases. The yield of VUS (class 3 mutations) is around 30% for gene panels testing between 40 and 50 genes and increases to around 40% if likely pathogenic variants (class 4 mutations) are also considered to be VUS [42]. In patients with signs of specific non-sarcomeric genetic causes of HCM, therefore genetic testing can be targeted. With new developments in diagnostic DNA testing and also increasing knowledge on tolerated DNA variants, we constantly have to reevaluate which test is best suited for which patient [42].

Disease Penetrance

HCM has long been regarded as a disease that mainly affects young people. It was thought that penetrance, i.e., the presence of LVH, was complete at approximately 20 years of age. Nowadays it is more and more recognized that not only symptoms but also hypertrophy can develop at any point in life.

Studies in carriers of a pathogenic variant show that disease penetrance is incomplete in adult life [43, 44]. The relationship between disease penetrance and the genotype (defined as the mutated gene or a specific variant within a gene) is still not completely resolved. Studies including a large number of carriers of a pathogenic variant show no difference in disease penetrance between carriers of different mutated genes [43].

Therapy

Management in HCM patients is directed toward control of symptoms, risk stratification for and prevention of SCD, and screening of relatives. Symptoms of dyspnea, angina, syncope, and fatigue are appraised and treated (Fig. 4.5) [4, 45]. Prophylactic pharmacological treatment in asymptomatic patients has not been proven to be effective in preventing progression of the disease. Drugs are often the only available treatment modality for symptomatic patients without LVOT obstruction. Negative inotropic agents like beta-blockers and calcium antagonists have shown to relieve symptoms. Beta-blockers decrease the heart rate which results in a prolongation of the diastole and relaxation phase of the heart and an increase in passive ventricular filling.

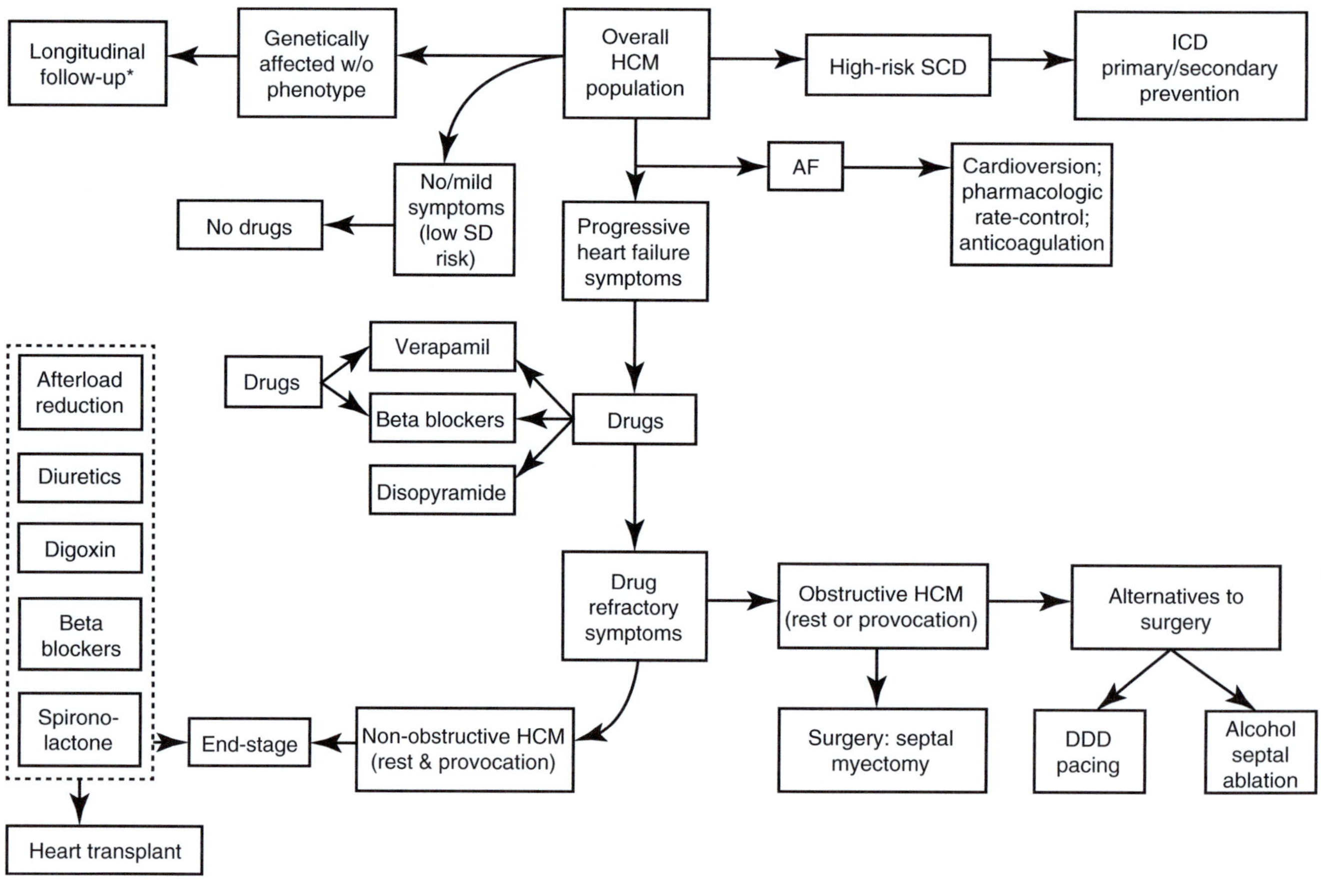

Fig. 4.5 Treatment strategies for patient subgroups within the broad clinical spectrum of HCM. *AF* atrial fibrillation, *DDD* dual-chamber, *ICD* implantable cardioverter defibrillator, *SD* sudden death. Figure derived from: American College of Cardiology/European Society of Cardiology clinical expert consensus document on hypertrophic cardiomyopathy. A report of the American College of Cardiology Foundation Task Force on Clinical Expert Consensus Documents and the European Society of Cardiology Committee for Practice Guidelines. Maron BJ et al.; Task Force on Clinical Expert Consensus Documents. American College of Cardiology; Committee for Practice Guidelines. European Society of Cardiology. J Am Coll Cardiol. 2003 Nov 5;42(9):1687–713

Besides, beta-blockers decrease LV contractibility and myocardial oxygen demand and can possibly reduce ischemia in myocardial microvessels. Verapamil, a calcium antagonist, also has favorable effects on symptoms by improving ventricular relaxation and filling. In patients with progressive heart failure symptoms with LVOT obstruction, disopyramide, a negative inotropic and type I-A antiarrhythmic drug, can be used. In end-stage HCM, load-reducing drugs (ACE inhibitors, angiotensin-II receptor blockers, diuretics, beta-blockers, or spironolactone) can be used to alleviate symptoms of systolic failure [4, 45].

In obstructive HCM, invasive septal reduction therapy is available if pharmacological treatment cannot alleviate symptoms. Septal myectomy and alcohol septal ablation can both be used in order to reduce the LVOT obstruction. Myectomy has low operative mortality and brings effective long-lasting improvement of symptoms. Alcohol septal ablation is a percutaneous catheter technique, in which the introduction of alcohol in the septal perforator branch of the left anterior descending coronary artery mimics septal myectomy. With the good selection of patients and in experienced hands, both therapies are successful in reducing LVOT obstruction and complaints with a low risk of complications [46]. Selection of the best therapy for a specific patient should be made based on the morphologic characteristics of the HCM (i.e., the amount of hypertrophy, associated mitral valve abnormalities), comorbidities of the patient, the presence of suitable septal arteries, and the availability of experienced thoracic surgeons and interventional cardiologists.

Indirect evidence suggests an association between exercise and SCD. Intense physical activity (e.g., sprinting) or systematic isometric exercise (e.g., heavy lifting) should be discouraged. HCM patients should be advised to avoid intense competitive sports and professional athletic careers. Bacterial endocarditis prophylaxis is recommended in obstructive HCM [4, 45].

Risk Stratification for SCD

In the past, HCM was seen as a disease with an ominous prognosis, because of severe symptoms and high rates of SCD (3–6% per year). These data, however, came from highly selected patient populations of severely affected patients treated in tertiary referral centers. These populations underrepresented clinically stable and asymptomatic patients. Recent reports with less referral bias indicate overall annual mortality rates from HCM of 1–2% (SCD and heart failure-related death). Annual mortality from SCD alone in HCM patients is 0.4–1% [47].

ICD Indications

Although the overall risk of SCD for HCM patients is low in absolute terms, a small subset of patients is at much higher risk of SCD. HCM patients, who survived ventricular fibrillation or symptomatic sustained ventricular tachycardia, are at high risk of SCD and should receive an implantable cardioverter defibrillator (ICD) for secondary prevention. ICDs for primary prevention in HCM patients are a challenge. Many clinical risk factors for SCD have been identified but their individual predictive value is low. In the ESC guidelines on HCM, it is advised to estimate a 5-year risk of SCD using the HCM Risk-SCD model (https://www.escardio.org/Guidelines/Clinical-Practice-Guidelines/Hypertrophic-Cardiomyopathy), which is based on a set of prognostic clinical variables [4, 48]. These clinical variables can be derived from the risk assessment which involves clinical (age, syncope) and family history of SCD, echocardiography, 48-h ambulatory ECG, and an exercise test. An ICD is not recommended if the estimated 5-year risk of SCD is <4% and other clinical features potentially associated with a risk of SCD are absent. In HCM patients with a calculated 5-year risk of SCD between 4 and 6%, there is a class IIb recommendation for the implantation of an ICD and in HCM patients with a risk ≥6% a class IIa indication. The HCM Risk-SCD model has not been evaluated in HCM patients <16 years, in professional athletes, in patients with a previous myectomy or alcohol septal ablation, and in patients with cardiac hypertrophy with a different etiology such as Anderson-Fabry disease.

In children, major risk factors for SCD are severe LVH, unexplained syncope, non-sustained ventricular tachycardia, and a family history of SCD. Cardiac hypertrophy in children is considered severe if ≥30 mm or a Z-score ≥6. In the presence of two or more risk factors, an ICD should be considered in children. If one risk factor is present, an individual approach with consideration of the risk and benefits of ICD implantation for the child and family should be followed [4].

In carriers of a pathogenic variant without LVH, the risk of SCD is very low and clinical evaluation can consist of ECG and echocardiography. If HCM becomes manifest, clinical assessments should include an assessment of the risk of SCD according to the HCM Risk-SCD model [4, 48].

Recommendations During Pregnancy and Delivery

The physiological changes during pregnancy are mostly tolerated well by asymptomatic or mildly symptomatic women with HCM. The hypertrophied LV can accommodate the rise in blood volume, cardiac output, and the reduction of systemic vascular resistance and blood pressure. The most common causes of complications are caused by diastolic dysfunction of the hypertrophied noncompliant LV, LVOT obstruction, and arrhythmias [49]. The maternal mortality rate is very low and limited to those patients with HCM who were significantly symptomatic before pregnancy, had impaired LV function before pregnancy, and/or had a high LVOT gradient [50, 51].

In known HCM patients, the risk of pregnancy should ideally be assessed and discussed with the patient before conception. Different classifications and risk scores have been developed to estimate maternal risk; most risk scores included the presence of LVOT obstruction as a risk factor. The modified World Health Organization (WHO) classification is the best available risk assessment model for estimating cardiovascular risk and should be used to assess the risk [4, 52, 53]. Risk assessment should include a detailed history, physical examination, and assessment of functional capacity and New York Heart Association (NYHA) functional class, electrocardiogram, and echocardiography [4, 53]. Exercise testing is used to assess functional capacity, heart rate response, and exercise-induced arrhythmias. Current cardiac medication and its use during pregnancy should be discussed with the patient. Some medications might need to be adjusted to prevent adverse fetal events

Follow-Up During Pregnancy

Development of heart failure symptoms is relatively uncommon during pregnancy, occurring in <5% of previously asymptomatic HCM patients and in 15% of the overall cohort. Clinical deterioration is twice as common in patients with LVOT obstruction compared to those without [51].

Women with a pathogenic variant without a cardiac phenotype don't need specific cardiac follow-up during their pregnancy.

Asymptomatic HCM patients with mild to moderate LVOT obstruction with or without medication, well-controlled arrhythmias, and maximal mildly reduced LV dysfunction are at low to moderate risk and should be assessed each trimester. Women with severe LVOT obstruction and symptoms despite medical therapy, poorly controlled arrhythmias, or moderate LV dysfunction have a high risk of complications and should be followed (bi) monthly in specialized centers, by a multidisciplinary team [50].

Management During Labor and Delivery

By the end of the second trimester, the multidisciplinary team should make a delivery plan. During labor, cardiac output is increased by catecholamine-induced increase in heart rate and stroke volume. Tachycardia will shorten the LV diastolic filling period, decrease preload, and increase LVOT obstruction. Venous return is impaired by the performance of the Valsalva maneuver during labor and delivery, and this might also increase LVOT obstruction. Substantial blood loss during delivery will also lead to reduction of venous return and thus increases LVOT obstruction. In a paper describing the association of cardiomyopathy with adverse cardiac events during delivery, one-fifth of the HCM patients experienced either heart failure or arrhythmias at delivery [54]. Asymptomatic women with mild disease may go into spontaneous labor, for others, a planned vaginal delivery is generally preferred. Compared to caesarean section, vaginal delivery is associated with less blood loss and lower infection risk. A caesarean section in general is indicated because of obstetric indications. There is no consensus on absolute contraindications for vaginal delivery, but in HCM patients with severe LVOT obstruction, severe heart failure, or preterm labor while on OAC, a caesarean section should be considered [4, 50]. In HCM patients with a high risk of arrhythmias, monitoring of the heart rate and rhythm should be considered. Epidural or spinal anesthesia should be used with caution, since vasodilatation and hypotension can induce or increase preexistent LVOT obstruction. Single-shot spinal anesthesia should be avoided [4, 50].

The use of prostaglandins like oxytocin for the induction of labor should only be given as a slow infusion, to avoid hypotension and tachycardia [50].

In the case of severe blood loss or hypotension, fluids should be used for volume replacement, and inotropes are relatively contraindicated in HCM because of the potential induction or aggravation of LVOT obstruction. When necessary, pure alpha-antagonists like phenylephrine are preferred.

Clinical observation after delivery should be continued for 24–48 h because of the increased risk of pulmonary edema due to fluid shifts postdelivery [4, 50].

Follow-Up Advices

HCM patients require lifelong follow-up to detect changes in phenotypic expression, symptoms, and risk of SCD. In stable patients a clinical evaluation including ECG, echocardiography, and 48-h ambulatory electrocardiography should be performed every 1–2 years. Symptom-limited exercise testing should be considered every 2–3 years. CMR evaluation may be considered every 5 years or earlier in case of progressive disease [4].

First-degree relatives in whom the genetic status is unknown should be seen with ECG and echocardiography every 1–2 years between the age of 10 and 20 years and every 2–5 years after the age of 20 years. Phenotype-negative carriers of a pathogenic variant should be seen every 2 years, including ECG and echocardiography, and every 1–2 years between 10 and 20 years [4, 45, 55].

Family Screening (Fig. 4.6)

Consensus documents and guidelines on HCM encourage screening of relatives in order to enable early detection of family members at risk. Identification of a disease-causing variant in a HCM patient (the proband) implies the opportunity of screening by means of predictive DNA testing in relatives. DNA testing for HCM, and especially predictive DNA testing in relatives, is becoming more common in most developed countries but is still uncommon in non-Western countries because health insurance does not cover the costs of DNA testing and/or because genetic counseling is unavailable. Instead, most of these countries use clinical modalities such as echocardiography and ECG to screen relatives on the presence of disease.

It is advised that before genetic testing, pretest genetic counseling is performed by a professional trained for this specific task working in a multidisciplinary team. This holds for probands as well as for relatives. Healthy children are advised to undergo clinical or predictive genetic testing starting from age 10, unless young children have been affected in their family or a non-sarcomeric genetic cause has been identified [4].

In a family where a definite pathogenic variant (class 5 variant) is detected, the most cost-efficient way to identify relatives at risk for HCM is by genetic cascade testing. First-degree relatives are often informed by the proband orally or using a family letter composed by the physician, about the possibility of predictive genetic testing. They can make an appointment for counseling where the pros and cons of genetic testing are discussed, after which a predictive DNA test can be performed [54, 56]. Relatives without the familial HCM variant can be reassured and don't need cardiac evaluation. Relatives who carry the familial HCM variant are referred for cardiac evaluation.

If no pathogenic variant can be detected in a proband with HCM or DNA diagnostics is not possible, first-degree relatives of HCM patients (and SCD victims in the family) still have a risk to develop HCM. DNA testing in these relatives is impossible; they are advised to undergo regular car-

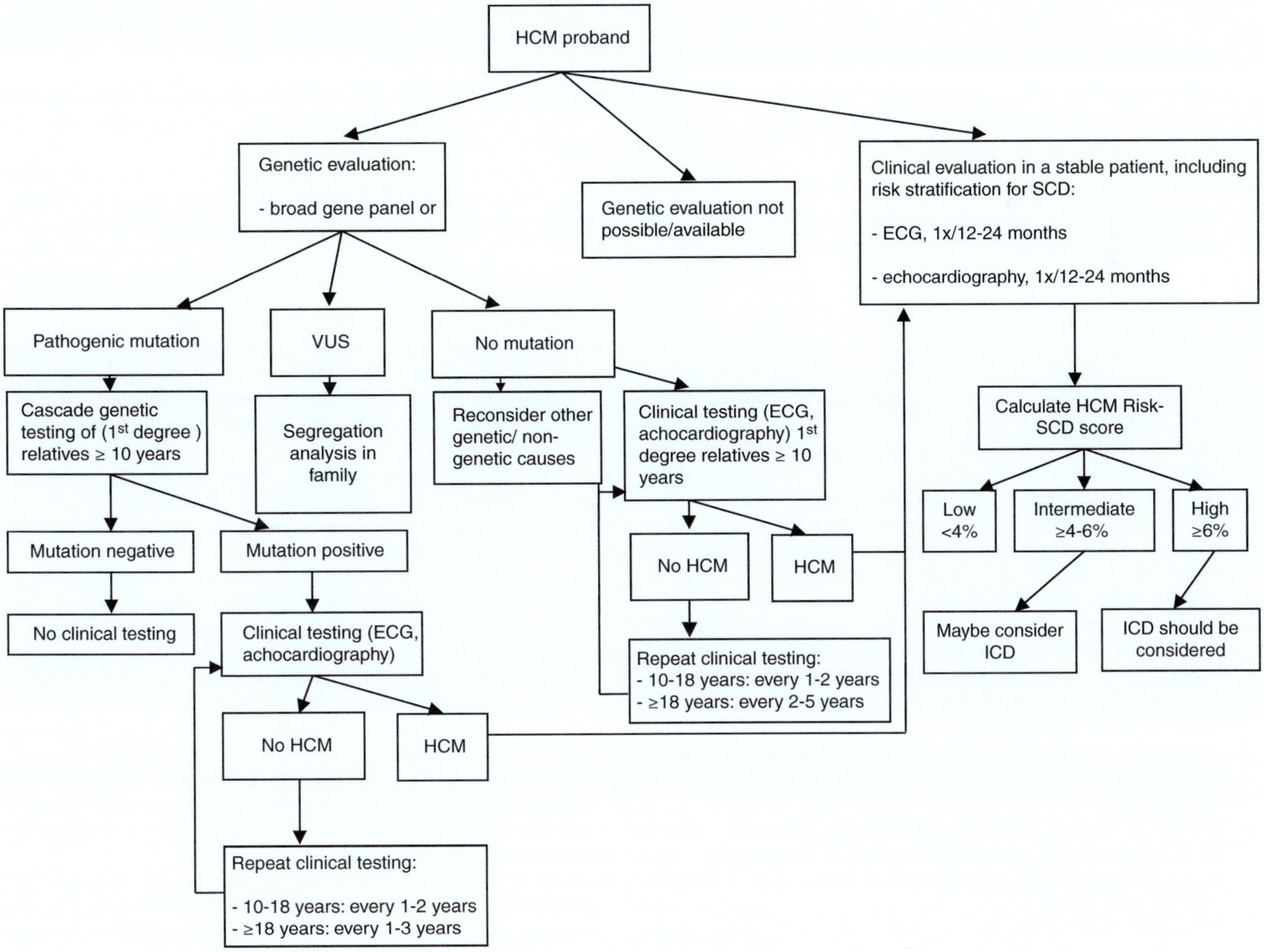

Fig. 4.6 Flowchart for clinical and genetic evaluation of HCM patients and their relatives

diac evaluations. If a variant of unknown significance (class 3 or 4 mutation) is detected in a proband, one can try to perform segregation analysis in the family. This can be done by genetic testing of all affected relatives, but often there are not enough available affected relatives to allow a mutation to be reclassified as clearly pathogenic. Testing non-affected relatives is of less value because of the age-dependent and incomplete disease penetrance of HCM. Another option is to offer relatives a combination of cardiac evaluation and genetic testing. This can be of value in class 4 variants (likely pathogenic). In class 3 variants, however, it is still unclear if this results in more variants being reclassified, while relatives can experience negative psychological effects if they are found to be a carrier of the variant even when they do not have a phenotype yet. If segregation is not possible or does not result in a reclassification of the DNA variant, first-degree relatives are advised to undergo regular cardiac evaluations just as in families where no mutation has been detected [4].

Take-Home Messages

1. Hypertrophic cardiomyopathy is the most common inherited cardiac disease.
2. Pathogenic sarcomeric variants are responsible for more than half of the HCM cases.
3. Genotype-phenotype correlations are weak.
4. Family screening, including genetic testing, is a cost-effective way to identify family members at risk.

References

1. Teare D. Asymmetrical hypertrophy of the heart in young adults. Br Heart J. 1958;20(1):1–8.
2. Coats CJ, Hollman A. Hypertrophic cardiomyopathy: lessons from history. Heart. 2008;94(10):1258–63.
3. Maron BJ, Gardin JM, Flack JM, Gidding SS, Kurosaki TT, Bild DE. Prevalence of hypertrophic cardiomyopathy in a general population of young adults. Echocardiographic analysis of 4111 subjects in the CARDIA study. Coronary artery risk development in (young) adults. Circulation. 1995;92(4):785–9.
4. Elliott PM, Anastasakis A, Borger MA, Borggrefe M, Cecchi F, Charron P, et al. ESC guidelines on diagnosis and management of hypertrophic cardiomyopathy: the task force for the diagnosis and management of hypertrophic cardiomyopathy of the European society of cardiology (ESC). Eur Heart J. 2014;35(39):2733–79.
5. Semsarian C, Ingles J, Maron MS, Maron BJ. New perspectives on the prevalence of hypertrophic cardiomyopathy. J Am Coll Cardiol. 2015;65(12):1249–54.
6. Kitaoka H, Doi Y, Casey SA, Hitomi N, Furuno T, Maron BJ. Comparison of prevalence of apical hypertrophic cardiomyopathy in Japan and the United States. Am J Cardiol. 2003;92(10):1183–6.
7. Maron BJ, Wolfson JK, Roberts WC. Relation between extent of cardiac muscle cell disorganization and left ventricular wall thickness in hypertrophic cardiomyopathy. Am J Cardiol. 1992;70(7):785–90.
8. Varnava AM, Elliott PM, Mahon N, Davies MJ, McKenna WJ. Relation between myocyte disarray and outcome in hypertrophic cardiomyopathy. Am J Cardiol. 2001;88(3):275–9.
9. Maron BJ, Wolfson JK, Epstein SE, Roberts WC. Intramural ("small vessel") coronary artery disease in hypertrophic cardiomyopathy. J Am Coll Cardiol. 1986;8(3):545–57.
10. van der Velden J, Tocchetti CG, Varricchi G, Bianco A, Sequeira V, et al. Metabolic changes in hypertrophic cardiomyopathies: scientific update from the Working Group of Myocardial Function of the European Society of Cardiology. Cardiovasc Res. 2018;114(10):1273–80.
11. Elliott P, Baker R, Pasquale F, Quarta G, Ebrahim H, Mehta AB, et al. Prevalence of Anderson-Fabry disease in patients with hypertrophic cardiomyopathy: the European Anderson-Fabry disease survey. Heart. 2011;97(23):1957–60.
12. Limongelli G, Masarone D, D'Alessandro R, Elliott PM. Mitochondrial diseases and the heart: an overview of molecular basis, diagnosis, treatment and clinical course. Futur Cardiol. 2012;8(1):71–88.
13. Wilkinson JD, Lowe AM, Salbert BA, Sleeper LA, Colan SD, Cox GF, et al. Outcomes in children with Noonan syndrome and hypertrophic cardiomyopathy: a study from the pediatric cardiomyopathy registry. Am Heart J. 2012;164(3):442–8.
14. Bhogal S, Ladia V, Sitwala P, Cook E, Bajaj K, Ramu V, et al. Cardiac amyloidosis: an updated review with emphasis on diagnosis and future directions. Curr Probl Cardiol. 2018;43(1):10–34.
15. Maron MS, Olivotto I, Zenovich AG, Link MS, Pandian NG, Kuvin JT, et al. Hypertrophic cardiomyopathy is predominantly a disease of left ventricular outflow tact obstruction. Circulation. 2006;114(21):2232–9.
16. Sanderson JE, Gibson DG, Brown DJ, Goodwin JF. Left ventricular filling in hypertrophic cardiomyopathy. An angiographic study. Br Heart J. 1977;39(6):661–70.
17. Olivotto I, Cecchi F, Casey SA, Dolara A, Traverse JH, Maron BJ. Impact of atrial fibrillation on the clinical course of hypertrophic cardiomyopathy. Circulation. 2001;104(21):2517–24.
18. Alfares AA, Kelly MA, McDermott G, Funke BH, Lebo MS, Baxter SB, et al. Results of clinical genetic testing of 2,912 probands with hypertrophic cardiomyopathy: expanded panels offer limited additional sensitivity. Genet Med. 2015;17(11):880–8.
19. Lekanne Deprez RH, Muurling-Vlietman JJ, Hruda J, Baars MJ, Wijnaendts LC, Stolte-Dijkstra I, et al. Two cases of severe neonatal hypertrophic cardiomyopathy caused by compound heterozygous mutations in the MYBPC3 gene. J Med Genet. 2006;43(10):829–32.
20. Girolami F, Ho CY, Semsarian C, Baldi M, Will ML, Baldini K, et al. Clinical features and outcome of hypertrophic cardiomyopathy associated with triple sarcomere protein gene mutations. J Am Coll Cardiol. 2010;55(14):1444–53.
21. Ingles J, Goldstein J, Thaxton C, Caleshu C, Corty EW, Crowley SB, et al. Evaluating the clinical validity of hypertrophic cardiomyopathy genes. Circ Genom Precis Med. 2019;12(2):e002460.
22. van Dijk SJ, Dooijes D, dos Remedios C, Michels M, Lamers JM, Winegrad S, et al. Cardiac myosin-binding protein C mutations and hyeprtrophic cardiomyopathy: haploinsufficiency, deranged phosphorylation, and cardiomyocyte dysfunction. Circulation. 2009;119(11):1473–83.
23. Marian AJ, Mares A Jr, Kelly DP, Yu QT, Abchee AB, Hill R, et al. Sudden cardiac death in hypertrophic cardiomyopathy. Variability in phenotypic expression of beta-myosin heavy chain mutations. Eur Heart J. 1995;16(3):368–76.
24. Anan R, Greve G, Thierfelder L, Watkins H, McKenna WJ, Solomon S, et al. Prognostic implications of novel beta cardiac myosin heavy chain gene mutations that cause familial hypertrophic cardiomyopathy. J Clin Invest. 1994;93(1):280–5.
25. Van Driest SL, Ackerman MJ, Ommen SR, Shakur R, Will ML, Nishimura RA, et al. Prevalence and severity of "benign" muta-

tions in the beta-myosin heavy chain, cardiac troponin T, and alpha-tropomyosin genes in hypertrophic cardiomyopathy. Circulation. 2002;106(24):3085–90.

26. Monserrat L, Gimeno-Blanes JR, Marin F, Hermida-Prieto M, Garcia-Honrubia A, Perez I, et al. Prevalence of fabry disease in a Cohort of 508 unrelated patients with hypertrophic cardiomyopathy. J Am Coll Cardiol. 50(25):2399–403.
27. Gollob MH, Green MS, Tang AS, Roberts R. PRKAG2 cardiac syndrome: familial ventricular preexcitation, conduction system disease, and cardiac hypertrophy. Curr Opin Cardiol. 2002;17(3):229–34.
28. Forissier JF, Richard P, Briault S, Ledeuil C, Dubourg O, Charbonnier B, et al. First description of germline mosaicism in familial hypertrophic cardiomyopathy. J Med Genet. 2000;37(2):132–4.
29. Watkins H, Thierfelder L, Hwang DS, McKenna W, Seidman JG, Seidman CE. Sporadic hypertrophic cardiomyopathy due to de novo myosin mutations. J Clin Invest. 1992;90(5):1666–71.
30. Alders M, Jongbloed R, Deelen W, van den Wijngaard A, Doevendans P, Ten Cate F, et al. The 2373insG mutation in the MYBPC3 gene is a founder mutation, which accounts for nearly one-fourth of the HCM cases in the Netherlands. Eur Heart J. 2003;24(20):1848–53.
31. Moolman-Smook JC, De Lange WJ, Bruwer EC, Brink PA, Corfield VA. The origins of hypertrophic cardiomyopathy-causing mutations in two South African subpopulations: a unique profile of both independent and founder events. Am J Hum Genet. 1999;65(5):1308–20.
32. Jaaskelainen P, Miettinen R, Karkkainen P, Toivonen L, Laakso M, Kuusisto J. Genetics of hypertrophic cardiomyopathy in eastern Finland: few founder mutations with benign or intermediary phenotypes. Ann Med. 2004;36(1):23–32.
33. Girolami F, Olivotto I, Passerini I, Zachara E, Nistri S, Re F, et al. A molecular screening strategy based on beta-myosin heavy chain, cardiac myosin binding protein C and troponin T genes in Italian patients with hypertrophic cardiomyopathy. J Cardiovasc Med (Hagerstown). 2006;7(8):601–7.
34. Dhandapany PS, Sadayappan S, Xue Y, Powell GT, Rani DS, Nallari P, et al. A common MYBPC3 (cardiac myosin binding protein C) variant associated with cardiomyopathies in South Asia. Nat Genet. 2009;41(2):187–91.
35. Zahka K, Kalidas K, Simpson MA, Cross H, Keller BB, Galambos C, et al. Homozygous mutation of MYBPC3 associated with severe infantile hypertrophic cardiomyopathy at high frequency among the Amish. Heart. 2008;94(10):1326–30.
36. Garneau NL, Wilusz J, Wilusz CJ. The highways and byways of mRNA decay. Nat Rev Mol Cell Biol. 2007;8(2):113–26.
37. Mearini G, Schlossarek S, Willis MS, Carrier L. The ubiquitin-proteasome system in cardiac dysfunction. Biochim Biophys Acta. 2008;1782(12):749–63.
38. Mogensen J, van Tintelen JP, Fokstuen S, Elliott P, van Langen IM, Meder B, et al. The current role of next-generation DNA sequencing in routine care of patients with hereditary cardiovascular conditions: a viewpoint paper of the European Society of Cardiology working group on myocardial and pericardial diseases and members of the European Society of Human Genetics. Eur Heart J. 2015;36(22):1367–70.
39. Chan PA, Duraisamy S, Miller PJ, Newell JA, McBride C, Bond JP, et al. Interpreting missense variants: comparing computational methods in human disease genes CDKN2A, MLH1, MSH2, MECP2, and tyrosinase (TYR). Hum Mutat. 2007;28(7):683–93.
40. Goldgar DE, Easton DF, Byrnes GB, Spurdle AB, Iversen ES, Greenblatt MS. Genetic evidence and integration of various data sources for classifying uncertain variants into a single model. Hum Mutat. 2008;29(11):1265–72.
41. Ingles J, McGaughran J, Scuffham PA, Atherton J, Semsarian C. A cost-effectiveness model of genetic testing for the evaluation of families with hypertrophic cardiomyopathy. Heart. 2012;98(8):625–30.
42. van Lint FHM, Mook ORF, Alders M, Bikker H, Lekanne Dit Deprez RH, Christiaans I. Large next-generation sequencing gene panels in genetic heart disease: yield of pathogenic variants and variants of unknown significance. Neth Heart J. 2019 Mar 7;27(6):304–9.
43. Christiaans I, Birnie E, Bonsel GJ, Mannens MM, Michels M, Majoor-Krakauer D, et al. Manifest disease, risk factors for sudden cardiac death, and cardiac events in a large nationwide cohort of predictively tested hypertrophic cardiomyopathy mutation carriers: determining the best cardiological screening strategy. Eur Heart J. 2011;32(9):1161–70.
44. van Velzen HG, Schinkel AFL, Baart SJ, Oldenburg RA, Frohn-Mulder IME, van Slegtenhorst MA, Michels M. Outcomes of contemporary family screening in hypertrophic cardiomyopathy. Circ Genom Precis Med. 2018;11(4):e001896.
45. Gersh BJ, Maron BJ, Bonow RO, Dearani JA, Fifer MA, Link MS, et al. ACCF/AHA guidelines for the diagnosis & treatment of HCM. Circulation. 2011;124:e783–831.
46. Vriesendorp PA, Liebregts M, Steggerda RC, Schinkel AF, Willems R, Ten Cate FJ, et al. Long-term outcomes after medical and invasive treatment in patients with hypertrophic cardiomyopathy. JACC Heart Fail. 2014;2(6):630–6.
47. Elliott PM, Gimeno JR, Thaman R, Shah J, Ward D, Dickie S, et al. Historical trends in reported survival rates in patients with hypertrophic cardiomyopathy. Heart. 2006;92(6):785–91.
48. O'Mahony C, Jichi F, Pavlou M, Monserrat L, Anastasakis A, Rapezzi C, et al. A novel clinical risk prediction model for sudden cardiac death in hypertrophic cardiomyopathy (HCM risk-SCD). Eur Heart J. 2014;35(30):2010–20.
49. Regitz-Zagrosek V, Blomstrom LC, Borghi C, et al. ESC guidelines on the management of cardiovascular diseases during pregnancy: the task force on the management of cardiovascular diseases during pregnancy of the European Society of Cardiology (ESC). Eur Heart J. 2011;32:3147–97.
50. Autore C, Conte MR, Piccininno M. Risk associated with pregnancy in hypertrophic cardiomyopathy. J Am Coll Cardiol. 2002;40:1864–9.
51. Lima V, Parikh P, Zhu J, et al. Association of cardiomyopathy with adverse cardiac events in pregnant women at the time of delivery. J Am Coll Cardiol. 2015;3:257–66.
52. Balci A, Sollie-Szarynska KM, van der Bijl AG, et al. Prospective validation and assessment of cardiovascular and offspring risks models for pregnant women with congenital heart disease. Heart. 2014;100:1373–81.
53. Stergiopoulous K, Shiang E, Bench T. Pregnancy in patients with pre-existing cardiomyopathies. J Am Coll Cardiol. 2011;58:337–50.
54. Christiaans I, Birnie E, Bonsel GJ, Wilde AAM, van Langen IM. Uptake of genetic counselling and predictive DNA testing in hypertrophic cardiomyopathy. Eur J Hum Genet. 2008;16(10):1201–7.
55. Charron P, Arad M, Arbustini E, Basso C, Bilinska Z, Elliott P, Helio T, Keren A, McKenna WJ, Monserrat L, Pankuweit S, Perrot A, Rapezzi C, Ristic A, Seggewiss H, van Langen I, Tavazzi L, European Society of Cardiology Working Group on Myocardial and Pericardial Diseases. Genetic counselling and testing in cardiomyopathies: a position statement of the European Society of Cardiology Working Group on myocardial and pericardial diseases. Eur Heart J. 2010 Nov;31(22):2715–26.
56. van der Roest WP, Pennings JM, Bakker M, van den Berg MP, van Tintelen JP. Family letters are an effective way to inform relatives about inherited cardiac disease. Am J Med Genet A. 2009;149a(3):357–63.

Dilated Cardiomyopathy

5

Jason R. Cowan, Karin Y. van Spaendonck-Zwarts,
and Ray E. Hershberger

Introduction

Dilated cardiomyopathy (DCM) is characterized by impaired left ventricular systolic function and left ventricular dilatation (see Section "Clinical Diagnosis"). Of many clinically detectable causes, reviewed below, DCM used here refers to dilated cardiomyopathy where all usual clinically detectable causes (except genetic) have been excluded. DCM can be asymptomatic but may present with heart failure, arrhythmia, embolus from mural thrombus, or sudden cardiac death. DCM, even when treated, has significant mortality. DCM is the most prevalent indication for heart transplantation.

The first classification of the cardiomyopathies was made in 1972 [1] and was reiterated by the World Health Organization (WHO) in 1980 [2], defining DCM as myocardial disease of unknown origin with impaired systolic function and dilatation of the left ventricle. The American Heart Association (AHA) followed the updated 1995 WHO definition [3] when it defined DCM as a disease of the myocardium characterized by ventricular chamber enlargement and systolic dysfunction with normal LV wall thickness [4]. The European Society of Cardiology (ESC) narrowed the definition to a myocardial disorder with left ventricular dilatation and left ventricular systolic dysfunction in the absence of abnormal loading conditions, like hypertension or valve disease, or coronary artery disease sufficient to cause global systolic impairment [5].

A revised definition of DCM was most recently proposed in a 2016 position statement of the ESC in which DCM is seen as a clinical spectrum with left ventricular dilatation, impaired left ventricular function, conduction disease, and arrhythmias. In this proposal, a new category of hereditary non-dilated cardiomyopathy (HNDC) was introduced as part of this spectrum, defined as left ventricular or biventricular global systolic dysfunction without dilatation not explained by abnormal loading conditions or coronary artery disease [6]. Preclinical phases of DCM were recognized, including isolated ventricular dilatation, which has been observed as an early sign of DCM in relatives [7].

The prevalence of DCM has not been formally evaluated with modern imaging methods. One early population-based study, conducted from 1975 to 1984, yielded an age- and sex-adjusted incidence of 6 per 100,000 person-years and a prevalence of 1 in 2700 [8]. This number is undoubtedly a substantial underestimate. A recent review used several approaches to conclude that DCM may be more than tenfold as prevalent at 1 in 250 [9].

DCM can be classified into idiopathic DCM (iDCM), DCM secondary to other causes, and syndromic DCM, a disorder with both cardiac and extra-cardiac features. Familial (fDCM) is defined when two or more closely related family members have DCM with all usual clinically detectable causes excluded [9, 10]. The European guidelines have also included unexplained sudden death before the age of 35 in a first-degree relative of a DCM patient as criteria to establish fDCM [10]. Nongenetic DCM can be secondary to a number of causes, including ischemic, structural, endocrine, toxicity,

J. R. Cowan
Dorothy M. Davis Heart and Lung Research Institute,
The Ohio State University College of Medicine,
Columbus, OH, USA

Divisions of Human Genetics, The Ohio State University College of Medicine, Columbus, OH, USA

K. Y. van Spaendonck-Zwarts
Department of Clinical Genetics, Amsterdam University Medical Centre, Amsterdam, The Netherlands

Genetic Health Queensland, Royal Brisbane and Women's Hospital, Herston, QLD, Australia

R. E. Hershberger (✉)
Dorothy M. Davis Heart and Lung Research Institute,
The Ohio State University College of Medicine,
Columbus, OH, USA

Divisions of Human Genetics, The Ohio State University College of Medicine, Columbus, OH, USA

Cardiovascular Medicine, Department of Internal Medicine,
The Ohio State University College of Medicine,
Columbus, OH, USA
e-mail: Ray.Hershberger@osumc.edu

H. F. Baars et al. (eds.), *Clinical Cardiogenetics*, https://doi.org/10.1007/978-3-030-45457-9_5

and environmental causes. Ischemic cause is excluded from idiopathic DCM definitions. Coronary artery disease should be excluded when assessing a DCM patient, especially in males over 40 years and females over 45 years and even at younger ages in the presence of significant coronary risk factors that include a strong family history of premature myocardial infarction, hypercholesterolemia, or cigarette smoking.

DCM can also occur as part of a neuromuscular or syndromic disease with extra-cardiac features, including metabolic, mitochondrial, and chromosomal disorders. This category is also genetic but differs from genetic DCM restricted to cardiac features with different genetic causes, disease courses, and epidemiology. Childhood-onset DCM has a more diverse etiology than adult-onset DCM and more frequently falls into the latter category.

In this chapter, the clinical aspects of DCM will first be covered. The focus will then shift to the clinical and molecular features of genetic DCM and family screening.

Clinical Presentation

Many DCM patients present from the fourth decade onwards [11] with presenting manifestations including heart failure (80–85%), arrhythmia (15%), and thromboembolism (1–2%). DCM may also be diagnosed postmortem in patients who died suddenly. Childhood-onset DCM also exists but is less common and has a diverse etiology and broader differential diagnosis.

Before modern-era treatment, reported mortality of DCM was 66% in 2 years [12]. With modern pharmaceutical and device therapy, this number has dropped to 20% in 5 years and 35% in 10 years [13, 14].

Etiology of DCM

DCM has a broad and mixed etiology with both genetic factors and nongenetic factors involved. An overview is given in Table 5.1. When no clinically detectable cause (except genetic) can be identified, DCM is called idiopathic (iDCM). Genetic causes are commonly identified in this category and clinical screening of family members to detect familial DCM (fDCM) has been recommended [15–18].

In most cases, genetic DCM has an autosomal dominant inheritance pattern, typically with age-dependent penetrance and variable expression. Rare, putatively causative variants have been identified in more than 50 genes. Despite the number of associated genes [19], and although recent advances in techniques have made it possible to test an increasing number of genes in patients in a diagnostic setting, a likely pathogenic genetic defect is identified in 30–40% of fDCM cases

Table 5.1 Classification of DCM

Main classification	Subclassification/etiology with some examples
Nongenetic DCM	Ischemic • Coronary artery disease (with or without infarction) Structural heart disease • Valvular, congenital, pressure, or volume overload Toxins • Chemotherapy (anthracyclines, alkylating agents, Trastuzumab), alcohol Infectious • Viral (e.g., HIV), other infectious etiology (e.g., Lyme) Autoimmune • SLE, noninfectious myocarditis Infiltrative • Amyloidosis, sarcoidosis Endocrine • Diabetes mellitus, hypo and hyperthyroidism, Cushing/Addison disease Metabolic • Thiamine or carnitine deficiency, hypocalcaemia, hypophosphatemia Other • Tachycardia, Kawasaki
Genetic DCM	Familial DCM, (apparently sporadic) idiopathic DCM, a subset of PPCM
DCM as part of a disorder with noncardiac features	Neuromuscular • Duchenne/Becker (*DMD*) • Myotonic dystrophy (DMPK) • Limb-girdle muscular dystrophy (*LMNA, SGCD, SGCB*) • Laing myopathy (*MYH7*) • Myofibrillar myopathy (*DES*) Syndromic/metabolic • Carnitine deficiency (*SLC22A5*) • Glycosylation disorders (*DOLK* or *PGM1*) • Alstrom syndrome (*ALMS1*) • Barth syndrome (*TAZ*) Mitochondrial • MIDD (maternally inherited diabetes and deafness) • Kearns-Sayre syndrome Chromosomal disorders • 1p36deletion syndrome

DCM divided in three categories, with subdivisions of each category and some examples of DCM causes

[20–22]. Apparently sporadic iDCM can also have a genetic cause [23–25], although whether this group has largely an underlying genetic basis has not yet been resolved; neither have its potential genetic mechanisms [9]. Part of this group may actually represent fDCM, underdiagnosed because of (age-related) low penetrance, the availability of only small families, or incomplete testing of relatives. The presence of more than one rare variant that may be relevant for disease in up to a third of patients from one DCM cohort [26] and in approximately one-fourth of families with lamin A/C (*LMNA*) variants in another cohort [27] suggests that oligogenic mechanisms may be at play.

DCM as part of a disorder with both cardiac and extra-cardiac features can be due to a neuromuscular disorder, inborn metabolism disorder, and malformation disorder. This category of DCM is more common in childhood-onset DCM. The age of onset and prognosis [28] differ between various forms of childhood-onset DCM, as do the potentially involved genes and inheritance patterns. Table 5.1 includes this category with some of the most relevant childhood-onset forms of DCM and the genes in which mutations cause disease. The origin of disease in this category of DCM remained elusive in two-thirds of these cases [28]. Introduction of genome-wide testing methods, like exome sequencing, has lowered this number to approximately 50% [29, 30]. In the rest of the chapter, the focus will be on adult-onset DCM.

Peripartum cardiomyopathy (PPCM) is defined as DCM without detectable clinical cause presenting during pregnancy or in the months following delivery [31]. Considerable debate remains regarding etiology, but a subset of PPCM has been shown to have a genetic cause [32–36]. Still, a comprehensive understanding of the etiology of all PPCM patients remains uncertain.

Myocarditis is an inflammatory disease of the myocardium and is of infectious, autoimmune, or, in many cases, unknown origin. It mostly resolves spontaneously but in some cases progresses to DCM. It has been postulated that myocarditis triggers disease onset in genetic DCM analogous to certain cardiotoxic chemotherapeutic agents that cause DCM [37, 38]. Whether a molecular genetic basis is relevant for susceptibility, onset, or progression remains to be explored.

Clinical Diagnosis

The diagnostic workup from clinical symptoms of DCM has been recently described [39]. In every step of the diagnostic process, information can be gathered that steers diagnosis toward one or more of the many different causes of DCM. Clinical characteristics that point to specific hereditary forms of DCM are covered in Section "Molecular Genetics."

Clinical discovery of DCM usually starts with cardiac symptoms, although, at times, DCM is identified serendipitously in a presymptomatic stage (e.g., with an abnormal preoperative ECG that leads to echocardiography). The next step is a complete medical history and physical examination. The personal and medical history should include known medical causes of DCM and assessment of environmental risk factors, including cancer chemotherapeutic agents, alcohol, drugs of abuse, and other possible environmental or work exposures. The patient's family history should be recorded, focusing on family members with a history of cardiomyopathy, heart failure, sudden cardiac death, cardiac transplantation, pacemaker or defibrillator implantation, stroke at early age, and skeletal muscle disease. If familial disease is present, the family history can help to determine the pattern of inheritance and may identify features specific to the cause of DCM in the particular family. Physical examination of the patient should be directed toward cardiac and extra-cardiac symptoms, such as skeletal muscle weakness. In children, physical examination should also include dysmorphic or syndromic features typical of childhood-onset DCM. Because family history is known to be insensitive to detect familial DCM, clinical screening of first-degree family members is recommended in all cases to detect evidence of asymptomatic DCM (see Section "Family Screening").

An electrocardiogram (ECG) is indicated for all cardiovascular evaluations. Certain ECG findings are more common in some genetic types of DCM, like atrioventricular conduction disease in *LMNA* [40]-, *FLNC* [41, 42]-, or *DES* [43]-induced DCM. Rhythm abnormalities may also be apparent.

Routine laboratory testing should be performed to assess disease severity and to identify other causes or exacerbating factors of left ventricular dysfunction and arrhythmias. Specifically, endocrine dysfunction can be identified (high or low thyroid hormone levels), and signs of infectious disease, metabolic dysfunction, and/or nutritional deficiencies can be found. Ischemic disease needs to be excluded, and, while a variety of noninvasive imaging modalities are available, a coronary angiography remains the gold standard.

Cardiac imaging is necessary to fully characterize the degree of left ventricular dilatation and left ventricular systolic dysfunction. Echocardiography is the most widely available imaging modality, which can be easily used to assess cardiac function and ventricular dimensions. Furthermore, echocardiography can implicate causes of left ventricular dysfunction, like valvular dysfunction, regional wall motion abnormalities suggestive of ischemic disease, or a thick septum suggestive of infiltrative diseases such as amyloidosis or sarcoidosis.

Most echocardiographic authorities have considered the lower limits of normal of the left ventricular ejection fraction (LVEF) to be 50%, from early M-mode echocardiographic studies [44] to more recent US consensus documents [45]. Larger population-based studies suggest that the lower limit of two standard deviations for adults is a LVEF of 52% [46, 47], although with modern imaging precision, this definition may be too stringent. Current heart failure guidelines define individuals with a LVEF between 40 and 49% as occupying a gray area between reduced and preserved function [48–50]. Assessment of LV size has been more challenging, with initial efforts devised using M-mode (one-dimensional) echocardiography for infants, children, and adults based on an equation derived from 93 younger and 136 older subjects [51]. These early efforts were updated with improved standards from a much larger cohort of 1099 adults without known cardiovascular disease using a height- and gender-based approach [52]. With proliferation of two-dimensional echocardiography (2D-echo) M-mode-derived 2D-guided measurements have been advocated. The recent US/European consensus statements use gender-based approaches and BSA to estimate LV dimensions [47].

Cardiac magnetic resonance (CMR) imaging can assess cardiac function and morphology with much greater accuracy than echocardiography. CMR can also be used for tissue characterization, which is helpful in the diagnosis of both ischemic cardiac disease (late gadolinium enhancement) and myocarditis (late gadolinium enhancement, T1- and T2-weighted images) [53, 54], amyloidosis, and sarcoidosis, and may be used to detect fibrofatty replacement commonly present in arrhythmogenic right ventricular cardiomyopathy (ARVC) that may present with left ventricular involvement.

Diagnostic procedures should be supplemented with genetic testing. This will be covered in Sections "Molecular Diagnostics" and "Molecular Genetics." The presence of DCM in relatives from families with fDCM is assessed according to less stringent criteria than in the index patient. These criteria will be covered in Section "Family Screening."

Clinical Therapy

Clinical management of DCM is pointed toward reducing symptoms and mortality and should be completed in accordance with ESC and ACCF/AHA guidelines [15, 49, 50, 55]. In short, therapy comprises ACE inhibitors or angiotensin receptor blockers and beta-blockers to prevent or treat heart failure and reduce morbidity and mortality in all patients, aldosterone receptor antagonists in patients with NYHA class II–IV HF and a LVEF of 35% or less to reduce morbidity and mortality, and diuretics to alleviate symptoms. In certain patients, further medical therapy may be considered. Exacerbating features such as ischemic disease or abnormal loading conditions, including hypertension and valvular disease, should be treated. Patients on maximal medical therapy may be considered for device therapy, for either reduction of symptoms (biventricular pacemaker for cardiac resynchronization therapy) or primary prevention of sudden cardiac death (implantable cardioverter defibrillator, ICD) to reduce mortality.

Depending on the cause of hereditary disease, one may augment therapy beyond usual guidelines. For instance, mutations in certain genes give rise to more arrhythmias than mutations in other genes. Especially in *LMNA* mutations, as initially recommended in the US HFSA guidelines in 2009 [56] and reiterated in 2018 [16], the presence of various risk factors [57] can guide early defibrillator device therapy.

Molecular Diagnostics

While genetic testing has been previously recommended for fDCM, US guidelines have recently also advocated for genetic testing of all iDCM cases, whether familial or sporadic [16, 17]. Genetic testing should be offered to all idiopathic DCM probands regardless of age. Children or infants with cardiomyopathy should be referred to expert centers for evaluation of syndromic forms of cardiomyopathy. Next-generation sequencing (NGS) has become widely available and has facilitated the almost universal use of panels of genes for NGS-based testing. NGS has also made it possible to routinely test for the most common genetic cause of DCM: truncating mutations in *TTN* [20, 23, 26, 58–60], a gene so large that NGS is necessary to make clinical testing feasible. The selection of genes used for DCM testing panels varies considerably but usually includes several dozen genes with varying degrees of evidence in support of their relevance for DCM (Table 5.2). Variants identified in genes with little evidence in support of their role in DCM in general should not be used for predictive testing. Stated simply, variants identified in genes of unknown significance are inevitably variants of unknown significance unless and until sufficient evidence has been accumulated for that gene to establish it as a legitimate cause of DCM. Rigorous curation of genetic causes of cardiomyopathy is carried out by the US-based, international effort, ClinGen, where both genes [204] and variants [205] are being curated for disease relevance.

If signs of neuromuscular disease are present, testing of particular genes with neuromuscular involvement increases the diagnostic yield of genetic testing [25]. As the etiology of childhood-onset DCM more often includes syndromic/metabolic and neuromuscular disease, with other genes involved than those tested in adult-onset DCM gene panels, the molecular diagnostic approach in these patients should be broader than in adult-onset DCM. Whole-exome/whole-genome sequencing (WES/WGS) is a good approach for childhood-onset DCM as sequencing gives information on more genes than those covered by gene panels, enables the discovery of *de novo* mutations and novel disease genes [206], and may lead to the identification of an unexpected underlying disorder.

A concern of NGS gene panels (and even more of whole-exome/whole-genome sequencing) is that, as more genes are tested, the number of identified variants of unknown significance (VUS) and, by extension, patients receiving inconclusive test results increases [207, 208]. Interpretation of the genetic data is a challenge, especially since most pathogenic variants are unique to a patient or his or her family - the exception being for a few founder mutations. Ideally, pathogenicity of a variant can be demonstrated by co-segregation of disease and variant, combined with prior available reports. Alternatively, functional analysis from *in vitro* data on the

Table 5.2 DCM-associated genes commonly covered by clinical genetic testing panels[a]

Gene	Protein	Disease associations/DCM-associated features	Known inheritance	MIM# DCM phenotype (associated inheritance)	Estimated fraction of iDCM
Sarcomere					
ACTC1 [61, 62]	Actin, alpha cardiac 1	DCM, HCM, LVNC, CHD	AD	613,424 (AD)	<0.01
ACTN2 [63–66]	Alpha actinin 2	DCM, HCM Heterogeneous phenotype, including LVNC, arrhythmia, and SCD	AD	612,158 (AD)	<0.01
ANKRD1 [67, 68]	Ankyrin repeat domain 1	DCM, HCM CSD, mild skeletal MD, or mild elevated CPK	AD	N/A	Unk
FLNC [41, 42, 69]	Filamin C	DCM, HCM, RCM, ARVC, myopathy CSD, arrhythmias, SCD	AD	N/A	0.02–0.04
MYBPC3 [24, 70–73]	Myosin-binding protein C	DCM, HCM, LVNC SCD	AD	615,396 (AD)	0.02
MYH6 [24, 70, 74]	Myosin heavy chain 6, alpha	DCM, HCM, CHD Late onset, CSD	AD	613,252 (Unk)	0.04
MYH7 [75–77]	Myosin heavy chain 7, beta	DCM, HCM, LVNC, myopathy Early onset, CSD	AD	613,426 (AD)	0.04
MYPN [70, 78, 79]	Myopalladin	DCM, HCM, RCM, myopathy	AD, AR	615,248 (AD)	0.03
NEBL [80, 81]	Nebulette	DCM, EFE	AD	N/A	Unk
TCAP [77, 82, 83]	Telethonin	DCM, HCM, LGMD	AD, AR	N/A	<0.01
TNNC1 [24, 70, 84]	Troponin C, slow	DCM, HCM	AD	611,879 (Unk)	<0.01
TNNI3 [24, 85, 86]	Troponin I	DCM, HCM, RCM	AD, AR	611,880 (AR) 613,286 (Unk)	<0.01
TNNT2 [70, 77, 84, 87–89]	Troponin T	DCM, HCM, RCM, LVNC	AD	601,494 (AD)	0.03
TPM1 [24, 90, 91]	Tropomyosin 1	DCM, HCM, LVNC	AD	611,878 (AD)	<0.01
TTN [22, 23, 58, 59, 92–95]	Titin	DCM, HCM, ARVC, LGMD, myopathy, MD	AD, AR	604,145 (Unk)	0.15–0.20 (truncating variants)
Cytoskeleton					
ALMS1 [96–98]	Alms 1	DCM, Alstrom syndrome	AR	N/A	Unk
CAV3 [99]	Caveolin 3	DCM, HCM, LQTS, LGMD, RMD, myopathy Reported in a family with RMD, CSD	AD, AR	N/A	Unk
CSRP3 [66, 77, 83]	Cysteine-rich protein 3	DCM, HCM	AD	607,482 (Unk)	<0.01
CRYAB [100, 101]	Crystallin, alpha 2	DCM, myopathy Late onset	AD, AR	615,184 (AD)	<0.01
DES [43, 70, 102–105]	Desmin	DCM, ARVC, RCM, LGMD, SCPNK, myopathy Myopathy or muscular weakness, CSD and arrhythmias, SCD	AD, AR	604,765 (Unk)	<0.01
DMD [62, 106–116]	Dystrophin	DCM, DMD, BMD	XL	302,045 (XL)	Unk
FHL2 [117]	Four-and-a-half LIM protein 2	DCM	Unk	N/A	Unk
FKRP [118]	Fukutin-related protein	DCM, LGMD, MDDG	AR	N/A	Unk
FKTN [119, 120]	Fukutin	DCM, LGMD, MDDG Early onset, muscle weakness	AR	611,615 (AR)	Unk
ILK [121]	Integrin-linked kinase	DCM	AD	N/A	<0.01
LDB3 [77, 122–124]	LIM domain binding 3	DCM, HCM, ARVC, LVNC, myopathy	AD	601,493 (AD)	<0.01

(continued)

Table 5.2 (continued)

Gene	Protein	Disease associations/DCM-associated features	Known inheritance	MIM# DCM phenotype (associated inheritance)	Estimated fraction of iDCM
NEXN [125]	Nexilin	DCM, HCM	AD, AR	613,122 (AD)	Unk
PDLIM3 [126]	PDZ and LIM domain protein 3	DCM	AD	N/A	<0.01
SGCD [127, 128]	Sarcoglycan, delta	DCM, LGMD	AR	606,685 (Unk)	<0.01
VCL [129]	Vinculin/Metavinculin	DCM, HCM, LVNC	AD	611,407 (Unk)	Unk
Nuclear envelope					
EMD [130]	Emerin	DCM, EDMD Reported in family with mild MD	XL	N/A	Unk
LMNA [131–134]	Lamin A/C	DCM, assorted laminopathies (see OMIM 150330) CSD, arrhythmias, skeletal muscle weakness, SCD	AD, AR	115,200 (AD)	0.06
TMEM43 [135]	Transmembrane protein 43	DCM, ARVC, EDMD	AD	N/A	Unk
TMPO [136, 137]	Thymopoietin	DCM	AD	N/A	Unk
Nucleus					
EYA4 [138]	Eyes absent 4	DCM Sensorineural hearing loss	AD	605,362 (AD)	Unk
GATAD1 [139, 140]	GATA zinc finger domain-containing protein 1	DCM	AR	614,672 (AR)	Unk
NKX2.5 [141–143]	NL2 homeobox 5	DCM, CHDs, congenital hypothyroidism Arrhythmias, SCD	AD	N/A	Unk
PRDM16 [144, 145]	PR domain-containing protein 16	DCM, LVNC Childhood onset	AD	615,373 (AD)	Unk
RBM20 [146–150]	RNA binding motif protein 20	DCM Arrhythmias, SCD	AD	613,172 (AD)	0.02 (hotspot), ? (non-hotspot)
TBX20 [151, 152]	T-box 20	DCM, CHDs	AD	N/A	Unk
Ion channel					
ABCC9 [153]	ATP-binding cassette, subfamily C, member 9	DCM, BrS, Cantu syndrome CSD, arrhythmias	AD	608,569 (AD)	<0.01
SCN5A [77, 154–160]	Sodium channel, voltage-gated type V, alpha	DCM, ARVC, BrS, LQTS, SSS, SIDS CSD, arrhythmias	AD	601,154 (AD)	0.02
Mitochondrial					
SDHA [161]	Succinate dehydrogenase complex, subunit A	DCM, LVNC, Leigh syndrome, mitochondrial complex II deficiency, paragangliomas Childhood onset	AR, AD,	613,642 (Unk)	Unk
TAZ [162–164]	Tafazzin	DCM, LVNC, Barth syndrome	XL	N/A	Unk
TXNRD2 [165]	Thioredoxin reductase 2	DCM, glucocorticoid deficiencyCSD	AR	N/A	Unk
Lysosomal					
LAMP2 [166–168]	Lysosome-associated membrane protein 2	DCM, HCM, Danon disease	XL	300,257 (XL)	Unk
Extracellular matrix					
LAMA4 [121]	Laminin, alpha 4	DCM	AD	615,235 (AD)	<0.01
Endoplasmic/sarcoplasmic reticulum					
DOLK [169]	Dolichol kinase	DCM, CDG type Im	AR	N/A	Unk
PLN [170–177]	Phospholamban	DCM, HCM, ARVC Early onset and mortality, arrhythmias	AD	609,909 (Unk)	<0.01
RYR2 [178]	Ryanodine receptor 2	DCM, LVNC, ARVC, CPVT Arrhythmias	AD	N/A	Unk

Table 5.2 (continued)

Gene	Protein	Disease associations/DCM-associated features	Known inheritance	MIM# DCM phenotype (associated inheritance)	Estimated fraction of iDCM
Desmosomal					
DSC2 [179, 180]	Desmocollin 2	DCM, ARVC/+keratoderma, woolly hair	AD, AR	N/A	Unk
DSG2 [180, 181]	Desmoglein 2	DCM, ARVC	AD	612,877 (Unk)	Unk
DSP [181–186]	Desmoplakin	DCM, ARVC, epidermolysis bullosa DCM with keratoderma, woolly hair, tooth agenesis	AD, AR	N/A	Unk
JUP [181, 187]	Plakoglobin	DCM, ARVC, Naxos disease	AD, AR	N/A	Unk
PKP2 [181, 188]	Plakophilin 2	DCM, ARVC	AD	N/A	Unk
Other					
BAG3 [189–196]	BCL2-associated anthanogene 3	DCM, myopathy Early onset, worse prognosis with nonsense variants	AD	613,881 (AD)	0.03
CHRM2 [197, 198]	Cholinergic receptor, muscarinic 2	DCM Earlier onset with milder disease	AD	N/A	Unk
LRRC10 [199–202]	Leucine-rich repeat-containing protein 10	DCMChildhood onset	AD	N/A	Unk
RAF1 [203]	Raf-1	DCM, HCM, Noonan syndrome, Noonan syndrome with multiple lentigines (NSML) Childhood onset	AD	615,916 (AD)	Unk

AD autosomal dominant, *AR* autosomal recessive, *ARVC* arrhythmogenic right ventricular cardiomyopathy, *BMD* Becker muscular dystrophy, *BrS* Brugada syndrome, *CDG* congenital disorder of glycosylation, *CHD* congenital heart defect, *CPK* creatine phosphokinase, *CSD* conduction system disease, *DCM* dilated cardiomyopathy, *DMD* Duchenne muscular dystrophy, *EDMD* Emery-Dreifuss muscular dystrophy, *EFE* endocardial fibroelastosis, *GR* growth retardation, *HCM* hypertrophic cardiomyopathy, *iDCM* idiopathic dilated cardiomyopathy, *LGMD* limb-girdle muscular dystrophy, *LQTS* long QT syndrome, *LVNC* left ventricular non-compaction, *MD* muscular dystrophy, *MDDG* muscular dystrophy-dystroglycanopathy, *MGA* methylglutaconic aciduria, *SCD* sudden cardiac death, *SCPNK* Scapuloperoneal syndrome, neurogenic, Kaeser type, *SIDS* sudden infant death syndrome, *SSS* sick sinus syndrome, *RCM* restrictive cardiomyopathy, *RMD* rippling muscle disease, *Unk* unknown, *XL* X-linked

[a]Includes DCM genes offered by at least three dilated cardiomyopathy multigene testing panels from the following genetic testing services: Invitae, Ambry Genetics, Fulgent Genetics, Prevention Genetics, GeneDx, EGL Genetics, Greenwood Genetics, Phosphorus Diagnostic LLC (as of Sept 26, 2018)

variant or affected gene may give information on how likely it is for the variant to cause disease. Finally, various software tools can be used to classify variants by assessing the effect of amino acid changes, splicing, and evolutionary variation. These software-based approaches should be interpreted with care, however, since their calls are merely predictions and for diagnostic purposes should only be used in concordance with other data.

Large reference databases, for instance the ExAC [209] and gnomAD [210] browsers, have recently emerged and are highly functional; however, large-scale sharing of identified variants in clearly defined DCM cohorts remains a work in progress [211]. The classification of variants has not been systematically applied between commercial testing laboratories or academic research groups, although guidelines have now been drafted by the American College of Medical Genetics and Genomics (ACMG) to aid in standardization of variant interpretation practices between laboratories [212]. Further, variant classifications can also change over time as more information on a particular variant is gathered. To be of value, variant databases need to be updated regularly. Ideally this requires continuous curation and worldwide collaboration. The US-based Clinical Genetics Resource (ClinGen) with its ClinVar database (http://www.ncbi.nlm.nih.gov/clinvar/) proposes to collect and collate such data and has recently started this effort [211].

Molecular Genetics

More than 50 genes have assertions of relevance for DCM, although not all have been robustly shown to cause DCM [19]. Genes with the most evidence in support of a causal relationship to DCM include *LMNA*, *RBM20*, *TTN*, *MYH7*, *PLN*, *TNNT2*, and a few others, with some having greater support due to the prevalence of founder mutations [20, 23, 25, 26]. Most genes putatively involved in DCM code for sarcomeric, Z-disk or cytoskeleton proteins, but, in

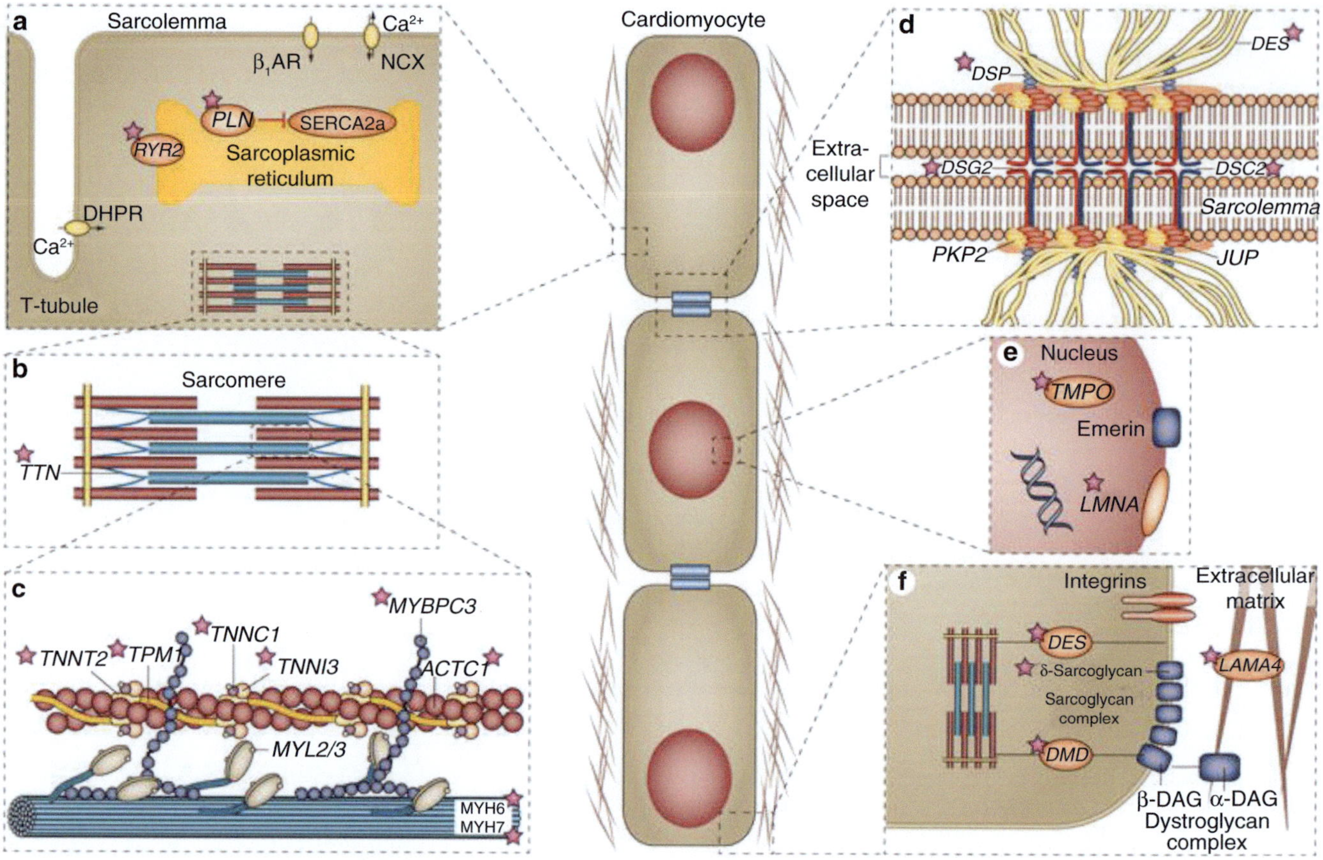

Fig. 5.1 Sarcomere/desmosome/cardiomyocyte structures (*Hershberger 2013*). Genes relevant to genetic DCM encode a diverse set of proteins. Some of the encoded proteins are illustrated in their cellular and molecular context and those in which a DCM-associated mutation has been identified in the coding sequence are indicated by a red star. (**a**) The cardiomyocyte membrane (sarcolemma), transverse (T) tubule, and sarcoplasmic reticulum. Mutations in the genes that encode the ryanodine receptor and phospholamban (*RYR2*, *PLN*), which are important proteins in the regulation of intracellular calcium, are known to cause DCM. (**b**, **c**) The sarcomere is the force-generating structure in cardiomyocytes and is comprised of several proteins including cardiac actin (ACTC1), myosin-binding protein C (MYBPC3), myosin heavy chains (MYH6, MYH7), myosin light chains (MYL2, MYL3), tropomyosin (TPM1), cardiac troponin C, troponin I, and troponin T (TNNC1, TNNI3, and TNNT2) and titin (*TTN*). (**d**) Desmosomal junctions, which assist in force transmission during muscle contraction. Variants in desmosomal proteins are associated with DCM, including desmin (DES), desmocollin-2 (DSC2), desmoglein-2 (DSG2), and desmoplakin (DSP). (**e**) The cardiomyocyte nucleus. Mutations in *LMNA*, which encodes the lamin A and C filaments of the protein structure associated with the inner nuclear membrane, and *TMPO* are associated with DCM. (**f**) Cardiomyocyte membrane and extracellular matrix proteins. Mutations in *LAMA4*, encoding an extracellular matrix protein, have been found in patients with DCM. The proteins encoded by *DES* and *DMD* are connected to the sarcomere and inner nuclear membrane by cytoskeletal filament protein ACTG1. Abbreviations: *β1AR* β1-adrenergic receptor, *DAG* dystrophin-associated glycoprotein, *DCM* dilated cardiomyopathy, *DHPR* dihydropyridine receptor (voltage-gated L-type calcium channel), *NCX* sodium/calcium exchanger, *SERCA2a* sarcoplasmic/endoplasmic reticulum Ca2+ ATPase 2a. (*Adapted from Hershberger 2013 with permission*)

contrast to HCM and ARVC, genes encoding proteins of diverse cardiomyocyte structures, functions, and pathways can be affected (Table 5.2 and Fig. 5.1). The pathophysiology through which variants in this diverse set of genes lead to DCM varies and is not known for all genes. Clinical overlap phenotypes at times occur in patients who have signs of DCM and another cardiomyopathy. This is understandable from a genetic point of view, as several DCM genes have been associated with one or more other cardiomyopathies (e.g., *MYH7* in DCM and HCM, *DSP* and *PLN* in DCM and ARVC [182, 183, 213], *NEBL* in DCM, HCM, and LVNC [80]). See also the respective chapters on these cardiomyopathies.

Familial DCM often has an autosomal dominant pattern of inheritance, but recessive [85], X-linked [106], and mitochondrial [214] inheritance patterns have also been reported. Missense mutations are most common, although in-frame insertions and deletions and frameshift, splice-site, and nonsense mutations also occur.

Penetrance of familial mutations in most cases is age-related, meaning that the probability that mutation carriers will develop the DCM phenotype increases with age.

Penetrance may also be incomplete. Even within one family, the phenotype in mutation carriers who do develop disease varies both in severity and clinical characteristics. For instance, one relative may develop structural cardiomyopathy while the other only develops conduction disease or arrhythmia. The cause for incomplete disease penetrance and varying disease expression is uncertain and largely unknown. One hypothesis suggests that multiple hit models comprised of one or more common or rare variants, likely in combination with environmental factors, may explain such phenotypic variation [26, 27]. This model implies a threshold for disease, requiring one or more factors to reach the threshold and cause disease. Environmental factors include general DCM risk factors, sex, blood pressure, activity level, drug and other toxicity exposure, and perhaps other specific physiologic or endocrine factors such as pregnancy or the postpartum state [215–222]. A recent study identifying more severe systolic impairment in *TTN*-truncating variant carriers who consume alcohol in excess [223] provides one example and highlights the interconnected roles of genetics and environmental factors in DCM.

TTN

Truncations in *TTN*, the gene encoding the sarcomeric protein titin, are to date the most common cause of fDCM, although it is not certain that all truncating variants affecting *TTN* cause DCM [59, 224]. Rare variants in *TTN* were first implicated in DCM in 2002 [92, 93] and the advent of NGS has made testing for mutations possible on large scale. The first study to report on the prevalence of truncating *TTN* variants reported these variants in 25% of fDCM patients [23]. Complicating matters, this study also reported truncating variants in *TTN* in healthy controls. As there are many isoforms of *TTN*, of which two are cardiac specific, not all truncating variants are disease causing. Filtering for variants that affect the cardiac isoforms still yields a prevalence of up to 22% [20, 22] and dramatically decreases the number of identified variants in controls [22, 225]. Whether all truncating *TTN* variants are pathogenic in cardiac specific isoforms has not yet been established [59, 224]. As prevalence and clinical outcomes in patients carrying *TTN* missense variants do not appear to differ from noncarrier patients [60], the potential role of *TTN* missense variants, which average 23 per individual, remains unclear.

LMNA

Variants in *LMNA*, coding for an inner nuclear envelope protein, are known to cause a distinctive form of DCM that may be characterized by progressive conduction system disease and supraventricular and ventricular arrhythmias as much as by contractile abnormalities. *LMNA* variants were first shown to cause DCM in families in 1999 [131], a study in which the association with conduction disease and arrhythmias was already suggested. Long-term follow-up demonstrated that disease penetrance in individuals with pathogenic *LMNA* variants is high and that these mutations are associated with high rates of heart failure, progressive conduction system disease requiring pacemakers, and malignant arrhythmias [40]. Because of this, ICD implementation may be considered even if usual guideline criteria (e.g., specifying LVEF of less than 35%) have not been met [15, 49, 50, 55] and should be guided more by the presence of the risk factors. These risk factors are non-sustained ventricular tachycardia, ejection fraction of less than 45% at first clinical contact or during follow-up, male sex, and non-missense mutations [57].

Other Genes

As depicted in Table 5.2, some genes are associated with certain clinical characteristics. The presence of these may inform genetic testing. In particular, some genes give rise to arrhythmias or conduction disease more often than others, with malignant phenotypes not only in patients with a mutation in *LMNA*, as discussed above, but also in patients with mutations in *RBM20* [146–148] or *FLNC* [42, 69].

Family Screening

Familial DCM and Affected Relatives

Obtaining a detailed family history of at least three generations is essential in patients with idiopathic DCM to detect evidence of familial disease. Furthermore, first-degree relatives should undergo clinical cardiac screening to exclude ventricular enlargement and systolic dysfunction or to detect signs of subclinical DCM, as further set out below.

Familial DCM is diagnosed when two or more individuals in a family have DCM and is suggestive if unexplained sudden death is documented before the age of 35 in a first-degree relative of a DCM patient [10].

In the US literature, the definition of DCM in family members has been the same as that for probands (LVEF <50% with left ventricular enlargement) [226]. Revised 2016 ESC diagnostic guidelines [6] recognize both reduced LVEF and unexplained left ventricular dilatation as independent major criteria, emphasizing the progressive clinical spectrum of DCM from preclinical to overt disease. Presence of a causative genetic variant in a relative is weighted similarly to other minor diagnostic criteria (arrhythmias, conduction disease, and other nonischemic imaging and myocardial abnormalities) and probable disease is suspected when one major criterion is present alongside at least one minor criterion or the causative genetic variant. If a relative has another clear cause for DCM features he or she is not considered as affected in the context of familial DCM [10].

Considering the varying phenotypic expression of known pathogenic variants and considerable age-dependent disease penetrance, variant classification in fDCM families as well as cardiac evaluation of patients may profit from less stringent criteria, as in the revised ESC guidelines. However, large, prospective, family-based DCM studies, accompanied by comprehensive genetic screening, are needed to validate these clinical criteria. Thus, thoughtful, thorough, and rigorous assembly of individual phenotype, pedigree, and genetic information by informed clinicians continues to be the mainstay of detection, assessment, and care for patients with possible genetic DCM. Even more relevant, no large multicenter or randomized clinical trials have been undertaken to halt disease progression in family members with findings consistent with early DCM.

Cardiac Screening of Relatives

Presymptomatic evaluation for DCM allows for early diagnosis [227, 228] and intervention, which may decrease morbidity and mortality. Cardiac evaluation should be performed in first-degree relatives of all DCM probands. Even if the family history is negative, fDCM is regularly found after cardiac screening in first-degree relatives. Evaluation should minimally include medical history, physical examination, ECG, and echocardiogram. Generally, in families with adult-onset fDCM, cardiac evaluation should be started in first-degree relatives at around 10–12 years of age and repeated every few years [16, 18, 56], with frequency in part derived from known genetic risk (positive genetic testing) or inferred genetic risk (a first-degree relative with DCM without informative genetic testing results). The findings at evaluation in an individual and disease characteristics specific to a family may influence the age at which evaluation should start and how frequent evaluations should take place in individual cases. The steps described in the text are also set out in a flowchart (Fig. 5.2).

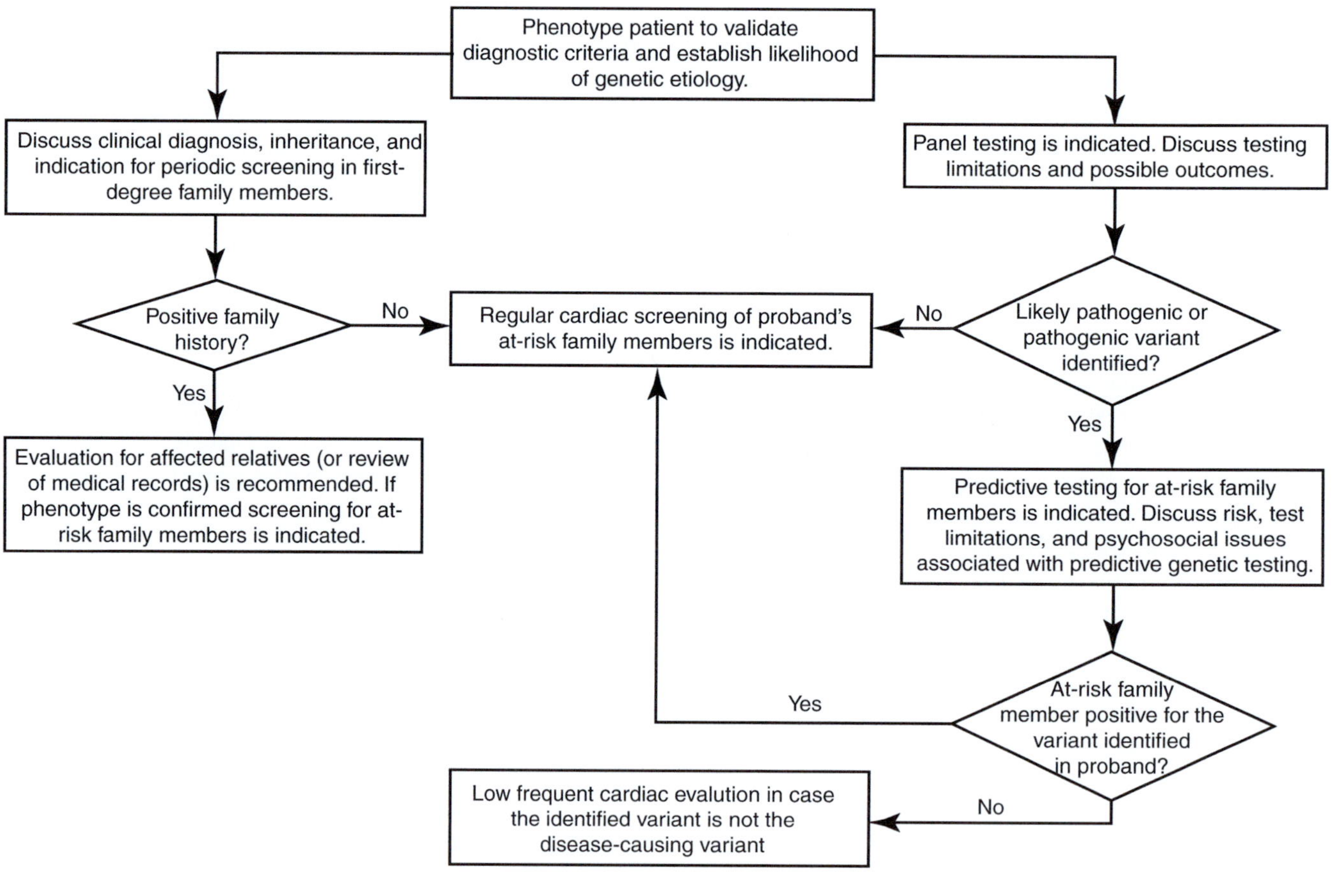

Fig. 5.2 Flowchart of family screening steps/decisions. The approach to the clinical evaluation and genetic testing of the relatives of a patient with DCM is shown. Not shown in this figure is the case when a variant of unknown significance (VUS) is identified in the patient or proband of the family. In this case, if additional affected family members are identified with family screening, efforts should be undertaken to attempt to move the VUS to a likely pathogenic or pathogenic classification

Genetic Testing Approach

Genetic testing in the proband will, in almost all cases, be performed by NGS by laboratories who offer a cardiomyopathy gene panel including several dozen or more genes (Table 5.2). When testing large numbers of genes, at times multiple rare variants in different DCM genes are identified. Variants may be categorized as pathogenic or likely pathogenic, a variant of unknown significance (VUS), or likely benign or benign, after the US ACMG approach to variant curation [212].

If a pathogenic or likely pathogenic variant is identified in the proband, testing affected relatives to show that the variant segregates in all those with DCM validates the premise that the identified variant indeed is the disease-causing allele. Subsequently, healthy relatives can be tested for the mutation to include or exclude them for regular cardiac evaluation. Mutation-positive relatives should be offered cardiac evaluation every 1–2 years. If the variant is still classified as likely pathogenic, not only should regular cardiac evaluation be offered to variant-positive relatives, but also low frequent cardiac evaluation should be offered to variant-negative relatives in case the identified variant is not the disease-causing variant.

If a VUS is identified in the proband, affected relatives may be tested for co-segregation of the variant and DCM. Nevertheless, most families are too small to be informative enough to reclassify a VUS. If a VUS segregates with DCM and the variant is reclassified as (likely) pathogenic, further genetic testing and clinical follow-up should be performed as described above. If a VUS remains classified as such only regular cardiac evaluation and not genetic testing should be offered to first-degree relatives.

If a likely benign or benign variant is identified, no further genetic testing is indicated and regular cardiac evaluation can be restricted to first-degree relatives. The identification of a benign or likely benign variant does not exclude the possibility of a genetic cause, as in familial disease a mutation is identified in only 40% of cases.

At times, relatives meeting a formal iDCM diagnosis will not carry the familial mutation. In a series of 19 *LMNA* pedigrees 6 were shown to have 1 or more family members who were negative for the familial *LMNA* variant, termed incomplete segregation pedigrees [132]. In five of the pedigrees the *LMNA* variant-negative members were shown to harbor pathogenic variants in other genes [27]. Such findings raise the question of how frequently variants from more than one gene are relevant in DCM. Individuals who do not carry a familial variant but exhibit the family DCM phenotype have traditionally been termed phenocopies, e.g., they show a resembling phenotype that has been considered due to another nongenetic cause. However, an alternative explanation is a multigene model, where more than one rare variant may be at play in an individual or a pedigree. This illustrates how important it is to test all affected relatives in a family and to perform cardiac evaluation in not only variant carriers but also in noncarriers if a variant is not pathogenic as described above and in the flowchart (Fig. 5.2).

It is essential that genetic counseling accompanies genetic testing. Further, since genetic testing and family evaluations touch many common ethical, medical, and psychosocial issues dealt with in clinical practice, it is recommended that genetic evaluations be performed by specialized cardiologists, clinical geneticists, and/or genetic counselors working in close collaboration. Patients and families should be informed that, although genetic testing can identify relatives at risk (thereby enabling early diagnosis and treatment), in the majority of cases a causative mutation will not be found and a VUS (uninformative for the family) may be identified. This latter situation, where no actionable genetic information can be derived from testing, is the case in more than half of the families with fDCM. For these families, testing cannot alleviate the uncertainty regarding genetic risk. Counseling should also cover that, at times, this uncertainty, perhaps exacerbated by continued clinical screening in asymptomatic individuals, may cause discomfort and undue concern. Also, if a causative mutation is found, the relatives who test positive for the mutation but are yet unaffected may have undue anxiety about the uncertainty of their prognosis and the timing of possible disease onset. This uncertainty may also influence individuals' eligibility for employment, mortgages, and life insurance as well as impact important life decisions such as whether to have children and what profession to choose.

Summary

Dilated cardiomyopathy is a complex cardiac disease characterized by left ventricular enlargement and systolic dysfunction. Etiology includes both genetic and nongenetic factors and age of onset and disease expression are variable. Clinical management aims to reduce symptoms and mortality and should be completed in accordance with ESC and ACCF/AHA guidelines. Rare causative variants have been identified in >50 genes, many of which overlap with other inherited cardiomyopathies, muscular dystrophies, and genetic syndromes. Children or infants with DCM should be referred for evaluation of syndromic forms of cardiomyopathy. Inheritance of non-syndromic DCM is usually autosomal dominant but can be autosomal recessive or X-linked. Identification of a disease-causing variant in a proband should spur targeted genetic testing in first-degree relatives, regardless of affected status. Genetic counseling should accompany all genetic testing and be provided as a vital component of collaborative patient care.

Take-Home Messages

- DCM is a disease with complex genetic and environmental etiology and high mortality.
- Genetic causes for DCM are common. A family history should be taken in all idiopathic DCM probands and their first-degree relatives should be offered clinical cardiac screening. Children or infants with DCM should be referred to expert centers for evaluation of syndromic forms of cardiomyopathy.
- If a (likely) pathogenic variant is identified in a DCM proband, first-degree relatives should be offered testing for that variant, regardless of age and affected status.
- The availability of sequencing panels with dozens of genes allows for more comprehensive testing of DCM probands; however, the need for stringency and expertise in the interpretation of rare variants becomes paramount.

References

1. Goodwin JF, Oakley CM. The cardiomyopathies. Br Heart J. 1972;34:545–52.
2. Report of the WHO/ISFC task force on the definition and classification of cardiomyopathies. Br Heart J. 1980;44:672–3.
3. Richardson P, McKenna W, Bristow M, Maisch B, Mautner B, O'Connell J, Olsen E, Thiene G, Goodwin J, Gyarfas I, Martin I, Nordet P. Report of the 1995 World Health Organization/International Society and federation of cardiology task force on the definition and classification of cardiomyopathies. Circulation. 1996;93:841–2.
4. Maron BJ, Towbin JA, Thiene G, Antzelevitch C, Corrado D, Arnett D, Moss AJ, Seidman CE, Young JB, American Heart A, Council on Clinical Cardiology HF, Transplantation C, Quality of C, Outcomes R, Functional G, Translational Biology Interdisciplinary Working G, Council on E. Prevention, contemporary definitions and classification of the cardiomyopathies: an American Heart Association Scientific Statement from the Council on Clinical Cardiology, Heart Failure and Transplantation Committee; Quality of Care and Outcomes Research and Functional Genomics and Translational Biology Interdisciplinary Working Groups; and Council on Epidemiology and Prevention. Circulation. 2006;113:1807–16.
5. Elliott P, Andersson B, Arbustini E, Bilinska Z, Cecchi F, Charron P, Dubourg O, Kuhl U, Maisch B, McKenna WJ, Monserrat L, Pankuweit S, Rapezzi C, Seferovic P, Tavazzi L, Keren A. Classification of the cardiomyopathies: a position statement from the European society of cardiology working group on myocardial and pericardial diseases. Eur Heart J. 2008;29:270–6.
6. Pinto YM, Elliott PM, Arbustini E, Adler Y, Anastasakis A, Bohm M, Duboc D, Gimeno J, de Groote P, Imazio M, Heymans S, Klingel K, Komajda M, Limongelli G, Linhart A, Mogensen J, Moon J, Pieper PG, Seferovic PM, Schueler S, Zamorano JL, Caforio AL, Charron P. Proposal for a revised definition of dilated cardiomyopathy, hypokinetic non-dilated cardiomyopathy, and its implications for clinical practice: a position statement of the ESC working group on myocardial and pericardial diseases. Eur Heart J. 2016;37:1850–8.
7. Michels VV, Moll PP, Miller FA, Tajik AJ, Chu JS, Driscoll DJ, Burnett JC, Rodeheffer RJ, Chesebro JH, Tazelaar HD. The frequency of familial dilated cardiomyopathy in a series of patients with idiopathic dilated cardiomyopathy. N Engl J Med. 1992;326:77–82.
8. Codd MB, Sugrue DD, Gersh BJ, Melton LJ 3rd. Epidemiology of idiopathic dilated and hypertrophic cardiomyopathy. A population-based study in Olmsted County, Minnesota, 1975–1984. Circulation. 1989;80:564–72.
9. Hershberger RE, Hedges DJ, Morales A. Dilated cardiomyopathy: the complexity of a diverse genetic architecture. Nat Rev Cardiol. 2013;10:531–47.
10. Mestroni L, Maisch B, McKenna WJ, Schwartz K, Charron P, Rocco C, Tesson F, Richter A, Wilke A, Komajda M. Guidelines for the study of familial dilated cardiomyopathies. Collaborative Research Group of the European Human and Capital Mobility Project on Familial Dilated Cardiomyopathy. Eur Heart J. 1999;20:93–102.
11. Elliott P, Charron P, Blanes JR, Tavazzi L, Tendera M, Konte M, Laroche C, Maggioni AP, Investigators ECRP. European cardiomyopathy pilot registry: EURO observational research programme of the European society of cardiology. Eur Heart J. 2016;37:164–73.
12. Fuster V, Gersh BJ, Giuliani ER, Tajik AJ, Brandenburg RO, Frye RL. The natural history of idiopathic dilated cardiomyopathy. Am J Cardiol. 1981;47:525–31.
13. Castelli G, Fornaro A, Ciaccheri M, Dolara A, Troiani V, Tomberli B, Olivotto I, Gensini GF. Improving survival rates of patients with idiopathic dilated cardiomyopathy in Tuscany over 3 decades: impact of evidence-based management. Circ Heart Fail. 2013;6:913–21.
14. Matsumura Y, Takata J, Kitaoka H, Kubo T, Baba Y, Hoshikawa E, Hamada T, Okawa M, Hitomi N, Sato K, Yamasaki N, Yabe T, Furuno T, Nishinaga M, Doi Y. Long-term prognosis of dilated cardiomyopathy revisited: an improvement in survival over the past 20 years. Circ J. 2006;70:376–83.
15. Yancy CW, Jessup M, Bozkurt B, Butler J, Casey DE Jr, Colvin MM, Drazner MH, Filippatos GS, Fonarow GC, Givertz MM, Hollenberg SM, Lindenfeld J, Masoudi FA, McBride PE, Peterson PN, Stevenson LW, Westlake C. 2017 ACC/AHA/HFSA focused update of the 2013 ACCF/AHA guideline for the management of heart failure: a report of the American College of Cardiology/American Heart Association Task Force on Clinical Practice Guidelines and the Heart Failure Society of America. Circulation. 2017;136:e137–61.
16. Hershberger RE, Givertz MM, Ho CY, Judge DP, Kantor PF, McBride KL, Morales A, Taylor MRG, Vatta M, Ware SM. Genetic evaluation of cardiomyopathy-a heart failure society of America practice guideline. J Card Fail. 2018;24:281–302.
17. Hershberger RE, Givertz MM, Ho CY, Judge DP, Kantor PF, McBride KL, Morales A, Taylor MRG, Vatta M, Ware SM, Practice AP, Guidelines C. Genetic evaluation of cardiomyopathy: a clinical practice resource of the American College of Medical Genetics and Genomics (ACMG). Genet Med. 2018;20:899–909.
18. Charron P, Arad M, Arbustini E, Basso C, Bilinska Z, Elliott P, Helio T, Keren A, McKenna WJ, Monserrat L, Pankuweit S, Perrot A, Rapezzi C, Ristic A, Seggewiss H, van Langen I, Tavazzi L, European Society of Cardiology Working Group on M, Pericardial D. Genetic counselling and testing in cardiomyopathies: a position statement of the European Society of Cardiology Working Group on myocardial and pericardial diseases. Eur Heart J. 2010;31:2715–26.
19. Posafalvi A, Herkert JC, Sinke RJ, van den Berg MP, Mogensen J, Jongbloed JD, van Tintelen JP. Clinical utility gene card for: dilated cardiomyopathy (CMD). Eur J Hum Genet. 2013;21:1185.
20. Akinrinade O, Ollila L, Vattulainen S, Tallila J, Gentile M, Salmenpera P, Koillinen H, Kaartinen M, Nieminen MS, Myllykangas S, Alastalo TP, Koskenvuo JW, Helio T. Genetics and genotype-phenotype correlations in Finnish patients with dilated cardiomyopathy. Eur Heart J. 2015;36:2327–37.

21. Lakdawala NK, Funke BH, Baxter S, Cirino AL, Roberts AE, Judge DP, Johnson N, Mendelsohn NJ, Morel C, Care M, Chung WK, Jones C, Psychogios A, Duffy E, Rehm HL, White E, Seidman JG, Seidman CE, Ho CY. Genetic testing for dilated cardiomyopathy in clinical practice. J Card Fail. 2012;18:296–303.
22. Roberts AM, Ware JS, Herman DS, Schafer S, Baksi J, Bick AG, Buchan RJ, Walsh R, John S, Wilkinson S, Mazzarotto F, Felkin LE, Gong S, JA MA, Cunningham F, Flannick J, Gabriel SB, Altshuler DM, Macdonald PS, Heinig M, Keogh AM, Hayward CS, Banner NR, Pennell DJ, O'Regan DP, San TR, de Marvao A, Dawes TJ, Gulati A, Birks EJ, Yacoub MH, Radke M, Gotthardt M, Wilson JG, O'Donnell CJ, Prasad SK, Barton PJ, Fatkin D, Hubner N, Seidman JG, Seidman CE, Cook SA. Integrated allelic, transcriptional, and phenomic dissection of the cardiac effects of titin truncations in health and disease. Sci Transl Med. 2015;7:270ra6.
23. Herman DS, Lam L, Taylor MR, Wang L, Teekakirikul P, Christodoulou D, Conner L, DePalma SR, McDonough B, Sparks E, Teodorescu DL, Cirino AL, Banner NR, Pennell DJ, Graw S, Merlo M, Di Lenarda A, Sinagra G, Bos JM, Ackerman MJ, Mitchell RN, Murry CE, Lakdawala NK, Ho CY, Barton PJ, Cook SA, Mestroni L, Seidman JG, Seidman CE. Truncations of titin causing dilated cardiomyopathy. N Engl J Med. 2012;366:619–28.
24. Hershberger RE, Norton N, Morales A, Li D, Siegfried JD, Gonzalez-Quintana J. Coding sequence rare variants identified in MYBPC3, MYH6, TPM1, TNNC1, and TNNI3 from 312 patients with familial or idiopathic dilated cardiomyopathy. Circ Cardiovasc Genet. 2010;3:155–61.
25. van Spaendonck-Zwarts KY, van Rijsingen IA, van den Berg MP, Lekanne Deprez RH, Post JG, van Mil AM, Asselbergs FW, Christiaans I, van Langen IM, Wilde AA, de Boer RA, Jongbloed JD, Pinto YM, van Tintelen JP. Genetic analysis in 418 index patients with idiopathic dilated cardiomyopathy: overview of 10 years' experience. Eur J Heart Fail. 2013;15:628–36.
26. Haas J, Frese KS, Peil B, Kloos W, Keller A, Nietsch R, Feng Z, Muller S, Kayvanpour E, Vogel B, Sedaghat-Hamedani F, Lim WK, Zhao X, Fradkin D, Kohler D, Fischer S, Franke J, Marquart S, Barb I, Li DT, Amr A, Ehlermann P, Mereles D, Weis T, Hassel S, Kremer A, King V, Wirsz E, Isnard R, Komajda M, Serio A, Grasso M, Syrris P, Wicks E, Plagnol V, Lopes L, Gadgaard T, Eiskjaer H, Jorgensen M, Garcia-Giustiniani D, Ortiz-Genga M, Crespo-Leiro MG, Deprez RH, Christiaans I, van Rijsingen IA, Wilde AA, Waldenstrom A, Bolognesi M, Bellazzi R, Morner S, Bermejo JL, Monserrat L, Villard E, Mogensen J, Pinto YM, Charron P, Elliott P, Arbustini E, Katus HA, Meder B. Atlas of the clinical genetics of human dilated cardiomyopathy. Eur Heart J. 2015;36:1123–35.
27. Cowan JR, Kinnamon DD, Morales A, Salyer L, Nickerson DA, Hershberger RE. Multigenic disease and bilineal inheritance in dilated cardiomyopathy is illustrated in nonsegregating LMNA pedigrees. Circ Genom Precis Med. 2018;11:e002038.
28. Towbin JA, Lowe AM, Colan SD, Sleeper LA, Orav EJ, Clunie S, Messere J, Cox GF, Lurie PR, Hsu D, Canter C, Wilkinson JD, Lipshultz SE. Incidence, causes, and outcomes of dilated cardiomyopathy in children. JAMA. 2006;296:1867–76.
29. Herkert JC, Abbott KM, Birnie E, Meems-Veldhuis MT, Boven LG, Benjamins M, du Marchie Sarvaas GJ, Barge-Schaapveld D, van Tintelen JP, van der Zwaag PA, Vos YJ, Sinke RJ, van den Berg MP, van Langen IM, Jongbloed JDH. Toward an effective exome-based genetic testing strategy in pediatric dilated cardiomyopathy. Genet Med. 2018;20:1374–86.
30. Luedde M, Ehlermann P, Weichenhan D, Will R, Zeller R, Rupp S, Muller A, Steen H, Ivandic BT, Ulmer HE, Kern M, Katus HA, Frey N. Severe familial left ventricular non-compaction cardiomyopathy due to a novel troponin T (TNNT2) mutation. Cardiovasc Res. 2010;86:452–60.
31. Sliwa K, Hilfiker-Kleiner D, Petrie MC, Mebazaa A, Pieske B, Buchmann E, Regitz-Zagrosek V, Schaufelberger M, Tavazzi L, van Veldhuisen DJ, Watkins H, Shah AJ, Seferovic PM, Elkayam U, Pankuweit S, Papp Z, Mouquet F, McMurray JJ, Heart Failure Association of the European Society of Cardiology Working Group on Peripartum C. Current state of knowledge on aetiology, diagnosis, management, and therapy of peripartum cardiomyopathy: a position statement from the Heart Failure Association of the European Society of Cardiology Working Group on peripartum cardiomyopathy. Eur J Heart Fail. 2010;12:767–78.
32. van Spaendonck-Zwarts KY, Posafalvi A, van den Berg MP, Hilfiker-Kleiner D, Bollen IA, Sliwa K, Alders M, Almomani R, van Langen IM, van der Meer P, Sinke RJ, van der Velden J, Van Veldhuisen DJ, van Tintelen JP, Jongbloed JD. Titin gene mutations are common in families with both peripartum cardiomyopathy and dilated cardiomyopathy. Eur Heart J. 2014;35:2165–73.
33. van Spaendonck-Zwarts KY, van Tintelen JP, van Veldhuisen DJ, van der Werf R, Jongbloed JD, Paulus WJ, Dooijes D, van den Berg MP. Peripartum cardiomyopathy as a part of familial dilated cardiomyopathy. Circulation. 2010;121:2169–75.
34. Ware JS, Li J, Mazaika E, Yasso CM, DeSouza T, Cappola TP, Tsai EJ, Hilfiker-Kleiner D, Kamiya CA, Mazzarotto F, Cook SA, Halder I, Prasad SK, Pisarcik J, Hanley-Yanez K, Alharethi R, Damp J, Hsich E, Elkayam U, Sheppard R, Kealey A, Alexis J, Ramani G, Safirstein J, Boehmer J, Pauly DF, Wittstein IS, Thohan V, Zucker MJ, Liu P, Gorcsan J 3rd, McNamara DM, Seidman CE, Seidman JG, Arany Z, Imac, Investigators I. Shared genetic predisposition in peripartum and dilated cardiomyopathies. N Engl J Med. 2016;374:233–41.
35. Kamiya CA, Yoshimatsu J, Ikeda T. Peripartum cardiomyopathy from a genetic perspective. Circ J. 2016;80:1684–8.
36. Lee YZJ, Judge DP. The role of genetics in peripartum cardiomyopathy. J Cardiovasc Transl Res. 2017;10:437–45.
37. van den Berg MP, van Spaendonck-Zwarts KY, van Veldhuisen DJ, Gietema JA, Postma A, van Tintelen JP. Familial dilated cardiomyopathy: another risk factor for anthracycline-induced cardiotoxicity? Eur J Heart Fail. 2010;12:1297–9.
38. Wasielewski M, van Spaendonck-Zwarts KY, Westerink ND, Jongbloed JD, Postma A, Gietema JA, van Tintelen JP, van den Berg MP. Potential genetic predisposition for anthracycline-associated cardiomyopathy in families with dilated cardiomyopathy. Open Heart. 2014;1:e000116.
39. Rapezzi C, Arbustini E, Caforio AL, Charron P, Gimeno-Blanes J, Helio T, Linhart A, Mogensen J, Pinto Y, Ristic A, Seggewiss H, Sinagra G, Tavazzi L, Elliott PM. Diagnostic work-up in cardiomyopathies: bridging the gap between clinical phenotypes and final diagnosis. A position statement from the ESC working group on myocardial and pericardial diseases. Eur Heart J. 2013;34:1448–58.
40. Pasotti M, Klersy C, Pilotto A, Marziliano N, Rapezzi C, Serio A, Mannarino S, Gambarin F, Favalli V, Grasso M, Agozzino M, Campana C, Gavazzi A, Febo O, Marini M, Landolina M, Mortara A, Piccolo G, Vigano M, Tavazzi L, Arbustini E. Long-term outcome and risk stratification in dilated cardiolaminopathies. J Am Coll Cardiol. 2008;52:1250–60.
41. Begay RL, Tharp CA, Martin A, Graw SL, Sinagra G, Miani D, Sweet ME, Slavov DB, Stafford N, Zeller MJ, Alnefaie R, Rowland TJ, Brun F, Jones KL, Gowan K, Mestroni L, Garrity DM, Taylor MR. FLNC gene splice mutations cause dilated cardiomyopathy. JACC Basic Transl Sci. 2016;1:344–59.
42. Ortiz-Genga MF, Cuenca S, Dal Ferro M, Zorio E, Salgado-Aranda R, Climent V, Padron-Barthe L, Duro-Aguado I, Jimenez-Jaimez J, Hidalgo-Olivares VM, Garcia-Campo E, Lanzillo C, Suarez-Mier MP, Yonath H, Marcos-Alonso S, Ochoa JP, Santome JL, Garcia-Giustiniani D, Rodriguez-Garrido JL, Dominguez F, Merlo M, Palomino J, Pena ML, Trujillo JP, Martin-Vila A, Stolfo

D, Molina P, Lara-Pezzi E, Calvo-Iglesias FE, Nof E, Calo L, Barriales-Villa R, Gimeno-Blanes JR, Arad M, Garcia-Pavia P, Monserrat L. Truncating FLNC mutations are associated with high-risk dilated and arrhythmogenic cardiomyopathies. J Am Coll Cardiol. 2016;68:2440–51.

43. van Spaendonck-Zwarts KY, van Hessem L, Jongbloed JD, de Walle HE, Capetanaki Y, van der Kooi AJ, van Langen IM, van den Berg MP, van Tintelen JP. Desmin-related myopathy. Clin Genet. 2011;80:354–66.
44. Pfisterer ME, Battler A, Zaret BL. Range of normal values for left and right ventricular ejection fraction at rest and during exercise assessed by radionuclide angiocardiography. Eur Heart J. 1985;6:647–55.
45. Radford MJ, Arnold JM, Bennett SJ, Cinquegrani MP, Cleland JG, Havranek EP, Heidenreich PA, Rutherford JD, Spertus JA, Stevenson LW, Goff DC, Grover FL, Malenka DJ, Peterson ED, Redberg RF, American College of C, American Heart Association Task Force on Clinical Data S, American College of Chest P, International Society for H, Lung T, Heart Failure Society of A. ACC/AHA key data elements and definitions for measuring the clinical management and outcomes of patients with chronic heart failure: a report of the American College of Cardiology/American Heart Association Task Force on Clinical Data Standards (Writing Committee to Develop Heart Failure Clinical Data Standards): developed in collaboration with the American College of Chest Physicians and the International Society for Heart and Lung Transplantation: endorsed by the Heart Failure Society of America. Circulation. 2005;112:1888–916.
46. Echocardiographic Normal Ranges Meta-Analysis of the Left Heart C. Ethnic-specific normative reference values for echocardiographic LA and LV size, LV mass, and systolic function: the EchoNoRMAL study. JACC Cardiovasc Imaging. 2015;8:656–65.
47. Lang RM, Badano LP, Mor-Avi V, Afilalo J, Armstrong A, Ernande L, Flachskampf FA, Foster E, Goldstein SA, Kuznetsova T, Lancellotti P, Muraru D, Picard MH, Rietzschel ER, Rudski L, Spencer KT, Tsang W, Voigt JU. Recommendations for cardiac chamber quantification by echocardiography in adults: an update from the American Society of Echocardiography and the European Association of Cardiovascular Imaging. Eur Heart J Cardiovasc Imaging. 2015;16:233–70.
48. Ponikowski P, Voors AA, Anker SD, Bueno H, Cleland JG, Coats AJ, Falk V, Gonzalez-Juanatey JR, Harjola VP, Jankowska EA, Jessup M, Linde C, Nihoyannopoulos P, Parissis JT, Pieske B, Riley JP, Rosano GM, Ruilope LM, Ruschitzka F, Rutten FH, van der Meer P, Authors/Task Force M, Document R. 2016 ESC Guidelines for the diagnosis and treatment of acute and chronic heart failure: the task force for the diagnosis and treatment of acute and chronic heart failure of the European Society of Cardiology (ESC). Developed with the special contribution of the heart failure association (HFA) of the ESC. Eur J Heart Fail. 2016;18:891–975.
49. Ponikowski P, Voors AA, Anker SD, Bueno H, Cleland JGF, Coats AJS, Falk V, Gonzalez-Juanatey JR, Harjola VP, Jankowska EA, Jessup M, Linde C, Nihoyannopoulos P, Parissis JT, Pieske B, Riley JP, Rosano GMC, Ruilope LM, Ruschitzka F, Rutten FH, van der Meer P, Group ESCSD. 2016 ESC guidelines for the diagnosis and treatment of acute and chronic heart failure: the task force for the diagnosis and treatment of acute and chronic heart failure of the European Society of Cardiology (ESC) developed with the special contribution of the heart failure association (HFA) of the ESC. Eur Heart J. 2016;37:2129–200.
50. Yancy CW, Jessup M, Bozkurt B, Butler J, Casey DE Jr, Drazner MH, Fonarow GC, Geraci SA, Horwich T, Januzzi JL, Johnson MR, Kasper EK, Levy WC, Masoudi FA, McBride PE, McMurray JJ, Mitchell JE, Peterson PN, Riegel B, Sam F, Stevenson LW, Tang WH, Tsai EJ, Wilkoff BL, American College of Cardiology F, American Heart Association Task Force on Practice G. 2013 ACCF/AHA guideline for the management of heart failure: a report of the American College of Cardiology Foundation/American Heart Association Task Force on Practice Guidelines. J Am Coll Cardiol. 2013;62:e147–239.
51. Henry WL, Gardin JM, Ware JH. Echocardiographic measurements in normal subjects from infancy to old age. Circulation. 1980;62:1054–61.
52. Vasan RS, Larson MG, Levy D, Evans JC, Benjamin EJ. Distribution and categorization of echocardiographic measurements in relation to reference limits: the Framingham heart study: formulation of a height- and sex-specific classification and its prospective validation. Circulation. 1997;96:1863–73.
53. Ferreira VM, Piechnik SK, Dall'Armellina E, Karamitsos TD, Francis JM, Ntusi N, Holloway C, Choudhury RP, Kardos A, Robson MD, Friedrich MG, Neubauer S. T(1) mapping for the diagnosis of acute myocarditis using CMR: comparison to T2-weighted and late gadolinium enhanced imaging. JACC Cardiovasc Imaging. 2013;6:1048–58.
54. Friedrich MG, Sechtem U, Schulz-Menger J, Holmvang G, Alakija P, Cooper LT, White JA, Abdel-Aty H, Gutberlet M, Prasad S, Aletras A, Laissy JP, Paterson I, Filipchuk NG, Kumar A, Pauschinger M, Liu P. International consensus group on cardiovascular magnetic resonance in M, cardiovascular magnetic resonance in myocarditis: a JACC white paper. J Am Coll Cardiol. 2009;53:1475–87.
55. McMurray JJ, Adamopoulos S, Anker SD, Auricchio A, Bohm M, Dickstein K, Falk V, Filippatos G, Fonseca C, Gomez-Sanchez MA, Jaarsma T, Kober L, Lip GY, Maggioni AP, Parkhomenko A, Pieske BM, Popescu BA, Ronnevik PK, Rutten FH, Schwitter J, Seferovic P, Stepinska J, Trindade PT, Voors AA, Zannad F, Zeiher A, Task Force for the D, Treatment of A, Chronic Heart Failure of the European Society of C, Bax JJ, Baumgartner H, Ceconi C, Dean V, Deaton C, Fagard R, Funck-Brentano C, Hasdai D, Hoes A, Kirchhof P, Knuuti J, Kolh P, McDonagh T, Moulin C, Popescu BA, Reiner Z, Sechtem U, Sirnes PA, Tendera M, Torbicki A, Vahanian A, Windecker S, McDonagh T, Sechtem U, Bonet LA, Avraamides P, Ben Lamin HA, Brignole M, Coca A, Cowburn P, Dargie H, Elliott P, Flachskampf FA, Guida GF, Hardman S, Iung B, Merkely B, Mueller C, Nanas JN, Nielsen OW, Orn S, Parissis JT, Ponikowski P, Guidelines ESCCfP. ESC guidelines for the diagnosis and treatment of acute and chronic heart failure 2012: the task force for the diagnosis and treatment of acute and chronic heart failure 2012 of the European Society of Cardiology. Developed in collaboration with the heart failure association (HFA) of the ESC. Eur J Heart Fail. 2012;14:803–69.
56. Hershberger RE, Lindenfeld J, Mestroni L, Seidman CE, Taylor MR, Towbin JA, Heart Failure Society of A. Genetic evaluation of cardiomyopathy - a Heart Failure Society of America practice guideline. J Card Fail. 2009;15:83–97.
57. van Rijsingen IA, Arbustini E, Elliott PM, Mogensen J, Hermans-van Ast JF, van der Kooi AJ, van Tintelen JP, van den Berg MP, Pilotto A, Pasotti M, Jenkins S, Rowland C, Aslam U, Wilde AA, Perrot A, Pankuweit S, Zwinderman AH, Charron P, Pinto YM. Risk factors for malignant ventricular arrhythmias in Lamin a/c mutation carriers a European cohort study. J Am Coll Cardiol. 2012;59:493–500.
58. Franaszczyk M, Chmielewski P, Truszkowska G, Stawinski P, Michalak E, Rydzanicz M, Sobieszczanska-Malek M, Pollak A, Szczygiel J, Kosinska J, Parulski A, Stoklosa T, Tarnowska A, Machnicki MM, Foss-Nieradko B, Szperl M, Sioma A, Kusmierczyk M, Grzybowski J, Zielinski T, Ploski R, Bilinska ZT. Titin truncating variants in dilated Cardiomyopathy - prevalence and genotype-phenotype correlations. PLoS One. 2017;12:e0169007.

59. Tabish AM, Azzimato V, Alexiadis A, Buyandelger B, Knoll R. Genetic epidemiology of titin-truncating variants in the etiology of dilated cardiomyopathy. Biophys Rev. 2017;9:207–23.
60. Begay RL, Graw S, Sinagra G, Merlo M, Slavov D, Gowan K, Jones KL, Barbati G, Spezzacatene A, Brun F, Di Lenarda A, Smith JE, Granzier HL, Mestroni L, Taylor M, Familial Cardiomyopathy R. Role of titin missense variants in dilated cardiomyopathy. J Am Heart Assoc. 2015;4(11):e002645.
61. Monserrat L, Hermida-Prieto M, Fernandez X, Rodriguez I, Dumont C, Cazon L, Cuesta MG, Gonzalez-Juanatey C, Peteiro J, Alvarez N, Penas-Lado M, Castro-Beiras A. Mutation in the alpha-cardiac actin gene associated with apical hypertrophic cardiomyopathy, left ventricular non-compaction, and septal defects. Eur Heart J. 2007;28:1953–61.
62. Olson TM, Michels VV, Thibodeau SN, Tai YS, Keating MT. Actin mutations in dilated cardiomyopathy, a heritable form of heart failure. Science. 1998;280:750–2.
63. Bagnall RD, Molloy LK, Kalman JM, Semsarian C. Exome sequencing identifies a mutation in the ACTN2 gene in a family with idiopathic ventricular fibrillation, left ventricular noncompaction, and sudden death. BMC Med Genet. 2014;15:99.
64. Chiu C, Bagnall RD, Ingles J, Yeates L, Kennerson M, Donald JA, Jormakka M, Lind JM, Semsarian C. Mutations in alpha-actinin-2 cause hypertrophic cardiomyopathy: a genome-wide analysis. J Am Coll Cardiol. 2010;55:1127–35.
65. Girolami F, Iascone M, Tomberli B, Bardi S, Benelli M, Marseglia G, Pescucci C, Pezzoli L, Sana ME, Basso C, Marziliano N, Merlini PA, Fornaro A, Cecchi F, Torricelli F, Olivotto I. Novel alpha-actinin 2 variant associated with familial hypertrophic cardiomyopathy and juvenile atrial arrhythmias: a massively parallel sequencing study. Circ Cardiovasc Genet. 2014;7:741–50.
66. Mohapatra B, Jimenez S, Lin JH, Bowles KR, Coveler KJ, Marx JG, Chrisco MA, Murphy RT, Lurie PR, Schwartz RJ, Elliott PM, Vatta M, McKenna W, Towbin JA, Bowles NE. Mutations in the muscle LIM protein and alpha-actinin-2 genes in dilated cardiomyopathy and endocardial fibroelastosis. Mol Genet Metab. 2003;80:207–15.
67. Duboscq-Bidot L, Charron P, Ruppert V, Fauchier L, Richter A, Tavazzi L, Arbustini E, Wichter T, Maisch B, Komajda M, Isnard R, Villard E, Network EHF. Mutations in the ANKRD1 gene encoding CARP are responsible for human dilated cardiomyopathy. Eur Heart J. 2009;30:2128–36.
68. Moulik M, Vatta M, Witt SH, Arola AM, Murphy RT, McKenna WJ, Boriek AM, Oka K, Labeit S, Bowles NE, Arimura T, Kimura A, Towbin JA. ANKRD1, the gene encoding cardiac ankyrin repeat protein, is a novel dilated cardiomyopathy gene. J Am Coll Cardiol. 2009;54:325–33.
69. Begay RL, Graw SL, Sinagra G, Asimaki A, Rowland TJ, Slavov DB, Gowan K, Jones KL, Brun F, Merlo M, Miani D, Sweet M, Devaraj K, Wartchow EP, Gigli M, Puggia I, Salcedo EE, Garrity DM, Ambardekar AV, Buttrick P, Reece TB, Bristow MR, Saffitz JE, Mestroni L, Taylor MRG, Filamin C. Truncation mutations are associated with arrhythmogenic dilated cardiomyopathy and changes in the cell-cell adhesion structures. JACC Clin Electrophysiol. 2018;4:504–14.
70. Zhao Y, Feng Y, Zhang YM, Ding XX, Song YZ, Zhang AM, Liu L, Zhang H, Ding JH, Xia XS. Targeted next-generation sequencing of candidate genes reveals novel mutations in patients with dilated cardiomyopathy. Int J Mol Med. 2015;36:1479–86.
71. Daehmlow S, Erdmann J, Knueppel T, Gille C, Froemmel C, Hummel M, Hetzer R, Regitz-Zagrosek V. Novel mutations in sarcomeric protein genes in dilated cardiomyopathy. Biochem Biophys Res Commun. 2002;298:116–20.
72. Ehlermann P, Weichenhan D, Zehelein J, Steen H, Pribe R, Zeller R, Lehrke S, Zugck C, Ivandic BT, Katus HA. Adverse events in families with hypertrophic or dilated cardiomyopathy and mutations in the MYBPC3 gene. BMC Med Genet. 2008;9:95.
73. Konno T, Shimizu M, Ino H, Matsuyama T, Yamaguchi M, Terai H, Hayashi K, Mabuchi T, Kiyama M, Sakata K, Hayashi T, Inoue M, Kaneda T, Mabuchi H. A novel missense mutation in the myosin binding protein-C gene is responsible for hypertrophic cardiomyopathy with left ventricular dysfunction and dilation in elderly patients. J Am Coll Cardiol. 2003;41:781–6.
74. Carniel E, Taylor MR, Sinagra G, Di Lenarda A, Ku L, Fain PR, Boucek MM, Cavanaugh J, Miocic S, Slavov D, Graw SL, Feiger J, Zhu XZ, Dao D, Ferguson DA, Bristow MR, Mestroni L. Alpha-myosin heavy chain: a sarcomeric gene associated with dilated and hypertrophic phenotypes of cardiomyopathy. Circulation. 2005;112:54–9.
75. Klaassen S, Probst S, Oechslin E, Gerull B, Krings G, Schuler P, Greutmann M, Hurlimann D, Yegitbasi M, Pons L, Gramlich M, Drenckhahn JD, Heuser A, Berger F, Jenni R, Thierfelder L. Mutations in sarcomere protein genes in left ventricular noncompaction. Circulation. 2008;117:2893–901.
76. Villard E, Duboscq-Bidot L, Charron P, Benaiche A, Conraads V, Sylvius N, Komajda M. Mutation screening in dilated cardiomyopathy: prominent role of the beta myosin heavy chain gene. Eur Heart J. 2005;26:794–803.
77. Hershberger RE, Parks SB, Kushner JD, Li D, Ludwigsen S, Jakobs P, Nauman D, Burgess D, Partain J, Litt M. Coding sequence mutations identified in MYH7, TNNT2, SCN5A, CSRP3, LBD3, and TCAP from 313 patients with familial or idiopathic dilated cardiomyopathy. Clin Transl Sci. 2008;1:21–6.
78. Duboscq-Bidot L, Xu P, Charron P, Neyroud N, Dilanian G, Millaire A, Bors V, Komajda M, Villard E. Mutations in the Z-band protein myopalladin gene and idiopathic dilated cardiomyopathy. Cardiovasc Res. 2008;77:118–25.
79. Purevjav E, Arimura T, Augustin S, Huby AC, Takagi K, Nunoda S, Kearney DL, Taylor MD, Terasaki F, Bos JM, Ommen SR, Shibata H, Takahashi M, Itoh-Satoh M, McKenna WJ, Murphy RT, Labeit S, Yamanaka Y, Machida N, Park JE, Alexander PM, Weintraub RG, Kitaura Y, Ackerman MJ, Kimura A, Towbin JA. Molecular basis for clinical heterogeneity in inherited cardiomyopathies due to myopalladin mutations. Hum Mol Genet. 2012;21:2039–53.
80. Perrot A, Tomasov P, Villard E, Faludi R, Melacini P, Lossie J, Lohmann N, Richard P, De Bortoli M, Angelini A, Varga-Szemes A, Sperling SR, Simor T, Veselka J, Ozcelik C, Charron P. Mutations in NEBL encoding the cardiac Z-disk protein nebulette are associated with various cardiomyopathies. Arch Med Sci. 2016;12:263–78.
81. Purevjav E, Varela J, Morgado M, Kearney DL, Li H, Taylor MD, Arimura T, Moncman CL, McKenna W, Murphy RT, Labeit S, Vatta M, Bowles NE, Kimura A, Boriek AM, Towbin JA. Nebulette mutations are associated with dilated cardiomyopathy and endocardial fibroelastosis. J Am Coll Cardiol. 2010;56:1493–502.
82. Hayashi T, Arimura T, Itoh-Satoh M, Ueda K, Hohda S, Inagaki N, Takahashi M, Hori H, Yasunami M, Nishi H, Koga Y, Nakamura H, Matsuzaki M, Choi BY, Bae SW, You CW, Han KH, Park JE, Knoll R, Hoshijima M, Chien KR, Kimura A. Tcap gene mutations in hypertrophic cardiomyopathy and dilated cardiomyopathy. J Am Coll Cardiol. 2004;44:2192–201.
83. Knoll R, Hoshijima M, Hoffman HM, Person V, Lorenzen-Schmidt I, Bang ML, Hayashi T, Shiga N, Yasukawa H, Schaper W, McKenna W, Yokoyama M, Schork NJ, Omens JH, McCulloch AD, Kimura A, Gregorio CC, Poller W, Schaper J, Schultheiss HP, Chien KR. The cardiac mechanical stretch sensor machinery involves a Z disc complex that is defective in a subset of human dilated cardiomyopathy. Cell. 2002;111:943–55.
84. Mogensen J, Murphy RT, Shaw T, Bahl A, Redwood C, Watkins H, Burke M, Elliott PM, McKenna WJ. Severe disease expression

of cardiac troponin C and T mutations in patients with idiopathic dilated cardiomyopathy. J Am Coll Cardiol. 2004;44:2033–40.
85. Murphy RT, Mogensen J, Shaw A, Kubo T, Hughes S, McKenna WJ. Novel mutation in cardiac troponin I in recessive idiopathic dilated cardiomyopathy. Lancet. 2004;363:371–2.
86. Carballo S, Robinson P, Otway R, Fatkin D, Jongbloed JD, de Jonge N, Blair E, van Tintelen JP, Redwood C, Watkins H. Identification and functional characterization of cardiac troponin I as a novel disease gene in autosomal dominant dilated cardiomyopathy. Circ Res. 2009;105:375–82.
87. Kamisago M, Sharma SD, DePalma SR, Solomon S, Sharma P, McDonough B, Smoot L, Mullen MP, Woolf PK, Wigle ED, Seidman JG, Seidman CE. Mutations in sarcomere protein genes as a cause of dilated cardiomyopathy. N Engl J Med. 2000;343:1688–96.
88. Menon SC, Michels VV, Pellikka PA, Ballew JD, Karst ML, Herron KJ, Nelson SM, Rodeheffer RJ, Olson TM. Cardiac troponin T mutation in familial cardiomyopathy with variable remodeling and restrictive physiology. Clin Genet. 2008;74:445–54.
89. Moller DV, Andersen PS, Hedley P, Ersboll MK, Bundgaard H, Moolman-Smook J, Christiansen M, Kober L. The role of sarcomere gene mutations in patients with idiopathic dilated cardiomyopathy. Eur J Hum Genet. 2009;17:1241–9.
90. Olson TM, Kishimoto NY, Whitby FG, Michels VV. Mutations that alter the surface charge of alpha-tropomyosin are associated with dilated cardiomyopathy. J Mol Cell Cardiol. 2001;33:723–32.
91. Probst S, Oechslin E, Schuler P, Greutmann M, Boye P, Knirsch W, Berger F, Thierfelder L, Jenni R, Klaassen S. Sarcomere gene mutations in isolated left ventricular noncompaction cardiomyopathy do not predict clinical phenotype. Circ Cardiovasc Genet. 2011;4:367–74.
92. Gerull B, Gramlich M, Atherton J, McNabb M, Trombitas K, Sasse-Klaassen S, Seidman JG, Seidman C, Granzier H, Labeit S, Frenneaux M, Thierfelder L. Mutations of TTN, encoding the giant muscle filament titin, cause familial dilated cardiomyopathy. Nat Genet. 2002;30:201–4.
93. Itoh-Satoh M, Hayashi T, Nishi H, Koga Y, Arimura T, Koyanagi T, Takahashi M, Hohda S, Ueda K, Nouchi T, Hiroe M, Marumo F, Imaizumi T, Yasunami M, Kimura A. Titin mutations as the molecular basis for dilated cardiomyopathy. Biochem Biophys Res Commun. 2002;291:385–93.
94. Tayal U, Newsome S, Buchan R, Whiffin N, Walsh R, Barton PJ, Ware JS, Cook SA, Prasad SK. Truncating variants in titin independently predict early arrhythmias in patients with dilated cardiomyopathy. J Am Coll Cardiol. 2017;69:2466–8.
95. Norton N, Li D, Rampersaud E, Morales A, Martin ER, Zuchner S, Guo S, Gonzalez M, Hedges DJ, Robertson PD, Krumm N, Nickerson DA, Hershberger RE, National Heart L. Blood institute GOESP, the exome sequencing project family studies project T, exome sequencing and genome-wide linkage analysis in 17 families illustrate the complex contribution of TTN truncating variants to dilated cardiomyopathy. Circ Cardiovasc Genet. 2013;6:144–53.
96. Long PA, Evans JM, Olson TM. Exome sequencing establishes diagnosis of Alstrom syndrome in an infant presenting with non-syndromic dilated cardiomyopathy. Am J Med Genet A. 2015;167A:886–90.
97. Mahamid J, Lorber A, Horovitz Y, Shalev SA, Collin GB, Naggert JK, Marshall JD, Spiegel R. Extreme clinical variability of dilated cardiomyopathy in two siblings with Alstrom syndrome. Pediatr Cardiol. 2013;34:455–8.
98. Bond J, Flintoff K, Higgins J, Scott S, Bennet C, Parsons J, Mannon J, Jafri H, Rashid Y, Barrow M, Trembath R, Woodruff G, Rossa E, Lynch S, Sheilds J, Newbury-Ecob R, Falconer A, Holland P, Cockburn D, Karbani G, Malik S, Ahmed M, Roberts E, Taylor G, Woods CG. The importance of seeking ALMS1 mutations in infants with dilated cardiomyopathy. J Med Genet. 2005;42:e10.
99. Catteruccia M, Sanna T, Santorelli FM, Tessa A, Di Giacopo R, Sauchelli D, Verbo A, Lo Monaco M, Servidei S. Rippling muscle disease and cardiomyopathy associated with a mutation in the CAV3 gene. Neuromuscul Disord. 2009;19:779–83.
100. Inagaki N, Hayashi T, Arimura T, Koga Y, Takahashi M, Shibata H, Teraoka K, Chikamori T, Yamashina A, Kimura A. Alpha B-crystallin mutation in dilated cardiomyopathy. Biochem Biophys Res Commun. 2006;342:379–86.
101. Pilotto A, Marziliano N, Pasotti M, Grasso M, Costante AM. Arbustini E, alphaB-crystallin mutation in dilated cardiomyopathies: low prevalence in a consecutive series of 200 unrelated probands. Biochem Biophys Res Commun. 2006;346:1115–7.
102. Brodehl A, Dieding M, Klauke B, Dec E, Madaan S, Huang T, Gargus J, Fatima A, Saric T, Cakar H, Walhorn V, Tonsing K, Skrzipczyk T, Cebulla R, Gerdes D, Schulz U, Gummert J, Svendsen JH, Olesen MS, Anselmetti D, Christensen AH, Kimonis V, Milting H. The novel desmin mutant p.A120D impairs filament formation, prevents intercalated disk localization, and causes sudden cardiac death. Circ Cardiovasc Genet. 2013;6:615–23.
103. Li D, Tapscoft T, Gonzalez O, Burch PE, Quinones MA, Zoghbi WA, Hill R, Bachinski LL, Mann DL, Roberts R. Desmin mutation responsible for idiopathic dilated cardiomyopathy. Circulation. 1999;100:461–4.
104. Otten E, Asimaki A, Maass A, van Langen IM, van der Wal A, de Jonge N, van den Berg MP, Saffitz JE, Wilde AA, Jongbloed JD, van Tintelen JP. Desmin mutations as a cause of right ventricular heart failure affect the intercalated disks. Heart Rhythm. 2010;7:1058–64.
105. Tesson F, Sylvius N, Pilotto A, Dubosq-Bidot L, Peuchmaurd M, Bouchier C, Benaiche A, Mangin L, Charron P, Gavazzi A, Tavazzi L, Arbustini E, Komajda M. Epidemiology of desmin and cardiac actin gene mutations in a European population of dilated cardiomyopathy. Eur Heart J. 2000;21:1872–6.
106. Towbin JA, Hejtmancik JF, Brink P, Gelb B, Zhu XM, Chamberlain JS, McCabe ER, Swift M. X-linked dilated cardiomyopathy. Molecular genetic evidence of linkage to the Duchenne muscular dystrophy (dystrophin) gene at the Xp21 locus. Circulation. 1993;87:1854–65.
107. Tang J, Song X, Ji G, Wu H, Sun S, Lu S, Li Y, Zhang C, Zhang H. A novel DMD splicing mutation found in a family responsible for X-linked dilated cardiomyopathy with hyper-CKemia. Medicine (Baltimore). 2018;97:e11074.
108. Nakamura A. X-linked dilated cardiomyopathy: a cardiospecific phenotype of dystrophinopathy. Pharmaceuticals (Basel). 2015;8:303–20.
109. Chamberlain RC, Smith EC, Campbell MJ. Novel rod domain duplication in dystrophin resulting in X-linked dilated cardiomyopathy. Pediatr Neurol. 2015;53:439–41.
110. Feng J, Yan JY, Buzin CH, Sommer SS, Towbin JA. Comprehensive mutation scanning of the dystrophin gene in patients with nonsyndromic X-linked dilated cardiomyopathy. J Am Coll Cardiol. 2002;40:1120–4.
111. Tasaki N, Yoshida K, Haruta SI, Kouno H, Ichinose H, Fujimoto Y, Urasawa N, Kawakami T, Taniguchi M, Kurushima S, Shimakura T. X-linked dilated cardiomyopathy with a large hot-spot deletion in the dystrophin gene. Intern Med. 2001;40:1215–21.
112. Franz WM, Muller M, Muller OJ, Herrmann R, Rothmann T, Cremer M, Cohn RD, Voit T, Katus HA. Association of nonsense mutation of dystrophin gene with disruption of sarcoglycan complex in X-linked dilated cardiomyopathy. Lancet. 2000;355:1781–5.
113. Ferlini A, Sewry C, Melis MA, Mateddu A, Muntoni F. X-linked dilated cardiomyopathy and the dystrophin gene. Neuromuscul Disord. 1999;9:339–46.

114. Ortiz-Lopez R, Li H, Su J, Goytia V, Towbin JA. Evidence for a dystrophin missense mutation as a cause of X-linked dilated cardiomyopathy. Circulation. 1997;95:2434–40.
115. Franz WM, Cremer M, Herrmann R, Grunig E, Fogel W, Scheffold T, Goebel HH, Kircheisen R, Kubler W, Voit T, et al. X-linked dilated cardiomyopathy. Novel mutation of the dystrophin gene. Ann N Y Acad Sci. 1995;752:470–91.
116. Muntoni F, Cau M, Ganau A, Congiu R, Arvedi G, Mateddu A, Marrosu MG, Cianchetti C, Realdi G, Cao A, et al. Brief report: deletion of the dystrophin muscle-promoter region associated with X-linked dilated cardiomyopathy. N Engl J Med. 1993;329:921–5.
117. Arimura T, Hayashi T, Matsumoto Y, Shibata H, Hiroi S, Nakamura T, Inagaki N, Hinohara K, Takahashi M, Manatsu SI, Sasaoka T, Izumi T, Bonne G, Schwartz K, Kimura A. Structural analysis of four and half LIM protein-2 in dilated cardiomyopathy. Biochem Biophys Res Commun. 2007;357:162–7.
118. Muller T, Krasnianski M, Witthaut R, Deschauer M, Zierz S. Dilated cardiomyopathy may be an early sign of the C826A Fukutin-related protein mutation. Neuromuscul Disord. 2005;15:372–6.
119. Arimura T, Hayashi YK, Murakami T, Oya Y, Funabe S, Arikawa-Hirasawa E, Hattori N, Nishino I, Kimura A. Mutational analysis of fukutin gene in dilated cardiomyopathy and hypertrophic cardiomyopathy. Circ J. 2009;73:158–61.
120. Murakami T, Hayashi YK, Noguchi S, Ogawa M, Nonaka I, Tanabe Y, Ogino M, Takada F, Eriguchi M, Kotooka N, Campbell KP, Osawa M, Nishino I. Fukutin gene mutations cause dilated cardiomyopathy with minimal muscle weakness. Ann Neurol. 2006;60:597–602.
121. Knoll R, Postel R, Wang J, Kratzner R, Hennecke G, Vacaru AM, Vakeel P, Schubert C, Murthy K, Rana BK, Kube D, Knoll G, Schafer K, Hayashi T, Holm T, Kimura A, Schork N, Toliat MR, Nurnberg P, Schultheiss HP, Schaper W, Schaper J, Bos E, Den Hertog J, van Eeden FJ, Peters PJ, Hasenfuss G, Chien KR, Bakkers J. Laminin-alpha4 and integrin-linked kinase mutations cause human cardiomyopathy via simultaneous defects in cardiomyocytes and endothelial cells. Circulation. 2007;116:515–25.
122. Arimura T, Hayashi T, Terada H, Lee SY, Zhou Q, Takahashi M, Ueda K, Nouchi T, Hohda S, Shibutani M, Hirose M, Chen J, Park JE, Yasunami M, Hayashi H, Kimura A. A cypher/ZASP mutation associated with dilated cardiomyopathy alters the binding affinity to protein kinase C. J Biol Chem. 2004;279:6746–52.
123. Vatta M, Mohapatra B, Jimenez S, Sanchez X, Faulkner G, Perles Z, Sinagra G, Lin JH, Vu TM, Zhou Q, Bowles KR, Di Lenarda A, Schimmenti L, Fox M, Chrisco MA, Murphy RT, McKenna W, Elliott P, Bowles NE, Chen J, Valle G, Towbin JA. Mutations in cypher/ZASP in patients with dilated cardiomyopathy and left ventricular non-compaction. J Am Coll Cardiol. 2003;42:2014–27.
124. Xing Y, Ichida F, Matsuoka T, Isobe T, Ikemoto Y, Higaki T, Tsuji T, Haneda N, Kuwabara A, Chen R, Futatani T, Tsubata S, Watanabe S, Watanabe K, Hirono K, Uese K, Miyawaki T, Bowles KR, Bowles NE, Towbin JA. Genetic analysis in patients with left ventricular noncompaction and evidence for genetic heterogeneity. Mol Genet Metab. 2006;88:71–7.
125. Hassel D, Dahme T, Erdmann J, Meder B, Huge A, Stoll M, Just S, Hess A, Ehlermann P, Weichenhan D, Grimmler M, Liptau H, Hetzer R, Regitz-Zagrosek V, Fischer C, Nurnberg P, Schunkert H, Katus HA, Rottbauer W. Nexilin mutations destabilize cardiac Z-disks and lead to dilated cardiomyopathy. Nat Med. 2009;15:1281–8.
126. Arola AM, Sanchez X, Murphy RT, Hasle E, Li H, Elliott PM, McKenna WJ, Towbin JA, Bowles NE. Mutations in PDLIM3 and MYOZ1 encoding myocyte Z line proteins are infrequently found in idiopathic dilated cardiomyopathy. Mol Genet Metab. 2007;90:435–40.
127. Tsubata S, Bowles KR, Vatta M, Zintz C, Titus J, Muhonen L, Bowles NE, Towbin JA. Mutations in the human delta-sarcoglycan gene in familial and sporadic dilated cardiomyopathy. J Clin Invest. 2000;106:655–62.
128. Bauer R, Hudson J, Muller HD, Sommer C, Dekomien G, Bourke J, Routledge D, Bushby K, Klepper J, Straub V. Does delta-sarcoglycan-associated autosomal-dominant cardiomyopathy exist? Eur J Hum Genet. 2009;17:1148–53.
129. Olson TM, Illenberger S, Kishimoto NY, Huttelmaier S, Keating MT, Jockusch BM. Metavinculin mutations alter actin interaction in dilated cardiomyopathy. Circulation. 2002;105:431–7.
130. Zhang M, Chen J, Si D, Zheng Y, Jiao H, Feng Z, Hu Z, Duan R. Whole exome sequencing identifies a novel EMD mutation in a Chinese family with dilated cardiomyopathy. BMC Med Genet. 2014;15:77.
131. Fatkin D, MacRae C, Sasaki T, Wolff MR, Porcu M, Frenneaux M, Atherton J, Vidaillet HJ Jr, Spudich S, De Girolami U, Seidman JG, Seidman C, Muntoni F, Muehle G, Johnson W, McDonough B. Missense mutations in the rod domain of the Lamin A/C gene as causes of dilated cardiomyopathy and conduction-system disease. N Engl J Med. 1999;341:1715–24.
132. Parks SB, Kushner JD, Nauman D, Burgess D, Ludwigsen S, Peterson A, Li D, Jakobs P, Litt M, Porter CB, Rahko PS, Hershberger RE. Lamin A/C mutation analysis in a cohort of 324 unrelated patients with idiopathic or familial dilated cardiomyopathy. Am Heart J. 2008;156:161–9.
133. Cowan J, Li D, Gonzalez-Quintana J, Morales A, Hershberger RE. Morphological analysis of 13 LMNA variants identified in a cohort of 324 unrelated patients with idiopathic or familial dilated cardiomyopathy. Circ Cardiovasc Genet. 2010;3:6–14.
134. Raharjo WH, Enarson P, Sullivan T, Stewart CL, Burke B. Nuclear envelope defects associated with LMNA mutations cause dilated cardiomyopathy and Emery-Dreifuss muscular dystrophy. J Cell Sci. 2001;114:4447–57.
135. Haywood AF, Merner ND, Hodgkinson KA, Houston J, Syrris P, Booth V, Connors S, Pantazis A, Quarta G, Elliott P, McKenna W, Young TL. Recurrent missense mutations in TMEM43 (ARVD5) due to founder effects cause arrhythmogenic cardiomyopathies in the UK and Canada. Eur Heart J. 2013;34:1002–11.
136. Taylor MR, Slavov D, Gajewski A, Vlcek S, Ku L, Fain PR, Carniel E, Di Lenarda A, Sinagra G, Boucek MM, Cavanaugh J, Graw SL, Ruegg P, Feiger J, Zhu X, Ferguson DA, Bristow MR, Gotzmann J, Foisner R, Mestroni L, Familial Cardiomyopathy Registry Research G. Thymopoietin (lamina-associated polypeptide 2) gene mutation associated with dilated cardiomyopathy. Hum Mutat. 2005;26:566–74.
137. Gotic I, Leschnik M, Kolm U, Markovic M, Haubner BJ, Biadasiewicz K, Metzler B, Stewart CL, Foisner R. Lamina-associated polypeptide 2alpha loss impairs heart function and stress response in mice. Circ Res. 2010;106:346–53.
138. Schonberger J, Wang L, Shin JT, Kim SD, Depreux FF, Zhu H, Zon L, Pizard A, Kim JB, Macrae CA, Mungall AJ, Seidman JG, Seidman CE. Mutation in the transcriptional coactivator EYA4 causes dilated cardiomyopathy and sensorineural hearing loss. Nat Genet. 2005;37:418–22.
139. Theis JL, Sharpe KM, Matsumoto ME, Chai HS, Nair AA, Theis JD, de Andrade M, Wieben ED, Michels VV, Olson TM. Homozygosity mapping and exome sequencing reveal GATAD1 mutation in autosomal recessive dilated cardiomyopathy. Circ Cardiovasc Genet. 2011;4:585–94.
140. Yang J, Shah S, Olson TM, Xu X. Modeling GATAD1-associated dilated cardiomyopathy in adult Zebrafish. J Cardiovasc Dev Dis. 2016;3:6.
141. Hanley A, Walsh KA, Joyce C, McLellan MA, Clauss S, Hagen A, Shea MA, Tucker NR, Lin H, Fahy GJ, Ellinor PT. Mutation of a

common amino acid in NKX2.5 results in dilated cardiomyopathy in two large families. BMC Med Genet. 2016;17:83.
142. Xu JH, Gu JY, Guo YH, Zhang H, Qiu XB, Li RG, Shi HY, Liu H, Yang XX, Xu YJ, Qu XK, Yang YQ. Prevalence and spectrum of NKX2-5 mutations associated with sporadic adult-onset dilated cardiomyopathy. Int Heart J. 2017;58:521–9.
143. Yuan F, Qiu XB, Li RG, Qu XK, Wang J, Xu YJ, Liu X, Fang WY, Yang YQ, Liao DN. A novel NKX2-5 loss-of-function mutation predisposes to familial dilated cardiomyopathy and arrhythmias. Int J Mol Med. 2015;35:478–86.
144. Arndt AK, Schafer S, Drenckhahn JD, Sabeh MK, Plovie ER, Caliebe A, Klopocki E, Musso G, Werdich AA, Kalwa H, Heinig M, Padera RF, Wassilew K, Bluhm J, Harnack C, Martitz J, Barton PJ, Greutmann M, Berger F, Hubner N, Siebert R, Kramer HH, Cook SA, MacRae CA, Klaassen S. Fine mapping of the 1p36 deletion syndrome identifies mutation of PRDM16 as a cause of cardiomyopathy. Am J Hum Genet. 2013;93:67–77.
145. Long PA, Evans JM, Olson TM. Diagnostic yield of whole exome sequencing in pediatric dilated cardiomyopathy. J Cardiovasc Dev Dis. 2017;4:11.
146. Brauch KM, Karst ML, Herron KJ, de Andrade M, Pellikka PA, Rodeheffer RJ, Michels VV, Olson TM. Mutations in ribonucleic acid binding protein gene cause familial dilated cardiomyopathy. J Am Coll Cardiol. 2009;54:930–41.
147. Li D, Morales A, Gonzalez-Quintana J, Norton N, Siegfried JD, Hofmeyer M, Hershberger RE. Identification of novel mutations in RBM20 in patients with dilated cardiomyopathy. Clin Transl Sci. 2010;3:90–7.
148. van den Hoogenhof MMG, Beqqali A, Amin AS, van der Made I, Aufiero S, Khan MAF, Schumacher CA, Jansweijer JA, van Spaendonck-Zwarts KY, Remme CA, Backs J, Verkerk AO, Baartscheer A, Pinto YM, Creemers EE. RBM20 mutations induce an arrhythmogenic dilated cardiomyopathy related to disturbed calcium handling. Circulation. 2018;138(13):1330–42.
149. Refaat MM, Lubitz SA, Makino S, Islam Z, Frangiskakis JM, Mehdi H, Gutmann R, Zhang ML, Bloom HL, MacRae CA, Dudley SC, Shalaby AA, Weiss R, McNamara DM, London B, Ellinor PT. Genetic variation in the alternative splicing regulator RBM20 is associated with dilated cardiomyopathy. Heart Rhythm. 2012;9:390–6.
150. Wells QS, Becker JR, Su YR, Mosley JD, Weeke P, D'Aoust L, Ausborn NL, Ramirez AH, Pfotenhauer JP, Naftilan AJ, Markham L, Exil V, Roden DM, Hong CC. Whole exome sequencing identifies a causal RBM20 mutation in a large pedigree with familial dilated cardiomyopathy. Circ Cardiovasc Genet. 2013;6:317–26.
151. Mittal A, Sharma R, Prasad R, Bahl A, Khullar M. Role of cardiac TBX20 in dilated cardiomyopathy. Mol Cell Biochem. 2016;414:129–36.
152. Qian L, Mohapatra B, Akasaka T, Liu J, Ocorr K, Towbin JA, Bodmer R. Transcription factor neuromancer/TBX20 is required for cardiac function in Drosophila with implications for human heart disease. Proc Natl Acad Sci U S A. 2008;105:19833–8.
153. Bienengraeber M, Olson TM, Selivanov VA, Kathmann EC, O'Cochlain F, Gao F, Karger AB, Ballew JD, Hodgson DM, Zingman LV, Pang YP, Alekseev AE, Terzic A. ABCC9 mutations identified in human dilated cardiomyopathy disrupt catalytic KATP channel gating. Nat Genet. 2004;36:382–7.
154. Amin AS. SCN5A-related dilated cardiomyopathy: what do we know? Heart Rhythm. 2014;11:1454–5.
155. Cheng J, Morales A, Siegfried JD, Li D, Norton N, Song J, Gonzalez-Quintana J, Makielski JC, Hershberger RE. SCN5A rare variants in familial dilated cardiomyopathy decrease peak sodium current depending on the common polymorphism H558R and common splice variant Q1077del. Clin Transl Sci. 2010;3:287–94.
156. Ge J, Sun A, Paajanen V, Wang S, Su C, Yang Z, Li Y, Wang S, Jia J, Wang K, Zou Y, Gao L, Wang K, Fan Z. Molecular and clinical characterization of a novel SCN5A mutation associated with atrioventricular block and dilated cardiomyopathy. Circ Arrhythm Electrophysiol. 2008;1:83–92.
157. Mann SA, Castro ML, Ohanian M, Guo G, Zodgekar P, Sheu A, Stockhammer K, Thompson T, Playford D, Subbiah R, Kuchar D, Aggarwal A, Vandenberg JI, Fatkin D. R222Q SCN5A mutation is associated with reversible ventricular ectopy and dilated cardiomyopathy. J Am Coll Cardiol. 2012;60:1566–73.
158. Mazzaccara C, Limongelli G, Petretta M, Vastarella R, Pacileo G, Bonaduce D, Salvatore F, Frisso G. A common polymorphism in the SCN5A gene is associated with dilated cardiomyopathy. J Cardiovasc Med (Hagerstown). 2018;19:344–50.
159. McNair WP, Ku L, Taylor MR, Fain PR, Dao D, Wolfel E, Mestroni L, Familial Cardiomyopathy Registry Research G. SCN5A mutation associated with dilated cardiomyopathy, conduction disorder, and arrhythmia. Circulation. 2004;110:2163–7.
160. Shen C, Xu L, Yang Z, Zou Y, Hu K, Fan Z, Ge J, Sun A. A1180V of cardiac sodium channel gene (SCN5A): is it a risk factor for dilated cardiomyopathy or just a common variant in Han Chinese? Dis Markers. 2013;35:531–5.
161. Levitas A, Muhammad E, Harel G, Saada A, Caspi VC, Manor E, Beck JC, Sheffield V, Parvari R. Familial neonatal isolated cardiomyopathy caused by a mutation in the flavoprotein subunit of succinate dehydrogenase. Eur J Hum Genet. 2010;18:1160–5.
162. Man E, Lafferty KA, Funke BH, Lun KS, Chan SY, Chau AK, Chung BH. NGS identifies TAZ mutation in a family with X-linked dilated cardiomyopathy. BMJ Case Rep. 2013;2013:bcr2012007529.
163. Bione S, D'Adamo P, Maestrini E, Gedeon AK, Bolhuis PA, Toniolo D. A novel X-linked gene, G4.5. is responsible for Barth syndrome. Nat Genet. 1996;12:385–9.
164. D'Adamo P, Fassone L, Gedeon A, Janssen EA, Bione S, Bolhuis PA, Barth PG, Wilson M, Haan E, Orstavik KH, Patton MA, Green AJ, Zammarchi E, Donati MA, Toniolo D. The X-linked gene G4.5 is responsible for different infantile dilated cardiomyopathies. Am J Hum Genet. 1997;61:862–7.
165. Sibbing D, Pfeufer A, Perisic T, Mannes AM, Fritz-Wolf K, Unwin S, Sinner MF, Gieger C, Gloeckner CJ, Wichmann HE, Kremmer E, Schafer Z, Walch A, Hinterseer M, Nabauer M, Kaab S, Kastrati A, Schomig A, Meitinger T, Bornkamm GW, Conrad M, von Beckerath N. Mutations in the mitochondrial thioredoxin reductase gene TXNRD2 cause dilated cardiomyopathy. Eur Heart J. 2011;32:1121–33.
166. Balmer C, Ballhausen D, Bosshard NU, Steinmann B, Boltshauser E, Bauersfeld U, Superti-Furga A. Familial X-linked cardiomyopathy (Danon disease): diagnostic confirmation by mutation analysis of the LAMP2gene. Eur J Pediatr. 2005;164:509–14.
167. Gourzi P, Pantou MP, Gkouziouta A, Kaklamanis L, Tsiapras D, Zygouri C, Constantoulakis P, Adamopoulos S, Degiannis D. A new phenotype of severe dilated cardiomyopathy associated with a mutation in the LAMP2 gene previously known to cause hypertrophic cardiomyopathy in the context of Danon disease. Eur J Med Genet. 2018;62(1):77–80.
168. Taylor MR, Ku L, Slavov D, Cavanaugh J, Boucek M, Zhu X, Graw S, Carniel E, Barnes C, Quan D, Prall R, Lovell MA, Mierau G, Ruegg P, Mandava N, Bristow MR, Towbin JA, Mestroni L, Familial Cardiomyopathy R. Danon disease presenting with dilated cardiomyopathy and a complex phenotype. J Hum Genet. 2007;52:830–5.
169. Lefeber DJ, de Brouwer AP, Morava E, Riemersma M, Schuurs-Hoeijmakers JH, Absmanner B, Verrijp K, van den Akker WM, Huijben K, Steenbergen G, van Reeuwijk J, Jozwiak A, Zucker N, Lorber A, Lammens M, Knopf C, van Bokhoven H, Grunewald S, Lehle L, Kapusta L, Mandel H, Wevers RA. Autosomal recessive dilated cardiomyopathy due to DOLK mutations results

from abnormal dystroglycan O-mannosylation. PLoS Genet. 2011;7:e1002427.
170. Fish M, Shaboodien G, Kraus S, Sliwa K, Seidman CE, Burke MA, Crotti L, Schwartz PJ, Mayosi BM. Mutation analysis of the phospholamban gene in 315 South Africans with dilated, hypertrophic, peripartum and arrhythmogenic right ventricular cardiomyopathies. Sci Rep. 2016;6:22235.
171. Young HS, Ceholski DK, Trieber CA. Deception in simplicity: hereditary phospholamban mutations in dilated cardiomyopathy. Biochem Cell Biol. 2015;93:1–7.
172. Lee TM, Addonizio LJ, Chung WK. Dilated cardiomyopathy due to a phospholamban duplication. Cardiol Young. 2014;24:953–4.
173. van der Zwaag PA, van Rijsingen IA, Asimaki A, Jongbloed JD, van Veldhuisen DJ, Wiesfeld AC, Cox MG, van Lochem LT, de Boer RA, Hofstra RM, Christiaans I, van Spaendonck-Zwarts KY, Lekanne dit Deprez RH, Judge DP, Calkins H, Suurmeijer AJ, Hauer RN, Saffitz JE, Wilde AA, van den Berg MP, van Tintelen JP. Phospholamban R14del mutation in patients diagnosed with dilated cardiomyopathy or arrhythmogenic right ventricular cardiomyopathy: evidence supporting the concept of arrhythmogenic cardiomyopathy. Eur J Heart Fail. 2012;14:1199–207.
174. Posch MG, Perrot A, Geier C, Boldt LH, Schmidt G, Lehmkuhl HB, Hetzer R, Dietz R, Gutberlet M, Haverkamp W, Ozcelik C. Genetic deletion of arginine 14 in phospholamban causes dilated cardiomyopathy with attenuated electrocardiographic R amplitudes. Heart Rhythm. 2009;6:480–6.
175. Medin M, Hermida-Prieto M, Monserrat L, Laredo R, Rodriguez-Rey JC, Fernandez X, Castro-Beiras A. Mutational screening of phospholamban gene in hypertrophic and idiopathic dilated cardiomyopathy and functional study of the PLN -42 C>G mutation. Eur J Heart Fail. 2007;9:37–43.
176. DeWitt MM, MacLeod HM, Soliven B, McNally EM. Phospholamban R14 deletion results in late-onset, mild, hereditary dilated cardiomyopathy. J Am Coll Cardiol. 2006;48:1396–8.
177. Schmitt JP, Kamisago M, Asahi M, Li GH, Ahmad F, Mende U, Kranias EG, MacLennan DH, Seidman JG, Seidman CE. Dilated cardiomyopathy and heart failure caused by a mutation in phospholamban. Science. 2003;299:1410–3.
178. Bhuiyan ZA, van den Berg MP, van Tintelen JP, Bink-Boelkens MT, Wiesfeld AC, Alders M, Postma AV, van Langen I, Mannens MM, Wilde AA. Expanding spectrum of human RYR2-related disease: new electrocardiographic, structural, and genetic features. Circulation. 2007;116:1569–76.
179. Gerull B, Kirchner F, Chong JX, Tagoe J, Chandrasekharan K, Strohm O, Waggoner D, Ober C, Duff HJ. Homozygous founder mutation in desmocollin-2 (DSC2) causes arrhythmogenic cardiomyopathy in the Hutterite population. Circ Cardiovasc Genet. 2013;6:327–36.
180. Posch MG, Posch MJ, Geier C, Erdmann B, Mueller W, Richter A, Ruppert V, Pankuweit S, Maisch B, Perrot A, Buttgereit J, Dietz R, Haverkamp W, Ozcelik C. A missense variant in desmoglein-2 predisposes to dilated cardiomyopathy. Mol Genet Metab. 2008;95:74–80.
181. Garcia-Pavia P, Syrris P, Salas C, Evans A, Mirelis JG, Cobo-Marcos M, Vilches C, Bornstein B, Segovia J, Alonso-Pulpon L, Elliott PM. Desmosomal protein gene mutations in patients with idiopathic dilated cardiomyopathy undergoing cardiac transplantation: a clinicopathological study. Heart. 2011;97:1744–52.
182. Rampazzo A, Nava A, Malacrida S, Beffagna G, Bauce B, Rossi V, Zimbello R, Simionati B, Basso C, Thiene G, Towbin JA, Danieli GA. Mutation in human desmoplakin domain binding to plakoglobin causes a dominant form of arrhythmogenic right ventricular cardiomyopathy. Am J Hum Genet. 2002;71:1200–6.
183. Yang Z, Bowles NE, Scherer SE, Taylor MD, Kearney DL, Ge S, Nadvoretskiy VV, DeFreitas G, Carabello B, Brandon LI, Godsel LM, Green KJ, Saffitz JE, Li H, Danieli GA, Calkins H, Marcus F, Towbin JA. Desmosomal dysfunction due to mutations in desmoplakin causes arrhythmogenic right ventricular dysplasia/cardiomyopathy. Circ Res. 2006;99:646–55.
184. Krishnamurthy S, Adhisivam B, Hamilton RM, Baskin B, Biswal N, Kumar M. Arrhythmogenic dilated cardiomyopathy due to a novel mutation in the desmoplakin gene. Indian J Pediatr. 2011;78:866–9.
185. Norgett EE, Hatsell SJ, Carvajal-Huerta L, Cabezas JC, Common J, Purkis PE, Whittock N, Leigh IM, Stevens HP, Kelsell DP. Recessive mutation in desmoplakin disrupts desmoplakin-intermediate filament interactions and causes dilated cardiomyopathy, woolly hair and keratoderma. Hum Mol Genet. 2000;9:2761–6.
186. Ramoglu MG, Ucar T, Ceylaner S, Atalay S, Tutar E. A novel mutation in the desmoplakin gene in two female siblings with a rare form of dilated cardiomyopathy: Carvajal syndrome. Anatol J Cardiol. 2017;18:435–6.
187. Pluess M, Daeubler G, Dos Remedios CG, Ehler E. Adaptations of cytoarchitecture in human dilated cardiomyopathy. Biophys Rev. 2015;7:25–32.
188. Klauke B, Gaertner-Rommel A, Schulz U, Kassner A, Zu Knyphausen E, Laser T, Kececioglu D, Paluszkiewicz L, Blanz U, Sandica E, van den Bogaerdt AJ, van Tintelen JP, Gummert J, Milting H. High proportion of genetic cases in patients with advanced cardiomyopathy including a novel homozygous Plakophilin 2-gene mutation. PLoS One. 2017;12:e0189489.
189. Arimura T, Ishikawa T, Nunoda S, Kawai S, Kimura A. Dilated cardiomyopathy-associated BAG3 mutations impair Z-disc assembly and enhance sensitivity to apoptosis in cardiomyocytes. Hum Mutat. 2011;32:1481–91.
190. Chami N, Tadros R, Lemarbre F, Lo KS, Beaudoin M, Robb L, Labuda D, Tardif JC, Racine N, Talajic M, Lettre G. Nonsense mutations in BAG3 are associated with early-onset dilated cardiomyopathy in French Canadians. Can J Cardiol. 2014;30:1655–61.
191. Fang X, Bogomolovas J, Wu T, Zhang W, Liu C, Veevers J, Stroud MJ, Zhang Z, Ma X, Mu Y, Lao DH, Dalton ND, Gu Y, Wang C, Wang M, Liang Y, Lange S, Ouyang K, Peterson KL, Evans SM, Chen J. Loss-of-function mutations in co-chaperone BAG3 destabilize small HSPs and cause cardiomyopathy. J Clin Invest. 2017;127:3189–200.
192. Feldman AM, Begay RL, Knezevic T, Myers VD, Slavov DB, Zhu W, Gowan K, Graw SL, Jones KL, Tilley DG, Coleman RC, Walinsky P, Cheung JY, Mestroni L, Khalili K, Taylor MR. Decreased levels of BAG3 in a family with a rare variant and in idiopathic dilated cardiomyopathy. J Cell Physiol. 2014;229:1697–702.
193. Fernlund E, Osterberg AW, Kuchinskaya E, Gustafsson M, Jansson K, Gunnarsson C. Novel genetic variants in BAG3 and TNNT2 in a Swedish family with a history of dilated cardiomyopathy and sudden cardiac death. Pediatr Cardiol. 2017;38:1262–8.
194. Franaszczyk M, Bilinska ZT, Sobieszczanska-Malek M, Michalak E, Sleszycka J, Sioma A, Malek LA, Kaczmarska D, Walczak E, Wlodarski P, Hutnik L, Milanowska B, Dzielinska Z, Religa G, Grzybowski J, Zielinski T, Ploski R. The BAG3 gene variants in Polish patients with dilated cardiomyopathy: four novel mutations and a genotype-phenotype correlation. J Transl Med. 2014;12:192.
195. Myers VD, Gerhard GS, McNamara DM, Tomar D, Madesh M, Kaniper S, Ramsey FV, Fisher SG, Ingersoll RG, Kasch-Semenza L, Wang J, Hanley-Yanez K, Lemster B, Schwisow JA, Ambardekar AV, Degann SH, Bristow MR, Sheppard R, Alexis JD, Tilley DG, Kontos CD, McClung JM, Taylor AL, Yancy CW, Khalili K, Seidman JG, Seidman CE, McTiernan CF, Cheung JY, Feldman AM. Association of variants in BAG3 with cardiomyopathy outcomes in African American individuals. JAMA Cardiol. 2018;3(10):929–38.

196. Norton N, Li D, Rieder MJ, Siegfried JD, Rampersaud E, Zuchner S, Mangos S, Gonzalez-Quintana J, Wang L, McGee S, Reiser J, Martin E, Nickerson DA, Hershberger RE. Genome-wide studies of copy number variation and exome sequencing identify rare variants in BAG3 as a cause of dilated cardiomyopathy. Am J Hum Genet. 2011;88:273–82.
197. Hou D, Chen Y, Liu J, Xu L, Zhang Z, Zhang J, Wang H, Wang X, Chen J, Zhao R, Hu A, Hakonarson H, Zhang L, Shen Y. Proteomics screen to reveal molecular changes mediated by C722G missense mutation in CHRM2 gene. J Proteome. 2013;89:39–50.
198. Zhang L, Hu A, Yuan H, Cui L, Miao G, Yang X, Wang L, Liu J, Liu X, Wang S, Zhang Z, Liu L, Zhao R, Shen Y. A missense mutation in the CHRM2 gene is associated with familial dilated cardiomyopathy. Circ Res. 2008;102:1426–32.
199. Brody MJ, Hacker TA, Patel JR, Feng L, Sadoshima J, Tevosian SG, Balijepalli RC, Moss RL, Lee Y. Ablation of the cardiac-specific gene leucine-rich repeat containing 10 (Lrrc10) results in dilated cardiomyopathy. PLoS One. 2012;7:e51621.
200. Brody MJ, Lee Y. The role of leucine-rich repeat containing protein 10 (LRRC10) in dilated cardiomyopathy. Front Physiol. 2016;7:337.
201. Qu XK, Yuan F, Li RG, Xu L, Jing WF, Liu H, Xu YJ, Zhang M, Liu X, Fang WY, Yang YQ, Qiu XB. Prevalence and spectrum of LRRC10 mutations associated with idiopathic dilated cardiomyopathy. Mol Med Rep. 2015;12:3718–24.
202. Woon MT, Long PA, Reilly L, Evans JM, Keefe AM, Lea MR, Beglinger CJ, Balijepalli RC, Lee Y, Olson TM, Kamp TJ. Pediatric dilated cardiomyopathy-associated LRRC10 (leucine-rich repeat-containing 10) variant reveals LRRC10 as an auxiliary subunit of cardiac L-type Ca(2+) channels. J Am Heart Assoc. 2018;7(3):e006428.
203. Dhandapany PS, Razzaque MA, Muthusami U, Kunnoth S, Edwards JJ, Mulero-Navarro S, Riess I, Pardo S, Sheng J, Rani DS, Rani B, Govindaraj P, Flex E, Yokota T, Furutani M, Nishizawa T, Nakanishi T, Robbins J, Limongelli G, Hajjar RJ, Lebeche D, Bahl A, Khullar M, Rathinavel A, Sadler KC, Tartaglia M, Matsuoka R, Thangaraj K, Gelb BD. RAF1 mutations in childhood-onset dilated cardiomyopathy. Nat Genet. 2014;46:635–9.
204. Disse S, Abergel E, Berrebi A, Houot A, Le Heuzey J, Diebold B, Guize L, Carpentier A, Corvol P, Jeunemaitre X. Mapping of a first locus for autosomal dominant myxomatous mitral-valve prolapse to chromosome 16p11.2-p12.1. Am J Hum Genet. 1999;65:1242–51.
205. Kelly MA, Caleshu C, Morales A, Buchan J, Wolf Z, Harrison SM, Cook S, Dillon MW, Garcia J, Haverfield E, JDH J, Macaya D, Manrai A, Orland K, Richard G, Spoonamore K, Thomas M, Thomson K, Vincent LM, Walsh R, Watkins H, Whiffin N, Ingles J, van Tintelen JP, Semsarian C, Ware JS, Hershberger R, Funke B. Adaptation and validation of the ACMG/AMP variant classification framework for MYH7-associated inherited cardiomyopathies: recommendations by ClinGen's inherited cardiomyopathy expert panel. Genet Med. 2018;20:351–9.
206. Almomani R, Verhagen JM, Herkert JC, Brosens E, van Spaendonck-Zwarts KY, Asimaki A, van der Zwaag PA, Frohn-Mulder IM, Bertoli-Avella AM, Boven LG, van Slegtenhorst MA, van der Smagt JJ, Van IWF, Timmer B, van Stuijvenberg M, Verdijk RM, Saffitz JE, du Plessis FA, Michels M, Hofstra RM, Sinke RJ, van Tintelen JP, Wessels MW, Jongbloed JD, van de Laar IM. Biallelic truncating mutations in ALPK3 cause severe pediatric cardiomyopathy. J Am Coll Cardiol. 2016;67:515–25.
207. Pugh TJ, Kelly MA, Gowrisankar S, Hynes E, Seidman MA, Baxter SM, Bowser M, Harrison B, Aaron D, Mahanta LM, Lakdawala NK, McDermott G, White ET, Rehm HL, Lebo M, Funke BH. The landscape of genetic variation in dilated cardiomyopathy as surveyed by clinical DNA sequencing. Genet Med. 2014;16:601–8.
208. Ouellette AC, Mathew J, Manickaraj AK, Manase G, Zahavich L, Wilson J, George K, Benson L, Bowdin S, Mital S. Clinical genetic testing in pediatric cardiomyopathy: is bigger better? Clin Genet. 2018;93:33–40.
209. Caforio A, Stewart J, McKenna W. Idiopathic dilated cardiomyopathy. BMJ. 1990;300:890–1.
210. Leiden J. The genetics of dilated cardiomyopathy--emerging clues to the puzzle. N Engl J Med. 1997;337:1080–1.
211. Rehm HL, Berg JS, Brooks LD, Bustamante CD, Evans JP, Landrum MJ, Ledbetter DH, Maglott DR, Martin CL, Nussbaum RL, Plon SE, Ramos EM, Sherry ST, Watson MS. ClinGen, ClinGen--the clinical genome resource. N Engl J Med. 2015;372:2235–42.
212. Richards S, Aziz N, Bale S, Bick D, Das S, Gastier-Foster J, Grody WW, Hegde M, Lyon E, Spector E, Voelkerding K, Rehm HL, Committee ALQA. Standards and guidelines for the interpretation of sequence variants: a joint consensus recommendation of the American College of Medical Genetics and Genomics and the Association for Molecular Pathology. Genet Med. 2015;17:405–24.
213. van Rijsingen IA, van der Zwaag PA, Groeneweg JA, Nannenberg EA, Jongbloed JD, Zwinderman AH, Pinto YM, Dit Deprez RH, Post JG, Tan HL, de Boer RA, Hauer RN, Christiaans I, van den Berg MP, van Tintelen JP, Wilde AA. Outcome in phospholamban R14del carriers: results of a large multicentre cohort study. Circ Cardiovasc Genet. 2014;7:455–65.
214. Zaragoza MV, Brandon MC, Diegoli M, Arbustini E, Wallace DC. Mitochondrial cardiomyopathies: how to identify candidate pathogenic mutations by mitochondrial DNA sequencing, MITOMASTER and phylogeny. Eur J Hum Genet. 2011;19:200–7.
215. Caforio AL, Marcolongo R, Jahns R, Fu M, Felix SB, Iliceto S. Immune-mediated and autoimmune myocarditis: clinical presentation, diagnosis and management. Heart Fail Rev. 2013;18:715–32.
216. Maisch B. Alcoholic cardiomyopathy : the result of dosage and individual predisposition. Herz. 2016;41:484–93.
217. Shakir DK, Rasul KI. Chemotherapy induced cardiomyopathy: pathogenesis, monitoring and management. J Clin Med Res. 2009;1:8–12.
218. Arany Z. Understanding peripartum cardiomyopathy. Annu Rev Med. 2018;69:165–76.
219. Koenig T, Hilfiker-Kleiner D, Bauersachs J. Peripartum cardiomyopathy. Herz. 2018;43(5):431–7.
220. Holloway CJ, Dass S, Suttie JJ, Rider OJ, Cox P, Cochlin LE, Jackson H, Fast AM, Johnson AW, Karamitsos TD, Neubauer S, Clarke K. Exercise training in dilated cardiomyopathy improves rest and stress cardiac function without changes in cardiac high energy phosphate metabolism. Heart. 2012;98:1083–90.
221. Pelliccia A, Culasso F, Di Paolo FM, Maron BJ. Physiologic left ventricular cavity dilatation in elite athletes. Ann Intern Med. 1999;130:23–31.
222. Fairweather D, Cooper LT Jr, Blauwet LA. Sex and gender differences in myocarditis and dilated cardiomyopathy. Curr Probl Cardiol. 2013;38:7–46.
223. Ware JS, Amor-Salamanca A, Tayal U, Govind R, Serrano I, Salazar-Mendiguchia J, Garcia-Pinilla JM, Pascual-Figal DA, Nunez J, Guzzo-Merello G, Gonzalez-Vioque E, Bardaji A, Manito N, Lopez-Garrido MA, Padron-Barthe L, Edwards E, Whiffin N, Walsh R, Buchan RJ, Midwinter W, Wilk A, Prasad S, Pantazis A, Baski J, O'Regan DP, Alonso-Pulpon L, Cook SA, Lara-Pezzi E, Barton PJ, Garcia-Pavia P. Genetic etiology for alcohol-induced cardiac toxicity. J Am Coll Cardiol. 2018;71:2293–302.
224. Akinrinade O, Alastalo TP, Koskenvuo JW. Relevance of truncating titin mutations in dilated cardiomyopathy. Clin Genet. 2016;90:49–54.

225. Akinrinade O, Koskenvuo JW, Alastalo TP. Prevalence of titin truncating variants in general population. PLoS One. 2015;10:e0145284.
226. Burkett EL, Hershberger RE. Clinical and genetic issues in familial dilated cardiomyopathy. J Am Coll Cardiol. 2005;45:969–81.
227. Baig MK, Goldman JH, Caforio AL, Coonar AS, Keeling PJ, McKenna WJ. Familial dilated cardiomyopathy: cardiac abnormalities are common in asymptomatic relatives and may represent early disease. J Am Coll Cardiol. 1998;31:195–201.
228. Mahon NG, Murphy RT, MacRae CA, Caforio AL, Elliott PM, McKenna WJ. Echocardiographic evaluation in asymptomatic relatives of patients with dilated cardiomyopathy reveals preclinical disease. Ann Intern Med. 2005;143:108–15.

Arrhythmogenic Cardiomyopathy

6

Moniek G. P. J. Cox, Anneline S. J. M. te Riele, and Richard N. W. Hauer

Introduction

Arrhythmogenic Cardiomyopathy (ACM) is a progressive heart muscle disease characterized histologically by fibrofatty replacement of ventricular myocardium. It is relatively rare, affecting approximately 1 in 1000 to 1 in 5000 people. Patients typically present with ventricular arrhythmias between the second and fourth decades of life. In early stages, ventricular arrhythmias originating from the right ventricle (RV) are most prominent, whereas usually in later stages, structural and functional abnormalities occur, eventually leading to heart failure. In all stages, ACM can be the cause of sudden death. However, sudden death most frequently occurs in adolescence, mainly in athletes. From autopsy studies, it is known that massive amounts of fibrofatty tissue can replace large parts of normal myocardium even in young teenagers (Fig. 6.1).

The largest subcategory of ACM is arrhythmogenic right ventricular cardiomyopathy (ARVC), in which the right ventricle is primarily involved [1–3]. Overt left ventricular (LV) involvement occurs in the later stages of this typical ARVC pattern [4]. Subforms of ACM with early biventricular or primarily LV involvement have also been described [4]. In addition, immunohistochemical analysis of human myocardial samples demonstrated that on a molecular (desmosomal) level, both ventricles are affected by the disease in all clinical subtypes [5]. Therefore, the term ACM is favored as a more appropriate terminology than ARVD, ARVC, ARVD/C, and ARVC/D. However, these terms are still being used by many authors, especially to denote the typical forms with apparently predominant RV involvement. All subforms of ACM are, similarly as classical ARVC, characterized by fibrofatty alteration, and are associated with ventricular arrhythmias.

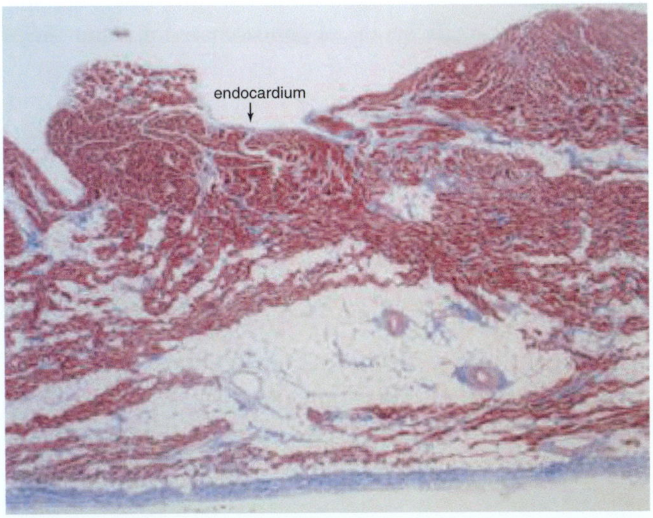

Fig. 6.1 Histology of right ventricle of a 13-year-old girl who died suddenly during exercise. AZAN staining (×400) with cardiac myocytes (red), collagen (blue), and adipocytes (*white*). Shown is the typical pattern of ACM with strands of fibrosis reaching all the way to the endocardium. Bundles of cardiac myocytes are embedded in between the fibrotic strands, particularly in the subendocardial layers. These interconnecting bundles of myocytes give rise to activation delay and reentrant circuits, the typical electrophysiologic substrate for ventricular arrhythmias in ACM

The first series of ACM patients was published in 1982, when it was called a disease in which "the right ventricular musculature is partially or totally absent and is replaced by fatty and fibrous tissue" [1]. At that time, the disease was thought to be a defect in RV development, was therefore classified as a "dysplasia" and called ARVD. In the years since then, increased insight into the development of the disease as well as the discovery of pathogenic mutations involved led to the current concept of ACM as a genetically determined "cardiomyopathy" [3, 6].

The molecular genetic era provided new insights into the pathophysiologic mechanism underlying ACM. The first disease-causing mutation was discovered in patients with the ACM subtype Naxos disease [7]. These patients carried an

Moniek G. P. J. Cox (✉) · Anneline S. J. M. te Riele
R. N. W. Hauer
Department of Cardiology, University Medical Center Utrecht, Utrecht, The Netherlands

Netherlands Heart Institute, Utrecht, The Netherlands

H. F. Baars et al. (eds.), *Clinical Cardiogenetics*, https://doi.org/10.1007/978-3-030-45457-9_6

autosomal recessive mutation in the gene encoding the desmosomal protein Plakoglobin (*JUP*). Its discovery pointed out research in the direction of other desmosomal genes. Desmosomes are proteins important for cell–cell adhesion and interaction, as will be discussed later on in more detail. Until 2004, evidence for genes underlying the autosomal dominantly inherited ACM had been very limited, with three genes and six loci being identified [8–16]. The Desmoplakin gene (*DSP*) was the first desmosomal protein gene mutation to be associated with the autosomal dominant form of ACM [16]. It was followed by the discovery of pathogenic mutations in desmosomal protein-encoding genes Plakophilin-2 (*PKP2*), Desmoglein-2 (*DSG2*), and Desmocollin-2 (*DSC2*) [17–19].

There are small series of autosomal dominant ACM being caused by mutations in non-desmosomal protein-encoding genes, such as genes encoding the cardiac ryanodine receptor (*RyR2*), the transforming growth factor-β3 gene (*TGFβ3*), and transmembrane protein 43 (*TMEM43*) [14, 15, 20]. In the Netherlands, a founder mutation in the gene encoding phospholamban (*PLN*) appears to be associated with a specific form of biventricular ACM [21]. In addition, pathogenic mutations in the genes encoding desmin (*DES*), Lamins A and C (*LMNA*), Titin (*TTN*), αT-catenin (*CTNNA3*), and Cadherin2 (*CDH2*), which binds plakophilin, have been identified in patients with a clinical diagnosis of ACM [22–25]. However, the causality of this last group of mutations to ACM is not always proven, specifically for *TTN* variants. Currently, mutations are discovered in up to 60% of ACM patients, mainly in desmosomal genes. In a cohort of more than 1000 ACM patients from The Netherlands and North America, *PKP2* mutations where the most prevalent, accounting for approximately 40% of pathogenic mutations [26].

Etiology/Pathophysiology: Theory of Desmosomal Dysfunction

Since pathogenic mutations in ACM patients are frequently found in genes encoding desmosomal proteins, hypotheses on the pathophysiologic mechanism underlying the disease are predominantly based on desmosomal dysfunction.

Together with adherens junctions and gap junctions, desmosomes form the intercalated disks. Intercalated disks enable the functional and structural integrity of cardiac myocytes and are located between cardiac myocytes at their longitudinal ends. Desmosomes are important for cell–cell adhesion and are predominantly found in tissues that experience mechanical stress: the heart and epidermis. They couple cytoskeletal elements to the plasma membrane at cell–cell adhesions. Desmosomes also protect other components of the intercalated disk from mechanical stress and are involved in structural organization of the intercalated disk. Figure 6.2 schematically represents the organization of the various proteins in the cardiac desmosome.

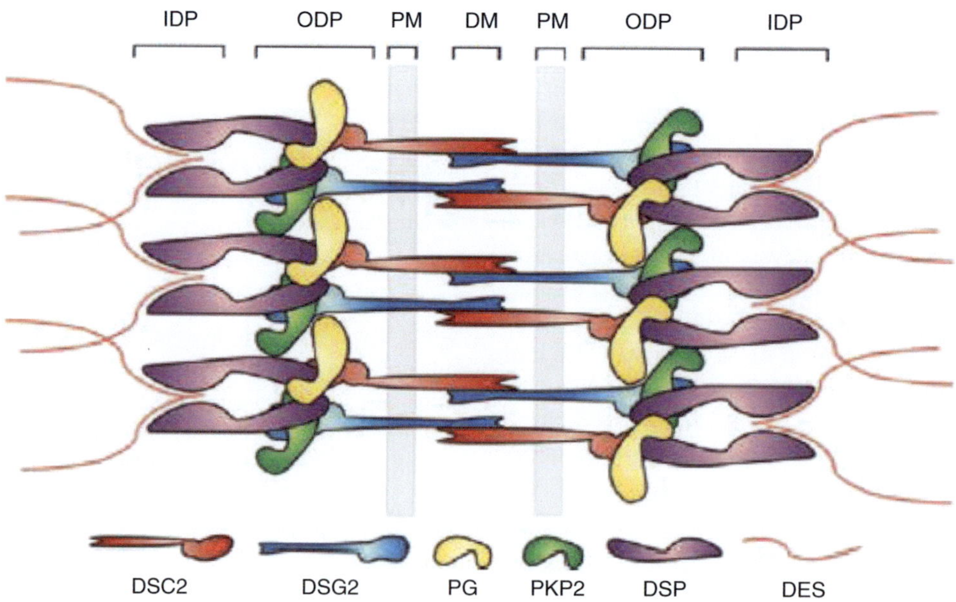

Fig. 6.2 Schematic representation of the molecular organization of cardiac desmosomes. The plasma membrane (PM) spanning proteins desmocollin-2 (DSC2) and desmoglein-2 (DSG2) interact in the extracellular space at the dense midline (DM). At the cytoplasmic side, they interact with plakoglobin (PG) and plakophilin-2 (PKP2) at the outer dense plaque (ODP). PKP2 and PG interact also with desmoplakin (DSP). At the inner dense plaque (IDP), the C-terminus of DSP anchors the intermediate filament desmin (DES). (Reprint with permission from Van Tintelen et al. Curr Opin Cardiol 2007)

Although the functions of different parts of the intercalated disk seem clear, the exact mechanism through which the mutations of desmosomal protein genes exactly cause disease remains to be elucidated. Various hypotheses, all based on the different functions of desmosomes, have been proposed.

First of all, genetic defects in a desmosomal protein are thought to lead to impairment in mechanical function provoking detachment of myocytes at the intercalated disks, particularly under the condition of mechanical stress (like that occurring during competitive sports activity). Such defective mechanical connection followed by mechanical and electrical uncoupling of cardiomyocytes leads to cell death with fibrofatty replacement. Interconnecting bundles of surviving myocardium embedded in the fibrofatty tissue lead to lengthening of conduction pathways (Fig. 6.1), and load mismatch. This results in marked activation delay, which is the pivotal mechanism for reentry and thereby ventricular tachycardia (VT). Previous invasive electrophysiologic studies have, by various mapping techniques, confirmed that sustained VT in patients with ACM is due to reentry circuits in areas of abnormal myocardium [27]. In this structural model, environmental factors such as exercise or inflammation from viral infection could aggravate impaired adhesion and accelerate disease progression. The right ventricle might be more vulnerable to disease than the left because of its thinner walls and its normal dilatory response to exercise.

Second, basic studies have shown that impairment of cell–cell adhesion due to changes in desmosomal components may affect amount and distribution of other intercalated disk proteins, including connexin43, the major protein-forming gap junctions in the ventricular myocardium [28, 29]. This was shown for DSP and JUP, but alterations in other desmosomal components such as PKP2, DSG2, and DSC2 are thought to have similar effects. Changes in number and function of gap junctions will diminish intercellular electrical coupling. This may contribute to intraventricular activation delay and the substrate for reentry.

The third hypothesis involves the canonical Wnt/β-catenin signaling pathway. Plakoglobin can localize both to the plasma membrane and the nucleus. It was demonstrated that disruption of desmoplakin frees plakoglobin from the plasma membrane allowing it to translocate to the nucleus and suppress canonical Wnt/β-catenin signaling. Suppression of Wnt signaling by plakoglobin nuclear localization could promote the differentiation to adipose tissue in the cardiac myocardium in patients with ACM [30].

Finally, redistribution of Nav1.5 due to reduced transportation of the channel toward the intercalated disk cell membrane appeared to be related to reduced PKP2 [31].

Clinical Presentation

ACM patients typically present between the second and fourth decade of life with VT originating from the right ventricle. However, in a minority of cases of sudden death, frequently already at a young age, is the first disease manifestation [32–34].

Classical Form of ACM, Also Defined as ARVC

Based on pathologic and patient follow-up studies, four different disease phases have been described for the classical form of ACM, which primarily affects the RV (Table 6.1).

1. Concealed phase in which clinical findings are frequently absent, although minor ventricular arrhythmias and subtle structural changes may be found. Although patients tend to be asymptomatic, they may nonetheless be at risk of sudden death, mainly during intense exercise.
2. The overt phase in which patients suffer from palpitations, syncope, and ventricular arrhythmias originating from the RV, ranging from isolated ventricular premature complexes to sustained VT and ventricular fibrillation (VF).
3. The third phase is characterized by RV failure due to progressive loss of myocardium with severe dilatation and systolic dysfunction, in the presence of preserved LV function.
4. Biventricular failure occurs due to LV involvement. This phase may mimic dilated cardiomyopathy (DCM) and may require cardiac transplantation.

Besides ventricular involvement, as indicated by histopathologic and macroscopic morphological as well as ventricular arrhythmias, the atria of the heart seem the be involved as well. A recent study demonstrated that compared

Table 6.1 Different phases of disease severity

Phase	Characteristics
1. Concealed	Asymptomatic patients with possibly only minor ventricular arrhythmia and subtle structural changes
	However, risk of sudden death
2. Overt	Symptoms due to LBBB VT or multiple premature complexes, with more obvious structural RV abnormalities
3. RV failure	With relatively preserved LV function
4. Biventricular	Significant overt LV involvement

LBBB left bundle branch block, *VT* ventricular tachycardia, *RV* right ventricle, *LV* left ventricle to healthy controls, patients with ARVC have enlarged atria with decreased function on functional cardiac magnetic resonance examination. RA and LA parameters predicted the incidence of atrial arrhythmias after adjusting for clinical and ventricular characteristics, which suggests atrial involvement in ARVC.

Other Forms of ACM

In the initially described classical form of ARVC, the RV is primarily affected with possibly (in a later stage) LV involvement. Two additional distinct patterns of disease have been identified by clinicogenetic characterization of families. These are the left dominant phenotype (also referred to as "left dominant arrhythmogenic cardiomyopathy," LDAC), with early and predominant LV manifestations as frequently seen in *DSP* mutation carriers, and the biventricular phenotype with equal involvement of both ventricles as seen in *TMEM43* and *PLN* mutation carriers.

Naxos Disease

All patients who homozygously carry the recessive *JUP* mutation for Naxos disease have diffuse palmoplantar keratosis and woolly hair in infancy [7]. Children usually have no cardiac symptoms, but may have ECG abnormalities and nonsustained ventricular arrhythmias [35]. The cardiac disease is 100% penetrant by adolescence, with symptomatic arrhythmias, ECG abnormalities, right ventricular structural alterations, and/or LV involvement. In one series of 26 patients followed for 10 years, 62% had structural progression of right ventricular abnormalities, and 27% developed heart failure due to LV involvement. Almost half of the patients developed symptomatic arrhythmias and the annual mortality rate was 5.3%, which is slightly higher than seen in autosomal dominant forms of classic ARVC. A minority of heterozygotes have minor ECG and structural changes, but clinically significant disease is not present.

Carvajal Syndrome

Carvajal syndrome is associated with a *DSP* gene mutation and is also a recessive disease manifested by woolly hair, epidermolytic palmoplantar keratoderma, and cardiomyopathy [36]. First patients diagnosed came from Ecuador. The cardiomyopathy part of Carvajal syndrome was first thought to be mainly left ventricular, mimicking dilated cardiomyopathy. A number of patients with Carvajal syndrome suffered from heart failure in their teenage years, resulting in early morbidity. However, further research revealed that it is characterized mainly by ventricular hypertrophy, ventricular dilatation, and discrete focal ventricular aneurysms. In the right ventricle, in particular, focal wall thinning and aneurysmal dilatation were identified in the triangle of dysplasia.

Clinical Diagnosis

Diagnosis of ACM can be very challenging and can only be made when all other diseases causing VT episodes and structural RV/LV abnormalities have been ruled out (see section on differential diagnosis). VF and sudden death may be the first manifestations of ACM, occurring especially in young patients (under 30 years of age). However, symptomatic ARVC patients present with sustained monomorphic VT with left bundle branch block morphology, thus originating from the RV, in the third or fourth decade of life. First disease presentation before the age of 11 years, as well as after the age of 65 is very rare [34]. The occurrence of VT episodes is usually driven by adrenergic stimulation and starts mainly during exercise or in the early recovery phase after exercise, especially during competitive endurance sports [37]. ACM is a disease that shows progression over time [38].

The gold standard for ACM diagnosis is the demonstration of fibrofatty replacement primarily of RV myocardium, determined at biopsy, surgery, or postmortem. Originally, predilection sites for these structural abnormalities were thought to be in the so-called triangle of dysplasia formed by the RV outflow tract (RVOT), the apex, and the subtricuspid region [1]. However, these observations were made mainly in patients with advanced overt disease. Recently, evidence was obtained that the disease process starts in the subepicardial layers of the subtricuspid area, or in the posterolateral LV wall. The RV apical area was only affected in advanced stages [39]. Endomyocardial biopsies can provide myocardium for histologic examination. However, biopsies have major limitations. Tissue sampling from the affected RV free wall is associated with a risk of perforation since this wall is usually thin, especially in ARVC patients. Sampling from the interventricular septum is relatively safe. However, the septum is histopathologically rarely affected in less advanced ACM stages. In addition, even in potentially affected areas, histology may be classified as normal because of the focal nature of the lesions. Finally, ACM starts in subepicardial and midmyocardial areas. Subendocardial layers are usually not affected in an early stage of the disease. Therefore, histologic diagnosis may be hampered by the nontransmural nature of endomyocardial biopsies. However, septal endomyocardial biopsy may be useful to diagnose cardiac sarcoid, a common differential diagnosis of ACM.

Since it is usually too hard to obtain material for histologic analysis, a set of clinically applicable criteria has been established for ACM diagnosis. These criteria were defined by a Task Force in 1994, and revised in 2010 [40, 41]. These consensus-based international Task Force Criteria (TFC) are considered the essential standard for clinical diagnosis worldwide. They include six different groups of clinical criteria:

Global or regional RV dysfunction and structural alterations, tissue characteristics, repolarization abnormalities, depolarization abnormalities, arrhythmias, and family history/genetics. Within these groups, diagnostic criteria were assigned major or minor according to their specificity for the disease. Every major criterion is scored as two points and every minor as one point. In total, four points have to be scored in order to fulfill ACM diagnosis, i.e., two major, one major plus two minor, or four minor criteria. From each different group, only one criterion can be counted for diagnosis, even when multiple criteria in one group are being fulfilled. These 2010 TFC are listed in Table 6.2. It should be kept in mind that these TFC are grafted on classical ARVC with pre-

Table 6.2 Diagnostic Task Force Criteria

2010 Task Force Criteria for ARVC Diagnosis[a]	
I. Global or regional dysfunction and structural alterations	*Major:* • By 2D echo. – Regional RV akinesia, dyskinesia, or aneurysm. – And one of the following (end diastole): PLAX RVOT ≥32 mm (corrected for body size [PLAX/BSA] ≥19 mm/m^2), PSAX ≥ 36 mm (corrected for body size (PSAX/BSA) ≥21 mm/m^2, or fractional area change ≤33%. • By MRI. – Regional RV akinesia or dyskinesia or dyssynchronous RV contraction. – And one of the following: ratio of RVEDV to BSA ≥110 mL/m^2 (male) or ≥ 100 mL/m^2 (female), or RV ejection fraction ≤40%. • By RV cine-angiography. – Regional RV akinesia, dyskinesia, or aneurysm. *Minor:* • By 2D echo. – Regional RV akinesia or dyskinesia. – And one of the following (end diastole): PLAX RVOT ≥29 mm to <32 mm (corrected for body size [PLAX/BSA] ≥16 mm/m^2 to <19 mm/m^2), PSAX ≥32 mm to <36 mm (corrected for body size (PSAX/BSA) ≥18 mm/m^2 to <21 mm/m^2, or fractional area change >33 to ≤40%. • By MRI. – Regional RV akinesia or dyskinesia or dyssynchronous RV contraction. – And one of the following: ratio of RVEDV to BSA ≥100 mL/m^2 to <110 mL/m^2 (male) or ≥ 90 mL/m^2 to <100 mL/m^2 (female), or RV ejection fraction >40 to ≤45%.
II. Tissue characterization of wall	*Major:* • Residual myocytes <60% by morphometric analysis (or <50% if estimated), with fibrous replacement of the RV free wall myocardium in ≥1 sample, with or without fatty replacement of tissue on endomyocardial biopsy. *Minor:* • Residual myocytes 60–75% by morphometric analysis (or 50–65% if estimated), with fibrous replacement of the RV free wall myocardium in ≥1 sample, with or without fatty replacement of tissue on endomyocardial biopsy.
III. Repolarization abnormalities	*Major:* • Inverted T waves in right precordial leads (V1, V2, V3) or beyond in individuals >14 years of age. *Minor:* • Inverted T waves in leads V1 and V2 in individuals >14 years of age or in V4, V5, V6. • Inverted T waves in leads V1, V2, V3, and V4 in individuals >14 years of age in the presence of complete right bundle branch block.
IV. Depolarization/conduction abnormalities	*Major:* • Epsilon wave (reproducible low-amplitude signals after the end of the QRS complex to onset of the T wave) in right precordial leads (V1, V2, V3). *Minor:* • Late potentials by SAECG in ≥1 of 3 parameters in the absence of QRS duration of ≥110 ms on the standard ECG. • Filtered QRS duration (fQRS) ≥114 ms. • Duration of terminal QRS <40 uV (low-amplitude signal duration) ≥38 ms. • Root mean square voltage of terminal 40 ms ≤20 uV. • Terminal activation duration ≥55 ms measured from the nadir of the S wave to the end of all depolarization deflections, including R', in V1, V2, or V3 in the absence of complete right bundle branch block.
V. Arrhythmias	*Major:* • Nonsustained or sustained ventricular tachycardia of left bundle branch block morphology with superior axis (negative or indeterminate QRS in leads II, III, and aVF and positive in lead aVL). *Minor:* • Nonsustained or sustained ventricular tachycardia of RVOT configuration, left bundle branch block morphology with inferior axis (positive QRS in II, III, and aVF and negative in aVL) or of unknown axis. • > 500 ventricular extrasystoles per 24 h (Holter).

(continued)

Table 6.2 (continued)

2010 Task Force Criteria for ARVC Diagnosis[a]	
VI. Family History	*Major:* • ACM confirmed in a first-degree relative who meets current TFC. • ACM confirmed pathologically at autopsy or surgery in a first-degree relative. • Identification of a pathogenic mutation categorized as associated or probably associated with ACM in the patient under evaluation.
	Minor: • History of ACM in a first- degree relative in whom it is not possible or practical to determine whether the family member meets current TFC. • Premature sudden death (<35 years of age) due to suspected ACM in a first-degree relative. • ACM confirmed pathologically or by current TFC in second-degree relative.

[a]These in 2010 revised criteria focus on classic arrhythmogenic right ventricular cardiomyopathy, although negative T waves in left precordial leads indicate left ventricular disease. *MRI* magnetic resonance imaging, *PLAX* parasternal long axis, *PSAX* parasternal short axis, *BSA* body surface area, *RV* right ventricle, *RVEDV* right ventricular end-diastolic volume, *SAECG* signal-averaged ECG, *ACM* arrhythmogenic cardiomyopathy, *TFC* task force criteria

dominant RV disease. In left-dominant ACM, however, their applicability may be hampered by absence of LV imaging and VT morphology criteria.

Specific examinations are recommended in all patients suspected of ACM. In all patients suspected of ACM, the following methods should be used at least: history and family history, physical examination, 12-lead ECG, 24 h Holter monitoring, exercise testing, and at least one imaging method, including magnetic resonance imaging (MRI) or transthoracic 2D-echocardiography with quantitative wall motion analysis. Since MRI combined with late gadolinium enhancement allows visualization of tissue alterations, as well as evaluation of morphology and function in a single investigation, this technique is particularly useful in ACM workup. In addition, imaging of tissue alteration is particularly useful in predominant LV disease with underestimation of TFC fulfillment. Because of non-unambiguous interpretation of the signal-averaged ECG (SAECG), this technique is questionable for ACM diagnosis and not universally used. Eventually, invasive tests are also available for diagnostic purposes: endomyocardial biopsy, RV cineangiography, and electrophysiologic testing. The next paragraphs give detailed information about the various diagnostic aspects summarized in Table 6.2.

ECG Criteria

Criteria on ECG changes have to be determined in sinus rhythm, and while off anti-arrhythmic drugs. ECG changes are detected in the large majority of ACM patients.

Depolarization Abnormalities

As explained above, RV activation delay is a hallmark of ACM. This delay is conveyed by the criteria of epsilon waves or prolonged terminal activation duration (TAD) in V1–3, and late potentials on signal-averaged ECG.

Epsilon waves are defined as low amplitude potentials after and clearly separated from the QRS complex, in at least one of V1–3 (Fig. 6.3) [42]. This highly specific major criterion is observed in only a small minority of patients, usually in advanced stages of the disease [43, 44]. In addition, recording of an epsilon wave is often questionable because of interpretation difficulties related to defining the end of the QRS complex and filter settings [45]. Of note, once epsilon waves are present, typically other (ECG) abnormalities are present and the diagnosis does not depend on epsilon waves by itself. TAD is defined from the nadir of the S-wave to the end of all depolarization deflections in V1–3, thereby covering all forms of RV activation delay, including epsilon waves [46]. TAD is considered prolonged when ≥55 ms. (Fig. 6.4) Since prolonged TAD is less specific for ACM, it counts as a minor criterion. Prolonged TAD can be present at early disease stages such as in non-symptomatic family members carrying a pathogenic mutation. Since both criteria are obtained from V1–3, predominantly delay in the RV outflow tract will be recorded. Thus, in the early stage of ACM with exclusively subtricuspid or LV involvement these criteria may be absent.

The detection of late potentials on SAECG is the surface counterpart of delayed activation or late potentials detected during mapping in electrophysiologic studies. They are frequently found in patients with documented VT. However, these late potentials can also be observed after myocardial infarction and other structural heart diseases. Due to this lack of specificity, it is considered a minor criterion. For all criteria on depolarization abnormalities, it is apparent that their finding will correlate with disease severity. For instance, a positive correlation has been found between late potentials and the extent of RV fibrosis, reduced RV systolic function, and significant morphological abnormalities on imaging [47–51].

Repolarization Abnormalities

Negative T-waves in leads V1–3 or beyond, in the absence of right bundle branch block (RBBB) are a major ECG criterion on repolarization abnormalities (see Fig. 6.3). They are the most frequently observed criterion. In the initial series reported by Marcus et al., this was detected in over 85% of

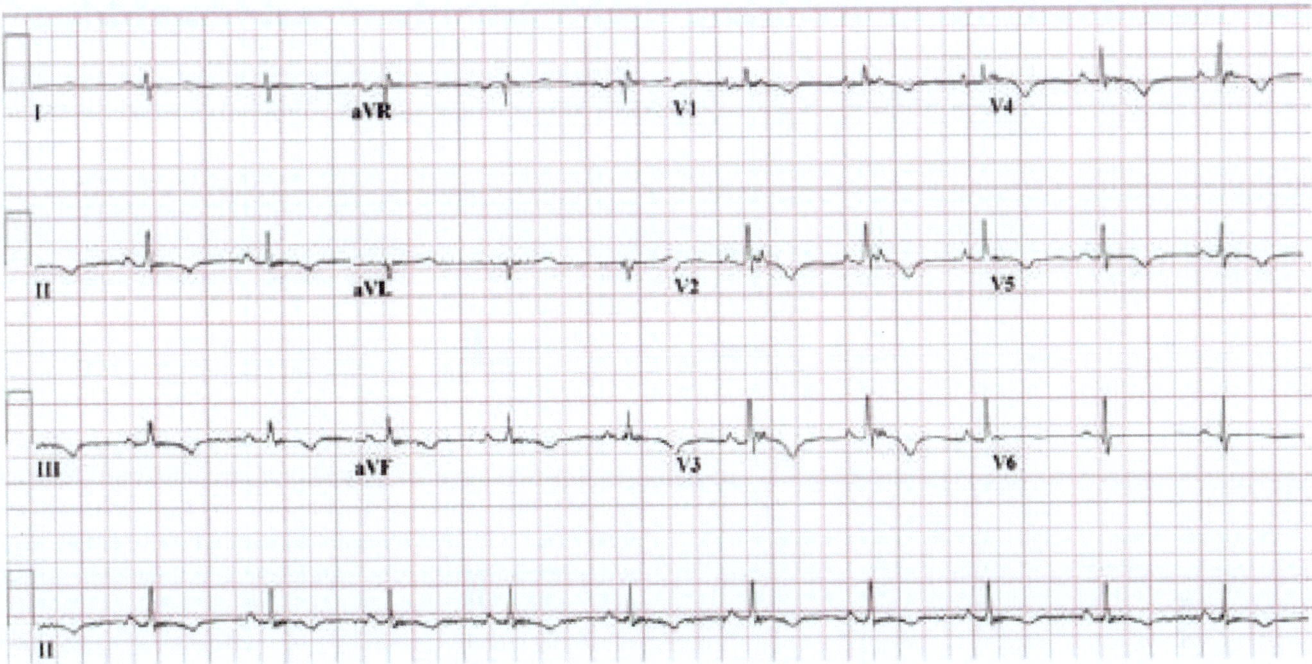

Fig. 6.3 Epsilon waves visible as late positive deflections in between the QRS complex and the T-wave in V1–3, and negative T-waves in V1–5. In addition, the terminal activation duration (TAD) is clearly prolonged

cases. Subsequent studies have reported variable prevalence of right precordial T-wave inversion, ranging from 19 to 94% [40, 43]. The lower percentages are often due to the evaluation of family members, while higher ones are seen in series consisting of unrelated index patients. T-wave inversion can be a normal feature of the ECG in children and early adolescence. Therefore, this finding is not considered pathogenic in persons aged 14 years and younger. Negative T-waves only in V1–2 are less specific for ACM and counted as a minor criterion. This is supposed to be a normal finding in women and people from African descent.

Although these negative T-waves were observed consistently in a series of evaluated ACM patients, T-wave inversions in the right precordial leads can also be observed in 1–3% of the healthy population aged 19–45 years, and in patients with RV overload, such as major pulmonary embolism and intracardial left to right shunt, or may develop following intracranial hemorrhage as a sign of adrenergic response to the cerebral insult.

In patients with RBBB, negative T-waves are common in V1–3. However, the presence of T-wave inversions in V4 or beyond is not physiologic even in the presence of complete RBBB, and thus considered as a minor criterion for ACM [52]. To facilitate fulfillment of ACM diagnosis in patients with LV involvement, recording of negative T-waves in V4-6 is also a minor criterion.

Arrhythmias

Ventricular arrhythmias range from premature ventricular complexes (PVCs) to sustained VT and VF [46, 52]. Because of the origin in the RV, QRS complexes of ventricular arrhythmias usually show a left bundle branch block (LBBB) morphology. Moreover, the QRS axis gives an indication of the VT origin, i.e., superior axis from the RV inferior wall, frequently the subtricuspid area, and inferior axis from the RV outflow tract (see Fig. 6.5). Since VT originating in the RV outflow tract is often idiopathic and benign, its occurrence in the setting of ACM gives only a minor criterion. On the contrary, a VT with LBBB morphology and superior axis is more specific for ACM and thus a major criterion. Patients with extensively affected RV may show multiple VT morphologies. LV involvement may give rise to VT with RBBB morphology (not part of 2010 TFC) [46].

VF is the mechanism of sudden death especially occurring in young people and athletes with ACM, who were often previously asymptomatic. In this subset of patients, VF may occur from deterioration of rapid monomorphic VT, or in a phase of acute disease progression, due to acute myocyte death and reactive inflammation [3]. In a recent study, the median age of presentation with SCD sudden cardiac death versus monomorphic VT in ACM was only 23 years and 36 years, respectively, suggesting a different arrhythmogenic mechanism [32].

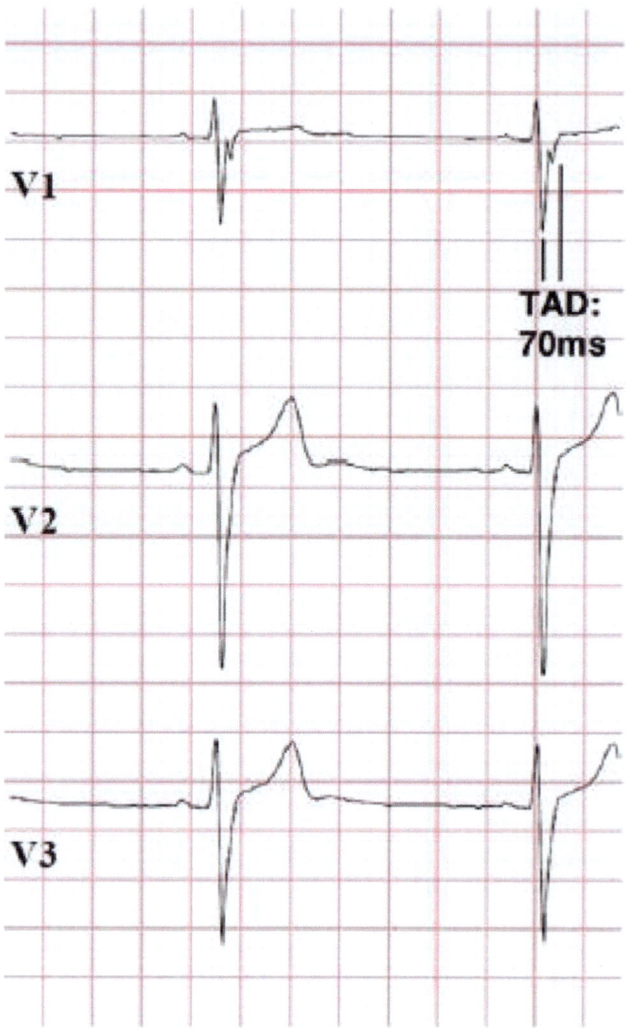

Fig. 6.4 Prolonged terminal activation duration (≥55 ms from nadir of S-wave to end of depolarization)

Global and/or Regional Dysfunction and Structural Alterations

Structural alterations can be evaluated by several imaging modalities, including echocardiography, cardiac magnetic resonance (CMR), and/or cineangiography. A detailed description of the pros and cons of these modalities for ACM evaluation is beyond the scope of this chapter and reviewed elsewhere [53]. In brief, the 2010 TFC grant major and minor criteria for echocardiography and CMR, which are defined by regional wall motion abnormalities (akinesia, dyskinesia, or aneurysm) combined with functional parameters (RV function and dilatation) (see Fig. 6.6). It is important to note that only akinesia (lack of motion), dyskinesia (systolic outward bulging), and aneurysms (both systolic and diastolic bulging) are considered to be diagnostic as wall motion abnormalities. Hypokinesia is not used anymore because of variable interpretation. Gadolinium late enhancement for tissue alteration analysis is not part of the current 2010 TFC, given the lack of specificity for ACM diagnosis [41]. As for cineangiography, RV wall motion abnormalities (dyskinesia, akinesia, or aneurysm) observed in at least two projections may also grant a major TFC. However, given the very suitable noninvasive alternatives, angiography is not routinely used and MRI (CMR) is the current gold standard for RV evaluation. While CT may be used to obtain additional information and rule out differentials, it is not included in the current TFC, given the lack of clinical studies investigating its value in ACM diagnosis.

Echocardiography is noninvasive, widely used, and often serves as the first-line imaging technique in evaluating patients suspected of ACM. Accurate evaluation of the RV by echocardiography, however, requires considerable expertise, since its complex geometry area complicates accurate interpretation. This may lead to over- as well as underdiagnosis of individuals with subtle structural disease [54]. With new echocardiographic modalities, such as three-dimensional echocardiography, deformation imaging, and tissue Doppler, sensitivity and specificity of echocardiography have increased, but these novel modalities are not included in the 2010 TFC yet.

CMR is an interesting technique for ACM evaluation, since it is multiplane, allows for morphologic and functional evaluation, but also has the unique possibility of visualizing the myocardium to characterize tissue composition. CMR serves as the gold standard for deriving RV volumes and function. However, MRI is expensive and not widely available and requires considerable expertise to prevent mis- or overdiagnosis of ACM [55]. Also, in ICD-carrying patients, this technique cannot always be applied. Cardiac MRI appears to be the most common cause of overdiagnosis of ACM, and physicians should therefore be very reluctant to diagnose ACM when structural abnormalities are only present on CMR [56, 57]. Furthermore, it is important to note that the presence of fat in the epi- and midmyocardial layers (without fibrosis) is often a nonspecific finding, sometimes referred to as cor adiposum, and should not be considered diagnostic of ACM.

Tissue Characterization

The gold standard for ACM diagnosis is the demonstration of fibrofatty replacement. Myocardial tissue for histologic examination is usually obtained by endomyocardial biopsy, autopsy, or from explanted hearts. However, for reasons outlined earlier, undirected endomyocardial biopsies are infrequently diagnostic. It had been included as a major criterion by the 2010 TFC since the finding of fibrofatty replacement was considered to strongly support any findings derived from other clinical investigations. The rather vague terminology of any “fibrofatty replacement of myocardium” has been quantified in the revised TFC. Diagnostic values according to the 2010 TFC are considered major if histomorphometric analysis of endomyocardial biopsies shows that the number

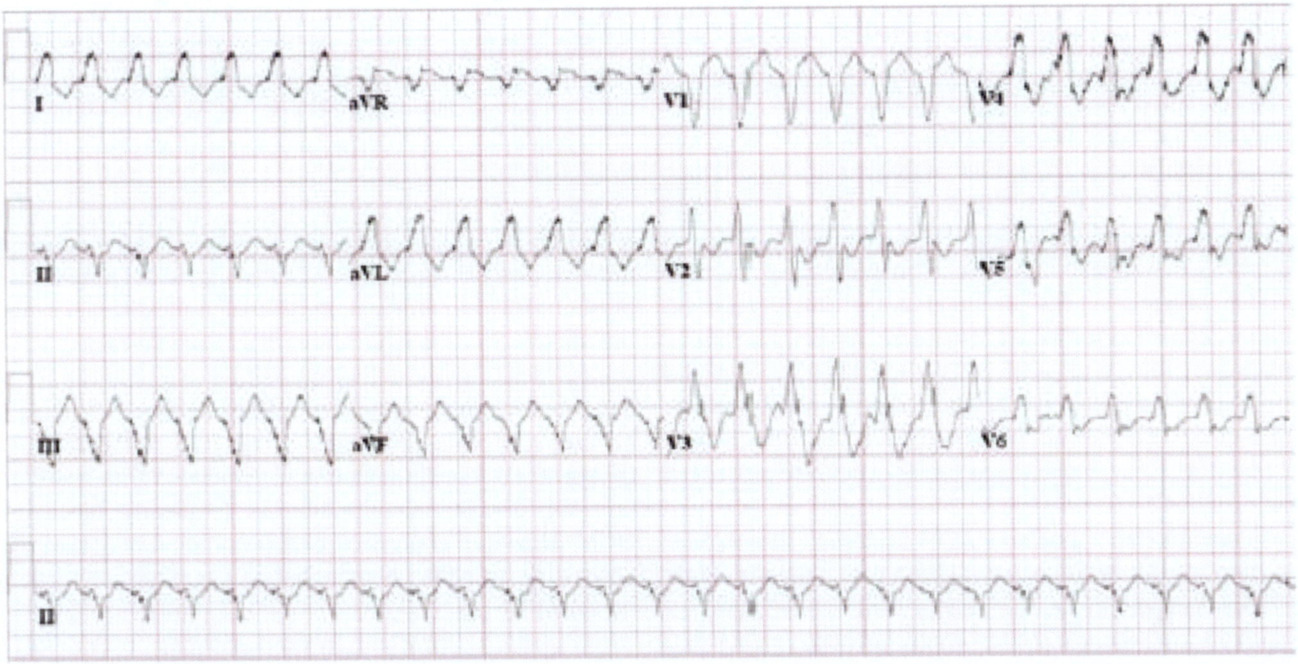

Fig. 6.5 ECG (25 mm/s) from a patient with classical arrhythmogenic right ventricular cardiomyopathy harboring a plakophilin-2 (*PKP2*) mutation. This ventricular tachycardia has an LBBB morphology and superior axis, thus originates from the inferior aspect of the right ventricle

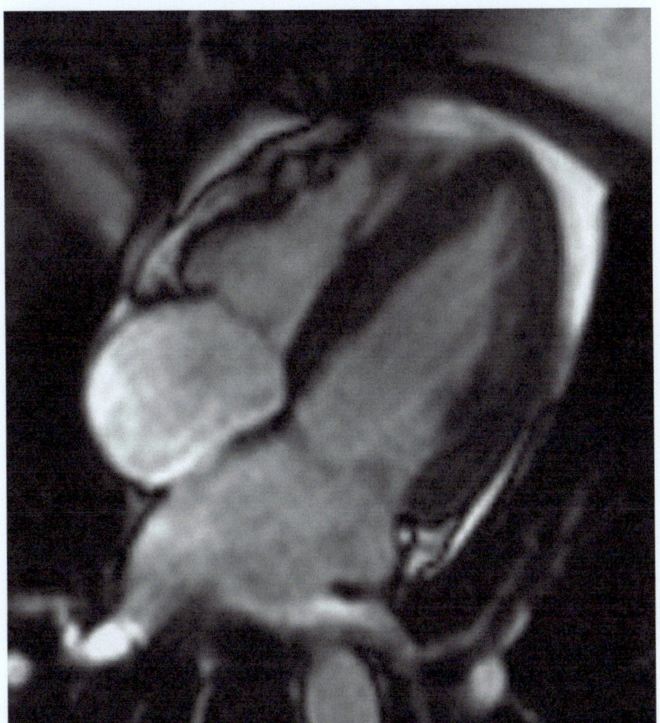

Fig. 6.6 Magnetic resonance imaging in a patient with arrhythmogenic right ventricular cardiomyopathy (*ARVC*) at the end of systole. Dyskinetic bulgings are clearly visible in the right ventricle free wall

of residual myocytes is below 60% or below 50% by estimation, with fibrous replacement of the RV-free wall in at least one sample, with or without fatty tissue replacement [58]. If the number of residual myocytes is higher but still below 75% (morphometric) or below 65% (estimated), only a minor criterion is fulfilled.

Family History

Already before the discovery of pathogenic mutations underlying the disease, it was recognized that ACM often runs in families. Having a family member with proven ACM is considered an increased risk for other family members to be affected. Therefore, having a first-degree relative who meets the 2010 TFC or who has ACM confirmed pathologically at autopsy or during surgery, or identification of a pathogenic mutation in the patient under evaluation, is included as a major diagnostic criterion. If there is a history of a first-degree relative being diagnosed with ACM, but it cannot be verified whether he or she does fulfill the 2010 TFC, only a minor criterion is counted. SCD of a family member under the age of 35 years, presumably but not proven to be due to ACM, is also a minor criterion [41].

Differential Diagnosis

Although diagnosis in an overt case of ACM is often not difficult, early and occasionally late stages of the disease may show similarities with other diseases. Especially differentiation from *idiopathic VT originating from the RV outflow tract* (RVOT) can be challenging. However, idiopathic RVOT VT is a benign nonfamilial condition, in which the ECG shows no depolarization or repolarization abnormalities, and no RV structural changes can be detected. Furthermore, VT episodes have a single morphology (LBBB morphology with inferior axis) and are usually not inducible by premature extrastimuli at programmed stimulation during electrophysiologic studies, since the mechanism of RVOT VT is abnormal automaticity or triggered activity [59, 60]. Thus, idiopathic RVOT VT may be inducible by regular burst pacing and isoproterenol infusion. It is important to differentiate idiopathic RVOT VT from ACM for several reasons. First, ACM has a known genetic etiology, which is not the case for idiopathic RVOT VT. Therefore, it has implications with regard to screening of family members. Second, the prognosis of idiopathic RVOT tachycardia is usually excellent with SCD occurring extremely rarely. Finally, in contrast to ACM, catheter ablation is usually a curative procedure in idiopathic RVOT VT.

Another disease mimicking ACM is *cardiac sarcoidosis*. Sarcoidosis is an inflammatory disease with unknown etiology, characterized by the presence of noncaseating granulomas in affected tissues; mainly lungs, but heart, skin, eyes, the reticuloendothelial system, kidneys, and central nervous system can also be affected. Cases in which only the heart seemed affected by the disease have been described. The prevalence of this condition varies in geographical regions (high prevalence in Japan), and the disease may also be familial and occurring in specific racial subgroups [61]. Clinical symptoms of cardiac involvement are present in approximately 5% of all patients with sarcoidosis.

Patients can present with clinical features similar to those of ACM including arrhythmias and SCD. One study that evaluated parameters that distinguish ACM from sarcoidosis showed that older age of symptom onset, presence of cardiovascular comorbidities, nonfamilial pattern of disease, PR interval prolongation, high-grade atrioventricular block, significant left ventricular dysfunction, myocardial delayed enhancement of the septum, and mediastinal lymphadenopathy should raise the suspicion for cardiac sarcoidosis. Cardiac sarcoidosis can only be diagnosed definitively by endomyocardial biopsy, when granulomas are visualized [62]. To strengthen differentiation from ACM, gadolinium-enhanced MRI may be beneficial by detecting located abnormalities in the septum, which is typical for sarcoidosis, but seldomly seen in ACM. Active foci of sarcoidosis can be visualized by positron emission tomography (PET) scan [63]. Therapy with corticosteroids is recommended for patients with a clear diagnosis of cardiac sarcoidosis. Treatment aims to control inflammation and fibrosis in order to maintain cardiac structure and function.

Also, any other form of *myocarditis* has to be excluded before diagnosis of ACM can be made. Myocarditis may arise from viral or other pathogenic exposure as well as toxic or immunologic insult. Cardiac MRI (particularly MRI with T2-weighted imaging) may be useful to visualize tissue edema, which is present in myocarditis but not in ACM. However, in general, endomyocardial biopsy is required to distinguish ACM from myocarditis. Some reports have suggested an overlap between ACM and viral myocarditis, rendering this differential diagnosis extremely difficult to exclude [64].

Especially in more advanced stages of the disease, when LV ejection fraction drops below 50%, ACM may mimic *dilated cardiomyopathy* (DCM). Patients with DCM usually present with heart failure or thromboembolic disease, including stroke. Since it is uncommon to have sustained VT or sudden death as the initial presenting symptom of DCM, patients with these symptoms should be first suspected of having ACM. Since in particular the *PLN* c.40_42delAGA (p.Arg14del) founder mutation is associated with heart failure, the disease manifestation is frequently labeled as DCM. However, expression of this mutation may start with ventricular arrhythmias years before hemodynamic deterioration [65].

Molecular Diagnosis

First of all, it has to be explicitly mentioned that ACM diagnosis cannot be made on results of DNA analysis only, as indicated in the paragraph on clinical diagnosis. Finding a pathogenic mutation in genes linked to ACM may only contribute as one major criterion of the 2010 TFC and most importantly guide cascade screening of the family.

Two patterns of inheritance have been described in ACM. The most common or classical form of ACM (i.e., ARVC) is inherited as an autosomal dominant trait. The rare Naxos disease and Carvajal syndrome are usually inherited autosomal recessively, although autosomal dominant forms have been described in these cardio-cutaneous syndromes. Table 6.3 summarizes the different genes involved in ACM with the corresponding phenotypes.

Autosomal Recessive ACM

In Naxos disease, the affected individuals were found to be homozygous for a 2 base pair deletion in the *JUP* gene [7]. The second autosomal recessive disease, Carvajal syndrome, is associated with a *DSP* gene mutation, and is manifested by woolly hair, epidermolytic palmoplantar keratoderma, and cardiomyopathy [49].

Autosomal Dominant ACM

Overall, mutations in the *PKP2* gene are most frequently observed in classic ARVC. Figure 6.7 shows the pedigree of

Table 6.3 Mutated genes with concurrent type of arrhythmogenic cardiomyopathy (*ACM*) (Modified from Van Tintelen et al. Curr Opin Cardiol 2007)

	Gene	Type of disease	Inheritance trait
Desmosomal	*PKP2*	Typical or classic ARVC	Autosomal dominant
	DSG2	Typical or classic ARVC	Autosomal dominant
	DSC2	Typical or classic ARVC	Autosomal dominant
	JUP	Naxos disease ARVC	Autosomal recessive Autosomal dominant
	DSP	Carvajal syndrome	Autosomal recessive
		Typical or classic ARVC	Autosomal dominant
	CTNNA3	LDAC ARVC	Autosomal dominant Autosomal dominant
Nondesmosomal	*RyR2*	CPVT	Autosomal dominant
		ARVC	Autosomal dominant
	TGF-β	Typical or classic ARVC	Autosomal dominant
	TMEM43 *PLN* *LMNA* *DES* *TTN*	Biventric ACM Biventric ACM Biventric ACM and LDAC Biventric ACM and LDAC ?	Autosomal dominant Autosomal dominant Autosomal dominant Autosomal dominant Autosomal dominant

CPVT catecholaminergic polymorphic VT, *LDAC* left dominant arrhythmogenic cardiomyopathy. See text for other abbreviations

a family with a *PKP2* mutation, showing an autosomal dominant inheritance pattern with incomplete penetrance and variable expressivity. Incomplete and age-dependent penetrance and clinical variability in ACM are well documented. In five studies from different countries, analyzing 56–149 ACM patients each, *PKP2* mutations were found in 11–51% of unrelated probands who fulfilled diagnostic TFC for ARVC [17, 66–69]. In a large combined study from the United States and the Netherlands, including 1001 ARVC probands and family members, pathogenic desmosomal and nondesmosomal mutations were identified in 63% of the 439 probands. In 46% of subjects, a single *PKP2* mutation was found [26]. In addition, multiple mutations were found in 4% of cases, which in the majority of subjects also included a *PKP2* mutation. In that large cohort, a total of 94 different desmosomal mutations (59 in *PKP2*) were observed. Thus, *PKP2* was mutated in approximately half of the included American and Dutch ACM patients.

Pathogenic mutations in the other desmosomal genes were much less common in the US–Dutch study: *DSG2* 4%, *DSC2* 1%, *JUP* 0.5%, and *DSP* 3% [26]. Although *PKP2* mutations are also frequently found in other ACM cohorts from other countries, the distribution of the different genes encoding desmosomal proteins is highly variable [70, 71]. In one Italian study including 134 desmosomal mutation carriers, *DSP* mutations were most frequent (39%) [72].

Mutations in *DSG2* and *DSC2* encoding transmembranous desmosomal proteins are associated with classic or typical ACM. *JUP* is primarily associated with the recessive Naxos disease, although a rare autosomal dominant form has been identified [73].

Mutations in the gene encoding the intracellular desmosomal component *DSP* lead to "classic ARVC" with a clini-

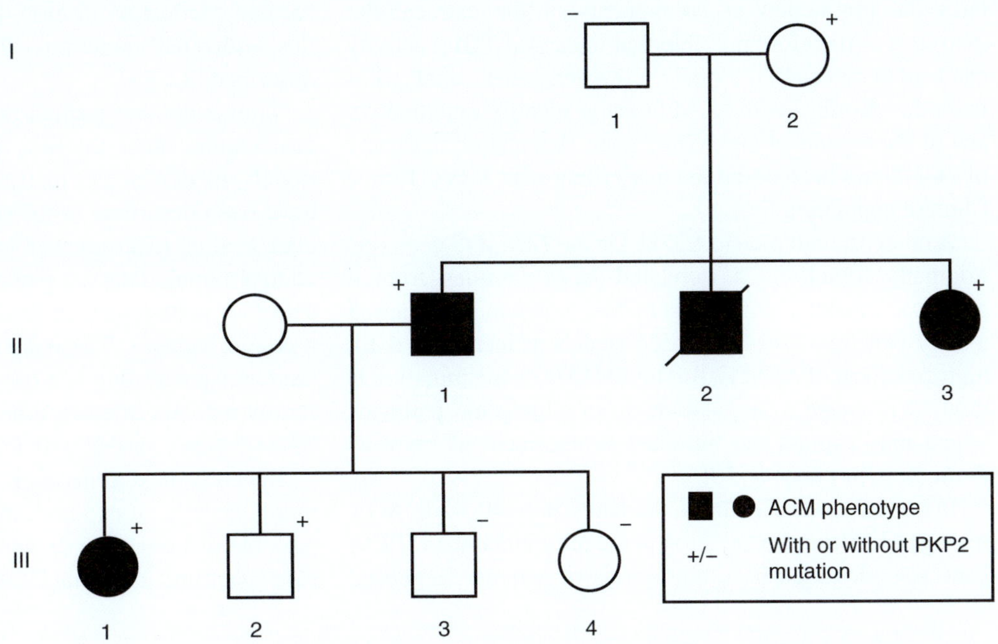

Fig. 6.7 Pedigree of family with classic arrhythmogenic right ventricular cardiomyopathy (*ARVC*) and plakophilin-2 (*PKP2*) mutation. This figure shows the variability in penetrance and clinical expression. Both the 72-year-old grandmother (I:2) and 20-year-old grandson (III:2) are free of any signs of disease, despite carrying the mutation. The proband (II:1) was resuscitated at age 35, his brother (II:2) died suddenly at age 18. Both the proband's sister (II:3) and daughter (III:1) were diagnosed with the disease due to a positive family history, ECG abnormalities, nonsustained VT, and RV structural abnormalities

cal presentation of VT, sudden death, and LV involvement as the disease progresses [16, 74, 75]. However, *DSP* mutations have also been associated with predominantly left-sided ACM and, as noted above, with autosomal recessive disease. A recent study showed that *DSP* mutation carriers are more prone to SCD, LV dysfunction, and heart failure [31].

Other, Nondesmosomal, Genes

Mutations in the gene encoding the cardiac ryanodine receptor *RyR2*, which is responsible for calcium release from the sarcoplasmic reticulum, have been described in one Italian ACM family [14]. Affected patients have exercise-induced polymorphic VT. Mutations in *RyR2* have primarily been associated with familial catecholaminergic polymorphic VT without ACM [76]. Although the general opinion is that *RyR2* mutations lead to catecholaminergic polymorphic VT, without structural abnormalities, the mutations in ACM have been advocated to act differently from those in familial polymorphic VT without ACM [76].

Transforming growth factor-β-3 (TGFβ3) regulates the production of extracellular matrix components and modulates expression of genes encoding desmosomal proteins. Its gene has been mapped to chromosome 14. Initial sequencing studies failed to identify any disease-causing mutations in the exonic regions of *TGFβ3*. This led to screening of the promoter and untranslated regions, where a mutation of the *TGFβ3* gene was found in all clinically affected members of a large family with ACM [15]. The mutation is predicted to produce an amino acid substitution in a short peptide with an inhibitory role in TGFβ3 regulation. The implication of these observations is that regulatory mutations resulting in overexpression of TGFβ3 may contribute to the development of ACM in these families. The TGFβ family of cytokines stimulates the production of components of the extracellular matrix. It is therefore possible that enhanced TGFβ activity can lead to myocardial fibrosis. However, genetic analysis of two other families with ACM failed to identify mutations in any of the regions of the *TGFβ3* gene. A mutation in exon 1 of *TGFβ3* has been described in a patient with ARVC from a Chinese population [76].

A missense mutation (p.S358L) in the *TMEM43* gene was originally found in 15 unrelated ACM families from a genetically isolated population in Newfoundland and caused a fully penetrant, sex-influenced (males at increased risk), high-risk form of ACM [20]. The *TMEM43* gene mutation is thought to cause dysregulation of an adipogenic pathway, which may explain the fibrofatty replacement of myocardium in ACM patients [76].

In the past decade, in the Netherlands, the c.40_42delAGA (p.Arg14del) founder mutation in the phospholamban (*PLN*) gene was identified in a large series of patients diagnosed with either DCM or ACM [21, 65, 77]. This specific *PLN* mutation was found in 5% of the 439 probands of the combined US–Dutch ACM cohort, and appeared to be the most frequently observed individual gene mutation [26]. Subsequently, the mutations were also discovered in other European countries and United States, Canada, and China. Onset of overt disease is usually later than in desmosomal mutation carriers. *PLN* is associated with ACM with more often biventricular (RV and LV) manifestation and LV dominant forms than most desmosomal mutations, although the histology of fibrofatty alteration is similar [65]. The pathophysiologic mechanism of the *PLN* mutation underlying ACM and specific phenotypic abnormalities is unknown yet. Hypotheses of PLN-mediated increased cytosolic calcium levels and thereby desmosome disassembly have been described [21]. In line with this hypothesis, it was recently shown that PLN expression is increased in myocardial tissue from patients with ACM independent of the underlying genetic mutation as compared to patients with DCM and healthy controls [78].

The gene-encoding lamins A and C, parts of the nuclear lamina, a protein network supporting the inner nuclear membrane, is believed to be involved in left dominant forms of ACM, although *LMNA* mutations have also been identified in patients fulfilling the ACM TFC [23, 79]. The patients and family members also demonstrate clinical features suggestive for a cardiac laminopathy, including conduction disease and atrial fibrillation.

Desmin is a large protein connected to the cardiac desmosome through desmoplakin. Mutations in *DES* have been identified in patients diagnosed with ACM including a large multigenerational family from Sweden [22, 80, 81]. The typical histological features of ACM were also found in these patients. Some of the patients also depict typical clinical desminopathy-related features like neuromuscular disease or cardiac conduction disease. Interestingly, in different families with *DES* mutations, RV involvement has also been described [82, 83].

Titin is another protein that is functionally linked to the desmosome, since the titin filament connects to the transitional junction at the intercalated disk. Mutations in *TTN* have been described in ACM [24]. Because rare *TTN* variants, leading to a truncated protein, can also be identified in control populations, its pathogenicity might be questioned. The *TTN* mutations identified in ACM have so far only been missense variants. These are even more difficult to interpret than variants leading to a truncated protein. However, in one family with six affected individuals with segregation of the *TTN* missense variant with the phenotype.

Recently, next-generation sequencing showed that sarcomeric genetic mutations/variants may be associated with possible or borderline diagnosis of ACM resulting in a disease spectrum, including DCM or phenocopies of ACM [84].

Therapy, Risk Stratification, and ICD Indications

Therapeutic options in patients with ACM include sports restriction, beta blockers, pharmacologic treatment of heart failure such as ACE-inhibitors, anti-arrhythmic drugs, catheter ablation, and implantation of a cardioverter defibrillator (ICD). Patients with VT have a favorable outcome when they are treated medically and therefore pharmacologic treatment is the first choice. This concerns not only patients who have presented with sustained VT but also patients and family members with nonsustained VT or >500 ventricular extrasystoles on 24 h Holter monitoring. Since ventricular arrhythmias and cardiac arrest occur frequently during or after physical exercise, or maybe triggered by catecholamines, anti-adrenergic β-blockers are recommended. Regarding anti-arrhythmic drugs, studies have shown that sotalol is particularly effective in patients with ACM. Alternatively, other β-receptor-blocking agents, amiodarone, and flecainide, have all been reported as useful [85]. Catheter ablation is an alternative in patients who are refractory to drug treatment and have frequently recurring VT episodes or ICD discharges. However, all reported results with exclusively endocardial approaches were mediocre, related to the technical difficulties of the procedure, the subepicardial onset of the disease, and disease progression. In recent years, results improved markedly in highly experienced centers by using a combined epicardial and endocardial approach nowadays reaching VT/VF-free survival rates of up to 80% at 2 years [86–89]. Yet, catheter ablation is considered as a palliative and not curative treatment option. Owing to disease progression, new VTs originating from different areas usually occur after a certain period of time [90, 91]. Interestingly, recent evidence has indicated that bilateral sympathectomy may serve as an effective treatment method for achieving arrhythmia control, even when all other treatment options including repeated catheter ablation have been exhausted [92]. Although anti-arrhythmic drugs and catheter ablation can significantly reduce VT burden, no prospective trials have been performed to demonstrate that these therapies will also prevent SCD.

A recent meta-analysis searched for predictors of arrhythmic risk in ACM [93]. Data of 45 different ACM cohorts were collected, containing 70 patients on average. The average proportion of arrhythmic events was 10.6% per year in patients with ACM and 3.7% per year in mutation carriers. Male sex, syncope, T-wave inversion beyond V3, RV dysfunction, and prior VT/VF consistently predicted ventricular arrhythmias in all populations studied.

ICD implantation is indicated in patients with a moderate (1–10% per year) to high risk (>10% risk per year) of SCD. As such, implantation of an ICD is warranted in ACM patients with aborted SCD or sustained VT for secondary prevention, and for primary prevention in those patients with risk factors for SCD as mentioned above. Recently, a prediction model was developed for the occurrence of VT in patients diagnosed with ACM, but no prior ventricular arrhythmias when diagnosed [94]. This model can assist in making the decision when to implant a primary prophylactic ICD.

If heart failure progresses toward end-stage disease or intractable ventricular arrhythmias occur despite optimal pharmacologic and ablative treatment, heart transplantation should be considered in this rather young population [95].

Despite growing registries and worldwide collaboration, data on mutation carrying patients are not sufficient to make mutation- or gene-specific risk stratifications or therapeutic advices. This is due to the relatively low numbers of patients, e.g. as compared to HCM populations, the limited numbers of events that occur in mutation carriers and the large variety of mutations leaving only small groups of patients per specific mutation.

Recommendations During Pregnancy and Delivery

Because ACM is relatively rare, no guidelines exist on pregnancy in this disease. The largest series of pregnant women with ACM consisted of 26 patients who had 39 pregnancies. Sustained VT occurred in 13%, all having a single episode during pregnancy. Heart failure, all new onset, complicated 5% of pregnancies. However, when comparing pregnant and nonpregnant female patients with ACM at similar ages, the likelihood of experiencing a first sustained VT or developing heart failure was not significantly increased during pregnancy. All pregnancies resulted in live-born infants without major obstetric concerns and all children were healthy at last follow-up. Of note, women taking β-blockers or experiencing major events during pregnancy had children with a significantly lower birth weight but who were otherwise healthy. Other smaller case series showed similar results. [9] Higher number of pregnancies did not seem to relate to a worse phenotype in women with AC. [96–98] These data suggest that it should be possible to manage pregnancy successfully in women with ACM. Before conception, antiarrhythmic drugs with low fetal toxicity should be chosen. ICD implantation, if indicated based on prepregnancy risk stratification, should be performed prior to pregnancy. Preconception assessment of biventricular structure and function is helpful since heart failure is more likely in those with structural abnormalities. LV dysfunction is associated with poor pregnancy outcomes in women with DCM and appears likely to be so for patients with ACM as well. Genetic counseling to discuss the heritable nature of ACM should be offered. Following recognition of pregnancy, discontinuation of medication with low fetal risk (e.g., β-blockers) is not advised. Vaginal delivery with cardiac monitoring is reasonable in many cases. For uneventful pregnancies, a 3-month postpartum visit followed by usual cardiac care is recommended as pregnancy is not expected to worsen long-term disease course [98].

References

1. Marcus FI, Fontaine GH, Guiraudon G, et al. Right ventricular dysplasia: a report of 24 adult cases. Circulation. 1982;65(2):384–98.
2. Corrado D, Basso C, Thiene G, et al. Spectrum of clinicopathologic manifestations of arrhythmogenic right ventricular cardiomyopathy/dysplasia: a multicenter study. J Am Coll Cardiol. 1997;30:1512–20.
3. Basso C, Thiene G, Corrado D, et al. Arrhythmogenic right ventricular cardiomyopathy: dysplasia, dystrophy, or myocarditis? Circulation. 1996;94:983–91.
4. Sen-Chowdhry S, Syrris P, Prasad SK, et al. Left-dominant arrhythmogenic cardiomyopathy: an underrecognized clinical entity. J Am Coll Cardiol. 2008;52:2175–87.
5. Asimaki A, Tandri H, Huang H, et al. A new diagnostic test for arrhythmogenic right ventricular cardiomyopathy. N Engl J Med. 2009;360:1075–64.
6. Richardson P, McKenna W, Bristow M, et al. Report of the 1995 World Health Organization/International Society and Federation of Cardiology Task Force on the Definition and Classification of cardiomyopathies. Circulation. 1996;93(5):841–2.
7. McKoy G, Protonotarios N, Crosby A, et al. Identification of a deletion in plakoglobin in arrhythmogenic right ventricular cardiomyopathy with palmoplantar keratoderma and woolly hair (Naxos disease). Lancet. 2000;355:2119–24.
8. Rampazzo A, Nava A, Miorin M, et al. ARVD4, a new locus for arrhythmogenic right ventricular cardiomyopathy, maps to chromosome 2 long arm. Genomics. 1997;45:259–63.
9. Ahmad F, Li D, Karibe A, et al. Localization of a gene responsible for arrhythmogenic right ventricular dysplasia to chromosome 3p23. Circulation. 1998;98:2791–5.
10. Li D, Ahmad F, Gardner MJ, et al. The locus of a novel gene responsible for arrhythmogenic right-ventricular dysplasia characterized by early onset and high penetrance maps to chromosome 10p12–p14. Am J Hum Genet. 2000;66:148–56.
11. Melberg A, Oldfors A, Blomstrom-Lundqvist C, et al. Autosomal dominant myofibrillar myopathy with arrhythmogenic right ventricular cardiomyopathy linked to chromosome 10q. Ann Neurol. 1999;46:684–92.
12. Rampazzo A, Nava A, Danieli GA, et al. The gene for arrhythmogenic right ventricular cardiomyopathy maps to chromosome 14q23–q24. Hum Mol Genet. 1994;3:959–62.
13. Severini GM, Krajinovic M, Pinamonti B, et al. A new locus for arrhythmogenic right ventricular dysplasia on the long arm of chromosome 14. Genomics. 1996;31:193–200.
14. Tiso N, Stephan DA, Nava A, et al. Identification of mutations in the cardiac ryanodine receptor gene in families affected with arrhythmogenic right ventricular cardiomyopathy type 2 (ARVD2). Hum Mol Genet. 2001;10(3):189–94.
15. Beffagna G, Occhi G, Nava A, et al. Regulatory mutations in transforming growth factor-beta3 gene cause arrhythmogenic right ventricular cardiomyopathy type 1. Cardiovasc Res. 2005;65:366–73.
16. Rampazzo A, Nava A, Malacrida S, et al. Mutation in human desmoplakin domain binding to plakoglobin causes a dominant form of arrhythmogenic right ventricular cardiomyopathy. Am J Hum Genet. 2002;71:1200–6.
17. Gerull B, Heuser A, Wichter T, et al. Mutations in the desmosomal protein plakophilin-2 are common in arrhythmogenic right ventricular cardiomyopathy. Nat Genet. 2004;36:1162–4.
18. Pilichou K, Nava A, Basso C, et al. Mutations in desmoglein-2 gene are associated to arrhythmogenic right ventricular cardiomyopathy. Circulation. 2006;113:1171–9.
19. Syrris P, Ward D, Evans A, et al. Arrhythmogenic right ventricular dysplasia/cardiomyopathy associated with mutations in the desmosomal gene desmocollin-2. Am J Hum Genet. 2006;79:978.
20. Merner ND, Hodgkinson KA, Haywood AF, et al. Arrhythmogenic right ventricular cardiomyopathy type 5 is a fully penetrant, lethal arrhythmic disorder caused by a missense mutation in the TMEM43 gene. Am J Hum Genet. 2008;82:809–21.
21. Van der Zwaag PA, van Rijsingen IA, Asimaki A, et al. Phospholamban R14del mutation in patients diagnosed with dilated cardiomyopathy or arrhythmogenic right ventricular cardiomyopathy: evidence supporting the concept of arrhythmogenic cardiomyopathy. Eur J Heart Fail. 2012;14:1199–207.
22. Van Tintelen JP, Van Gelder IC, Asimaki A, et al. Severe cardiac phenotype with right ventricular predominance in a large cohort of patients with a single missense mutation in the DES gene. Heart Rhythm. 2009;6:1574–83.
23. Quarta G, Syrris P, Ashworth M, et al. Mutations in the Lamin A/C gene mimic arrhythmogenic right ventricular cardiomyopathy. Eur Heart J. 2012;33:1128–36.
24. Taylor M, Graw S, Sinagra G, et al. Genetic variation in titin in arrhythmogenic right ventricular cardiomyopathy-overlap syndromes. Circulation. 2011;124:876–85.
25. Van Hengel J, Calore M, Bauce B, et al. Mutations in the area composita protein αT-catenin are associated with arrhythmogenic right ventricular cardiomyopathy. Eur Heart J. 2013;34:201–10.
26. Groeneweg JA, Bhonsale A, James CA, et al. Clinical presentation, long-term follow-up, and outcomes of 1001 arrhythmogenic right ventricular dysplasia/cardiomyopathy patients and family members. Circ Cardiovasc Genet. 2015 Jun;8(3):437–46.
27. Ellison KE, Friedman PL, Ganz LI, Stevenson WG. Entrainment mapping and radiofrequency catheter ablation of ventricular tachycardia in right ventricular dysplasia. J Am Coll Cardiol. 1998;32:724–8.
28. Saffitz JE. Dependence of electrical coupling on mechanical coupling in cardiac myocytes: insights gained from cardiomyopathies caused by defects in cell-cell connections. Ann N Y Acad Sci. 2005;1047:336–44.
29. Kaplan SR, Gard JJ, Carvajal-Huerta L, Ruiz-Cabezas JC, Thiene G, Saffitz JE. Structural and molecular pathology of the heart in Carvajal syndrome. Cardiovasc Pathol. 2004;13(1):26–32.
30. Garcia-Gras E, Lombardi R, Giocondo MJ, et al. Suppression of canonical Wnt/beta-catenin signaling by nuclear plakoglobin recapitulates phenotype of arrhythmogenic right ventricular cardiomyopathy. J Clin Invest. 2006;116:2012–21.
31. Cerrone M, Noorman M, Lin X, et al. Sodium current deficit and arrhythmogenesis in a murine model of plakophilin-2 haploinsufficiency. Cardiovasc Res. 2012;95:460–8.
32. Bhonsale A, Groeneweg JA, James CA, et al. Impact of genotype on clinical course in arrhythmogenic right ventricular dysplasia/cardiomyopathy-associated mutation carriers. Eur Heart J. 2015;36:847–55.
33. Quarta G, Muir A, Pantazis A, et al. Familial evaluation in arrhythmogenic right ventricular cardiomyopathy: impact of genetics and revised task force criteria. Circulation. 2011;123:2701–9.
34. Te Riele AS, James CA, Sawant AC, et al. Arrhythmogenic right ventricular dysplasia/cardiomyopathy in the pediatric population: clinical characterization and comparison with adult-onset disease. J Am Coll Cardiol EP. 2015;1:551–60.
35. Protonotarios N, Tsatsopoulou A, Anastasakis A, et al. Genotype-phenotype assessment in autosomal recessive arrhythmogenic right

ventricular cardiomyopathy (Naxos disease) caused by a deletion in plakoglobin. J Am Coll Cardiol. 2001;38(5):1477–84.
36. Norgett EE, Hatsell SJ, Carvajal-Huerta L, et al. Recessive mutation in desmoplakin disrupts desmoplakin-intermediate filament interactions and causes dilated cardiomyopathy, woolly hair and keratoderma. Hum Mol Genet. 2000;9:2761–6.
37. Ruwald AC, Marcus F, Estes NA 3rd, et al. Association of competitive and recreational sport participation with cardiac events in patients with arrhythmogenic right ventricular cardiomyopathy: results from the North American multidisciplinary study of arrhythmogenic right ventricular cardiomyopathy. Eur Heart J. 2015;36:1735–43.
38. Saguner AM, Ganahl S, Kraus A, et al. Electrocardiographic features of disease progression in arrhythmogenic right ventricular cardiomyopathy/dysplasia. BMC Cardiovasc Disord. 2015;15:4.
39. Te Riele A, James CA, Philips B, et al. Mutation-positive arrhythmogenic right ventricular dysplasia/cardiomyopathy: the triangle of dysplasia displaced. J Cardiovasc Electrophysiol. 2013;24:1311–20.
40. McKenna WJ, Thiene G, Nava A, et al. Diagnosis of arrhythmogenic right ventricular dysplasia/cardiomyopathy. Task Force of the Working Group Myocardial and Pericardial Disease of the European Society of Cardiology and of the Scientific Council on Cardiomyopathies of the International Society and Federation of Cardiology. Br Heart J. 1994;71:215–8.
41. Marcus FI, McKenna WJ, Sherrill D, et al. Diagnosis of arrhythmogenic right ventricular cardiomyopathy/dysplasia: proposed modification of the task force criteria. Eur Heart J. 2010;31:806–14.
42. Fontaine G, Umemura J, Di Donna P, Tsezana R, Cannat JJ, Frank R. Duration of QRS complexes in arrhythmogenic right ventricular dysplasia. A new non-invasive diagnostic marker. Ann Cardiol Angeiol (Paris). 1993;42:399–405.
43. Peters S, Trümmel M. Diagnosis of arrhythmogenic right ventricular dysplasia-cardiomyopathy: value of standard ECG revisited. Ann Noninvasive Electrocardiol. 2003;8:238–45.
44. Pinamonti B, Sinagra G, Salvi A, et al. Left ventricular involvement in right ventricular dysplasia. Am Heart J. 1992;123:711–24.
45. Platonov PG, Calkins H, Hauer RN, Corrado D, Svendsen JH, Wichter T, Biernacka EK, Saguner AM, Te Riele AS, Zareba W. High interobserver variability in the assessment of epsilon waves: Implications for diagnosis of arrhythmogenic right ventricular cardiomyopathy/dysplasia. Heart Rhythm. 2016 Jan;13(1):208–16.
46. Cox MG, Nelen MR, Wilde AA, et al. Activation delay and VT parameters in arrhythmogenic right ventricular dysplasia/cardiomyopathy: toward improvement of diagnostic ECG criteria. J Cardiovasc Electrophysiol. 2008;19:775–81.
47. Saguner AM, Ganahl S, Baldinger SH, et al. Usefulness of electrocardiographic parameters for risk prediction in arrhythmogenic right ventricular dysplasia. Am J Cardiol. 2014;113:1728–34.
48. Nasir K, Rutberg J, Tandri H, Berger R, Tomaselli G, Calkins H. Utility of SAECG in arrhythmogenic right ventricle dysplasia. Ann Noninvasive Electrocardiol. 2003;8:112–20.
49. Oselladore L, Nava A, Buja G, et al. Signal-averaged electrocardiography in familial form of arrhythmogenic right ventricular cardiomyopathy. Am J Cardiol. 1995;75:1038–41.
50. Turrini P, Angelini A, Thiene G, et al. Late potentials and ventricular arrhythmias in arrhythmogenic right ventricular cardiomyopathy. Am J Cardiol. 1999;83:1214–9.
51. Tannawuttiwat T, Te Riele AS, Philips B, et al. Electroanatomic correlates of depolarization abnormalities in arrhythmogenic right ventricular dysplasia/cardiomyopathy. J Cardiovasc Electrophysiol. 2016;27:443–52.
52. Jain R, Dalal D, Daly A, et al. Electrocardiographic features of arrhythmogenic right ventricular dysplasia. Circulation. 2009;120:477–87.
53. Te Riele ASJM, Tandri H, Sanborn DM, Bluemke DA. Noninvasive multimodality imaging in ARVD/C. JACC Cardiovasc Imaging. 2015 May;8(5):597–611.
54. Teske AJ, Cox MG, Te Riele AS, et al. Early detection of regional functional abnormalities in asymptomatic arrhythmogenic right ventricular dysplasia/cardiomyopathy mutation carriers. J Am Soc Echocardiogr. 2012;25:997–1006.
55. Borgquits R, Haugaa KH, Gilljam T, et al. The diagnostic performance of imaging methods in ARVC using the 2010 task force criteria. Eur Heart J Cardiovasc Imaging. 2014;15:1219–25.
56. Bluemke DA, Krupinski EA, Ovitt T, et al. MR imaging of arrhythmogenic right ventricular cardiomyopathy: morphologic findings and interobserver reliability. Cardiology. 2003;99:153–62.
57. Tandri H, Calkins H, Nasir K, et al. Magnetic resonance imaging findings in patients meeting task force criteria for arrhythmogenic right ventricular dysplasia. J Cardiovasc Electrophysiol. 2003;14:476–82.
58. Basso C, Ronco F, Marcus F, et al. Quantitative assessment of endocardial biopsy in arrhythmogenic cardiomyopathy/dysplasia: an in vitro validation of diagnostic criteria. Eur Heart J. 2008;29:2760–71.
59. Lerman BB, Stein KM, Markowitz SM. Idiopathic right ventricular outflow tract tachycardia: a clinical approach. PACE. 1996;19:2120–37.
60. Markowitz SM, Litvak BL, Ramirez de Arellano EA, et al. Adenosine-sensitive ventricular tachycardia, right ventricular abnormalities delineated by magnetic resonance imaging. Circulation. 1997;96:1192–200.
61. Thomas KW, Hunninghake GW. Sarcoidosis. JAMA. 2003;289:3300–3.
62. Ladyjanskaja GA, Basso C, Hobbelink MG, et al. Sarcoid myocarditis with ventricular tachycardia mimicking ARVD/C. J Cardiovasc Electrophysiol. 2010;21:94–8.
63. Blankstein R, Osborne M, Naya M, et al. Cardiac positron emission tomography enhances prognostic assessment of patients with suspected cardiac sarcoidosis. J Am Coll Cardiol. 2014;63:329–36.
64. Tanawuttiwat T, Sager SJ, Hare JM, Myerburg RJ, et al. Myocarditis and ARVC/D: variants or mimics? Heart Rhythm. 2013;10:1544–8.
65. Groeneweg JA, van der Zwaag PA, Jongbloed JD, et al. Left-dominant arrhythmogenic cardiomyopathy in a large family: associated desmosomal or nondesmosomal phenotype? Heart Rhythm. 2013;10:548–59.
66. Syrris P, Ward D, Asimaki A, et al. Clinical expression of plakophilin-2 mutations in familial arrhythmogenic right ventricular cardiomyopathy. Circulation. 2006;113:356–64.
67. Dalal D, Molin LH, Piccini J, et al. Clinical features of arrhythmogenic right ventricular dysplasia/cardiomyopathy associated with mutations in plakophilin-2. Circulation. 2006;113:1641–9.
68. Van Tintelen JP, Entius MM, Bhuiyan ZA, et al. Plakophilin-2 mutations are the major determinant of familial arrhythmogenic right ventricular dysplasia/cardiomyopathy. Circulation. 2006;113:1650–8.
69. Cox MG, van der Zwaag PA, van der Werf C, et al. Arrhythmogenic right ventricular dysplasia/cardiomyopathy: pathogenic desmosome mutations in index-patients predict outcome of family screening: Dutch ARVD/C genotype-phenotype follow-up study. Circulation. 2011;123:2690–700.
70. Watkins DA, Hendricks N, Shaboodien G, et al. Clinical features, survival experience, and profile of plakophylin-2 gene mutations in participants of the arrhythmogenic right ventricular cardiomyopathy registry of South Africa. Heart Rhythm. 2009;6(11 Suppl):S10–7.
71. Van Tintelen JP, Hofstra RM, Wiesfeld AC, et al. Molecular genetics of arrhythmogenic cardiomyopathy: emerging horizon? Curr Opin Cardiol. 2007;22:185–92.
72. Rigato I, Bauce B, Rampazzo A, et al. Compound and digenic heterozygosity predicts lifetime arrhythmic outcome and sudden cardiac death in desmosomal gene-related. Circ Cardiovasc Genet. 2013;6:533–42.

73. Syrris P, Ward D, Asimaki A, et al. Desmoglein-2 mutations in arrhythmogenic right ventricular cardiomyopathy: a genotype-phenotype characterization of familial disease. Eur Heart J. 2007;28:581–8.
74. Bauce B, Basso C, Rampazzo A, et al. Clinical profile of four families with arrhythmogenic right ventricular cardiomyopathy caused by dominant desmoplakin mutations. Eur Heart J. 2005;26:1666–75.
75. Sen-Chowdhry S, Syrris P, McKenna WJ. Desmoplakin disease in arrhythmogenic right ventricular cardiomyopathy: early genotype-phenotype studies. Eur Heart J. 2005;26:1582–4.
76. Rampazzo A, Beffagna G, Nava A, et al. Arrhythmogenic right ventricular cardiomyopathy type 1 (ARVD1): confirmation of locus assignment and mutation screening of four candidate genes. Eur J Hum Genet. 2003;11:69–76.
77. Groeneweg JA, van der Zwaag PA, Olde Nordkamp LR, et al. Arrhythmogenic right ventricular dysplasia/cardiomyopathy according to revised 2010 task force criteria with inclusion of non-desmosomal phospholamban mutation carriers. Am J Cardiol. 2013;112:1197–206.
78. Akdis D, Medeiros-Domingo A, Gaertner-Rommel A, et al. Myocardial expression profiles of candidate molecules in patients with arrhythmogenic right ventricular cardiomyopathy/dysplasia compared to those with dilated cardiomyopathy and healthy controls. Heart Rhythm. 2016;13:731–41.
79. Forleo LMNA, Forleo C, Carmosino M, Resta N, et al. Clinical and functional characterization of a novel mutation in lamin a/c gene in a multigenerational family with arrhythmogenic cardiac laminopathy. PLoS One. 2015;10:e0121723.
80. Klauke B, Kossmann S, Gaertner A, et al. De novo desmin-mutation N116S is associated with arrhythmogenic right ventricular cardiomyopathy. Hum Mol Genet. 2010;19:4595–607.
81. Hedberg C, Melberg A, Kuhl A, et al. Autosomal dominant myofibrillar myopathy with arrhythmogenic right ventricular cardiomyopathy 7 is caused by a DES mutation. Eur J Hum Genet. 2012;20:984–5.
82. Ross SE, Hemati N, Longof KA, et al. Inhibition of adipogenesis by Wnt signaling. Science. 2000;289:950–3.
83. Van Spaendonck-Zwarts KY, van Hessem L, Jongbloed JD, et al. Desmin-related myopathy. Clin Genet. 2011;80:354–66.
84. Medeiros-Domingo A, et al. Arrhythmogenic right ventricular cardiomyopathy: implications of next-generation sequencing in appropriate diagnosis. Europace. 2016;
85. Wichter T, Paul TM, Eckardt L, et al. Arrhythmogenic right ventricular cardiomyopathy. Antiarrhythmic drugs, catheter ablation, or ICD? Herz. 2005;30:91–101.
86. Corrado D, Wichter T, Link MS, et al. Treatment of arrhythmogenic cardiomyopathy/dysplasia: an international task force consensus statement. Circulation. 2015;132:441–53.
87. Corrado D, Wichter T, Link MS, et al. Treatment of arrhythmogenic cardiomyopathy/dysplasia: an international task force consensus statement. Eur Heart J. 2015;36:3227–37.
88. Garcia FC, Bazan V, Zado ES, et al. Epicardial substrate and outcome of epicardial ablation of ventricular tachycardia in arrhythmogenic right ventricular cardiomyopathy/dysplasia. Circulation. 2009;120:366–75.
89. Philips B, te Riele AS, Sawant A, et al. Outcomes and ventricular recurrence characteristics after epicardial ablation of ventricular tachycardia in arrhythmogenic right ventricular dysplasia/cardiomyopathy. Heart Rhythm. 2015;12(4):716–25.
90. Santangeli P, Zado ES, Supple GE, et al. Long-term outcome with catheter ablation for ventricular tachycardia in patients with arrhythmogenic right ventricular cardiomyopathy. Circ Arrhythm Electrophysiol. 2015;8:1413–21.
91. Dalal D, Jain R, Tandri H, et al. Long-term efficacy of catheter ablation of ventricular tachycardia in patients with arrhythmogenic right ventricular dysplasia/cardiomyopathy. J Am Coll Cardiol. 2007;50:432–40.
92. Schwartz PJ, De Ferrari GM, Pugliese L. Cardiac sympathetic denervation 100 years later: Jonnesco would have never believed it. Int J Cadiol. 2017;237:25–8.
93. Bosman LP, Sammani A, James CA, et al. Predicting arrhythmic risk in arrhythmogenic right ventricular cardiomyopathy: a systematic review and meta-analysis. Heart Rhythm. 2018;15(7):1097–107.
94. Cadrin-Tourigny J, Bosman LP, Nozza A, et al. A new prediction model for ventricular arrhythmias in arrhythmogenic right ventricular cardiomyopathy. Eur Heart J. 2019;40:1850–8.
95. DePasquale EC, Cheng RK, Deng MC, et al. Survival after heart transplantation in patients with arrhythmogenic right ventricular cardiomyopathy. J Card Fail. 2017;23(2):107–12.
96. Hodes AR, Tichnell C, Te Riele AS, et al. Pregnancy course and outcomes in women with arrhythmogenic right ventricular cardiomyopathy. Heart. 2016;102(4):303–12.
97. Bauce B, Daliento L, Frigo G, et al. Pregnancy in women with arrhythmogenic right ventricular cardiomyopathy/dysplasia. EJOG. 2006;127(2):186–9.
98. Castrini AI, Lie OH, Leren IS, et al. Eur Heart J Cardiovasc Imaging. 2019;20:192–8.

Left Ventricular Noncompaction

7

Yvonne M. Hoedemaekers and Tjeerd Germans

Introduction

Description of disease

Noncompaction of the left ventricle (LV) or left ventricular noncompaction (LVNC) was first described by Feldt et al. in 1969 [1] is a hereditary cardiomyopathy which is genetically heterogeneous and is characterized by prominent trabeculations on the luminal surface of the left ventricular apex, the lateral wall and, rarely, the interventricular septum in association with deep recesses that extend into the ventricular wall, which do not communicate with the coronary circulation. With cardiac imaging, LVNC is defined by the ratio of non-compact and compact myocardium, see Table 7.1, It is associated with a clinical triad of heart failure, arrhythmias and/or thrombo-embolic events [2, 3]. LVNC occurs in non-isolated and isolated forms.

The non-isolated forms of LVNC are more frequent in childhood and co-occur with congenital heart disease, or may be part of a malformation or chromosomal syndrome [10]. Also, LVNC is frequently observed in patients with neuromuscular disorders.

Isolated forms of LVNC are most prevalent in adults and have been associated with mutations in *sarcomere* genes that are also involved in hypertrophic cardiomyopathy (HCM), dilated cardiomyopathy (DCM) and restrictive cardiomyopathy (RCM) [11].

Clinical presentation of LVNC ranges from a coincidental finding in asymptomatic in adults to severe congenital forms resulting in symptoms very early in life, depending on co-existing cardiac phenotype [10, 12, 13].

LVNC was classified by the American Heart Association (AHA) as a separate primary, genetic cardiomyopathy, based on the predominant myocardial involvement and genetic aetiology [14]. The European Society of Cardiology (ESC)

Table 7.1 Diagnostic criteria for LVNC

Diagnostic criteria for LVNC
Echocardiographic criteria
I. Chin et al. [4].
Focusing on trabeculae localized at the LV apex on the parasternal short axis and apical views and on LV free-wall thickness at end-diastole LVNC is defined by a ratio of X/Y ≤ 0.5 with
X = distance from the epicardial surface to the trough of the trabecular recess
Y = distance from the epicardial surface to the peak of the trabeculation
II. Jenni et al. [2].
1. An excessively thickened left ventricular myocardial wall with a two-layered structure consisting of a compact epicardial layer (C) and a noncompacted endocardial layer (NC) of prominent trabeculations and deep intertrabecular recesses.
2. A maximal NC/C ratio > 2, measured at the parasternal short axis in end systole.
3. Colour Doppler evidence of deep perfused intertrabecular recesses.
4. Absence of coexisting cardiac anomalies.
III. Stollberger et al. [5]
1. More than three trabeculations protruding from the left ventricular wall, apical to the papillary muscles and visible in a single image
2. Perfusion of the intertrabecular spaces from the ventricular cavity visualized on colour Doppler imaging
Cardiovascular magnetic resonance
I. Petersen et al. [6].
A maximal NC/C ratio > 2.3, measured on a long axis view in end diastole
II. Jacquier et al. [7].
Trabeculated mass percentage of total LV mass > 20% on stack of short-axis LV slices in end diastole
III. Stacey et al. [8].
A maximal NC/C ratio > 2.0 in end systole on a short axis non-apical slice.
IV. Captur et al. [9].
Fractional dimension >1.392 of apical third of left ventricle in end diastole

Y. M. Hoedemaekers (✉)
Department of Clinical Genetics, Radboudumc, Radboud University Nijmegen, Nijmegen, The Netherlands
e-mail: yvonne.hoedemaekers@radboudumc.nl

T. Germans
Department of Cardiology, Northwest Clinics Alkmaar, Amsterdam University Medical Centres, Amsterdam, The Netherlands
e-mail: t.germans@amsterdamumc.nl

H. F. Baars et al. (eds.), *Clinical Cardiogenetics*, https://doi.org/10.1007/978-3-030-45457-9_7

considers LVNC as unclassified, due to the lack of consensus whether LVNC may be regarded as a distinct form of cardiomyopathy or a non-specific morphological trait that is shared by different cardiomyopathies like ACM, HCM, DCM and RCM, or by congenital heart diseases [15, 16].

The nomenclature of this form of cardiomyopathy in literature varies widely. It has been referred to as left ventricular noncompaction (LVNC), noncompaction cardiomyopathy (NCCM), noncompaction of the left ventricular myocardium (NCLVM), left ventricular hypertrabeculation (LVHT), spongiform cardiomyopathy, embryonic myocardium, honeycombed myocardium, persisting myocardial sinusoids, myocardial dysgenesis, ventricular dysplasia or spongy myocardium.

Prevalence

Estimates of prevalence of LVNC were derived from large retrospective studies of patients referred for echocardiography. In 1997, Ritter et al. identified LVNC in 17 of 37,555 (0.045%) patients who underwent echocardiographic evaluation [17]. Similarly, in 2006, Aras et al. reported a prevalence of 0.14% in over 42,000 patients and in 2008 Sandhu identified definite or possible LVNC in 13/4929 (0.26%) patients referred for echocardiography [18, 19]. Prevalence was much higher (3.7%) in patients with an LV ejection fraction ≤45% [18]. Depending on the diagnostic criteria applied, even higher prevalences of LVNC (15.8% by Belanger; 23.6% by Kohli) were reported, indicating that LVNC may be more prevalent than previously thought [3, 20]. In 2013, a study among athletes revealed that 8% fulfilled echocardiographic criteria for LVNC [21]. A substantial proportion of individuals is asymptomatic, suggesting that true prevalence of LVNC may be higher, because asymptomatic individuals may go unnoticed in the studies of cardiologic patients [3, 11]. In a large study on childhood cardiomyopathies, LVNC was the most frequent cardiomyopathy after DCM and HCM, with an estimated prevalence of 9% in paediatric cardiomyopathies [22].

Aetiology/Pathophysiology

The aetiology of LVNC is rapidly being unravelled as more and more genetic defects in different genes are found, indicating that LVNC is genetically heterogeneous.

There is evidence that some forms of isolated LVNC are part of a spectrum of cardiomyopathies, including hypertrophic, dilated and restrictive cardiomyopathy. A shared aetiology consisting of genetic defects in the same sarcomere genes, sometimes even with identical mutations, has been found in these types of cardiomyopathy [11]. The phenotypic variability of cardiomyopathies within families, including variability in age of onset and severity of clinical presentation, might be explained by additional modifying factors, additional genetic variants or defects, or may depend on yet unidentified exogenous and/or systemic factors. Genetic defects in LVNC are discussed further on in the molecular diagnosis section.

Mutations in different genes associated with LVNC affect different mechanisms in the cardiomyocyte leading to changes that may individually cause LVNC or lead to a common cellular disturbance resulting in LVNC. Cellular growth and differentiation signalling pathways are thought to be involved in LVNC pathogenesis [23–26].

Mutations in sarcomere genes may exert their effect through defective force generation (either by a dominant-negative mechanism where the mutant protein acts as a "poison polypeptide" or by haplo-insufficiency resulting in less protein); mutated cytoskeletal proteins may lead to a defective force transmission; mutations in ATP-regulatory genes cause myocardial energy deficits and a fourth possible mechanism is abnormal calcium homeostasis either due to changes in calcium availability or myofibrillar sensitivity for calcium [20, 22–24, 27]. The development of LVNC features might be a compensatory response to dysfunction in one of these mechanisms.

The variable phenotypic expression of gene mutations leading to different types of cardiomyopathy is the net result of a complex interplay between the genetic defect, post transcriptional molecular processes, modifying genes and external factors. The localization of the mutations within the gene may partly explain phenotypic diversity, but also a "dose-effect" may be important; the extent of the defective mechanism may determine which phenotype ultimately develops.

Pathology

Macroscopy

The noncompacted endocardial layer of the myocardium comprises excessively numerous and prominent trabeculations with deep intertrabecular recesses that extend into the compacted myocardial layer. The apical and mid-ventricular segments of the left ventricular inferior and lateral wall are predominantly affected [28, 29]. In a pathoanatomical study of LVNC, Burke et al. described the morphology and microscopy of 14 paediatric LVNC cases. The macroscopic appearance varied from anastomosing trabeculae to a relatively smooth endocardial surface, with narrow openings of the recesses to the ventricular cavity. Three types of recess patterns were distinguished: (1) anastomosing broad trabeculae; (2) coarse trabeculae resembling multiple papillary muscles; and (3) interlacing smaller muscle bundles or relatively smooth endocardial surface with compressed invaginations, identified primarily microscopically (Fig. 7.1). In this study,

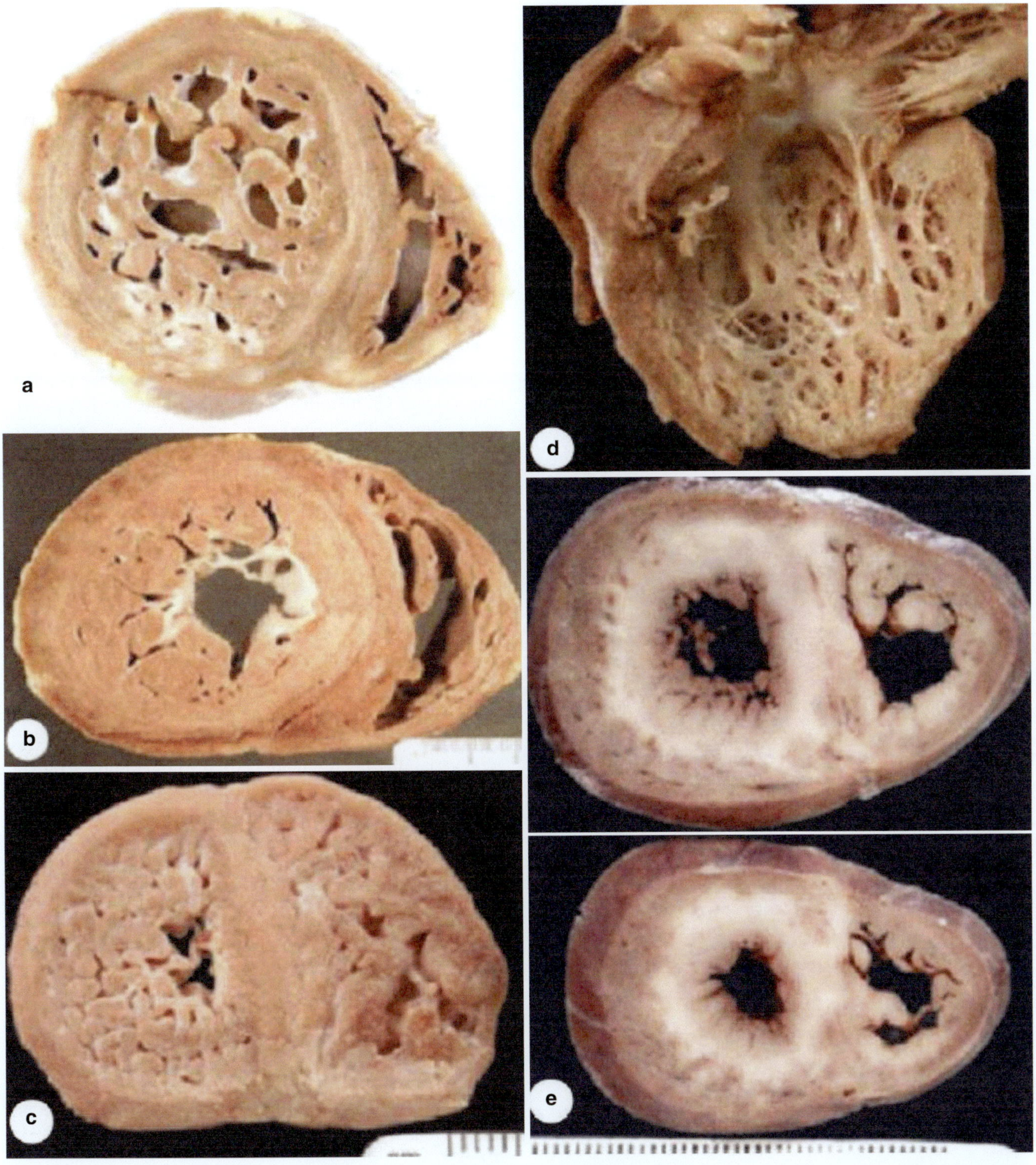

Fig. 7.1 LVNC gross pathology with a variety of LVNC patterns: (**a**) Anastomosing broad trabeculae. (**b**) Coarse trabeculae resembling multiple papillary muscles. (**c**) Interlacing smaller muscle bundles resembling a sponge. (**d**) Trabeculae viewed en face. (**e**) Subtle LVNC on gross section requires histological confirmation (Reproduced from Burke et al. [28] with permission)

no morphological differences were found between isolated and nonisolated LVNC [28].

In 1987, in an autopsy study of 474 normal hearts of all ages, it was found that prominent trabeculations may be observed in as many as 68% of the hearts, although more than three trabeculations were only identified in 3.4% [30].

Microscopy

Two patterns of myocardial structure in the superficial noncompacted layer in LVNC have been described by Burke et al. (1) anastomosing muscle bundles forming irregularly branching endocardial recesses with a staghorn-like appearance and (2) multiple small papillary muscles, resulting in an irregular surface appearance (Fig. 7.2). In most patients, these patterns overlapped. Endocardial fibrosis with prominent elastin deposition was found in all 14 cases and subendocardial replacement fibrosis, consistent with microscopic ischaemic infarcts, was present in 10; right ventricular involvement was identified in 6 cases [28].

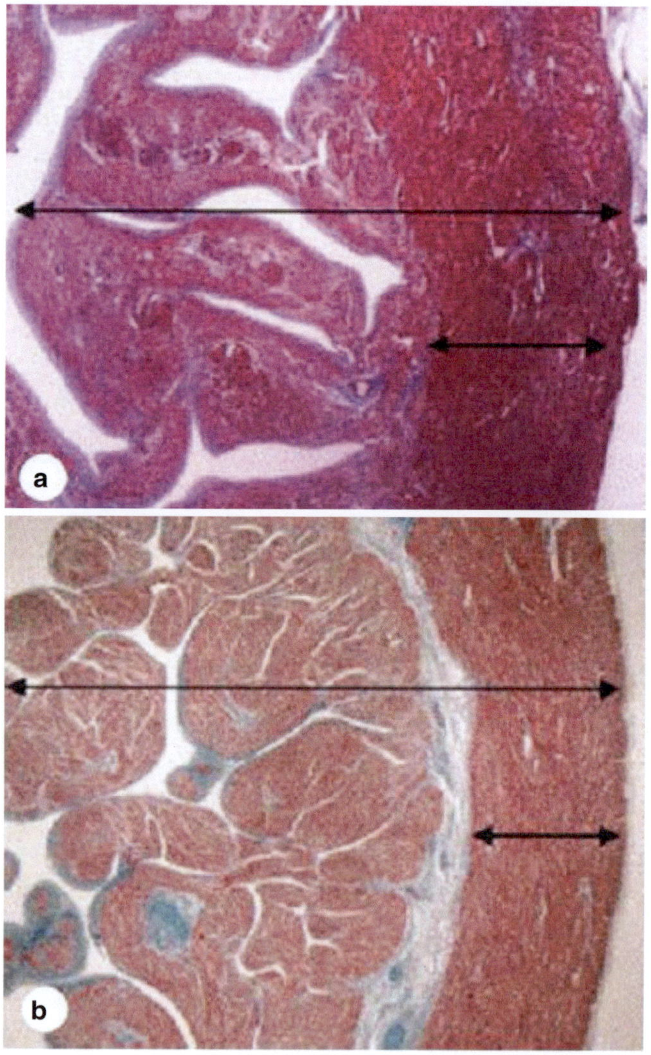

Fig. 7.2 Histological features in LVNC. The ratio of noncompact versus compact myocardium is larger than 2. (**a**) Relatively smooth endocardial surface (*left*) with anastomosing broad trabeculae. (**b**) Polypoid pattern of trabeculae; prominent fibrous band separating the noncompact from the compact myocardium (Reproduced from Burke et al. [28] with permission)

Histological examination in another study showed that ventricular endocardium covered the recesses in continuity with the LV cavity and identified ischaemic lesions in the thickened endocardium and the prominent trabeculae. Interstitial fibrosis ranged from being absent to severe. No fibre disarray was identified in any of these cases. Signs of chronic inflammation and abnormalities of intramyocardial blood vessels were present in some patients [2].

Freedom et al. proposed two criteria for the pathological diagnosis of LVNC: (1) absence of well-formed LV papillary muscles and (2) histological verification of more than 50% penetration of invaginated endocardial recesses towards the epicardial surface. The endothelium that covers the recesses extends close to the surface of the compact layer. The recesses neither communicate nor connect with the coronary circulation [31].

Clinical Presentation

Heart failure is among the most frequent presentations of LVNC, followed by supraventricular and ventricular arrhythmias, including sudden cardiac death and thrombo-embolic events. However, as in other cardiomyopathies, there is a great variability in presentation, even within families, ranging from a fully asymptomatic course to severe heart failure necessitating cardiac transplantation. The age of presentation is also highly variable varying from prenatal and neonatal diagnosis to diagnosis at the age of 94 years [13, 32, 33]. Prenatal diagnostic imaging more often detects bilateral ventricular hypertrophy/hypertrabeculations than the typical left ventricular morphologic changes observed postnatally and in adults [11]. The fourth to fifth decade is the median age at diagnosis in adult-isolated LVNC. Many patients remain asymptomatic, in whom isolated LVNC is an incidental finding or diagnosed in a family screening programme. Symptomatic patients may present with symptoms of dyspnoea, fatigue (atypical) chest pain and/or (pre) syncope. LVNC may also present as a peripartum cardiomyopathy [12, 34]. Review of the literature revealed a male to female ratio of almost 2:1 [35]. This gender difference cannot be fully explained by the occurrence of X-linked forms of LVNC.

Different arrhythmias and conduction disorders may occur in LVNC patients (Table 7.2) [36]. None of these arrhythmias is characteristic or pathognomonic for LVNC. Thrombo-embolic events may include stroke (cerebrovascular event or transient ischaemic attack), peripheral embolism and mesenterial thrombosis.

Table 7.2 Arrhythmia and conduction disorders associated with left ventricular noncompaction (LVNC)

Arrhythmia/conduction disorders associated with LVNC	References
Atrial fibrillation	[5, 37, 38]
Atrioventricular nodal re-entrant tachycardia	[39]
Bigemini ventricular extra systole	[40]
Complete atrioventricular block	[1, 41–43]
Complete left bundle branch block	[40, 44]
Early repolarization	[11]
Giant P-waves and focal atrial tachycardia	[45]
Long QT syndrome 2	[46]
Narrow QRS complex	[47–49]
Persistent atrial standstill	[50]
Sick sinus syndrome	[51, 52]
Sinus bradycardia	[52–55]
Supraventricular tachyarrhythmia	[10, 37, 40, 56, 57]
Ventricular fibrillation	[41, 47, 58]
Ventricular tachycardia	[10, 44, 47, 53, 59]
Wolff–Parkinson–White syndrome	[4, 10, 37, 40, 53]

Clinical Diagnosis

Diagnosis of LVNC remains challenging on two-dimensional transthoracic echocardiography and/or cardiac magnetic resonance imaging (CMR) (Table 7.1). Improvements in cardiac imaging techniques have led to increased recognition and diagnosis of LVNC. Figure 7.3 displays echocardiographic and cardiac MRI images of two LVNC patients, showing the abnormal segmental trabeculations as the hallmark of this entity.

Features of noncompaction observed in cardiology patients and normal controls still illustrate the necessity of defining criteria in order to accurately differentiate between normal physiological trabecularization and LVNC [20].

In 1990, the first diagnostic criteria for LVNC by Chin et al. were derived from the observations in eight LVNC patients [4]. These diagnostic criteria defined LVNC by the ratio of the distance from the epicardial surface to the trough of the trabecular recess (X) to the distance from the epicardial surface to the peak of the trabeculations (Y), with ratio $X/Y \leq 0.5$.

More than a decade later, Jenni et al. proposed new diagnostic criteria for isolated LVNC, consisting of four echocardiographic features: (1) an excessively thickened left ventricular myocardial wall with a two-layered structure consisting of a compact epicardial layer (C) and a noncompacted endocardial layer (NC) of prominent trabeculations and deep intertrabecular recesses; (2) a maximal end-systolic *NC/C ratio* > 2, measured at the parasternal short axis; (3) colour-Doppler evidence of deeply perfused intertrabecular recesses; (4) absence of coexisting cardiac anomalies [2]. For this study, they used seven patients with isolated LVNC in whom the heart could be anatomically evaluated with 10 DCM patients and 9 LVH transplant patients. Maximum non-compacted ratio found in the DCM patients was 2.0. Therefore, the end-systolic ratio of 2.0 was defined [11].

In 2002, Stollberger et al. proposed other diagnostic criteria for LVNC, wherein the diagnosis was a function of the number of trabeculations (>3) protruding from the left ventricular wall, apically to the papillary muscles and visible in a single image plane with obligatory perfusion of the intertrabecular spaces from the ventricular cavity visualized on colour-Doppler imaging [5]. With CMR, criteria to diagnose LVNC were first reported by Petersen et al. A noncompacted/compacted ratio (NC/C) of >2.3, measured in end diastole on long-axis views, was found to distinguish LVNC from various forms of cardiomyopathies and athletes hearts with a sensitivity of 86% and specificity of 99% [6]. Jacquier et al. proposed to express the trabeculated left ventricular mass as a percentage of total LV mass measured on a stack of short-axis views with CMR in end diastole. They deemed a trabeculated mass above 20% diagnostic for LVNC [7]. Other diagnostic criteria used in CMR are described by Stacey et al., who determined that a maximal noncompacted/compacted ratio >2.0 in a non-apical short axis in end systole was diagnostic for LVNC [8]. Captur et al. used fractal analysis considering a fractional dimension >1.392 in the apical third of the LV to be diagnostic for LVNC [9].

However, when applying above mentioned criteria in large-scale observational studies, diagnosis of LVNC tended to be as high as 23% in DCM patients using the echocardiographic criteria, and up to 4–13% in asymptomatic, low-risk general populations using the CMR criteria proposed by Petersen, Jacuier and Stacey [20, 60], suggesting that current diagnostic criteria might still lack specificity, further refinement of diagnosis/classification of LVNC is required as proposed by Belanger et al. and Arbustini et al. (Table 7.3).

Belanger et al. proposed such a classification system of LVNC by dividing noncompaction into four categories (none, mild, moderate and severe) according to noncompaction to compaction ratio and the size of the noncompaction area [3]. This classification scheme used the following criteria: (1) absence of congenital heart disease, hypertrophic or infiltrative cardiomyopathy, and coronary artery disease; (2) evidence of prominent trabeculations in the apex in any view (noncompacted to compacted ratio does not require to be >2); (3) concentration of the noncompacted area in the apex and (4) blood flow through the area of noncompaction.

Arbustini et al. divided LVNC into seven groups, according to current knowledge and terminology [61]. The first group consists of idiopathic LVNC, with normal systolic and

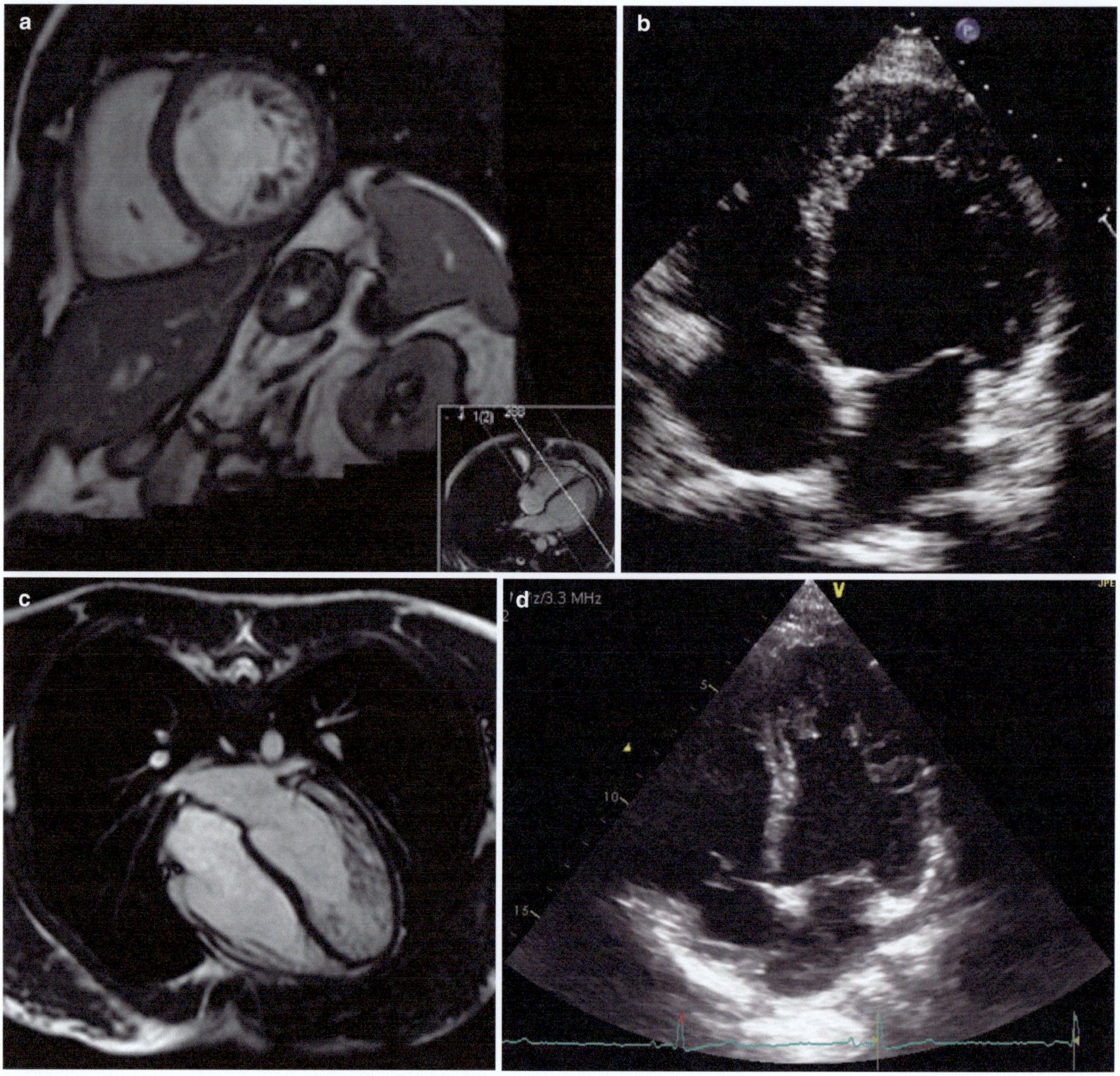

Fig. 7.3 (**a**, **b**) Cardiac MRI and echocardiography of a 43-year-old patient illustrating a two-layered myocardium with prominent intertrabecular recesses. (**c, d**) Cardiac MRI and echocardiography, four-chamber view each, of a 15-year-old patient with LVNC

diastolic function and normal dimensions. The second group is LVNC with LV dilatation and dysfunction at onset, therefore as such LVNC cardiomyopathy. The third is the group of LVNC also fulfilling diagnostic criteria for ACM, DCM, HCM or RCM. The fourth group consists of LVNC with congenital heart defects. The fifth group is the group of syndromes associated with LVNC. The sixth group is acquired and potentially reversible LVNC and the seventh group consists of right ventricular noncompaction, with or without LVNC.

Differential Diagnosis

The definitive diagnosis of LVNC relies on the morphological features of the LV myocardium observed on echocardiography, MRI, CT or LV angiography. The variability in the extent of physiological trabecularization may complicate distinction of LVNC from normal physiological left ventricular trabeculations. Especially in the area around the base of the papillary muscles of the mitral valve, more trabeculations may be present. However, in the normal heart, there is no

Table 7.3 Proposed LVNC classification systems

Belanger et al. [3]		
	NC/C ratio	LVNC area (cm^2)
1. None	0	0
2. Mild	>0 and < 1	≥0 and < 2.5
3. Moderate	≥1 and < 2	≥2.5 and < 5.0
4. Severe	≥2	≥5.0
Criteria used		
I. Absence of congenital heart disease, hypertrophic or infiltrative cardiomyopathy and coronary artery disease.		
II. Evidence of prominent trabeculations in the apex in any view.		
III. Concentration of the noncompacted area in the apex.		
IV. Blood flow through the area of noncompaction.		
Arbustini et al. [61]		
1. Idiopathic LVNC with normal systolic and diastolic function and normal dimensions.		
2. LVNC with LV dilatation and dysfunction at onset (LVNC cardiomyopathy or noncompaction cardiomyopathy).		
3. LVNC also fulfilling diagnostic criteria for ACM, DCM, HCM or RCM.		
4. LVNC with congenital heart defects.		
5. Syndromal LVNC.		
6. Acquired and potentially reversible LVNC.		
7. Right ventricular noncompaction, with or without LVNC.		

Table 7.4 Differential diagnosis of LVNC

Acquired LVNC	Hypertension
	Ischaemic heart disease Sickle cell anaemia Pregnancy Athletes Chronic renal failure
Dilated cardiomyopathy	
Hypertrophic cardiomyopathy	
Arrhythmogenic cardiomyopathy	
Neuromuscular disorders	
Syndromal LVNC	
Chromosomal abnormalities	

excessive segmental thickening (due to hypertrabeculation) like in LVNC and the thickness of these physiological trabeculations does not exceed the thickness of the compact layer. Also, the area of noncompaction is larger in LVNC than in physiological trabeculations [3].

Secondary forms of (acquired) LVNC may be the result of hypertension, chronic volume or pressure overload, ischaemic heart disease or extreme physical activity (i.e. athletes), leading to hypertrabecularization. These are referred to as pseudo-left ventricular noncompaction or LVNC mimicry. Hypertensive patients are diagnostically challenging, because of the occurrence of LV hypertrophy due to hypertension. Further studies are needed to confirm whether excessive trabeculation is more prevalent in specific ethnic groups, as suggested by one study [20].

Furthermore, dilated, hypertrophic and ischaemic cardiomyopathy may be mistaken for LVNC or vice versa, due to prominent trabeculations or abnormal myocardial thickening. Neuromuscular disorders, syndromes and chromosomal abnormalities (Tables 7.4 and 7.5) should be considered in the differential diagnosis of nonisolated LVNC, especially when LVNC occurs in patients with dysmorphism, growth retardation or skeletal muscle weakness.

Molecular Diagnosis

Over the years many genes have been associated with LVNC, with *MYH7* as the most prevalent genetic cause. An overview of the genes associated with LVNC is given in Table 7.5.

Molecular Defects in LVNC

Isolated LVNC has been associated with mutations in 27 different genes (Table 7.5). Defects in sarcomere genes have been identified to be the most prevalent genetic cause occurring in approximately 30% of all patients with isolated LVNC [11, 23].

Over 40 different mutations in sarcomere genes encoding thick (*MYH7*), intermediate (*MYBPC3*) and thin filaments (*TNNT2*, *TNNI3*, *TPM1*, *ACTC*) have been described. In particular in *MYH7*, the most frequent LVNC-associated gene, accounting for up to 21% of isolated LVNC [11, 23]. *MYH7* mutations currently associated with LVNC cluster in the ATPase active site of the head region in the N-terminal part of MYH7. This is an evolutionary well-conserved region of MYH7. As the ATPase active site is required for normal force production, impaired force generation might play a role in the aetiology of LVNC. Mutations in this region have been associated with LVNC with or without Ebstein anomaly [79, 94]. Other *MYH7* mutations (30%) were found in the C-terminal rod-region of the MYH7 protein that plays an important role in the formation of the core of the thick filament. Mutations in this region of the gene are more commonly associated with skeletal myopathies. Relatively few cardiomyopathy mutations are situated in this region.

With the availability of targeted cardiomyopathy panels (next-generation sequencing) more genes are and will be associated with LVNC, but as these data are still unpublished they are not mentioned here. Complex genotypes will become more common when more genes are analysed per patient.

Multiple or compound/double heterozygous mutations were identified in 25% of the children and in 10% of the adult LVNC patients [11]. In hypertrophic cardiomyopathy, complex genotypes have been described in 7% [95]. In HCM, double heterozygosity for truncating sarcomere mutations has been previously associated with severe congenital forms mostly inherited in an autosomal recessive mode [69, 96–99]. Nonsarcomere genetic causes for isolated LVNC include mutations in the calcium-handling

Table 7.5 Genes associates with left ventricular noncompaction (LVNC)

Gene	Locus; inheritance	Protein	Other associated disorders	References
ABCC9	12p12.1; AD	ATP-binding cassette subfamily C, member 9	AF, DCM Hypertrichotic osteochondrodysplasia (Cantu syndrome)	[62]
ACTC1	15q14; AD	α-Cardiac actin	DCM, HCM Congenital myopathy with fibre-type disproportion	[11, 12, 63]
ACTN2	1q43; AD	α-Actinin	DCM, HCM	[64]
CASQ2	1p13.3-p11; AD, AR	Calsequestrin	CPVT, HCM	[11, 65, 66]
DMPK	19q13.32; AD	Dystrophia myotonica protein kinase	Myotonic dystrophy 1	[67, 68]
DSP	6p24.3; AD	Desmoplakin	ACM, DCM, epidermolysis bullosa, keratosis palmoplantaris striata, skin fragility—Woolly hair syndrome	[69]
DTNA	18q12.1-q12.2; AD	α-Dystrobrevin		[70, 71]
GLA	Xq22.1; XL	α -galactosidase	Fabry disease	[72, 73]
HCN4	15q24.1; AD	Hyperpolarization-activated cyclic nucleotid-gated potassium channel 4	BrS, SSS	[52, 55]
KCNH2	7q35-q36; AD	Potassium voltage-gated channel, subfamily H, member 2	LQTS2, SQTS	[46]
LAMP2	Xq24; XL	Lysosome-associated membrane protein 2	Danon disease	[74]
LDB3[a]	10q22.2-q23.3; AD	LIM-domain binding protein	DCM Late-onset distal myopathy Myofibrillar myopathy	[11, 71, 75, 76]
LMNA	1q21.2; AD	Lamin A/C	DCM, RCM Emery–Dreifuss muscular dystrophy Lipodystrophy Werner syndrome Hutchinson–Gilford progeria Limb-girdle muscular dystrophy 1B Charcot–Marie–Tooth 2B1	[11, 77, 78]
MIB1	18q11.2; AD	Mindbomb drosophila homolog 1	LVNC	[55]
MYBPC3	11p11.2; AD	Cardiac myosin-binding protein C	DCM, HCM	[11, 23]
MYH7	14q12; AD	β-Myosin heavy chain	DCM, HCM, RCM Myosin storage myopathy Distal myopathy Scapuloperoneal myopathy	[11, 12, 23, 61, 79]
NKX2.5	5q35.1; AD	NK2 homeobox 5	Hypoplastic left heart syndrome; ventricular septal defect; atrial septal defect; Fallot; congenital hypothyroidism	[25]
PLEKHM2	1p36.21; AD	Pleckstrin homology domain-containing protein, family M, member 2	DCM, LVNC	[80]
PLN	6q22.1; AD	Phospholamban	ACM, DCM, HCM	[11, 66]
PKP2	12p11.21; AD, AR	Plakophillin 2	ACM	[81]
PRDM16	1p36; AD	PR domain-containing protein 16	DCM, Del1p36 syndrome	[82]
RYR2	1q43; AD	Ryanodine receptor 2	CPVT, ACM	[83, 84]
SCN5A	3p21; AD	Sodium channel type 5 α-subunit	BrS, DCM, LQTS3, SSS Familial heart block Paroxysmal ventricular fibrillation Cardiac conduction defect	[85]
TAZ[b]	Xq28; XL	Taffazin	Barth syndrome DCM	[11, 70, 71, 75, 86–93]
TNNI3	19p13.4; AD	Cardiac troponin I	DCM, HCM, RCM	[11]
TNNT2	1q32; AD	Cardiac troponin T	DCM, HCM, RCM	[11, 12, 23]
TPM1	15q22.1; AD	A-tropomyosin	DCM, HCM	[11, 23]

[a]Cypher/ZASP

[b]G4.5

ACM arrhythmogenic cardiomyopathy, *AF* atrial fibrillation, *BrS* Brugada syndrome, *CPVT* catecholaminergic polymorphic ventricular tachycardia, *DCM* dilated cardiomyopathy, *HCM* hypertrophic cardiomyopathy, *LQTS* long QT syndrome, *LVNC* left ventricular noncompaction, *RCM* restrictive cardiomyopathy, *SSS* sick sinus syndrome, *SQTS* short QT syndrome genes calsequestrin (*CASQ2*) and phospholamban (*PLN*), in taffazin (*TAZ*), α-dystrobrevin (*DTNA*), lamin A/C (*LMNA*) and LIM domain binding 3 (*LDB3*), potassium voltage-gated channel (*KCNH2*) and sodium channel type 5 (*SCN5A*) genes. However, mutations in these genes were only rare causes of LVNC in single families.

The absence of a mutation in approximately half of familial LVNC could be explained by phenotype assignment errors, the involvement of other yet unidentified genes, the presence of mutations in non-analysed gene sequences and incomplete sensitivity of the methods used.

Genotype–Phenotype Correlations

Molecular studies of LVNC have thus far shown that there are few recurrent mutations. Therefore, it is difficult to establish genotype–phenotype correlations. Additionally, intrafamilial phenotypic variability complicates predictions based on an identified mutation. The presence of multiple (truncating) sarcomere mutations in an individual appears to result in a more severe phenotype with childhood onset [11, 69]. Multiple mutations identified in adults mostly also comprise involvement of a nonsarcomere gene. Adult patients with multiple mutations seem to have more symptoms than adults with a single mutation [11].

Isolated LVNC

The first hypothesis on the pathogenesis of LVNC stemmed from observations that the morphology of LVNC was reminiscent of the embryonic stages of cardiac development. Consequently, it was postulated that LVNC could be the result from an arrest of compaction of myocardial fibres [4, 100, 101]. Figure 7.4 illustrates the striking resemblance between LVNC and the physiological embryonic noncompaction in the 8th–10th embryonic week. However, the possible mechanisms causing this arrest remain unclear. Epicardium-derived cells are thought to play an important role in myocardial architecture and in the development of noncompaction [102, 103]. Mutations in genes involved in myocardial genesis like peroxisome proliferator activator receptor binding protein (*PBP*), jumonji (*JMJ*), FK506-binding protein (*FKBP12*), transcription factor specificity protein (*Sp3*), homeobox factor *NKX2.5*, bone morphogenetic protein 10 (*BMP10*) lead to congenital LVNC in knock out mice [104–109]. However, apart from the NKX2.5 gene, in human LVNC, no mutations in these genes have been described.

Until now, there is very little insight into factors that influence the variability in age at onset and severity of symptoms of LVNC, or any other familial form of cardiomyopathy.

In the majority of patients, LVNC is diagnosed in adulthood, similar to ACM, HCM, DCM and RCM, which are rarely congenital. Of course, it could be that in LVNC, the lesions detected in adult patients were present from birth on, but remained unnoticed until symptoms developed and high-resolution cardiac imaging techniques were applied. However, the detection of sarcomere defects in LVNC patients may suggest otherwise, since mutations in sarcomere genes are known to cause late-onset HCM and DCM. Similarly, sarcomere mutations might lead to late-onset LVNC. Longitudinal cardiologic studies of unaffected carriers of pathogenic mutations are necessary to provide insight on whether noncompaction may develop later in life. The pathogenetic mechanism(s) of sarcomere defects in cardiomyopathies are not fully understood. It is possible that the pathological myocardial changes in the adult-onset sarcomere-related cardiomyopathies are caused by a compensatory response to impaired myocyte function resulting from mutations in the sarcomere genes [27, 110].

Nonisolated LVNC

LVNC has been observed in a number of neuromuscular disorders, metabolic and mitochondrial disease, congenital malformations and chromosomal syndromes.

Some of these disorders may share pathogenetic mechanisms with LVNC. Alternatively, LVNC might be secondary to other cardiac malformations or other malformations or even vice versa. Another possibility is that the co-occurrence is coincidental. Congenital heart malformations for instance are relatively frequent (birth prevalence 0.008) and may therefore occasionally coincide with LVNC without a mutual aetiology.

Congenital Heart Disease

The co-occurrence of congenital heart disease and noncompaction is predominantly observed in children. Tsai et al. showed that 78% of 46 children with LVNC had a congenital heart defect [10]. Nevertheless, congenital heart defects and LVNC also co-occur in adults [12]. The large number of structural heart malformations reported in association with noncompaction is presented in Table 7.6, indicating that septal defects, patent ductus arteriosus and Ebstein's anomaly are the most prevalent congenital heart defects in LVNC.

Increasingly, *congenital cardiac malformations* (septal defects, Ebstein anomaly, patent ductus arteriosus, Fallot's tetralogy, aortic coarctation and aortic aneurysms) are being reported in familial cardiomyopathies (HCM, DCM and LVNC) linked to sarcomere mutations, suggesting that these specific sarcomere defects may have been involved in car-

Table 7.6 Congenital heart disease associated with left ventricular noncompaction (LVNC)

Congenital heart disease in LVNC	Proportion of CHD		References
	In LVNC studies[a]	Case reports	
Aberrant origin of right/left subclavian artery	1/12 (8%)	1	[40, 111]
Absent aortic valve		1	[112]
Anomalous pulmonary venous return	2/26 (8%)		[28, 40]
Aortic coarctation	6/204 (3%)		[10, 11, 37, 40, 113]
Aortico-left ventricular tunnel		1	[114]
Aortic stenosis	2/46 (4%)	2	[10, 31, 115]
Aortopulmonary window	1/21 (5%)		[37]
Atrial septal defect	22/135 (16%)	3	[10, 11, 37, 54, 79, 116]
Atrio-ventricular diverticulum		1	[117]
Bicuspid aortic valves	3/64 (5%)	3	[10, 37, 118, 119]
Bicuspid pulmonary valve	1/14 (7%)		[28]
Cardiac aneurysms		4	[43, 120–122]
Coronary ostial stenosis	1/14 (7%)		[28]
Cor triatriatum	1/46 (2%)		[10]
Dextrocardia	2/58 (3%)	1	[1, 10, 40]
Dextro malposed great arteries	1/12 (8%)		[40]
Dextroversion		1	[123]
Double inlet left ventricle	1/46 (2%)		[10]
Double orifice mitral valve		4	[124–126]
Double outlet right ventricle	1/54 (2%)		[113]
Ebstein's anomaly	11/130 (8%)	14	[10, 11, 54, 61, 127–132]
Fallot's tetralogy	1/71 (1%)	1	[11, 111]
Hypoplastic left heart syndrome	3/54 (6%)		[113]
Hypoplastic right ventricle	3/58 (5%)		[10, 40]
Isomerism of the left atrial appendage	4/66 (6%)	8	[31, 40, 113, 133]
Left-sided superior vena cava	1/46 (2%)		[10]
Mitral valve atresia		1	[112]
Mitral valve cleft	2/54 (4%)	1	[43, 113]
Mitral valve dysplasia	2/14 (14%)		[28]
Mitral valve prolapse	1/46 (2%)		[10]
Patent ductus arteriosus	16/182 (9%)	1	[10, 11, 54, 113]
Persistent left superior vena cava	1/14 (7%)	1	[28, 122]
Pulmonary atresia	6/125 (5%)	1	[11, 54, 113]
Pulmonary valve dysplasia	2/14 (14%)		[28]
Pulmonary stenosis	4/97 (4%)	1	[11, 28, 40, 54]
Single ventricle	1/12 (8%)	1	[40, 134]
Subaortic membrane	2/55 (4%)		[113]
Transposition of the great arteries	1/46 (2%)	1	[10, 135]
Tricuspid atresia	2/54 (4%)		[113]
Tricuspid valve dysplasia	1/14 (7%)		[28]
Ventricular septal defect	23/218 (11%)	3	[1, 10, 11, 28, 37, 40, 113, 115, 122]

[a]Cumulative number of LVNC patients with congenital heart defect (CHD) described in one or more LVNC studies

diac morphogenesis [11, 63, 79, 136–139]. But since there is rarely more than one patient with a congenital heart defect, even in families with multiple cardiomyopathy patients, the association of sarcomere defects and heart defects still requires further exploration.

Neuromuscular Disease

Similar to HCM and DCM, LVNC has been associated with neuromuscular disorders. Stollberger and Finsterer identified LVNC-like morphological features in Duchenne and Becker muscular dystrophy and in myotonic dystrophy (see chapter *Neuromuscular disorders*) [140–142]. The gene mutated in Duchenne and Becker muscular dystrophy is a part of the dystrophin complex, a complex of muscle membrane-associated proteins, connecting the cytoskeleton to the surrounding extracellular matrix and may also play a role in cell signalling. The dystrophin gene is expressed in skeletal and cardiac myocytes. Other genes previously associated with neuromuscular disorders, like adult-onset myofibrillar myopathy (*LDB3* or *Cypher/ZASP*), limb-girdle muscular dystrophy (LGMD) (*LMNA*), scapuloperoneal myopathy (*MYH7*), myosin storage distal myopathy (*MYH7*) and Barth syndrome (*TAZ*) have recently been associated with isolated LVNC (Table 7.5). ZASP, lamin A and C, β-myosin heavy chain and taffazin are all expressed in cardiac and skeletal muscle tissue. ZASP has a function in cytoskeletal assembly. Mutations in ZASP can lead to DCM and to skeletal myopathy. Lamin A and C, proteins situated in the nuclear membrane, play an important role in maintaining nuclear architecture. *LMNA* mutations have been described in three LVNC patients [11, 77, 78]. In one of them, there was familial limb-girdle muscular dystrophy (LGMD) as well as DCM [11]. Over 200 mutations have been described in *LMNA*, causing over 20 different phenotypes, including isolated DCM, LGMD, Emery–Dreifuss muscular dystrophy, Hutchinson–Gilford progeria, partial lipodystrophy and peripheral neuropathy. For many of the phenotypes, there is no clear genotype–phenotype correlation, phenotypes may overlap and different phenotypes are associated with single mutations. Up to 25% of patients with an LMNA mutation may remain free from manifest cardiac disease [143].

Syndromes

LVNC can occur as part of a syndrome in combination with dysmorphic features and other congenital malformations. When there are other congenital defects or when there are dysmorphic features in a patient, one of the listed syndromes in Table 7.7 or one of the chromosomal defects in Table 7.8 could be considered in the differential diagnosis.

Table 7.7 Syndromes associated with left ventricular noncompaction (LVNC)/hypertrabeculation

Syndrome	Gene	Inheritance	Features	References
Barth syndrome/3-methylglutaconic aciduria	*TAZ*	XR	Growth retardation, DCM, skeletal myopathy, intermittent lactic acidemia, granulocytopenia, recurrent infections	[70, 71, 75, 86–93, 144]
Branchio-oto-renal syndrome I/ Melnick Fraser syndrome	*EYA1*	AD	Long narrow face; hearing loss (sensory/conductive/mixed); preauricular pits; microtia; cup-shaped ears; lacrimal duct stenosis; cleft palate; bifid uvula; branchial cleft fistulas/cysts; renal dysplasia/aplasia; polycystic kidneys; vesico-ureteric reflux	[145]
Coffin–Lowry syndrome	*RSK2*	XD	Short stature; weight <3rd percentile; microcephaly; coarse facies with prominent brow, chin and ears; sensorineural hearing loss; downslant; hypertelorism; heavy, arched eyebrows; broad nose with thick alae nasi and nasal septum; anteverted nostrils; large mouth; thick everted lower lip; narrow, high palate; hypodontia, malocclusion, pectus excavatum/carinatum; mitral insufficiency; inguinal hernia; uterine prolapse; skeletal abnormalities; loose skin; straight, coarse hair; mental retardation; hypotonia; seizures	[146]
Congenital adrenal hypoplasia	*NR0B1*	XR	Failure to thrive; hypogonadotropic hypogonadism; cryptorchidism; hyperpigmentation; primary adrenocortical failure; adrenal insufficiency; gluco-mineralocorticoid insufficiency; salt-wasting; delayed puberty	[147]
Contractural arachnodactyly/ Beals syndrome	*FBN2*	AD	Marfanoid habitus; micrognathia; frontal bossing; crumpled ear helices; ectopia lentis; high-arched palate; septal defects; bicuspid aortic valve; mitral valve prolapse; patent ductus arteriosus; aortic root dilatation; pectus carinatum; kyphoscoliosis; hip/knee/elbow contractures; arachnodactyly; ulnar deviation of fingers; talipes equinovarus; hypoplastic calf muscles; motor development delay	[148]
Cornelia de Lange syndrome I	*NIPBL*	AD	Short stature; microcephaly; long philtrum; micrognathia; low-set ears; sensorineural hearing loss; synophrys; myopia; long curly eyelashes; ptosis; anteverted nostrils; depressed nasal bridge; cleft lip/palate; thin upper lip; widely spaced teeth; congenital heart defect; pyloric stenosis; hypoplastic male genitalia; structural renal anomalies; phocomelia; oligodactyly; syndactyly of second and third toes; single transverse palmar crease; cutis marmorata; hirsutism; low posterior hair line; mental retardation; language delay; automutilation	[37]
Holt Oram syndrome	*TBX5*	AD	ASD; VSD; HLHS; PDA; absent pectoralis major muscle; pectus excavatum/carinatum; vertebral anomalies; thoracic scoliosis; absent, bifid or triphalangeal thumb; carpal bone anomalies; phocomelia of upper extremity, radial-ulnar anomalies; asymmetric involvement	[149]
Leopard syndrome	*PTPN11* *RAF1*	AD	Short stature; triangular face; low-set ears; sensorineural hearing loss; hypertelorism; ptosis; epicanthal folds; broad flat nose; cleft palate; short neck; pulmonic stenosis; HCM; subaortic stenosis; complete heart block; bundle branch block; winged scapulae; hypospadias; absent/hypoplastic ovary; unilateral renal agenesis; spina bifida occulta; dark lentigines (mostly neck and trunk); café-au-lait spots	[150]
Melnick Needles osteodysplasty	*FLNA*	XD	Short stature; micrognathia; large ears; hypertelorism; exophthalmos; cleft palate; misaligned teeth; long neck; mitral/tricuspid valve prolapse; LVNC; pulmonary hypertension; pectus excavatum; omphalocele; hydronephrosis; tall vertebrae; bowing of humerus/radius/ulna/tibia; short distal phalanges of the fingers; pes planus; coarse hair; delayed motor development; hoarse voice	[151]

(continued)

Table 7.7 (continued)

Syndrome	Gene	Inheritance	Features	References
Nail Patella syndrome	*LMX1B*	AD	Short stature; sensorineural hearing loss; ptosis; cataract; cleft lip/palate; malformed sternum; hypoplasia of first ribs; glomerulanephritis; renal failure; scoliosis; elbow deformities; hypoplastic or absent patella; clinodactyly; talipes equinovarus; longitudinal ridging nails; slow nail growth; koilonychias; anonychia; aplasia pectaralis minor/biceps/triceps/quadriceps	[152]
Noonan syndrome	*PTPN11*[a] *KRAS* *SOS1* *RAF1*	AD	Short stature; triangular face; low-set ears; hypertelorism; downslanting palpebral fissures; epicanthal folds; myopia; micrognathia; high-arched palate; low posterior hairline; webbed neck; septal defects; pulmonic stenosis; patent ductus arteriosus; pectus carinatum superiorly/pectus excavatum inferiorly; cryptorchidism; clinodactyly; woolly hair; mental retardation (mild); bleeding tendency; malignant schwannoma	[153]
Roifman syndrome		XR	Short-trunk dwarfism; long philtrum; strabismus; narrow and downslanting palpebral fissures; long eyelashes; retinal dystrophy; narrow upturned nose; LVNC; hepato-splenomegaly; spondylo-epiphyseal dysplasia; eczema; hyperconvex nails; hypotonia; (mild) mental retardation; hypogonadotropic hypogonadism; recurrent infections; antibody deficiency	[154]
Sotos syndrome	*NSD1*	AD	Length $\geq$ 97th percentile in early adolescence; adult height often normal; macrocephaly; frontal bossing, prognathism; pointed chin; conductive hearing loss; downslant; nystagmus; strabismus; high arched palate; premature tooth eruption; tooth agenesis; ASD; VSD; PDA; advanced bone age; large hands and feet; developmental delay/variable mental retardation; neonatal hypotonia; seizures; poor coordination; behavioural problems	[155]
Syndromic microphtalmia/MIDAS syndrome (MIcrophtalmia, dermal aplasia, Sclerocornea)	*HCCS*	XD	Short stature; microcephaly; hearing loss; microphthalmia; sclerocornea; cataract; iris coloboma; retinopathy; septal defects; cardiac conduction defects; cardiomyopathy; overriding aorta; anteriorly placed anus; hypospadias; linear skin defects; corpus callosum agenesis; hydrocephalus; mental retardation; seizures	[156, 157]

AD autosomal dominant, *XD* X-linked dominant, *XR* X-linked recessive.
[a]most frequently involved genes

Table 7.8 Chromosomal defects associated with left ventricular noncompaction (LVNC)

Chromosomal defects	Features	References
Deletion		
1p36	Microcephaly; sensorineural hearing loss; deep-set eyes; flat nose; cleft lip/palate; cardiomyopathy; septal defects; patent ductus arteriosus; dilated aortic root; feeding problems; gastro-oesophageal reflux; short fifth finger and clinodactyly; mental retardation (severe); seizures; hypotonia	[82, 158–162]
1q43-q43	Microcephaly; upslanting palpebral fissures; epicanthus, broad nasal bridge, micrognathia; low-set ears; bow-shaped upper lip; widely spaced teeth; short webbed neck; congenital heart defects; mental retardation (severe); speech impairment; seizures; corpus callosum agenesis	[163]
5q35.1q35.3	Facial hirsutism; synophrys; downslanting palpebral fissures; atrial septal defect and patent ductus arteriosus; LVNC with sick sinus syndrome and second degree heart block; feeding problems; gastro-oesophageal reflux; joint hypermobility	[164]
7p14.3p14.1	Ventricular septal defect, atrial septal defect, aortic valve dysplasia, mental retardation, sacral fistula, growth retardation, microcephaly, facial dysmorphism	[162]
18p subtelomeric deletion	Oesophageal atresia, otodysplasia, short stature, deafness, mental retardation, facial dysmorphism	[162]
22q11.2	Velo-cardio-facial syndrome: Short stature; microcephaly; retrognathia; narrow palpebral fissures; square nasal root; prominent tubular nose; cleft palate; velopharyngeal insufficiency; congenital heart defect (85%): Ventricular septal defect; Fallot's tetralogy; inguinal/umbilical hernia; slender hands and digits; learning disability; mental retardation; schizophrenia; bipolar disorder	[147, 162]

(continued)

Table 7.8 (continued)

Chromosomal defects	Features	References
Numeric		
4q trisomy/1q monosomy	Senile-like appearance; narrow palpebral fissures; telecanthus; epicanthus; broad nasal bridge; low-set ears; long philtrum; dimple below lower lip; anteriorly displaced anus; rocker-bottom feet; mental retardation; hypotonia, hypoplastic corpus callosum	[165]
Trisomy 13	Microcephaly; hypotelorism; cleft lip/palate; coloboma; low-set ears; septal defects; patent ductus arteriosus	[166]
	Polydactyly; overlapping fingers; mental retardation (severe); hypotonia; seizures	
Trisomy 21	Short stature; brachycephaly; flat facial profile; conductive hearing loss; epicanthal folds; upslant; iris brushfield spots; protruding tongue; congenital heart malformation; duodenal atresia; Hirschsprung disease; joint laxity; single transverse palmar crease; excess nuchal skin; mental retardation; hypothyroidism; leukaemia	[11, 113]
Mosaic trisomy 22	Microcephaly; hypertelorism; preauricular pits/tags; low-set ears; micrognathia, long philtrum; septal defects; double aortic arch; clinodactyly; hypoplastic nails; hemiatrophy; mental retardation	[167]
45,X0 (including mosaics)	Turner syndrome: Short stature; short webbed neck; low hair line; broad nasal bridge; low-set ears; congenital heart defects: Aortic coarctation; bicuspid aortic valves; aortic dilatation; lymph-edema of hands and feet; renal abnormalities: Single horseshoe kidney; renal vascular abnormalities; delayed puberty; amenorrhea; infertility; hypothyroidism	[162, 168, 169]
Translocation		
Robertsonian t13;14	Ventricular septal defect, mental retardation, linear cutaneous achromic lesions, growth retardation, toe syndactyly (II–III), facial dysmorphism	[162]
Loci		
6p24.3–21.1	LVNC; bradycardia; pulmonary valve stenosis; atrial septal defect; left bronchial isomerism; azygous continuation of the inferior vena cava; polysplenia; intestinal malrotation	[54]
11p15	LVNC; mild pulmonary stenosis; mild mitral valve prolapse; atrial septal defect	[170]

Mitochondrial Disorders

Mitochondrial disorders often lead to multi-organ disease, including central and peripheral nervous system, eyes, heart, kidney and endocrine organs. One of the cardiac features observed in mitochondrial disease is LVNC. Cardiac features may be the first or only feature in patients suffering from a mitochondrial disorder. In a study of 113 paediatric patients with mitochondrial disease, LVNC was identified in 13% [171]. Pignatelli et al. showed that 5 of the 36 paediatric LVNC patients who underwent a skeletal muscular biopsy, had morphologic and biochemical evidence for a mitochondrial defect, including a partial deficiency of complex I–III of the mitochondrial respiratory chain [147]. Mutations in mitochondrial DNA (mtDNA) and in nuclear DNA have been identified in the mitochondrial disorders associated with LVNC [172, 173].

Diagnostic Work-up

Work-up of an LVNC patient should focus on identifying the underlying cause either genetic or other (Table 7.9).

Therapy

Treatment and follow-up of LVNC largely depend on co-existent cardiomyopathy. When DCM is present, treatment with ACE inhibitors and β-Blockers should be initiated as soon as symptomatic heart failure with reduced left ventricular ejection fraction (HFrEF) occurs [175].

An important issue is the use of prophylactic anticoagulants, in view of frequent thrombo-embolic events. The early case reports and case series emphasized the high risk of thromboembolism and advised routine anticoagulation therapy. However, recent long-term follow-up studies found no association between the presence and/or extent of hypertrabularization/noncompaction and risk of trombo-embolic events [176–178]. Therefore, the mere presence of noncompaction does not seem to be an independent risk factor for trombo-embolic events in DCM patients [47, 176, 179].

When selecting candidates for cardiac resynchronization therapy (CRT) according to current guidelines for CRT, this therapy has also been shown to be effective in LVNC patients, with reported response rates >50% [180].

Heart transplantation has been performed in some LVNC patients with severe heart failure [36, 55, 69, 181]. Left ventricular restoration surgery has been reported successful in a single patient [182]. Treatment with an implantable cardioverter defibrillator (ICD) will be discussed later.

Risk Stratification and Indications for ICD Implantation

Patients at the highest risk for sudden death are patients who previously experienced (aborted) cardiac arrest, ventricular fibrillation and sustained VF. Family history of sudden death, unexplained syncope (especially during exercise), abnormal

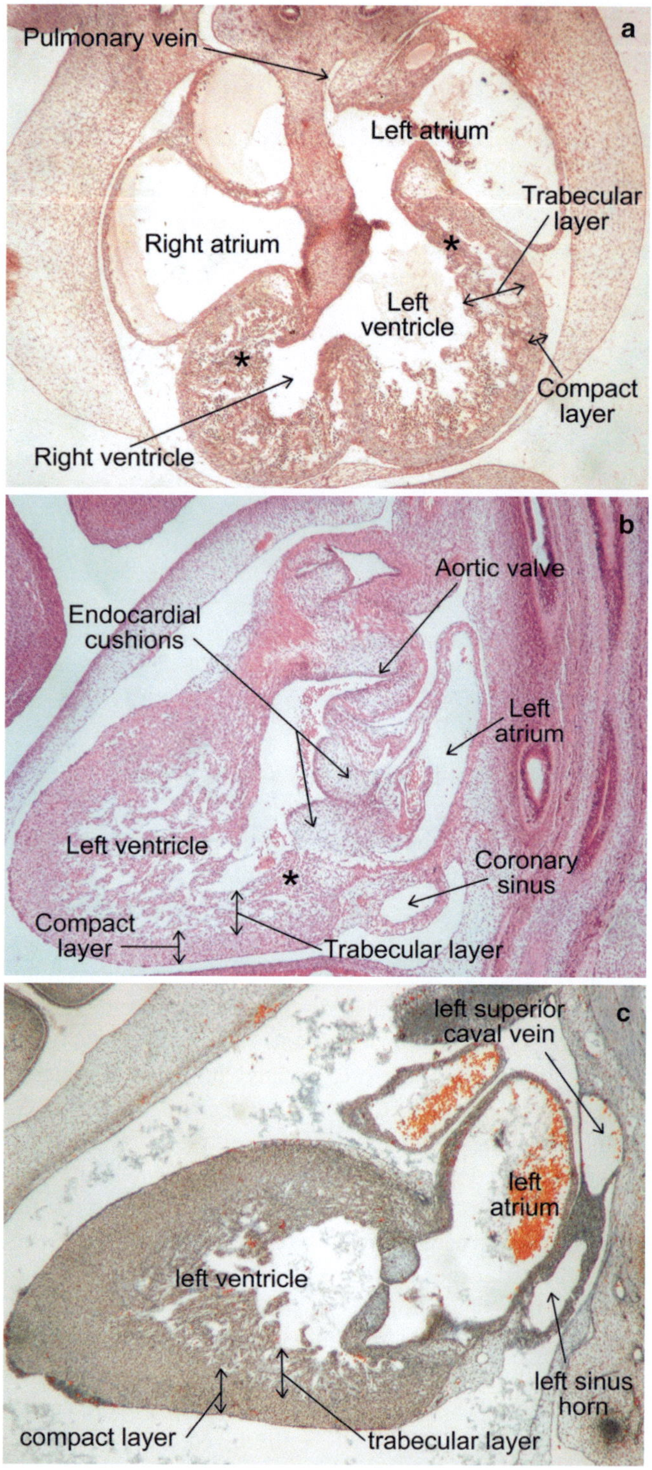

Fig. 7.4 Human embryos at Carnegie stage 16 (**a**), stage 18 (**b**) and after closing of the embryonic interventricular foramen (**c**). During development, there is an extensive trabecular layer forming the greater part of the ventricular wall thickness compared to the extent of the compact layer. The trabecular layer becomes compacted and forms the papillary muscles of the atrioventricular valves (*asterisks*) (Reproduced from Freedom et al. [31] with permission)

Table 7.9 Proposed diagnostic work-up of a newly identified index patient with LVNC (modified from the ACCF/AHA guidelines for the diagnosis and management of heart failure in adults) [174]

History	Chest pain; palpitations; intake of alcohol, cocaine, medication; chemotherapy; radiation; deficiencies
Family history	Cardiomyopathy; conduction disease, arrhythmia, sudden cardiac or unexplained death; neuromuscular disease
ECG	Conduction disease; arrhythmia; sick sinus syndrome; prolonged QT; Q-waves; hypertrophy (see also Table 7.2)
Echocardiography	Congenital heart disease; Jenni criteria; left ventricular ejection fraction
Laboratory	Complete blood count; serum electrolytes; blood urea nitrogen serum creatinine, fasting blood glucose, lipids, liver function tests thyroid function, CRP, iron status, creatine kinase, noradrenaline cortisol, growth hormone
Viral workup	Antibodies: Coxsackie-; influenza-; adeno-; echo-; cytomegalo-;human immunodeficiency virus
CMR	Myocardial infarction; infiltrative disease; myocarditis; dilated or hypertrophic cardiomyopathy, late gadolinium enhancement, NC/C ratio
Coronary angiography/ myocardial perfusion scintigraphy	Coronary artery disease
Mitochondrial workup	When signs of mitochondrial disorder (e.g. myopathy; deafness; diabetes; encephalopathy; stroke-like episodes; ophthalmoplegia; retinopathy
Neurologic examination	When signs of neuromuscular disease or when family history is positive for neuromuscular disease
Genetic counselling	Preferably for all cases
Genetic testing	Core panel when available; when unavailable ACTC1, MYBPC3, MYH7, TNNI3, TNNT2 and TPM1 (see also Fig. 7.5)

blood pressure response during exercise tests, frequent premature ventricular beats on the resting ECG and/or nonsustained ventricular tachycardia on Holter monitoring and significantly impaired left ventricular function may be considered risk factors. The results from longitudinal studies and the understanding of underlying disease mechanisms will hopefully help to gain more insight into the risk factors and allow more appropriate risk stratification.

Regular ICD indications include primary and secondary prevention. For secondary prevention, i.e. after a previous episode of aborted cardiac death or collapse due to sustained VT or VF, current ICD guidelines advise ICD implantation.

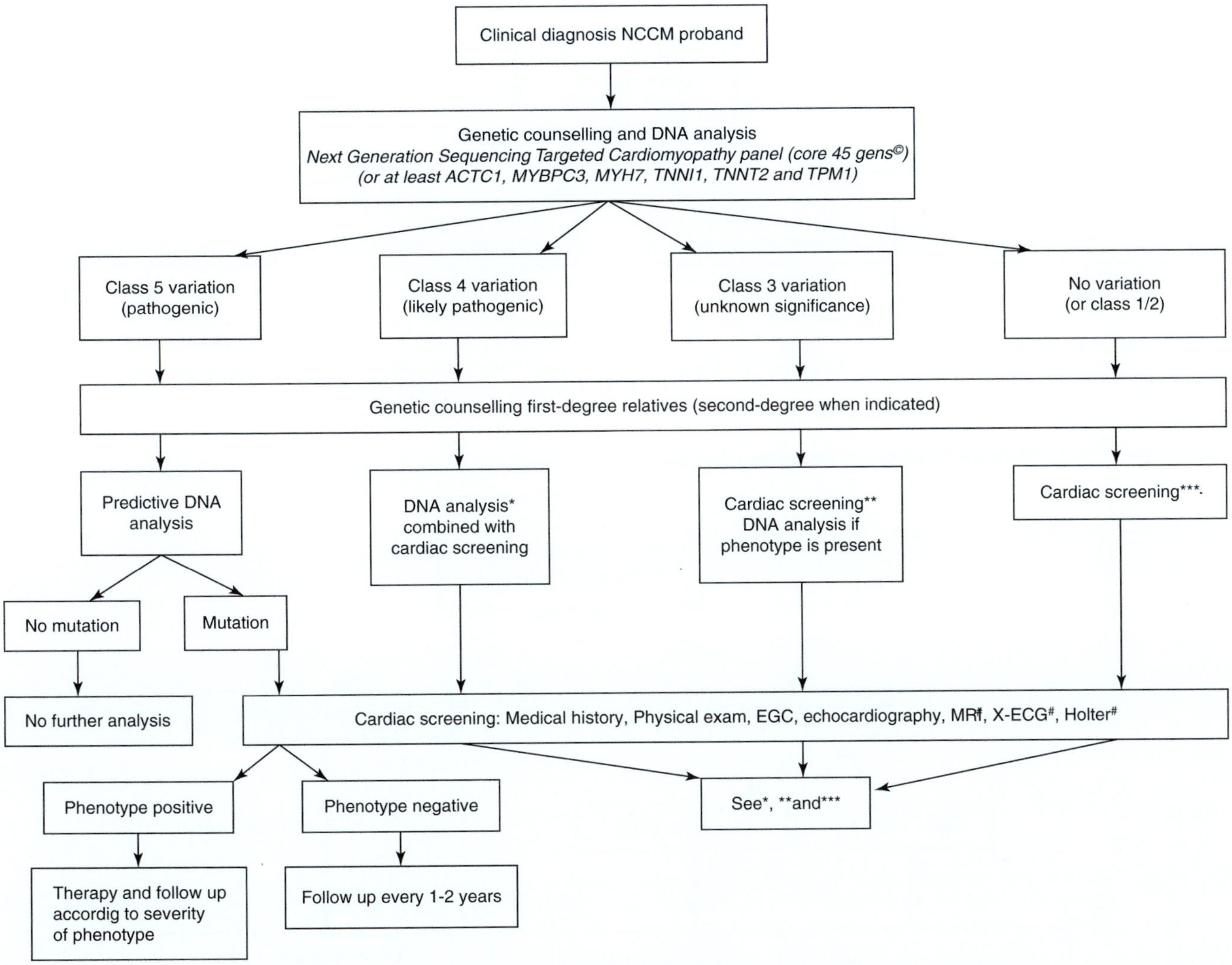

Fig. 7.5 Flowchart for family screening in LVNC including ∗likely pathogenic variants (class 4), ∗∗variants of unknown significance (class 3) and ∗∗∗no variants or class 1 or 2 variants; # if clinically indicated; @ core panel: *ACTC1, ACTN2, ANKRD1, BAG3, CALR3, CAV3, CRYAB, CSRP3, CTNNA3, DES, DSC2, DSG2, DSP, EMD, FHL1, GLA, JPH2, JUP, LAMA4, LAMP2, LMNA, LDB3, MIB1, MYBPC3, MYH6, MYH7, MYL2, MYL3, MYOZ2, MYPN, NEXN, PKP2, PLN, PRDM16, PRKAG2, RBM20, SCN5A, TAZ, TCAP, TMEM43, TNNC1, TNNI3, TNNT2, TPM1, TTN, TTR, VCL*

In the Rotterdam LVNC cohort of 67 patients, an ICD was indicated in 42% according to current ICD guidelines ($n = 28$; 21 primary and 7 for secondary prevention). After long-term follow-up, appropriate ICD therapy occurred only in patients in whom ICD was implanted for secondary prevention ($n = 3$). Inappropriate ICD therapy occurred in 33% of the patients with primary prevention and in 29% of the patients with secondary prevention [183]. In another study, follow-up of 12 patients who received an ICD showed overall appropriate therapy in 42% in primary and secondary prevention combined. In primary prevention, 25% of ICD therapy was appropriate as opposed to 50% in secondary prevention [56]. In a recent long-term follow-up study, there was no significant difference between HCM, DCM and LVNC patients with regard to appropriate and inappropriate discharge of ICDs implanted in these patient groups [184].

Prognosis

Initially, LVNC was reported to have a grave prognosis. However, the application of new imaging techniques allowing diagnosing LVNC in asymptomatic individuals suggests that the first observations were influenced by selection of the most severely affected individuals. In children, age is not a predictor of the outcome [185]. New York Heart Association Class III or higher and presence of cardiovascular complications do seem to be a strong predictor [186]. It

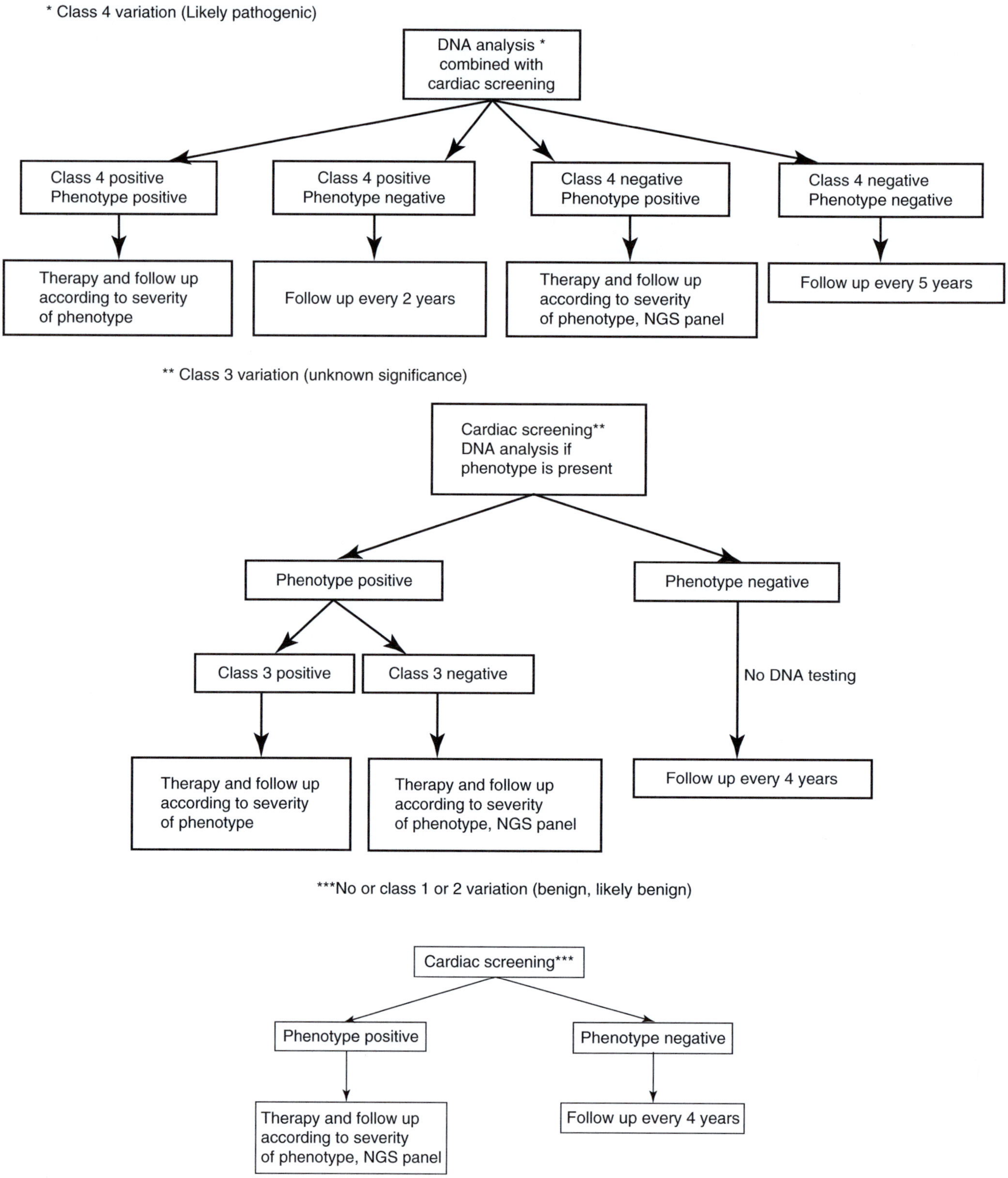

Fig. 7.5 (continued)

has become clear that prognosis of LVNC is as variable as the prognosis in other cardiomyopathies. Even in those with presentation in early childhood, gradual improvement in cardiac function may be observed, although in others evolvement to severe heart failure requiring heart transplantation does occur.

LVNC patients in whom contrast-enhanced myocardial areas are present on CMR seem to have worse prognosis compared to LVNC patients without contrast-enhanced myocardial areas [187]. Also, LVNC patients with DCM have worse prognosis compared to patients with HCM or sporadic LVNC [188]. In contrast, genotype-negative LVNC patients without overt cardiomyopathy have excellent prognosis [178]. Malignant arrhythmias leading to sudden cardiac death and heart failure are the main indicators of poor prognosis, also in children [189]. The establishment of appropriate risk stratification will be an important issue in the near future in order to identify patients at risk and to help prevent sudden cardiac death.

Recommendations During Pregnancy and Delivery

Maternal risk in LVNC largely depends on the severity of the concomitant cardiomyopathy and/or congenital heart disease. According to ESC guidelines, patients who are at highest risk for cardiac events (modified WHO class IV) have a maternal event risk of 40–100%, this should be considered a contra-indication for pregnancy. However, when pregnant, patients should be offered counselling and should be referred to an expert centre with close monthly follow-up. These group of patients encompasses LVNC patients with peripartum cardiomyopathy with any residual LV functional impairment, LVEF <30% or NYHA class III–IV or severe mitral valve or aortic valve stenosis. LVNC patients with moderate risk for cardiac events (modified WHO class II–III) have a maternal event rate of 10–19% and should be offered counselling and should be monitored bimonthly in a referral centre. Examples of cardiac disease that are associated with LVNC in this WHO class are patients with HCM, patients with moderate mitral valve or aortic valve disease, AVSD and repaired coarctation [190].

Follow-Up Advice

The indication for cardiologic follow-up depends on individual symptoms and cardiac abnormalities. In asymptomatic patients with preserved LV function, annual or biannual cardiologic follow-up is recommended, including ECG and echocardiography. When indicated, 24-h-Holter monitoring and exercise testing could also be included in the follow-up. Importantly, LNVC patients in whom one or more genetic mutation(s) were found tended to have a worse prognosis than patients with sporadic forms of LVNC and may justify more strict follow-up [179].

Family Screening

Molecular and Cardiologic Family Screening

Familial LVNC has been estimated to occur in 18–71% of adults with isolated LVNC, mostly consistent with an autosomal dominant mode of inheritance, indicating the importance of informing and examining relatives of patients with isolated LVNC [4, 11, 19, 147, 191–194]. Since extensive family studies showed that the majority of affected relatives are asymptomatic, cardiologic evaluation should include all adult relatives irrespective of medical history. Obviously, taking a family history is by itself insufficient to identify familial disease, given the high frequency of asymptomatic disease in families [11]. In families where a pathogenic mutation has been identified, relatives can be offered predictive DNA analysis. In families without a pathogenic mutation, cardiac family screening remains the method of choice to identify relatives at risk of developing symptomatic cardiomyopathy, who may benefit from early treatment. In families where a variant (class 3 or 4) is identified, DNA analysis and cardiologic screening are advised as depicted in Fig. 7.5.

Apart from LVNC, other cardiomyopathies may co-occur within families, like hypertrophic and dilated cardiomyopathy, so cardiac screening should aim at identifying all cardiomyopathies. Cardiac screening of relatives may show minor abnormalities not fulfilling LVNC criteria, which may be difficult to differentiate from normal physiologic trabecularization. Hypothetically, these minor abnormalities might develop into LVNC eventually. Longitudinal studies of patients with mild LVNC features are needed to investigate the natural history of these forms of noncompaction.

The proposed strategies for the molecular and cardiologic evaluation of LVNC are depicted in the flowchart in Fig. 7.5. Extensive genetic screening, preferably with a targeted cardiomyopathy gene panel, may lead to the identification of a molecular defect in over 40% of isolated LVNC patients and in half of these patients an *MYH7* mutation is found [11].

When no targeted panel is available, *MYH7* gene sequencing should be considered as an initial approach, being the most prevalent cause for LVNC in adults and children. Further molecular analysis of the other genes within the LVNC spectrum, which quantitatively have a relatively modest contribution to LVNC morbidity, may be considered when no mutation in *MYH7* can be identified. Sarcomere gene analysis is also warranted in paediatric patients, given the high percentage of sarcomere mutations in this group.

When an adult or paediatric patient is severely affected, screening for a second molecular defect is advised, given the high frequency of multiple mutations in LVNC.

Summary

LVNC is a relatively new, genetically heterogeneous, cardiomyopathy. Clinical presentation and prognosis range from asymptomatic disease with no or slow progression, to severe disabling, rapidly progressive cardiac failure. Initial presentation includes the triad of heart failure (potentially lethal) arrhythmias and/or thrombo-embolism. In adults, the majority of LVNC is isolated.

The first clinical presentation of LVNC may occur at all ages, even prenatally. In childhood, clinical features are often more severe and LVNC is frequently associated with congenital heart defects. The echocardiographic diagnostic criteria as proposed by Jenni et al. are convenient in daily practice and currently the most widely applied. The general cardiac guidelines for chronic heart failure and ICDs are suitable and applicable to the LVNC population.

In as much as 40% of isolated LVNC, molecular testing may yield a genetic defect, mostly in sarcomere genes. The *MYH7* gene is the most prevalent disease gene. The nonisolated forms of LVNC are caused by a range of different (rare) genetic defects. Until now, in half of familial isolated LVNC, the genetic defect remains unknown. Genetic defects in a large number of sarcomere and other cardiomyopathy genes and in genes primarily associated with skeletal myopathies indicate that LVNC may result from a wide range of pathophysiologic mechanisms.

Shared genetic defects and familial aggregation of LVNC, HCM and DCM indicate that LVNC may be part of a broad spectrum of cardiomyopathies.

The genetic aetiology of LVNC requires that patients and their relatives are offered genetic testing and counselling. This may include (predictive) molecular analysis of relatives, when applicable, and/or cardiac evaluation of at-risk relatives, even when they are as yet asymptomatic.

Take-Home Messages

LVNC is regarded as a morphological trait and defined by a specific ratio between noncompacted and compact myocardium. When found in patients with DCM, it is defined as an LVNC cardiomyopathy, which is a difficult (clinical) diagnosis and is genetic/hereditary in the majority of cases.

Sarcomere gene defects (especially in *MYH7*) are the most frequent cause of genetic isolated LVNC.

Treatment consists of standard heart failure care and prevention of arrhythmia.

Prognosis is highly variable, even within families depending on the underlying cardiomyopathy.

Relatives at risk may be asymptomatic, warranting active screening and follow up of first-degree relatives.

References

1. Feldt RH, Rahimtoola SH, Davis GD, Swan HJ, Titus JL. Anomalous ventricular myocardial patterns in a child with complex congenital heart disease. Am J Cardiol. 1969;23(5):732–4.
2. Jenni R, Oechslin E, Schneider J, Attenhofer Jost C, Kaufmann PA. Echocardiographic and pathoanatomical characteristics of isolated left ventricular non-compaction: a step towards classification as a distinct cardiomyopathy. Heart. 2001;86(6):666–71.
3. Belanger AR, Miller MA, Donthireddi UR, Najovits AJ, Goldman ME. New classification scheme of left ventricular noncompaction and correlation with ventricular performance. Am J Cardiol. 2008;102(1):92–6.
4. Chin TK, Perloff JK, Williams RG, Jue K, Mohrmann R. Isolated noncompaction of left ventricular myocardium. A study of eight cases. Circulation. 1990;82(2):507–13.
5. Stollberger C, Finsterer J, Blazek G. Left ventricular hypertrabeculation/noncompaction and association with additional cardiac abnormalities and neuromuscular disorders. Am J Cardiol. 2002;90(8):899–902.
6. Petersen SE, Selvanayagam JB, Wiesmann F, Robson MD, Francis JM, Anderson RH, et al. Left ventricular non-compaction: insights from cardiovascular magnetic resonance imaging. J Am Coll Cardiol. 2005;46(1):101–5.
7. Jacquier A, Thuny F, Jop B, Giorgi R, Cohen F, Gaubert JY, et al. Measurement of trabeculated left ventricular mass using cardiac magnetic resonance imaging in the diagnosis of left ventricular non-compaction. Eur Heart J. 2010;31(9):1098–104.
8. Stacey RB, Andersen MM, St Clair M, Hundley WG, Thohan V. Comparison of systolic and diastolic criteria for isolated LV noncompaction in CMR. JACC. 2013;6(9):931–40.
9. Captur G, Muthurangu V, Cook C, Flett AS, Wilson R, Barison A, et al. Quantification of left ventricular trabeculae using fractal analysis. J Cardiovasc Magn Reson. 2013;15:36. Epub 2013/05/15
10. Tsai SF, Ebenroth ES, Hurwitz RA, Cordes TM, Schamberger MS, Batra AS. Is left ventricular noncompaction in children truly an isolated lesion? Pediatr Cardiol. 2009;30:597–602.
11. Hoedemaekers YM, Caliskan K, Michels M, Frohn-Mulder I, van der Smagt JJ, Phefferkorn JE, et al. The importance of genetic counseling, DNA diagnostics, and cardiologic family screening in left ventricular noncompaction cardiomyopathy. Circ Cardiovasc Genet. 2010;3(3):232–9.
12. Hoedemaekers YM, Caliskan K, Majoor-Krakauer D, van de Laar I, Michels M, Witsenburg M, et al. Cardiac {beta}-myosin heavy chain defects in two families with non-compaction cardiomyopathy: linking non-compaction to hypertrophic, restrictive, and dilated cardiomyopathies. Eur Heart J. 2007;28(22):2732–7.
13. Moura C, Hillion Y, Daikha-Dahmane F, Eydoux P, Fallet C, Oury JF, et al. Isolated non-compaction of the myocardium diagnosed in the fetus: two sporadic and two familial cases. Cardiol Young. 2002;12(3):278–83.
14. Maron BJ, Towbin JA, Thiene G, Antzelevitch C, Corrado D, Arnett D, et al. Contemporary definitions and classification of the cardiomyopathies: an American Heart Association scientific statement from the Council On Clinical Cardiology, Heart Failure And Transplantation Committee; Quality of Care and Outcomes Research and Functional Genomics and Translational Biology

Interdisciplinary Working Groups; and Council on Epidemiology and Prevention. Circulation. 2006;113(14):1807–16.
15. Elliott P, Andersson B, Arbustini E, Bilinska Z, Cecchi F, Charron P, et al. Classification of the cardiomyopathies: a position statement from the European Society of Cardiology Working Group on Myocardial and Pericardial Diseases. Eur Heart J. 2008;29(2):270–6.
16. Stacey AF, Gill TK, Price K, Warmington R, Taylor AW. Unpaid informal caregivers in South Australia: population characteristics, prevalence and age-period-cohort effects 1994–2014. PLoS One. 2016;11(9):e0161994.
17. Ritter M, Oechslin E, Sutsch G, Attenhofer C, Schneider J, Jenni R. Isolated noncompaction of the myocardium in adults. Mayo Clin Proc. 1997;72(1):26–31.
18. Sandhu R, Finkelhor RS, Gunawardena DR, Bahler RC. Prevalence and characteristics of left ventricular noncompaction in a community hospital cohort of patients with systolic dysfunction. Echocardiography (Mount Kisco NY). 2008;25(1):8–12.
19. Aras D, Tufekcioglu O, Ergun K, Ozeke O, Yildiz A, Topaloglu S, et al. Clinical features of isolated ventricular noncompaction in adults long-term clinical course, echocardiographic properties, and predictors of left ventricular failure. J Card Fail. 2006;12(9):726–33.
20. Kohli SK, Pantazis AA, Shah JS, Adeyemi B, Jackson G, McKenna WJ, et al. Diagnosis of left-ventricular non-compaction in patients with left-ventricular systolic dysfunction: time for a reappraisal of diagnostic criteria? Eur Heart J. 2008;29(1):89–95.
21. Gati S, Chandra N, Bennett RL, Reed M, Kervio G, Panoulas VF, et al. Increased left ventricular trabeculation in highly trained athletes: do we need more stringent criteria for the diagnosis of left ventricular non-compaction in athletes? Heart. 2013;99(6):401–8.
22. Nugent AW, Daubeney PE, Chondros P, Carlin JB, Cheung M, Wilkinson LC, et al. The epidemiology of childhood cardiomyopathy in Australia. N Engl J Med. 2003;348(17):1639–46.
23. Hoedemaekers YM, Cohen-Overbeek TE, Frohn-Mulder IM, Dooijes D, Majoor-Krakauer DF. Prenatal ultrasound diagnosis of MYH7 non-compaction cardiomyopathy. Ultrasound Obstet Gynecol. 2013;41(3):336–9.
24. Nannenberg EA, Michels M, Christiaans I, Majoor-Krakauer D, Hoedemaekers YM, van Tintelen JP, et al. Mortality risk of untreated myosin-binding protein C-related hypertrophic cardiomyopathy: insight into the natural history. J Am Coll Cardiol. 2011;58(23):2406–14.
25. Zhang W, Chen H, Qu X, Chang CP, Shou W. Molecular mechanism of ventricular trabeculation/compaction and the pathogenesis of the left ventricular noncompaction cardiomyopathy (LVNC). Am J Med Genet C Semin Med Genet. 2013;163C(3):144–56.
26. Stacey G, Holland K. Graduate entry nurse education: a challenge or opportunity for the future of the profession? Nurse Educ Pract. 2017;22:A1–2.
27. Fatkin D, Graham RM. Molecular mechanisms of inherited cardiomyopathies. Physiol Rev. 2002;82(4):945–80.
28. Burke A, Mont E, Kutys R, Virmani R. Left ventricular noncompaction: a pathological study of 14 cases. Hum Pathol. 2005;36(4):403–11.
29. Hughes SE, McKenna WJ. New insights into the pathology of inherited cardiomyopathy. Heart. 2005;91(2):257–64.
30. Boyd MT, Seward JB, Tajik AJ, Edwards WD. Frequency and location of prominent left ventricular trabeculations at autopsy in 474 normal human hearts: implications for evaluation of mural thrombi by two-dimensional echocardiography. J Am Coll Cardiol. 1987;9(2):323–6.
31. Freedom RM, Yoo SJ, Perrin D, Taylor G, Petersen S, Anderson RH. The morphological spectrum of ventricular noncompaction. Cardiol Young. 2005;15(4):345–64.
32. Ozkutlu S, Bostan O, Karagoz T, Deren O, Tekinalp G. Prenatal diagnosis of isolated non-compaction of the ventricular myocardium: study of six cases. Pediatr Int. 2007;49(2):172–6.
33. Sato Y, Matsumoto N, Matsuo S, Yoda S, Iida K, Kunimasa T, et al. Isolated noncompaction of the ventricular myocardium in a 94-year-old patient: depiction at echocardiography and magnetic resonance imaging. Int J Cardiol. 2007;119(1):e32–4.
34. Bahl A, Swamy A, Sharma Y, Kumar N. Isolated noncompaction of left ventricle presenting as peripartum cardiomyopathy. Int J Cardiol. 2006;109(3):422–3.
35. Stollberger C, Finsterer J. Left ventricular hypertrabeculation/noncompaction. J Am Soc Echocardiogr. 2004;17(1):91–100.
36. Michels M, Soliman OI, Phefferkorn J, Hoedemaekers YM, Kofflard MJ, Dooijes D, et al. Disease penetrance and risk stratification for sudden cardiac death in asymptomatic hypertrophic cardiomyopathy mutation carriers. Eur Heart J. 2009;30(21):2593–8.
37. Fazio G, Pipitone S, Iacona MA, Marchi S, Mongiovi M, Zito R, et al. The noncompaction of the left ventricular myocardium: our paediatric experience. J Cardiovasc Med (Hagerstown, MD). 2007;8(11):904–8.
38. Sajeev CG, Francis J, Shanker V, Vasudev B, Abdul Khader S, Venugopal K. Young male with isolated noncompaction of the ventricular myocardium presenting with atrial fibrillation and complete heart block. Int J Cardiol. 2006;107(1):142–3.
39. Enriquez SG, Entem FR, Cobo M, Olalla JJ. Uncommon etiology of syncope in a patient with isolated ventricular noncompaction. Pacing Clin Electrophysiol. 2007;30(4):577–9.
40. Ozkutlu S, Ayabakan C, Celiker A, Elshershari H. Noncompaction of ventricular myocardium: a study of twelve patients. J Am Soc Echocardiogr. 2002;15(12):1523–8.
41. Celiker A, Kafali G, Dogan R. Cardioverter defibrillator implantation in a child with isolated noncompaction of the ventricular myocardium and ventricular fibrillation. Pacing Clin Electrophysiol. 2004;27(1):104–8.
42. Taniguchi M, Hioka T, Maekawa K, Takagagi K, Shoji K, Yoshida K. Adult case of isolated ventricular noncompaction discovered by complete atrioventricular block. Circ J. 2004;68(9):873–5.
43. Dagdeviren B, Eren M, Oguz E. Noncompaction of ventricular myocardium, complete atrioventricular block and minor congenital heart abnormalities: case report of an unusual coexistence. Acta Cardiol. 2002;57(3):221–4.
44. Okubo K, Sato Y, Matsumoto N, Kunimasa T, Kasama S, Sano Y, et al. Cardiac resynchronization and cardioverter defibrillation therapy in a patient with isolated noncompaction of the ventricular myocardium. Int J Cardiol. 2008;136:e66–8.
45. Zhou Y, Zhang P, Zhou Q, Guo J, Xu Y, Li X. Giant P waves and focal atrial tachycardia in a patient with ventricular noncompaction. Int J Cardiol. 2008;123(2):210–2.
46. Ogawa K, Nakamura Y, Terano K, Ando T, Hishitani T, Hoshino K. Isolated non-compaction of the ventricular myocardium associated with long QT syndrome. Circ J. 2009;73(11):2169–72.
47. Oginosawa Y, Nogami A, Soejima K, Aonuma K, Kubota S, Sato T, et al. Effect of cardiac resynchronization therapy in isolated ventricular noncompaction in adults: follow-up of four cases. J Cardiovasc Electrophysiol. 2008;19(9):935–8.
48. Saito K, Ibuki K, Yoshimura N, Hirono K, Watanabe S, Watanabe K, et al. Successful cardiac resynchronization therapy in a 3-year-old girl with isolated left ventricular non-compaction and narrow QRS complex. Circ J. 2009;73(11):2173–7.
49. Kubota S, Nogami A, Sugiyasu A, Kasuya K. Cardiac resynchronization therapy in a patient with isolated noncompaction of the left ventricle and a narrow QRS complex. Heart Rhythm. 2006;3(5):619–20.
50. El Menyar AA, Gendi SM. Persistent atrial standstill in noncompaction cardiomyopathy. Pediatr Cardiol. 2006;27(3):364–6.

51. Ozkutlu S, Onderoglu L, Karagoz T, Celiker A, Sahiner UM. Isolated noncompaction of left ventricular myocardium with fetal sustained bradycardia due to sick sinus syndrome. Turk J Pediatr. 2006;48(4):383–6.
52. Schweizer PA, Schroter J, Greiner S, Haas J, Yampolsky P, Mereles D, et al. The symptom complex of familial sinus node dysfunction and myocardial noncompaction is associated with mutations in the HCN4 channel. J Am Coll Cardiol. 2014;64(8):757–67.
53. Celiker A, Ozkutlu S, Dilber E, Karagoz T. Rhythm abnormalities in children with isolated ventricular noncompaction. Pacing Clin Electrophysiol. 2005;28(11):1198–202.
54. Wessels MW, De Graaf BM, Cohen-Overbeek TE, Spitaels SE, de Groot-de Laat LE, Ten Cate FJ, et al. A new syndrome with noncompaction cardiomyopathy, bradycardia, pulmonary stenosis, atrial septal defect and heterotaxy with suggestive linkage to chromosome 6p. Hum Genet. 2008;122(6):595–603.
55. Milano A, Vermeer AM, Lodder EM, Barc J, Verkerk AO, Postma AV, et al. HCN4 mutations in multiple families with bradycardia and left ventricular noncompaction cardiomyopathy. J Am Coll Cardiol. 2014;64(8):745–56.
56. Kobza R, Jenni R, Erne P, Oechslin E, Duru F. Implantable cardioverter-defibrillators in patients with left ventricular noncompaction. Pacing Clin Electrophysiol. 2008;31(4):461–7.
57. Fazio G, Corrado G, Pizzuto C, Zachara E, Rapezzi C, Sulafa AK, et al. Supraventricular arrhythmias in noncompaction of left ventricle: is this a frequent complication? Int J Cardiol. 2008;127(2):255–6.
58. Sato Y, Matsumoto N, Takahashi H, Imai S, Yoda S, Kasamaki Y, et al. Cardioverter defibrillator implantation in an adult with isolated noncompaction of the ventricular myocardium. Int J Cardiol. 2006;110(3):417–9.
59. Sato Y, Matsumoto N, Matsuo S, Imai S, Yoda S, Tani S, et al. Subendomyocardial perfusion abnormality and necrosis detected by magnetic resonance imaging in a patient with isolated noncompaction of the ventricular myocardium associated with ventricular tachycardia. Cardiovasc Revasc Med. 2009;10(1):66–8.
60. Weir-McCall JR, Yeap PM, Papagiorcopulo C, Fitzgerald K, Gandy SJ, Lambert M, et al. Left ventricular noncompaction: anatomical phenotype or distinct cardiomyopathy? J Am Coll Cardiol. 2016;68(20):2157–65.
61. Arbustini E, Favalli V, Narula N, Serio A, Grasso M. Left ventricular noncompaction: a distinct genetic cardiomyopathy? J Am Coll Cardiol. 2016;68(9):949–66.
62. Waldmuller S, Schroeder C, Sturm M, Scheffold T, Imbrich K, Junker S, et al. Targeted 46-gene and clinical exome sequencing for mutations causing cardiomyopathies. Mol Cell Probes. 2015;29(5):308–14.
63. Monserrat L, Hermida-Prieto M, Fernandez X, Rodriguez I, Dumont C, Cazon L, et al. Mutation in the alpha-cardiac actin gene associated with apical hypertrophic cardiomyopathy, left ventricular non-compaction, and septal defects. Eur Heart J. 2007;28(16):1953–61.
64. Hoorntje ET, van Spaendonck-Zwarts KY, Te Rijdt WP, Boven L, Vink A, van der Smagt JJ, et al. The first titin (c.59926 + 1G > a) founder mutation associated with dilated cardiomyopathy. Eur J Heart Fail. 2018;20(4):803–6.
65. Egan KR, Ralphe JC, Weinhaus L, Maginot KR. Just sinus bradycardia or something more serious? Case Rep Pediatr. 2013;2013:736164.
66. Landstrom AP, Ackerman MJ. Beyond the cardiac myofilament: hypertrophic cardiomyopathy-associated mutations in genes that encode calcium-handling proteins. Curr Mol Med. 2012;12(5):507–18.
67. Finsterer J. Cardiogenetics, neurogenetics, and pathogenetics of left ventricular hypertrabeculation/noncompaction. Pediatr Cardiol. 2009;30(5):659–81.
68. Finsterer J, Stollberger C, Wegmann R, Janssen LA. Acquired left ventricular hypertrabeculation/noncompaction in myotonic dystrophy type 1. Int J Cardiol. 2009;137(3):310–3.
69. Wessels MW, Herkert JC, Frohn-Mulder IM, Dalinghaus M, van den Wijngaard A, de Krijger RR, et al. Compound heterozygous or homozygous truncating MYBPC3 mutations cause lethal cardiomyopathy with features of noncompaction and septal defects. Eur J Hum Genet. 2015;23(7):922–8.
70. Ichida F, Tsubata S, Bowles KR, Haneda N, Uese K, Miyawaki T, et al. Novel gene mutations in patients with left ventricular noncompaction or Barth syndrome. Circulation. 2001;103(9):1256–63.
71. Xing Y, Ichida F, Matsuoka T, Isobe T, Ikemoto Y, Higaki T, et al. Genetic analysis in patients with left ventricular noncompaction and evidence for genetic heterogeneity. Mol Genet Metab. 2006;88(1):71–7.
72. Azevedo O, Gaspar P, Sa Miranda C, Cunha D, Medeiros R, Lourenco A. Left ventricular noncompaction in a patient with fabry disease: overdiagnosis, morphological manifestation of fabry disease or two unrelated rare conditions in the same patient? Cardiology. 2011;119(3):155–9.
73. Stollberger C, Finsterer J, Voigtlander T, Slany J. Is left ventricular hypertrabeculation/ noncompaction a cardiac manifestation of Fabry's disease? Zeitschrift fur Kardiologie. 2003;92(11):966–9.
74. Van Der Starre P, Deuse T, Pritts C, Brun C, Vogel H, Oyer P. Late profound muscle weakness following heart transplantation due to Danon disease. Muscle Nerve. 2013;47(1):135–7.
75. Marziliano N, Mannarino S, Nespoli L, Diegoli M, Pasotti M, Malattia C, et al. Barth syndrome associated with compound hemizygosity and heterozygosity of the TAZ and LDB3 genes. Am J Med Genet. 2007;143(9):907–15.
76. Vatta M, Mohapatra B, Jimenez S, Sanchez X, Faulkner G, Perles Z, et al. Mutations in Cypher/ZASP in patients with dilated cardiomyopathy and left ventricular non-compaction. J Am Coll Cardiol. 2003;42(11):2014–27.
77. Hermida-Prieto MML, Castro-Beiras A, et al. Familial dilated cardiomyopathy and isolated left ventricular noncompaction associated with Lamin A/C gene mutations. Am J Cardiol. 2004;94:50–4.
78. Rankin J, Auer-Grumbach M, Bagg W, Colclough K, Nguyen TD, Fenton-May J, et al. Extreme phenotypic diversity and nonpenetrance in families with the LMNA gene mutation R644C. Am J Med Genet. 2008;146A(12):1530–42.
79. Budde BS, Binner P, Waldmuller S, Hohne W, Blankenfeldt W, Hassfeld S, et al. Noncompaction of the ventricular myocardium is associated with a De novo mutation in the beta-myosin heavy chain gene. PLoS One. 2007;2(12):e1362.
80. Muhammad E, Levitas A, Singh SR, Braiman A, Ofir R, Etzion S, et al. PLEKHM2 mutation leads to abnormal localization of lysosomes, impaired autophagy flux and associates with recessive dilated cardiomyopathy and left ventricular noncompaction. Hum Mol Genet. 2015;24(25):7227–40.
81. Ramond F, Janin A, Di Filippo S, Chanavat V, Chalabreysse L, Roux-Buisson N, et al. Homozygous PKP2 deletion associated with neonatal left ventricle noncompaction. Clin Genet. 2017;91(1):126–30.
82. Arndt AK, Schafer S, Drenckhahn JD, Sabeh MK, Plovie ER, Caliebe A, et al. Fine mapping of the 1p36 deletion syndrome identifies mutation of PRDM16 as a cause of cardiomyopathy. Am J Hum Genet. 2013;93(1):67–77.
83. Campbell MJ, Czosek RJ, Hinton RB, Miller EM. Exon 3 deletion of ryanodine receptor causes left ventricular noncompaction, wors-

ening catecholaminergic polymorphic ventricular tachycardia, and sudden cardiac arrest. Am J Med Genet. 2015;167A(9):2197–200.
84. Ohno S, Omura M, Kawamura M, Kimura H, Itoh H, Makiyama T, et al. Exon 3 deletion of RYR2 encoding cardiac ryanodine receptor is associated with left ventricular non-compaction. Europace. 2014;16(11):1646–54.
85. Shan L, Makita N, Xing Y, Watanabe S, Futatani T, Ye F, et al. SCN5A variants in Japanese patients with left ventricular noncompaction and arrhythmia. Mol Genet Metab. 2008;93(4):468–74.
86. Bione S, D'Adamo P, Maestrini E, Gedeon AK, Bolhuis PA, Toniolo D. A novel X-linked gene, G4.5. is responsible for Barth syndrome. Nat Genet. 1996;12(4):385–9.
87. Bleyl SB, Mumford BR, Brown-Harrison MC, Pagotto LT, Carey JC, Pysher TJ, et al. Xq28-linked noncompaction of the left ventricular myocardium: prenatal diagnosis and pathologic analysis of affected individuals. Am J Med Genet. 1997;72(3):257–65.
88. Bleyl SB, Mumford BR, Thompson V, Carey JC, Pysher TJ, Chin TK, et al. Neonatal, lethal noncompaction of the left ventricular myocardium is allelic with Barth syndrome. Am J Hum Genet. 1997;61(4):868–72.
89. Brady AN, Shehata BM, Fernhoff PM. X-linked fetal cardiomyopathy caused by a novel mutation in the TAZ gene. Prenat Diagn. 2006;26(5):462–5.
90. Chen R, Tsuji T, Ichida F, Bowles KR, Yu X, Watanabe S, et al. Mutation analysis of the G4.5 gene in patients with isolated left ventricular noncompaction. Mol Genet Metab. 2002;77(4):319–25.
91. Cortez-Dias N, Varela MG, Sargento L, Brito D, Almeida A, Cerqueira R, et al. Left ventricular non-compaction: a new mutation predisposing to reverse remodeling? Rev Port Cardiol. 2009;28(2):185–94.
92. Kenton AB, Sanchez X, Coveler KJ, Makar KA, Jimenez S, Ichida F, et al. Isolated left ventricular noncompaction is rarely caused by mutations in G4.5, alpha-dystrobrevin and FK binding Protein-12. Mol Genet Metab. 2004;82(2):162–6.
93. Yen TY, Hwu WL, Chien YH, Wu MH, Lin MT, Tsao LY, et al. Acute metabolic decompensation and sudden death in Barth syndrome: report of a family and a literature review. Eur J Pediatr. 2008;167(8):941–4.
94. Klaassen S, Probst S, Oechslin E, Gerull B, Krings G, Schuler P, et al. Mutations in sarcomere protein genes in left ventricular noncompaction. Circulation. 2008;117(22):2893–901.
95. Morita H, Rehm HL, Menesses A, McDonough B, Roberts AE, Kucherlapati R, et al. Shared genetic causes of cardiac hypertrophy in children and adults. N Engl J Med. 2008;358(18):1899–908.
96. Alsters S, Wong L, Peferoen L, Niessen HWM, Bikker H, Elting MW, et al. Fatal neonatal hypertrophic cardiomyopathy caused by compound heterozygous truncating MYBPC3 mutation. Netherland Heart J. 2019;27(5):282–3.
97. Lekanne Deprez RH, Muurling-Vlietman JJ, Hruda J, Baars MJ, Wijnaendts LC, Stolte-Dijkstra I, et al. Two cases of severe neonatal hypertrophic cardiomyopathy caused by compound heterozygous mutations in the MYBPC3 gene. J Med Genet. 2006;43(10):829–32.
98. Van Driest SL, Vasile VC, Ommen SR, Will ML, Tajik AJ, Gersh BJ, et al. Myosin binding protein C mutations and compound heterozygosity in hypertrophic cardiomyopathy. J Am Coll Cardiol. 2004;44(9):1903–10.
99. Zahka K, Kalidas K, Simpson MA, Cross H, Keller BB, Galambos C, et al. Homozygous mutation of MYBPC3 associated with severe infantile hypertrophic cardiomyopathy at high frequency among the Amish. Heart. 2008;94(10):1326–30.
100. Oechslin EN, Attenhofer Jost CH, Rojas JR, Kaufmann PA, Jenni R. Long-term follow-up of 34 adults with isolated left ventricular noncompaction: a distinct cardiomyopathy with poor prognosis. J Am Coll Cardiol. 2000;36(2):493–500.
101. Sedmera D, Pexieder T, Vuillemin M, Thompson RP, Anderson RH. Developmental patterning of the myocardium. Anat Rec. 2000;258(4):319–37.
102. Lie-Venema H. The role of epicardium-derived cells (EPDCs) in the development of non-compaction cardiomyopathy. Florence International Course on Advances in Cardiomyopathies - 5th meeting of the European Myocardial and Pericardial Disease WG of the ESC; 22/24 May 2008; Florence Italy 2008.
103. Lie-Venema H, van den Akker NM, Bax NA, Winter EM, Maas S, Kekarainen T, et al. Origin, fate, and function of epicardium-derived cells (EPDCs) in normal and abnormal cardiac development. ScientificWorldJournal. 2007;7:1777–98.
104. Breckenridge RA, Anderson RH, Elliott PM. Isolated left ventricular non-compaction: the case for abnormal myocardial development. Cardiol Young. 2007;17(2):124–9.
105. Crawford SE, Qi C, Misra P, Stellmach V, Rao MS, Engel JD, et al. Defects of the heart, eye, and megakaryocytes in peroxisome proliferator activator receptor-binding protein (PBP) null embryos implicate GATA family of transcription factors. J Biol Chem. 2002;277(5):3585–92.
106. Lee Y, Song AJ, Baker R, Micales B, Conway SJ, Lyons GE. Jumonji, a nuclear protein that is necessary for normal heart development. Circ Res. 2000;86(9):932–8.
107. Shou W, Aghdasi B, Armstrong DL, Guo Q, Bao S, Charng MJ, et al. Cardiac defects and altered ryanodine receptor function in mice lacking FKBP12. Nature. 1998;391(6666):489–92.
108. van Loo PF, Mahtab EA, Wisse LJ, Hou J, Grosveld F, Suske G, et al. Transcription factor Sp3 knockout mice display serious cardiac malformations. Mol Cell Biol. 2007;27(24):8571–82.
109. Chai W, Hoedemaekers Y, van Schaik RH, van Fessem M, Garrelds IM, Saris JJ, et al. Cardiac aldosterone in subjects with hypertrophic cardiomyopathy. J Renin-Angiotensin-Aldosterone Syst. 2006;7(4):225–30.
110. Lombardi R, Betocchi S. Aetiology and pathogenesis of hypertrophic cardiomyopathy. Acta Paediatr Suppl. 2002;91(439):10–4.
111. Tunaoglu FS, Kula S, Olgunturk R, Ozturk G. Noncompaction with arcus aorta anomalies. Turk J Pediatr. 2003;45(4):363–6.
112. Niwa K, Ikeda F, Miyamoto H, Nakajima H, Ando M. Absent aortic valve with normally related great arteries. Heart Vessel. 1987;3(2):104–7.
113. Ali SK. Unique features of non-compaction of the ventricular myocardium in Arab and African patients. Cardiovasc J Afr. 2008;19(5):241–5.
114. Vijayalakshmi IB, Chitra N, Prabhu Deva AN. Use of an Amplatzer duct occluder for closing an aortico-left ventricular tunnel in a case of noncompaction of the left ventricle. Pediatr Cardiol. 2004;25(1):77–9.
115. Tatu-Chitoiu A, Bradisteanu S. A rare case of biventricular non-compaction associated with ventricular septal defect and descendent aortic stenosis in an young man. Eur J Echocardiogr. 2006;9(2):306–8.
116. Song ZZ. A combination of right ventricular hypertrabeculation/noncompaction and atrial septal defect. Int J Cardiol. 2009;148(2):e25–7.
117. Salazar Gonzalez JJ, Rite Montanes S, Asso Abadia A, Pueo Crespo E, Salazar Gonzalez E, Placer Peralta LJ. Miocardio ventricular no compacto aislado [Isolated non-compaction of the ventricular myocardium]. Anales espanoles de pediatria. 2002;57(6):570–3.
118. Cavusoglu Y, Ata N, Timuralp B, Gorenek B, Goktekin O, Kudaiberdieva G, et al. Noncompaction of the ventricular myocardium: report of two cases with bicuspid aortic valve demonstrating poor prognosis and with prominent right ventricular involvement. Echocardiography (Mount Kisco NY). 2003;20(4):379–83.

119. Cavusoglu Y, Aslan R, Birdane A, Ozbabalik D, Ata N. Noncompaction of the ventricular myocardium with bicuspid aortic valve. Anadolu Kardiyol Derg. 2007;7(1):88–90.
120. Sato Y, Matsumoto N, Yoda S, Inoue F, Kunimoto S, Fukamizu S, et al. Left ventricular aneurysm associated with isolated noncompaction of the ventricular myocardium. Heart Vessel. 2006;21(3):192–4.
121. Cavusoglu Y, Tunerir B, Birdane A, Timuralp B, Ata N, Gorenek B, et al. Transesophageal echocardiographic diagnosis of ventricular noncompaction associated with an atrial septal aneurysm in a patient with dilated cardiomyopathy of unknown etiology. Can J Cardiol. 2005;21(8):705–7.
122. Unlu M, Ozeke O, Kara M, Yesillik S. Ruptured sinus of Valsalva aneurysm associated with noncompaction of the ventricular myocardium. Eur J Echocardiogr. 2008;9(2):311–3.
123. Friedman MA, Wiseman S, Haramati L, Gordon GM, Spevack DM. Noncompaction of the left ventricle in a patient with dextroversion. Eur J Echocardiogr. 2007;8(1):70–3.
124. Gorgulu S, Celik S, Eksik A, Tezel T. Double-orifice mitral valve associated with nonisolated left ventricular noncompaction—a case report. Angiology. 2004;55(6):707–10.
125. Sugiyama H, Hoshiai M, Toda T, Nakazawa S. Double-orifice mitral valve associated with noncompaction of left ventricular myocardium. Pediatr Cardiol. 2006;27(6):746–9.
126. Wang XX, Song ZZ. A combination of left ventricular noncompaction and double orifice mitral valve. Cardiovasc Ultrasound. 2009;7:11.
127. Betrian Blasco P, Gallardo AE. Ebstein's anomaly and left ventricular noncompaction association. Int J Cardiol. 2007;119(2):264–5.
128. Ilercil A, Barack J, Malone MA, Barold SS, Herweg B. Association of noncompaction of left ventricular myocardium with Ebstein's anomaly. Echocardiography (Mount Kisco NY). 2006;23(5):432–3.
129. Sinkovec M, Kozelj M, Podnar T. Familial biventricular myocardial noncompaction associated with Ebstein's malformation. Int J Cardiol. 2005;102(2):297–302.
130. Arslan S, Gurlertop HY, Gundogdu F, Senocak H. Left ventricular noncompaction and mid-caviter narrowing associated with Ebstein's anomaly: three-dimensional transthoracic echocardiographic image. Int J Cardiol. 2007;115(1):e52–5.
131. Attenhofer Jost CH, Connolly HM, Warnes CA, O'Leary P, Tajik AJ, Pellikka PA, et al. Noncompacted myocardium in Ebstein's anomaly: initial description in three patients. J Am Soc Echocardiogr. 2004;17(6):677–80.
132. Bagur RH, Lederlin M, Montaudon M, Latrabe V, Corneloup O, Iriart X, et al. Images in cardiovascular medicine. Ebstein anomaly associated with left ventricular noncompaction. Circulation. 2008;118(16):e662–4.
133. Friedberg MK, Ursell PC, Silverman NH. Isomerism of the left atrial appendage associated with ventricular noncompaction. Am J Cardiol. 2005;96(7):985–90.
134. Vanpraagh R, Ongley PA, Swan HJ. Anatomic types of single or common ventricle in man. Morphologic and geometric aspects of 60 necropsied cases. Am J Cardiol. 1964;13:367–86.
135. Dogan R, Dogan OF, Oc M, Duman U, Ozkutlu S, Celiker A. Noncompaction of ventricular myocardium in a patient with congenitally corrected transposition of the great arteries treated surgically: case report. Heart Surg Forum. 2005;8(2):E110–3.
136. Guo DC, Pannu H, Tran-Fadulu V, Papke CL, Yu RK, Avidan N, et al. Mutations in smooth muscle alpha-actin (ACTA2) lead to thoracic aortic aneurysms and dissections. Nat Genet. 2007;39(12):1488–93.
137. Wessels MW, Willems PJ. Mutations in sarcomeric protein genes not only lead to cardiomyopathy but also to congenital cardiovascular malformations. Clin Genet. 2008;74(1):16–9.
138. Xin B, Puffenberger E, Tumbush J, Bockoven JR, Wang H. Homozygosity for a novel splice site mutation in the cardiac myosin-binding protein C gene causes severe neonatal hypertrophic cardiomyopathy. Am J Med Genet. 2007;143A(22):2662–7.
139. Zhu L, Vranckx R, Khau Van Kien P, Lalande A, Boisset N, Mathieu F, et al. Mutations in myosin heavy chain 11 cause a syndrome associating thoracic aortic aneurysm/aortic dissection and patent ductus arteriosus. Nat Genet. 2006;38(3):343–9.
140. Finsterer J, Stollberger C. Spontaneous left ventricular hypertrabeculation in dystrophin duplication based Becker's muscular dystrophy. Herz. 2001;26(7):477–81.
141. Finsterer J, Stollberger C, Feichtinger H. Noncompaction in Duchenne muscular dystrophy: frustrated attempt to create a compensatory left ventricle? Cardiology. 2006;105(4):223–5.
142. Finsterer J, Stollberger C, Wegmann R, Jarius C, Janssen B. Left ventricular hypertrabeculation in myotonic dystrophy type 1. Herz. 2001;26(4):287–90.
143. Malhotra R, Mason PK. Lamin A/C deficiency as a cause of familial dilated cardiomyopathy. Curr Opin Cardiol. 2009;24(3):203–8.
144. D'Adamo P, Fassone L, Gedeon A, Janssen EA, Bione S, Bolhuis PA, et al. The X-linked gene G4.5 is responsible for different infantile dilated cardiomyopathies. Am J Hum Genet. 1997;61(4):862–7.
145. Stollberger C, Finsterer J. Noncompaction in Melnick Fraser syndrome. Pacing Clin Electrophysiol. 2007;30(8):1047 author reply 8.
146. Facher JJ, Regier EJ, Jacobs GH, Siwik E, Delaunoy JP, Robin NH. Cardiomyopathy in Coffin-Lowry syndrome. Am J Med Genet. 2004;128A(2):176–8.
147. Pignatelli RH, McMahon CJ, Dreyer WJ, Denfield SW, Price J, Belmont JW, et al. Clinical characterization of left ventricular noncompaction in children: a relatively common form of cardiomyopathy. Circulation. 2003;108(21):2672–8.
148. Matsumoto T, Watanabe A, Migita M, Gocho Y, Hayakawa J, Ogawa S, et al. Transient cardiomyopathy in a patient with congenital contractural arachnodactyly (Beals syndrome). Journal of Nippon Medical School = Nihon Ika Daigaku zasshi. 2006;73(5):285–8.
149. Ross SB, Bagnall RD, Yeates L, Sy RW, Semsarian C. Holt-Oram syndrome in two families diagnosed with left ventricular noncompaction and conduction disease. HeartRhythm Case Rep. 2018;4(4):146–51.
150. Limongelli G, Pacileo G, Marino B, Digilio MC, Sarkozy A, Elliott P, et al. Prevalence and clinical significance of cardiovascular abnormalities in patients with the LEOPARD syndrome. Am J Cardiol. 2007;100(4):736–41.
151. Wong JA, Bofinger MK. Noncompaction of the ventricular myocardium in Melnick-Needles syndrome. Am J Med Genet. 1997;71(1):72–5.
152. Finsterer J, Stollberger C, Kopsa W. Noncompaction on cardiac MRI in a patient with nail-patella syndrome and mitochondriopathy. Cardiology. 2003;100(1):48–9.
153. Amann G, Sherman FS. Myocardial dysgenesis with persistent sinusoids in a neonate with Noonan's phenotype. Pediatric Pathol. 1992;12(1):83–92.
154. Mandel K, Grunebaum E, Benson L. Noncompaction of the myocardium associated with Roifman syndrome. Cardiol Young. 2001;11(2):240–3.
155. Martinez HR, Belmont JW, Craigen WJ, Taylor MD, Jefferies JL. Left ventricular noncompaction in Sotos syndrome. Am J Med Genet. 2011;155A(5):1115–8.
156. Happle R, Daniels O, Koopman RJ. MIDAS syndrome (microphthalmia, dermal aplasia, and sclerocornea): an X-linked phenotype distinct from Goltz syndrome. Am J Med Genet. 1993;47(5):710–3.

157. Kherbaoui-Redouani L, Eschard C, Bednarek N, Morville P. Aplasie cutanee congenitale, defaut de compaction du ventricule gauche et troubles du rythme cardiaque graves: un nouveau cas de syndrome MLS (microphtalmia with linear skin defects) [Cutaneous aplasia, non compaction of the left ventricle and severe cardiac arrhythmia: a new case of MLS syndrome (microphtalmia with linear skin defects)]. Arch Pediatr. 2003;10(3):224–6.
158. Battaglia A, Hoyme HE, Dallapiccola B, Zackai E, Hudgins L, McDonald-McGinn D, et al. Further delineation of deletion 1p36 syndrome in 60 patients: a recognizable phenotype and common cause of developmental delay and mental retardation. Pediatrics. 2008;121(2):404–10.
159. Cremer K, Ludecke HJ, Ruhr F, Wieczorek D. Left-ventricular non-compaction (LVNC): a clinical feature more often observed in terminal deletion 1p36 than previously expected. Eur J Med Genet. 2008;51(6):685–8.
160. Saito S, Kawamura R, Kosho T, Shimizu T, Aoyama K, Koike K, et al. Bilateral perisylvian polymicrogyria, periventricular nodular heterotopia, and left ventricular noncompaction in a girl with 10.5-11.1 Mb terminal deletion of 1p36. Am J Med Genet. 2008;146A(22):2891–7.
161. Thienpont B, Mertens L, Buyse G, Vermeesch JR, Devriendt K. Left-ventricular non-compaction in a patient with monosomy 1p36. Eur J Med Genet. 2007;50(3):233–6.
162. Stacey D, Redlich R, Buschel A, Opel N, Grotegerd D, Zaremba D, et al. TNF receptors 1 and 2 exert distinct region-specific effects on striatal and hippocampal grey matter volumes (VBM) in healthy adults. Genes Brain Behav. 2017;16(3):352–60.
163. Kanemoto N, Horigome H, Nakayama J, Ichida F, Xing Y, Buonadonna AL, et al. Interstitial 1q43-q43 deletion with left ventricular noncompaction myocardium. Eur J Med Genet. 2006;49(3):247–53.
164. Pauli RM, Scheib-Wixted S, Cripe L, Izumo S, Sekhon GS. Ventricular noncompaction and distal chromosome 5q deletion. Am J Med Genet. 1999;85(4):419–23.
165. De Rosa G, Pardeo M, Bria S, Caresta E, Vasta I, Zampino G, et al. Isolated myocardial non-compaction in an infant with distal 4q trisomy and distal 1q monosomy. Eur J Pediatr. 2005;164(4):255–6.
166. McMahon CJ, Chang AC, Pignatelli RH, Miller-Hance WC, Eble BK, Towbin JA, et al. Left ventricular noncompaction cardiomyopathy in association with trisomy 13. Pediatr Cardiol. 2005;26(4):477–9.
167. Wang JC, Dang L, Mondal TK, Khan A. Prenatally diagnosed mosaic trisomy 22 in a fetus with left ventricular non-compaction cardiomyopathy. Am J Med Genet. 2007;143A(22):2744–6.
168. Altenberger H, Stollberger C, Finsterer J. Isolated left ventricular hypertrabeculation/noncompaction in a Turner mosaic with male phenotype. Acta Cardiol. 2009;64(1):99–103.
169. van Heerde M, Hruda J, Hazekamp MG. Severe pulmonary hypertension secondary to a parachute-like mitral valve, with the left superior caval vein draining into the coronary sinus, in a girl with Turner's syndrome. Cardiol Young. 2003;13(4):364–6.
170. Sasse-Klaassen S, Probst S, Gerull B, Oechslin E, Nurnberg P, Heuser A, et al. Novel gene locus for autosomal dominant left ventricular noncompaction maps to chromosome 11p15. Circulation. 2004;109(22):2720–3.
171. Scaglia F, Towbin JA, Craigen WJ, Belmont JW, Smith EO, Neish SR, et al. Clinical spectrum, morbidity, and mortality in 113 pediatric patients with mitochondrial disease. Pediatrics. 2004;114(4):925–31.
172. Finsterer J, Bittner R, Bodingbauer M, Eichberger H, Stollberger C, Blazek G. Complex mitochondriopathy associated with 4 mtDNA transitions. Eur Neurol. 2000;44(1):37–41.
173. Finsterer J, Stollberger C, Schubert B. Acquired left ventricular hypertrabeculation/noncompaction in mitochondriopathy. Cardiology. 2004;102(4):228–30.
174. Hunt SA. ACC/AHA 2005 guideline update for the diagnosis and management of chronic heart failure in the adult: a report of the American College of Cardiology/American Heart Association task force on practice guidelines (writing committee to update the 2001 guidelines for the evaluation and management of heart failure). J Am Coll Cardiol. 2005;46(6):e1–82.
175. Ponikowski P, Voors AA, Anker SD, Bueno H, Cleland JGF, Coats AJS, et al. 2016 ESC guidelines for the diagnosis and treatment of acute and chronic heart failure: the task force for the diagnosis and treatment of acute and chronic heart failure of the European Society of Cardiology (ESC)developed with the special contribution of the Heart Failure Association (HFA) of the ESC. Eur Heart J. 2016;37(27):2129–200.
176. Amzulescu MS, Rousseau MF, Ahn SA, Boileau L, de Meester de Ravenstein C, Vancraeynest D, et al. Prognostic impact of Hypertrabeculation and noncompaction phenotype in dilated cardiomyopathy: a CMR study. JACC. 2015;8(8):934–46.
177. Andreini D, Pontone G, Bogaert J, Roghi A, Barison A, Schwitter J, et al. Long-term prognostic value of cardiac magnetic resonance in left ventricle noncompaction: a prospective multicenter study. J Am Coll Cardiol. 2016;68(20):2166–81.
178. Ivanov A, Dabiesingh DS, Bhumireddy GP, Mohamed A, Asfour A, Briggs WM, et al. Prevalence and prognostic significance of left ventricular noncompaction in patients referred for cardiac magnetic resonance imaging. Circ Cardiovasc Imaging. 2017;10(9):e006174.
179. van Waning JI, Caliskan K, Hoedemaekers YM, van Spaendonck-Zwarts KY, Baas AF, Boekholdt SM, et al. Genetics, clinical features, and long-term outcome of noncompaction cardiomyopathy. J Am Coll Cardiol. 2018;71(7):711–22.
180. Bertini M, Balla C, Pavasini R, Boriani G. Efficacy of cardiac resynchronization therapy in patients with isolated ventricular noncompaction with dilated cardiomyopathy: a systematic review of the literature. J Cardiovasc Med (Hagerstown, MD). 2018;19(7):324–8.
181. Kovacevic-Preradovic T, Jenni R, Oechslin EN, Noll G, Seifert B, Attenhofer Jost CH. Isolated left ventricular noncompaction as a cause for heart failure and heart transplantation: a single center experience. Cardiology. 2009;112(2):158–64.
182. Shimamoto T, Marui A, Yamanaka K, Shikata N, Tambara K, Ikeda T, et al. Left ventricular restoration surgery for isolated left ventricular noncompaction: report of the first successful case. J Thorac Cardiovasc Surg. 2007;134(1):246–7.
183. Caliskan KTD, Hoedemaekers YM, Ten Cate FJ, Jordaens L, Szili TT. Implantable cardioverter-defibrillators for primary and secondary prevention in patients with noncompaction cardiomyopathy. J Am Coll Card. 2009;53(10, supplement 1):A136.
184. Caliskan KYS, Schinkel A, Constantinescu A, Michels M, Manintveld O, Szili-Torok T, Theuns D. Long-term outcome of noncompaction cardiomyopathy patients with implantable cardioverter-defibrillators compared with patients with dilated or hypertrophic cardiomyopathy. J Am Coll Card. 2017;69(11 supplement):33745–2.
185. Michels M, Soliman OI, Kofflard MJ, Hoedemaekers YM, Dooijes D, Majoor-Krakauer D, et al. Diastolic abnormalities as the first feature of hypertrophic cardiomyopathy in Dutch myosin-binding protein C founder mutations. JACC. 2009;2(1):58–64.
186. Stacey G. The international development of second degree graduate entry nursing. Nurse Educ Pract. 2016;. Epub 2017/01/17
187. Grigoratos C, Barison A, Ivanov A, Andreini D, Mazurkiewicz L, et al. Meta-analysis of the prognostic role of late Gadolinium enhancement and global systolic impairment in left ventricular noncompaction. JACC. 2019;12(11):2141–51.
188. van Waning JI, Caliskan K, Michels M, Schinkel AFL, Hirsch A, Dalinghaus M, et al. Cardiac phenotypes, genetics, and risks

in familial noncompaction cardiomyopathy. J Am Coll Cardiol. 2019;73(13):1601–11.

189. Stacey D, Pritchard C. An ecological study of excess winter mortality in England and deprivation. Public Health. 2016;141:207–9.

190. Regitz-Zagrosek V, Roos-Hesselink JW, Bauersachs J, Blomstrom-Lundqvist C, Cifkova R, De Bonis M, et al. 2018 ESC guidelines for the management of cardiovascular diseases during pregnancy. Eur Heart J. 2018;39(34):3165–241.

191. Espinola-Zavaleta N, Soto ME, Castellanos LM, Jativa-Chavez S, Keirns C. Non-compacted cardiomyopathy: clinical-echocardiographic study. Cardiovasc Ultrasound. 2006;4:35.

192. Ichida F, Hamamichi Y, Miyawaki T, Ono Y, Kamiya T, Akagi T, et al. Clinical features of isolated noncompaction of the ventricular myocardium: long-term clinical course, hemodynamic properties, and genetic background. J Am Coll Cardiol. 1999;34(1):233–40.

193. Lofiego C, Biagini E, Pasquale F, Ferlito M, Rocchi G, Perugini E, et al. Wide spectrum of presentation and variable outcomes of isolated left ventricular non-compaction. Heart. 2007;93(1):65–71.

194. Murphy RT, Thaman R, Blanes JG, Ward D, Sevdalis E, Papra E, et al. Natural history and familial characteristics of isolated left ventricular non-compaction. Eur Heart J. 2005;26(2):187–92.

8 Restrictive Cardiomyopathy

R. L. Braam and J. G. Post

Introduction

According to a position statement of the European Society of Cardiology, cardiomyopathies can be classified as dilated, hypertrophic, arrhythmogenic, restrictive and 'unclassified' [1]. Restrictive cardiomyopathy (RCM) is probably the least common type [1]. In RCM, ventricular filling is impeded because of increased stiffness of the myocardium, causing a rapid increase in ventricular pressure upon only small increases in volume [1]. Biventricular chamber size, wall thickness and systolic function are usually normal or near-normal until later stages of the disease [2, 3].

RCM constitutes a heterogeneous group of disorders [4]. RCM can result from an inherited or acquired disease [2]. RCM may result from various systemic disorders, in particular amyloidosis, sarcoidosis, carcinoid heart disease, scleroderma and anthracycline toxicity (Table 8.1) [1].

Hypertensive and hypertrophic cardiomyopathy (HCM) must be excluded [3]. In infiltrative processes, wall thickness may be increased [3]. In Western countries, the most common cause of RCM is amyloidosis. Clinically differentiation from constrictive pericarditis (CP) can be challenging [4]. In genetic forms of RCM autosomal dominant as well as recessive inheritance have been reported [4].

Table 8.1 Classification of restrictive cardiomyopathy (RCM)

I. Infiltrative
1. Sarcoidosis
2. Amyloidosis *Acquired:* AL (Ig light chain); AA (acute phase protein SAA); 'senile' (wild-type TTR) *Inherited:* mutated TTR
3. Hemochromatosis *Acquired:* Frequent blood transfusions (e.g. in patients with Thalassemia major, etc.) *Inherited:* Mutated HFE (and rare other genes)
II. Primary genetic RCM
III. Lysosomal storage diseases
1. Fabry disease
2. Gaucher disease
3. Glycogen storage diseases (Pompe, Danon, PRKAG2-WPW)
4. Mucopolysaccharidoses
IV. Cardiovascular causes
Acquired/multifactorial: Diabetes mellitus, autoimmune, Scleroderma/systemic sclerosis *Inherited:* Pseudoxanthoma elasticum, progeria
V. Endo(myo)cardial causes
1. Endomyocardial fibrosis
2. Endocardial fibroelastosis
3. Hypereosinophilic syndromes (e.g. eosinophilic leukaemia, drug related etc.)
VI. Cancer related
1. Treatment related (drugs and radiotherapy)
2. Metastatic (including carcinoid)

Clinical Presentation and Diagnosis

Heart failure is the most common initial manifestation [3]. Also, exercise intolerance, fatigue and lower extremity oedema may occur [3]. Echocardiography will show normal right and left ventricular function. A restrictive diastolic filling pattern with biatrial enlargement will usually be present. Advanced stages of RCM are characterized by a typical restrictive physiology with a mitral inflow E/A ratio > 2.5, deceleration time (DT) of E velocity < 150 ms, isovolumic relaxation time (IVRT) < 50 ms, decreased septal and lateral e' velocities (3–4 cm/s), E/e' ratio > 14, as well as a markedly increased left atrial (LA) volume index (>50 mL/m^2) [5]. This advanced restrictive pattern is associated with the worst prognosis [5]. Wall thickness is usually normal.

Cardiac magnetic resonance imaging (CMR) is a very powerful diagnostic tool [3, 5]. Delayed myocardial enhancement can be found in at least one-third of all cases of RCM [3, 6]. The pattern of delayed enhancement can help to dif-

R. L. Braam (✉)
Gelre Hospitals, Apeldoorn, The Netherlands
e-mail: r.braam@gelre.nl

J. G. Post
Gelre Hospitals, Apeldoorn, The Netherlands

University Medical Center Utrecht, Utrecht, The Netherlands

H. F. Baars et al. (eds.), *Clinical Cardiogenetics*, https://doi.org/10.1007/978-3-030-45457-9_8

ferentiate between e.g. Fabry disease, amyloidosis, endomyocardial fibrosis (EMF) and sarcoidosis [5]. The presence of delayed enhancement also has prognostic impact. Computed tomography (CT) can help to detect thickening and calcification of the pericardium associated with CP [5].

Cardiac catheterization will show elevation of right- and left-sided filling pressures along with reduction in cardiac index [3]. Right atrial pressure is elevated, x and y descents are prominent [3, 7]. A restrictive filling pattern is characterized by a so-called dip-and-plateau or square root sign. There is a rapid early decrease in ventricular pressure at the onset of diastole, followed by a rapid increase to a plateau in early diastole [8, 9]. Endomyocardial biopsy can be helpful to diagnose the cause of RCM. CMR has diminished the need of performing an endomyocardial biopsy [3]. A recent series from Johns Hopkins showed that right ventricular biopsy was diagnostic in 29% of patients with unexplained RCM [10].

Differentiation from Constrictive Pericarditis

As stated before differentiating RCM from CP can be challenging from a clinical viewpoint. Because the treatment for these two entities is completely different, making the right diagnosis is of great importance. In CP, the pericardium is thickened, fibrous, and sometimes calcified. CP can be seen in patients after cardiac surgery and in patients who received chest irradiation for treatment of a malignancy [3, 11]. In patients with RCM, the reduction in chamber compliance is the result of a myocardial process, whereas in patients with CP external constraint is the central problem [3]. Echocardiography, CMR and cardiac catheterization can help to make the distinction between the two diseases. Patients with CP exhibit exaggerated interventricular dependence and dissociation between intracardiac and intrathoracic pressures during respiration [12]. In CP with inspiration, the lower intrathoracic pressure is transmitted to the pulmonary veins, but not to the encased left atrium, therefore reducing the pressure gradient and venous return to the left heart. As the intracardiac volume is fixed by the encased pericardium, venous return increases to the right heart through the inferior vena cava because this vessel enters the right atrium directly from the abdomen and is not exposed to the intrathoracic pressure changes [12]. This exaggerated interventricular dependence can be studied using echocardiography, CMR and during invasive hemodynamic measurements, Fig. 8.1. In patients with RCM end-diastolic filling pressures are elevated and a square root sign is present, however there is no enhanced ventricular interdependence, with parallel changes in LV and RV pressure during inspiration and expiration [13]. Thus, respiratory flow variation is absent in RCM, but is frequently noted in constrictive pericarditis [3].

Of the echocardiographic imaging parameters, the most useful one to distinguish between the two conditions is tissue Doppler imaging. A normal tissue Doppler e' velocity (>8 cm/s) indicates normal LV relaxation and virtually excludes RCM [14].

Echocardiography can detect pericardial thickening, but CMR and CT are better. CMR has excellent accuracy (93%) for detection of pericardial thickening >4 mm [15]. Myocardial delayed enhancement, indicative of myocardial inflammation or fibrosis, is classically absent in CP [13]. Real-time, free-breathing image acquisition can be performed using CMR, to assess ventricular septal motion during respiration possible.

Chest radiography may demonstrate calcification of the pericardium, best assessed on the lateral view, but this finding is only seen in approximately one-quarter of patients with CP [16].

Frequently, pericardial calcification not recognized on chest X-ray is identified on CT [16]. Normal pericardial thickness is <2 mm [17]. Although a pathologically thickened pericardium (>4 mm) is highly suggestive of CP, lack of this finding should not be used in isolation to exclude the diagnosis, because pericardial thickness is normal in 18% of patients with CP [18].

Brain natriuretic peptide (BNP) can be elevated in both RCM and CP. Patients with RCM tend to have higher BNP values, however there is significant overlap [19].

Table 8.2 summarizes important criteria that can be used to differentiate between CP and RCM.

General Treatment of RCM

The treatment depends on the underlying cause of RCM. In general, in the case of congestive symptoms diuretics can be used. However, because stroke volume can decline rapidly in case of RCM when hypovolemia occurs, the use of loop diuretics should be monitored strictly [3]. Sodium restriction and fluid restriction can be advised. Atrial fibrillation and other supraventricular arrhythmias should be treated using rhythm control rather than rate control to improve stroke volume [3].

Several disorders that can manifest as RCM will now be addressed in more detail.

Infiltrative Causes of RCM

Sarcoidosis

Sarcoidosis is a systemic granulomatous disease of unknown aetiology [20]. Cardiac sarcoidosis generally occurs in association with other manifestations of the systemic disease, but solitary cardiac symptomatology does occur [4].

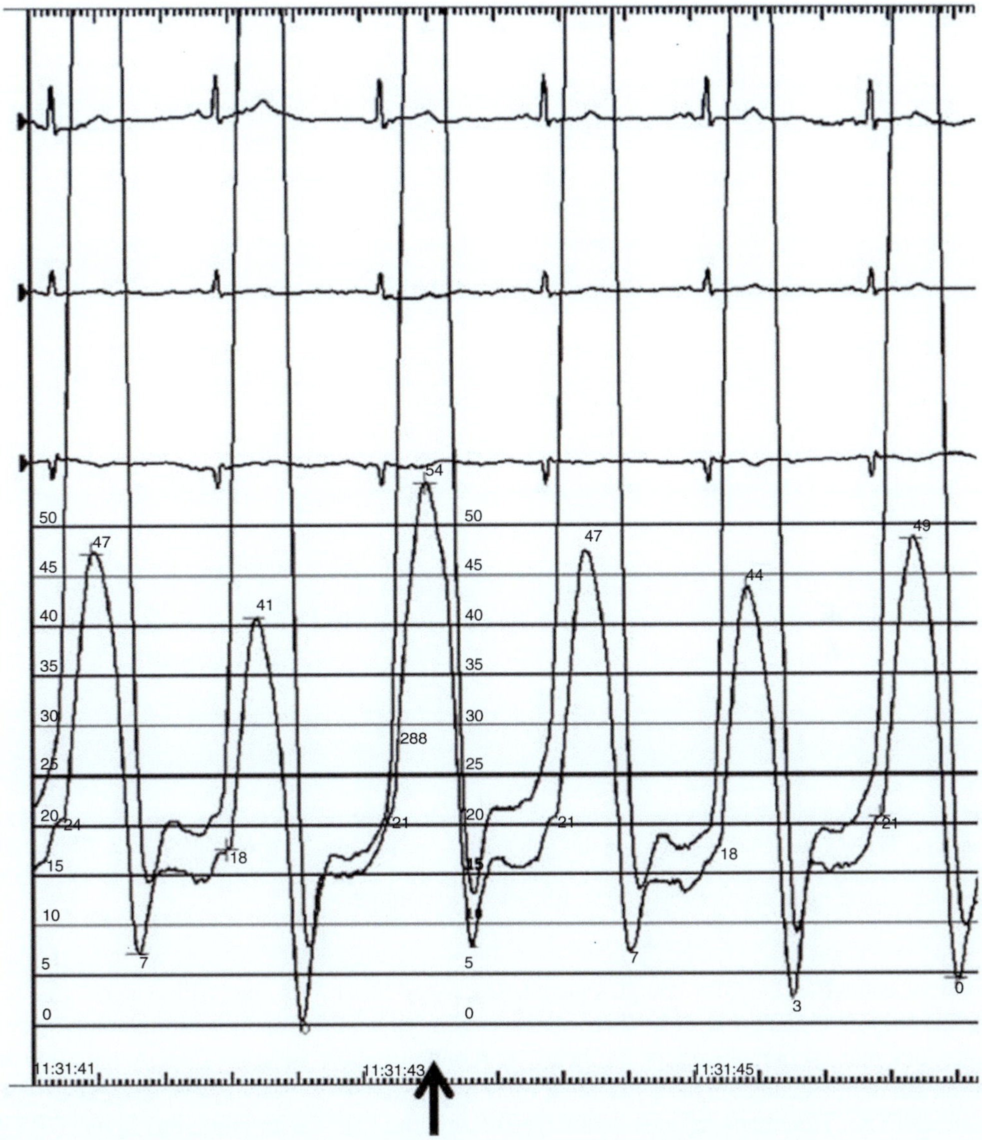

Fig. 8.1 A snapshot of a hemodynamic tracing of a patient with tuberculous constrictive pericarditis in whom a pericardectomy subsequently had to be performed. A square root sign is noticed, further there is interventricular dependence: right ventricular pressure increases during inspiration (arrow), peak left ventricular pressure is not shown here

Table 8.2 Important criteria that can be used to differentiate between CP and RCM

Criteria	Favours Constriction	Favours Restriction
Increased pericardial thickness on CT/MRI	X	
e′ velocity decreased on echocardiography		X
Increased respiratory variation of transmitral flow and septal shift on echocardiography	X	
Enhanced respiratory ventricular interdependence demonstrated with cardiac MRI or during invasive hemodynamic measurements	X	
Abnormal myocardial delayed enhancement on cardiac MRI		X

Adapted from Figure 10, ref. [13]

Cardiac infiltration by sarcoid granulomas may result in increased stiffness of the heart, with overt features of RCM. In addition, systolic dysfunction, conduction abnormalities and arrhythmias may be seen [4]. The role of genetic factors is supported by familial clustering, increased concordance in monozygotic twins and ethnic clustering [2, 4]. Genome-wide association studies have found the butyrophilin-like 2 (BTNL2), annexin A11 and RAB23 genes to be associated with sarcoidosis [2].

Cardiac Amyloidosis

Cardiac amyloidosis (CA) is frequently challenging to diagnose. As the diagnosis and treatment of CA will be covered in full detail in a separate chapter, only a few points will be made here. Concentric thickened heart walls in the absence of known hypertension or valvular disease and low-to-

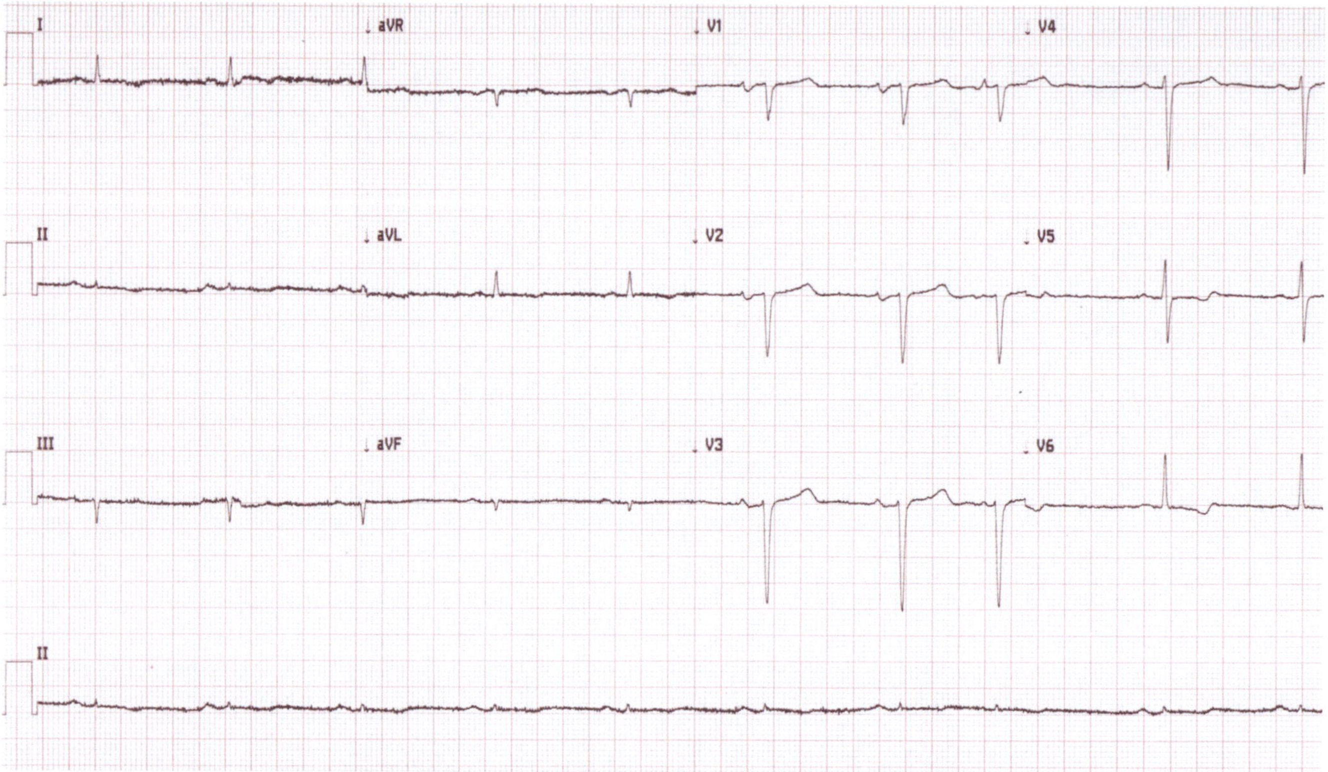

Fig. 8.2 Electrocardiogram of a patient with cardiac amyloidosis (AL) showing low voltages QRS complexes in the limb leads, being one of the most common electrocardiogram abnormalities in AL cardiac amyloidosis (occurring in approximately 50%), it is less common in the other forms of cardiac amyloidosis, being reported in approximately 25% of patients with familial disease and in approximately 40% of patients with senile cardiac amyloidosis

normal voltage in the QRS complex despite thickened heart walls suggest CA [2], Fig. 8.2. There are two main types of amyloid that commonly affect the heart: immunoglobulin light chain associated amyloid (AL) and transthyretin amyloid (ATTR). Treatment depends on the type of amyloid [3].

Hemochromatosis

Hemochromatosis can cause a cardiomyopathy due to iron overload. It is characterized in early stages by RCM, which progresses to an end-stage dilated cardiomyopathy [21]. Excess iron accumulation can be due to increased gastro-intestinal absorption or high parenteral iron administration, due to frequent red blood cell transfusions, e.g. in patients with thalassemia major and sickle cell disease [21]. Excess of iron leads to formation of reactive oxygen-free radicals causing damage to proteins [21]. Iron deposition in the heart begins in the epicardium, extending finally to the endocardium.

Hereditary hemochromatosis (HH) can be caused by mutations of genes involved in iron metabolism, which cause iron overload due to increased gastro-intestinal absorption [21]. There are four types of HH. Type 1 HH is an autosomal recessive disorder linked to mutations in the HFE gene that encodes a protein involved in controlling gastro-intestinal absorption of iron. Type 2 HH is associated with mutations of the HFE2 gene that encodes for homojuvelin [21]. Homojuvelin interacts with hepcidin, a key regulator of circulating iron. A mutation in the gene coding for hepcidin (HAMP) can also cause type 2 HH. Type 3 HH is associated with mutations in the TfR2 gene that encodes for transferrin receptor 2. Type 4 HH is caused by mutations in the SLC40A1 gene, which codes for ferroportin, a protein involved in iron efflux [21].

Clinical Features

Type 1 and 4 hemochromatosis usually manifest during the fourth or fifth decades of life, whereas type 2 typically presents by the second decade [21]. The onset of type 3 is usually intermediate between types 1 and 2. The typical triad of hemochromatosis consists of cirrhosis, skin bronzing and diabetes mellitus.

Diagnostic Evaluation

Indicators of iron overload are a plasma transferrin saturation >55% and serum ferritin >200 (for women) or 300 ng/ml (for men). Genetic screening for mutations in the HFE gene is widely available.

Echocardiography can be used to screen patients for iron overload cardiomyopathy [21]. Unlike most infiltrative cardiomyopathies LV wall thickness is not increased [21]. Impaired diastolic LV function is an early finding. Advanced-stage disease is characterized by left and right ventricular dilatation and reduced left ventricular ejection fraction (LVEF) (the dilated phenotype) or, alternatively, by restrictive LV filling with left atrial and right ventricular dilatation, increased pulmonary artery pressure and preserved LVEF (the restrictive phenotype) [22]. CMR can quantitate the amount of iron load. Iron has a paramagnetic effect, shortening the T2-weighted relaxation time. T2∗ relaxation is more sensitive than T2- or T1-based imaging for iron overload cardiomyopathy [23]. In RCM due to iron overload, T2∗ values are typically <20 ms [21]. A T2∗ value <10 ms is indicative of severe iron overload and predicts subsequent risk of heart failure [23].

Treatment

The mainstay of treatment is phlebotomy [21]. Iron chelation therapy is an option when phlebotomy is not feasible [21]. Potential new therapies are antioxidants and calcium-channel antagonists [21].

Primary Genetic RCM

Whereas RCM in adults is mostly symptomatic ('secondary') to underlying disease, RCM in children is most likely 'primary' caused by mutations in sarcomeric protein genes [24]. When familial, RCM is often part of a phenotypic variable spectrum of cardiomyopathies [25].

The classification of cardiomyopathies is subject to discussion. In 2006, a writing committee of the American Heart Association distinguishes primary and secondary causes [26]. When secondary the heart muscle is involved in a systemic disease. A cardiomyopathy is classified as primary when the disease affects (almost) exclusively the heart muscle. An even more strict 'primary' definition would be that the disease originates in the heart muscle. This would exclude cardio-specific infections and leave little room for causes other than genetic. 'Primary genetic' would then be a tautology.

Most genes associated with primary RCM have a direct role in the sarcomere. There have been few reports on RCM caused by mutations in genes involved in the intermediate filaments (IF) desmin and lamin A/C, which attach the sarcomere to the cytoskeleton. There are no mutations specific to RCM. Sarcomeric genes mainly cause HCM and to a lesser extend DCM. Mutations in the IF genes almost exclusively give rise to DCM. Taking this genetic background into account one could argue that primary RCM is equal to HCM without thickening of the myocardium. This is corroborated by the finding that in primary RCM the thickness of myocardium is often in the high range, but not exceeding the upper limit of what is considered normal. Other common features are gadolinium late enhancement on CMR. Also, disarray of cardiomyocytes is seen in endomyocardial biopsy.

Many reports describe primary genetic RCM as childhood disease leading to serious or fatal consequences. HCM most often has its debut at young adult age. The age difference between primary RCM (assuming it to be a subtype of HCM) and HCM may be explained by two factors. Firstly, RCM at adult age is most often secondary (infiltrative, tumour-related, etc.). Primary genetic RCM does occur at adult age, but is outnumbered by the secondary causes. Secondly, the severe expression of primary RCM compared to HCM suggests the existence of a second hit. This may be in the other allele of the same gene or in an independent second gene. Caleshu et al reported on two patients with RCM [24]. One with terminal heart failure at 22 years of age. She was homozygous for an MYL3 mutation and heterozygous for an MYL2 mutation. Her mother was a double heterozygote for the MYL3 and MYL2 mutations and had no symptoms of cardiomyopathy. The inclined conclusion is that homozygosity of the MYL3 mutation is the cause of the RCM. The second patient (pre-transplantation at age 35) was homozygous for a mutation in TPM1. Her heterozygous father was diagnosed with HCM at age 42. The requirement of a second hit clinically presents as a recessive mode of inheritance, whereas HCM causing mutations are typically autosomal dominant. On the other hand, there is compelling evidence of dominantly acting mutations causing RCM. The BAG Pro209Leu mutation by itself causes childhood RCM, be it associated with myofibrillar myopathy [27]. As the severe consequences prohibit offspring the BAG mutation always occurs *de novo* (so the locus is a mutation 'hot spot'). One recurrence was reported as a consequence of somatic mosaicism in the father [28]. *De novo* dominant mutations causing childhood RCM also occur in TNNI3 [25, 29]. Mogensen et al. reviewed the TNNI3 gene to be the most prevalent mutated gene in primary RCM [25]. In the only familial case they describe the RCM mixed with HCM. Another gene repeatedly reported to be involved in primary RCM is FLNC, both as a *de novo* mutation with childhood onset and dominantly inherited in families with adult onset [30, 31].

The genes with the highest mutation rate in HCM, MYH7 and MYBPC3, are much less frequent in RCM. For MYH7, there are few if any recent publications. Wu et al. describe a family with three affected members and one solitary index with RCM caused by a nonsense mutation in MYBPC3 [32].

Brodehl et al. report a CRYAB mutation in a German brother and sister who were diagnosed with RCM at age 19 and 28. Both were also carrier of a rare RBM20 variant. The possibility of a compound heterozygous cause of the RCM (fitting a 'recessive' double hit) was not considered [33]. An MYPN nonsense mutation was described in two siblings who underwent heart transplantation because of RCM at age 19 and 22. Their mother, carrier of the mutation, was unaffected, shedding doubt on the MYPN mutation to be the solitary cause [34].

Three genes, classically associated with DCM rather than HCM, have been tossed to cause primary RCM: TTN, LMNA and DES. By means of linkage analysis, Peled et al. found a TTN missense mutation in a three-generation family [35]. Four family members were severely affected, five carrying the same haplotype were healthy. Seventeen genes and one locus were excluded because of lack of segregation. Since TTN missense mutations are very common (as much as one in four individuals) and as many family members were affected as unaffected further evidence is needed to adopt the TTN gene in the list of genes associated with RCM. Paller et al. describe an LMNA frameshift mutation which is no doubt pathogenic, including an atrioventricular (AV) conduction defect and progressive skeletal muscle weakness [36]. The mother and sister were carrier of the mutation, had bradycardia and conduction defects, but no RCM (neither DCM). The authors state that an alternative, more precise description of this patient's phenotype would be 'mildly depressed LVEF and prominent restrictive features'. Nevertheless, the phenotype at least closely resembles the classical RCM phenotype. Publication of further families is awaited. Arbustini et al. describe nine patients in four families with a DES mutation [37]. Eight of nine patients had an AV block. LVEFs were below normal (40–50%), ventricular sizes were normal (LVEDD 40–56 mm). Three of four mutations were dominant (one *de novo*), one mutation was recessive with three unaffected heterozygotes, including the parents. Because of the presence in both LMNA and DES families, it is tempting to hypothesize that RCM caused by mutations in IF genes is somehow dependent on the presence of AV conduction disturbances. Then the description of primary RCM being 'HCM without hypertrophy' needs to be extended with 'or can be evoked by an AV block' especially when caused by an IF mutation (e.g. LMNA or DES).

Lysosomal Storage Diseases

Fabry Disease

Fabry disease (FD) is a lysosomal storage disease resulting from a deficiency of α-galactosidase A, which leads to the accumulation of globotriaosylceramide in skin, eye, heart, kidney, brain, vascular and nervous systems [38]. Males tend to develop more severe symptoms, than females [38]. Clinical symptoms include painful extremities related to peripheral neuropathy, angiokeratoma, adiaphoresis, corneal opacities, auditory disturbance, renal disease, cerebrovascular disease, cardiac hypertrophy and arrhythmia [38]. A cardiac variant of FD (cardiac FD), whose manifestations are limited to the heart is reported and patients with this variant type of the disease have residual a-Gal A activity, whereas it is (nearly) absent in classic Fabry disease [39]. Therefore, screening for FD is advised in patients even if classic FD symptoms are missing.

FD is the second most prevalent lysosomal storage disease after Gaucher disease. The disease is caused by mutations in the GLA gene [40]. The gene is located on the X chromosome (Xq22.1 region), explaining the male predominance. Several hundred mutations in the gene have been identified [4].

The prevalence of Fabry disease is estimated to range from 1:17,000 to 1:117,000 males in Caucasians [4]. Cardiac involvement may lead to (concentric) ventricular hypertrophy, conduction defects, coronary artery disease, valve insufficiencies and aortic root dilatation [4].

Echocardiography is a useful tool for screening, diagnosing and follow-up evaluation in FD. The most frequent morphological pattern in FD is concentric left ventricular hypertrophy (LVH), but concentric remodelling, asymmetric septal hypertrophy, eccentric or normal pattern are also observed occasionally [38]. LV enlargement and diffuse hypokinesia with posterior wall thinning, mimicking a dilated phase of hypertrophic cardiomyopathy, is seen in more advanced stage of FD. Left ventricular posterior wall thinning is an important echocardiographic finding that precedes heart failure and cardiac death in patients with FD [38]. Approximately 50% of patients with FD show myocardial enhancement on late Gadolinium imaging in the basal inferolateral left ventricular wall, usually involving the mid and subepicardial part of the myocardial wall [41]. Low native T1 values (prior to contrast administration) are postulated to indicate sphingolipid accumulation in FD [42]. In a recent study it has been shown that in patients with FD and LVH, myocardial strain (measured by global longitudinal strain) reduces with hypertrophy, storage (measured by a low T1), ECG abnormalities and scar (measured by LGE). In early disease (LVH negative), global longitudinal strain impairs as native T1 reduces.

A definitive diagnosis can be made based on a low plasma α-galactosidase A level in males or by analysis of the GLA gene [4].

FD can be treated using enzyme replacement therapy (ERT), which consists of the regular intravenous infusion of a recombinant enzyme formulation [43]. Studies comparing ERT to placebo show significant results in regard to microvascular endothelial deposits of globotriaosylceramide and in pain-related quality of life [43]. If ERT is started before myocardial fibrosis has developed, a long-term improvement of myocardial morphology, function and exercise capacity can be achieved [44].

Another treatment option is oral chaperone therapy with migalastat (Amicus Therapeutics) [45]. Migalastat

(1-deoxygalactonojirimycin) is an oral small molecule chaperone that stabilizes endogenous GLA enzyme and supports proper folding in the endoplasmic reticulum, leads to increased endogenous enzymatic GLA activity in the lysosomes of patients with an amenable mutation [45]. These are missense mutations that result in reduced enzymatic activity, caused by misfolding of the enzyme, which the chaperone can correct [44]. There are at least 359 amenable and 706 nonamenable mutations (on the basis of an in vitro test in human embryonic kidney cells), according to a list published by Amicus, which markets migalastat www.galafoldamenabilitytable.com, updated 16th May 2018) [44]. Recently therapeutic cardiac goals for patients with FD have been established [45].

Gaucher Disease

Although Gaucher disease (GD) is the most common lysosomal storage disease, it very rarely affects the heart (only subtype 3, occurring 1 in 200,000) [4]. This is an autosomal recessive disease attributable to deficiency of β-glucocerebrosidase. The glucocerebrosidase gene is located on chromosome 1q21, and more than 180 distinct mutations are known [40]. There are three forms of the disease and in types 2 and 3, neurological manifestations are present. In type 1, hepatosplenomegaly, bone marrow disease and skeletal abnormalities are present. Cardiac manifestations are rare [4].

Glycogen Storage Disease

Disorders of glycogen metabolism most often affect the liver and skeletal muscle, where glycogen is most abundant [4] (see also Chap. 22). To date, 12 subforms of glycogen storage disease (GSD) have been identified. The physiologic importance of a given enzyme determines the clinical manifestations of the disease.

In general, hypoglycaemia, hepatomegaly and skeletal muscle weakness and easy fatigability are the predominant clinical features [4]. In GSD type II (Pompe disease) and IIa (Danon disease), cardiac involvement may occur. The classic infantile form is characterized by cardiomyopathy and severe generalized muscular hypotonia [4]. The tongue may be enlarged. Hepatomegaly also may be present and is usually due to heart failure. Pompe disease is an autosomal recessive disorder with considerable allelic heterogeneity. The defect is attributable to deficiency of the lysosomal enzyme acid α-glucosidase. The gene (GAA) is located at 17q25.3 [40]. There are >150 mutations including nonsense, gene rearrangements and splicing defects [40]. Complete absence of enzyme activity results in early onset of severe disease, whereas residual enzyme activity is seen in patients with adult-onset disease [40].

Danon disease is a lysosomal storage disease caused by deficiency of lysosome-associated membrane protein 2 (LAMP2) [40]. The gene is located at Xq24, and >60 mutations have been reported [40]. It is an X-linked dominant disease. Once glucose enters the cell, it is either used for energy production or stored as glycogen. Excess glycogen is broken down in lysosomes, but with LAMP2 defects glycogen accumulates in cardiac myocytes leading to the appearance of vacuoles.

The usual clinical presentation is the result of disease in skeletal and cardiac muscle with or without intellectual deficiency. Males are more severely affected and present at a younger age than females. Females usually have a more benign course but there are reports of sudden cardiac death in women.

The usual findings include LVH in males (HCM phenocopy) with extreme hypertrophy noted in some cases (maximum wall thickness as high as 65 mm) [40]. Follow-up of these cases showed the subsequent development of LV dilatation and depression of LVEF. Some patients can also present with a dilated cardiomyopathy. Wolf–Parkinson–White (WPW) syndrome occurs in both males and females, though with a much higher frequency in males. It is important to consider Danon disease in patients with unexplained (concentric) LVH [40]. There is no specific treatment. For patients with WPW syndrome, catheter ablation is usually effective. Implantable cardiac defibrillator can be life-saving because of the danger of sudden cardiac death. With progressive LV dysfunction, cardiac transplantation should be considered.

Mucopolysaccharidoses

The mucopolysaccharidoses (MPS) are lysosomal storage disorders caused by the deficiency of enzymes required for the stepwise breakdown of glycosaminoglycans (GAGs), previously known as mucopolysaccharides [4]. Fragments of partially degraded GAGs accumulate in the lysosomes, resulting in cellular dysfunction and clinical abnormalities. These are rare conditions, with an estimated total incidence of all types of MPS of approximately 1 in 20,000 live births. *Hurler* syndrome is the severe form of MPS I and is characterized by a broad spectrum of clinical problems including skeletal abnormalities, hepatosplenomegaly and severe intellectual deficiency [46]. The incidence is approximately 1 in 100,000 births.

Cardiovascular abnormalities are most frequently seen in MPS types I, II and VI [40]. Cardiac abnormalities become apparent between birth and 5 years of age. These include cardiomyopathy, endocardial fibroelastosis and valvular regurgitation, which on itself or combined may lead to heart failure. GAG storage within blood vessels causes irregular and diffuse narrowing of the coronary arteries and irregular lesions of the aorta. Coronary artery disease is often unrecognized until autopsy examination; it should be considered in affected patients with cardiac problems. ERT with laronidase was approved for all phenotypes of MPS I in 2003 in

Europe and the United States [47]. Mucopolysaccharidosis II (*Hunter* syndrome) is caused by a deficiency of iduronate 2-sulfatase (IDS), which results in the storage of heparan and dermatan sulphate. MPS II is caused by mutations in the gene encoding for IDS, which is located on chromosome Xq28. Although the disorder is X-linked, cases in females have been reported on rare occasions [4].

Cardiovascular Causes of RCM

Pseudoxanthoma Elasticum

Pseudoxanthoma elasticum (PXE) is an autosomal recessive disorder with ectopic mineralization. PXE manifests with characteristic skin findings, ocular involvement and cardiovascular problems [46]. It may lead to peripheral and coronary arterial occlusive disease as well as gastrointestinal bleedings [4].

The classic forms of PXE are due to loss-of-function mutations in the ATP-Binding Cassette Family C Member 6 (ABCC6) gene, which encodes the ABCC6 protein, a putative transmembrane efflux transporter expressed primarily in the liver [46, 48]. This disorder leads to deposition of calcium hydroxyapatite in various connective tissues.

The precise prevalence of PXE is estimated to be around 1 in 50,000, with a carrier frequency of 1:150–300 [48]. In a study of 19 patients, it was found that systolic function was normal, but diastolic parameters were abnormal in seven patients [4, 49]. Explanations for these abnormalities could be silent myocardial ischaemia due to early coronary involvement and/or the direct consequences of ultrastructural defects of the elastic tissue of the heart [49].

Recently, treatment of PXE with the bisphophonate etidronate has been shown to reduce arterial calcification and subretinal neovascularization events [50].

Scleroderma/Systemic Sclerosis

In systemic sclerosis (SSc), there is often involvement of the pericardium, myocardium, conduction system and vasculature [51]. Patchy myocardial fibrosis as a result of recurrent vasospasm of small vessels may lead to the clinical picture of RCM [4]. Extensive fibrosis may be seen in patients with a long history of Raynaud phenomenon [4]. Significant cardiac involvement in SSc portends a poor prognosis. The relative risk of developing SSc is 1.6% in families with a history of SSc and 0.026% in the general population [52]. SSc is not the result of a single mutation but rather results from multiple genetic variants that predispose individuals to developing SSc [52]. Class II HLA genes have the highest statistically significant association with SSc; in particular, genetic polymorphisms in HLA-DQA1, HLA-DQB1, HLA-DPB1 and HLA-DRB1 have been associated with SSc in more than five different studies. Many of the different genes associated with SSc are also found in non-HLA loci [52].

Endo(Myo)Cardial Causes of RCM

Endomyocardial Fibrosis, Endocardial Fibroelastosis and Hypereosinophilic Syndromes

The most common form of endomyocardial disease is EMF, other forms are endocardial fibroelastosis (EF) and hypereosinophilic syndromes (HES).

EMF was initially described in Uganda and is the most common cause of RCM worldwide. It is commonly seen in equatorial countries and accounts for a substantial percentage of heart failure cases [21]. Malnutrition, parasitic infections and genetic factors have been proposed as aetiological factors [21]. Echocardiography in patients with EMF typically shows small ventricles, normal wall thickness, dilated atria and valvular dysfunction [21]. CMR can help to confirm the presence of a left ventricular cavitary thrombus. Management consists of sodium and fluid restriction, diuretics and aspirin or anticoagulation in case of intracardiac thrombi [21].

EF is characterized by diffuse thickening of the left ventricular endocardium [21]. Two forms have been described: a dilated form (DCM phenotype) and an RCM phenotype in which the LV cavity is small. A familial pattern is seen in the majority. This disease is very rare and may respond to surgery [21].

Eosinophils usually combat parasites and participate in hypersensitivity and allergic responses. Eosinophilia can be due to parasitic infections, malignancies, eosinophilic leukaemia, allergic drug reactions or idiopathic causes [53]. Cardiac damage can result from eosinophilia [54]. In HES affecting the heart (formerly known as Loeffler's endocarditis) damage to the endothelium and myocardium is caused by highly active biological substances [21]. Most patients diagnosed with HES are between 20 and 50 years of age. Eosinophilic heart disease has been categorized in three phases: an acute necrotic phase; an intermediate phase with thrombus formation and a fibrotic phase characterized by impaired cardiac function, heart failure due to RCM with also damage to chordal structures leading to mitral and tricuspid regurgitation [21]. CMR can reliably detect the different phases of the disease, Fig. 8.3 [55].

Treatment can be effective in the early stages of disease [21]. Corticosteroids alone or in combination with cytolytic therapies (hydroxyurea, interferon-alpha) have been shown to improve the acute necrotic phase of disease [21, 56]. The role for systemic anticoagulation in patients with intracardiac thrombi is controversial because treatment failures are common [21].

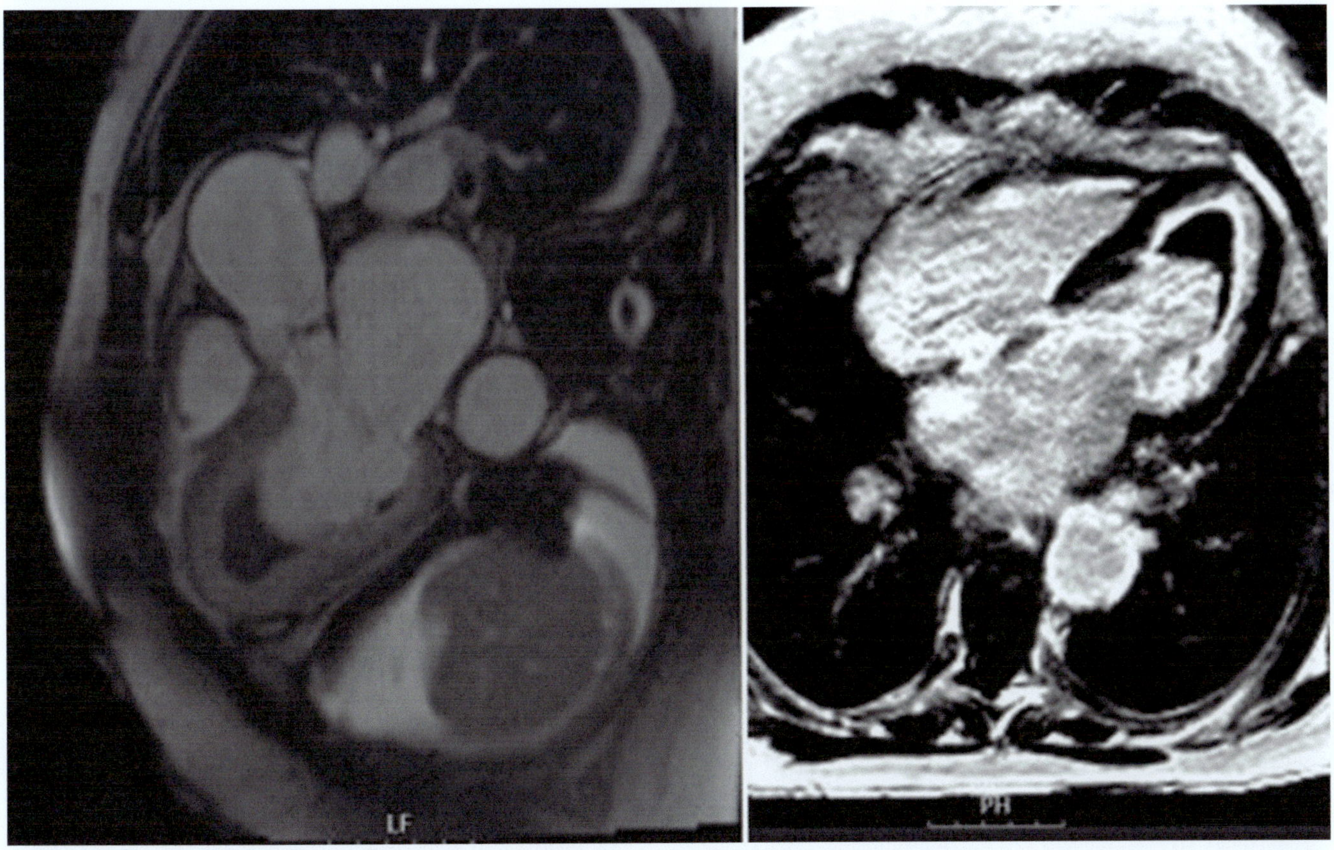

Fig. 8.3 A cardiac MRI showing an apical thrombus in the left ventricle (left panel) and extended subendocardial late enhancement (right panel) in a patient with histologically proven hypereosinophilic syndrome

Cancer-Related Causes of RCM

Radiation-Induced Heart Disease

Radiation therapy can cause accelerated coronary artery disease, valvular dysfunction, RCM, aortopathy and constrictive pericarditis [21]. Especially in patients with high doses of radiation (>30 Gray) effects can be seen. Radiation-induced heart disease typically occurs after a latent period of 10–15 years [21]. Radiation-related RCM is due to inflammation, microvascular injury and replacement fibrosis. Management of established disease is symptomatic and consists of diuretics to control volume overload [21].

Approach to a Patient Suspected of RCM

The main diagnostic work-up will consist of an extensive medical history with particular focus on issues like cancer, including leukaemia, medication, chronic diseases (infections, diabetes, autoimmune), anaemia, both in past and present. A detailed family history, with focus on the presence of (cardio)myopathies, can give additional clues. A thorough echocardiographic examination should be performed, often extended with CMR and if indicated a PET-CT scan. Laboratory investigations should include a serum-free light chain assay and determination of ferritin and transferrin saturation levels. A cardiogenetic panel (including sarcomeric, lysosomal, TTR, HFE, ABCC6 (PXE)) should be considered and in some cases an endomyocardial biopsy. With increasing availability and reducing costs genetic analysis might become the investigation of first choice, especially at young age. After the age of 50, with a family history negative for heart failure below 60, infiltrative causes are by far the most common cause and need to be excluded thoroughly.

Summary

RCM represents a heterogeneous group of diseases. In RCM ventricular filling is impeded because of increased stiffness of the myocardium, causing a rapid increase in ventricular pressure upon only small increases in volume. Biventricular chamber size, wall thickness and systolic function are usually normal or near-normal until later stages of the disease. Differentiation form constrictive pericarditis is important but can be challenging. RCM can result from an inherited or acquired disease. Besides general supportive measures, treatment of RCM depends on the underlying cause of RCM. Searching for the underlying cause is of utmost importance, since for several disorders more or less effective treatment options are currently available.

Take-Home Messages

- When confronted with a patient with heart failure and (near) normal wall thickness and systolic function, be aware of RCM.
- RCM represents a heterogeneous group of disorders, both acquired and inherited.
- In a patient with RCM extensive diagnostic evaluation is indicated to look for an underlying cause.
- Besides general supportive treatment options for heart failure in RCM, in selected cases disease targeted treatment is possible.

References

1. Elliott P, Andersson B, Arbustini E, et al. Classification of the cardiomyopathies: a position statement from the European society of cardiology working group on myocardial and pericardial diseases. Eur Heart J. 2008;29:270–6.
2. Muchtar E, Blauwet LA, Gertz MA. Restrictive cardiomyopathy. genetics, pathogenesis, clinical manifestations, diagnosis, and therapy. Circ Res. 2017;121:819–37.
3. Pereira N, Grogan M, Dec GW. Spectrum of restrictive and infiltrative cardiomyopathies. part 1 of a 2-part series. J Am Coll Cardiol. 2018;71:1130–48.
4. Kirkels JH, de Jonge N. Restrictive cardiomyopathy. Chapter 8. In: Baars HF, Doevendans PAFM, Houweling AC, van Tintelen JP, editors. Clinical cardiogenetics. 2nd ed. Cham: Springer; 2016.
5. Habib G, Bucciarelli-Ducci C, Caforio ALP, et al. Multimodality Imaging in Restrictive Cardiomyopathies: an EACVI expert consensus document In collaboration with the "Working Group on myocardial and pericardial diseases" of the European Society of Cardiology. Endorsed by The Indian Academy of Echocardiography. Eur Heart J Cardiovasc Imaging. 2017;18:1090–1.
6. Cheng H, Zhao S, Jiang S, et al. The relative atrial volume ratio and late gadolinium enhancement provide additive information to differentiate constrictive pericarditis from restrictive cardiomyopathy. J Cardiovasc Magn Reson. 2011;13:15.
7. Lorell BH, Grossman W. Profiles in constrictive pericarditis, restrictive cardiomyopathy, and cardiac tamponade. Chapter 33. In: Baim DS, Grossman W, editors. Grossman's cardiac catheterization, angiography, and intervention. 6th ed. Philadelphia: Lippincott Williams & Wilkins; 2000. p. 829–50.
8. Kushwaha SS. Restrictive cardiomyopathy. Chapter 99. In: Murphy JG, Lloyd MA, editors-in-chief. Mayo Clinic Cardiology. Concise textbook. 4th ed. Rochester, MN/New York: Mayo Clinic Scientific Press/Oxford University Press; 2013. p. 892–7.
9. Kushwaha SS, Fallon JT, Fuster V. Restrictive cardiomyopathy. N Engl J Med. 1997;336:267–76.
10. Bennett MK, Gilotra NA, Harrington C, et al. Evaluation of the role of endomyocardial biopsy in 851 patients with unexplained heart failure from 2000-2009. Circ Heart Fail. 2013;6:676–84.
11. Hutchison SJ. Chapter 9. Pericardial constriction. In: pericardial diseases. Clinical diagnostic imaging atlas. Philadelphia, PA: Saunders, Elsevier; 2009.
12. Garcia MJ. Constrictive pericarditis versus restrictive cardiomyopathy. J Am Coll Cardiol. 2016;67:2061–76.
13. Geske JB, Anavekar NS, Nishimura RA, et al. Differentiation of constriction and restriction. Complex cardiovascular hemodynamics. J Am Coll Cardiol. 2016;68:2329–47.
14. Rajagopalan N, Garcia MJ, Rodriguez L, et al. Comparison of new Doppler echocardiographic methods to differentiate constrictive pericardial heart disease and restrictive cardiomyopathy. Am J Cardiol. 2001;87:86–94.
15. Masui T, Finck S, Higgins CB. Constrictive pericarditis and restrictive cardiomyopathy: evaluation with MR imaging. Radiology. 1992;182:369–73.
16. Ling LH, Oh JK, Breen JF, et al. Calcific constrictive pericarditis: is it still with us? Ann Intern Med. 2000;132:444–50.
17. Bull RK, Edwards PD, Dixon AK. CT dimensions of the normal pericardium. Br J Radiol. 1998;71:923–5.
18. Talreja DR, Edwards WD, Danielson GK, et al. Constrictive pericarditis in 26 patients with histologically normal pericardial thickness. Circulation. 2003;108:1852–7.
19. Sengupta PP, Krishnamoorthy VK, Abhayaratna WP, et al. Comparison of usefulness of tissue Doppler imaging versus brain natriuretic peptide for differentiation of constrictive pericardial disease from restrictive cardiomyopathy. Am J Cardiol. 2008;102:357–62.
20. Kusano KF, Satomi K. Diagnosis and treatment of cardiac sarcoidosis. Heart. 2016;102(3):184–90.
21. Pereira NL, Grogan M, Dec GW. Spectrum of restrictive and infiltrative cardiomyopathies: part 2 of a 2-part series. J Am Coll Cardiol. 2018;71(10):1149–66.
22. Kremastinos DT, Farmakis D. Iron overload cardiomyopathy in clinical practice. Circulation. 2011;124:2253–63.
23. Kirk P, Roughton M, Porter JB, et al. Cardiac T2∗ magnetic resonance for prediction of cardiac complications in thalassemia major. Circulation. 2009;120:1937–9.
24. Caleshu C, Sakhuja R, Nussbaum RL, et al. Furthering the link between the sarcomere and primary cardiomyopathies: restrictive cardiomyopathy associated with multiple mutations in genes previously associated with hypertrophic or dilated cardiomyopathy. Am J Med Genet A. 2011;155A(9):2229–35.
25. Mogensen J, Hey T, Lambrecht S. A systematic review of phenotypic features associated with cardiac troponin I mutations in hereditary cardiomyopathies. Can J Cardiol. 2015;31(11):1377–85.
26. Maron BJ, Towbin JA, Thiene G, et al. Contemporary definitions and classification of the cardiomyopathies. Circulation. 2006;113(14):1807–16.
27. Schänzer A, Rupp S, Gräf S, et al. Dysregulated autophagy in restrictive cardiomyopathy due to Pro209Leu mutation in BAG3. Mol Genet Metab. 2018;123(3):388–99.
28. Odgerel Z, Sarkozy A, Lee HS, et al. Inheritance patterns and phenotypic features of myofibrillar myopathy associated with a BAG3 mutation. Neuromuscul Disord. 2010;20(7):438–42.
29. Kaski JP, McKenna WJ, Elliott PM, et al. Idiopathic restrictive cardiomyopathy in children is caused by mutations in cardiac sarcomere protein genes. Heart. 2008;94(11):1478–84.
30. Tucker NR, McLellan MA, Hu D et al. Novel mutation in FLNC (filamin C) causes familial restrictive cardiomyopathy. Circ Cardiovasc Genet. 2017;10(6).
31. Schubert J, Tariq M, Geddes G, et al. Novel pathogenic variants in filamin C identified in pediatric restrictive cardiomyopathy. Hum Mutat. 2018;39(12):2083–96.
32. Wu W, Lu CX, Wang YN, et al. Novel phenotype-genotype correlations of restrictive cardiomyopathy with MYBPC3 gene mutations tested by NGS. J Am Heart Assoc. 2015;10:4(7).
33. Brodehl A, Gaertner-Rommel A, Klauke B, et al. The novel αB-crystallin (CRYAB) mutation p.D109G causes restrictive cardiomyopathy. Hum Mutat. 2017;38(8):947–52.
34. Huby AC, Mendsaikhan U, Takagi K, et al. Disturbance in Z-disk mechanosensitive proteins induced by a persistent mutant myopalladin causes familial restrictive cardiomyopathy. J Am Coll Cardiol. 2014;64(25):2765–76.

35. Peled Y, Gramlich M, Yoskovitz G, et al. Titin mutation in familial restrictive cardiomyopathy. Int J Cardiol. 2014;171(1):24–30.
36. Paller MS, Martin CM, Pierpont ME. Restrictive cardiomyopathy: an unusual phenotype of a lamin A variant. ESC Heart Fail. 2018;5(4):724–6.
37. Arbustini E, Pasotti M, Pilotto A, et al. Desmin accumulation restrictive cardiomyopathy and atrioventricular block associated with desmin gene defects. Eur J Heart Fail. 2006;8(5):477–83.
38. Yuasa T, Takenaka T, Higuchi K. Fabry disease. J Echocardiogr. 2017;15:151–7.
39. Nakao S, Takenaka T, Maeda M, et al. An atypical variant of Fabry's disease in men with left ventricular hypertrophy. N Engl J Med. 1995;333:288–93.
40. Nagueh SF. Anderson-Fabry disease and other lysosomal storage disorders. Circulation. 2014;130(13):1081–90.
41. Bogaert J, Taylor AM. Heart muscle disease. In: Bogaert J et al., editors. Clinical cardiac MRI. Berlin: Springer; 2012.
42. Vijapurapu R, Nordin S, Baig S, et al. Global longitudinal strain, myocardial storage and hypertrophy in Fabry disease. Heart 2018; 1–7. https://doi.org/10.1136/heartjnl-2018-313699.
43. El Dib R, Gomaa H, Carvalho RP, et al. Enzyme replacement therapy for Anderson-Fabry disease. Cochrane Database Syst Rev. 2016;7:CD006663. https://doi.org/10.1002/14651858.CD006663.pub4.
44. Lenders M, Brand E. Effects of enzyme replacement therapy and antidrug antibodies in patients with Fabry disease. JASN. 2018;29(9):2265–78.
45. Wanner C, Arad M, Baron R, et al. European expert consensus statement on therapeutic goals in Fabry disease. Mol Genet Metab. 2018;124(3):189–203.
46. Uitto J, Bercovitch L, Terry SF, et al. Pseudoxanthoma elasticum: progress in diagnostics and research towards treatment. Summary of the 2010 PXE International Research Meeting. Am J Med Genet A. 2011;155(7):1517–26. https://doi.org/10.1002/ajmg.a.34067.
47. Eisengart JB, Rudser KD, Xue Y, et al. Long-term outcomes of systemic therapies for Hurler syndrome: an international multicenter comparison. Genet Med. 2018; https://doi.org/10.1038/gim.2018.29. [Epub ahead of print]
48. Kranenburg, G., Baas AF, de Jong PA, et al. The prevalence of Pseudoxanthoma elasticum: revised estimations based on genotyping in a high vascular risk cohort. Eur J Med Genet. 2018. https://doi.org/10.1016/j.ejmg.2018.05.020.
49. Nguyen LD, Terbah M, Daudon P, Martin L. Left ventricular systolic and diastolic function by echocardiogram in pseudoxanthoma elasticum. Am J Cardiol. 2006;97:1535–7.
50. Kranenburg G, de Jong PA, Bartstra JW. Etidronate for prevention of ectopic mineralization in patients with Pseudoxanthoma elasticum. J Am Coll Cardiol. 2018;71:1117–26.
51. Parks JL, Taylor MH, Parks LP. Systemic sclerosis and the heart. Rheum Dis Clin N Am. 2014;40:87–102.
52. Angiolilli C, Marut W, van der Kroef M, et al. New insights into the genetics and epigenetics of systemic sclerosis. Nat Rev Rheumatol. 2018;14(11):657–73.
53. Weller PF, Bubley GJ. The idiopathic hypereosinophilic syndrome. Blood. 1994;83:2759–79.
54. Cheung CC, Constantine M, Ahmadi A, et al. Eosinophilic myocarditis. Am J Med Sci. 2017;354(5):486–92.
55. Syed IS, Martinez WM, Feng DL, et al. Cardiac magnetic resonance imaging of eosinophilic endomyocardial disease. Int J Cardiol. 2008;126:e50–2.
56. Butterfield JH, Weiler CR. Treatment of hypereosinophilic syndromes—the first 100 years. Semin Hematol. 2012;49:182–91.

Metabolic Cardiomyopathy

9

Aleš Linhart

Introduction

Inborn errors of metabolism (IEM) represent a large end heterogeneous group of diseases caused by a variety of genetic causes. Most important cardiomyopathy-causing diseases include the following groups of metabolic defects [1, 2]:

- *Disorders of amino acid and organic acid metabolism* (e.g. β-ketothiolase deficiency, tyrosinemia or oxalosis) [3–5].
- *Disorders of fatty acid metabolism* represented by carnitine transport defects (systemic primary or muscle carnitine deficiency), and fatty acid oxidation defects (e.g. by very long-chain or long-chain acyl-CoA dehydrogenase deficiency) [6].
- *Lysosomal storage diseases (LSDs)* a heterogeneous group of diseases where cardiac involvement is found in disorders of glycogen, mucopolysaccharide and glycosphingolipid lysosomal metabolism. The glycogen storage diseases (GSDs) overlap in part with LSDs as Danon and Pompe disease, causing cardiac hypertrophy and failure, can be categorized in both LSDs and GSDs. Among LSDs, mucopolysaccharidoses (MPS) and Anderson Fabry disease (AFD) are known to cause cardiomyopathy and/or valvular involvement. Although some cardiac abnormalities were described in other LSDs such as Gaucher disease, most patients with this particular disorder show no sign of cardiac involvement [7, 8].
- *Glycogen storage diseases (GSDs)* may be characterized either by lysosomal or extralysosomal glycogen storage. Most diseases are characterized by skeletal myopathy. Lysosomal storage with cardiac involvement includes Danon and infantile Pompe disease. An example of systemic diseases with cardiac involvement is Cori disease (debrancher enzyme deficiency) [9]. In contrast, an isolated cardiac involvement characterized by hypertrophic cardiomyopathy with AV conduction abnormalities and preexcitation pattern on ECG is present in PRKAG2 cardiomyopathy caused by mutations in the gene encoding the gamma-2 regulatory subunit of AMP-activated protein kinase (AMPK) [10].

A. Linhart (✉)
First Faculty of Medicine, Charles University,
General University Hospital, Prague, Czech Republic
e-mail: ales.linhart@vfn.cz

Incidence and Prevalence

Traditionally, the overall IEM incidence is estimated to be around 1:4000 newborns. However, recent studies applying genetic screening for different diseases indicate that the real incidence may be substantially higher. However, interpretation of newborn screenings should be done with caution since many detected mutations may be benign variants or variants causing mild and/or late-onset phenotypes [11, 12].

So far, more than 1000 IEM were described in the literature. Of these, about 5% are believed to be associated with some cardiac involvement. In paediatric patients, IEM is believed to cause about one-fourth of cases of hypertrophic cardiomyopathy. Most of infantile HCM cases are due to infantile Pompe disease.

In adults, the prevalence of IEMs among patients with cardiomyopathies is rapidly decreasing to numbers below 5%. Literature data about the prevalence should be interpreted with caution as many mutations found in targeted screening programs of HCM patients were not properly considering the pathogenicity of the mutations and the prevalence may be overestimated. For example, in Fabry disease, the reasonable estimate of the disease prevalence in HCM cohorts is only about 1% although numbers as high as 12% were reported in the past [2, 12].

Among paediatric DCM patients, IEMs are encountered with a lower frequency (below 10%). A substantial proportion of the cases are represented by oxidative phosphorylation defects. In adult patients, IEMs are believed to be rare. However, some patients with burnt-out cardiomyopathies may be affected for example by Danon disease [13].

H. F. Baars et al. (eds.), *Clinical Cardiogenetics*, https://doi.org/10.1007/978-3-030-45457-9_9

Aetiology/Pathophysiology

The biochemical aetiology may be described on the basis of the biochemical defect (fatty acid metabolism, amino acid metabolism), or by the affected organelle (lysosomal storage, mitochondrial disease). In most cases, the underlying metabolic defect is due to a missing or dysfunctional enzyme. However, in some diseases, the defect may concern activator proteins, proteins necessary for intracellular trafficking such as lysosomal membrane proteins (LAMP2 deficiency—Danon disease), or regulatory proteins (abnormal activation of AMPK by a mutation in gamma-2 regulatory subunit in PRKAG2 cardiomyopathy) [1, 2, 14].

Cardiomyopathy caused by IEMs may be induced by different mechanisms affecting the cardiac muscle usually in combination. The disorders characterized by the accumulation of large macromolecules (glycogen, glycolipids, triglycerides) may lead to disruption of normal sarcomere structure and loss of its function. In addition, mechanical storage is always associated with profound functional changes. The second mechanism includes either direct or indirect impairment of energy production and handling within the cells. The inadequate energy supply is almost always provoking compensatory changes in the form of hypertrophy. However, in case of profound energy deficiency pro-apoptotic signals may be triggered leading to cellular death and replacement fibrosis. The latter mechanism may be caused also by toxic metabolic products provoking changes in intracellular homeostasis (e.g. pH maintenance) and increasing the oxidative stress which in turn damages the oxidative metabolism and worsens the energy deficiency [15].

Phenotypical manifestation is believed to reflect the prevailing mechanism—hypertrophy develops mostly as a compensatory mechanism but may be in part due to the storage itself. In several storage diseases, such as AFD, a genuine muscular hypertrophy contributes to the muscular mass increase to a bigger extent as compared to the amount of stored material. In contrast apoptosis (or necrosis in most severe cases) provokes subsequent inflammatory and fibrotic changes leading either to systolic dysfunction or severely impaired ventricular filling. Valvular changes in MPS are initially caused by storage of glycosaminoglycans (GAGs), lysosomal storage is also found in valvular fibroblasts in AFD patients [16].

Clinical Presentation

The phenotypical manifestation of IEMs is heterogeneous. Many diseases are characterized by a hypertrophic cardiomyopathy (HCM) phenotype with or without subsequent deterioration of systolic dysfunction to a burnt-out HCM pattern. In others, the phenotype may be characterized from early stages rather as a dilated cardiomyopathy (DCM). In early stages, IEMs lead only rarely to a restrictive cardiomyopathy (RCM) phenotype. However, a restrictive filling pattern may develop in advanced stages of many cardiomyopathies.

Many IEMs cause infantile forms of cardiomyopathy (Pompe disease, primary carnitine deficiency). However, several diseases become apparent only in adolescents (Danon disease) or even in adult age (AFD). In spite of variable clinical manifestations, the age of onset represents an important criterium in the differential diagnosis [17, 18].

Electrophysiological manifestations are frequent in many cardiomyopathies caused by IEMs. Glycogen storage diseases and AFD lead frequently to PR shortening with or without a preexcitation pattern. AV conduction disturbances develop in later stages of many metabolic cardiomyopathies. Many other arrhythmias develop in many cases of advanced cardiomyopathies. However, some arrhythmias could develop even in absence of clinically detectable structural changes (e.g. in carnitine deficiency or in fatty acid oxidation defects).

Valvular involvement is typically seen in mucopolysaccharidoses and to a lesser extent in AFD [19].

Examples of Inborn Errors of Metabolism Associated with Cardiac Involvement

Disorders of Amino Acid and Organic Acid Metabolism

Defects in amino acid and organic acid metabolism are causing cardiomyopathy relatively rarely. Out of the listed diseases, cardiac involvement is most predominant in *primary hyperoxaluria (PH)*. The disease is inherited as an autosomal recessive trait. The metabolic defect involves glyoxylate metabolism that causes increased production of oxalate.

PH is caused by mutations in three different genes that encode enzymes involved in glyoxylate metabolism: type I, alanine–glyoxylate aminotransferase (*AGXT*); type II, glyoxylate reductase/hydroxypyruvate reductase (*GRHPR*); type III, 4-hydroxy-2-oxoglutarate aldolase (*HOGA1*). The overwhelming majority is represented by PH type 1 (almost 80% of all cases). The estimated prevalence ranges between 1 and 3 per 1 million people [20].

The stored substance in PH is oxalate produced from the excess of glyoxylate. PH has multisystemic manifestations with kidney involvement by urolithiasis and nephrocalcinosis. Kidney impairment further decreases oxalate excretion which accumulates within skin, skeletal system, retina, vessels and myocardium. Cardiomyopathy is present in about one-third of affected individuals and is characterized by LVH, left atrial dilatation and arrhythmias including AV conduction defects. Occasionally, restrictive cardiomyopathy was reported. Cardiac involvement is at least partially reversible after kidney and liver transplantation [5, 21].

Disorders of Fatty Acid Metabolism

Carnitine Transport Defects

Carnitine is an essential molecule for the transfer of long-chain fatty acids across the mitochondrial membrane to allow subsequent beta-oxidation. Carnitine deficiency states include the primary defect, genetically caused and involving directly the high-affinity carnitine transporter and secondary carnitine deficiency induced by other inherited or acquired metabolic defects.

Primary carnitine deficiency (PCD, also reported as carnitine uptake defect, carnitine transporter deficiency, systemic carnitine deficiency), is an autosomal recessive disorder caused by numerous mutations of *SLC22A5,* a gene encoding the high-affinity carnitine transporter OCTN2 in the plasma membrane. More than 60 mutations in the SLC22A5 gene (5q31.1 locus) have been found. The incidence of PCD is about 1:40,000 with an approximate 1% carrier prevalence in the general population (high incidence was reported in Faroe Islands while a lower incidence was found in the United States—1:142,000 by newborn screening) [22].

Defects of the OCNT2 transporter protein result in urinary carnitine loss, low circulating carnitine levels and intracellular carnitine depletion resulting in defective fatty acid oxidation. Resulting in impairment of energy generation and reduced ketogenesis that becomes more apparent during fasting or stress. In addition, the defect induces an accumulation of long-chain fatty acids in the cytoplasm of affected tissues. The clinical manifestation is ranging from relatively benign or asymptomatic course of the disease to severe cardiac manifestations in early childhood. Metabolic clinical symptoms usually appear as episodes of hypoketotic hypoglycemia, hepatomegaly and muscle weakness. Cardiac disease is associated with intracellular lipid accumulation and fibrosis clinically appearing as dilated or hypertrophic cardiomyopathy with congestive heart failure and/or arrhythmias. The most common presentation occurring in about two-third of infantile cases is DCM or HCM which may become apparent in early childhood (1–4 years). In late-onset phenotypes, cardiomyopathy appears to be less frequent. However, cases presenting with various arrhythmias were reported. Sudden cardiac death may be the first manifestation in otherwise asymptomatic adult individuals. Resting ECG may show short QT interval with peaked T waves [23].

Heterozygotes for PCD can have decreased carnitine transport activity and reduced plasma carnitine levels and can develop benign cardiac hypertrophy. Some cases have been associated with arrhythmias responding to carnitine treatment.

The clinical diagnosis of PCD is based on the finding of severe reduction of plasma or tissue carnitine levels (at least five to ten times lower than in healthy controls—<5 or 8 μM, normal 25–50 μM) with reduced renal reabsorption (<90%) in presence of normal renal function and no abnormalities in urine organic acids or impairment of fatty acid oxidation (both potentially causing secondary carnitine deficiency), confirmed defects of carnitine transport in fibroblasts, and improvements with carnitine supplementation. Tandem mass spectrometry (MS/MS) from dry blood spots combined with genetic diagnosis using next-generation sequencing was shown to be effective in newborn screening programs. The sequencing method is relevant since about 15% of mutations are within non-exonic regions [24].

Treatment is based on L-carnitine supplementation using high doses of 100–400 mg/kg/day. It has been shown to rapidly improve cardiomyopathy and muscle weakness as well as manifestations linked to fasting ketogenesis. The dose of carnitine should be adapted according to plasma carnitine level measurement. In case of treatment interruption, the disease usually reappears within a very short time.

Secondary carnitine deficiencies may be hereditary or acquired. Secondary carnitine deficiency can be caused by a number of organic acidemias, defects of fatty acid oxidation and the carnitine cycle.

Other disturbances of carnitine system include *carnitine palmitoyltransferase defects* which represent a disorder of carnitine-related transport of long-chain fatty acids. Cardiomyopathy was described as one of the manifestations in infantile and neonatal CPT 2 deficiencies. Another rare condition causing cardiac structural involvement and arrhythmias is *carnitine/acylcarnitine translocase deficiency* [25].

Fatty Acid Oxidation Defects

Fatty acid oxidation (FAO) is an essential metabolic pathway for energy production particularly in presence of high-demand conditions. The process involves multiple mechanisms including fatty acid uptake and activation, carnitine and beta-oxidation cycle and electron transfer system. Multiple diseases resulting from fatty acid oxidation defects have been described. In a broader sense, these include also above-mentioned carnitine transport defects and defects of oxidative phosphorylation usually listed among mitochondrial diseases [26].

Fatty acid beta-oxidation taking place within the mitochondria may be affected by either intramitochondrial β-oxidation defects of long-chain fatty acids affecting membrane-bound enzymes, or β-oxidation defects of short- and medium-chain fatty acids affecting enzymes of the mitochondrial matrix. At least 20 separate transport proteins and enzymes are required for activation and breakdown of fatty acids via FAO. Since under normal physiological conditions, FAO provides up to 70% ATP for cardiac contraction, many defects lead to cardiomyopathy. Almost all FAO disorders are inherited as autosomal recessive diseases usually manifesting early in infants and children. The large phenotypical spectrum may include growth retardation, neuropathies, skeletal myopathy, liver failure, lactacidemia, hypoglycaemia and premature death. FAO disorders were shown to cause about 25% of paediatric HCM and DCM and may manifest with arrhythmias as well. However, later onset forms can occur as well usually presenting as neuropathy, myopathy and/or cardiac involvement with rhythm disturbances. More specifically, very long-chain acyl-CoA dehydrogenase deficiency—VLCAD and multiple acyl-CoA dehydrogenase deficiency (glutaric academic type II)—MCAD were shown to cause predominantly HCM, while long-chain 3-hydroxyacyl-CoA dehydrogenase deficiency—LCHAD may cause either HCM or DCM [27].

The diagnosis in children requires a large spectrum of laboratory tests including routine analysis up to assessments of acylcarnitine levels, organic acids, plasma carnitine, acylcarnitines and urine acylglycine analysis. The definitive diagnosis could be done by mutation analysis or measurement of specific enzyme activity.

Currently, there is no specific treatment for FAO defects. Common measures include reduction in fat intake, and avoidance of prolonged fasting. Liver transplant may be considered in patients without significant neurological and systemic involvement.

Lysosomal Storage Diseases (LSDs)

Anderson Fabry disease (AFD) is an X-linked syndrome caused by the deficiency of alpha-galactosidase A (AGALA). AFD belongs to a larger group of LSDs—sphingolipidoses. The metabolic defect results in the accumulation of neutral glycosphingolipids, primarily globotriaosylceramide (Gb_3), in various organs and tissues (Fig. 9.1). Deacylated form of Gb_3 (lyso-Gb3, globotriaosylsphingosine) was found to be

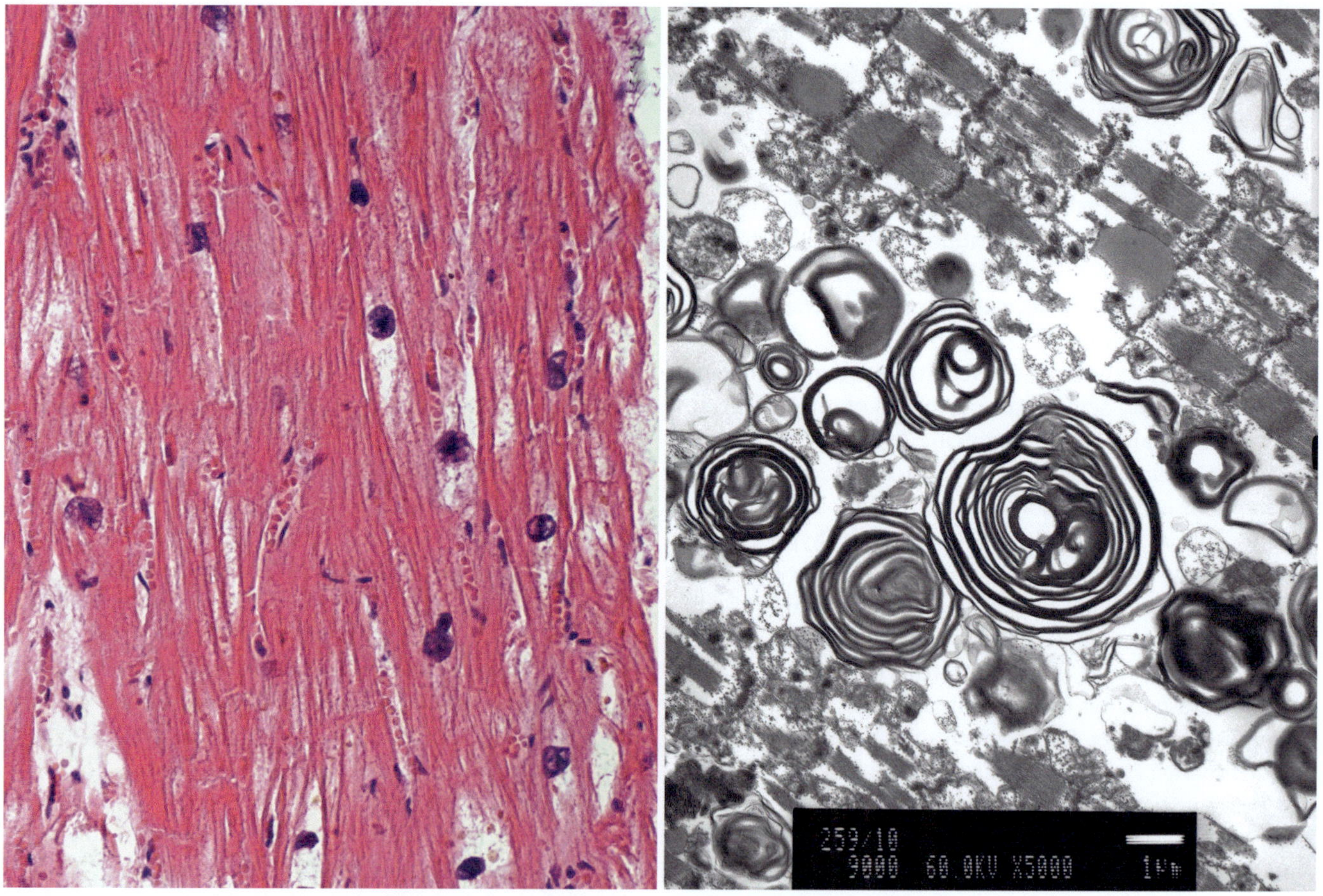

Fig. 9.1 Histological changes in Anderson Fabry disease. Left panel: Haematoxylin and eosin staining showing storage (perinuclear vacuoles) and hypertrophy of cardiomyocytes. Of note, the hypertrophy is predominantly due to sarcomere thickening, storage contributes to a lesser extent. Right panel: Electron microscopy showing typical lamellar structures ("zebra bodies") containing the stored substance—globotriaosylceramiide (Gb3)

closely linked to the disease severity and may play a causal role in the development of cellular and organ damage.

The disease is caused by a mutation within GLA gene located q22.1 region of the X chromosome. Until now, more than 1000 mutations were described. The frequency of AFD based on neonatal screening studies is ranging from less than 1:1000 (founder's effect in Taiwan) up to 1:3500 or more. However, many mutations retrieved by the neonatal screening have unknown clinical significance or may lead to mild clinical course (late-onset variants). The incidence of the classical phenotype is estimated to 1 in 30,000–40,000 live male births. Females are usually less affected than males. However, due to random X-chromosome inactivation, women with highly skewed inactivation patterns may have clinical manifestations as severe as their male counterparts [28, 29].

The classical phenotype of AFD is multisystemic. The earliest manifestations include neuropathic pain, hypohidrosis, appearance of cutaneous lesions (angiokeratomas—Fig. 9.2) and gastrointestinal symptoms in children and adolescents. Kidney involvement (proteinuria, renal failure) appears first as microalbuminuria and may become apparent from the second or third decade of life. Neurological involvement includes appearance of white matter lesions, premature strokes, vertigo and hearing impairment. Ocular changes include cornea verticillata (Fig. 9.3), tortuous vessels and Fabry posterior cataract [30].

Cardiac involvement usually manifests during the third or fourth decade of life (later in women) and includes development of HCM, posterolateral fibrosis, heart failure due to impaired left ventricular filling, and arrhythmias (chronotropic incompetence, atrial fibrillation, AV conduction abnormalities, malignant arrhythmias) (Figs. 9.4, 9.5, 9.6 and 9.7). ICDs should be considered in patients with advanced disease keeping in mind that ICD indication criteria developed for HCM are not applicable [31, 32].

In some patients, the disease remains limited to one organ and leads to "variant" late-onset manifestation usually appearing as cardiac hypertrophy, arrhythmias and failure. Many of the variant manifestations are found in patients with missense mutations and some preserved residual enzyme activity [33].

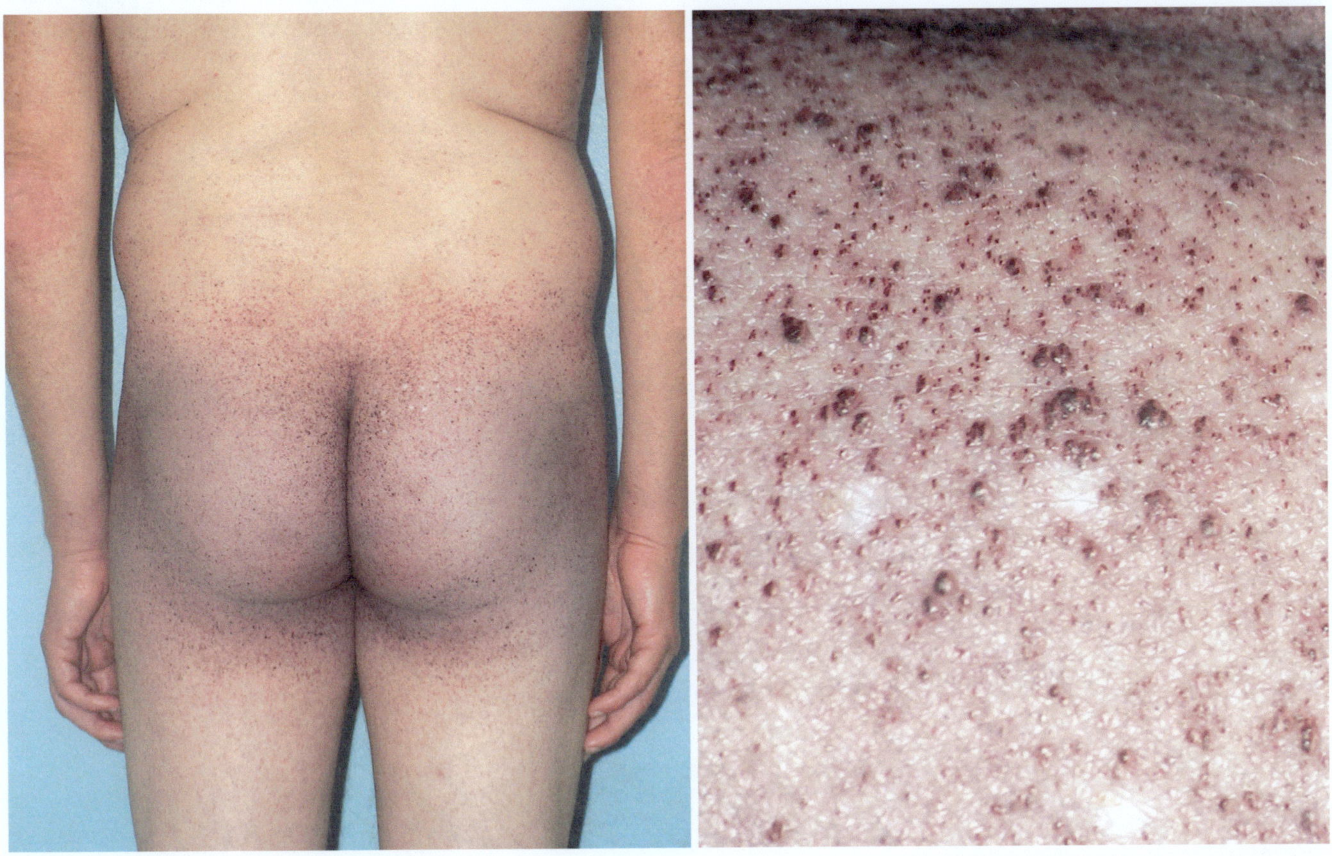

Fig. 9.2 Angiokeratomas represent a typical cutaneous finding in multisystemic or "classical" AFD phenotype. These reddish maculopapular spots are distributed primarily within the bathing trunk of the body, on genitalia, around the umbilicus and on extensor surfaces of upper limbs. The appearance of angiokeratomas occurs namely in male patients within the first and more so the second decade of life. In later onset variants and in women angiokeratomas may never develop. The lesions do not respond to enzyme replacement therapy

The diagnosis of AFD is established by an assessment of AGALA activity in male patients (e.g. within leukocytes or plasma, dry blood-spot testing methods are available). In some females, the enzyme activity may be borderline or normal. Therefore, GLA gene sequencing seems to be the most straightforward diagnostic approach in women with disease suspicion. Some screening strategies are using lyso-Gb_3 assessment to identify affected women before proceeding to gene sequencing. In the last decade, it became obvious that several mutations originally associated with the disease are in fact benign polymorphisms or cause only pseudodeficiency. In presence of VUS, organ biopsy (skin, kidney, heart) should be considered before initiating the treatment [34–36].

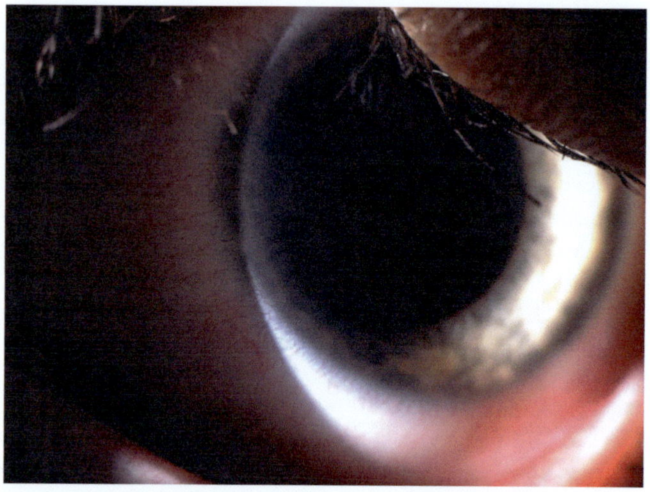

Fig. 9.3 Cornea verticillata represents a typical ocular finding in AFD. These spoke-like corneal opacities may be also seen after amiodarone and chloroquine prolonged administration

Enzyme replacement therapy (ERT) is widely available represented by two preparations available on the EU market (agalsidase alfa and agalsidase beta). Both enzymes are administered in a short bi-weekly infusion at different doses (agalsidase alfa 0.2 mg/kg/EOW, agalsidase beta 1.0 mg/kg/EOW). ERT was shown to reduce the progression of kidney disease, decrease peripheral pain and improve gastrointestinal symptoms. Cardiac structural changes regress to a lesser extent but long-term stabilization may be achieved in many cases. Data from two global registries are suggesting an improved survival and decreased rate of clinical complications [37, 38].

Recently a pharmacological chaperone stabilizing the misfolded enzyme—migalastat—was approved for the clinical use in EU. Migalastat, a low-molecular-weight iminosugar, is effective only in patients with amenable mutations allowing a synthesis of a functional but misfolded enzyme. It binds to the active site of the enzyme and facilitates the proper trafficking to lysosomes where it dissociates and allows α-galactosidase to catabolize accumulated substrates. First trials have shown significant improvements in LVH [39, 40].

Several novel enzymes (e.g. plant-derived pegylated pegunigalsidase alfa), substrate reduction therapies (lucera-

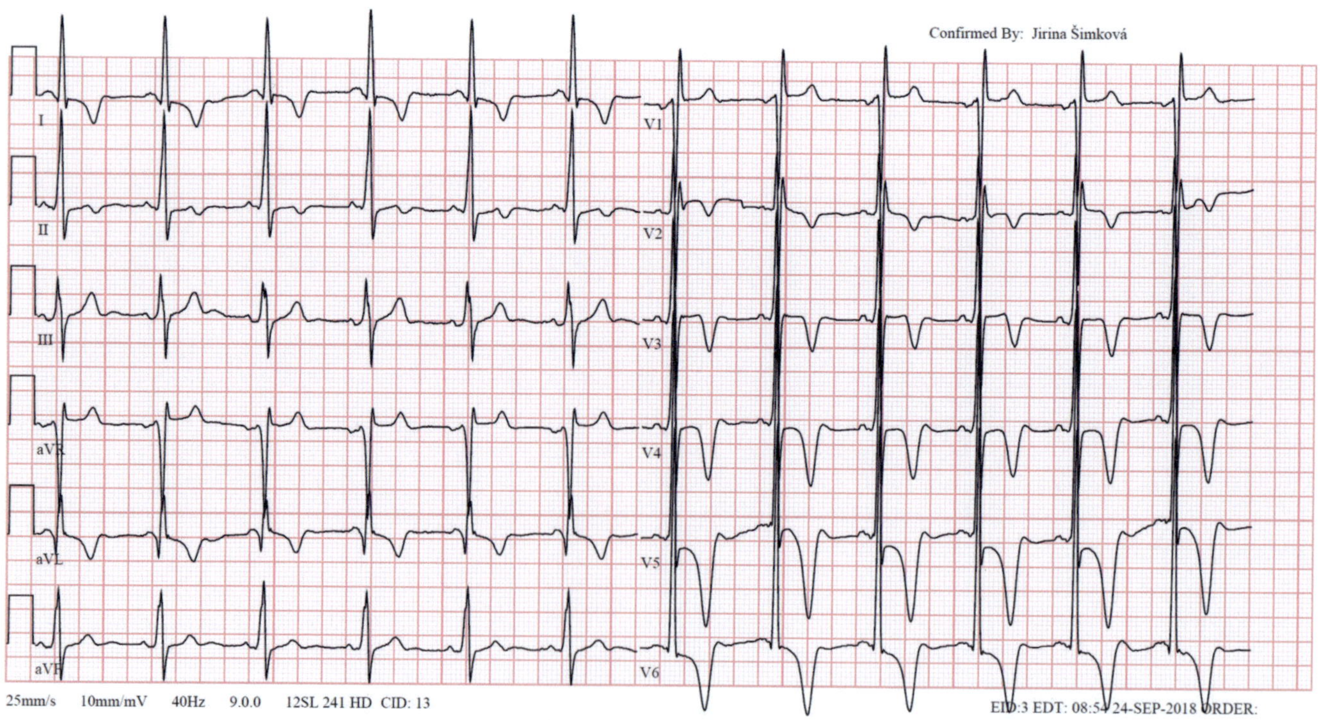

Fig. 9.4 Typical ECG from a male AFD patient showing PR interval shortening, right bundle branch block pattern, signs of LV hypertrophy and marked diffuse repolarization changes. Short PR interval is not due to pre-excitation. Repolarization changes are usually present in patients with pronounced left ventricular hypertrophy and fibrosis

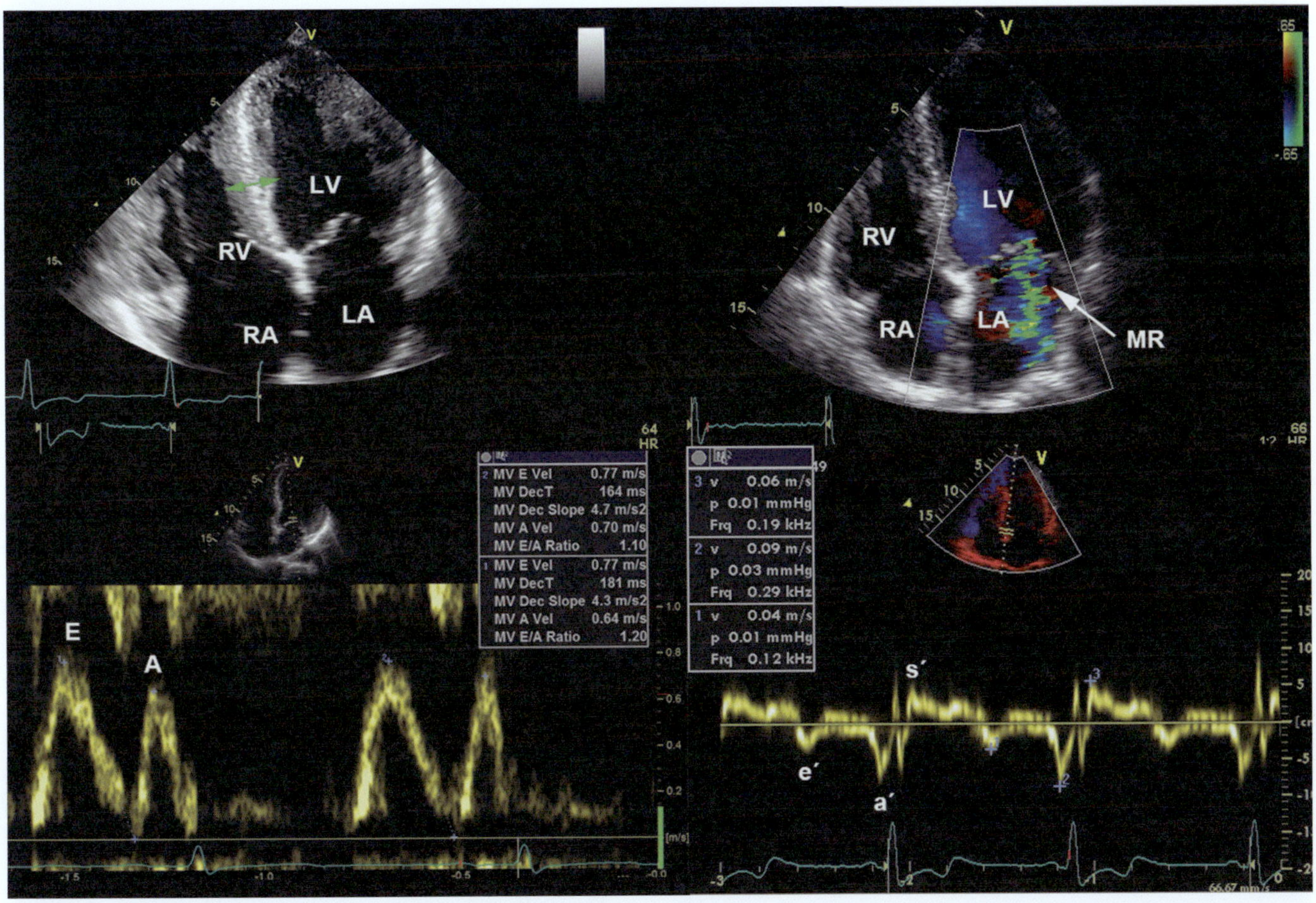

Fig. 9.5 Echocardiographic findings in AFD demonstrating the presence of left (and to a lesser extent also right) ventricular hypertrophy, mild-to-moderate mitral regurgitation due to valvular changes and impaired (pseudonormal) left ventricular filling pattern

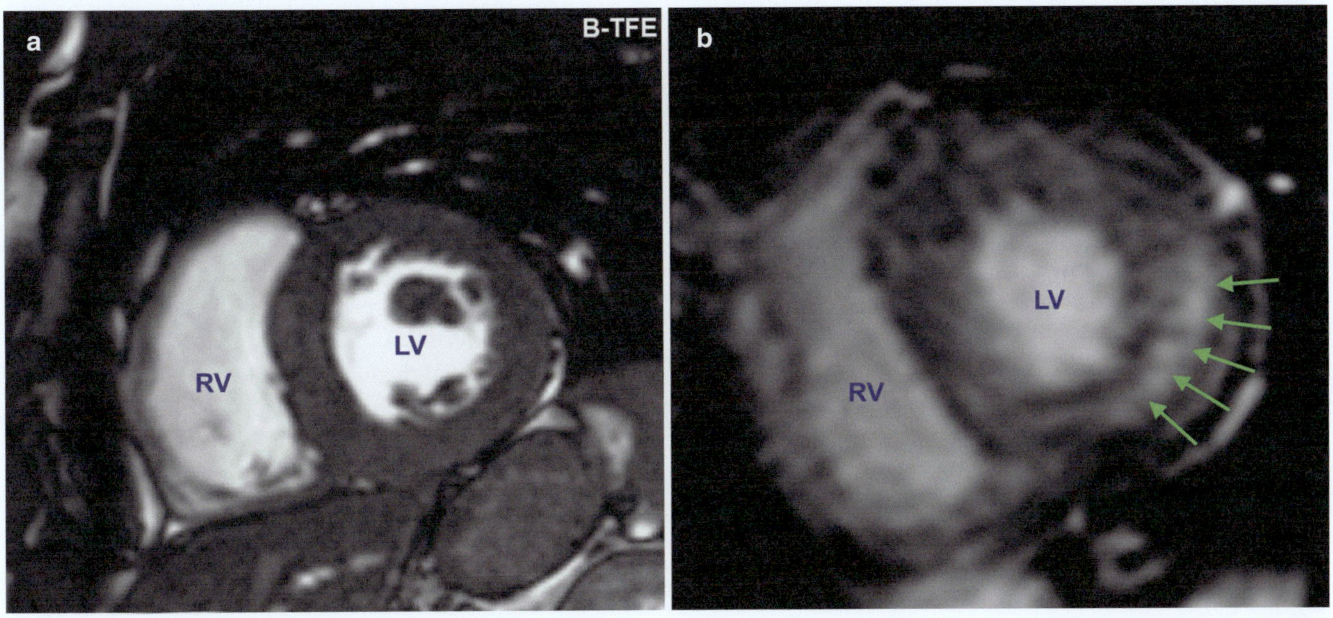

Fig. 9.6 Cardiac MRI findings in AFD showing diffuse left ventricular hypertrophy (left panel) and replacement fibrosis demonstrated by late gadolinium enhancement (right panel—green arrows) distributed in a typical localization for AFD, affecting midwall layer of the posterolateral basal left ventricular segments

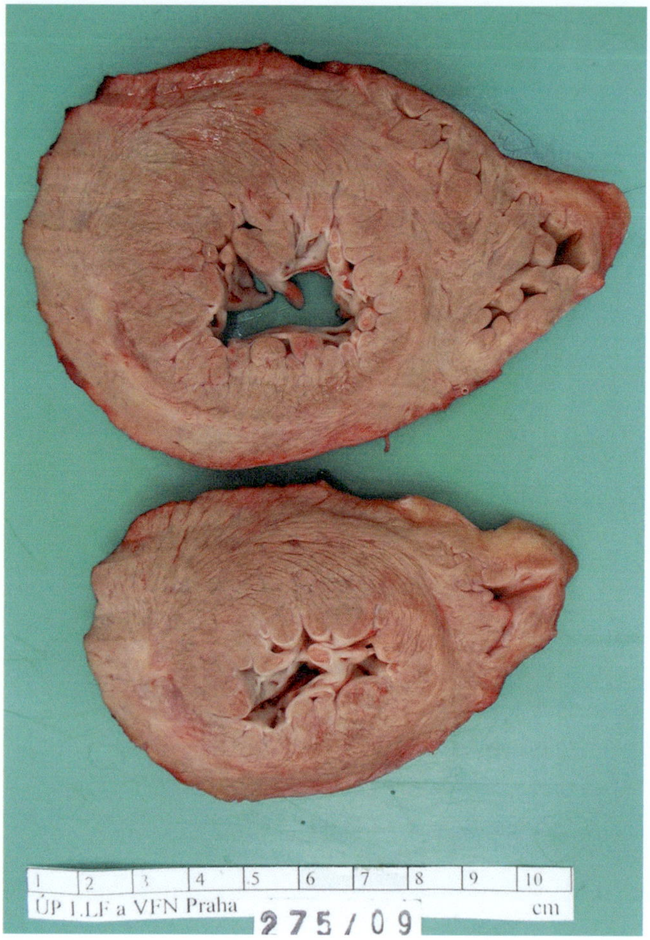

Fig. 9.7 Autopsy finding from a 52-year-old male AFD patient dying from congestive heart failure after cardiac surgery. Of note are the excessive hypertrophy and apparent fibrosis

stat and venglustat inhibiting glucosylceramide synthase) and genetic treatments (using ex vivo or in vivo gene editing) are being developed and tested in clinical trials [41–43].

Mucopolysaccharidoses (MPS) represent a group of LSDs caused by the absence of functional enzymes that degrade glycosaminoglycans (GAGs). Genetic causes are known for defects in 11 enzymes and the disease is divided in seven main clinical types. The estimated incidence is 1:25,000 newborns [44, 45].

The deficiency leads to progressive systemic deposition of GAGs and results in multi-organ involvement. The clinical manifestation depends on the deposited GAG type and the specific enzyme mutation present. Based on the severity and age at onset, some of the MPS syndromes have been categorized into slowly and rapidly progressing subtypes. Cardiac involvement has been described in all MPS syndromes [46]. In particular, it appears common in:

- MPS I—divided into three subtypes based on severity of symptoms: Hurler (MPS I H), Hurler–Scheie (MPS I HS) and Scheie (MPS I S). Hurler disease is the most severe while Scheie disease is the mildest form. MPS I is caused by deficiency of α-L-iduronidase and inherited as a recessive disease encoded by IDUA gene located on 4p16.3 chromosome region [47, 48].
- MPS II—Hunter syndrome and X-linked disease caused by iduronate sulfatase (IDS) deficiency encoded by IDS gene located on Xq28 chromosome region. The incidence of MPS II is ranging from 1 in 100,000–150,000 male births. Heterozygous female carriers may develop mild-to-moderate symptoms in case of skewed X-chromosome inactivation.
- MPS IV Morquio syndrome (Morquio–Brailsford syndrome)—This syndrome has two forms, Morquio A and Morquio B; MPS IVA is caused by a defect in the GALNS gene (16q24, galactosamine-6 sulfatase), MPS IV B involves a malfunction of the GLB1 gene (3p22, beta-galactosidase). The incidence is estimated at between 1 in 200,000 and 1 in 300,000 live births [49, 50].
- MPS VI—Maroteaux–Lamy syndrome, an autosomal recessive syndrome caused by N-acetylgalactosamine-4-sulfatase deficiency encoded by ARSB gene located on 5q14.1 chromosome region [51, 52].
- MPS VII—Sly syndrome, an autosomal recessive very rare disease caused by beta-glucuronidase deficiency. The causative gene has been located on 7q21–q22 and more than 40 mutations have been identified [53, 54].

The multisystemic involvement usually appears relatively early in life. The cardiac pathology often develops earlier in life in individuals with more rapidly progressing types of MPS. However, there are also mild cases that are discovered during adolescence or adulthood following presentation with skeletal abnormalities (thoracic kyphosis, growth retardation) and/or valvular disease.

Systemic abnormalities found in MPS include growth retardation, dysmorphic facial characteristics, skeletal and joint deformities (dysostosis multiplex), central nervous system involvement (mental retardation, spinal cord compression, increased intracranial pressure, hearing impairment) and ocular (corneal clouding, retinal degeneration and blindness). In some patients, respiratory difficulties develop and patients may suffer from gastrointestinal pathology (hepatosplenomegaly, bowel dysfunction) and umbilical or inguinal hernias. Premature death in untreated MPS syndromes is most commonly a result of respiratory compromise and cardiac disease.

Cardiac abnormalities include valve thickening and dysfunction (mitral and aortic valves are more severely involved than right heart valves). Mitral valve appears to be involved more often than the aortic. Although the disease may result in stenotic lesions, most patients suffer from regurgitations (Fig. 9.8). The management of valvular disease is complicated by the high risk of general anaesthesia and related spinal cord injuries [55, 56].

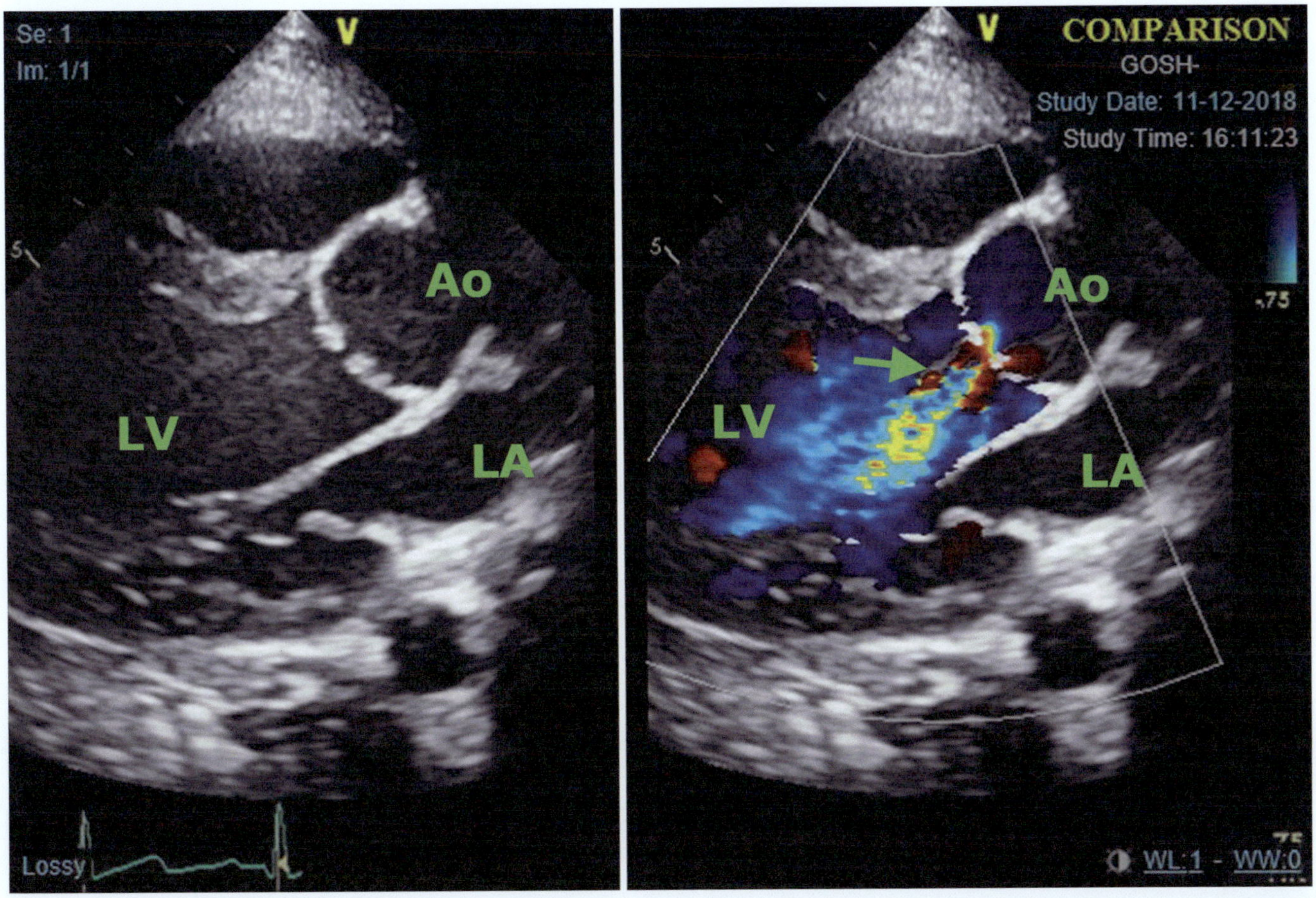

Fig. 9.8 Echocardiographic finding from a patient with Morquio syndrome with aortic valve involvement and aortic regurgitation (arrow) (courtesy J. Marek, Great Ormond Street Hospital, London, UK)

Cardiac hypertrophy and diastolic dysfunction have been repeatedly described. Later stages may progress into LV dilatation and dysfunction. Conduction abnormalities including high-degree AV block develops due to conduction system infiltration [57].

Although very premature coronary disease has been described in all types of MPS, it appears most common in MPS I and MPS II. Stenotic or occlusive lesions are caused by progressive diffuse intimal proliferation from GAGs deposition within large epicardial coronary arteries. The disease may emerge silently but may result in significant left ventricular impairment due to ischaemia [58].

The first laboratory screening test for an MPS disorder is a urine test for GAGs. Although abnormal values suggest with high probability the presence of an MPS disorder, negative results do not fully exclude the diagnosis.

A definitive diagnosis is made by assessment enzymatic activity for the respective disease either in serum, white blood cells or fibroblasts from skin biopsy, and genetic testing. Prenatal diagnosis is possible from amniocentesis and chorionic villus sampling [59].

Current therapeutic strategies differ according to the type of MPS and include valvular surgery, ERT or haematopoietic stem cell transplantation [60, 61]. Although stem cell transplantation results in regression of cardiac hypertrophy and prevents cardiac function deterioration, it has little if any effect on already existing valvular lesions. ERT using human recombinant enzyme by regular intravenous infusion is approved for MPS I (laronidase), MPS II (idursulfase), MPS IVA (elosulfase alfa), MPS VI (galsulfase) and MPS VII (vestronidase alfa-vjbk) [62]. Similarly to stem cell transplantation, beneficial effects of ERT on the myocardium were observed while limited data are suggesting stabilization or regression of valvular involvement. This may be in part due to the fact that ERT is often started relatively late (after several years of disease progression). Documented cases with very early treatment beginning are suggesting that ERT may prevent or substantially delay the cardiac disease development [63, 64].

Glycogen Storage Diseases (GSDs)

Glycogen storage diseases may be caused by different defects of glycogen synthesis and degradation. Glycogen itself is a branched glucose polymer serving as a rapid source of deposited energy for muscle tissue. The degradation of glycogen is linked to the lysosome. Therefore, some GSDs may be classified as lysosomal storage diseases while others induce little or no lysosomal storage [65].

Disease manifestations are caused either by energetic deficiency due to inability to use the glycogen during fasting or exercise or by toxic effects of the accumulated glycogen. In addition, the deposits induce disturbances in cellular architecture, affect cellular biophysical properties and impair lysosomal or mitochondrial function. The condition leads to development of hypertrophy with variable and progressive degree of systolic dysfunction. Electrophysiological abnormalities include accelerated conduction at the early stage followed by development of AV blocks and/or other arrhythmias [8].

Pompe disease or glycogen storage disease type II (GSD II) is an autosomal recessive disorder caused by a mutation in acid alpha-glucosidase (GAA also known as acid maltase) gene leading to the corresponding enzyme deficiency. The gene is located on 17q25.3 region. The estimated incidence is ranging from 1:14,000 to 1:300,000 newborns depending on the ethnicity (combined incidence estimate about 1:40,000) [66].

In Pompe disease, the glycogen accumulates mainly in lysosomes affecting multiple organs with predominant involvement of skeletal, cardiac and smooth muscle cells.

The disease is classified by age of onset, organ involvement, severity and progression rate. Severity of the disease depends on the age of onset and extent of muscular involvement. The clinical tableau is dominated by muscular weakness and hypotonia, respiratory and cardiac failure. The heart is particularly severely affected by cardiomegaly due to HCM in infantile-onset Pompe disease (Fig. 9.9). In contrast later onset forms typically involve skeletal muscles without severe cardiomyopathy [67].

The cardiac hypertrophy in infantile-onset Pompe disease is affecting both ventricles. Wall thickening is usually very prominent and may be associated with outflow tract obstruction. ECG pattern shows broad and high-voltage QRS complexes often accompanied by signs of pre-excitation. This type of disorder often presents in the first 2 months of life with hypotonia, generalized muscle weakness, cardiomyopathy, feeding difficulties, failure to thrive, respiratory distress and hearing loss. Without ERT, the classic infantile-onset Pompe disease results in death in the first year of life. The non-classic variant of infantile-onset Pompe disease and

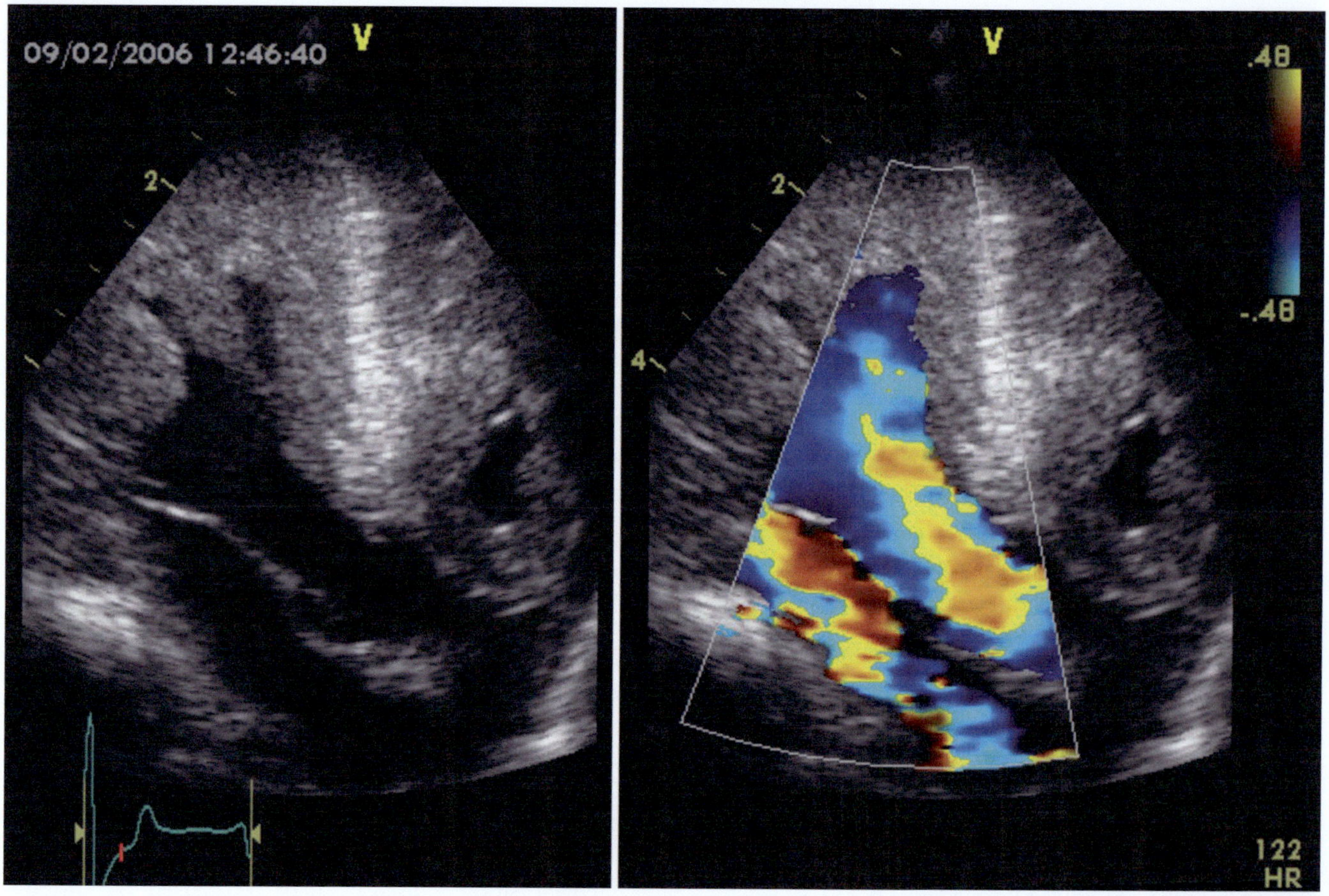

Fig. 9.9 Echocardiography obtained in a newborn patient affected by Pompe disease. The image is dominated by a massive left ventricular hypertrophy. Colour Doppler mapping demonstrates a significant mitral regurgitation (courtesy J. Marek, Great Ormond Street Hospital, London, UK)

late-onset (juvenile and adult-onset) Pompe disease are characterized by proximal muscle weakness and respiratory insufficiency usually without clinically significant cardiac involvement [68, 69].

The diagnosis is based on the evidence of absence (infantile-onset) or substantially reduced (late-onset) GAA activity in tissues such as skin fibroblasts, muscle biopsy or leukocytes (more precisely isolated lymphocytes). In addition, dry blood spot tests are available for screening purposes. Muscle biopsy shows presence of vacuoles staining positive for glycogen that may involve not only lysosomes but may extend to cytoplasm as well. Glc4 may be used as biomarker. More than 100 mutations have been identified some of them showing regional or ethnic predominance [70].

Substantial improvements have been reported in infantile type of Pompe disease using ERT by alglucosidase alfa, particularly in subjects not developing antibodies against the protein. As in Fabry disease, the research continues having as target development of more efficient enzymes, chaperones and gene therapies [71–73].

Danon disease is also known as lysosomal glycogen-storage disease with normal acid maltase. It is an X-linked disease caused by a deficiency of lysosomal-associated membrane protein-2 (LAMP-2 also known as CD107b), which increases the autophagic flux. Alternative splicing of the gene produces three isoforms of which the LAMP-2B is associated with Danon disease. About 70 different mutations were identified, all affecting at least the 2B isoform. Immunohistochemical staining shows absent LAMP2 protein [74].

In Danon disease, the cytoplasm of skeletal muscles and myocardium becomes filled with vacuoles containing autophagic material and glycogen [75]. The excessive intra-sarcomeric glycogen accumulation is responsible for the severe myocardial hypertrophy and preexcitation pattern (in spite of the characteristic ECG pattern, the preexcitation nature of this finding has been recently disputed) (Fig. 9.10) [76, 77]. The cellular defect is causing an elevation in oxidative stress and leading to apoptosis and extensive fibrosis in later stages of the disease [78, 79].

The age of onset and severity of manifestation are variable. Due to X-linked type of inheritance, the disease is milder and begins later in affected women than in men. In classically affected men, the disease develops in the second decade of life. In most cases, it's course is rapidly progressive leading to death between the second and third decades. Isolated cardiac involvement has been repeatedly described. Missense mutations may lead to milder forms of the disease [80].

The typical phenotype of Danon disease usually includes cardiomyopathy, skeletal myopathy and mental retardation

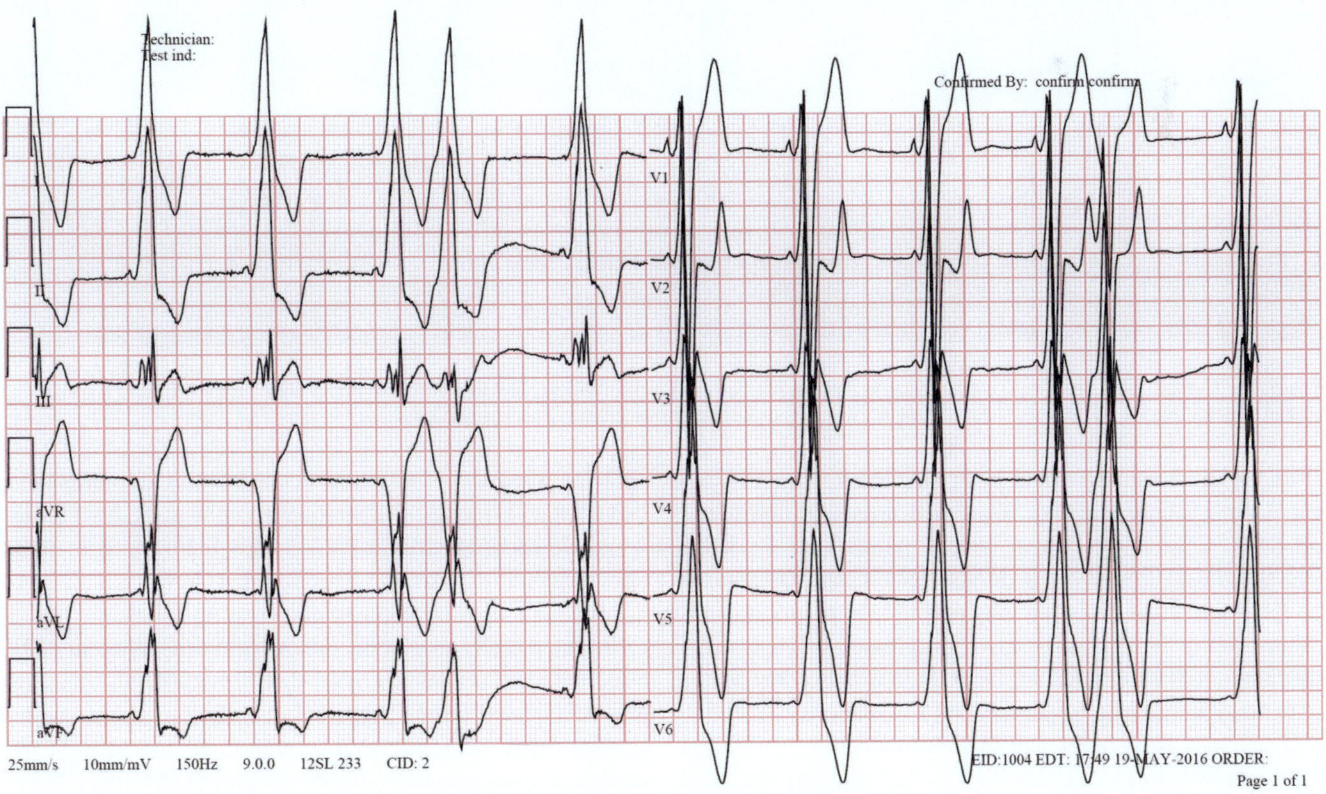

Fig. 9.10 ECG tracing from a 17-year-old male patient affected by Danon disease. Of note are the short PR interval and WPW preexcitation pattern

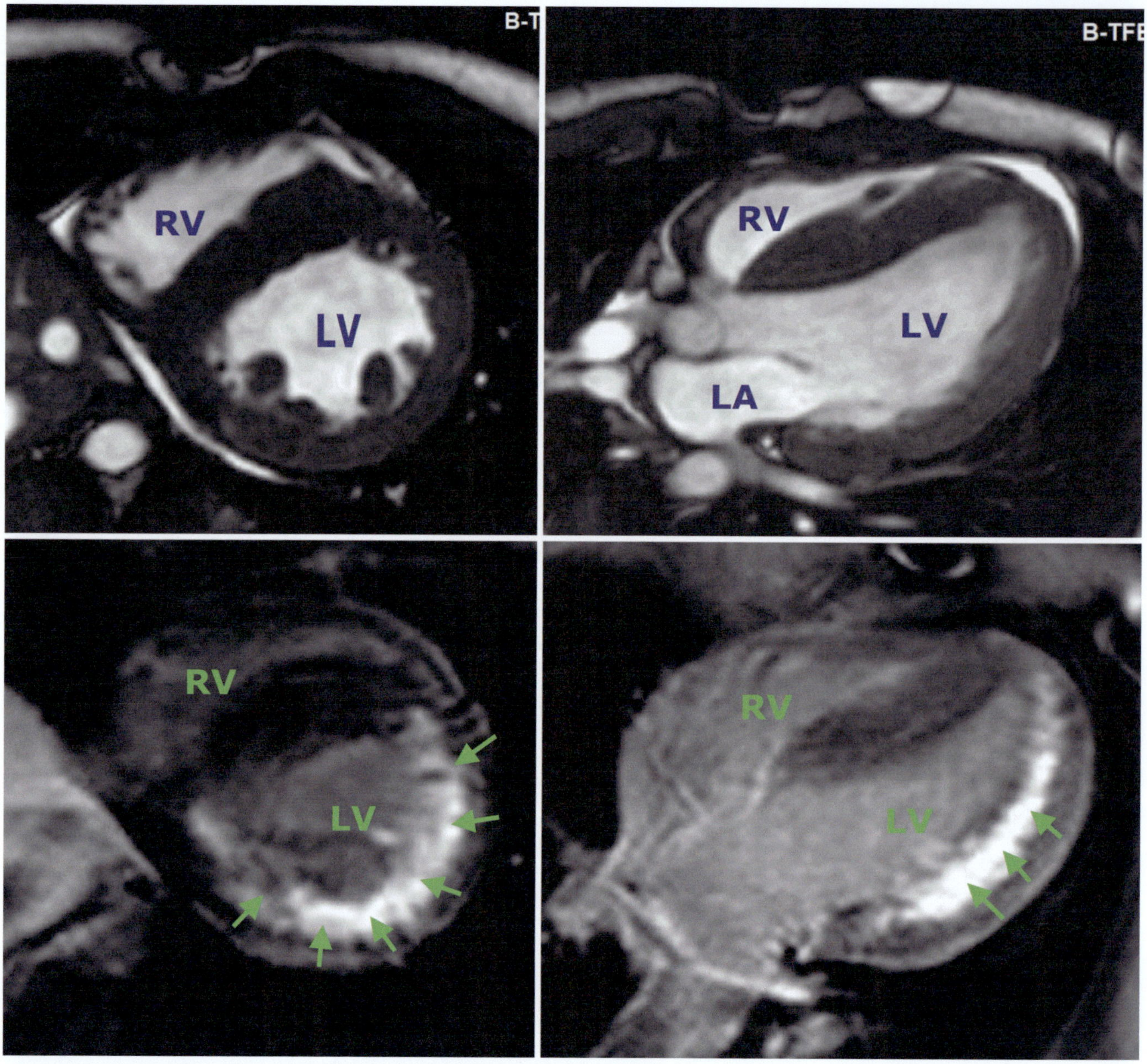

Fig. 9.11 Cardiac MRI from a 17-year-old male patient affected by Danon disease showing diffuse homogenous left ventricular hypertrophy (upper panels). Extensive fibrosis is demonstrated by late gadolinium enhancement (lower panels)

(Fig. 9.11). Classical patients have elevated serum CPK levels, lactate, abnormal liver functional tests and natriuretic peptides. Cardiac symptoms include palpitations, syncope and shortness of breath or sudden cardiac death. Depending on the stage of the disease it may resemble hypertrophic cardiomyopathy but in many cases progresses to ventricular dysfunction with congestive heart failure and complicates with arrhythmias [81, 82].

Diagnosis is complex and includes evidence of elevated CPK and liver functional tests as first-line assessments. Acid maltase level assessment show normal levels and exclude Pompe disease. Muscle biopsy confirms the diagnosis by showing typical cytoplasmic accumulation of autophagic vacuoles and immunohistochemistry showing LAMP2 protein deficiency. The diagnosis is completed by genetic mutation analysis of LAMP2 gene which is now part of most hypertrophic cardiomyopathy gene testing panels.

So far, there is no specific treatment for the inherent metabolic defect. The management should include all measures preventing heart failure progression, arrhythmias and sudden cardiac death. ICD implantation should be considered early particularly in cases with extensive fibrosis [83–85].

PRKAG2 cardiomyopathy, sometimes described as PRKAG2 syndrome, is caused by mutations in the gene encoding for the 5′ adenosine monophosphate-activated protein kinase (AMPK), specifically for its γ2 regulatory subunit (PRKAG2) [86].

The enzyme is involved in regulation of cellular energy handling. AMPK dysfunction associated with the disease alters myocyte glucose and fatty acid uptake, storage and mobilization and causes storage of glycogen and amylopectin. Due to this feature, the cardiomyopathy is often classified among glycogen storage disorders [87].

The gene encoding PRKAG2 is located on 7q36.1 locus. Most mutations described so far were missense. The inheritance pattern is autosomal dominant [88, 89].

The exact prevalence and incidence of the disease remain unknown. Although the disease may be rare among unselected patients with HCM, it was frequently found among those with AV conduction abnormalities. The onset of symptoms is variable and ranges from childhood to fourth or fifth decade of life. The most severe mutation c.1592G>A (Arg531Gln) may even lead to death within first months of life. Systemic manifestations including skeletal myopathy are relatively rare [90].

The cardiomyopathy associated with PRKAG2 is usually hypertrophic with progressive development of diastolic and eventually systolic heart failure. Moreover, the syndrome often comprises supraventricular tachycardias (atrial flutter and/or fibrillation), and preexcitation pattern on ECG with proven accessory pathways on electrophysiological studies. In later stages of the disease, atrioventricular conduction deteriorates leading to AV blocks of variable degrees. Many patients suffer from symptoms related to chronotropic incompetence either due to AV blocks or to sinus bradycardia. Sudden cardiac death may complicate the disease irrespective of presence or absence of severe LVH [91].

The diagnosis is based on clinical manifestations and genetic testing. There is no specific treatment for PRKAG2 cardiomyopathy.

Summary

Metabolic cardiomyopathies represent phenocopies of either hypertrophic, dilated or restrictive cardiomyopathies. Although as individual diseases they may be considered as rare disorders, their overall incidence is relatively high and inborn metabolic errors may be responsible for a substantial proportion of cardiomyopathies, particularly in paediatric patients. In many diseases, the metabolic defect leads to systemic manifestations with other organ involvement (skin, bones, liver, central or peripheral nervous system) which may be more apparent than cardiac structural and functional changes. However, many later onset phenotypes may be restricted to the cardiac muscle. Therefore, metabolic diseases should be always considered during the diagnostic process.

Take-Home Message

In presence of cardiomyopathy of unknown cause, all efforts should be made to identify the underlying mechanism. Among early-onset infantile diseases, Pompe disease, several types of MPS and primary carnitine deficiency represent potentially treatable conditions. In adults, Anderson Fabry disease and transthyretin amyloidosis could be effectively treated as well. Therefore, the knowledge of associated systemic manifestations is essential, and these conditions should be considered in diagnostic panels for respective cardiomyopathies.

References

1. Sweet ME, Mestroni L, Taylor MRG. Genetic infiltrative cardiomyopathies. Heart Fail Clin. 2018;14(2):215–24.
2. Cox GF. Diagnostic approaches to pediatric cardiomyopathy of metabolic genetic etiologies and their relation to therapy. Prog Pediatr Cardiol. 2007;24(1):15–25.
3. Fukao T, Sasai H, Aoyama Y, Otsuka H, Ago Y, Matsumoto H, Abdelkreem E. Recent advances in understanding beta-ketothiolase (mitochondrial acetoacetyl-CoA thiolase, T2) deficiency. J Hum Genet. 2019;64(2):99–111.
4. Arora N, Stumper O, Wright J, Kelly DA, McKiernan PJ. Cardiomyopathy in tyrosinaemia type I is common but usually benign. J Inherit Metab Dis. 2006;29(1):54–7.
5. Lorenzo V, Torres A, Salido E. Primary hyperoxaluria. Nefrologia. 2014;34(3):398–412.
6. Merritt JL 2nd, Norris M, Kanungo S. Fatty acid oxidation disorders. Ann Transl Med. 2018;6(24):473.
7. Nair V, Belanger EC, Veinot JP. Lysosomal storage disorders affecting the heart: a review. Cardiovasc Pathol. 2019;39:12–24.
8. Linhart A, Cecchi F. Common presentation of rare diseases: left ventricular hypertrophy and diastolic dysfunction. Int J Cardiol. 2018;257:344–50.
9. Arbustini E, Di Toro A, Giuliani L, Favalli V, Narula N, Grasso M. Cardiac phenotypes in hereditary muscle disorders: JACC state-of-the-art review. J Am Coll Cardiol. 2018;72(20):2485–506.
10. Akhtar M, Elliott P. The genetics of hypertrophic cardiomyopathy. Glob Cardiol Sci Pract. 2018;2018(3):36.
11. Lipshultz SE, Sleeper LA, Towbin JA, Lowe AM, Orav EJ, Cox GF, Lurie PR, McCoy KL, McDonald MA, Messere JE, Colan SD. The incidence of pediatric cardiomyopathy in two regions of the United States. N Engl J Med. 2003;348(17):1647–55.
12. Doheny D, Srinivasan R, Pagant S, Chen B, Yasuda M, Desnick RJ. Fabry Disease: prevalence of affected males and heterozygotes with pathogenic GLA mutations identified by screening renal, cardiac and stroke clinics, 1995-2017. J Med Genet. 2018;55(4):261–8.
13. Towbin JA, Lowe AM, Colan SD, Sleeper LA, Orav EJ, Clunie S, Messere J, Cox GF, Lurie PR, Hsu D, Canter C, Wilkinson JD, Lipshultz SE. Incidence, causes, and outcomes of dilated cardiomyopathy in children. JAMA. 2006;296(15):1867–76.

14. Thevenon J, Laurent G, Ader F, Laforêt P, Klug D, Duva Pentiah A, Gouya L, Maurage CA, Kacet S, Eicher JC, Albuisson J, Desnos M, Bieth E, Duboc D, Martin L, Réant P, Picard F, Bonithon-Kopp C, Gautier E, Binquet C, Thauvin-Robinet C, Faivre L, Bouvagnet P, Charron P, Richard P. High prevalence of arrhythmic and myocardial complications in patients with cardiac glycogenosis due to PRKAG2 mutations. Europace. 2017;19(4):651–9.
15. Platt FM, Boland B, van der Spoel AC. The cell biology of disease: lysosomal storage disorders: the cellular impact of lysosomal dysfunction. J Cell Biol. 2012;199(5):723–34.
16. Burke MA, Cook SA, Seidman JG, Seidman CE. Clinical and Mechanistic Insights Into the Genetics of Cardiomyopathy. J Am Coll Cardiol. 2016;68(25):2871–86.
17. Vasilescu C, Ojala TH, Brilhante V, Ojanen S, Hinterding HM, Palin E, Alastalo TP, Koskenvuo J, Hiippala A, Jokinen E, Jahnukainen T, Lohi J, Pihkala J, Tyni TA, Carroll CJ, Suomalainen A. Genetic basis of severe childhood-onset cardiomyopathies. J Am Coll Cardiol. 2018;72(19):2324–38.
18. Lipshultz SE, Cochran TR, Briston DA, Brown SR, Sambatakos PJ, Miller TL, Carrillo AA, Corcia L, Sanchez JE, Diamond MB, Freundlich M, Harake D, Gayle T, Harmon WG, Rusconi PG, Sandhu SK, Wilkinson JD. Pediatric cardiomyopathies: causes, epidemiology, clinical course, preventive strategies and therapies. Future Cardiol. 2013;9(6):817–48.
19. Linhart A, Palecek T, Bultas J, Ferguson JJ, Hrudová J, Karetová D, Zeman J, Ledvinová J, Poupetová H, Elleder M, Aschermann M. New insights in cardiac structural changes in patients with Fabry's disease. Am Heart J. 2000;139(6):1101–8.
20. Lieske JC, Monico CG, Holmes WS, Bergstralh EJ, Slezak JM, Rohlinger AL, Olson JB, Milliner DS. International registry for primary hyperoxaluria. Am J Nephrol. 2005;25(3):290–6.
21. Salido E, Pey AL, Rodriguez R, Lorenzo V. Primary hyperoxalurias: disorders of glyoxylate detoxification. Biochim Biophys Acta. 2012;1822(9):1453–64.
22. Wilcken B, Wiley V, Sim KG, Carpenter K. Carnitine transporter defect diagnosed by newborn screening with electrospray tandem mass spectrometry. J Pediatr. 2001;138(4):581–4.
23. Fu L, Huang M, Chen S. Primary carnitine deficiency and cardiomyopathy.Korean. Circ J. 2013;43(12):785–92.
24. Frigeni M, Balakrishnan B, Yin X, Calderon FRO, Mao R, Pasquali M, Longo N. Functional and molecular studies in primary carnitine deficiency. Hum Mutat. 2017;38(12):1684–99.
25. Guertl B, Noehammer C, Hoefler G. Metabolic cardiomyopathies. Int J Exp Pathol. 2000;81(6):349–72.
26. Vishwanath VA. Fatty acid beta-oxidation disorders: a brief review. Ann Neurosci. 2016;23(1):51–5.
27. Kang E, Kim YM, Kang M, Heo SH, Kim GH, Choi IH, Choi JH, Yoo HW, Lee BH. Clinical and genetic characteristics of patients with fatty acid oxidation disorders identified by newborn screening. BMC Pediatr. 2018;18(1):103.
28. Mehta A, Ricci R, Widmer U, Dehout F, Garcia de Lorenzo A, Kampmann C, Linhart A, Sunder-Plassmann G, Ries M, Beck M. Fabry disease defined: baseline clinical manifestations of 366 patients in the Fabry Outcome Survey. Eur J Clin Invest. 2004;34(3):236–242.
29. Echevarria L, Benistan K, Toussaint A, Dubourg O, Hagege AA, Eladari D, Jabbour F, Beldjord C, De Mazancourt P, Germain DP. X-chromosome inactivation in female patients with Fabry disease. Clin Genet. 2016;89(1):44–54.
30. Linhart A, Elliott PM. The heart in Anderson-Fabry disease and other lysosomal storage disorders. Heart. 2007;93(4):528–35.
31. Linhart A, Kampmann C, Zamorano JL, Sunder-Plassmann G, Beck M, Mehta A, Elliott PM, European FOS Investigators. Cardiac manifestations of Anderson-Fabry disease: results from the international Fabry outcome survey. Eur Heart J. 2007;28(10):1228–35.
32. Militaru S, Ginghina C, Popescu BA, Saftoiu A, Linhart A, Jurcut R. Multimodality imaging in Fabry cardiomyopathy: from early diagnosis to therapeutic targets. Eur Heart J Cardiovasc Imaging. 2018;19(12):1313–22.
33. Germain DP, Brand E, Burlina A, Cecchi F, Garman SC, Kempf J, Laney DA, Linhart A, Maródi L, Nicholls K, Ortiz A, Pieruzzi F, Shankar SP, Waldek S, Wanner C, Jovanovic A. Phenotypic characteristics of the p.Asn215Ser (p.N215S) GLA mutation in male and female patients with Fabry disease: a multicenter Fabry Registry study. Mol Genet Genomic Med. 2018. https://doi.org/10.1002/mgg3.389.
34. Nowak A, Mechtler T, Kasper DC, Desnick RJ. Correlation of Lyso-Gb3 levels in dried blood spots and sera from patients with classic and Later-Onset Fabry disease. Mol Genet Metab. 2017;121(4):320–4.
35. Kramer J, Weidemann F. Biomarkers for diagnosing and staging of Fabry disease. Curr Med Chem. 2018;25(13):1530–7.
36. Smid BE, van der Tol L, Cecchi F, Elliott PM, Hughes DA, Linthorst GE, Timmermans J, Weidemann F, West ML, Biegstraaten M, Lekanne Deprez RH, Florquin S, Postema PG, Tomberli B, van der Wal AC, van den Bergh Weerman MA, Hollak CE. Uncertain diagnosis of Fabry disease: consensus recommendation on diagnosis in adults with left ventricular hypertrophy and genetic variants of unknown significance. Int J Cardiol. 2014;177(2):400–8.
37. Germain DP, Elliott PM, Falissard B, Fomin VV, Hilz MJ, Jovanovic A, Kantola I, Linhart A, Mignani R, Namdar M, Nowak A, Oliveira JP, Pieroni M, Viana-Baptista M, Wanner C, Spada M. The effect of enzyme replacement therapy on clinical outcomes in male patients with Fabry disease: a systematic literature review by a European panel of experts. Mol Genet Metab Rep. 2019;19:100454.
38. Wanner C, Arad M, Baron R, Burlina A, Elliott PM, Feldt-Rasmussen U, Fomin VV, Germain DP, Hughes DA, Jovanovic A, Kantola I, Linhart A, Mignani R, Monserrat L, Namdar M, Nowak A, Oliveira JP, Ortiz A, Pieroni M, Spada M, Tylki-Szymańska A, Tøndel C, Viana-Baptista M, Weidemann F, Hilz MJ. European expert consensus statement on therapeutic goals in Fabry disease. Mol Genet Metab. 2018;124(3):189–203.
39. Ortiz A, Germain DP, Desnick RJ, Politei J, Mauer M, Burlina A, Eng C, Hopkin RJ, Laney D, Linhart A, Waldek S, Wallace E, Weidemann F, Wilcox WR. Fabry disease revisited: management and treatment recommendations for adult patients. Mol Genet Metab. 2018;123(4):416–27.
40. Hughes DA, Nicholls K, Shankar SP, Sunder-Plassmann G, Koeller D, Nedd K, Vockley G, Hamazaki T, Lachmann R, Ohashi T, Olivotto I, Sakai N, Deegan P, Dimmock D, Eyskens F, Germain DP, Goker-Alpan O, Hachulla E, Jovanovic A, Lourenco CM, Narita I, Thomas M, Wilcox WR, Bichet DG, Schiffmann R, Ludington E, Viereck C, Kirk J, Yu J, Johnson F, Boudes P, Benjamin ER, Lockhart DJ, Barlow C, Skuban N, Castelli JP, Barth J, Feldt-Rasmussen U. Oral pharmacological chaperone migalastat compared with enzyme replacement therapy in Fabry disease: 18-month results from the randomised phase III ATTRACT study. J Med Genet. 2017;54(4):288–96.
41. Welford RWD, Mühlemann A, Garzotti M, Rickert V, Groenen PMA, Morand O, Üçeyler N, Probst MR. Glucosylceramide synthase inhibition with lucerastat lowers globotriaosylceramide and lysosome staining in cultured fibroblasts from Fabry patients with different mutation types. Hum Mol Genet. 2018;27(19):3392–403.
42. Guérard N, Morand O, Dingemanse J. Lucerastat, an iminosugar with potential as substrate reduction therapy for glycolipid storage disorders: safety, tolerability, and pharmacokinetics in healthy subjects. Orphanet J Rare Dis. 2017;12(1):9.
43. Germain DP, Hughes DA, Nicholls K, Bichet DG, Giugliani R, Wilcox WR, Feliciani C, Shankar SP, Ezgu F, Amartino H, Bratkovic D, Feldt-Rasmussen U, Nedd K, Sharaf El Din U, Lourenco CM, Banikazemi M, Charrow J, Dasouki M, Finegold D,

Giraldo P, Goker-Alpan O, Longo N, Scott CR, Torra R, Tuffaha A, Jovanovic A, Waldek S, Packman S, Ludington E, Viereck C, Kirk J, Yu J, Benjamin ER, Johnson F, Lockhart DJ, Skuban N, Castelli J, Barth J, Barlow C, Schiffmann R. Treatment of Fabry's disease with the pharmacologic chaperone migalastat. N Engl J Med. 2016;375(6):545–55.

44. Khan SA, Peracha H, Ballhausen D, Wiesbauer A, Rohrbach M, Gautschi M, Mason RW, Giugliani R, Suzuki Y, Orii KE, Orii T, Tomatsu S. Epidemiology of mucopolysaccharidoses. Mol Genet Metab. 2017;121(3):227–40.
45. Muenzer J. Overview of the mucopolysaccharidoses. Rheumatology (Oxford). 2011;50 Suppl 5:v4–12.
46. Braunlin E, Wang R. Cardiac issues in adults with the mucopolysaccharidoses: current knowledge and emerging needs. Heart. 2016;102(16):1257–62.
47. Soliman OI, Timmermans RG, Nemes A, Vletter WB, Wilson JH, ten Cate FJ, Geleijnse ML. Cardiac abnormalities in adults with the attenuated form of mucopolysaccharidosis type I. J Inherit Metab Dis. 2007;30(5):750–7.
48. Wraith JE, Jones S. Mucopolysaccharidosis type I. Pediatr Endocrinol Rev. 2014;12(Suppl 1):102–6.
49. Hendriksz CJ, Berger KI, Giugliani R, Harmatz P, Kampmann C, Mackenzie WG, Raiman J, Villarreal MS, Savarirayan R. International guidelines for the management and treatment of Morquio A syndrome. Am J Med Genet A. 2015;167A(1):11–25.
50. Lin HY, Chuang CK, Chen MR, Lin SM, Hung CL, Chang CY, Chiu PC, Tsai WH, Niu DM, Tsai FJ, Lin SJ, Hwu WL, Lin JL, Lin SP. Cardiac structure and function and effects of enzyme replacement therapy in patients with mucopolysaccharidoses I, II, IVA and VI. Mol Genet Metab. 2016;117(4):431–7.
51. Kampmann C, Lampe C, Whybra-Trümpler C, Wiethoff CM, Mengel E, Arash L, Beck M, Miebach E. Mucopolysaccharidosis VI: cardiac involvement and the impact of enzyme replacement therapy. J Inherit Metab Dis. 2014;37(2):269–76.
52. Braunlin E, Rosenfeld H, Kampmann C, Johnson J, Beck M, Giugliani R, Guffon N, Ketteridge D, Sá Miranda CM, Scarpa M, Schwartz IV, Leão Teles E, Wraith JE, Barrios P, Dias da Silva E, Kurio G, Richardson M, Gildengorin G, Hopwood JJ, Imperiale M, Schatz A, Decker C, Harmatz P, MPS VI Study Group. Enzyme replacement therapy for mucopolysaccharidosis VI: long-term cardiac effects of galsulfase (Naglazyme®) therapy. J Inherit Metab Dis. 2013;36(2):385–94.
53. Montaño AM, Lock-Hock N, Steiner RD, Graham BH, Szlago M, Greenstein R, Pineda M, Gonzalez-Meneses A, Çoker M, Bartholomew D, Sands MS, Wang R, Giugliani R, Macaya A, Pastores G, Ketko AK, Ezgü F, Tanaka A, Arash L, Beck M, Falk RE, Bhattacharya K, Franco J, White KK, Mitchell GA, Cimbalistiene L, Holtz M, Sly WS. Clinical course of sly syndrome (mucopolysaccharidosis type VII). J Med Genet. 2016;53(6):403–18.
54. McCafferty EH, Scott LJ. Vestronidase alfa: a review in mucopolysaccharidosis VII. BioDrugs. 2019;33(2):233–40.
55. Hack HA, Walker R, Gardiner P. Anaesthetic implications of the changing management of patients with mucopolysaccharidosis. Anaesth Intensive Care. 2016;44(6):660–8.
56. Walker R, Belani KG, Braunlin EA, Bruce IA, Hack H, Harmatz PR, Jones S, Rowe R, Solanki GA, Valdemarsson B. Anaesthesia and airway management in mucopolysaccharidosis. J Inherit Metab Dis. 2013;36(2):211–9.
57. Braunlin EA, Harmatz PR, Scarpa M, Furlanetto B, Kampmann C, Loehr JP, Ponder KP, Roberts WC, Rosenfeld HM, Giugliani R. Cardiac disease in patients with mucopolysaccharidosis: presentation, diagnosis and management. J Inherit Metab Dis. 2011;34(6):1183–97.
58. Braunlin E, Orchard PJ, Whitley CB, Schroeder L, Reed RC, Manivel JC. Unexpected coronary artery findings in mucopolysaccharidosis. Report of four cases and literature review. Cardiovasc Pathol. 2014;23(3):145–51.
59. Boffi L, Russo P, Limongelli G. Early diagnosis and management of cardiac manifestations in mucopolysaccharidoses: a practical guide for paediatric and adult cardiologists. Ital J Pediatr. 2018;44(Suppl 2):122.
60. Muenzer J, Wraith JE. Clarke LA; International Consensus Panel on Management and Treatment of Mucopolysaccharidosis I. Mucopolysaccharidosis I: management and treatment guidelines. Pediatrics. 2009;123(1):19–29.
61. Aldenhoven M, Wynn RF, Orchard PJ, O'Meara A, Veys P, Fischer A, Valayannopoulos V, Neven B, Rovelli A, Prasad VK, Tolar J, Allewelt H, Jones SA, Parini R, Renard M, Bordon V, Wulffraat NM, de Koning TJ, Shapiro EG, Kurtzberg J, Boelens JJ. Long-term outcome of Hurler syndrome patients after hematopoietic cell transplantation: an international multicenter study. Blood. 2015;125(13):2164–72.
62. Laraway S, Mercer J, Jameson E, Ashworth J, Hensman P, Jones SA. Outcomes of long-term treatment with laronidase in patients with mucopolysaccharidosis type I. J Pediatr. 2016;178:219–26.e1.
63. Concolino D, Deodato F, Parini R. Enzyme replacement therapy: efficacy and limitations. Ital J Pediatr. 2018;44(Suppl 2):120
64. Muenzer J. Early initiation of enzyme replacement therapy for the mucopolysaccharidoses. Mol Genet Metab. 2014;111(2):63–72.
65. Hicks J, Wartchow E, Mierau G. Glycogen storage diseases: a brief review and update on clinical features, genetic abnormalities, pathologic features, and treatment. Ultrastruct Pathol. 2011;35(5):183–96.
66. Kishnani PS, Steiner RD, Bali D, Berger K, Byrne BJ, Case LE, Crowley JF, Downs S, Howell RR, Kravitz RM, Mackey J, Marsden D, Martins AM, Millington DS, Nicolino M, O'Grady G, Patterson MC, Rapoport DM, Slonim A, Spencer CT, Tifft CJ, Watson MS. Pompe disease diagnosis and management guideline. Genet Med. 2006;8(5):267–88.
67. Bembi B, Cerini E, Danesino C, Donati MA, Gasperini S, Morandi L, Musumeci O, Parenti G, Ravaglia S, Seidita F, Toscano A, Vianello A. Diagnosis of glycogenosis type II. Neurology. 2008;71(23 Suppl 2):S4–11.
68. Chan J, Desai AK, Kazi ZB, Corey K, Austin S, Hobson-Webb LD, Case LE, Jones HN, Kishnani PS. The emerging phenotype of late-onset Pompe disease: a systematic literature review. Mol Genet Metab. 2017;120(3):163–72.
69. Boentert M, Florian A, Dräger B, Young P, Yilmaz A. Pattern and prognostic value of cardiac involvement in patients with late-onset Pompe disease: a comprehensive cardiovascular magnetic resonance approach. J Cardiovasc Magn Reson. 2016;18(1):91.
70. Fayssoil A. Cardiomyopathy in Pompe's disease. Eur J Intern Med. 2008;19(1):57–9.
71. Schoser B, Stewart A, Kanters S, Hamed A, Jansen J, Chan K, Karamouzian M, Toscano A. Survival and long-term outcomes in late-onset Pompe disease following alglucosidase alfa treatment: a systematic review and meta-analysis. J Neurol. 2017;264(4):621–30.
72. Joanne M, Skye N, Tracy M. The effectiveness of enzyme replacement therapy for juvenile-onset Pompe disease: a systematic review. J Inherit Metab Dis. 2019;42(1):57–65.
73. Vita G, Vita GL, Musumeci O, Rodolico C, Messina S. Genetic neuromuscular disorders: living the era of a therapeutic revolution. Part 2: diseases of motor neuron and skeletal muscle. Neurol Sci. 2019;40(4):671–81.
74. D'souza RS, Levandowski C, Slavov D, Graw SL, Allen LA, Adler E, Mestroni L, Taylor MR. Danon disease: clinical features, evaluation, and management. Circ Heart Fail. 2014;7(5):843–9.
75. Nascimbeni AC, Fanin M, Angelini C, Sandri M. Autophagy dysregulation in Danon disease. Cell Death Dis. 2017;8(1):e2565.

76. Konrad T, Sonnenschein S, Schmidt FP, Mollnau H, Bock K, Ocete BQ, Münzel T, Theis C, Rostock T. Cardiac arrhythmias in patients with Danon disease. Europace. 2017;19(7):1204–10.
77. Sternick EB, Oliva A, Magalhães LP, Gerken LM, Hong K, Santana O, Brugada P, Brugada J, Brugada R. Familial pseudo-Wolff-Parkinson-White syndrome. J Cardiovasc Electrophysiol. 2006;17(7):724–32.
78. Arad M. Cardiac Danon disease: insights and challenges. Int J Cardiol. 2017;245:211–2.
79. Rowland TJ, Sweet ME, Mestroni L, Taylor MR. Danon disease - dysregulation of autophagy in a multisystem disorder with cardiomyopathy. J Cell Sci. 2016;129(11):2135–43.
80. Brambatti M, Caspi O, Maolo A, Koshi E, Greenberg B, Taylor MRG, Adler ED. Danon disease: gender differences in presentation and outcomes. Int J Cardiol. 2019;286:92–8.
81. Konrad T, Sonnenschein S, Schmidt FP, Mollnau H, Bock K, Ocete BQ, Münzel T, Theis C, Rostock T. Cardiac arrhythmias in patients with Danon disease. Europace. 2017;19(7):1204–10.
82. Boucek D, Jirikowic J, Taylor M. Natural history of Danon disease. Genet Med. 2011;13:563–8.
83. Stokes MB, Taylor AJ, McLean CA, D'Arcy CE, Mariani JA. Severe left ventricular hypertrophy and marked cardiac fibrosis in Danon disease. Int J Cardiol. 2016;221:14–6.
84. Ng KM, Mok PY, Butler AW, Ho JC, Choi SW, Lee YK, Lai WH, Au KW, Lau YM, Wong LY, Esteban MA, Siu CW, Sham PC, Colman A, Tse HF. Amelioration of X-linked related autophagy failure in Danon disease with DNA methylation inhibitor. Circulation. 2016;134(18):1373–89.
85. Finsterer J, Stöllberger C, Maeztu C. Sudden cardiac death in neuromuscular disorders. Int J Cardiol. 2016;203:508–15.
86. Zaha VYL. Amp-activated protein kinase regulation and biological actions in the heart. Circ Res. 2012;111:800–14.
87. Hedberg-Oldfors C, Oldfors A. Polyglucosan storage myopathies. Mol Aspects Med. 2015;46:85–100.
88. Murphy RT, Mogensen J, McGarry K, Bahl A, Evans A, Osman E, Syrris P, Gorman G, Farrell M, Holton JL, Hanna MG, Hughes S, Elliott PM, Macrae CA, McKenna WJ. Adenosine monophosphate-activated protein kinase disease mimicks hypertrophic cardiomyopathy and Wolff-Parkinson-White syndrome: natural history. J Am Coll Cardiol. 2005;45(6):922–30.
89. Gollob MH, Green MS, Tang AS, Gollob T, Karibe A, Ali Hassan AS, Ahmad F, Lozado R, Shah G, Fananapazir L, Bachinski LL, Roberts R. Identification of a gene responsible for familial Wolff-Parkinson-White syndrome. N Engl J Med. 2001;344(24):1823–31.
90. Porto AG, Brun F, Severini GM, Losurdo P, Fabris E, Taylor MRG, Mestroni L, Sinagra G. Clinical spectrum of PRKAG2 syndrome. Circ Arrhythm Electrophysiol. 2016;9(1):e003121.
91. Arad M, Maron BJ, Gorham JM, Johnson WH Jr, Saul JP, Perez-Atayde AR, Spirito P, Wright GB, Kanter RJ, Seidman CE, Seidman JG. Glycogen storage diseases presenting as hypertrophic cardiomyopathy. N Engl J Med. 2005;352(4):362–72.

Cardiac Amyloidosis

10

Liza S. M. Wong and Daniel P. Judge

Introduction

Cardiac amyloidosis is the most common form of infiltrative cardiomyopathy [1]. Historically, there were no effective therapies, and the prognosis was accordingly very grim. Improved understanding of the pathogenesis of this condition has facilitated better therapeutic options, which should lead to earlier diagnoses and better outcomes. This chapter addresses the etiology, pathogenesis, and clinical presentations of cardiac amyloidosis. It will also include traditional therapies, novel pharmacologic strategies, and electrophysiological implications for cardiac amyloidosis.

The most common forms of amyloid affecting the heart are caused by aggregation of immunoglobulin light chains (AL) or transthyretin (ATTR). Nomenclature for amyloidosis typically uses letters corresponding to the mutant protein. When immunoglobulin light chains are deposited as amyloid, it is called AL. When transthyretin deposits as amyloid, the proper designation is ATTR. While deposition of serum amyloid protein A (AA) due to chronic inflammation may be seen with noncardiac manifestations, it rarely causes meaningful cardiac dysfunction. ATTR is caused either by destabilizing mutations, which occur throughout the *TTR* gene, or in the absence of a detectable *TTR* mutation. These are referred to as ATTRmut (or ATTRm) and ATTRwt, respectively [2]. ATTRwt was traditionally called "senile" amyloid, but younger ages and its lack of ubiquitous prevalence among older people make this term inappropriate. Other rare inherited forms of amyloid are shown in Table 10.1. Familial amyloidosis was traditionally divided into two separate categories: familial amyloid polyneuropathy (FAP) and familial amyloid cardiomyopathy (FAC). However, with improved understanding that these two conditions are part of the same spectrum, many now consider them to be one single disease [3].

Nomenclature for specific mutations throughout the *TTR* gene, transthyretin, traditionally refers to amino acid positions that were determined from early protein studies performed on the mature form, without including the first 20 residues that are cleaved as a signal peptide [2]. Accordingly, a common mutation that causes familial amyloid polyneuropathy is usually called V30M or Val30Met; when referring to the same mutation with HUGO nomenclature, it is called p.Val50Met.

Etiology/Pathophysiology

All forms of amyloidosis have a common mechanistic etiology, which is related to misfolded protein in a form that is generally insoluble. Dense insoluble proteins clump together as fibrils, which accumulate in tissues throughout the body. Conditions that favor misfolding of the protein, such as production of a monoclonal immunoglobulin free light chain at high levels, oxidative stress, or destabilizing mutations, can facilitate the initiation and propagation of amyloidosis. These proteins typically exist in a steady state favoring the most stable form, but once an unstable subset develops, its deposition in tissue is usually irreversible.

Transthyretin is synthesized in the liver, choroid plexus, and retina [4]. This protein is also known as "prealbumin," because it is smaller than albumin and its position on gel electrophoresis of serum proteins is prior to albumin, the most common serum protein. Its role in serum is to serve as a carrier protein, transporting complexes with retinol (vitamin A) and thyroid hormone.

Some mutations cause amyloid to deposit predominantly in the heart, while others affect peripheral and autonomic nerves at earlier ages [3]. Many questions persist about the mechanisms for tissue tropism. To date, some of the processes contributing to initial denaturation of the proteins involved in amyloidosis are known, but the mechanism whereby the heart

L. S. M. Wong (✉)
Amsterdam, The Netherlands
e-mail: l.wong@vumc.nl

D. P. Judge
Charleston, SC, USA
e-mail: judged@musc.edu

H. F. Baars et al. (eds.), *Clinical Cardiogenetics*, https://doi.org/10.1007/978-3-030-45457-9_10

Table 10.1 Genes in which pathogenic variants predispose to amyloidosis

AA	Serum amyloid protein A
AANP	Atrial natriuretic peptide; also called Isolated Atrial Amyloid
AApoA-I	Apolipoprotein AI
AApoA-IV	Apolipoprotein AIV
AGel	Gelsolin
AL	Monoclonal immunoglobulin light chains
ALECT2	Leukocyte chemotactic factor 2
ALys	Lysozyme
ATTR	Transthyretin (mutant or wild type, depending on the presence/absence of a TTR mutation)

Table 10.2 Clinical hallmarks of amyloidosis

Cardiac manifestations
• Atrial fibrillation
• Concentric biventricular hypertrophy
• Conduction delay on ECG
• Coronary arterial obstruction
• Disproportionately low voltage on ECG
• Heart failure, diastolic or combined with systolic
• Increased echodensity and thickness of the atria
• Increased echodensity and thickness of the cardiac valves
• Pericardial effusion
Extra-cardiac manifestations
• Ascites
• Autonomic neuropathy
• Carpal tunnel syndrome
• Constipation, diarrhea, malabsorption
• Enlargement of the tongue with dental indentations
• Hematuria from amyloid infiltration in the bladder
• Periorbital purpura
• Peripheral neuropathy
• Peripheral edema
• Pleural effusion
• Ruptured biceps tendon

either actively or passively accumulates amyloid is not known. Once a nidus of amyloid exists, additional progression seems to occur even if the underlying problem is removed. For instance, for people with ATTRmut, a liver transplant removes the source of mutant protein, yet disease will often progress with deposition of wild-type TTR protein [5].

Missense substitutions of nearly every amino acid in the small TTR protein are associated with ATTR, with the exception of an apparently benign polymorphism occurring at the sixth codon after cleavage of 20 amino acids from the N-terminal of the pro-protein [6]. Certain mutations in *TTR* are more common among different ethnicities. The most frequently diagnosed mutation worldwide is Val30Met, affecting many people in both Portugal and Brazil, with probably a separate founder mutation at the same site arising in Japan. For unknown genetic or environmental reasons, people with this same mutation in Sweden tend to have later onset with milder disease [7]. A founder mutation arising early in Donegal Ireland (Thr60Ala) is also seen in North America among some individuals with Donegal Irish ancestry. The mutation that is probably the most prevalent worldwide is Val122Ile. The average age of onset is approximately 70 years. Its later onset and reduced penetrance contrast with earlier onset Val30Met in the Portuguese-type Val30Met, leading to fewer people recognized to have amyloid with the Val122Ile mutation. The Val122Ile mutation has been traced to a founder population in West Africa [8]. The prevalence of the Val122Ile mutation in North America is 3.4%, and homozygosity for this mutation also occurs. Somewhat surprisingly, the age of onset or severity of disease in the homozygotes is not much different, according to an analysis of one small cohort and literature review [9]. Among 13 new homozygotes and 11 whose information was determined from prior reports, the age at first symptoms was approximately 10 years earlier.

Pathophysiology of Heart Failure in Cardiac Amyloidosis

With progressively worsening left ventricular hypertrophy (LVH), the LV cavity typically gets smaller. Despite preserved ejection fraction (EF), the stroke volume declines and the cardiac output becomes directly proportional to heart rate within the physiologic spectrum. Fast heart rates are usually poorly tolerated due to LV stiffness, but slow heart rates usually cause worsening heart failure. The earliest signs on echocardiography include diffuse LVH with thickening of the heart valves and the atrial septum. With time and progressive accumulation of amyloid in the heart, the LVEF declines, though the apex is spared. In contrast with dilated cardiomyopathy (DCM), neurohormonal antagonism with ACE-inhibitors, angiotensin receptor blockers, and beta-blockers is poorly tolerated.

Clinical Presentation

Cardiac amyloidosis can present itself with a variety of symptoms, partly depending on the stage of the disease at first presentation. Table 10.2 includes many of the phenotypic hallmarks. In general, the accumulation of amyloid proteins in the extracellular matrix of the myocardium results in increased ventricular wall thickness, resulting in diastolic dysfunction and eventually a restrictive cardiomyopathy. This manifests most commonly as congestive heart failure, including edema, dyspnea, and ascites. When systolic function also becomes impaired, low cardiac output may lead to forward failure. Also, low blood pressure or orthostasis might be present, not only due to systolic heart failure but also due to autonomic dysfunction [10].

Angina pectoris in absence of epicardial obstructive coronary artery disease has also been recognized in cardiac amyloidosis [11–13]. Aside from potential obstructive coronary artery disease in epicardial large vessels, cardiac ischemia in cardiac amyloidosis potentially originates from microvascular dysfunction. Autopsy studies have shown amyloid depositions not only in the interstitium between cardiomyocytes but also in the perivascular regions and in the intima media of coronary vessels [14, 15]. In a prospective study, 21 cardiac amyloidosis patients without epicardial obstructive coronary artery disease underwent a vasodilator stress positron emission tomography test and were compared to 10 patients with left ventricular hypertrophy due to hypertensive cardiomyopathy [12]. In the cardiac amyloidosis patients, various degrees of regional cardiac ischemia were seen, whereas the group with hypertensive cardiomyopathy did not show regional perfusion defects. Furthermore, mean rest myocardial blood flow, stress myocardial blood flow, and coronary flow reserve—all indicators of coronary microvascular function—were significantly lower in the cardiac amyloidosis group, even after correction for wall thickness differences. These results indicate that the microvascular dysfunction in cardiac amyloidosis is not solely due to increased wall thickness and indicators of coronary microvascular function were inversely related to myocardial mass in the amyloidosis patients [12].

Conduction disorders are a common feature of cardiac amyloidosis. Early pathology studies reported direct infiltration of amyloid in the conduction system as well as its diffuse fibrosis [16, 17]. Sinoatrial node dysfunction, chronotropic incompetence, bundle branch blocks, and various degrees of atrioventricular blocks can be present in cardiac amyloidosis [18, 19]. In addition to bradyarrhythmias, patients with cardiac amyloidosis often have frequent ventricular ectopy, although this rarely proceeds to ventricular tachycardia. The most common tachyarrhythmia in people with cardiac amyloidosis is atrial fibrillation. Its management is challenged by poor tolerance of medications that slow AV conduction, although amyloid deposits will slow AV conduction in later phases of the disease.

Cardiac thromboembolism has been reported in patients with cardiac amyloidosis. One cause is the frequent prevalence of atrial fibrillation. However, cardiac thromboembolism in the absence of documented atrial fibrillation has also been described. In an autopsy study of hearts with amyloidosis, intracardiac thrombus was found in as many as 33% of the examined hearts, with the majority of the thrombi located in the atria and only sporadically in the ventricles. The prevalence of intracardiac thrombi was not different between patients with and without documented atrial fibrillation. The precise mechanism for intracardiac thrombi in the absence of atrial fibrillation is unknown. Some have suggested that endothelial dysfunction or hypercoagulability is the contributing factors [20, 21], however, decreased mechanical atrial activity despite normal sinus rhythm may also be a factor [22, 23]. Currently in daily practice, no routine diagnostic evaluations are made in cardiac amyloidosis patients for the detection of intracardiac thrombi. The potential risks and benefits of prophylactic oral anticoagulants in sinus rhythm are unknown and further research may contribute to better insights on this topic.

Diagnostic Tests

Several testing modalities can be useful for confirming a diagnosis of cardiac amyloidosis, when it is suspected. Figure 10.1 shows an algorithm for diagnostic testing, and additional information about commonly used tests is included below.

Electrocardiography

The most common abnormal finding in cardiac amyloidosis is low ECG voltage in the limb leads. This phenomenon occurs in approximately 50–60% in AL amyloidosis patients, but this is less common in the other forms of amyloidosis, being present in approximately 30% of the familial amyloidosis patients and 40% of the patients with senile amyloidosis [24]. Although an ECG may not achieve diagnostic criteria for low QRS voltage, there is usually discordance between the presence of LVH on imaging and the absence of LVH on ECGs. Other abnormal ECG findings include various degrees of atrioventricular block, atrial fibrillation, pseudo-infarction, nonspecific intraventricular delay, and ventricular tachycardia, but naturally none of these findings is specific for amyloidosis [25].

Echocardiography

One of the most characteristic signs of cardiac amyloidosis with echocardiography is diffuse increase in wall thickness. The increased wall thickness is not due to myocyte hypertrophy, but due to accumulation of amyloid proteins in the extracellular matrix. However, the term left ventricular hypertrophy has widely been adopted. Mostly, it is symmetrical and involves the left ventricle; however, the right ventricle, atrial walls, and valves can also be thickened [26]. The "sparkling aspect" of the myocardium due to accumulation of amyloid proteins is frequently described as a typical sign of amyloidosis [27, 28]. However, the diagnostic value of this sign has been challenged, as other causes of hypertrophy can also cause this phenomenon and the sensitivity and specificity have been shown to be low in a few studies [29, 30]. It can however be the trigger to consider the diagnosis of cardiac amyloidosis in a patient.

Diastolic function is often impaired. In early stages of cardiac amyloidosis, it might be the first and only sign. In

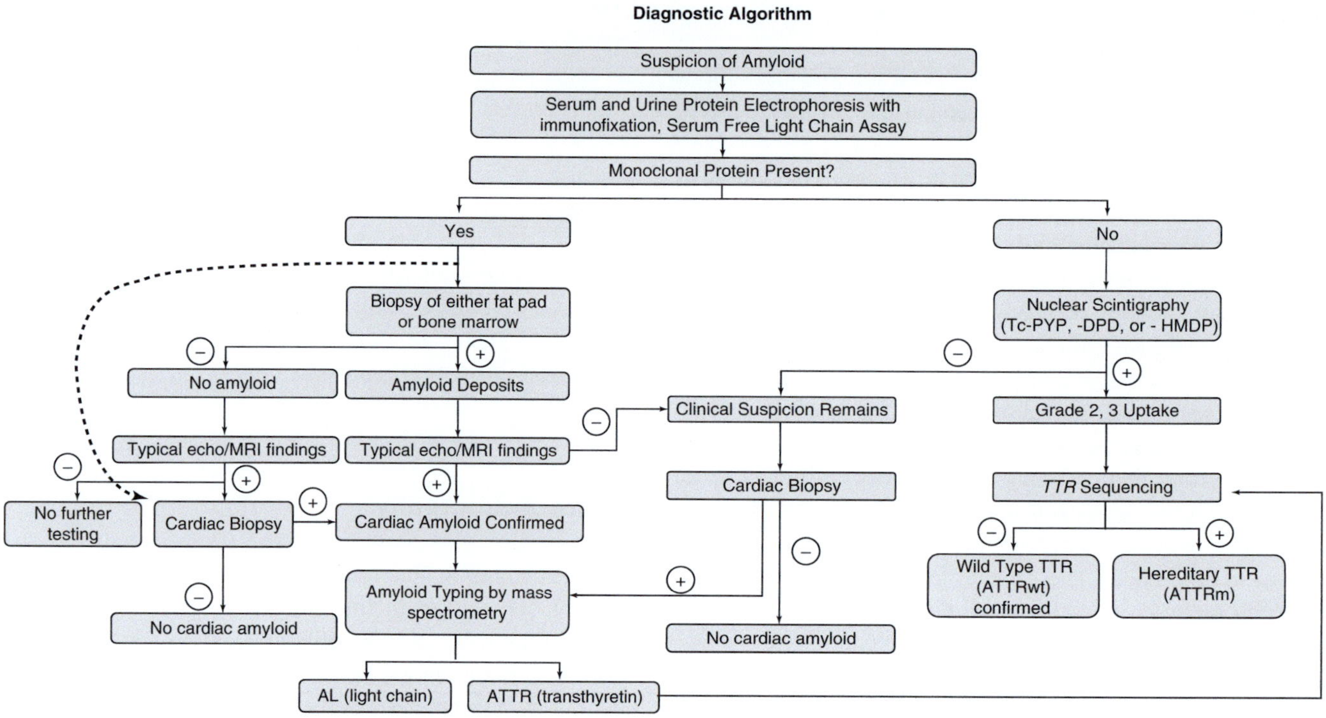

Fig. 10.1 Diagnostic algorithm for cardiac amyloid: This proposed approach for making the diagnosis of cardiac amyloid begins with testing for monoclonal gammopathy. If present with suspicion for cardiac amyloid, a biopsy must be obtained, either of noncardiac tissue (such as an abdominal fat pad), or of the right ventricle of the heart. Dotted lines indicate optional pathways

later stages, diastolic function can become more severe, in the worst case resulting in a restrictive cardiomyopathy. Biatrial dilatation is often visible in this stage.

Ventricular dysfunction spans the spectrum from diastolic dysfunction in the earliest stages to impaired systolic function affecting both the left and right ventricles in later stages. Pericardial effusion can be present; however, it is likely to be mild and only rarely causes tamponade [31–34]. Due to decreased contractility and factors noted above, intracardiac thrombi may also occur. The majority are located in the atria, however, in cases of severely impaired systolic ventricular function, ventricular thrombi may also be present.

More recently, tissue Doppler imaging and tissue speckle tracking have been of interest in relation to cardiac amyloidosis. Tissue Doppler imaging and tissue speckle tracking are techniques in which segmental myocardial deformation is assessed. Investigations have shown that longitudinal deformation is impaired in an early stage of cardiac amyloidosis [35]. In particular, longitudinal impairment in the basal and mid-ventricular segments is more pronounced than in the apical parts and this specific pattern is associated with a high sensitivity and specificity for cardiac amyloidosis [36, 37]. Similar results were obtained using tissue speckle tracking [38, 39]. In conclusion, echocardiography is a useful tool to assess the presence of cardiac amyloidosis in an easily accessible and noninvasive manner.

Cardiac Magnetic Resonance Imaging

Cardiac MRI (CMR) is an excellent method to evaluate cardiac amyloidosis. Its higher spatial resolution compared to echocardiography allows for detailed review of the morphology as well as the function of the heart. Also, the assessment of late gadolinium enhancement (LGE) is of high added value. Gadolinium accumulates in the areas of fibrotic tissue and enters damaged cardiomyocytes. In cardiac amyloidosis, where the extracellular matrix has expanded due to accumulation of the amyloid proteins, diffuse LGE can be seen. Also, the so-called nulling of the myocardium in the LGE sequences can be difficult [40, 41]. Nulling is the determination of the optimal settings (specifically: the inversion time) of the LGE sequence, which renders the myocardium dark (Fig. 10.2).

Another CMR parameter that contributes greatly to the distinction between left ventricular hypertrophy due to cardiac amyloidosis or other causes is the T1 relaxation time. CMR signals are determined by differences in magnetic properties of different tissues, reflected by T1 and T2 relaxation times. T1 relaxation time of the myocardium in cardiac amyloidosis is greatly increased due to its altered composition. Instead of consisting mainly of myocytes, and to much lesser extent vessels and extracellular matrix, the extracellular matrix in the myocardium increases greatly from amyloid infiltration, leading to an increased T1 relaxation time.

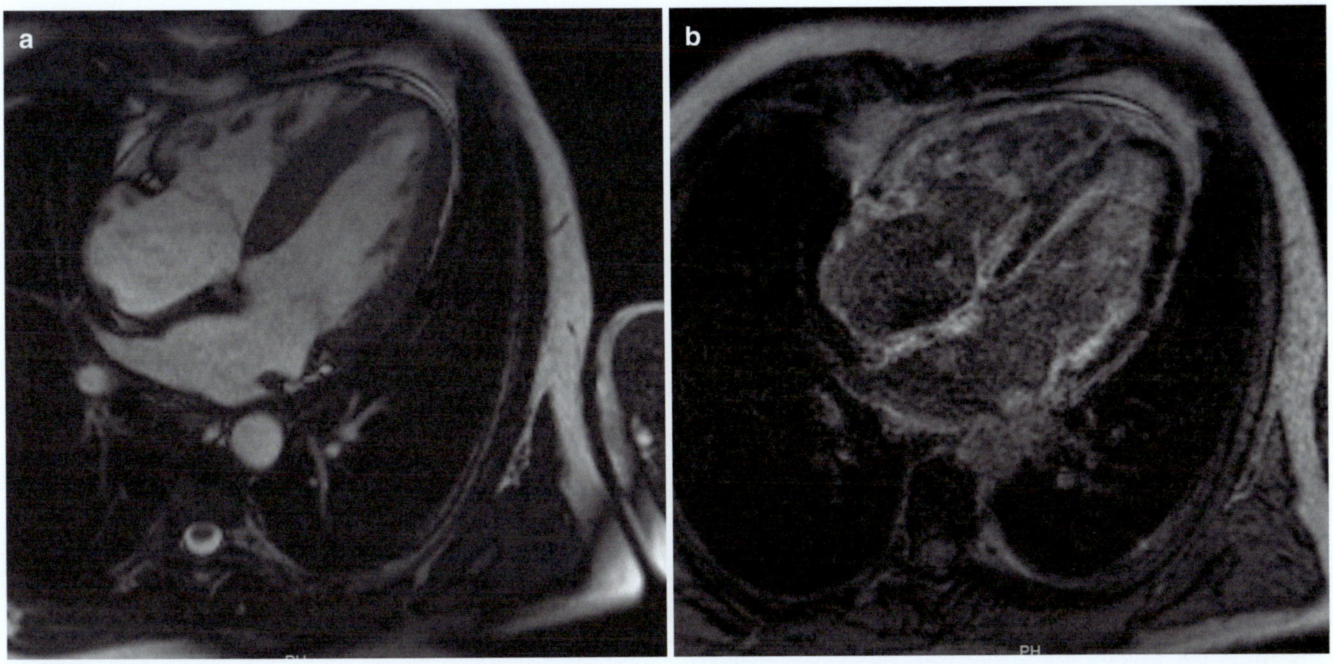

Fig. 10.2 Image of amyloid: (**a**) A four-chamber image of the heart of a patient with cardiac amyloidosis, obtained by cardiac MRI, showing left ventricular hypertrophy. (**b**) The same four-chamber image showing diffuse late gadolinium enhancement, indicating increased extracellular tissue, due to accumulation of amyloid proteins

A specific application of assessing the T1 relaxation time before and after gadolinium contrast injection is the estimation of the extracellular matrix by applying the T1 relaxation times of blood and myocardium before and after gadolinium injection in a mathematical model [42]. It has been shown that an estimated ECV of >40% is highly predictive of cardiac amyloidosis [43, 44].

Nuclear Imaging Techniques

While all of the other imaging techniques can contribute to diagnosing cardiac amyloidosis, they cannot differentiate between the different types of amyloidosis. In recent years, nuclear imaging has been recognized to have both high sensitivity and specificity for ATTR cardiac amyloid in the absence of a monoclonal gammopathy or skewed ratio of kappa/lambda free immunoglobulin light chains. It should be considered diagnostic for ATTR in the absence of either a monoclonal gammopathy or abnormal kappa/lambda free light chain ratio [45]. Nuclear imaging using tracers ^{99m}Tc-DPD (technetium-3,3-diphophono-1,2-propranodicarboxylic acid) and ^{99m}Tc-PYP (technetium pyrophosphate) in single-photon emission computed tomography (SPECT) have been evaluated in their properties to identify ATTR amyloidosis. ^{99m}Tc-DPD has been proven to be highly sensitive in identifying ATTR amyloidosis; however, it has also been described to have lower specificity since uptake has also been reported in AL amyloidosis, although much lower than in ATTR amyloidosis [45, 46]. Interestingly, using ^{99m}Tc-DPD in nuclear imaging seems to identify cardiac ATTR amyloidosis before any echocardiographic evidence was detectable [47]. Other studies using ^{99m}Tc-PYP as a tracer have shown a high sensitivity and specificity to distinguish amyloidosis from other causes of heart failure [48] and moreover, using not only the dichotomous outcome presence or absence of uptake but the extent of uptake (expressed as the ratio of uptake in the myocardium vs. the whole ventricular cavity), it was able to distinguish ATTR from AL amyloidosis [48]. The use of positron emission tomography (PET) imaging has also been investigated, however, data are scarce and the definitely added value needs to be further explored.

One should consider amyloidosis on the basis of clinical symptoms, LVH by echo or CMR, and particularly when there is discordant lack of LVH on ECG. AL amyloid should next be considered on the basis of a monoclonal gammopathy by immunofixation electrophoresis of serum and urine, as well as testing for immunoglobulin kappa and lambda free light chains. If a monoclonal gammopathy or skewed free light chain ratio is present, then a biopsy of affected tissue is necessary to establish the diagnosis. Without a monoclonal gammopathy, nuclear cardiac imaging (Tc-DPD, −PYP, or −HMDP) imaging should be used to test for ATTR. An uptake ratio for the nuclear tracer in the heart vs. contralateral ribs of ≥2.0 is considered diagnostic for ATTR cardiac amyloid. If ATTR is diagnosed, then TTR genetic testing should be performed to discern ATTRmut from ATTRwt.

Histological Diagnosis

With the development of imaging techniques in order to establish cardiac amyloidosis in combination with investigations aimed at detecting extracardiac amyloidosis (e.g., bone marrow biopsy, fat biopsy), the role of endomyocardial biopsy has declined. However, in case of suspicion of cardiac amyloidosis but failure to establish extracardiac amyloidosis, endomyocardial biopsy is still very valuable. Most commonly, Congo red staining is used for visualizing amyloid deposition. Amyloid deposits may be found anywhere in the heart. Most typically they are found in the myocardial interstitium of the ventricles, but also in the atria. However, because amyloid due to atrial natriuretic peptide (AANP) frequently occurs in the atrium, conclusive evidence for ventricular amyloid (either by imaging or ventricular biopsy) is necessary before making this diagnosis. Vascular involvement is not uncommon, especially in AL amyloidosis. While involvement of the epicardial coronary arteries is not usually associated with significant stenosis, obstructive microvascular amyloidosis has been associated with angina pectoris. Accumulation of amyloid proteins on the surface of the valves is also a well-known feature of cardiac amyloidosis [26].

When an endomyocardial biopsy shows amyloid, immunostaining for immunoglobulin light chains and transthyretin may both be positive, and assigning a definitive diagnosis of AL or ATTR on this basis may be limited. Fortunately, liquid chromatography and mass spectrometry can more definitively determine the subtype. Use of mass spectrometry is now considered routine in making the diagnosis, and it sometimes will identify mutant peptides of transthyretin, if present. However, if ATTR is determined by mass spectrometry, TTR genetic testing should be used to clarify the etiology (ATTRmut or ATTRwt) [49].

Therapy for Cardiac Amyloidosis

The therapy for cardiac amyloidosis comprises a dual approach: treating cardiac symptoms and treating the underlying disease.

Heart Failure Therapy

The medical therapy of heart failure secondary to cardiac amyloidosis differs from the conventional therapy for other forms of heart failure. There is little evidence for the safety and efficacy of conventional heart failure drugs in patients with cardiac amyloidosis. Loop diuretics are the most prominent therapy for treating heart failure due to cardiac amyloidosis. Due to elevated intracardiac pressures and diastolic dysfunction, volume overload occurs and causes symptoms of heart failure. Loop diuretics are often needed to maintain a euvolemic state. Other common drug strategies used in other forms of systolic chronic heart failure, like ACE inhibitors/ARBs and beta-blockers, have never been proven effective for cardiac amyloidosis. Moreover, ACE inhibitors and/or ARBs can potentially be harmful for patients with cardiac amyloidosis, because they can worsen (orthostatic) hypotension, because hearts with cardiac amyloid typically cannot augment stroke volume in response to vasodilation. Although they are beneficial in other forms of heart failure, beta-blockers might be harmful in cardiac amyloidosis since stroke volume is somewhat fixed in restrictive heart failure, and the cardiac output is highly dependent on the heart rate in severe cardiac amyloidosis. Digoxin and calcium channel blockers may bind to cardiac amyloid and cause toxicity despite normal circulating levels in blood. However, a recent report suggests that some patients may tolerate digoxin if their renal function and serum drug levels are closely monitored [50].

In summary, treatment of heart failure in cardiac amyloidosis is aimed at maintaining euvolemic state, and loop diuretics with restriction of sodium and fluid intake are paramount. Other conventional heart failure drugs have not been proven safe or effective and might even be harmful.

Cardiac Transplantation

From epidemiological studies, it has become clear that prognosis in amyloidosis patients is severely impaired if there is cardiac involvement, compared to patients without cardiac involvement [51]. This applies to AL amyloidosis, as well as ATTR amyloidosis. For patients with cardiac AL amyloidosis, the median overall survival has been reported to be as short as 7 months, whereas, for patients with amyloidosis without cardiac involvement, it was 40–94 months [51]. It is not surprising, therefore, that heart transplantation has come to mind as a potential effective treatment for cardiac amyloidosis patients. However, there are many pitfalls, which will be discussed here. Because the etiology and subsequently the treatment for AL and ATTR amyloidosis are very different, both types of amyloidosis will be discussed separately.

AL Amyloidosis and Heart Transplantation

In AL amyloidosis, the abnormal amyloid protein that accumulates in the heart and other organs originates from monoclonal plasma cells. The primary treatment goal is therefore reduction of the monoclonal plasma cell population, which is most often accomplished by systemic chemotherapy. If a heart transplantation is intended, there is a need for robust collaboration between hematologists and cardiologists. The appropriate sequence would be chemotherapy, followed by heart transplantation, if possible. Subsequently, the last step is conditioning chemotherapy and autologous bone marrow transplantation. With this strategy, the recurrence of amyloid in the transplanted heart is diminished.

One of the first studies to report short- and long-term outcomes after heart transplantation in AL amyloidosis patients (with cardiac involvement) showed a 1-year survival of only 59% among 17 transplanted patients. However, there was a pronounced difference in survival of AL amyloidosis patients who did and did not receive posttransplant chemotherapy. Patients who received posttransplant chemotherapy showed a 1- and 5-year survival of 71 and 36%, respectively. Comparably, patients who did not receive posttransplant chemotherapy showed a 1- and 5-year survival of 50 and 20%. Recurrence of amyloid deposits in the transplanted heart was also seemingly higher and occurred at much earlier time point in patients who did not receive posttransplant chemotherapy compared to those who did receive posttransplant chemotherapy [52]. However, it should be noted that chemotherapeutic agents directed against plasma cells have improved over the years. More recent studies of long-term outcomes after heart transplantation for cardiac amyloidosis are more optimistic, given that patients underwent the full cycle of induction chemotherapy, heart transplantation, and subsequently posttransplant chemotherapy and autologous stem cell transplantation. One- and 5-year survival have been reported at 82 and 65% respectively in a study conducted between 2008 and 2013 [53]. Another study reported a 1- and 7-year survival at 100 and 60%, respectively [54], and other studies reported comparable results [55–57].

These results deem more hopeful perspectives for AL amyloidosis patients with cardiac involvement. However, it must be noted that in the light of donor shortage, the selection of patients eligible for cardiac transplant is very strict, and cardiac transplantation is only feasible for a very limited group of patients. Evaluation of eligibility for heart transplantation involves an intensive cooperation among several specialists to assess the extracardiac organ involvement. Multiple myeloma and involvement of other organ systems (gastrointestinal, liver, kidney involvement) may be a contraindication for heart transplantation. Other predisposing factors causing an impairment in posttransplant mobility and rehabilitation, for example, severe neuropathy due to amyloidosis, will limit feasibility for transplantation [58]. Even so, the lucky few that are deemed eligible for heart transplantation face long waiting lists and will likely deteriorate to a state beyond being able to undergo the transplantation or die before receiving a cardiac transplant.

ATTR Amyloidosis and Heart/Liver Transplantation

In ATTR amyloidosis, the liver produces abnormal amyloid proteins either due to an inherited genetic mutation (ATTRmut) or, as previously noted, without a mutation (ATTRwt). In general, patients with ATTRwt amyloidosis are often older than patients with AL type or ATTRmut. Since the liver is the source of the abnormal protein, orthotopic liver transplantations were the first type of transplantation considered as a therapy for ATTRmut amyloidosis. Later, combined heart and liver transplantation has been explored. Although ATTRwt itself is not a contraindication for transplantation, the average age of onset of disease tends to be higher than for the other forms of amyloidosis, and old age can be a contraindication for heart transplantation [59]. Because the liver in patients with ATTRwt produces normal TTR, orthotopic liver transplant would not be effective therapy.

People with certain *TTR* mutations fare better with liver transplant than with other mutations [5]. The Val30Met mutation, for instance, typically responds well to liver transplant when performed prior to diffuse systemic involvement or severe autonomic dysfunction. Later conduction block and LVH can occur, and patients with liver transplant for ATTR should continue with posttransplant cardiac surveillance for amyloid. In contrast, the Thr60Ala mutation usually has severe multiorgan involvement, and most transplant programs decline these patients for isolated liver transplant. The use of novel disease-modifying therapies posttransplant is currently under investigation, as noted below.

The long-term outcomes of liver or liver/heart transplantations vary greatly depending on the clinical status of the patient pretransplantation and the type of mutation. The 5-year survival for various mutation types in larger studies has been reported between 62 and 82% [60, 61]. In general, it is safe to say that patients with ATTR amyloidosis with cardiac involvement have better prognosis when not only a liver transplantation, but a combined liver/heart transplantation was performed.

In conclusion, organ transplantation has been accepted as an established therapy for amyloidosis patients that yields reasonable long-term results. Careful selection of eligible patients must be performed and requires an intensive multidisciplinary approach. Considering the scarceness of organs, however, it must certainly not be regarded as a "routine therapy" and it must be borne in mind that even if a patient is placed on the waiting list for transplantation, the chances of receiving a heart transplant are limited.

Novel Treatment Strategies for ATTR

Emerging therapies directed at the underlying cause of ATTR can be divided into three categories: stabilizing the TTR tetramer, silencing the TTR gene, and removing ATTR from diseased tissues with antibodies. The idea of stabilizing the tetramer to halt progression of this disease originated with an insightful observation regarding a stabilizing gain-of-function mutation (Thr119Met), which very rarely occurs in one of two copies of this gene, while the other TTR gene copy contains a destabilizing mutation (Val30Met) [62]. Individuals with both mutations have marked delay in onset and decline in severity, in comparison with people who have the destabilizing mutation alone. In vitro studies showed that increasing the concentration of the stabilizing monomer coordinately improves the stability of the tetramer [62].

There is good evidence that at least four drugs stabilize the TTR tetramer: diflunisal, tafamidis, tolcapone, and AG10. Diflunisal was developed as a nonsteroidal anti-inflammatory drug (NSAID), and its ability to stabilize TTR was recognized much later. Although not approved by any regulatory agencies for the treatment of amyloidosis, a multicenter double-blinded, placebo-controlled trial showed that it reduced progression of familial amyloid polyneuropathy (FAP) due to TTR mutations [63]. Its use in patients with heart failure is challenging, since its properties as an NSAID may cause fluid retention and renal dysfunction. Tafamidis was developed to have the same stabilizing effect without the properties of an NSAID [64]. Early studies showed its ability to slow the progression of FAP [65, 66]. More recently, a large multicenter double-blinded, placebo-controlled trial compared tafamidis 80 mg daily, 20 mg daily, and placebo (2:1:2) in patients with ATTR cardiac amyloid, including ATTRmut and ATTRwt [67]. Over 30 months, treatment with tafamidis in either dose led to decrease in all-cause mortality, lower rate of cardiovascular-related hospitalizations, lower rate of decline in distance on 6-min walk test, and lower rate of decline in quality-of-life scores, as compared to treatment with placebo. Furthermore, tafamidis was tolerated well, with similar incidence of adverse events as placebo [67].

Tolcapone is a catechol-O-methyltransferase (COMT) inhibitor, which was developed as a medication to treat Parkinson's Disease [68]. After a few treated patients developed severe liver toxicity (with three fatalities), this drug was removed from the market in many countries, but it was returned with dire warnings regarding the need for close liver monitoring. A chemical screen identified tolcapone for its ability to bind to the TTR tetramer in human plasma and to stabilize it [69]. A clinical trial will investigate its safety and efficacy in patients with ATTR.

The fourth pharmacologic stabilizer is currently called AG10, identified from a chemical screen for its ability to stabilize the TTR tetramer [70]. Phase 1 studies showed good human tolerability, and a phase 2 trial in people with ATTRmut and ATTRwt also showed good safety and tolerability, along with elevation of serum TTR levels as a marker of biological effect. A large multicenter double-blinded, placebo-controlled trial is planned for the near future.

TTR silencers work to interfere with hepatic synthesis of transthyretin. Two medications in this category have recently been tested in multicenter randomized, double-blinded, placebo-controlled clinical trials: patisiran and inotersen [71, 72]. Patisiran is considered an RNA-interfering drug, and inotersen is considered an antisense oligonucleotide. Both of these trials exclusively enrolled patients with ATTRmut (not ATTRwt). Each trial demonstrated efficacy in dramatically reducing the serum level of TTR, with median reductions in serum levels by approximately 80%. Both trials were successful by achieving their primary end points, which included stabilization of neuropathy without appreciable progression of neuropathic limitations. Although both trials focused on familial amyloid polyneuropathy, some participants in each study had cardiomyopathy or mild heart failure due to cardiac amyloidosis. Since both trials focused their primary endpoint on measures of neuropathic impairment, it is difficult to draw conclusions about their ability to treat ATTR cardiomyopathy. In theory, reduced production of hepatic TTR should help any affected organ system, except the brain and retinas. Future clinical trials investigating TTR silencers should focus on ATTR cardiomyopathy, ideally with both ATTRmut and ATTRwt.

Therapies designed to stabilize the TTR tetramer or reduce production of this protein will ideally halt worsening, but are not likely to remove amyloid directly from the heart. In contrast, another therapeutic strategy seeks to do so by triggering antibody-mediated destruction of the amyloid plaques without harming the affected organs involved with amyloid. One approach targets a common component of all subtypes of amyloid, serum amyloid P-component (SAP). This protein can first be removed from serum with (R)-1-[6-[(R)-2-carboxy-pyrrolidin-1-yl]-6-oxo-hexanoyl] pyrrolidine-2-carboxylic acid (CPHPC), then a humanized monoclonal IgG1 anti-SAP antibody is used to activate macrophage destruction of the SAP-containing amyloid deposits in tissues [73]. Another such treatment is called PRX004, a monoclonal antibody designed to target and clear misfolded TTR protein that is present in tissues affected by ATTR amyloidosis. Neither of these treatments is approved for use in humans, and both are in clinical trials.

Cardioverter Defibrillators in Cardiac Amyloid

In its later stages, cardiac amyloid typically manifests with refractory heart failure. Although ventricular ectopy is commonly seen, sudden cardiac death due to tachyarrhythmia is unusual. This may be due to diffuse slowing of conduction mediated by deposits of amyloid fibrils throughout the heart. One retrospective study investigated 45 people with cardiac amyloid who received an ICD, 38 (84%) of whom had no prior syncope [74]. This was a mixed cohort with 27% AL amyloid and the remainder with ATTR (60% ATTRmut and 13% ATTRwt). With average follow-up of 17 months, 27% had at least one appropriate ICD therapy, although transplant-free survival remained quite low, with 60% transplant-free survival over this 17-month interval [74]. With newer therapies on the horizon, use of a primary-prevention cardioverter-defibrillator is reasonable to consider, but data are lacking to support this use more broadly.

Pregnancy and Family Screening

The age of onset for AL amyloid and most forms of ATTR amyloid is usually postmenopausal in women, who tend to present later with amyloid than men. That aside, there are genotypes (i.e., Val30Met) with earlier onset that becomes relevant for women who may carry this mutation and consider pregnancy. Because the earlier onset forms of ATTRmut typically affect peripheral nerves more prominently than the heart, pregnancy does not impose increased risk of heart failure in this rare circumstance. There are no published trials or case reports of women who have heart failure from cardiac amyloid during pregnancy.

As with any genetic disease, preimplantation genetic diagnosis (PGD) is an option to prevent disease transmission to subsequent generations. For some mutations in TTR, such as Val30Met or Thr60Ala, the penetrance is relatively high and the challenges of PGD are more relevant than for other mutations with later onset and probably low penetrance (i.e., Val122Ile). PGD has been reported for ATTR, and its use should be included in discussions with patients with this condition who are considering pregnancy [75].

Genetic counseling with discussion of risk to family members is a critical part of caring for individuals and families with familial forms of amyloid. The majority of people with ATTRmut have dominant mutations, though homozygotic mutations also occur, usually without much difference from those with heterozygotic mutations. Genetic testing for first-degree relatives of affected patients should be offered at ages when the familial mutation tends to occur, or earlier if desired for family planning purposes.

Summary and Take-Home Message

Cardiac amyloidosis is the most common form of infiltrative cardiomyopathy, with substantial morbidity and mortality. Some forms are hereditary, whereas other forms are not. Recognition of cardiac amyloidosis, especially in early stages, can be challenging and often requires multimodality imaging techniques. Throughout the years the understanding of the pathophysiology has deepened and subsequently, more effective treatment aimed at the underlying cause of amyloidosis has been developed, leading to improved prognosis. Since cardiac amyloidosis is a symptom of an underlying disease causing amyloid overload, a multidisciplinary approach toward treatment is recommended, and, in the familial forms of amyloidosis, genetic counseling and genetic testing should be offered.

References

1. Falk RH. Diagnosis and management of the cardiac amyloidoses. Circulation. 2005;112(13):2047–60.
2. Sipe JD, Benson MD, Buxbaum JN, Ikeda S-i, Merlini G, MJM S, et al. Amyloid fibril proteins and amyloidosis: chemical identification and clinical classification International Society of Amyloidosis 2016 Nomenclature Guidelines. Amyloid. 2016;23(4):209–13.
3. Rapezzi C, Quarta CC, Obici L, Perfetto F, Longhi S, Salvi F, et al. Disease profile and differential diagnosis of hereditary transthyretin-related amyloidosis with exclusively cardiac phenotype: an Italian perspective. Eur Heart J. 2013;34(7):520–8.
4. Ton V-K, Mukherjee M, Judge DP. Transthyretin cardiac amyloidosis: pathogenesis, treatments, and emerging role in heart failure with preserved ejection fraction. Clin Med Insights Cardiol. 2014;8(s1). https://doi.org/10.4137/CMC.S15719
5. Benson MD. Liver transplantation and transthyretin amyloidosis. Muscle Nerve. 2013;47(2):157–62.
6. Jacobson DR, Alves IL, Saraiva MJ, Thibodeau SN, Buxbaum JN. Transthyretin Ser 6 gene frequency in individuals without amyloidosis. Hum Genet. 1995;95(3):308–12.
7. Klaassen SHC, Tromp J, Nienhuis HLA, van der Meer P, van den Berg MP, Blokzijl H, et al. Frequency of and prognostic significance of cardiac involvement at presentation in hereditary transthyretin-derived amyloidosis and the value of N-terminal pro-B-type natriuretic peptide. Am J Cardiol. 2018;121(1):107–12.
8. Jacobson DR, Alexander AA, Tagoe C, Garvey WT, Williams SM, Tishkoff S, et al. The prevalence and distribution of the amyloidogenic transthyretin (TTR) V122I allele in Africa. Mol Genet Genomic Med. 2016;4(5):548–56.
9. Reddi HV, Jenkins S, Theis J, Thomas BC, Connors LH, Van Rhee F, et al. Homozygosity for the V122I mutation in transthyretin is associated with earlier onset of cardiac amyloidosis in the African American population in the seventh decade of life. J Mol Diagn. 2014;16(1):68–74.
10. Algalarrondo V, Eliahou L, Thierry I, Bouzeman A, Dasoveanu M, Sebag C, et al. Circadian rhythm of blood pressure reflects the severity of cardiac impairment in familial amyloid polyneuropathy. Arch Cardiovasc Dis. 2012;105(5):281–90.
11. Al Suwaidi J, Velianou JL, Gertz MA, Cannon RO 3rd, Higano ST, Holmes DR Jr, et al. Systemic amyloidosis presenting with angina pectoris. Ann Intern Med. 1999;131(11):838–41.
12. Dorbala S, Vangala D, Bruyere J Jr, Quarta C, Kruger J, Padera R, et al. Coronary microvascular dysfunction is related to abnormalities in myocardial structure and function in cardiac amyloidosis. JACC Heart Fail. 2014;2(4):358–67.
13. Mueller PS, Edwards WD, Gertz MA. Symptomatic ischemic heart disease resulting from obstructive intramural coronary amyloidosis. Am J Med. 2000;109(3):181–8.
14. Hongo M, Yamamoto H, Kohda T, Takeda M, Kinoshita O, Uchikawa S, et al. Comparison of electrocardiographic findings in patients with AL (primary) amyloidosis and in familial amyloid

polyneuropathy and anginal pain and their relation to histopathologic findings. Am J Cardiol. 2000;85(7):849–53.
15. Modesto KM, Dispenzieri A, Gertz M, Cauduro SA, Khandheria BK, Seward JB, et al. Vascular abnormalities in primary amyloidosis. Eur Heart J. 2007;28(8):1019–24.
16. James TN, Birk RE. Pathology of the cardiac conduction system in polyarteritis nodosa. Arch Intern Med. 1966;117(4):561–7.
17. Ridolfi RL, Bulkley BH, Hutchins GM. The conduction system in cardiac amyloidosis. Clinical and pathologic features of 23 patients. Am J Med. 1977;62(5):677–86.
18. Mathew V, Olson LJ, Gertz MA, Hayes DL. Symptomatic conduction system disease in cardiac amyloidosis. Am J Cardiol. 1997;80(11):1491–2.
19. Reisinger J, Dubrey SW, Lavalley M, Skinner M, Falk RH. Electrophysiologic abnormalities in AL (primary) amyloidosis with cardiac involvement. J Am Coll Cardiol. 1997;30(4):1046–51.
20. Berghoff M, Kathpal M, Khan F, Skinner M, Falk R, Freeman R. Endothelial dysfunction precedes C-fiber abnormalities in primary (AL) amyloidosis. Ann Neurol. 2003;53(6):725–30.
21. Yood RA, Skinner M, Rubinow A, Talarico L, Cohen AS. Bleeding manifestations in 100 patients with amyloidosis. JAMA. 1983;249(10):1322–4.
22. Dubrey S, Pollak A, Skinner M, Falk RH. Atrial thrombi occurring during sinus rhythm in cardiac amyloidosis: evidence for atrial electromechanical dissociation. Br Heart J. 1995;74(5):541–4.
23. Plehn JF, Southworth J, Cornwell GG 3rd. Brief report: atrial systolic failure in primary amyloidosis. N Engl J Med. 1992;327(22):1570–3.
24. Rapezzi C, Merlini G, Quarta CC, Riva L, Longhi S, Leone O, et al. Systemic cardiac amyloidoses: disease profiles and clinical courses of the 3 main types. Circulation. 2009;120(13):1203–12.
25. Cyrille NB, Goldsmith J, Alvarez J, Maurer MS. Prevalence and prognostic significance of low QRS voltage among the three main types of cardiac amyloidosis. Am J Cardiol. 2014;114(7):1089–93.
26. Maleszewski JJ. Cardiac amyloidosis: pathology, nomenclature, and typing. Cardiovasc Pathol. 2015;24(6):343–50.
27. Rahman JE, Helou EF, Gelzer-Bell R, Thompson RE, Kuo C, Rodriguez ER, et al. Noninvasive diagnosis of biopsy-proven cardiac amyloidosis. J Am Coll Cardiol. 2004;43(3):410–5.
28. Bhandari AK, Nanda NC. Myocardial texture characterization by two-dimensional echocardiography. Am J Cardiol. 1983;51(5):817–25.
29. Simons M, Isner JM. Assessment of relative sensitivities of noninvasive tests for cardiac amyloidosis in documented cardiac amyloidosis. Am J Cardiol. 1992;69(4):425–7.
30. Hongo M, Kono J, Yamada H, Misawa T, Tanaka M, Nakatsuka T, et al. Doppler echocardiographic assessments of left ventricular diastolic filling in patients with amyloid heart disease. J Cardiol. 1991;21(2):391–401.
31. Yuda S, Hayashi T, Yasui K, Muranaka A, Ohnishi H, Hashimoto A, et al. Pericardial effusion and multiple organ involvement are independent predictors of mortality in patients with systemic light chain amyloidosis. Intern Med. 2015;54(15):1833–40.
32. Kuprian M, Mount G. Acute cardiac tamponade in light-chain amyloidosis. BMJ Case Rep. 2014. https://doi.org/10.1136/bcr-2013-200248
33. Navarro JF, Rivera M, Ortuno J. Cardiac tamponade as presentation of systemic amyloidosis. Int J Cardiol. 1992;36(1):107–8.
34. Brodarick S, Paine R, Higa E, Carmichael KA. Pericardial tamponade, a new complication of amyloid heart disease. Am J Med. 1982;73(1):133–5.
35. Lindqvist P, Olofsson BO, Backman C, Suhr O, Waldenstrom A. Pulsed tissue Doppler and strain imaging discloses early signs of infiltrative cardiac disease: a study on patients with familial amyloidotic polyneuropathy. Eur J Echocardiogr. 2006;7(1):22–30.
36. Koyama J, Ray-Sequin PA, Falk RH. Longitudinal myocardial function assessed by tissue velocity, strain, and strain rate tissue Doppler echocardiography in patients with AL (primary) cardiac amyloidosis. Circulation. 2003;107(19):2446–52.
37. Bellavia D, Pellikka PA, Dispenzieri A, Scott CG, Al-Zahrani GB, Grogan M, et al. Comparison of right ventricular longitudinal strain imaging, tricuspid annular plane systolic excursion, and cardiac biomarkers for early diagnosis of cardiac involvement and risk stratification in primary systematic (AL) amyloidosis: a 5-year cohort study. Eur Heart J Cardiovasc Imaging. 2012;13(8):680–9.
38. Sun JP, Stewart WJ, Yang XS, Donnell RO, Leon AR, Felner JM, et al. Differentiation of hypertrophic cardiomyopathy and cardiac amyloidosis from other causes of ventricular wall thickening by two-dimensional strain imaging echocardiography. Am J Cardiol. 2009;103(3):411–5.
39. Quarta CC, Solomon SD, Uraizee I, Kruger J, Longhi S, Ferlito M, et al. Left ventricular structure and function in transthyretin-related versus light-chain cardiac amyloidosis. Circulation. 2014;129(18):1840–9.
40. Pandey T, Jambhekar K, Shaikh R, Lensing S, Viswamitra S. Utility of the inversion scout sequence (TI scout) in diagnosing myocardial amyloid infiltration. Int J Cardiovasc Imaging. 2013;29(1):103–12.
41. Di Bella G, Pizzino F, Minutoli F, Zito C, Donato R, Dattilo G, et al. The mosaic of the cardiac amyloidosis diagnosis: role of imaging in subtypes and stages of the disease. Eur Heart J Cardiovasc Imaging. 2014;15(12):1307–15.
42. Dabir D, Child N, Kalra A, Rogers T, Gebker R, Jabbour A, et al. Reference values for healthy human myocardium using a T1 mapping methodology: results from the International T1 Multicenter cardiovascular magnetic resonance study. J Cardiovasc Magn Reson. 2014;16:69.
43. Banypersad SM, Sado DM, Flett AS, Gibbs SD, Pinney JH, Maestrini V, et al. Quantification of myocardial extracellular volume fraction in systemic AL amyloidosis: an equilibrium contrast cardiovascular magnetic resonance study. Circ Cardiovasc Imaging. 2013;6(1):34–9.
44. Mongeon FP, Jerosch-Herold M, Coelho-Filho OR, Blankstein R, Falk RH, Kwong RY. Quantification of extracellular matrix expansion by CMR in infiltrative heart disease. JACC Cardiovasc Imaging. 2012;5(9):897–907.
45. Aljaroudi WA, Desai MY, Tang WH, Phelan D, Cerqueira MD, Jaber WA. Role of imaging in the diagnosis and management of patients with cardiac amyloidosis: state of the art review and focus on emerging nuclear techniques. J Nucl Cardiol. 2014;21(2):271–83.
46. Rapezzi C, Quarta CC, Guidalotti PL, Longhi S, Pettinato C, Leone O, et al. Usefulness and limitations of 99mTc-3,3-diphosphono-1,2-propanodicarboxylic acid scintigraphy in the aetiological diagnosis of amyloidotic cardiomyopathy. Eur J Nucl Med Mol Imaging. 2011;38(3):470–8.
47. Rapezzi C, Quarta CC, Guidalotti PL, Pettinato C, Fanti S, Leone O, et al. Role of (99m)Tc-DPD scintigraphy in diagnosis and prognosis of hereditary transthyretin-related cardiac amyloidosis. JACC Cardiovasc Imaging. 2011;4(6):659–70.
48. Yamamoto Y, Onoguchi M, Haramoto M, Kodani N, Komatsu A, Kitagaki H, et al. Novel method for quantitative evaluation of cardiac amyloidosis using (201)TlCl and (99m)Tc-PYP SPECT. Ann Nucl Med. 2012;26(8):634–43.
49. Brown EE, Lee YZJ, Halushka MK, Steenbergen C, Johnson NM, Almansa J, et al. Genetic testing improves identification of transthyretin amyloid (ATTR) subtype in cardiac amyloidosis. Amyloid. 2017;24(2):92–5.
50. Muchtar E, Gertz MA, Kumar SK, Lin G, Boilson B, Clavell A, et al. Digoxin use in systemic light-chain (AL) amyloidosis: contra-indicated or cautious use? Amyloid. 2018;25(2):86–92.
51. Wechalekar AD, Schonland SO, Kastritis E, Gillmore JD, Dimopoulos MA, Lane T, et al. A European collaborative study of

treatment outcomes in 346 patients with cardiac stage III AL amyloidosis. Blood. 2013;121(17):3420–7.
52. Dubrey SW, Burke MM, Hawkins PN, Banner NR. Cardiac transplantation for amyloid heart disease: the United Kingdom experience. J Heart Lung Transplant. 2004;23(10):1142–53.
53. Davis MK, Kale P, Liedtke M, Schrier S, Arai S, Wheeler M, et al. Outcomes after heart transplantation for amyloid cardiomyopathy in the modern era. Am J Transplant. 2015;15(3):650–8.
54. Dey BR, Chung SS, Spitzer TR, Zheng H, Macgillivray TE, Seldin DC, et al. Cardiac transplantation followed by dose-intensive melphalan and autologous stem-cell transplantation for light chain amyloidosis and heart failure. Transplantation. 2010;90(8):905–11.
55. Lacy MQ, Dispenzieri A, Hayman SR, Kumar S, Kyle RA, Rajkumar SV, et al. Autologous stem cell transplant after heart transplant for light chain (Al) amyloid cardiomyopathy. J Heart Lung Transplant. 2008;27(8):823–9.
56. Gillmore JD, Goodman HJ, Lachmann HJ, Offer M, Wechalekar AD, Joshi J, et al. Sequential heart and autologous stem cell transplantation for systemic AL amyloidosis. Blood. 2006;107(3):1227–9.
57. Sattianayagam PT, Gibbs SD, Pinney JH, Wechalekar AD, Lachmann HJ, Whelan CJ, et al. Solid organ transplantation in AL amyloidosis. Am J Transplant. 2010;10(9):2124–31.
58. Sousa M, Monohan G, Rajagopalan N, Grigorian A, Guglin M. Heart transplantation in cardiac amyloidosis. Heart Fail Rev. 2017;22(3):317–27.
59. Bradshaw SH, Veinot JP. Cardiac amyloidosis: what are the indications for transplant? Curr Opin Cardiol. 2012;27(2):143–7.
60. Suhr OB, Larsson M, Ericzon BG, Wilczek HE, Investigators FAs. Survival after transplantation in patients with mutations other than Val30Met: extracts from the FAP World Transplant Registry. Transplantation. 2016;100(2):373–81.
61. Careddu L, Zanfi C, Pantaleo A, Loforte A, Ercolani G, Cescon M, et al. Combined heart-liver transplantation: a single-center experience. Transpl Int. 2015;28(7):828–34.
62. Hammarström P, Schneider F, Kelly JW. Trans-suppression of misfolding in an amyloid disease. Science. 2001;293(5539):2459–62.
63. Berk JL, Suhr OB, Obici L, et al. Repurposing diflunisal for familial amyloid polyneuropathy: a randomized clinical trial. JAMA. 2013;310(24):2658–67.
64. Bulawa CE, Connelly S, DeVit M, Wang L, Weigel C, Fleming JA, et al. Tafamidis, a potent and selective transthyretin kinetic stabilizer that inhibits the amyloid cascade. Proc Natl Acad Sci. 2012;109(24):9629–34.
65. Coelho T, Maia LF, Martins da Silva A, Waddington Cruz M, Planté-Bordeneuve V, Lozeron P, et al. Tafamidis for transthyretin familial amyloid polyneuropathy. A randomized, controlled trial. Neurology. 2012;79(8):785–92.
66. Merlini G, Planté-Bordeneuve V, Judge DP, Schmidt H, Obici L, Perlini S, et al. Effects of tafamidis on transthyretin stabilization and clinical outcomes in patients with non-Val30Met transthyretin amyloidosis. J Cardiovasc Transl Res. 2013;6(6):1011–20.
67. Maurer MS, Schwartz JH, Gundapaneni B, Elliott PM, Merlini G, Waddington-Cruz M, et al. Tafamidis treatment for patients with transthyretin amyloid cardiomyopathy. N Engl J Med. 2018;379(11):1007–16.
68. Borges N. Tolcapone in Parkinson's disease: liver toxicity and clinical efficacy. Expert Opin Drug Saf. 2005;4(1):69–73.
69. Sant'Anna R, Gallego P, Robinson LZ, Pereira-Henriques A, Ferreira N, Pinheiro F, et al. Repositioning tolcapone as a potent inhibitor of transthyretin amyloidogenesis and associated cellular toxicity. Nat Commun. 2016;7:10787.
70. Alhamadsheh MM, Connelly S, Cho A, Reixach N, Powers ET, Pan DW, et al. Potent kinetic stabilizers that prevent transthyretin-mediated cardiomyocyte proteotoxicity. Sci Transl Med. 2011;3(97):97ra81.
71. Adams D, Gonzalez-Duarte A, O'Riordan WD, Yang C-C, Ueda M, Kristen AV, et al. Patisiran, an RNAi therapeutic, for hereditary transthyretin amyloidosis. N Engl J Med. 2018;379(1):11–21.
72. Benson MD, Waddington-Cruz M, Berk JL, Polydefkis M, Dyck PJ, Wang AK, et al. Inotersen treatment for patients with hereditary transthyretin amyloidosis. N Engl J Med. 2018;379(1):22–31.
73. Richards DB, Cookson LM, Berges AC, Barton SV, Lane T, Ritter JM, et al. Therapeutic clearance of amyloid by antibodies to serum amyloid P component. N Engl J Med. 2015;373(12):1106–14.
74. Hamon D, Algalarrondo V, Gandjbakhch E, Extramiana F, Marijon E, Elbaz N, et al. Outcome and incidence of appropriate implantable cardioverter-defibrillator therapy in patients with cardiac amyloidosis. Int J Cardiol. 2016;222:562–8.
75. Carvalho F, Sousa M, Fernandes S, Silva J, Saraiva MJ, Barros A. Preimplantation genetic diagnosis for familial amyloidotic polyneuropathy (FAP). Prenat Diagn. 2001;21(12):1093–9.

11 Mitochondrial Cardiomyopathies

Andreas C. Blank, Johannes M. P. J. Breur, Sabine A. Fuchs, Klaas Koop, and Annette F. Baas

Introduction

Mitochondria play a pivotal role in the metabolism of the human body. Most importantly, in a process called oxidative phosphorylation (OXPHOS), mitochondria produce most of the cellular energy to power all forms of biological processes.

Mutations in nuclear and mitochondrial DNA can cause mitochondrial dysfunction leading to primary mitochondrial diseases (PMD). This chapter focuses on PMD with cardiac involvement.

PMD can present with few or many symptoms in almost every organ system, at any moment from birth into adulthood.

Cardiac abnormalities are present in up to 60% of patients with PMD [1] and can be fatal if not properly recognized and managed.

When considering the age at presentation, the following prevalence (per 100,000 individuals) can be assumed: 5–15 patients with childhood-onset PMD and 10–15 patients with adult-onset PMD [2].

Recently several excellent reviews have been published on mitochondrial disease in general [2–5] as well as on cardiac involvement in mitochondrial disease [6–9].

Etiology

Mitochondria are present in all nucleated cells of the human body. They fulfill a pivotal role in various metabolic pathways, calcium signaling, and apoptosis. However, their main function is the production of cellular energy, stored in adenosine triphosphate (ATP), in a process called oxidative phosphorylation (OXPHOS). OXPHOS encompasses the transfer of electrons to oxygen by the mitochondrial respiratory chain. The respiratory chain consists of a series of protein complexes (complex I-IV) in the inner mitochondrial membrane, assisted by two mobile electron carriers, ubiquinone (coenzyme Q10) and cytochrome C [2]. Finally, the respiratory chain generates a proton gradient that drives ATP production by ATP synthase (complex V). Figure 11.1 provides a schematic overview of mitochondrial structure and OXPHOS.

About 1500 proteins are required for normal mitochondrial function; only around 100 are directly involved in OXPHOS. Most of these proteins are encoded by nuclear DNA, but some (approximately 1%) are encoded by mitochondrial DNA (mtDNA). The mtDNA consists of 16.6 kb circular double-stranded DNA, encoding 13 proteins essential for OXPHOS (complex I, III, IV, and V) and 24 different RNAs [6].

Mutations in nuclear or mitochondrial DNA can cause mitochondrial dysfunction leading to PMD, either by directly affecting the proteins involved in OXPHOS, but also through dysfunction of mtDNA maintenance, fissure and fusion, defects of mitochondrial DNA translation and protein synthesis, and impaired synthesis of cofactors of vitamins [5].

Because of the two types of genomes, hundreds of proteins and myriad of biochemical processes involved, PMD represent a group of diseases that are characterized by clinical, biochemical, and genetic heterogeneity. They can affect any organ system, at any age, with any inheritance pattern. Typically, PMD is progressive conditions that affect one or more organs with high energy demand (brain, heart, muscle, kidney, liver, eyes).

Clinical Presentation

Cardiologists become involved in the clinical care for patients with PMD either in case of cardiac symptoms as the presenting feature of PMD or to evaluate cardiac involvement in a patient with a known/suspected PMD.

A. C. Blank (✉) · Johannes M. P. J. Breur
S. A. Fuchs · K. Koop
Division Pediatrics, Wilhelmina Children's Hospital, University Medical Center Utrecht, Utrecht, The Netherlands
e-mail: A.C.Blank@umcutrecht.nl

A. F. Baas
Department of Genetics, University Medical Center Utrecht, Utrecht, The Netherlands

H. F. Baars et al. (eds.), *Clinical Cardiogenetics*, https://doi.org/10.1007/978-3-030-45457-9_11

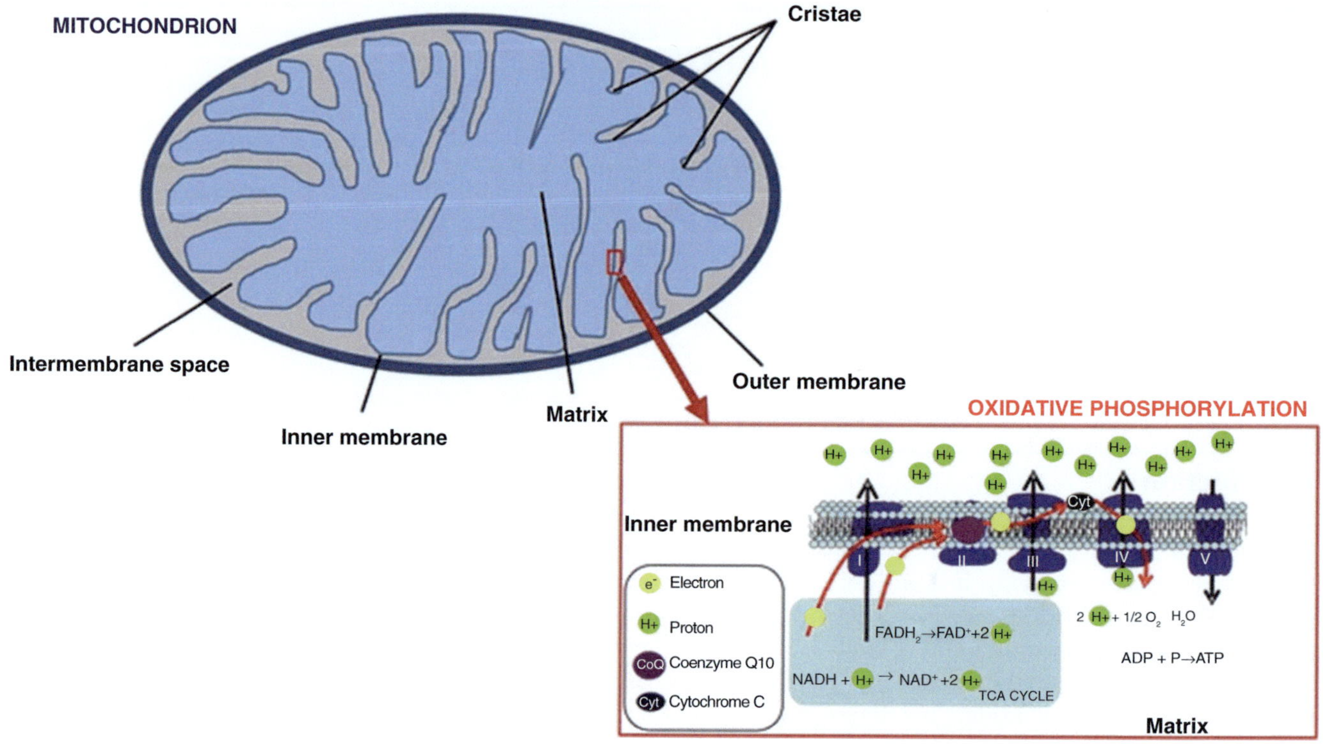

Fig. 11.1 Schematic overview of mitochondrial structure and oxidative phosphorylation (OXPHOS). Reproduced with permission from [10]

Although PMD can present at any moment from birth into late adulthood, there are roughly two age peaks of presentation. The first peak occurs in the first 3 years of life. The second peak spans from the last years of adolescence into early adulthood.

Early childhood-onset PMD is generally severe with multi-system involvement. Patients typically have hypotonia, feeding problems, failure to thrive, exercise intolerance, seizures, and encephalopathy [2]. PMD in adolescents and adults is also characterized by multi-system involvement, although single-organ infestation might occur, for example, isolated eye involvement in Leber hereditary optic neuropathy (LHON) [2]. Cardiac involvement is seen in 40% of children [11] and 31% of adults [12] at first presentation, with cardiomyopathy, arrhythmias, and conduction defects being the three main cardiac disease manifestations.

Patients may be asymptomatic or might present with symptoms of exercise intolerance, dyspnea, chest pain, palpitations, syncope, and occasionally, sudden death (see case presentation, Fig. 11.2).

Cardiac symptoms may be the only presenting sign, but signs of other system involvement should be actively looked for. Nervous system involvement is common with the following neurological symptoms: developmental delay or regression, hypotonia, seizures, irritability, microcephaly, abnormal reflexes, muscle weakness, vision and hearing disturbances, spasticity, dystonia/dyskinesia, and ataxia. Figure 11.3 provides an overview of all clinical manifestations of PMD.

In the era before widespread and early use of genetic diagnostics, some clinical mitochondrial syndromes could be recognized by the constellation of clinical symptoms. Some of these syndromes are characterized by prominent cardiac involvement. Well-known examples are Barth syndrome, Sengers syndrome, and MELAS. Now that genetic techniques have advanced, new mutations causing mitochondrial disease are continuously being discovered. Moreover, it is now clear that the genetic background of the known "classical" mitochondrial syndromes is diverse, with multiple genes leading to the same clinical syndrome (e.g., Leigh syndrome can be caused by mutations in more than 70 different genes), and mutations in the same gene can lead to a spectrum of clinical phenotypes.

Because of this diversity, it is not possible to describe the "typical" clinical presentation of PMDs. Instead, we will illustrate some of the hallmarks of mitochondrial disease using one of the classical mitochondrial syndromes, MELAS. A list of classical syndromes with cardiac involvement is shown in Table 11.1.

MELAS

Mitochondrial encephalopathy, lactic acidosis, and stroke-like episodes (MELAS) are caused by an mtDNA mutation affecting—in most cases—the gene that encodes the mitochondrial leucine transfer RNA.

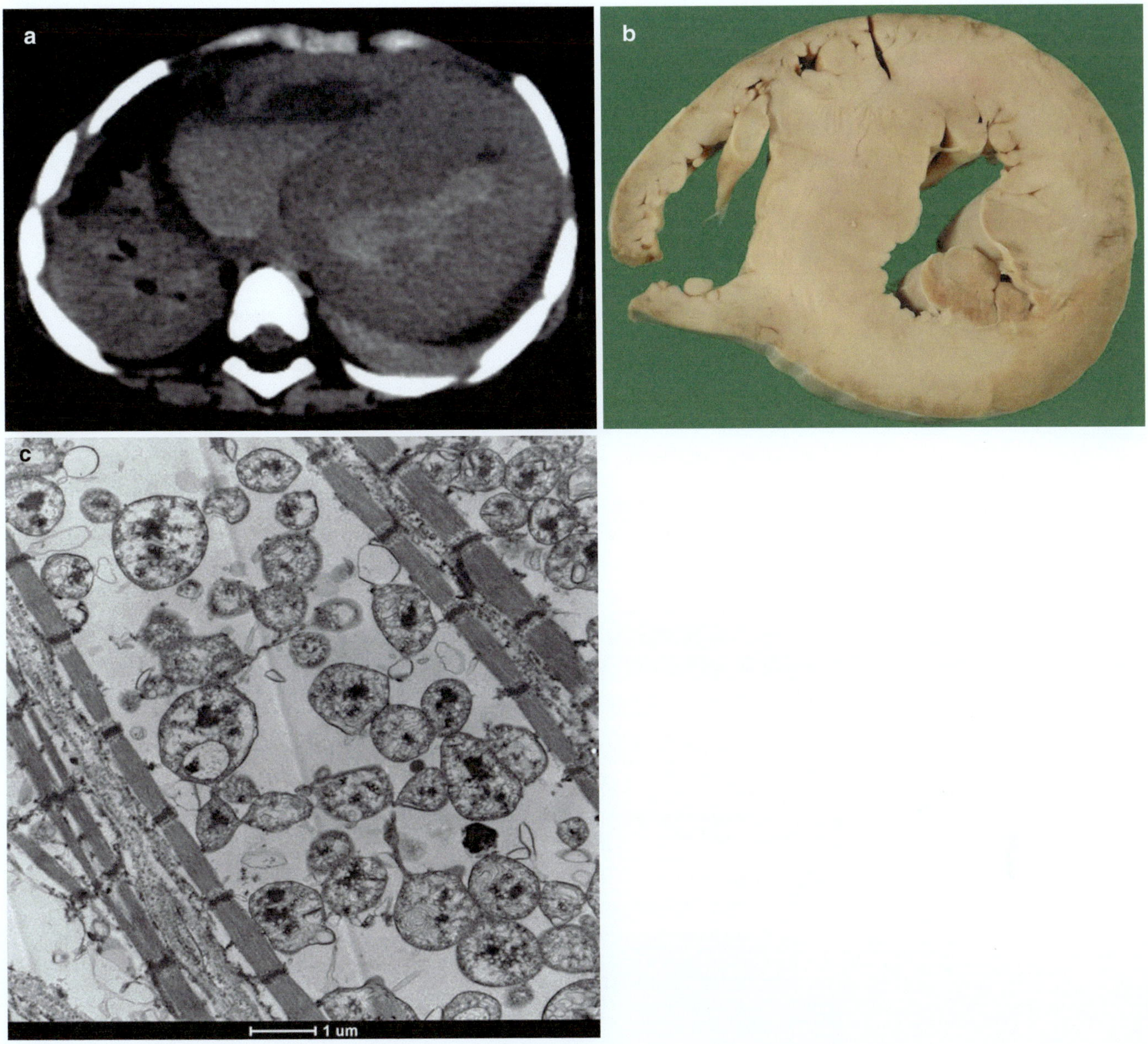

Fig. 11.2 Case presentation. (**a**) Postmortem CT thorax, (**b**) Short axis slice autopsy heart, (**c**) Postmortem electron microscopy of heart muscle

A 15-month-old girl presented in shock at the emergency department of a local hospital. Resuscitation was not successful, and the girl died. Autopsy showed mild facial dysmorphia (broad nasal bridge, upturned nasal tip), mild liver enlargement due to steatosis, and an extreme enlarged heart with severe left ventricular hypertrophy and mild right ventricular hypertrophy (Fig. 11.2a, b). Electron microscopy of heart muscle revealed swollen mitochondria (Fig. 11.2c). In the week before presentation the girl was not "feeling well" and cried easily. One day before presentation the girl drank less well and had fewer wet diapers. The parents were healthy, family history was unremarkable (paternal grandfather had hypercholesterolemia), pregnancy and birth were normal. The girl had a history of mild feeding problems (could not drink large volumes, could not tolerate solid food, even when mashed), and normal motor development. Her speech development was mildly delayed since she babbled but did not use words.

Trio-WES identified a homozygous missense mutation c.467T-G in the MRPL44 gene, resulting in p. Leu156Arg substitution. ClinVar search revealed that the mutation was described earlier in two patients, daughters of non-consanguineous Finnish parents, with HCM and liver steatosis [33]. Patient 1 died of cardiac failure upon a respiratory infection at the age of 6 months, whereas patient 2 was an asymptomatic adolescent. The MRPL44 gene was shown to encode a protein in the large subunit of the mitochondrial ribosome. In patient fibroblasts, decreased MRLP44 affected assembly of the large ribosomal subunit leading to OXPHOS/RC complex IV deficiency [33].

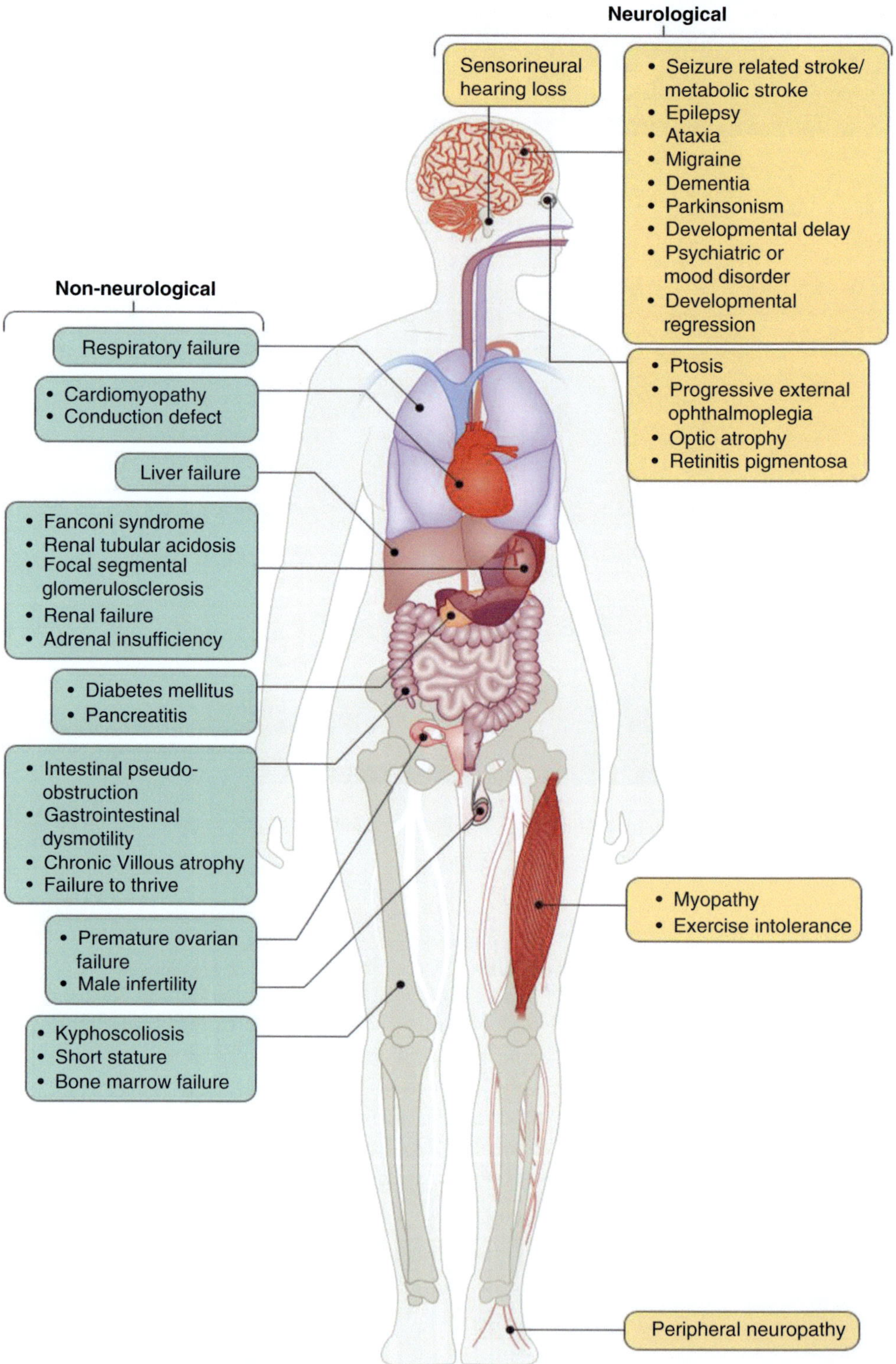

Fig. 11.3 Clinical presentations of primary mitochondrial diseases. Reproduced with permission from [2]

Patients often have normal development initially, but typically present with symptoms including headache, vomiting, and seizures between 2 and 10 years of age. Seizures may be accompanied or followed by stroke-like episodes resulting in hemiparesis or cortical blindness. These transient, but recurrent episodes can lead to chronic impairment and eventually encephalopathy. Events may be triggered by infections.

Eventually, other organ systems will be involved with exercise intolerance, muscle weakness, progressive hearing impairment, developmental delay, short stature, gastrointes-

Table 11.1 Clinical syndromes of primary mitochondrial disease with cardiac involvement

Clinical syndrome	Age of onset	Extra-cardiac clinical features	Cardiac features	Genetic basis	Reference
Barth syndrome	Infancy	Myopathy Neutropenia Short stature	In 70%: most often DCM, often with EFE, also LVNC, rarely HCM VT, VF Low threshold for ICD if symptoms or EPS suggest VT	nDNA, *TAZ* gene on X-chromosome	[9]
Leigh syndrome (subacute necrotizing encephalopathy)	Infancy	Ataxia Encephalopathy Seizures Failure to thrive Intention tremor Hypotonia Lactic acidosis Myopathy Optic atrophy Nystagmus Psychomotor delay	HCM, DCM Bradycardia Ventricular preexcitation	mtDNA and nDNA, many mutations	[13]
Sengers syndrome	Infancy	Congenital cataract Myopathy Lactic acidosis Almost always fatal!	HCM, DCM Ventricular preexcitation	nDNA, homozygous or compound heterozygous mutations in *AGK* gene	[9]
Mitochondrial encephalomyopathy, lactic acidosis and stroke-like episodes (MELAS)	Childhood to adulthood	Diabetes mellitus Seizures Exercise intolerance Lactic acidosis Hearing loss Myopathy Short stature Stroke-like episodes Sudden death	In 50%: HCM, without LVOTO, later DCM, LVNC, RCM First-degree AV block IV conduction block Ventricular preexcitation (in ~15%) PVC's (>15/h) SCD	mtDNA, point mutations (m.3243A>G in 80%; m.3256C>T, m.3271T>C, m.4332G>A, m.135513G>A, m.13514A>G)	[9, 12, 13]
Myoclonus, epilepsy and ragged red fibers (MERRF)	Childhood to adolescence	Ataxia Seizures Hearing loss Myopathy Myoclonus Spasticity	In 40%: HCM, DCM, HiCM Ventricular preexcitation	mtDNA, point mutations (m.8344A>G most common; m.8356T>C, m.12147G>A)	[9, 13]
Neuropathy, ataxia and retinitis pigmentosa (NARP)	Childhood to adulthood	Ataxia Dementia Seizures Hearing loss Myopathy Peripheral neuropathy Vision loss	HCM	mtDNA, point mutations (m.8993T>G, m.8933T>C)	[9, 13]

(continued)

Table 11.1 (continued)

Clinical syndrome	Age of onset	Extra-cardiac clinical features	Cardiac features	Genetic basis	Reference
Kearns–Sayre syndrome (KSS)	Adolescence	Ataxia Deafness Delayed puberty Diabetes mellitus Ophtalmoplegia Myopathy Renal dysfunction Short stature Sudden death in ~10%	In >50%: HCM, DCM First- to third-degree AV block IV conduction block: mostly LAHB, RBBB Ventricular preexcitation SCD in up to 20% AFib Low threshold for PM implantation, this may precipitate TdP, consider preventive ICD placement	mtDNA, single large heteroplasmic deletion	[9, 12–14]
Leber hereditary optic neuropathy (LHON)	Adolescence to adulthood	Central scotoma Optic atrophy Postural tremor Peripheral neuropathy Multiple sclerosis-like illness	HCM, LVNC Ventricular preexcitation	mtDNA, point mutations, homoplasmic (m.11778G>A, m.14484T>C, m.3460A>G)	[9, 13, 15]
Chronic progressive external ophtalmoplegia (CPEO)	Adulthood	Dysphagia Exercise intolerance Hearing loss Myopathy Opthalmoplegia Parkinsonism Ptosis	HCM	mtDNA and nDNA, many mutations	[13]
Maternally inherited diabetes and deafness (MIDD)	Adulthood	Diabetes Exercise intolerance Hearing loss Muscular atrophy Myopathy Renal failure	HCM Ventricular preexcitation	mtDNA	[13]

AGK acylglycerol kinase, *AFib* atrial fibrillation, *DCM* dilated cardiomyopathy, *EFE* endocardial fibroelastosis, *HCM* hypertrophic cardiomyopathy, *HiCM* histiocytoid cardiomyopathy, *ICD* implantable cardiac defibrillator, *LAHB* left anterior hemiblock, *LVNC* left ventricular non-compaction, *RCM* restrictive cardiomyopathy, *SCD* sudden cardiac death, *TdP* torsade de pointes, *VT* ventricular tachycardia, *VF* ventricular fibrillation

tinal dysmotility, nephropathy, and diabetes mellitus as possible manifestations.

Cardiac manifestations include arrhythmias, conduction defects, and cardiomyopathy, mostly of the hypertrophic type.

Disease severity is dependent on the level of mutation load in the involved tissues (see section Molecular Diagnosis) which may lead to different clinical presentation of phenotype, even among affected family members.

Curative therapy is not available. Supportive therapy includes supplementation of arginine (precursor of nitrogen oxide that may prevent or ameliorate stroke-like episodes), CoQ10 and carnitine. In contrast, valproic acid as antiepileptic drug, as well as aminoglycoside antibiotics should be avoided.

Clinical Diagnosis

The diagnostic process starts with a detailed history and family history followed by a systematic physical examination. Signs of multisystem involvement should be actively searched for. Mitochondrial disease should be suspected when ≥2 organs are involved. In addition to cardiac and neurological involvement look for:

- gastrointestinal involvement: feeding difficulties, vomiting, failure to thrive
- liver involvement: (neonatal) cholestasis, elevated serum liver enzymes, hypoglycemia
- renal involvement: elevated serum creatinine, albuminuria, hematuria, aciduria

- endocrinological involvement: elevated serum glucose, decreased thyroid function

Figure 11.3 provides an overview of all clinical manifestations of PMD.

Additionally, history taking should focus on deterioration, prolonged clinical course, or excessive symptoms associated with energy-consuming periods or triggers (e.g., infectious diseases, vaccinations, exercise).

Special attention should be given to the possibility of maternal inheritance. Consanguinity should be noted.

A comprehensive physical examination, including evaluation by an ophthalmologist and neurologist, should be performed in case of suspected PMD. Based on the findings, this can be supplemented by vision and hearing tests, development or exercise tests, and/or imaging of liver, spleen, kidney, and brain.

Cardiac evaluation includes 12-lead electrography (ECG) and transthoracic echocardiography. The echocardiogram should examine ventricular wall thickness, ventricular cavity size, left ventricular (LV) systolic and diastolic function, LV outflow obstruction (LVOTO), and valve abnormalities [16]. In the case of a poor echo window, other imaging modalities as transesophageal echocardiography, cardiac magnetic resonance (CMR), or cardiac computed tomography (CT) should be considered.

Hypertrophic cardiomyopathy (HCM) is the most common form of cardiomyopathy, followed by dilated cardiomyopathy (DCM) and left ventricular non-compaction (LVNC). Rarely, restrictive or histiocytoid cardiomyopathy is encountered.

Hypertrophic cardiomyopathy is diagnosed if imaging reveals unexplained left ventricular wall thickening >15 mm or >+2 Z-score (interventricular septum and/or left ventricular posterior wall). HCM in PMD is typically characterized by concentric hypertrophy without LVOTO. The development of LV systolic dysfunction is more common than in sarcomeric HCM [7]. Very rarely, asymmetric hypertrophy, right ventricular hypertrophy, or LVOTO due to systolic anterior motion of the mitral valve (SAM) or mid-left ventricular cavity obstruction can be seen [1]. In borderline cases, myocardial deformation imaging with speckle tracking may detect subclinical cardiac involvement. CMR is the gold standard for the evaluation of LV and RV function and for detection of fibrosis (when combined with late gadolinium enhancement (LGE)). The pattern and extent of LGE might point into the direction of a specific PMD. For example, MELAS patients have focal intramural LGE diffusely distributed over all LV segments [17].

Dilated cardiomyopathy is less often seen, in approximately 30% of all cases with cardiomyopathy, and is defined by the presence of unexplained left ventricular (LV) dilatation with LV end-diastolic volumes or diameters (>+2 Z-score) and systolic dysfunction. DCM often develops as a secondary consequence of preexisting HCM [9].

Twelve-lead ECG will show abnormalities in 68% of all cases [1] with T-wave inversion (negative T wave in V6) being the most common ECG abnormality, sometimes found as first sign of cardiac involvement [7]. Other abnormal ECG findings are all degrees of atrioventricular (AV) block, left or right bundle branch block, left anterior hemiblock, nonspecific intraventricular conduction delay, ventricular preexcitation, prolonged corrected QT interval, left ventricular hypertrophy (LVH), pathologic Q waves, and ST-segment depression. Where patients with CPEO/KSS typically show right bundle branch block with T-wave inversion, MELAS patients have pathologic Q waves, LVH, left bundle branch block, and ST/T changes [17]. Holter ECG will facilitate the diagnosis of conduction defects and arrhythmias.

Patients with ventricular preexcitation may develop AV-reentry tachycardia or atrial fibrillation. Other arrhythmias found in patients with PMD are premature ventricular contractions, ventricular tachycardia, and ventricular fibrillation.

Although a detailed clinical evaluation will help to support the diagnosis of a PMD, it is difficult to make a definitive diagnosis without the help of molecular and genetic investigations. With the improvement of genetic techniques, genetic evaluation has claimed a prominent place in the diagnostic process and should be considered early or even upfront. The case presentation (Fig. 11.2) illustrates how genetic techniques help to elucidate PMD as a cause of hypertrophic cardiomyopathy.

Specific laboratory findings associated with mitochondrial dysfunction involve elevated lactate concentrations in plasma (although easily falsely elevated by blood withdrawal or pre-analysis conditions) and cerebrospinal fluid (more specific). Among metabolic analyses, abnormal urinary organic acids (lactate, tricarboxylic acid cycle intermediates) and elevated plasma amino acids (alanine, proline) and pipecolinic acid may be found. To further screen for organ dysfunction and to evaluate other differential diagnostic possibilities, basic laboratory tests should also include acid–base status, hematology, basic chemistry (ammonia, CK, CK–MB, transaminases, renal function tests, basic hormone screens). Basic metabolic analysis should involve screening for other disorders in energy metabolism (fatty acid oxidation disorders, glycogen storage disorders), storage diseases, and congenital disorders of glycosylation.

The diagnosis of PMD can be further supported by abnormal findings in an oral glucose tolerance test or muscle biopsy. However, these tests are invasive and time-consuming, and do not yield a molecular/genetic diagnosis. In this era of genetic technological possibilities, we therefore advocate genetic testing (specific gene, gene-panel, or untargeted (whole exome/genome sequencing) early in the diagnostic process, especially in acute settings.

When the diagnosis is not straightforward, especially in acute or life-threatening disease, tissue biopsy should be considered, also for further biological elucidation of potentially novel genetic defects. Skin biopsies are easy to obtain with local anesthesia. However, the disease phenotype of PMDs is not always apparent in fibroblasts. More invasive diagnostic procedures (muscle biopsy or other tissues depending on the clinical signs) should be considered in parallel with genetic testing if urgent diagnosis is needed.

If PMD is suspected, a metabolic specialist should be consulted, together with other specialists, depending on the organ systems affected. Often these will include neurologists, geneticists, ophthalmologists, ENT specialists, and physiotherapists.

The Mitochondrial Medicine Society provided a consensus statement on the diagnosis of mitochondrial disease [18].

Differential Diagnosis

The differential diagnosis of multi-system involvement is broad and comprises other metabolic disorders, systemic autoimmune rheumatic disease, systemic infections, malignancies, and intoxications. The diagnosis of specific cardiac phenotypes might narrow the list of potential causes. HCM is caused by mutations in genes encoding sarcomere proteins, inborn errors of metabolism, neuromuscular disorders, and syndromic diseases. DCM is caused by myocarditis, mutations in genes encoding sarcomere proteins, neuromuscular disorders, drugs, toxins, nutritional deficiencies, electrolyte disturbances, endocrine disease, and autoimmune disease.

From the inborn errors of metabolism fatty acid oxidation disorders (FAO), storage disorders, disorders of glycosylation, and PRKAG2 syndrome should be considered.

FAO, especially long-chain 3-hydroxyacyl-CoA dehydrogenase deficiency (LCHADD) and very long-chain acyl-CoA dehydrogenase deficiency (VLCADD), may present with arrhythmias, cardiomyopathy, and sudden cardiac arrest. Storage disorders, especially Pompe (GSD 2) and Danon disease, may show HCM, ventricular preexcitation, multisystem involvement, and developmental delay. Congenital disorders of glycosylation can present with HCM in combination with pericardial effusion, sometimes leading to cardiac tamponade. PRKAG2 syndrome is characterized by HCM, ventricular preexcitation, arrhythmias, and high-grade AV block.

Molecular Diagnosis

Inheritance

In mitochondrial disease, different modes of inheritance are observed, as the mtDNA is exclusively maternally inherited and diseases due to nDNA mutations follow a Mendelian inheritance pattern (i.e., autosomal dominant (AD), autosomal recessive (AR), and X-linked (XL)). The maternal inheritance pattern of mtDNA defects is a result of the fact that the mammalian egg contains about 100,000 copies mitochondrial mtDNA, while the sperm head only contains approximately 100 copies.

DNA Testing

When a patient is suspected of a mitochondrial disease based on clinical presentation, biochemical screening, and/or histopathological studies, DNA analysis of both the mtDNA and nDNA should be considered. If a maternal inheritance pattern is observed, mtDNA should be analyzed. Since the load of mutated mtDNA may vary between tissues, different input materials can be considered, including blood, urine, and saliva. When the inheritance pattern is unsure, both the mtDNA and the genes of the nDNA encoding mitochondrial proteins should be sequenced. In the era of next-generation sequencing, for the nDNA genes, targeted panels, as well as whole-exome sequencing (WES), are available. For variant interpretation, it is highly recommended to simultaneously test the parents of the proband (trio-WES).

Genotype–Phenotype Correlations

The mtDNA can be identical, defined as homoplasmy, or a mixture of two or more types, defined as heteroplasmy. Most mutations in the mtDNA are present in a subset of mtDNA copies, and therefore the cell contains a mixture of normal and mutant mitochondria (heteroplasmy). When the cell divides, the mitochondria are randomly distributed. Therefore, the percentage of mutant mtDNA can differ in different organs and tissues. As a result, the phenotype of mitochondrial disease can be very heterogeneous. The phenotype of mitochondrial disease caused by nDNA mutations is generally more homogeneous, however, as in most genetic diseases, variable expression is usually observed. Due to the rare prevalence and the many different genes involved, genotype–phenotype studies in mitochondrial disease due to nDNA mutations are hampered.

Therapy

General Management

The Mitochondrial Medicine Society has provided consensus statements on the management of mitochondrial disease

[18, 31]. In general, there is no curative therapy available and management is mainly supportive. Because of the multi-organ involvement of PMD therapy is best provided by a multidisciplinary team. The current treatment options (reviewed in [19]) are symptomatic treatment (e.g., physiotherapy for hypotonia, cardiac pacing for conduction defects), exercise, diet, and the use of agents to improve mitochondrial function and to ameliorate the effects of mitochondrial dysfunction. These agents act in various ways: CoQ10, riboflavin, and thiamine enhance mitochondrial OXPHOS function, creatine provides an energy buffer, vitamin C, vitamin E, lipoic acid, cysteine donors, and EPI-743 act as antioxidant, amino acids such as arginine and citrulline restore nitric oxide production, elamipretide protects cardiolipin and bezafibrate, epicatechin, and RTA 408 enhance mitochondrial biogenesis [19]. Idebenone, a CoQ10 analog, has been shown beneficial in the treatment of Leber hereditary optic neuropathy (LHON). Since the field of mitochondrial disease is advancing rapidly a mitochondrial expertise center may be contacted to inform about (upcoming trials of) new therapies.

Though some treatment options (e.g., supplementation with thiamin, riboflavin, biotin, and CoQ10) can be employed empirically to all (critically ill) patients with PMD [20]), others are guided by a specific molecular diagnosis. For example, ketogenic diet is advised in mitochondrial diseases caused by complex I defects.

Another aim in the management of mitochondrial disease is the prevention of clinical exacerbations. Patients with mitochondrial disease can develop metabolic dysregulation during and after anesthesia, operations, and intercurrent illness. Preoperative fasting should be minimized, and patients should be provided with enough intravenous glucose to maintain normoglycemia. Caution must be used with various certain inhalation anesthetics, muscle relaxants, and propofol (reviewed by [21]).

Beside anesthetic medication, other classes of drugs can aggravate mitochondrial disease, and should be used with caution. Examples include antiepileptics as valproic acid, topiramate and vigabatrin, aminoglycoside antibiotics, the antidiabetic metformin, the beta-blockers carvedilol, metoprolol [22] and propranolol, the class III anti-arrhythmic amiodarone and statins [21].

Management of Cardiac Involvement

The therapy of mitochondrial cardiomyopathies follows the current guidelines [23, 24], and comprises a combination of diuretics, an angiotensin-converting enzyme inhibitor, and a beta-blocker. Choosing the right beta-blocker for a patient with PMD is difficult. As mentioned earlier, the beta-blockers carvedilol, metoprolol, and propranolol are reported to inhibit mitochondrial function. In vitro data showed a correlation to lipophilicity [25]. The high-lipophilic beta-blocker propranol caused the highest inhibition. The low-lipophilic atenolol showed no inhibition, making it a safe first choice. Cardiac device therapy should follow the current guidelines [26].

Risk Stratification

In childhood-onset PMD, mortality is higher in younger patients and in those with cardiomyopathy. Holmgren et al. described 71% mortality in patients with cardiomyopathy compared to 26% in those without [27]. When measured at the age of 16 years, Scaglia et al. observed 16% survival in patients with cardiomyopathy, and 95% in patients without cardiomyopathy [11]. Age at first symptoms is a major prognostic factor for mortality. Infants presenting before 6 months of age have a tenfold increased risk of mortality compared with those presenting later [28].

For HCM a risk model/calculator has been developed in Europe comprising age at evaluation, family history of SCD, maximal LV wall thickness, fractional shortening, left atrial diameter, maximal LV outflow tract gradient, non-sustained ventricular tachycardia, and unexplained syncope [23]. Unfortunately, this model/calculator has not been validated for pediatric patients (<16 years) and for patients with metabolic and syndromic HCM. Norris et al. found the following imaging findings associated with increased SCD in childhood: increased left atrial size, increased mitral E/E′ ratio, reduced global longitudinal strain, and increased LGE [29].

Recommendations During Pregnancy and Delivery

Women with mitochondrial disease are likely to experience a variable clinical course before, during, and after pregnancy with an increased risk for cardiac deterioration, preterm delivery, preeclampsia, and toxicity from magnesium sulfate (given for preeclampsia) [30].

General and Specific Recommendations, ICD Recommendations, Follow-Up Advice

The following recommendations are derived from the Patient care standards of the Mitochondrial Medicine Society [31].

1. Care at a tertiary center with metabolic and cardiology expertise in mitochondrial diseases is preferred.
2. Follow-up evaluation should include clinical assessment, blood pressure measurement, ECG, and echocardiography every 12 months for at least 3 years.

- Earlier follow-up is suggested for those with new-onset cardiac symptoms or those at higher risk.
- Extension of this 12-month interval may be considered after consultation of a clinician experienced in the management of cardiac involvement. However, if the patient is stable for 3 years, ECG and echocardiography may be extended to every 2–3 years with return to yearly follow-up (or more frequently) if cardiac deterioration is suspected.
- In asymptomatic mutation carriers, the interval of follow-up should be according to their risk of developing disease.

3. 24- to 48-hour ECG monitoring should be obtained every 1–2 years for all patients at high risk of preexcitation syndrome/conduction disease, patients with severely impaired left ventricular systolic function (left ventricular ejection-fraction <35%), patients with paroxysmal symptoms suggestive of cardiac involvement (palpitations), and patients with left ventricular systolic or diastolic dysfunction.
   - More frequent monitoring is needed in patients with large-scale mtDNA deletions due to the high risk of heart block and either of two of the more common pathogenic mtDNA mutations (m.3243A>G and m.8344A>G) owing to the high risk of ventricular preexcitation.
   - Ablation should be considered in supraventricular tachycardia, Wolff–Parkinson–White syndrome, or any arrhythmia potentially treatable by this technique.
   - A low threshold for pacemaker implantation is needed to prevent cardiac death. Pacemakers can be combined with implantable defibrillator if needed. An implantable cardioverter defibrillator is indicated in patients at risk of sudden death, when the left ventricle wall thickness is >30 mm, and in patients with ventricular tachycardia (sustained and non-sustained).
4. Cardiac magnetic resonance imaging is indicated in patients with inconclusive echocardiographic images to identify structural remodeling, to quantify abnormalities more precisely prior to starting a treatment and when invasive therapies like septal myectomy are considered.
5. Other cardiovascular risk factors should be assessed and treated accordingly.
6. Exercise testing and/or stress echocardiography should be performed under close monitoring to assess functional capacity, response to therapy, and exercise-induced dynamic left ventricular outflow tract obstruction. This test should not be performed in all patients; the potential health risks (exercise intolerance, metabolic decompensation) should be weighed against the expected benefits of such a test.
7. If physical activity is possible, the intensity of the physical activity should be prescribed by the cardiology team, according to the limitations of their cardiac function.
8. In the setting of end-stage heart failure, transplantation may be considered. Decisions to list a patient for transplant should be taken in the light of other comorbidities and the known natural history of the specific mitochondrial disease.

Family Screening

Cascade Molecular Screening

When a molecular defect is identified it is essential to analyze close relatives in order to identify other family members at risk of PMD. Depending on the inheritance pattern, different family members can qualify for predictive DNA testing. For instance, if an mtDNA mutation is identified, only individuals in the maternal line are selected and children of male carriers do not require a DNA test. If biallelic mutations are identified in an autosomal recessive gene, siblings can be analyzed.

In case of a variant of unknown significance (VUS) close family members can be analyzed in order to obtain more information about its character. For instance, a de novo variant in a proband in an autosomal dominant gene is often considered likely pathogenic if the parents do not show signs of disease. Also demonstrating that a VUS and a pathogenic mutation in the same autosomal recessive gene are biallelic and carried by both parents may raise suspicion of pathogenicity of the VUS.

Cascade Clinical Screening

When mitochondrial disease is still highly suspected and no causative mutation is identified in the proband, clinical evaluation may be considered in first-degree relatives. This may involve biochemical screening, including the determination of plasma lactate and amino acids, blood glucose, urine organic acids, depending on the abnormalities found in the proband. If cardiomyopathy is the main feature in the proband, periodic cardiological evaluations should be considered.

Follow-Up Advice

When mitochondrial disease is identified in a family member, in general similar follow-up advice as to the proband is given.

Family Planning

Once the pathogenic mutation has been identified in an affected family member in the nDNA, prenatal testing and preimplantation genetic diagnosis for PMD are possible. Interpretation of prenatal diagnostic results is complex in PMD due to an mtDNA mutation because the mutational load in the tissues sampled (i.e., amniocytes and chorionic villi) may not correspond to that of the fetal tissues. Moreover, the mutational load may shift in utero or after birth as a result of random mitotic segregation. For de novo mtDNA point mutations, recurrence risks are low and prenatal testing can be offered. Prenatal testing is also an option for female carriers with low mutational load [32]. Using preimplantation genetic diagnosis, embryos with a mutant load below a mutation-specific or general expression threshold of 18% can be transferred [32].

Alternatively, oocyte donation will prevent the transmission of mtDNA.

Summary

Primary mitochondrial diseases (PMD) are caused by mitochondrial dysfunction due to mutations in nuclear or mitochondrial DNA. Cardiac involvement is present in the majority of patients with cardiomyopathy, arrhythmias, and conduction defects being most prevalent. Hypertrophic cardiomyopathy is the most frequently encountered cardiomyopathy in PMD but also dilated cardiomyopathy and left ventricular non-compaction can occur. Cardiac symptoms may be the presenting sign of PMD or can be found when screening patients with suspected PMD. Early-onset PMD (0–3 years) is generally more severe with multi-organ involvement than late-onset PMD (adolescence/early adulthood).

Where PMD like Barth syndrome, Sengers syndrome, and MELAS used to be clinical diagnoses, DNA analysis plays an increasingly important role early in the diagnostic process and should be performed as soon as PMD or a mitochondrial cardiomyopathy is suspected. Since mitochondria, and thus mutant mitochondrial DNA, are randomly distributed during the cell cycle, disease and phenotype may vary greatly.

Treatment for mitochondrial cardiomyopathies is mainly supportive and comprises a combination of diuretics, an angiotensin-converting enzyme inhibitor, a beta-blocker, preferably atenolol, and cardiac device therapy. Furthermore, an increasing number of supplements are being used to improve mitochondrial function and to ameliorate the effects of mitochondrial dysfunction. Despite supportive therapy mortality in mitochondrial cardiomyopathy remains high (up to 84%) and is inversely related to age at presentation.

Take-Home Message

Mitochondrial cardiomyopathies are rare but highly lethal, especially when diagnosed early in life. They are always part of a primary mitochondrial disease and should be considered in patients with multi-organ involvement. DNA analysis is key in establishing the correct diagnosis. Therapy is mainly supportive.

References

1. Limongelli G, Tome-Esteban M, Dejthevaporn C, Rahman S, Hanna MG, Elliott PM. Prevalence and natural history of heart disease in adults with primary mitochondrial respiratory chain disease. Eur J Heart Fail. 2010;12:114–21.
2. Gorman GS, Chinnery PF, DiMauro S, Hirano M, Koga Y, McFarland R, Suomalainen A, Thorburn DR, Zeviani M, Turnbull DM. Mitochondrial diseases. Nat Rev Dis Prim. 2016;2:1–23.
3. Davison JE, Rahman S. Recognition, investigation and management of mitochondrial disease. Arch Dis Child. 2017;102(11):1082–90.
4. Muraresku CC, McCormick EM, Falk MJ. Mitochondrial disease: advances in clinical diagnosis, management, therapeutic development, and preventative strategies. Curr Genet Med Rep. 2018;6:62–72.
5. Rahman J, Rahman S. Mitochondrial medicine in the omics era. Lancet. 2018;391:2560–74.
6. El-Hattab AW, Scaglia F. Mitochondrial Cardiomyopathies. Front Cardiovasc Med. 2016;3:1–9.
7. Limongelli G, Masarone D, Pacileo G. Education in heart mitochondrial disease and the heart. Heat. 2017; 103(5):390–8.
8. Enns GM. Pediatric mitochondrial diseases and the heart. Curr Opin Pediatr. 2017;29(5):541–51.
9. Keogh MJ, Steele HE, Chinnery PF. Mitochondrial cardiovascular diseases. In: Kumar D, Elliott P, editors. Cardiovascular genetics and genomics. Cham: Springer; 2018. p. 239–58.
10. McCormick EM, Muraresku CC, Falk MJ. Mitochondrial genomics: a complex field now coming of age. Curr Genet Med Rep. 2018;6:52–61.
11. Scaglia F. Clinical spectrum, morbidity, and mortality in 113 pediatric patients with mitochondrial disease. Pediatrics. 2004;114:925–31.
12. Wahbi K, Bougouin W, Béhin A, et al. Long-term cardiac prognosis and risk stratification in 260 adults presenting with mitochondrial diseases. Eur Heart J. 2015;36:2886–93.
13. Hsu YHR, Yogasundaram H, Parajuli N, Valtuille L, Sergi C, Oudit GY. MELAS syndrome and cardiomyopathy: linking mitochondrial function to heart failure pathogenesis. Heart Fail Rev. 2016;21:103–16.
14. Khambatta S, Nguyen DL, Beckman TJ, Wittich CM. Kearns-Sayre syndrome: a case series of 35 adults and children. Int J Gen Med. 2014;7:325–32.
15. Govindaraj P, Khan NA, Rani B, et al. Mitochondrial DNA variations associated with hypertrophic cardiomyopathy. Mitochondrion. 2014;16:65–72.
16. Cardim N, Galderisi M, Edvardsen T, et al. Role of multimodality cardiac imaging in the management of patients with hypertrophic cardiomyopathy: an expert consensus of the European Association of Cardiovascular Imaging Endorsed by the Saudi Heart Association. Eur Heart J Cardiovasc Imaging. 2015;16:280.
17. Florian A, Ludwig A, Stubbe-Dräger B, Boentert M, Young P, Waltenberger J, Rösch S, Sechtem U, Yilmaz A. Characteristic cardiac phenotypes are detected by cardiovascular magnetic resonance in patients with different clinical phenotypes and genotypes of mitochondrial myopathy. J Cardiovasc Magn Reson. 2015;17:1–11.
18. Parikh S, Goldstein A, Koenig MK, et al. Diagnosis and management of mitochondrial disease: a consensus statement from the Mitochondrial Medicine Society. Genet Med. 2015;17:689–701.
19. El-Hattab AW, Zarante AM, Almannai M, Scaglia F. Therapies for mitochondrial diseases and current clinical trials. Mol Genet Metab. 2017;122:1–9.

20. Distelmaier F, Haack TB, Wortmann SB, Mayr JA, Prokisch H. Treatable mitochondrial diseases: cofactor metabolism and beyond. Brain. 2017;140:e11.
21. Finsterer J, Segall L. Drugs interfering with mitochondrial disorders. Drug Chem Toxicol. 2010;33:138–51.
22. Samuels C, Koenig MK, Hernandez M. Mitochondrial disorder aggravated by metoprolol. Case Rep Pediatr. 2016;2016:1–3.
23. Zamorano JL, Anastasakis A, Borger MA, et al. 2014 ESC guidelines on diagnosis and management of hypertrophic cardiomyopathy: the task force for the diagnosis and management of hypertrophic cardiomyopathy of the European Society of Cardiology (ESC). Eur Heart J. 2014;35:2733–79.
24. Ponikowski P, Voors AA, Anker SD, et al. 2016 ESC Guidelines for the diagnosis and treatment of acute and chronic heart failure. Eur J Heart Fail. 2016;18:891–975.
25. Dreisbach AW, Greif RL, Lorenzo BJ, Reidenberg MM. Lipophilic beta-blockers inhibit rat skeletal muscle mitochondrial respiration. Pharmacology. 1993;47:295–9.
26. Brignole M, Auricchio A, Baron-Esquivias G, et al. 2013 ESC Guidelines on cardiac pacing and cardiac resynchronization therapy: the Task Force on cardiac pacing and resynchronization therapy of the European Society of Cardiology (ESC). Developed in collaboration with the European Heart Rhythm Association. Eur Heart J. 2013;34:2281–329.
27. Holmgren D, Wåhlander H, Eriksson BO, Oldfors A, Holme E, Tulinius M. Cardiomyopathy in children with mitochondrial disease: clinical course and cardiological findings. Eur Heart J. 2003;24:280–8.
28. Debray F-G, Lambert M, Chevalier I, Robitaille Y, Decarie J-C, Shoubridge EA, Robinson BH, Mitchell GA. Long-term outcome and clinical spectrum of 73 pediatric patients with mitochondrial diseases. Pediatrics. 2007;119:722–33.
29. Norrish G, Cantarutti N, Pissaridou E, Ridout DA, Limongelli G, Elliott PM, Kaski JP. Risk factors for sudden cardiac death in childhood hypertrophic cardiomyopathy: a systematic review and meta-analysis. Eur J Prev Cardiol. 2017;24:1220–30.
30. Say RE, Whittaker RG, Turnbull HE, McFarland R, Taylor RW, Turnbull DM. Mitochondrial disease in pregnancy: a systematic review. Obstet Med. 2011;4:90–4.
31. Parikh S, Goldstein A, Karaa A, et al. Patient care standards for primary mitochondrial disease: a consensus statement from the Mitochondrial Medicine Society. Genet Med. 2017; https://doi.org/10.1038/gim.2017.107.
32. Smeets HJM, Sallevelt SCEH, Dreesen JCFM, de Die-Smulders CEM, de Coo IFM. Preventing the transmission of mitochondrial DNA disorders using prenatal or preimplantation genetic diagnosis. Ann N Y Acad Sci. 2015;1350:29–36.
33. Carroll CJ, Isohanni P, Pöyhönen R, et al. Whole-exome sequencing identifies a mutation in the mitochondrial ribosome protein MRPL44 to underlie mitochondrial infantile cardiomyopathy. J Med Genet. 2013;50:151–9.

Part III

Inherited Arrhythmia Syndromes

12 Long QT Syndrome

Yanushi D. Wijeyeratne and Elijah R. Behr

Introduction

Long QT syndrome (LQTS) predisposes to life-threatening ventricular arrhythmias and sudden death. It is an inherited arrhythmia syndrome leading to prolongation of the repolarisation phase of the cardiac action potential. It may manifest as lengthening of the heart rate-corrected QT interval (QTc) on the surface electrocardiogram (ECG).

LQTS was first described as an autosomal recessive form with sensorineural deafness, the Jervell and Lange-Nielsen syndrome, and the autosomal dominant form, the Romano-Ward syndrome [1–3]. It was not until the 1990s that the molecular basis of the condition began to unravel through linkage studies and the subsequent identification of mutations in specific genes that encode cardiac ion channels [4–8].

The prevalence of LQTS amongst Caucasians is estimated to be 1:2000–1:2500 based upon a large study of neonatal ECGs and targeted genetic testing in nearly 45,000 Italian infants [9]. The clinically diagnosed prevalence in the general population is however likely to be less than 1:2000. This is because of incomplete penetrance with a large proportion of mutation carriers remaining asymptomatic throughout life and escaping detection. In others, the first presentation may be a fatal cardiac arrhythmia and the diagnosis made post-mortem. Indeed, LQTS is one of the most common causes of autopsy-negative sudden death, also known as sudden arrhythmic death syndrome (SADS), accounting for up to 20% of cases [10–12]. Patients with LQTS have been identified worldwide, although there is a paucity of cases reported amongst black ethnic groups [13].

This chapter will review the clinical presentation of LQTS, its diagnosis, and principles of management in the context of recent clinical advances and molecular genetics, with a focus on the most common forms of LQTS—LQT1, LQT2, and LQT3.

Aetiology/Pathophysiology

LQTS is most frequently caused by loss-of-function mutations of genes encoding cardiac potassium channels responsible for I_{Ks} and I_{Kr}, the slow and rapid rectifying currents, resulting in reduced outward potassium currents and a longer action potential duration (APD). The ion channel dysfunction is secondary to two distinct biophysical mechanisms. One is the failure of assembly and trafficking of the channel to the cell membrane resulting in haploinsufficiency. The other is successful trafficking to the membrane of defective channels with a dominant-negative effect (where channel α-subunits are organised in tetramers and mutant protein acts antagonistically to the wild-type protein). Gain-of-function mutations affecting the cardiac sodium channel and its interacting proteins may lengthen the plateau phase of the APD by increasing the late inward sodium current (late I_{Na}), whilst gain-of-function mutations affecting the calcium channel (I_{CaL}) may also occasionally be associated. Figure 12.1 depicts some of the cardiac ion channels and other proteins involved in different inherited arrhythmia syndromes, though not all of these are implicated in LQTS [14].

Molecular Genetics

Advances in molecular genetics over the past 20 years have led to the discovery of mutations in a total of 15 genes causing LQTS and have provided insights into underlying molecular mechanisms. A mutation is identified in 80–85% of definite LQTS cases, but 15–20% of LQTS cases remain genetically elusive (no pathogenic variant identified despite standard clinical genetic testing).

Y. D. Wijeyeratne · E. R. Behr (✉)
Cardiovascular Medicine, Cardiology Clinical Academic Group, St. George's, University of London, London, UK

St. George's University Hospitals NHS Foundation Trust, London, UK
e-mail: ebehr@sgul.ac.uk

H. F. Baars et al. (eds.), *Clinical Cardiogenetics*, https://doi.org/10.1007/978-3-030-45457-9_12

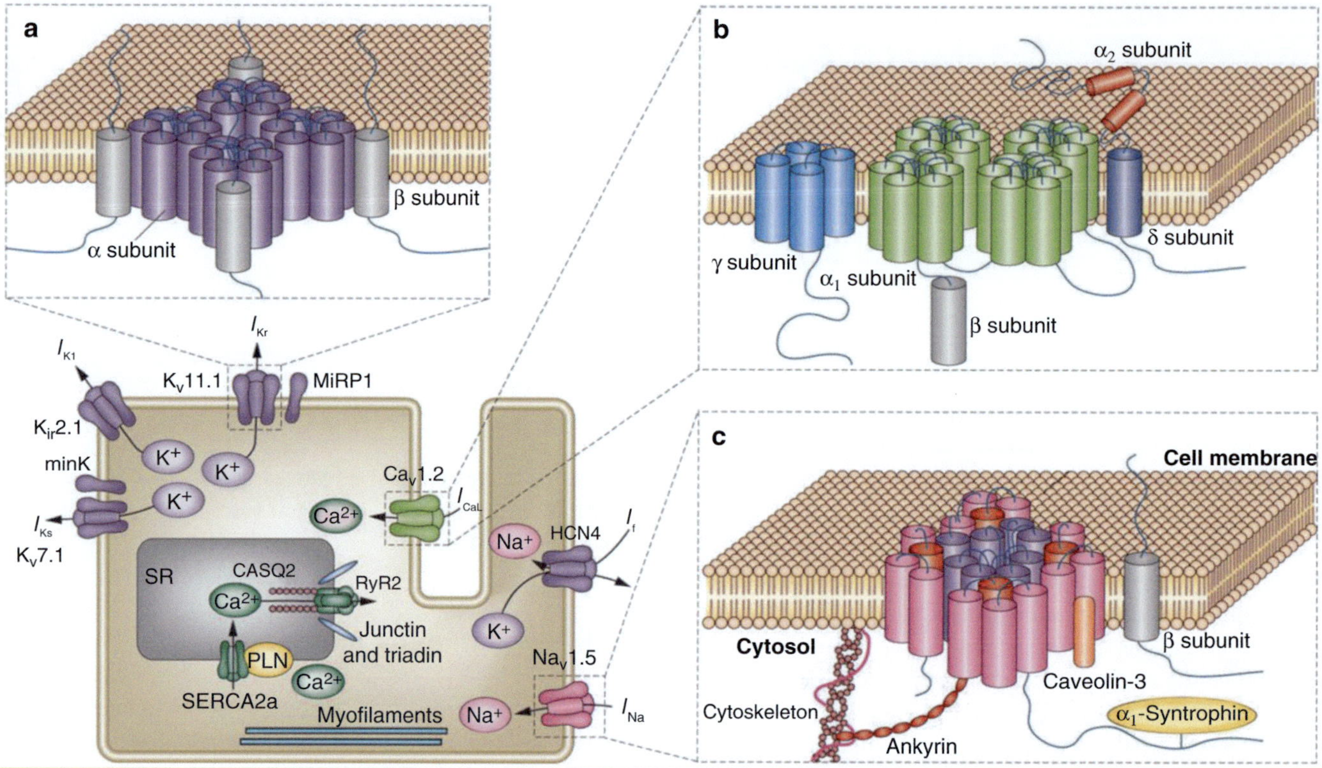

Fig. 12.1 Mutations in the ion channel encoding genes lead to the aberrant function of the respective proteins and to different cardiac channelopathies. (**a**) Potassium (I_{Kr}), (**b**) calcium (I_{CaL}), and (**c**) sodium (I_{Na}) channel structures and subunits are shown. Abbreviations: *CASQ2* calsequestrin-2, *PLN* cardiac phospholamban, *RyR2* ryanodine receptor 2, *SERCA2a* sarcoplasmic/endoplasmic reticulum calcium ATPase 2a, *SR* sarcoplasmic reticulum. Reproduced with permission from Wilde and Behr [14]

LQT1, LQT2, and LQT3, caused by mutations in *KCNQ1*, *KCNH2*, and *SCN5A* respectively, account for over 90% of genetically confirmed LQTS. Genes encoding β-subunits, membrane scaffolding proteins, or proteins interacting with cardiac ion channels have been implicated in some rarer types of LQTS and have only been identified in a few families or isolated individuals [14, 15].

More than 70% of cases of LQTS are caused by missense mutations, whilst the remainder comprise frameshift (10%) and splice-site mutations and in-frame insertions and deletions [16, 17]. Most reported mutations are exonic (in coding regions of the gene), but non-coding mutations that affect allele expression and larger genomic rearrangements have been described [18].

Table 12.1 summarises the genes known to cause LQTS.

Mechanisms of Arrhythmia in LQTS

Polymorphic ventricular tachycardia (polymorphic), or torsades de pointes (TdP), is the classical ventricular arrhythmia associated with LQTS. TdP can be self-limiting causing syncope, but it can also rapidly deteriorate into ventricular fibrillation (VF) and cardiac arrest.

TdP is typically triggered by a ventricular extrasystole. Accentuated spatial dispersion of repolarisation within the ventricular myocardium can lead to a unidirectional block in conduction. This can set the stage for re-entry, which forms the arrhythmic substrate. The ventricular extrasystole initiating the re-entry may either be pause-dependent, or it may be triggered in the absence of a preceding pause [21, 22].

Pause-dependent TdP typically occurs in LQT2 but can also occur in LQT3 [22]. It is initiated by 'early afterdepolarisations' (EAD) that develop under conditions of prolonged cellular repolarisation [23, 24]. Acceleration of an initially slow heart rate or a short-long-short sequence of preceding R-R intervals may then trigger EADs [22, 25]. The prolonged plateau phase of the action potential, together with enhancement of the sodium-calcium exchange current, allows for the reactivation of the L-type calcium current before repolarisation is complete, thereby generating the EAD [23]. In contrast, early animal models suggested that TdP in LQT1 may be triggered by 'delayed afterdepolarisations' (DAD) secondary to intracellular calcium overload at higher heart rates, as a result of blockade of the slowly activating delayed rectifier potassium current (I_{Ks}). Data from a canine wedge preparation also showed that in the presence of I_{Ks} block, β-adrenoceptor stimulation accentuates transmural

Table 12.1 The genes implicated in LQTS

LQTS subtype	Gene	Locus	Frequency (%)	Affected protein	Physiological role	Predominantly affected current	Functional effect
LQT1	*KCNQ1*	11p15.5-p15.4	40–55	Kv7.1	α-Subunit	I_{Ks}	Loss of function
LQT2	*KCNH2*	7q36.1	30–45	Kv11.1	α-Subunit	I_{Kr}	Loss of function
LQT3	*SCN5A*	3p22.2	5–10	Nav1.5	α-Subunit	I_{Na}	Gain of function
LQT4	*ANK2*	4q25-q26	<1	ANK2	Scaffolding	I_{Na} and others	Loss of function
LQT5	*KCNE1*	21q22.12	<1	MinK	β-Subunit	I_{Ks}	Loss of function
LQT6[a]	*KCNE2*	21q22.11	<1	MIRP1	β-Subunit	I_{Kr}	Loss of function
LQT7	*KCNJ2*	17q24.3	<1	Kir2.1	α-Subunit	I_{K1}	Loss of function
LQT8	*CACNA1C*	12p13.33	<1	CaV1.2	α-Subunit	I_{Ca}	Gain of function
LQT9[a]	*CAV3*	3p25.3	<1	Caveolin 3	Scaffolding	I_{Na}	Gain of function?
LQT10	*SCN4B*	11q23.3	<1	Navβ4	β-Subunit	I_{Na}	Loss of function
LQT11	*AKAP9*	7q21.2	<1	Yotiao	ChIP	I_{Ks}	Loss of function
LQT12	*SNTA1*	20q11.21	<1	Syntrophin α1	ChIP	I_{Na}	Loss of function
LQT13	*KCNJ5*	11q24.3	<1	Kir3.4	Transmembrane domain	I_{KACh}	Loss of function
LQT14	*CALM1*	14q32.11	<1	Calmodulin	Ca^{2+} binding protein	–	Loss of function
LQT15	*CALM2*	2p21	<1	Calmodulin	Ca^{2+} binding protein	–	Loss of function

[a]Conflicting data [19, 20]

dispersion of the APD [21]. More recent data from yet another animal model indicates that TdP in LQT1 may be initiated by focal excitations in the right ventricular wall, which may be triggered by either DADs or EADs, and maintained by complex biventricular excitation dynamics [26].

Atrial arrhythmias, particularly atrial fibrillation, are more frequent at younger ages in LQTS compared to the general population. Abnormal atrial repolarisation and refractoriness may contribute to the pathogenesis of atrial fibrillation [27–29].

Clinical Presentation

The principal clinical presentations of LQTS constitute arrhythmic events and distinct ECG features which may be detected incidentally or as a consequence of family screening. Symptomatic individuals may present with syncope (unexplained loss of consciousness without warning or preceding neurological symptoms), documented ventricular arrhythmias (VT/VF), and/or cardiac arrest. On evaluation, every effort must be made to distinguish true cardiac syncope from other likely aetiologies not relevant to a diagnosis of LQTS, although making such a distinction may often be challenging.

Genotype-Phenotype Correlation

The typical phenotypic features of LQTS may vary depending on the genotype.

LQT1 patients have a high risk of developing ventricular arrhythmias with physical exertion (particularly swimming or diving) or emotional stress. The I_{Ks} current is normally activated by adrenergic stress, thereby shortening ventricular repolarisation during fast heart rates. Reduced I_{Ks} in LQT1 leads to an abnormal response to adrenergic stimulation with inadequate action potential shortening at higher heart rates. This is manifest as a progressive prolongation of the QTc during exercise and early recovery [22, 25]. The increase in risk with swimming and diving may be related to increased cardiac vagal tone and peripheral sympathetically driven vasoconstriction known as the 'dive reflex' [30].

Arrhythmic events in LQT2 are particularly associated with auditory stimuli, particularly sudden loud noises such as alarm clocks. The I_{Kr} current is modulated by α- and β-adrenergic stimulation, leading to an increased incidence of arrhythmias during sudden stress or auditory stimuli [31].

In LQT3, increased late inward sodium current (late I_{Na}) during the plateau phase of the action potential results in prolongation of repolarisation that is particularly marked at slow heart rates. The highest risk of arrhythmias in LQT3 patients is during sleep, and their corrected QTc intervals typically shorten with exercise. It has been proposed that as a result of the persistence of the late inward sodium current (I_{Na}) in LQT3, Na^+ accumulates in the cardiomyocyte at faster heart rates, lowering the Na^+ gradient and thereby I_{Na}. The effect of this reduction would most apparent in the plateau phase of the action potential, leading to a shortening of APD at faster heart rates [32]. In addition, the normal I_{Ks} current in LQT2 and LQT3 may provide protection against ventricular arrhythmias during physical exercise [33, 34]. A number of

LQT3 mutations may also be associated with phenotypic variability and cause an overlap phenotype with Brugada syndrome and progressive cardiac conduction defect due to accompanying reduced current density and/or peak current [35, 36]. Table 12.2 summarises some of the unique features of LQT1–LQT3.

Incomplete penetrance is common in LQTS with concealed mutation-positive carriers who have neither clinical symptoms nor electrocardiographic features of LQTS [13]. Such genotype-phenotype mismatch may be due to age- and gender-related penetrance, genetic modifiers, or environmental factors. More recently, it has been proposed that differences in autonomic function may also contribute to variation in phenotype between carriers of the same mutation [37].

Natural History

The occurrence of the initial cardiac event appears to be related to age, sex, and the severity of QT prolongation. In particular, male children and female adults are at greater risk. Early data suggested that genotype may also predict risk. For example, early registry data indicated a higher incidence of lethal events in LQT3 despite therapy, especially at the first episode [38]. Cardiac events occur earlier in LQT1 males than females, and LQT1 patients typically experience cardiac events at a younger age, with the majority experiencing their first event (syncope, resuscitated cardiac arrest, or sudden death) by the age of 20 years [34]. Other data, however, have suggested that LQT2 and LQT3 patients have the highest incidence of first cardiac event under the age of 40 years (42–45%) compared to LQT1 (30%) [39]. The most recent data from the long QT registry suggest however that whilst the gene affected in an individual may influence the incidence of cardiac events, it plays less of a role in overall arrhythmic mortality than the above main factors. The exception is the female LQT2 carrier who is at higher risk than other genotypes [40, 41].

The overall 10-year mortality of untreated, symptomatic LQTS patients is estimated at nearly 50% [42].

Table 12.2 Typical features of LQT1, LQT2, and LQT3

	LQT1	LQT2	LQT3
Typical circumstances of cardiac events	Physical exertion/ swimming	Sudden loud noise	Sleep
Events in childhood	++	+	Rare
Events <40 years	+++	++	++
Typical T-wave morphology	Broad-based and prolonged	Low amplitude, wide, notched and/or bifid	Long isoelectric segment with late-appearing T wave
QTc shortening with exercise	Reduced	Normal	Accentuated
Efficacy of beta-blockers	+++	++	++

Clinical Diagnosis

Diagnostic Criteria: Taskforce Criteria and Expert Opinion

Figure 12.2 summarises the current HRS/EHRA/APHRS consensus recommendations for the diagnosis of LQTS. The international consensus risk score for probability of LQTS is summarised in Table 12.3. ESC guidelines that were published in 2015 recommended less stringent clinical diagnostic criteria (LQTS risk score > 3; QTc ≥ 480 ms on repeated ECGs, or QTc ≥ 460 ms on repeated ECGs with unexplained syncope) [45]. The presence of an unequivocally pathogenic LQTS mutation is sufficient to make the diagnosis according to both guidelines.

Electrocardiographic Features of LQTS

Prolongation of the heart rate-corrected QT (QTc) interval is the hallmark of LQTS, but the QTc will vary and patients

Expert Consensus Recommendations on LQTS Diagnosis

1. LQTS is diagnosed:
   a) in the presence of an LQTS risk score ≥3.5 (Table 3) in the absence of a secondary cause for QT prolongation and/or
   b) in the presence of an unequivocally pathogenic mutation in one of the LQTS genes or
   c) in the presence of a QT interval corrected for heart rate using Bazett's formula (QTc) ≥500 ms in repeated 12-lead electrocardiogram (ECG) and in the absence of a secondary cause for QT prolongation.

2. LQTS can be diagnosed in the presence of a QTc between 480–499 ms in repeated 12-lead ECGs in a patient with unexplained syncope in the absence of a secondary cause for QT prolongation and in the absence of a pathogenic mutation.

Fig. 12.2 Current HRS/EHRA/APHRS Expert Consensus Recommendations on LQTS Diagnosis. (Reproduced with permission from Priori et al. [13])

with prolonged QTc can intermittently be within normal limits. Other features to look for on the ECG include T-wave morphology, T-wave alternans, and evidence of sinus node dysfunction.

QT Interval

The QT interval is defined as the time between the onset of the QRS complex and the end of the T wave. The end of the T wave has classically been defined as the intersection of a tangent to the steepest slope of the last limb of the T wave and the baseline, in lead II or V5/V6 (see Fig. 12.3) [46]. However, this method is not without its shortcomings, and it is easy to overestimate or underestimate the slope of the tangent. An alternative method is to use the visual end of the T wave (see Fig. 12.4). A recent study has suggested only a small difference between the two methods and good reproducibility in expert hands [47]. With either method, the end of the T wave can be difficult to determine in the presence of certain T-wave morphologies, or if U waves are present and merge with the terminal part of the T wave. Generally, if the U wave is of low amplitude compared to the T wave, it is unlikely to be part of the T wave and should not be measured (see Fig. 12.3). If both waves are of similar amplitude with a biphasic or notched appearance, then the U wave can be included in the measurement (see Fig. 12.4b) [48]. The only exception is Andersen-Tawil syndrome where the QT/U wave is routinely measured [49].

The measured QT interval is then corrected for heart rate: the QTc interval. QTc is most commonly calculated using the Bazett's formula (QT interval/$\sqrt{[\text{R-R interval}]}$) or occasionally Fridericia's (QT interval/$\sqrt[3]{[\text{R-R interval}]}$), Framingham, or Hodges formulae [50]. Ideally, the QT and RR intervals are measured on at least three separate beats and the mean values taken to minimise error due to sinus arrhythmia. Atrial fibrillation further complicates the time correction due to rhythm irregularity. Automated QTc measurements can be taken as a guide, but it is important that the QT interval is measured manually by a clinician with suitable expertise. Bazett's formula leads to an underestimation of the QTc at slow heart rates, whilst at fast heart rates there is under-correction of the QT interval leading to an overestimated QTc.

Furthermore, interventricular conduction delay and bundle branch block may lead to overestimation of the QTc interval. In left bundle branch block (LBBB), it has been proposed that a 'modified QTc' can be calculated to correct

Table 12.3 Schwartz LQTS risk score [43]. (Reproduced with permission from Schwartz and Ackerman [44])

			Points
Electrocardiographic findings[a]			
A	QTc[b]	≥480 ms	3
		460–479 ms	2
		450–459 ms (male)	1
B	QTc[b] fourth minute of recovery from exercise stress test ≥480 ms		1
C	Torsades de pointes[c]		2
D	T-wave alternans		1
E	Notched T wave in three leads		1
F	Low heart rate for age[d]		0.5
Clinical history			
A	Syncope	With stress	2
		Without stress	1
B	Congenital deafness		0.5
Family history			
A	Family members with definite LQTS[e]		1
B	Unexplained sudden cardiac death below age 30 amongst immediate family members[e]		0.5

Score: ≤1 point: low probability of LQTS. 1.5–3 points: intermediate probability of LQTS. ≥3.5 points: high probability

[a]In the absence of medications or disorders known to affect these electrocardiographic features

[b]QTc calculated by Bazett's formula where QTc = QT/$\sqrt{RR}$

[c]Mutually exclusive

[d]Resting heart rate below the second percentile for age

[e]The same family member cannot be counted in *A* and B

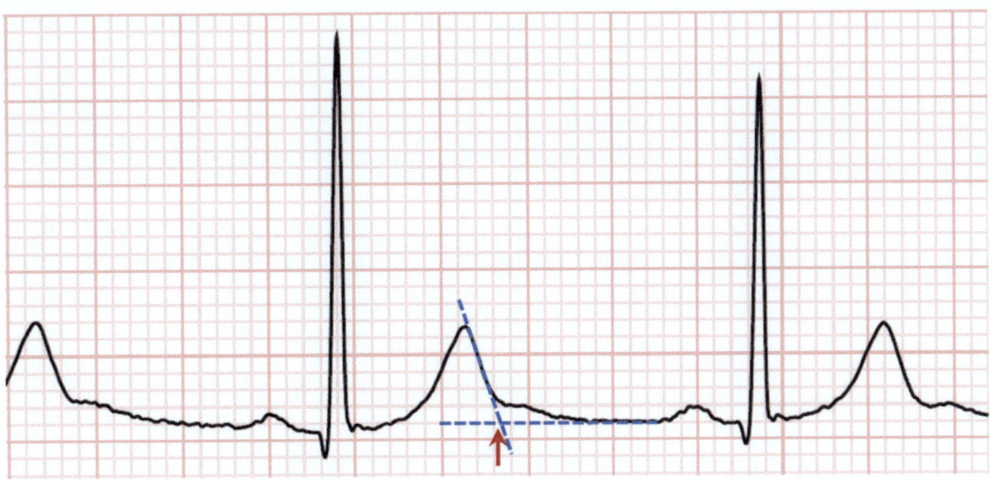

Fig. 12.3 Determining the end of the T wave using the tangent method

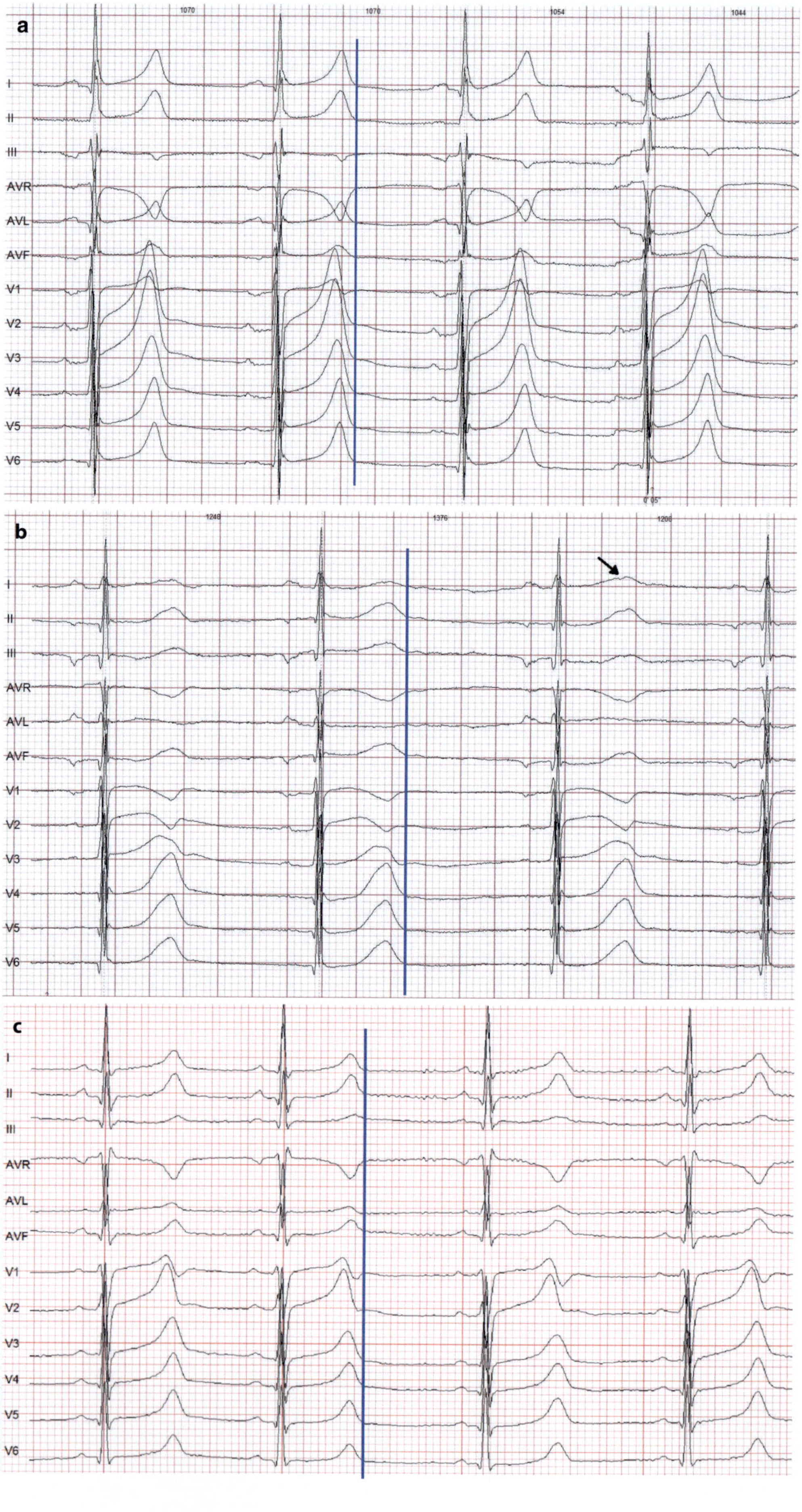

Fig. 12.4 Typical LQTS ECGs. (**a**) LQT1. (**b**) LQT2. The arrow shows a notched T wave, not to be mistaken for a U wave, and the whole T wave should be included in measurement. (**c**) LQT3. The vertical blue lines indicate the end of the T wave for measuring the QT interval

for the QRS prolongation, but this was based on a small study where 60 patients with sinus rhythm and narrow QRS underwent electrophysiological study with ventricular pacing at the right ventricular apex and right ventricular outflow tract to simulate LBBB [51]. Whilst the same methods as described above are applied when calculating the corrected QT interval, it is important that the physician is aware that there may be an overestimate of the QTc interval [52–56].

There is considerable overlap of QTc intervals between unaffected individuals and LQTS patients in families and the general population. Many genetically confirmed LQTS patients may have QTc within the normal range due to variable penetrance: 30–40% of genotype-positive LQT1 patients, approximately 20% of LQT2 patients, and 10% of LQT3 patients do not have overt QT prolongation on the baseline ECG [39]. As a result, QTc on the surface ECG alone is not sufficient to diagnose LQTS in the vast majority of patients. An exception is if QTc is <400 ms which has a negative predictive value of nearly 100%, and QTc > 480 ms has a high positive predictive value. In primary care, LQTS should be suspected if QTc > 460 ms in a child under the age of 15 years, if QTc > 450 ms in an adult male, or if QTc > 470 ms in an adult female, and the patient should be referred for further evaluation [57]. Investigators studying a large cohort of genotype-positive and genotype-negative LQTS family members have proposed suitable cut-offs based on age and gender for the likelihood of carrying pathogenic variants responsible for LQTS [47]. This remains to be validated in other LQTS populations or the general population.

T-Wave Morphology

In addition to QTc prolongation, there are changes in T-wave morphology in LQTS, with some morphologies being characteristically associated with mutations in certain genes. LQT1 (*KCNQ1*) is characterised by broad-based, often peaked T waves; LQT2 (*KCNH2*) by low-amplitude, sometimes notched, T waves; and LQT3 (*SCN5A*) by late-onset T waves of normal duration and amplitude with a long isoelectric ST segment [58]. These characteristic morphologies, however, may not always be present and can even overlap [59]. Examples of LQT1, LQT2, and LQT3 ECGs are shown in Fig. 12.4.

T-Wave Alternans

T-wave alternans is a beat-to-beat variation in the T-wave morphology and ST segment secondary to regional heterogeneity of repolarisation. Macroscopic T-wave alternans is one of the diagnostic criteria for LQTS and is a marker of high cardiac electrical instability. T-wave alternans may be present at rest but more commonly appears during periods of emotional stress or physical exertion [60]. It is associated with a propensity to life-threatening ventricular arrhythmias and high risk of cardiac events as it can precede TdP [61]. More recently, microvolt T-wave alternans, calculated from 24 h continuous 12-lead ECG recordings, was shown to be prevalent in LQTS patients and a marker of arrhythmia risk [62].

Post-Ectopic QT Prolongation

QT prolongation is common in post-ectopic sinus beats. QT prolongation of post-ectopic sinus beats >480 ms should raise suspicion of LQTS which may be more apparent in LQT2 [63].

Figure 12.5 illustrates post-ectopic QT prolongation in LQTS.

Sinus Node Dysfunction

Long sinus pauses or inappropriate sinus bradycardia indicative of sinus node dysfunction may be seen in patients with LQT3 [35, 64]. Incomplete penetrance of sinus node dysfunction in LQT3 may be manifest as exaggerated sinus arrhythmia, heart rates slower than would be expected for age in infants and children, or inappropriate sinus bradycardia.

Clinical Evaluation

The standard evaluation includes a thorough clinical history, ECG, Echo, and 24 h ECG, ideally by a cardiologist with expertise. Provocative tests for QT prolongation such as QT measurement during change from a supine to standing position, exercise testing, or an epinephrine infusion have been proposed, but the clinical validity of these tests is yet to be fully determined [13]. The recovery phase of exercise does appear to offer the best additional value and has been included in the LQTS risk score [43, 44, 65, 66]. The exercise test thus should be a standard part of clinical evaluation.

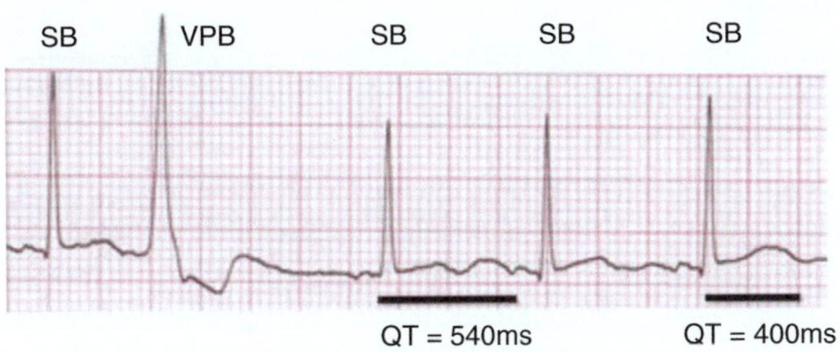

Fig. 12.5 Post-ectopic QT prolongation in LQTS. *SB* spontaneous beat and *VPB* ventricular premature beat

LQTS can be overdiagnosed by physicians with less experience in the condition. In one study, diagnostic concordance was present in less than one third of patients diagnosed with LQTS and subsequently referred to a tertiary centre for second opinion [48]. Comprehensive evaluation by a cardiologist with expertise in electrophysiology and inherited cardiac conditions working in close association with a clinical geneticist and genetic counsellor is recommended. Such a setting would provide the optimal facilities for accurate diagnosis and holistic management of patients suspected to have LQTS, as well as their families.

Clinical History and Examination

A thorough history of relevant symptoms must be taken, with emphasis on distinguishing the aetiology of any syncopal episode by eliciting details of any unexplained collapses or loss of consciousness at all ages. Personal or family history of unexplained road traffic accidents or drowning incidents should raise suspicion of syncope. Furthermore, a note should be made of any family history of epilepsy or sudden infant death. If there have been any sudden deaths in the family, every effort must be taken to (1) find out the circumstances of the death, (2) obtain any ante-mortem ECGs, (3) obtain the post-mortem report, and (4) find out if a specialist cardiac autopsy was carried out to confirm if it was a sudden arrhythmic death syndrome (SADS) death [67]. A physical examination should be carried out to look for any features described in "Clinical Evaluation".

ECG

The baseline 12-lead ECG must be carefully evaluated as described in section "Clinical Evaluation", and a 12-lead ECG should be repeated at each follow-up appointment for dynamic evaluation.

Cardiac Imaging

Cardiac structural abnormalities are excluded using transthoracic echocardiography and, if there is any doubt, cardiac MRI.

Holter

Ambulatory ECG, or Holter, monitoring over a 24 or 48 h period can provide information on QT intervals over a 24 or 48 h period. However, there is insufficient data on the normal range for maximum QTc on a Holter, and QTc intervals detected on Holter alone are insufficient to diagnose LQTS. Supportive diagnostic features on Holter monitoring include T-wave morphology, as well as features of electrical instability such as T-wave alternans that can indicate higher risk [68, 69]. Holter recordings have shown that LQT1 patients have more frequent QTc prolongation during the day compared to night-time, but this variation is much less marked in LQT2 [70]. In LQT3, the QT prolongation is often more pronounced at night-time [71].

Lying/Standing ECG

Patients with LQTS tend to have inadequate shortening of QTc in response to the sudden heart rate accelerations provoked by standing, resulting in QTc prolongation that can persist even after the heart rate returns to baseline. This can be present in both LQT1 and LQT2. This test can be carried out conveniently using continuous ECG recordings to measure the QTc in the supine position, on standing quickly, and for 5 min afterwards. The normal values for this test have, however, not been agreed, and its diagnostic value is still unclear [72–74]. Figure 12.6 illustrates QT prolongation on standing in an LQT1 patient.

Exercise ECG

Exercise testing can be useful to measure exercise-induced QT prolongation during exercise and in early recovery, particularly in LQT1 patients who will have relative QTc prolongation with exercise. The QTc prolongation is most readily measured in early recovery and measurement of QTc in the fourth minute of recovery can be used for the diagnosis of LQTS amongst relatives of affected individuals and in probands where it forms part of the Schwartz score [43, 65, 66]. Figure 12.7 shows ECGs of an LQTS patient on exercise.

LQT1 is also associated with a diminished chronotropic response to exercise. In LQT2, there are normal QT shortening with exercise and a normal chronotropic response. Conversely, in LQT3, QT shortening with exercise is often exaggerated [32]. Exercise-induced ventricular ectopy is uncommon in LQTS and should raise the suspicion of CPVT, particularly if there is exercise-induced bigeminy [75].

Epinephrine Challenge

This provocation test can be useful to unmask QTc prolongation in concealed LQT1 [76]. The characteristic T-wave morphology in LQT2 (notched T wave) may also appear with epinephrine challenge, potentially unmasking concealed LQT2 [77]. There are two widely used protocols for this challenge [78, 79]. Induction of TdP or VF is unusual. The utility of epinephrine challenge in routine clinical practice is debatable, however, as noncarriers can also show QTc prolongation, and in our experience, false positives outside of familial testing are common [80].

Differential Diagnosis

When making the diagnosis of LQTS, structural heart disease must be excluded using transthoracic echocardiography and, if necessary, cardiac magnetic resonance imaging

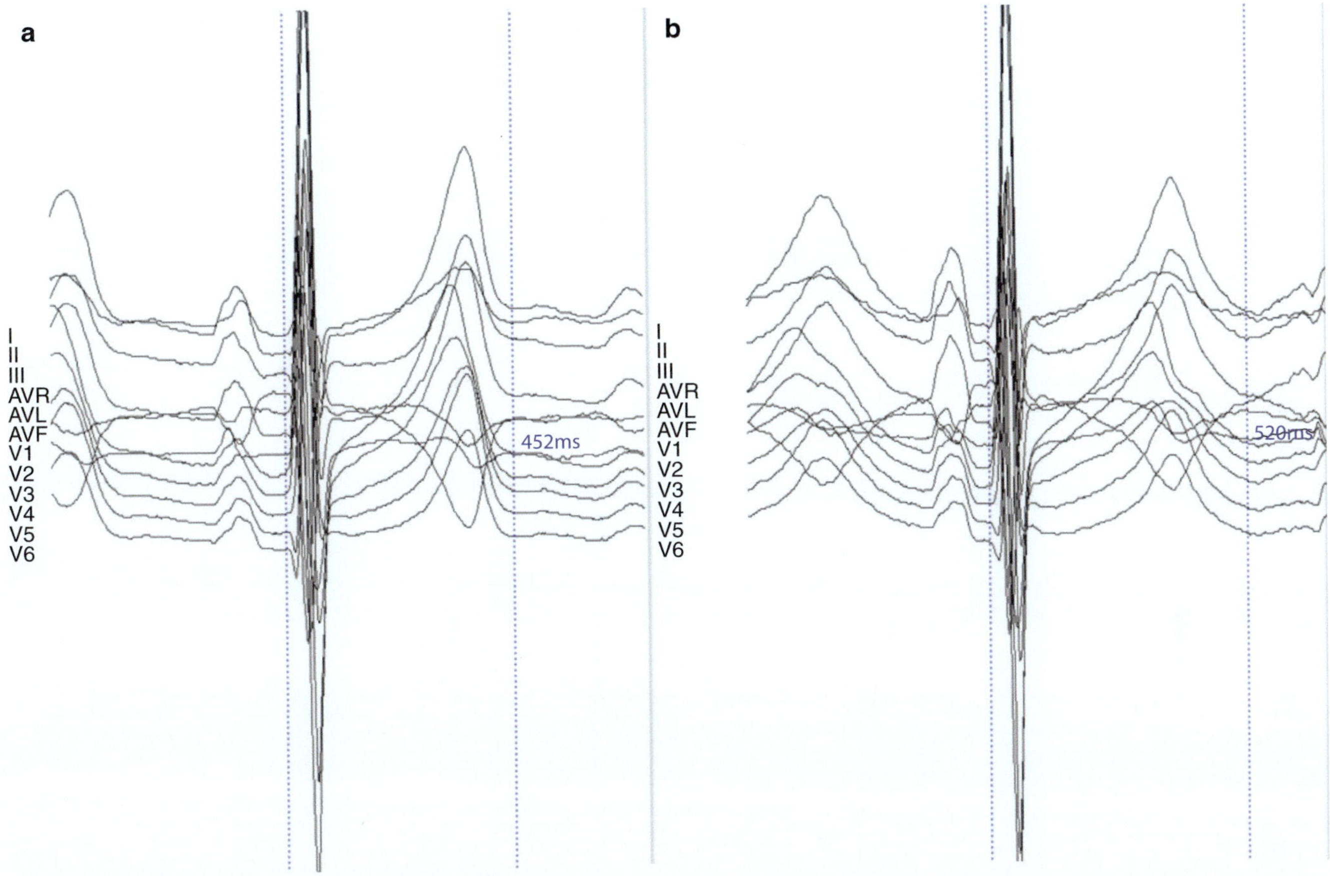

Fig. 12.6 (**a**) Lying-standing ECG with overlapping complexes of a single beat demonstrating QT prolongation during an orthostatic challenge in an LQT1 female patient. (**a**) Lying ECG QT = 452 ms. (**b**) ECG 20 s after standing QT = 520 ms

(MRI). Several hereditary and acquired cardiomyopathies can cause intrinsic prolongation of QTc [81–83].

Other conditions that need to be considered, particularly in symptomatic patients with a borderline QTc interval, include vasovagal syncope, catecholaminergic polymorphic ventricular tachycardia (CPVT), and epilepsy. In particular, increased ventricular ectopy on exercise in a patient with normal or borderline QTc should raise suspicion of CPVT.

Syncope with seizure activity can be misdiagnosed as epilepsy, whilst in other cases, absences secondary to epilepsy can be misdiagnosed as cardiac syncope. Therefore, if unclear, a neurological opinion can be helpful. Other differential diagnoses for a syncopal episode include vasovagal syncope that may be preceded by postural changes or associated with other physiological circumstances such as micturition, emotion, dehydration, or environmental factors such as external stressors or heat. Taking a thorough history of the symptoms and the circumstances, including collateral history, examination (e.g. looking for postural changes in blood pressure), and undertaking a tilt test if required, can help ascertain if the reported event should be considered as a cardiac event, i.e. whether the patient is having symptomatic LQTS.

A careful history should be taken to exclude acquired long QT syndrome secondary to QT-prolonging drugs or electrolyte abnormalities secondary to intercurrent illness, metabolic disorders, or eating disorders. Drugs that cause QT prolongation are numerous including cardiac and non-cardiac agents. In approximately 10% of cases of drug-induced TdP, the congenital LQTS may be uncovered [84, 85]. Electrolyte abnormalities that will cause QTc prolongation include hypokalaemia, hypomagnesaemia, and hypocalcaemia. Other situations causing prolonged QTc to be aware of include hypothermia and hypothyroidism.

Table 12.4 summarises other diagnoses to be considered when making a diagnosis of LQTS.

Multisystem Disorders

Several multisystem disorders have been described with LQTS. Jervell and Lange-Nielsen syndrome is associated with congenital deafness and may be caused by autosomal recessive mutations in *KCNQ1* or *KCNE1*. Affected individuals may be either homozygotes (same mutation in both alleles) or compound heterozygotes (two different mutated

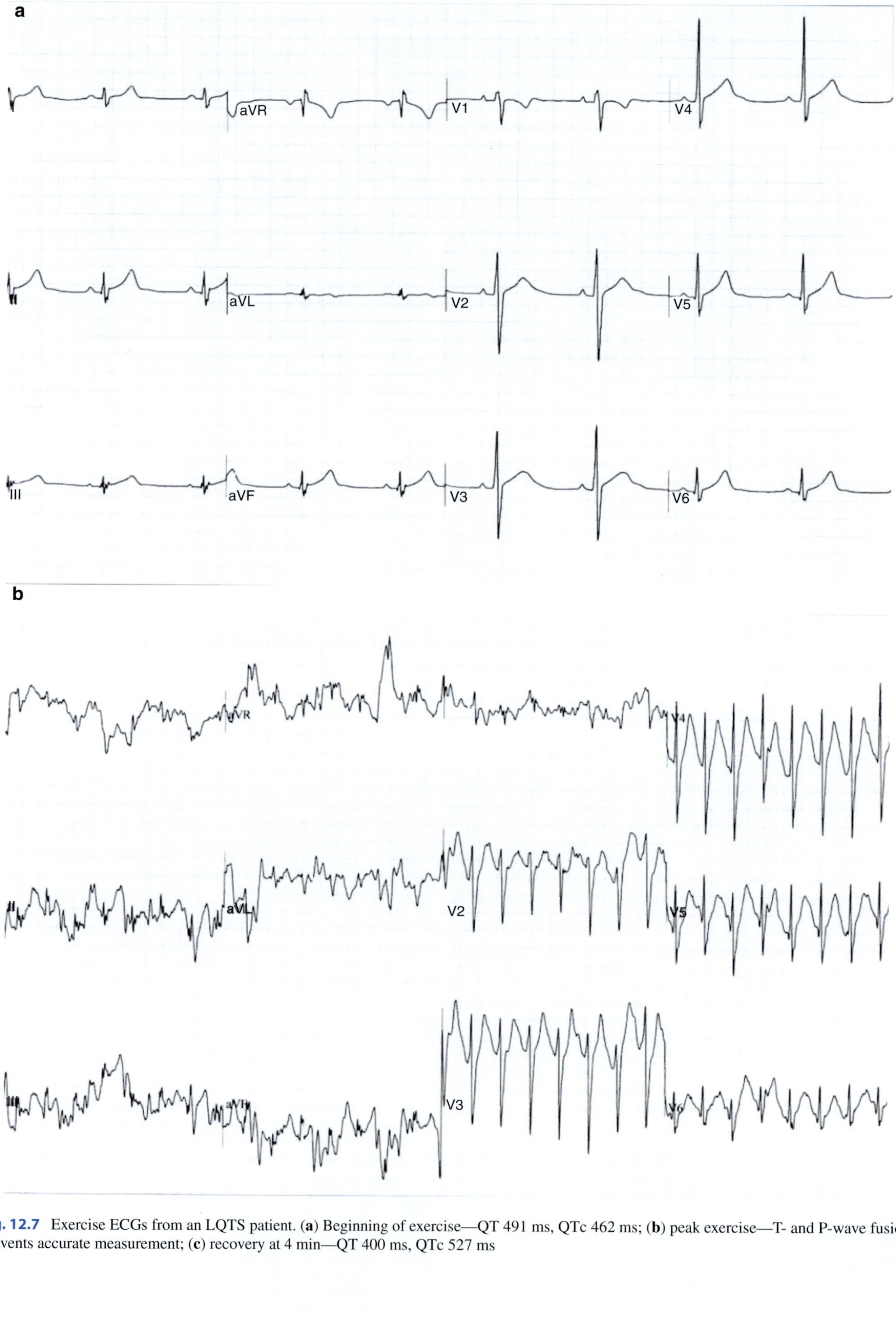

Fig. 12.7 Exercise ECGs from an LQTS patient. (**a**) Beginning of exercise—QT 491 ms, QTc 462 ms; (**b**) peak exercise—T- and P-wave fusion prevents accurate measurement; (**c**) recovery at 4 min—QT 400 ms, QTc 527 ms

c

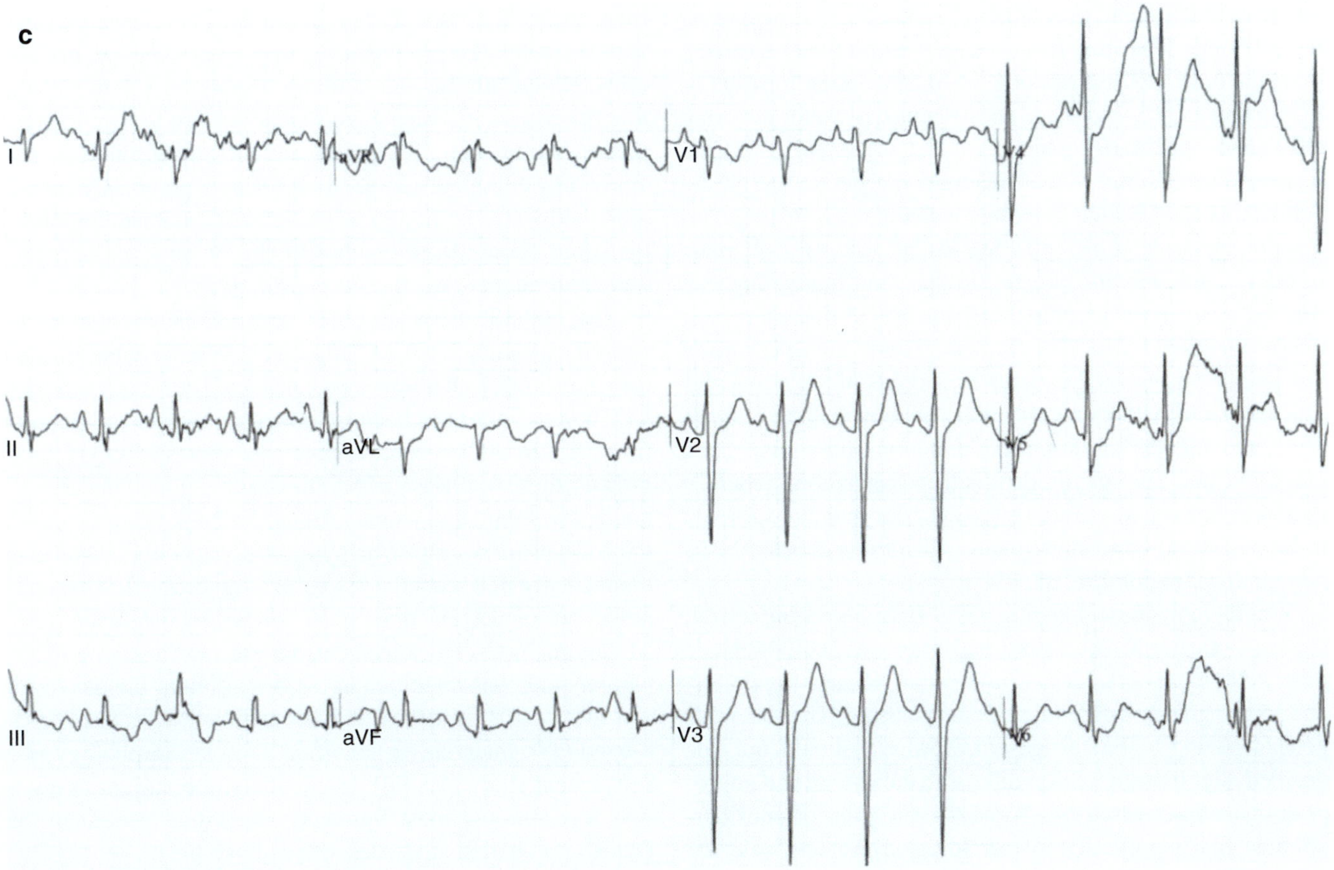

Fig. 12.7 (continued)

Table 12.4 Summary of differential diagnoses in LQTS

Cardiomyopathy	Both inherited and acquired cardiomyopathy can be associated with prolonged QTc
Other inherited arrhythmia syndromes	CPVT with borderline QTc can mimic LQTS
Drug-induced prolonged QTc	Several drugs can prolong QTc. These can be found at qtdrugs.org [85]
Electrolyte disturbances	Electrolyte disturbances associated with intercurrent illness, metabolic disorders, or eating disorders can mimic LQTS
Neurological conditions	Epilepsy
Environmental or physiological circumstances	Hypothermia

alleles) and usually have a more malignant phenotype [86–88]. Mutations in *KCNJ2* (LQT7) cause Andersen-Tawil Syndrome which is associated with neurological and musculoskeletal abnormalities as well as QT prolongation with marked U waves. Its main extracardiac features include minor facial abnormalities and periodic hypokalaemic paralysis [89, 90]. Mutations in *CACNA1C* (LQT8) are responsible for Timothy syndrome that results in multisystem defects in addition to prolonged cardiac repolarisation. These include developmental delay, autism, congenital heart defects, cutaneous syndactyly, and distinctive facial features [91]. Timothy syndrome is extremely rare: fewer than 20 individuals have been reported worldwide, and survival beyond childhood is unusual.

Molecular Diagnosis

Clinical assessment by a cardiologist with expertise in assessing the likelihood of LQTS and genetic counselling by suitably trained professionals are essential prerequisites to genetic testing. Implications of genetic testing for the patient as well as the family and the option of not testing must be discussed. Other issues that should be covered during genetic counselling include implications on lifestyle, job prospects, and health insurance. The possibility of finding 'unclassified variants' or 'variants of uncertain significance' (VUS) and the resultant psychological consequences and the importance of informing relatives need to be discussed. The patient should understand that a negative genetic test does not rule out the diagnosis.

Genetic testing can be in the form of either cascade screening of a single known pathogenic variant that was found in the proband or a targeted gene panel to investigate the proband. This may consist of a limited panel focusing upon the most well-understood genes accounting for LQT1–LQT3 and LQT5–LQT6 or an all-inclusive panel covering all known associated genes (see below) enabled by the increased availability of next-generation sequencing (NGS). Whilst this has resulted in more detailed genetic testing over a short timescale, it has also led to the discovery of many novel variants that are 'private' to that family meaning that they have not been identified elsewhere and therefore their diagnostic value may be limited. These are then often labelled as unclassified variants or variants of unknown significance until pathogenicity can be established (see Section "Age and Gender"). 'Founder' mutations have also been identified that are specific to distinct populations where a mutation has occurred in a single ancestor and has survived to be passed down to subsequent generations clustered in a geographical region [36, 92, 93].

Whole-genome sequencing (WGS) is becoming faster, cheaper, and more accessible and may eventually replace other NGS methods such as whole-exome sequencing (WES) due to the greater range of analyses possible. The extent of genetic testing to be carried out, however, should only be decided after thorough discussion with the patient and appropriate genetic counselling. An additional point of consideration is the opportunity to test for appropriately selected non-LQTS genes. This can even lead to the correct diagnosis in selected cases. For example, in one study, over 5% of patients with negative LQTS genetic testing who were tested for RyR2 mutations were found to be mutation-positive and diagnosed subsequently with CPVT [94].

Unclassified Variants and Importance of Genotype-Phenotype Correlation

Establishing the pathogenicity of variants is crucial as genetic screening has become an important tool in family screening. Identification of a VUS leads to diagnostic uncertainty with potential adverse psychological and economic consequences to patients and families. Many studies implicating genetic variants with pathogenicity have relied on small control sample data without necessarily showing genotype-phenotype co-segregation [95, 96]. A study of the Exome Variant Server in 2012, however, identified a much higher prevalence of previously LQTS-associated variants than expected in exome data from population studies, suggesting that caution must be exercised when interpreting the pathogenicity of variants in individuals and families [97]. In a further Danish population study, 33 genetic variants that were previously reported in LQTS patients were identified in 243 individuals from a sample of 7000 individuals from the general population. Ten variants were identified in eight or more individuals included in this study. There were no associations with QTc prolongation, history of syncope, or mortality. Interestingly, the authors report that half of the identified variants also had functional studies supporting pathogenicity. The 33 variants called into question in this study only comprise <2.5% of all variants previously associated with LQTS; however, these studies raise important questions about the true pathogenicity of some variants previously thought to be disease-causing [95].

The classifications of LQT6 and LQT9, thought to be caused by mutations in KCNE2 and CAV3, have been called into question. High allelic frequencies of previously reported LQT6 mutations have been found within the general population [20]. In the largest available case series of LQT6 individuals, there was a lack of familial segregation of phenotype, and it was found that where a single KCNE2 variant was felt to be the primary culprit, arrhythmic events only occurred in the presence of a secondary stressor, suggesting that the classification of LQT6 may need to be reconsidered [20]. Mutations in CAV3 causing LQTS are rare, and one of the variants that was identified in 2006 that led to the discovery of LQT9, CAV3 p.T78M, did not associate with either prolonged QTc intervals or abnormal T-wave morphology in a subsequent study [19, 98]. Incidentally, the variant in question was also the most frequently identified variant in the Danish population study described above [95].

Thus, given the potential uncertainties that can arise with genetic testing, it is essential that these services are provided in expert centres where cardiologists with expertise in inherited heart disease, genetic counsellors, and clinical geneticists, preferably with cardiac expertise, work closely as a team. Where an unclassified variant is found, it will not add to the diagnosis. Further analysis of the variant must be made by testing more family members with and without the phenotype to establish linkage. If further resources are available, in vitro studies can help understand the functional significance of a particular variant and add to the knowledge base.

Genetic Modifiers

Genetic loci, tagged by single nucleotide polymorphisms (SNPs), both in LQTS-associated genes as well as other genes, have been shown to be associated with QTc in the general population [99–102]. These are thought to influence variable penetrance and incomplete expression in some pedigrees. For example, variants in the NOS1AP gene in chromosome 1 have been shown to be associated with increased risk of sudden death in a South African population harbouring a founder mutation in *KCNQ1* [92]. More recently, NOS1AP SNPs were shown to be strongly associated with QTc interval in patients with LQT2. There was also a trend for effect on risk of cardiac events in these patients. Furthermore, common genetic variations at *KCNQ1* were shown to be associated with risk of LQTS [103]. At this time, these markers have not entered into routine clinical guidelines.

Risk Stratification

A critical aspect of management in LQTS is the prevention of sudden death. Accurate risk stratification can be challenging; however, there are certain clinical and genetic markers that can facilitate risk assessment.

Age and Gender

In LQT1, male gender is independently associated with a higher risk of cardiac events before the age of 15 years, but beyond this age, gender risk reversal has been observed with adult females being at higher risk. In LQT2 too, females aged 16 years and older are at higher risk of cardiac events than males [104, 105]. LQT1 males who are asymptomatic at a young age are at low risk of becoming symptomatic later in life, whereas females, especially those with LQT2, remain at risk of having their first cardiac event even after the age of 40 years. In females aged 40–60 years, the LQTS-related risk of sudden death remains higher than in unaffected females, but the LQTS-related risk in males of this age group is lower. The exact mechanisms of gender differences are unclear but may be due to environmental or hormonal factors [13, 40, 106, 107]. Recent data suggest that oestradiol plays an important role in I_{Kr} trafficking [108].

Physiological States

Effects of exercise, emotion, and rest in different LQTS genotypes are described in Section "Diagnostic Criteria: Taskforce Criteria and Expert Opinion".

Pregnancy appears to affect the risk of cardiac events in LQTS although data are limited. The risk of arrhythmias is reduced during pregnancy, possibly secondary to hormonal factors. However, the risk is increased 10–20% during the post-partum period in LQT2 patients and is most marked in the first 9 months post-partum, with approximately 1 in 10 female LQT2 probands experiencing their first cardiac event in the post-partum period. Apart from hormonal factors, environmental factors including sleep deprivation, emotional stress, and noise (crying of the baby) may contribute to risk [109–111].

Family History

Early data indicated that the severity of a proband's presentation did not influence risk in first-degree relatives [112]. A family history of multiple cardiac arrests can be indicative of higher risk; however, sudden death in one sibling does not predict risk of cardiac arrest [113]. In view of these data, sudden death in one first-degree relative is not, by itself, an indication for implantation of an implantable cardioverter-defibrillator (ICD) in a surviving affected family member unless there are other features of risk [13].

Symptoms

Data from the International LQTS Registry indicates that a history of syncope over time is a powerful predictor of risk with different implications depending on age. The risk of recurrent cardiac events is higher in children with syncope or a cardiac arrest before the age of 7 years, even if they are on appropriate medical therapy. Furthermore, infants who have had a cardiac event before the age of 1 year are at especially high risk of further lethal arrhythmias [114]. Adolescents who have had one syncopal event over the preceding 24 months have a 12-fold increased risk of recurrence compared to asymptomatic teenagers with the condition. Two or more syncopal events over the preceding 24 months are associated with an 18-fold increased risk. If the event is more remote, then the increase in risk is threefold. In adults, a previous syncopal event before the age of 18 years is not associated with increased risk, provided there have not been any further events. Syncope after the age of 18 years is then associated with a fivefold increase in risk [40, 104]. Patients who have recurrent cardiac events despite preventative lifestyle measures and appropriate medical therapy are at increased risk regardless of age [13].

QTc Interval

There is often marked variability in the QTc interval when serial ECGs are measured over time. It has been suggested that the maximum QTc measured on follow-up ECGs at any one time provides incremental prognostic information beyond the baseline measurement [115]. However, this needs to be further validated. Nonetheless, the more prolonged a resting QTc interval is, the greater the arrhythmic risk is. The estimated risk of life-threatening arrhythmic events has been shown to increase by 15% per 10 millisecond increase in QTc duration, regardless of LQT1–LQT13 genotype (see Fig. 12.8) [116]. Patients exceeding a QTc of 500 ms have a 3.3-fold increased risk of cardiac events, and the risk increases to 6.3-fold when QTc is >550 ms. [40] In adolescents, QTc > 530 ms is associated with a particular increase in risk with an adjusted hazard ratio of 2.3 [104]. Concealed mutation-positive carriers who are asymptomatic and have normal QTc intervals have a relatively low risk of arrhythmic events although this is still greater than noncarriers [13, 117].

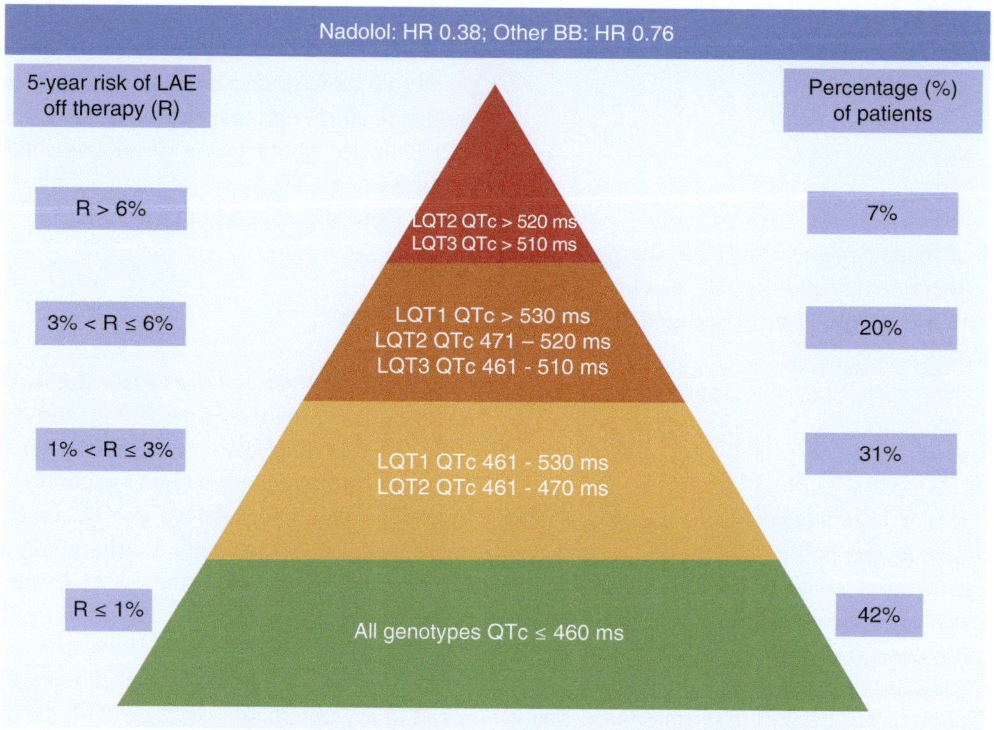

Fig. 12.8 Visualisation of 5-year risk of life-threatening arrhythmic events (LAEs) by genotype and QTc interval before and after therapy according to models derived from the patient population of the present study. The column to the left indicates the cut-off of the 5-year risk of LAEs that corresponds to each color-coded group of patients characterised by QTc duration and genotype (from green (lower risk) to red (higher risk)). The column to the right indicates the percentage of patients in each color-coded category present in the cohort. The bar on the top shows the HR of patients treated with nadolol (HR: 0.38) and other BBs (selective BBs and propranolol; HR: 0.76) and can be used to estimate the residual risk for each group of patients when treated with BBs. *BB* beta-blocker, *HR* hazard ratio, *LAEs* life-threatening arrhythmic events. (Reproduced with permission from Mazzanti et al. [116])

Genotype

Certain subtypes of LQTS, such as the Jervell and Lange-Nielsen syndrome (homozygous or compound heterozygous LQT1 and LQT5) and the Timothy syndrome (LQT8), have a high risk of malignant ventricular arrhythmias at an early age and have a poor prognosis. Other compound and multiple mutation carriers also seem to be at elevated risk [87, 118, 119]. Initial evidence had suggested that LQT2 and LQT3 are associated with a higher risk of sudden death than LQT1 [39]. Although subsequent larger studies have indicated however that genotype locus is of less utility other than LQT2 females being of moderately higher risk, a more recent longitudinal study of 1710 LQTS patients followed up over a median period of 7 years showed that, at any QTc duration, patients with LQT2 and LQT3 have a greater risk of life-threatening arrhythmic events compared to LQT1 patients (30% and 57% greater risk, respectively) [40, 41]. Further, it was shown that, for each genotype, the 5-year risk of life-threatening arrhythmias increases with increasing QTc. This is illustrated in Fig. 12.9.

Studies have since focused on the biophysical consequences of specific mutations. In LQT1, mutations in the pore region of the potassium channel Kv7.1 are associated with a higher frequency of cardiac events, as opposed to mutations in the C-terminal region that are associated with a milder phenotype [17]. Furthermore, missense and dominant-negative mutations are also associated with an increase in risk. The dominant-negative *KCNQ1 A341V* mutation causes a particularly severe phenotype [13, 120]. In LQT2, mutations in the pore-forming region are associated with a more severe phenotype [121]. In addition, evidence is growing that additional genetic variants can modify the clinical phenotype of known pathogenic mutations [122–125]. Common variants known to modulate the QT interval in the general population have been associated with longer QT intervals and clinical severity [92, 126]. These newer genetic risk stratifiers have not been incorporated into clinical practice as yet, pending further confirmation in larger populations with longitudinal data.

Management/Therapy

There is a paucity of randomised controlled trials on the management of LQTS owing to the low prevalence of the condition and variable penetrance. Current guidelines are

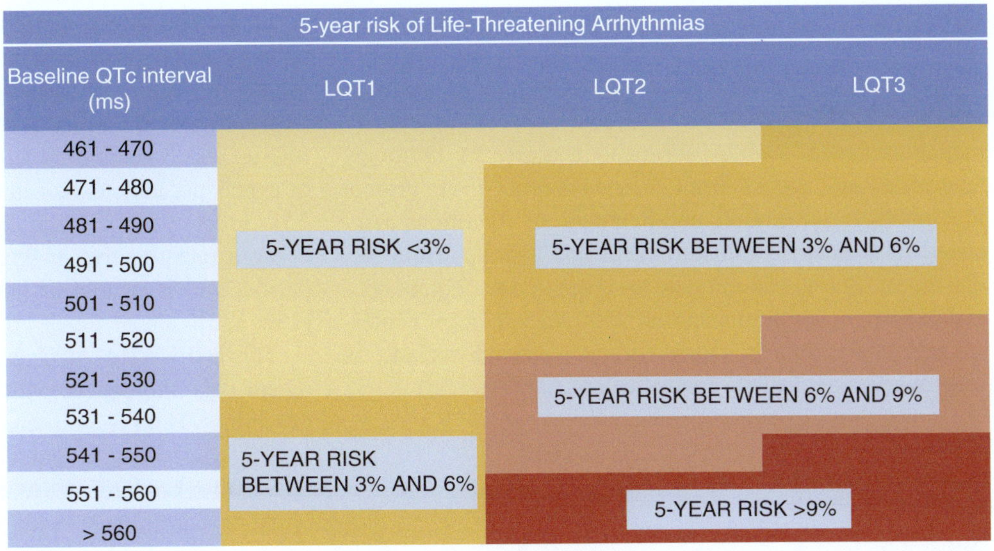

Fig. 12.9 Visualisation of the 5-year relative risk for patients with each genotype and for each QTc duration. The four colours group patients within the same 5-year risk of life-threatening arrhythmic events. This scheme can be used to personalise the risk estimate of patients at diagnosis in the absence of beta-blocker therapy and to estimate the risk of life-threatening arrhythmic events in patients who are not compliant with treatment. (Reproduced with permission from Mazzanti et al. [116])

Expert Consensus Recommendations on management of LQTS

Class I Recommendations:

1. The following lifestyle changes are recommended in all patients with a diagnosis of LQTS:
   a) Avoidance of QT-prolonging drugs (www.crediblemeds.org/new-drug-list/)
   b) Identification and prompt correction of dehydration/electrolyte abnormalities (hypokalaemia, hypomagnesaemia, hypocalcaemia) that may occur during diarrhoea, vomiting, metabolic conditions, imbalanced diets for weight loss or eating disorders.
   c) Avoidance and prompt treatment of hyperthermia, including training-related heat exhaustion in athletes
   d) Avoidance of genotype-specific triggers for arrhythmias (strenuous swimming, especially in LQT1, and exposure to loud noises in LQT2 patients).
2. Beta-blockers are recommended for patients with a clinical diagnosis of LQTS
3. ICD implantation with the use of beta blockers is recommended for patients with a diagnosis of LQTS who are survivors of a cardiac arrest.
4. Left cardiac sympathetic denervation (LCSD) is recommended for high-risk patients with a diagnosis of LQTS in whom:
   a) Implantable cardioverter defibrillator (ICD) therapy is contraindicated or refused and/or
   b) Beta-blockers are either not effective in preventing syncope/arrhythmias, not tolerated, not accepted or contraindicated.
5. All LQTS patients who wish to engage in competitive sports should be referred to a clinical expert for evaluation of risk.

Class IIa Recommendations:

7. Beta-blockers should be considered in carriers of a causative LQTS mutation and normal QT interval
8. ICD implantation in addition to beta-blockers should be considered in patients with a diagnosis of LQTS who experience recurrent syncope and/or VT while on adequate beta-blocker therapy.
8. LCSD can be useful in patients with a diagnosis of LQTS who experience breakthrough events while on therapy with beta-blockers/ICD.

Class IIb recommendations

9. Sodium channel blockers can be useful, as add-on therapy, for LQT3 patients with a QTc >500 ms who shorten their QTc by >40 ms following an acute oral drug test with one of these compounds.
10. ICD implantation may be considered in addition to beta-blocker therapy in asymptomatic carriers of a pathogenic mutation in KCNH2 or SCN5A

Fig. 12.10 Amalgamation of current expert consensus guidelines on the management of LQTS. (Adapted from Priori et al. [13, 45], [127, 128])

based on data from large registries and tertiary centre experience.

Determination of the appropriate management strategy is dependent on the risk assessment—patients with a higher lifetime risk of life-threatening arrhythmic events should be managed more aggressively than those who are considered to be at lower risk. Figure 12.10 summarises the current consensus guidelines on the management of LQTS.

Lifestyle

Patients should be advised of lifestyle changes that can minimise risk. LQT2 patients can minimise exposure to arrhythmogenic triggers such as abrupt loud noises by removing telephones and clocks from their bedrooms [34]. Prompt identification, prevention, and treatment of conditions associated with electrolyte disturbances and hypokalaemia (eg. diarrhoeal illness) can mitigate arrhythmic risk. Patient education and good communication with other medical professionals involved in their care (primary care physicians, as well as other specialists) are critical.

Drugs to Avoid

Patients and all healthcare professionals involved in their care need to be aware of drugs to avoid in LQTS. These include antiarrhythmic agents such as amiodarone, disopyramide, and sotalol; antimicrobials such as erythromycin and ciprofloxacin; and psychotropic drugs. A full list of drugs that prolong the QTc interval is beyond the scope of this chapter and is available on crediblemeds.org [85].

Competitive Sports

The 2005 and 2008 Bethesda Conference guidelines and the ESC consensus recommendations first addressed the risk of sudden cardiac death during sport for athletes with LQTS [129]. The Bethesda guidelines recommended that regardless of QTc or underlying genotype, all competitive sport should be restricted in LQTS patients who have previously experienced a cardiac event that could have been attributed to LQTS. Furthermore, asymptomatic patients with baseline QTc prolongation were advised to restrict low-intensity sport. If they were an LQT3 carrier, they were then allowed to participate in more intensive sport. Asymptomatic patients with concealed LQTS (i.e. genotype-positive/phenotype-negative) were allowed to participate in competitive sport, with the exception of competitive swimming for concealed *KCNQ1* mutation carriers (LQT1). Patients with an ICD or permanent pacemaker were be advised to avoid contact sport to prevent traumatic damage to the implanted device system [130].

The ESC guidelines were much more restrictive and recommended that anyone with a definitive diagnosis of LQTS after comprehensive evaluation should be restricted from all competitive sport, regardless of the presence/absence of any arrhythmic events. The recommended QTc cut-off values for using as a trigger for further evaluation were also much lower in the 2005 ESC guidelines [129, 131]

In 2012, a single-centre retrospective study of over 350 athletes who chose to continue competitive sport against guideline recommendations demonstrated a low rate of LQTS-triggered cardiac events during sport. The mean follow-up was 5 years (650 athlete-years), and the overall rate of events per athlete-year in this study was 0.003 (1 event in 331 athlete-years). Limitations of this study, apart from being a retrospective analysis, include the short follow-up period, and it is unclear how generalisable the results are [132, 133].

The 2015 AHA/ACC guidelines were driven by these recent data and concur with the 2013 HRS/EHRA/APHRS guidelines. Both recommend that all athletes with suspected LQTS who wish to pursue competitive sports must be referred for comprehensive evaluation by an electrophysiologist or cardiologist with expertise in managing LQTS patients. The AHA/ACC guidelines go further however in liberalising the approach to managing any patient with suspected or diagnosed with LQTS. Initially, these athletes should be advised to abstain from all competitive sport until:

1. They have had appropriate comprehensive evaluation of their risk by a suitable expert.
2. The patient and family have received appropriate counselling and education on minimising risk.
3. The patient has been asymptomatic on therapy for at least 3 months [127, 128].

Unlike earlier guidelines, it is now recommended that asymptomatic patients with concealed LQTS (i.e. genotype-positive/phenotype-negative) may participate in competitive sport once they have had comprehensive cardiac evaluation, as long as they follow appropriate precautionary measures (Fig. 12.1: Lifestyle changes). Facilities that need to be in place before such participation include (1) availability of an automatic external defibrillator at the sports venue and (2) establishment of an emergency action plan with the patient's school/club/team officials [127]. Asymptomatic patients with borderline QTc prolongation but no other high risk features may also participate in competitive sport after thorough expert evaluation if appropriate precautionary measures as described above are in place [13]. There is clearly conflict with current European guidelines, and a global consensus is still required.

In 2017, a 4-year follow-up study amongst 440 competitive athletes with implanted ICDs (of whom 20% had LQTS and 46% had a preimplantation history of VT/VF), LQTS was not a variable associated with receiving an appropriate shock, and the proportion receiving an appropriate shock during competition/practice was found to be similar to that during other physical activities [134]. Longer-term follow-up of larger numbers of athletes with LQTS is awaited. There is increased recognition of the need for shared decision-making following an individual athlete's comprehensive evaluation in an Inherited Cardiac Conditions specialist centre, rather than a simple yes-or-no approach [135].

Drug Therapies

It is recommended that all affected patients with LQTS are treated with beta-blockers unless there is a contraindication to beta-blocker use. Mutation carriers with concealed LQTS should be offered beta-blocker therapy although evidence of efficacy is limited. Beta-blockers are particularly effective in LQT1 and, provided that compliance is good, can be sufficient to provide adequate protection against arrhythmic risk in LQT1 [136, 137]. Beta-blockers are thought to act by reducing intracellular calcium overload, thereby minimising the arrhythmogenic substrate for re-entry.

Long-acting non-selective drugs such as nadolol or sustained release propranolol are preferred for ease of administration (once or twice daily) and to avoid wide fluctuations in serum drug concentrations. Recent follow-up data on over 1700 Italian patients have shown that, in all genotypes, only nadolol reduced the arrhythmic risk compared to no therapy (Fig. 12.8) [116].

Beta-blockers that could potentially increase sinus node recovery time and prolong sinus cycle length, such as bisoprolol or metoprolol, are less preferred, particularly in LQT3 patients who have evidence of sinus node dysfunction [138]. It is recommended that patients are maintained on the maximum tolerated dose for age and weight. Abrupt discontinuation of beta-blockers must be avoided if at all possible due to upregulation of beta receptors whilst on treatment. In principle, beta-blockers should be continued during and after pregnancy [13]. Whilst beta-blockers may cause intrauterine growth restriction, neonatal hypoglycaemia, and bradycardia, the decision to continue treatment during pregnancy must take into account arrhythmic risk. Detailed discussion with the patient is essential, but the general experience has been reassuring especially if the foetus and neonate are closely monitored for side effects of beta-blockade.

Phenotypic variability in LQT3 can make clinical management challenging. The sodium channel blocker mexiletine reduces the late I_{Na} in LQT3 and has been shown to be effective in reducing the QTc interval and arrhythmic risk in some LQT3 mutations although the data available is limited [139–142]. The late I_{Na} blocker ranolazine has also been shown to be useful in LQT3, but at present, its therapeutic role is less certain [143–145]. In silico models and patient-specific models of disease induced pluripotent stem cell-derived cardiomyocytes have been used to investigate tailored therapies to suit phenotype, but the clinical applicability of such approaches is currently limited [146].

ICD Indications

ICD implantation is appropriate for selected patients who are at high risk of sudden cardiac death (see Fig. 12.10). ICD implantation is, however, an invasive treatment strategy, and the lifetime risk of complications is not insignificant, especially when implanted in younger patients. Careful consideration of benefits vs risks and appropriate counselling taking into account overall risk and patient preference are essential. TdP is often self-limiting, but an ICD discharge in a conscious patient may trigger further arrhythmias due to the adrenergic surge, leading to an 'electrical storm' (recurrent episodes of VT/VF in a 24 h period). Programming should therefore be directed at minimising the chances of shocks to conscious patients by extending time to therapy as well as avoiding inappropriate shocks. These can otherwise leave patients with devastating psychological consequences [13, 147, 148].

ICD implantation is indicated for secondary prevention in any LQTS patient who has been resuscitated from a cardiac arrest (see Fig. 12.10). Very-high-risk patients, such as those carrying two or more LQTS mutations (compound heterozygotes) or homozygotes, including those with Jervell and Lange-Nielsen syndrome, should be considered for prophylactic ICD implantation at an early age. ICD implantation should also be strongly considered in any LQTS patient with cardiac syncope whilst on appropriate beta-blocker therapy, but there should be a very high threshold to implant ICD in an asymptomatic patient. [13]

The addition of an atrial lead to an ICD system provides several potential benefits. In LQT2, where the onset of TdP is preceded by a pause, a pacemaker with appropriate pause-preventing algorithms can prevent the onset of TdP and minimise the need for ICD therapy. Dual-chamber devices can provide atrial pacing to LQT3 patients with sinus node dysfunction. If a pacemaker is required LQTS, implanting an ICD with appropriate pacing modes may be the most appropriate strategy to prevent the need to have a further procedure if a device upgrade is needed in the future. This needs to be balanced with the potential for higher risk of defibrillator lead failure. Beta-blocker therapy should be continued following device implantation [13, 148].

Surgical Options

Left cardiac sympathetic denervation (LCSD) involves the removal of the first four thoracic ganglia and has a significant antiarrhythmic effect in patients with LQTS [149]. The precise mechanism of the therapeutic effect is not fully understood. Some patients may have paradoxically increased QTc post-LCSD, but these effects are often transient and not associated with risk of arrhythmia [150, 151]. The procedure may be undertaken through a thoracotomy but is increasingly performed as a video-assisted minimally invasive procedure.

LCSD is useful in reducing arrhythmic risk in patients who are intolerant of beta-blockers or if they have refractory symptoms on beta-blockers. This procedure can also be useful in high-risk infants or children where it would be desirable to avoid ICD implantation for as long as possible due to the physical size of the patient. The most common complication is Horner's syndrome.

Recommendations during Pregnancy and Delivery

Evidence on the optimal management of LQTS during pregnancy and delivery is limited. Close cardiac follow-up by a specialist with expertise in the management of LQTS and adherence to medical therapy in the post-partum period is important, particularly if there is evidence of QTc prolongation compared to pre-pregnancy or if QTc is >500 ms. Current ESC guidelines recommend that non-selective beta-blockers should be continued throughout pregnancy and during the post-partum period (at least 40 weeks after delivery) [152]. Exceptions may be LQTS patients without prior syncope or TdP or any other risk profile, for whom a selective beta-blocker may be chosen.

Follow-Up Advice

The frequency of follow-up should be guided by the initial risk assessment and age. High-risk patients need to be followed up closely on at least an annual basis, whilst low-risk patients can be followed up less frequently, for example, every other year. Testing can include a resting ECG and exercise test. Children should be followed at least annually during development and puberty, especially girls, as there is age-dependent evolution of risk and beta-blocker therapy will need to be up-titrated with increasing weight. Changes in genetic technology and family findings may indicate the need for review of relatives as required.

Figure 12.11 summarises the recommended approach to be taken when evaluating and managing an index case presenting to the clinic.

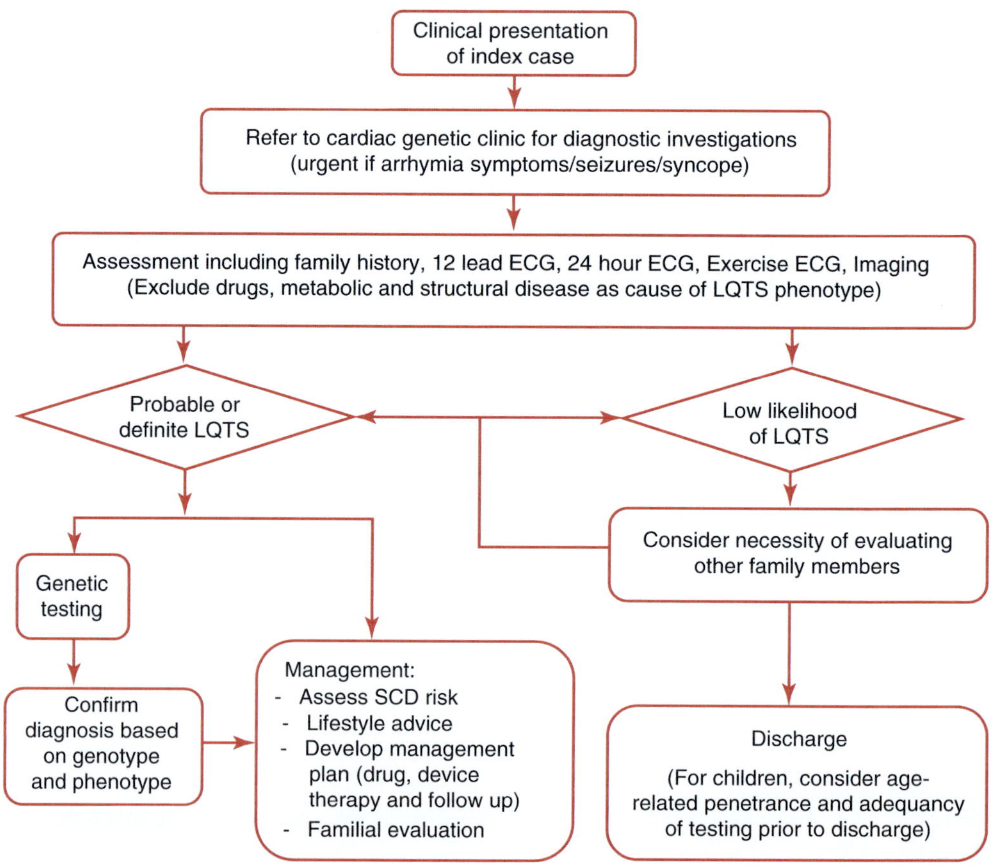

Fig. 12.11 Flowchart summarising the recommended approach to be taken when evaluating and managing an index case presenting to the clinic. (Adapted from Association of Inherited Cardiac Conditions, UK [153])

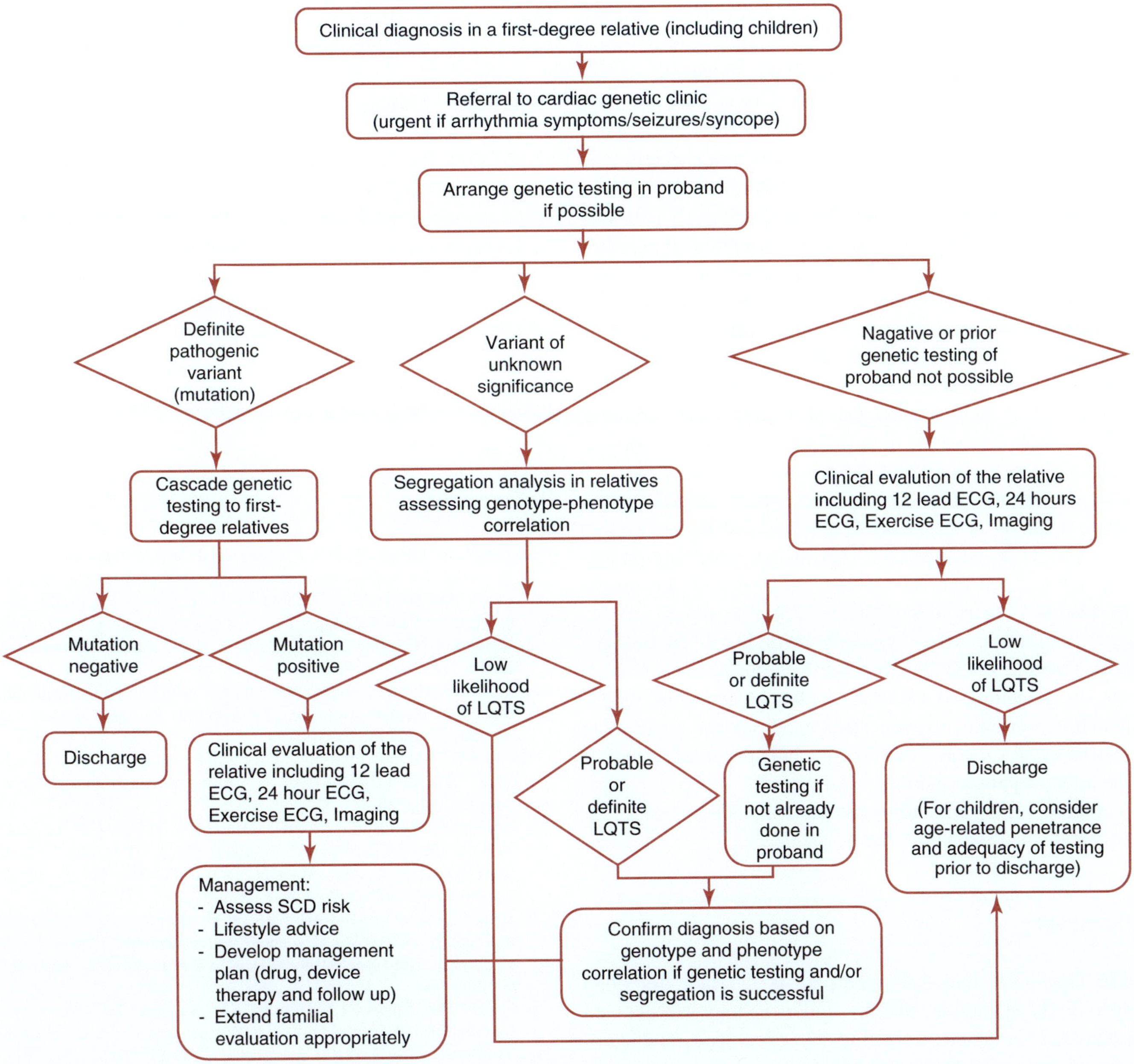

Fig. 12.12 Flowchart summarising the recommended approach to be taken when evaluating and managing a family member of an LQTS patient presenting to clinic. (Adapted from Association of Inherited Cardiac Conditions, UK [153])

Family Screening

Cascade Molecular Screening

Identification of a pathogenic mutation in the index patient (proband) enables cascade genetic screening of other family members, starting with first-degree relatives. Cascade genetic screening enables the identification of affected family members with a single test, including very young children. Thereby, asymptomatic mutation carriers can be easily identified, and preventative measures can be started in a timely manner. Unaffected family members can be reassured and safely discharged from further follow-up. However, this is only possible when a clear pathogenic variant has been identified.

Cascade Clinical Screening and Follow-Up Advice

Upon making the diagnosis of LQTS in a proband, immediate steps must be taken to arrange clinical screening of the family incorporating genetic screening if a pathogenic mutation has been identified in the proband. If the latter is the case, then this can be used early on to exclude negative relatives from further testing and discharge them from the clinic. Otherwise, a clinical assessment should be carried out by or at least discussed with an appropriately experienced specialist in inherited cardiac conditions. There should be systematic evaluation of first-degree blood relatives, with a focus on symptomatic relatives and obligate carriers. A focused but thorough medical history should be obtained from each relative and a physical examination performed. Resting 12-lead and exercise ECGs are a fundamental part of screening. Following this, a transthoracic echocardiogram may be performed to confirm a structurally normal heart [154]. If any suspicions of structural abnormalities are raised on echocardiography, cardiac MRI could be considered. If there is no suspicion of LQTS, the individual can be safely discharged from further follow-up. If, however, clinical screening is negative but it is not possible to carry out cascade genetic testing due to the absence of a clearly pathogenic mutation in the proband, reassessment for age-related penetrance may be important. This applies particularly in pre-pubertal and peri-pubertal children and/or if a child is unable to undertake full exercise testing until they are older.

A multidisciplinary approach involving a cardiologist with expertise in LQTS, a paediatric cardiologist for managing the screening of children, a clinical geneticist, and a genetic counsellor, together with facilities for appropriate psychosocial support, is critical for holistic management of the affected patient and their family.

Figure 12.12 summarises the recommended approach to be taken when evaluating family members.

Summary

The congenital long QT syndrome is the first described arrhythmia syndrome, and its understanding has evolved remarkably as genetic technology has developed. Its diagnosis and management can be challenging, and expert evaluation is recommended if the diagnosis is suspected. Nonetheless, guidelines for diagnosis, risk stratification, and the prevention of sudden death are increasingly well-defined, and genetic information is playing an ever more important role. Expert physicians are progressively more comfortable with their patients undertaking normal lifestyle activities including sports. Whilst ICD therapy is a crucial component of management, improved utilisation of beta-blockers, LCSD, and unconventional medications can minimise its usage. The future promises the potential for mutation-specific and genetic modifier-guided risk assessment. Patient-specific models of disease in the form of induced pluripotent stem cell-derived cardiomyocytes raise the possibility of tailoring therapies and novel agents to suit the phenotype. Of all the cardiac genetic disorders, the era of personalised medicine for LQTS patients is closest to hand.

Take Home Message

- LQT1, LQT2, and LQT3, caused by mutations in *KCNQ1*, *KCNH2*, and *SCN5A*, account for over 90% of genetically confirmed LQTS.
- Diagnosis of LQTS can be challenging—refer for expert evaluation if the diagnosis is suspected.
- The hallmark of management constitutes accurate risk assessment, prevention of cardiac events, and timely screening of family members at risk.

Acknowledgements The authors gratefully acknowledge VN Batchvarov for the assistance with preparing Fig. 12.4.

References

1. Jervell A, Lange-Nielsen F. Congenital deaf-mutism, functional heart disease with prolongation of the Q-T interval and sudden death. Am Heart J. 1957;54(1):59–68. http://www.ncbi.nlm.nih.gov/pubmed/13435203
2. Romano C, Gemme G, Pongiglione R. Rare cardiac arrythmias of the pediatric age. II. Syncopal attacks due to paroxysmal ventricular fibrillation (presentation of 1st case in Italian pediatric literature). Clin Pediatr (Bologna). 1963;45:656–83. http://www.ncbi.nlm.nih.gov/pubmed/14158288
3. Ward OC. A new familial cardiac syndrome in children. J Irish Med Assoc. 1964;54:103–6. http://www.ncbi.nlm.nih.gov/pubmed/14136838
4. Keating M, Atkinson D, Dunn C, Timothy K, Vincent GM, Leppert M. Linkage of a cardiac arrhythmia, the long QT syndrome, and the Harvey ras-1 gene. Science. 1991;252(5006):704–6. http://www.ncbi.nlm.nih.gov/pubmed/1673802
5. Jiang C, Atkinson D, Towbin JA, et al. Two long QT syndrome loci map to chromosomes 3 and 7 with evidence for further heterogeneity. Nat Genet. 1994;8(2):141–7. https://doi.org/10.1038/ng1094-141.
6. Curran ME, Splawski I, Timothy KW, Vincent GM, Green ED, Keating MT. A molecular basis for cardiac arrhythmia: HERG mutations cause long QT syndrome. Cell. 1995;80(5):795–803. http://www.ncbi.nlm.nih.gov/pubmed/7889573
7. Wang Q, Shen J, Splawski I, et al. SCN5A mutations associated with an inherited cardiac arrhythmia, long QT syndrome. Cell. 1995;80(5):805–11. http://www.ncbi.nlm.nih.gov/pubmed/7889574
8. Wang Q, Curran ME, Splawski I, et al. Positional cloning of a novel potassium channel gene: KVLQT1 mutations cause cardiac arrhythmias. Nat Genet. 1996;12(1):17–23. https://doi.org/10.1038/ng0196-17.
9. Schwartz PJ, Stramba-Badiale M, Crotti L, et al. Prevalence of the congenital long-QT syndrome. Circulation. 2009;120(18):1761–7. https://doi.org/10.1161/CIRCULATIONAHA.109.863209.
10. Tester DJ, Ackerman MJ. Postmortem long QT syndrome genetic testing for sudden unexplained death in the young. J Am Coll Cardiol. 2007;49(2):240–6. https://doi.org/10.1016/j.jacc.2006.10.010.
11. Behr ER, Dalageorgou C, Christiansen M, et al. Sudden arrhythmic death syndrome: familial evaluation identifies inherit-

able heart disease in the majority of families. Eur Heart J. 2008;29(13):1670–80. https://doi.org/10.1093/eurheartj/ehn219.
12. Papadakis M, Raju H, Behr ER, et al. Sudden cardiac death with autopsy findings of uncertain significance: potential for erroneous interpretation. Circ Arrhythm Electrophysiol. 2013;6(3):588–96. https://doi.org/10.1161/CIRCEP.113.000111.
13. Priori SG, Wilde AA, Horie M, et al. HRS/EHRA/APHRS expert consensus statement on the diagnosis and management of patients with inherited primary arrhythmia syndromes: document endorsed by HRS, EHRA, and APHRS in may 2013 and by ACCF, AHA, PACES, and AEPC in June 2013. Heart Rhythm. 2013;10(12):1932–63. https://doi.org/10.1016/j.hrthm.2013.05.014.
14. Wilde AAM, Behr ER. Genetic testing for inherited cardiac disease. Nat Rev Cardiol. 2013;10(10):571–83. https://doi.org/10.1038/nrcardio.2013.108.
15. Ackerman MJ, Priori SG, Willems S, et al. HRS/EHRA expert consensus statement on the state of genetic testing for the channelopathies and cardiomyopathies this document was developed as a partnership between the Heart Rhythm Society (HRS) and the European heart rhythm association (EHRA). Heart Rhythm. 2011;8(8):1308–39. https://doi.org/10.1016/j.hrthm.2011.05.020.
16. Splawski I, Shen J, Timothy KW, et al. Spectrum of mutations in long-QT syndrome genes. KVLQT1, HERG, SCN5A, KCNE1, and KCNE2. Circulation. 2000;102(10):1178–85. http://www.ncbi.nlm.nih.gov/pubmed/10973849
17. Moss AJ, Shimizu W, Wilde AAM, et al. Clinical aspects of type-1 long-QT syndrome by location, coding type, and biophysical function of mutations involving the KCNQ1 gene. Circulation. 2007;115(19):2481–9. https://doi.org/10.1161/CIRCULATIONAHA.106.665406.
18. Tester DJ, Benton AJ, Train L, Deal B, Baudhuin LM, Ackerman MJ. Prevalence and spectrum of large deletions or duplications in the major long QT syndrome-susceptibility genes and implications for long QT syndrome genetic testing. Am J Cardiol. 2010;106(8):1124–8. https://doi.org/10.1016/j.amjcard.2010.06.022.
19. Hedley PL, Kanters JK, Dembic M, et al. The role of CAV3 in long-QT syndrome: clinical and functional assessment of a caveolin-3/Kv11.1 double heterozygote versus caveolin-3 single heterozygote. Circ Cardiovasc Genet. 2013;6(5):452–61. https://doi.org/10.1161/CIRCGENETICS.113.000137.
20. Roberts JD, Krahn AD, Ackerman MJ, et al. Loss-of-Function KCNE2 Variants: True Monogenic Culprits of Long-QT Syndrome or Proarrhythmic Variants Requiring Secondary Provocation? Circ Arrhythm Electrophysiol. 2017;10(8):e00528. https://doi.org/10.1161/CIRCEP.117.005282.
21. Burashnikov A, Antzelevitch C. Block of I(Ks) does not induce early afterdepolarization activity but promotes beta-adrenergic agonist-induced delayed afterdepolarization activity. J Cardiovasc Electrophysiol. 2000;11(4):458–65. http://www.ncbi.nlm.nih.gov/pubmed/10809500
22. Tan HL, Bardai A, Shimizu W, et al. Genotype-specific onset of arrhythmias in congenital long-QT syndrome: possible therapy implications. Circulation. 2006;114(20):2096–103. https://doi.org/10.1161/CIRCULATIONAHA.106.642694.
23. Viswanathan PC, Rudy Y. Pause induced early afterdepolarizations in the long QT syndrome: a simulation study. Cardiovasc Res. 1999;42(2):530–42.
24. Antzelevitch C. M cells in the human heart. Circ Res. 2010;106(5):815–7. https://doi.org/10.1161/CIRCRESAHA.109.216226.
25. Burashnikov A, Antzelevitch C. Acceleration-induced action potential prolongation and early afterdepolarizations. J Cardiovasc Electrophysiol. 1998;9(9):934–48.
26. Kim TY, Kunitomo Y, Pfeiffer Z, et al. Complex excitation dynamics underlie polymorphic ventricular tachycardia in a transgenic rabbit model of long QT syndrome type 1. Heart Rhythm. 2015;12(1):220–8. https://doi.org/10.1016/j.hrthm.2014.10.003.
27. Johnson JN, Tester DJ, Perry J, Salisbury BA, Reed CR, Ackerman MJ. Prevalence of early-onset atrial fibrillation in congenital long QT syndrome. Heart Rhythm. 2008;5(5):704–9. https://doi.org/10.1016/j.hrthm.2008.02.007.
28. Zellerhoff S, Pistulli R, Mönnig G, et al. Atrial arrhythmias in long-QT syndrome under daily life conditions: a nested case control study. J Cardiovasc Electrophysiol. 2009;20(4):401–7. https://doi.org/10.1111/j.1540-8167.2008.01339.x.
29. Mandyam MC, Soliman EZ, Alonso A, et al. The QT interval and risk of incident atrial fibrillation. Heart Rhythm. 2013;10(10):1562–8. https://doi.org/10.1016/j.hrthm.2013.07.023.
30. Batra AS, Silka MJ. Mechanism of sudden cardiac arrest while swimming in a child with the prolonged QT syndrome. J Pediatr. 2002;141(2):283–4. https://doi.org/10.1067/mpd.2002.126924.
31. Thomas D, Kiehn J, Katus HA, Karle CA. Adrenergic regulation of the rapid component of the cardiac delayed rectifier potassium current, I(Kr), and the underlying hERG ion channel. Basic Res Cardiol. 2004;99(4):279–87. https://doi.org/10.1007/s00395-004-0474-7.
32. Schwartz PJ, Priori SG, Locati EH, et al. Long QT syndrome patients with mutations of the SCN5A and HERG genes have differential responses to Na+ channel blockade and to increases in heart rate. Implications for gene-specific therapy. Circulation. 1995;92(12):3381–6. http://www.ncbi.nlm.nih.gov/pubmed/8521555
33. Priori SG, Barhanin J, Hauer RN, et al. Genetic and molecular basis of cardiac arrhythmias; impact on clinical management. Study group on molecular basis of arrhythmias of the working group on arrhythmias of the european society of cardiology. Eur Heart J. 1999;20(3):174–95. http://www.ncbi.nlm.nih.gov/pubmed/10082151
34. Schwartz PJ, Priori SG, Spazzolini C, et al. Genotype-phenotype correlation in the long-QT syndrome: gene-specific triggers for life-threatening arrhythmias. Circulation. 2001;103(1):89–95. http://www.ncbi.nlm.nih.gov/pubmed/11136691
35. Makita N, Behr E, Shimizu W, et al. The E1784K mutation in SCN5A is associated with mixed clinical phenotype of type 3 long QT syndrome. J Clin Invest. 2008;118(6):2219–29. https://doi.org/10.1172/JCI34057.
36. Postema PG, Van den Berg M, Van Tintelen JP, et al. Founder mutations in the Netherlands: SCN5a 1795insD, the first described arrhythmia overlap syndrome and one of the largest and best characterised families worldwide. Neth Heart J. 2009;17(11):422–8. http://www.ncbi.nlm.nih.gov/pubmed/19949711
37. Porta A, Girardengo G, Bari V, et al. Autonomic control of heart rate and QT interval variability influences arrhythmic risk in long QT syndrome type 1. J Am Coll Cardiol. 2015;65(4):367–74. https://doi.org/10.1016/j.jacc.2014.11.015.
38. Zareba W, Moss AJ, Schwartz PJ, et al. Influence of genotype on the clinical course of the long-QT syndrome. International long-QT syndrome registry research group. N Engl J Med. 1998;339(14):960–5. https://doi.org/10.1056/NEJM199810013391404.
39. Priori SG, Schwartz PJ, Napolitano C, et al. Risk stratification in the long-QT syndrome. N Engl J Med. 2003;348(19):1866–74. https://doi.org/10.1056/NEJMoa022147.
40. Sauer AJ, Moss AJ, McNitt S, et al. Long QT syndrome in adults. J Am Coll Cardiol. 2007;49(3):329–37. https://doi.org/10.1016/j.jacc.2006.08.057.
41. Migdalovich D, Moss AJ, Lopes CM, et al. Mutation and gender-specific risk in type 2 long QT syndrome: implications for risk stratification for life-threatening cardiac events in patients with long QT syndrome. Heart Rhythm. 2011;8(10):1537–43. https://doi.org/10.1016/j.hrthm.2011.03.049.

42. Chiang CE, Roden DM. The long QT syndromes: genetic basis and clinical implications. J Am Coll Cardiol. 2000;36(1):1–12. http://www.ncbi.nlm.nih.gov/pubmed/10898405
43. Schwartz PJ, Crotti L. QTc behavior during exercise and genetic testing for the long-QT syndrome. Circulation. 2011;124(20):2181–4. https://doi.org/10.1161/CIRCULATIONAHA.111.062182.
44. Schwartz PJ, Ackerman MJ. The long QT syndrome: a transatlantic clinical approach to diagnosis and therapy. Eur Heart J. 2013;34(40):3109–16. https://doi.org/10.1093/eurheartj/eht089.
45. Priori SG, Blomström-Lundqvist C, Mazzanti A, et al. 2015 ESC guidelines for the management of patients with ventricular arrhythmias and the prevention of sudden cardiac death: the task force for the management of patients with ventricular arrhythmias and the prevention of sudden cardiac death of the Europe. Eur Heart J. 2015;36(41):2793–867. https://doi.org/10.1093/eurheartj/ehv316.
46. Lepeschkin E, Surawicz B. The measurement of the Q-T interval of the electrocardiogram. Circulation. 1952;6(3):378–88. http://www.ncbi.nlm.nih.gov/pubmed/14954534
47. Vink AS, Neumann B, Lieve KVV, et al. Determination and interpretation of the QT interval. Circulation. 2018;138:2345–58.
48. Taggart NW, Haglund CM, Tester DJ, Ackerman MJ. Diagnostic miscues in congenital long-QT syndrome. Circulation. 2007;115(20):2613–20. https://doi.org/10.1161/CIRCULATIONAHA.106.661082.
49. Kukla P, Biernacka EK, Baranchuk A, Jastrzebski M, Jagodzinska M. Electrocardiogram in Andersen-Tawil syndrome. New electrocardiographic criteria for diagnosis of type-1 Andersen-Tawil syndrome. Curr Cardiol Rev. 2014;10(3):222–8. http://www.ncbi.nlm.nih.gov/pubmed/24827800
50. Luo S, Michler K, Johnston P, Macfarlane PW. A comparison of commonly used QT correction formulae: the effect of heart rate on the QTc of normal ECGs. J Electrocardiol. 2004;37(Suppl):81–90. http://www.ncbi.nlm.nih.gov/pubmed/15534815
51. Bogossian H, Frommeyer G, Ninios I, et al. New formula for evaluation of the QT interval in patients with left bundle branch block. Heart Rhythm. 2014;11(12):2273–7. https://doi.org/10.1016/j.hrthm.2014.08.026.
52. Viskin S, Rosovski U, Sands AJ, et al. Inaccurate electrocardiographic interpretation of long QT: the majority of physicians cannot recognize a long QT when they see one. Heart Rhythm. 2005;2(6):569–74. https://doi.org/10.1016/j.hrthm.2005.02.011.
53. Postema PG, De Jong JSSG, Van der Bilt IAC, Wilde AAM. Accurate electrocardiographic assessment of the QT interval: teach the tangent. Heart Rhythm. 2008;5(7):1015–8. https://doi.org/10.1016/j.hrthm.2008.03.037.
54. Hibino S, Ueda N, Horiba M, et al. Detection of QT prolongation through approximation of the T wave on Gaussian mixture modeling. Circ J. 2013;77(11):2728–35. http://www.ncbi.nlm.nih.gov/pubmed/23986028
55. Chiladakis J, Kalogeropoulos A, Koutsogiannis N, et al. Optimal QT/JT interval assessment in patients with complete bundle branch block. Ann Noninvasive Electrocardiol. 2012;17(3):268–76. https://doi.org/10.1111/j.1542-474X.2012.00528.x.
56. Cobos MA. Assessment of QT and JT intervals in bundle branch block: a new formula. Circulation. 2013;128:A176.
57. Goldenberg I, Moss AJ, Zareba W. QT interval: how to measure it and what is "normal". J Cardiovasc Electrophysiol. 2006;17(3):333–6. https://doi.org/10.1111/j.1540-8167.2006.00408.x.
58. Moss AJ, Zareba W, Benhorin J, et al. ECG T-wave patterns in genetically distinct forms of the hereditary long QT syndrome. Circulation. 1995;92(10):2929–34. http://www.ncbi.nlm.nih.gov/pubmed/7586261
59. Zhang L, Timothy KW, Vincent GM, et al. Spectrum of ST-T-wave patterns and repolarization parameters in congenital long-QT syndrome: ECG findings identify genotypes. Circulation. 2000;102(23):2849–55. http://www.ncbi.nlm.nih.gov/pubmed/11104743
60. Kop WJ, Krantz DS, Nearing BD, et al. Effects of acute mental stress and exercise on T-wave alternans in patients with implantable cardioverter defibrillators and controls. Circulation. 2004;109(15):1864–9. https://doi.org/10.1161/01.CIR.0000124726.72615.60.
61. Zareba W, Moss AJ, le Cessie S, Hall WJ. T wave alternans in idiopathic long QT syndrome. J Am Coll Cardiol. 1994;23(7):1541–6. http://www.ncbi.nlm.nih.gov/pubmed/8195511
62. Takasugi N, Goto H, Takasugi M, et al. Prevalence of microvolt T-wave Alternans in patients with long QT syndrome and its association with torsade de pointes. Circ Arrhythm Electrophysiol. 2016;9(2):e003206. https://doi.org/10.1161/CIRCEP.115.003206.
63. Reiffel AJ, Reiffel JA. QT prolongation following ectopic beats: initial data regarding the upper limit of normal with possible implications for antiarrhythmic therapy and concealed (unexpressed) long QT. J Atr Fibrillation. 2009;1(5):113. https://doi.org/10.4022/jafib.113.
64. Veldkamp MW, Wilders R, Baartscheer A, Zegers JG, Bezzina CR, Wilde AAM. Contribution of sodium channel mutations to bradycardia and sinus node dysfunction in LQT3 families. Circ Res. 2003;92(9):976–83. https://doi.org/10.1161/01.RES.0000069689.09869.A8.
65. Horner JM, Horner MM, Ackerman MJ. The diagnostic utility of recovery phase QTc during treadmill exercise stress testing in the evaluation of long QT syndrome. Heart Rhythm. 2011;8(11):1698–704. https://doi.org/10.1016/j.hrthm.2011.05.018.
66. Sy RW, van der Werf C, Chattha IS, et al. Derivation and validation of a simple exercise-based algorithm for prediction of genetic testing in relatives of LQTS probands. Circulation. 2011;124(20):2187–94. https://doi.org/10.1161/CIRCULATIONAHA.111.028258.
67. de Noronha SV, Behr ER, Papadakis M, et al. The importance of specialist cardiac histopathological examination in the investigation of young sudden cardiac deaths. Europace. 2014;16(6):899–907. https://doi.org/10.1093/europace/eut329.
68. Lupoglazoff JM, Denjoy I, Berthet M, et al. Notched T waves on Holter recordings enhance detection of patients with LQt2 (HERG) mutations. Circulation. 2001;103(8):1095–101. http://www.ncbi.nlm.nih.gov/pubmed/11222472
69. Seethala S, Singh P, Shusterman V, Ribe M, Haugaa KH, Němec J. QT adaptation and intrinsic QT variability in congenital long QT syndrome. J Am Heart Assoc. 2015;4(12):e002395. https://doi.org/10.1161/JAHA.115.002395.
70. Page A, Aktas MK, Soyata T, Zareba W, Couderc J-P. "QT clock" to improve detection of QT prolongation in long QT syndrome patients. Heart Rhythm. 2016;13(1):190–8. https://doi.org/10.1016/j.hrthm.2015.08.037.
71. van den Berg MP, Haaksma J, Veeger NJGM, Wilde AAM. Diurnal variation of ventricular repolarization in a large family with LQT3-Brugada syndrome characterized by nocturnal sudden death. Heart Rhythm. 2006;3(3):290–5. https://doi.org/10.1016/j.hrthm.2005.11.023.
72. Viskin S, Postema PG, Bhuiyan ZA, et al. The response of the QT interval to the brief tachycardia provoked by standing: a bedside test for diagnosing long QT syndrome. J Am Coll Cardiol. 2010;55(18):1955–61. https://doi.org/10.1016/j.jacc.2009.12.015.
73. Aziz PF, Wieand TS, Ganley J, et al. Genotype- and mutation site-specific QT adaptation during exercise, recovery, and postural changes in children with long-QT syndrome. Circ Arrhythm Electrophysiol. 2011;4(6):867–73. https://doi.org/10.1161/CIRCEP.111.963330.
74. Adler A, van der Werf C, Postema PG, et al. The phenomenon of "QT stunning": the abnormal QT prolongation provoked by standing persists even as the heart rate returns to normal in patients with

long QT syndrome. Heart Rhythm. 2012;9(6):901–8. https://doi.org/10.1016/j.hrthm.2012.01.026.
75. Horner JM, Ackerman MJ. Ventricular ectopy during treadmill exercise stress testing in the evaluation of long QT syndrome. Heart Rhythm. 2008;5(12):1690–4. https://doi.org/10.1016/j.hrthm.2008.08.038.
76. Vyas H, Hejlik J, Ackerman MJ. Epinephrine QT stress testing in the evaluation of congenital long-QT syndrome: diagnostic accuracy of the paradoxical QT response. Circulation. 2006;113(11):1385–92. https://doi.org/10.1161/CIRCULATIONAHA.105.600445.
77. Khositseth A, Hejlik J, Shen W-K, Ackerman MJ. Epinephrine-induced T-wave notching in congenital long QT syndrome. Heart Rhythm. 2005;2(2):141–6. https://doi.org/10.1016/j.hrthm.2004.11.008.
78. Ackerman MJ, Khositseth A, Tester DJ, Hejlik JB, Shen W-K, Porter CJ. Epinephrine-induced QT interval prolongation: a gene-specific paradoxical response in congenital long QT syndrome. Mayo Clin Proc. 2002;77(5):413–21. https://doi.org/10.4065/77.5.413.
79. Shimizu W, Noda T, Takaki H, et al. Epinephrine unmasks latent mutation carriers with LQT1 form of congenital long-QT syndrome. J Am Coll Cardiol. 2003;41(4):633–42. http://www.ncbi.nlm.nih.gov/pubmed/12598076
80. Krahn AD, Healey JS, Chauhan VS, et al. Epinephrine infusion in the evaluation of unexplained cardiac arrest and familial sudden death: from the cardiac arrest survivors with preserved ejection fraction registry. Circ Arrhythm Electrophysiol. 2012;5(5):933–40. https://doi.org/10.1161/CIRCEP.112.973230.
81. Johnson JN, Grifoni C, Bos JM, et al. Prevalence and clinical correlates of QT prolongation in patients with hypertrophic cardiomyopathy. Eur Heart J. 2011;32(9):1114–20. https://doi.org/10.1093/eurheartj/ehr021.
82. Madias C, Fitzgibbons TP, Alsheikh-Ali AA, et al. Acquired long QT syndrome from stress cardiomyopathy is associated with ventricular arrhythmias and torsades de pointes. Heart Rhythm. 2011;8(4):555–61. https://doi.org/10.1016/j.hrthm.2010.12.012.
83. Gray B, Ingles J, Medi C, Semsarian C. Prolongation of the QTc interval predicts appropriate implantable cardioverter-defibrillator therapies in hypertrophic cardiomyopathy. JACC Heart Fail. 2013;1(2):149–55. https://doi.org/10.1016/j.jchf.2013.01.004.
84. Behr ER, Roden D. Drug-induced arrhythmia: pharmacogenomic prescribing? Eur Heart J. 2013;34(2):89–95. https://doi.org/10.1093/eurheartj/ehs351.
85. Arizona Center for Education and Research on Therapeutics (AZCERT). crediblemeds.org. 2016.
86. Neyroud N, Tesson F, Denjoy I, et al. A novel mutation in the potassium channel gene KVLQT1 causes the Jervell and Lange-Nielsen cardioauditory syndrome. Nat Genet. 1997;15(2):186–9. https://doi.org/10.1038/ng0297-186.
87. Westenskow P, Splawski I, Timothy KW, Keating MT, Sanguinetti MC. Compound mutations: a common cause of severe long-QT syndrome. Circulation. 2004;109(15):1834–41. https://doi.org/10.1161/01.CIR.0000125524.34234.13.
88. Goldenberg I, Moss AJ, Zareba W, et al. Clinical course and risk stratification of patients affected with the Jervell and Lange-Nielsen syndrome. J Cardiovasc Electrophysiol. 2006;17(11):1161–8. https://doi.org/10.1111/j.1540-8167.2006.00587.x.
89. Tawil R, Ptacek LJ, Pavlakis SG, et al. Andersen's syndrome: potassium-sensitive periodic paralysis, ventricular ectopy, and dysmorphic features. Ann Neurol. 1994;35(3):326–30. https://doi.org/10.1002/ana.410350313.
90. Sansone V, Griggs RC, Meola G, et al. Andersen's syndrome: a distinct periodic paralysis. Ann Neurol. 1997;42(3):305–12. https://doi.org/10.1002/ana.410420306.
91. Splawski I, Timothy KW, Sharpe LM, et al. Ca(V)1.2 calcium channel dysfunction causes a multisystem disorder including arrhythmia and autism. Cell. 2004;119(1):19–31. https://doi.org/10.1016/j.cell.2004.09.011.
92. Crotti L, Monti MC, Insolia R, et al. NOS1AP is a genetic modifier of the long-QT syndrome. Circulation. 2009;120(17):1657–63. https://doi.org/10.1161/CIRCULATIONAHA.109.879643.
93. Takahashi K, Shimizu W, Miyake A, Nabeshima T, Nakayashiro M, Ganaha H. High prevalence of the SCN5A E1784K mutation in school children with long QT syndrome living on the Okinawa islands. Circ J. 2014;78(8):1974–9. http://www.ncbi.nlm.nih.gov/pubmed/24871449
94. Tester DJ, Kopplin LJ, Will ML, Ackerman MJ. Spectrum and prevalence of cardiac ryanodine receptor (RyR2) mutations in a cohort of unrelated patients referred explicitly for long QT syndrome genetic testing. Heart Rhythm. 2005;2(10):1099–105. https://doi.org/10.1016/j.hrthm.2005.07.012.
95. Ghouse J, Have CT, Weeke P, et al. Rare genetic variants previously associated with congenital forms of long QT syndrome have little or no effect on the QT interval. Eur Heart J. 2015;36(37):2523–9. https://doi.org/10.1093/eurheartj/ehv297.
96. Mogensen J, van Tintelen JP, Fokstuen S, et al. The current role of next-generation DNA sequencing in routine care of patients with hereditary cardiovascular conditions: a viewpoint paper of the European Society of Cardiology working group on myocardial and pericardial diseases and members of the Europ. Eur Heart J. 2015;36(22):1367–70. https://doi.org/10.1093/eurheartj/ehv122.
97. Refsgaard L, Holst AG, Sadjadieh G, Haunsø S, Nielsen JB, Olesen MS. High prevalence of genetic variants previously associated with LQT syndrome in new exome data. Eur J Hum Genet. 2012;20(8):905–8. https://doi.org/10.1038/ejhg.2012.23.
98. Vatta M, Ackerman MJ, Ye B, et al. Mutant caveolin-3 induces persistent late sodium current and is associated with long-QT syndrome. Circulation. 2006;114(20):2104–12. https://doi.org/10.1161/CIRCULATIONAHA.106.635268.
99. Nolte IM, Wallace C, Newhouse SJ, et al. Common genetic variation near the phospholamban gene is associated with cardiac repolarisation: meta-analysis of three genome-wide association studies. PLoS One. 2009;4(7):e6138. https://doi.org/10.1371/journal.pone.0006138.
100. Arking DE, Pfeufer A, Post W, et al. A common genetic variant in the NOS1 regulator NOS1AP modulates cardiac repolarization. Nat Genet. 2006;38(6):644–51. https://doi.org/10.1038/ng1790.
101. Pfeufer A, Sanna S, Arking DE, et al. Common variants at ten loci modulate the QT interval duration in the QTSCD study. Nat Genet. 2009;41(4):407–14. https://doi.org/10.1038/ng.362.
102. Newton-Cheh C, Eijgelsheim M, Rice KM, et al. Common variants at ten loci influence QT interval duration in the QTGEN study. Nat Genet. 2009;41(4):399–406. https://doi.org/10.1038/ng.364.
103. Kolder ICRM, Tanck MWT, Postema PG, et al. Analysis for genetic modifiers of disease severity in patients with long-QT syndrome type 2. Circ Cardiovasc Genet. 2015;8(3):447–56. https://doi.org/10.1161/CIRCGENETICS.114.000785.
104. Hobbs JB, Peterson DR, Moss AJ, et al. Risk of aborted cardiac arrest or sudden cardiac death during adolescence in the long-QT syndrome. JAMA. 2006;296(10):1249–54. https://doi.org/10.1001/jama.296.10.1249.
105. Goldenberg I, Moss AJ, Peterson DR, et al. Risk factors for aborted cardiac arrest and sudden cardiac death in children with the congenital long-QT syndrome. Circulation. 2008;117(17):2184–91. https://doi.org/10.1161/CIRCULATIONAHA.107.701243.
106. Locati EH, Zareba W, Moss AJ, et al. Age- and sex-related differences in clinical manifestations in patients with congenital long-QT syndrome: findings from the international LQTS registry. Circulation. 1998;97(22):2237–44. http://www.ncbi.nlm.nih.gov/pubmed/9631873

107. Goldenberg I, Moss AJ, Bradley J, et al. Long-QT syndrome after age 40. Circulation. 2008;117(17):2192–201. https://doi.org/10.1161/CIRCULATIONAHA.107.729368.
108. Anneken L, Baumann S, Vigneault P, et al. Estradiol regulates human QT-interval: acceleration of cardiac repolarization by enhanced KCNH2 membrane trafficking. Eur Heart J. 2016;37(7):640–50. https://doi.org/10.1093/eurheartj/ehv371.
109. Khositseth A, Tester DJ, Will ML, Bell CM, Ackerman MJ. Identification of a common genetic substrate underlying postpartum cardiac events in congenital long QT syndrome. Heart Rhythm. 2004;1(1):60–4. https://doi.org/10.1016/j.hrthm.2004.01.006.
110. Seth R, Moss AJ, McNitt S, et al. Long QT syndrome and pregnancy. J Am Coll Cardiol. 2007;49(10):1092–8. https://doi.org/10.1016/j.jacc.2006.09.054.
111. Meregalli PG, Westendorp ICD, Tan HL, Elsman P, Kok WEM, Wilde AAM. Pregnancy and the risk of torsades de pointes in congenital long-QT syndrome. Neth Heart J. 2008;16(12):422–5. http://www.ncbi.nlm.nih.gov/pubmed/19127321
112. Kimbrough J, Moss AJ, Zareba W, et al. Clinical implications for affected parents and siblings of probands with long-QT syndrome. Circulation. 2001;104(5):557–62. http://www.ncbi.nlm.nih.gov/pubmed/11479253
113. Kaufman ES, McNitt S, Moss AJ, et al. Risk of death in the long QT syndrome when a sibling has died. Heart Rhythm. 2008;5(6):831–6. https://doi.org/10.1016/j.hrthm.2008.02.029.
114. Spazzolini C, Mullally J, Moss AJ, et al. Clinical implications for patients with long QT syndrome who experience a cardiac event during infancy. J Am Coll Cardiol. 2009;54(9):832–7. https://doi.org/10.1016/j.jacc.2009.05.029.
115. Goldenberg I, Mathew J, Moss AJ, et al. Corrected QT variability in serial electrocardiograms in long QT syndrome: the importance of the maximum corrected QT for risk stratification. J Am Coll Cardiol. 2006;48(5):1047–52. https://doi.org/10.1016/j.jacc.2006.06.033.
116. Mazzanti A, Maragna R, Vacanti G, et al. Interplay between genetic substrate, QTc duration, and arrhythmia risk in patients with long QT syndrome. J Am Coll Cardiol. 2018;71(15):1663–71. https://doi.org/10.1016/j.jacc.2018.01.078.
117. Goldenberg I, Horr S, Moss AJ, et al. Risk for life-threatening cardiac events in patients with genotype-confirmed long-QT syndrome and normal-range corrected QT intervals. J Am Coll Cardiol. 2011;57(1):51–9. https://doi.org/10.1016/j.jacc.2010.07.038.
118. Itoh H, Shimizu W, Hayashi K, et al. Long QT syndrome with compound mutations is associated with a more severe phenotype: a Japanese multicenter study. Heart Rhythm. 2010;7(10):1411–8. https://doi.org/10.1016/j.hrthm.2010.06.013.
119. Mullally J, Goldenberg I, Moss AJ, et al. Risk of life-threatening cardiac events among patients with long QT syndrome and multiple mutations. Heart Rhythm. 2013;10(3):378–82. https://doi.org/10.1016/j.hrthm.2012.11.006.
120. Crotti L, Spazzolini C, Schwartz PJ, et al. The common long-QT syndrome mutation KCNQ1/A341V causes unusually severe clinical manifestations in patients with different ethnic backgrounds: toward a mutation-specific risk stratification. Circulation. 2007;116(21):2366–75. https://doi.org/10.1161/CIRCULATIONAHA.107.726950.
121. Moss AJ, Zareba W, Kaufman ES, et al. Increased risk of arrhythmic events in long-QT syndrome with mutations in the pore region of the human ether-a-go-go-related gene potassium channel. Circulation. 2002;105(7):794–9. http://www.ncbi.nlm.nih.gov/pubmed/11854117
122. Crotti L, Lundquist AL, Insolia R, et al. KCNH2-K897T is a genetic modifier of latent congenital long-QT syndrome. Circulation. 2005;112(9):1251–8. https://doi.org/10.1161/CIRCULATIONAHA.105.549071.
123. Duchatelet S, Crotti L, Peat RA, et al. Identification of a KCNQ1 polymorphism acting as a protective modifier against arrhythmic risk in long-QT syndrome. Circ Cardiovasc Genet. 2013;6(4):354–61. https://doi.org/10.1161/CIRCGENETICS.113.000023.
124. de Villiers CP, van der Merwe L, Crotti L, et al. AKAP9 is a genetic modifier of congenital long-QT syndrome type 1. Circ Cardiovasc Genet. 2014;7(5):599–606. https://doi.org/10.1161/CIRCGENETICS.113.000580.
125. Earle N, Yeo Han D, Pilbrow A, et al. Single nucleotide polymorphisms in arrhythmia genes modify the risk of cardiac events and sudden death in long QT syndrome. Heart Rhythm. 2014;11(1):76–82. https://doi.org/10.1016/j.hrthm.2013.10.005.
126. Tomás M, Napolitano C, De Giuli L, et al. Polymorphisms in the NOS1AP gene modulate QT interval duration and risk of arrhythmias in the long QT syndrome. J Am Coll Cardiol. 2010;55(24):2745–52. https://doi.org/10.1016/j.jacc.2009.12.065.
127. Ackerman MJ, Zipes DP, Kovacs RJ, Maron BJ. Eligibility and disqualification recommendations for competitive athletes with cardiovascular abnormalities: task force 10: the cardiac Channelopathies: a scientific statement from the American Heart Association and American College of Cardiology. J Am Coll Cardiol. 2015;66(21):2424–8. https://doi.org/10.1016/j.jacc.2015.09.042.
128. Zipes DP, Link MS, Ackerman MJ, Kovacs RJ, Myerburg RJ, Estes NAM. Eligibility and disqualification recommendations for competitive athletes with cardiovascular abnormalities: task force 9: arrhythmias and conduction defects: a scientific statement from the American Heart Association and American College of Cardiology. J Am Coll Cardiol. 2015;66(21):2412–23. https://doi.org/10.1016/j.jacc.2015.09.041.
129. Pelliccia A, Zipes DP, Maron BJ. Bethesda conference #36 and the European Society of Cardiology Consensus Recommendations revisited a comparison of U.S. and European criteria for eligibility and disqualification of competitive athletes with cardiovascular abnormalities. J Am Coll Cardiol. 2008;52(24):1990–6. https://doi.org/10.1016/j.jacc.2008.08.055.
130. Maron BJ, Zipes DP. Introduction: eligibility recommendations for competitive athletes with cardiovascular abnormalities-general considerations. J Am Coll Cardiol. 2005;45(8):1318–21. https://doi.org/10.1016/j.jacc.2005.02.006.
131. Pelliccia A, Fagard R, Bjørnstad HH, et al. Recommendations for competitive sports participation in athletes with cardiovascular disease: a consensus document from the study group of sports cardiology of the working group of cardiac rehabilitation and exercise physiology and the working Group of my. Eur Heart J. 2005;26(14):1422–45. https://doi.org/10.1093/eurheartj/ehi325.
132. Johnson JN, Ackerman MJ. Competitive sports participation in athletes with congenital long QT syndrome. JAMA. 2012;308(8):764–5. https://doi.org/10.1001/jama.2012.9334.
133. Johnson JN, Ackerman MJ. Return to play? Athletes with congenital long QT syndrome. Br J Sports Med. 2013;47(1):28–33. https://doi.org/10.1136/bjsports-2012-091751.
134. Lampert R, Olshansky B, Heidbuchel H, et al. Safety of sports for athletes with implantable Cardioverter-defibrillators: long-term results of a prospective multinational registry. Circulation. 2017;135(23):2310–2. https://doi.org/10.1161/CIRCULATIONAHA.117.027828.
135. Baggish AL, Ackerman MJ, Lampert R. Competitive sport participation among athletes with heart disease: a call for a paradigm shift in decision making. Circulation. 2017;136(17):1569–71. https://doi.org/10.1161/CIRCULATIONAHA.117.029639.
136. Vincent GM, Schwartz PJ, Denjoy I, et al. High efficacy of beta-blockers in long-QT syndrome type 1: contribution of noncompliance and QT-prolonging drugs to the occurrence of beta-blocker treatment "failures". Circulation. 2009;119(2):215–21. https://doi.org/10.1161/CIRCULATIONAHA.108.772533.

137. Goldenberg I, Bradley J, Moss A, et al. Beta-blocker efficacy in high-risk patients with the congenital long-QT syndrome types 1 and 2: implications for patient management. J Cardiovasc Electrophysiol. 2010;21(8):893–901. https://doi.org/10.1111/j.1540-8167.2010.01737.x.
138. Wilde AAM, Ackerman MJ. Beta-blockers in the treatment of congenital long QT syndrome: is one beta-blocker superior to another? J Am Coll Cardiol. 2014;64(13):1359–61. https://doi.org/10.1016/j.jacc.2014.06.1192.
139. Ruan Y, Liu N, Napolitano C, Priori SG. Therapeutic strategies for long-QT syndrome: does the molecular substrate matter? Circ Arrhythm Electrophysiol. 2008;1(4):290–7. https://doi.org/10.1161/CIRCEP.108.795617.
140. Funasako M, Aiba T, Ishibashi K, et al. Pronounced shortening of QT interval with Mexiletine infusion test in patients with type 3 congenital long QT syndrome. Circ J. 2016;80(2):340–5. https://doi.org/10.1253/circj.CJ-15-0984.
141. Mazzanti A, Maragna R, Faragli A, et al. Gene-specific therapy with Mexiletine reduces arrhythmic events in patients with long QT syndrome type 3. J Am Coll Cardiol. 2016;67(9):1053–8. https://doi.org/10.1016/j.jacc.2015.12.033.
142. Mazzanti A, Maragna R, Napolitano C, Priori SG. Reply: did mutation type affect the efficacy of Mexiletine observed in patients with LQTS type 3? J Am Coll Cardiol. 2017;69(2):248–9. https://doi.org/10.1016/j.jacc.2016.09.981.
143. Moss AJ, Zareba W, Schwarz KQ, Rosero S, McNitt S, Robinson JL. Ranolazine shortens repolarization in patients with sustained inward sodium current due to type-3 long-QT syndrome. J Cardiovasc Electrophysiol. 2008;19(12):1289–93. https://doi.org/10.1111/j.1540-8167.2008.01246.x.
144. Huang H, Priori SG, Napolitano C, O'Leary ME, Chahine M. Y1767C, a novel SCN5A mutation, induces a persistent Na+ current and potentiates ranolazine inhibition of Nav1.5 channels. Am J Physiol Heart Circ Physiol. 2011;300(1):H288–99. https://doi.org/10.1152/ajpheart.00539.2010.
145. Chorin E, Hu D, Antzelevitch C, et al. Ranolazine for congenital long-QT syndrome type III: experimental and long-term clinical data. Circ Arrhythm Electrophysiol. 2016;9(10):e004370. https://doi.org/10.1161/CIRCEP.116.004370.
146. Paci M, Passini E, Severi S, Hyttinen J, Rodriguez B. Phenotypic variability in LQT3 human induced pluripotent stem cell-derived cardiomyocytes and their response to antiarrhythmic pharmacologic therapy: an in silico approach. Hear Rhythm. 2017;14(11):1704–12. https://doi.org/10.1016/j.hrthm.2017.07.026.
147. Schwartz PJ, Spazzolini C, Priori SG, et al. Who are the long-QT syndrome patients who receive an implantable cardioverter-defibrillator and what happens to them?: data from the European long-QT syndrome implantable Cardioverter-defibrillator (LQTS ICD) registry. Circulation. 2010;122(13):1272–82. https://doi.org/10.1161/CIRCULATIONAHA.110.950147.
148. Kusumoto FM, Calkins H, Boehmer J, et al. HRS/ACC/AHA expert consensus statement on the use of implantable cardioverter-defibrillator therapy in patients who are not included or not well represented in clinical trials. J Am Coll Cardiol. 2014;64(11):1143–77. https://doi.org/10.1016/j.jacc.2014.04.008.
149. Schwartz PJ, Priori SG, Cerrone M, et al. Left cardiac sympathetic denervation in the management of high-risk patients affected by the long-QT syndrome. Circulation. 2004;109(15):1826–33. https://doi.org/10.1161/01.CIR.0000125523.14403.1E.
150. Desimone CV, Bos JM, Bos KM, et al. Effects on repolarization using dynamic QT interval monitoring in long-QT patients following left cardiac sympathetic denervation. J Cardiovasc Electrophysiol. 2015;26(4):434–9. https://doi.org/10.1111/jce.12609.
151. Schneider AE, Bos JM, Ackerman MJ. Effect of left cardiac sympathetic denervation on the electromechanical window in patients with either type 1 or type 2 long QT syndrome: a pilot study. Congenit Heart Dis. February 2016;11:437. https://doi.org/10.1111/chd.12332.
152. Regitz-Zagrosek V, Roos-Hesselink JW, Bauersachs J, et al. 2018 ESC guidelines for the management of cardiovascular diseases during pregnancy. Eur Heart J. 2018;39(34):3165–241. https://doi.org/10.1093/eurheartj/ehy340.
153. AICC. Association of Inherited Cardiac Conditions – Pathways. http://theaicc.org/?page_id=55. Published 2018.
154. Mellor G, Behr ER. Sudden Unexplained Death – Treating the Family. Arrhythmia Electrophysiol Rev. 2014;3(3):156–60. https://doi.org/10.15420/aer.2014.3.3.156.

Short QT Syndrome

13

Christian Wolpert and Eric Schulze-Bahr

Introduction

In 2000, Gussak et al. first described an idiopathic short QT interval associated with atrial fibrillation (AF) in one family and sudden death in an unrelated individual [1]. A few years later, Gaita et al. reported the association of a short QT interval and sudden cardiac death in two unrelated European families [2]. A variety of mutations in different genes most likely causative for a novel primary electrical heart disease termed short QT syndrome (SQTS) were identified until this day. The very first reported mutations caused either a gain of function of cardiac potassium channels I_{Kr}, I_{Ks} and I_{K1} or a loss of function in the cardiac L-type calcium channel (I_{Ca}) [3–10]. Meanwhile, new mutations have been reported recently resulting in different alterations of ion channel activity.

Clinical Presentation

The clinical presentation of patients with SQTS is heterogeneous. The first comprehensive data were presented by Giustetto et al. from the EUROSHORT registry [10]. A total of 29 patients (21 m, 8 f) were studied. Eighteen out of twenty-nine were symptomatic at the time of enrolment. Nine of the patients had a history of cardiac arrest, six had suffered syncope, and seven had documented atrial flutter or atrial fibrillation [10]. The onset of symptoms was highly variable ranging from the age of 4 months up to the age of 62 years, and it was distributed over all decades of life. Sudden cardiac death (SCD) occurred in the youngest patient at the age of 4 months. Thus, SQTS represented also a new potential cause for the sudden infant death syndrome (SIDS).

C. Wolpert · E. Schulze-Bahr (✉)
Klinikum Ludwigsburg, Department of Medicine – Cardiology, Ludwigsburg, Germany

Institut für Genetik von Herzerkrankungen (IfGH), Universitätsklinikum Münster (UKM), Münster, Germany
e-mail: christian.wolpert@rkh-kliniken.de

Mazzanti and co-workers studied a population of 47 probands who were referred to the database for cardiac arrest (n = 19), syncope (n = 9), family history of sudden death (n = 2) or an incidentally found short QTc interval [11]. Twelve subjects had a family history of sudden death in the young, and four had multiple victims in their family (2.5 ± 0.6.) Of note, the QTc interval among the asymptomatic individuals, the sudden death victims and patients with syncope did not differ significantly. The age at the time of syncope or sudden death was also comparable with 21 ± 11 vs 25 ± 13 years. The QTc interval in those, in whom a mutation was identified, was significantly shorter (300 vs 335 ms). There was no difference in the likelihood of sudden death between mutation-positive and mutation-negative probands.

Villafane and co-workers published an international series of 21 paediatric SQTS patients [12, 13]. The median age was 15 years. Fifty-six percent (84% males) of the patients were symptomatic for syncope (n = 4) or sudden death (n = 6). Sixteen patients had either a personal or family history of sudden death. The rate of atrial fibrillation was high for this young cohort with 4/21 patients. It is important to note that some of these children were part of the other patient populations such as the first publication on the *KCNH2* gene mutation [12].

A gene mutation can be identified in only 24%. Eleven of 21 patients received an ICD, two patients received an appropriate shock, and in 64% of the patients, inappropriate shocks were observed. The authors applied the Gollob score [14] and observed that asymptomatic individuals with a Gollob score of <5 were asymptomatic for ventricular tachycardia or ventricular fibrillation (VT/VF) or sudden death and syncope over a 6-year follow-up. In a Japanese series of five Japanese unrelated families, symptoms were AF in two, ventricular fibrillation (VF) in two, sudden death in three patients and severe bradycardia in one newborn. The QTc in this series was between 280 and 340 ms, i.e. somewhat longer than in patients with SQT1 [15, 16]. Recently, Hu et al. presented a population of 18 members of 7 unrelated families from different countries who suffered

H. F. Baars et al. (eds.), *Clinical Cardiogenetics*, https://doi.org/10.1007/978-3-030-45457-9_13

from a *KCNH2*-Thr618Ile mutation. Eighteen members of these seven families had suffered sudden cardiac death. The penetrance was 100% in all carriers. The QTc interval in this cohort was 294.1 ± 23.8 ms in probands and 313.2 ± 23.8 ms in all carriers [17].

Triggers of VF

There is only little reported about the circumstances of symptoms and sudden death in patients with a short QT syndrome. In the first series published by Giustetto et al., there were three with symptoms during sleep, three at rest and three during definite effort, and the remainder was either unknown or in two during normal daily activity. This means that there is not a common trigger for arrhythmias as sees as in catecholaminergic polymorphic ventricular tachycardia (CPVT; trigger: exercise) or in long QT syndrome (LQTS; stress or exercise) [10]. Mazzanti et al. reported on 20 patients of whom 10 experienced multiple events. Twenty occurred during rest, three while eating and two while driving; three events only were seen during emotional stress and two during effort. This speaks against an adrenergic stimulation as a trigger for VF as general mechanism [11].

Clinical Diagnosis of SQTS and Prevalence

After 18 years since its first clinical description, there are recommendations in the guidelines for the lower limit of the QTc interval and, subsequently, criteria for the diagnosis for SQTS. The basis for these limits is derived from all the available clinical reports, which is limited by the low total number of individuals worldwide that have been identified with an SQTS. In all publications, the QTc interval is reported to be constantly short. However, there may be an SQTS with only intermittent abbreviation of the QTc interval such as in LQTS, where a minority of patients present with a long QTc interval only under certain conditions. However, there are no reports yet.

What Is a Normal QTc Interval?

In the general population, heart rate-corrected QT intervals (QTc intervals) follow a Gaussian normal distribution [18–25]. Normal QTc intervals were proposed as QTc intervals within two standard deviations from the mean. Thus, 95% of the QTc intervals of the general population are "normal". QTc shorter than the 2.5th percentile were defined as "short". Following this calculation, QTc of <350 ms for men and QTc < 360 ms for women are considered as short. In large population-based studies, the prevalence of such a short QT interval was analysed. Within an Italian predominantly male cohort, the prevalence of a QTc < 360 ms was 0.5%. Anttonen et al. analysed a population of 10,822 subjects and found short QTc intervals of <340 ms in 0.4% of the subjects [18]. Very short QTc intervals <320 ms were seen in 0.1% of the cases. Both patients with a short and a very short QTc interval had no cardiac events [8]. In a Japanese cohort of 12,149 subjects, 0.01% exhibited a QTc interval within the 2.5th percentile (men QTc < 354 ms; females <364 ms) and only 3 male subjects a QTc of <300 ms [19]. In another analysis of 19,153 subjects undergoing biannual health examinations in the follow-up program in Hiroshima and Nagasaki since 1958, the prevalence for a short QT interval (QTc < 350 ms) was 0.01% [13]. Kobza et al. found a similar low prevalence of 0.01% of QTc intervals <320 ms in 41,767 male army conscripts [21].

A recent report on an ECG population sample among 1.7 million persons yielded a QTc of less than 300 ms in 2.7 in 100,000. The risk of dying in a period of 8.3 years of follow-up was increased 2.6-fold [23].

The hallmark of diagnosis is a short QT interval in baseline ECG. QTc intervals of <350 ms for males and < 360 ms for females should gain attention and warrant further clinical work-up. In coincidence with the clinical symptoms such as atrial fibrillation, sudden cardiac death, family history of SQTS or sudden cardiac death or syncope, the diagnosis of SQTS can be established.

Overall, the prevalence of SQTS can be estimated at around 1: 10,000.

The electrocardiogram of the first patients identified with an SQTS (SQT1 subtype) showed very short QT intervals and in addition short QT intervals corrected for heart rate (QTc < 300 ms). (Figs. 13.1 and 13.2) The patients identified as SQT2–SQT5 subtypes exhibited QTc values up to 360 ms. The ECG in SQT1–SQT3 patients showed tall, symmetrical and asymmetrical peaked T waves especially in the precordial chest leads (Fig. 13.2). In SQT3, the T wave has a less steep ascending part and a steep downslope. In most cases, an ST segment is absent with the T wave originating directly from the S wave. Another finding in SQTS is a prolonged T_{peak}–T_{end} interval. Anttonen et al. compared the J-point-T_{peak} interval in symptomatic patients with SQTS, probands with a short QT interval and a control group of subjects with normal QT interval [26]. Symptomatic patients with SQTS had significantly shorter J-point-T_{peak} intervals and higher corrected T_{peak}–T_{end}/QTc ratios compared to asymptomatic probands with a short QT interval and subjects with a normal QT interval. Patients diagnosed with SQT4 and SQT5 on the basis of a mutation in the cardiac calcium channel exhibit shorter than normal QT intervals of 330–360 ms, which is relatively longer than in SQT1–SQT3. These patients additionally show ST-segment elevation diagnostic of Brugada syndrome either spontaneously or after the administration of intravenous ajmaline [5].

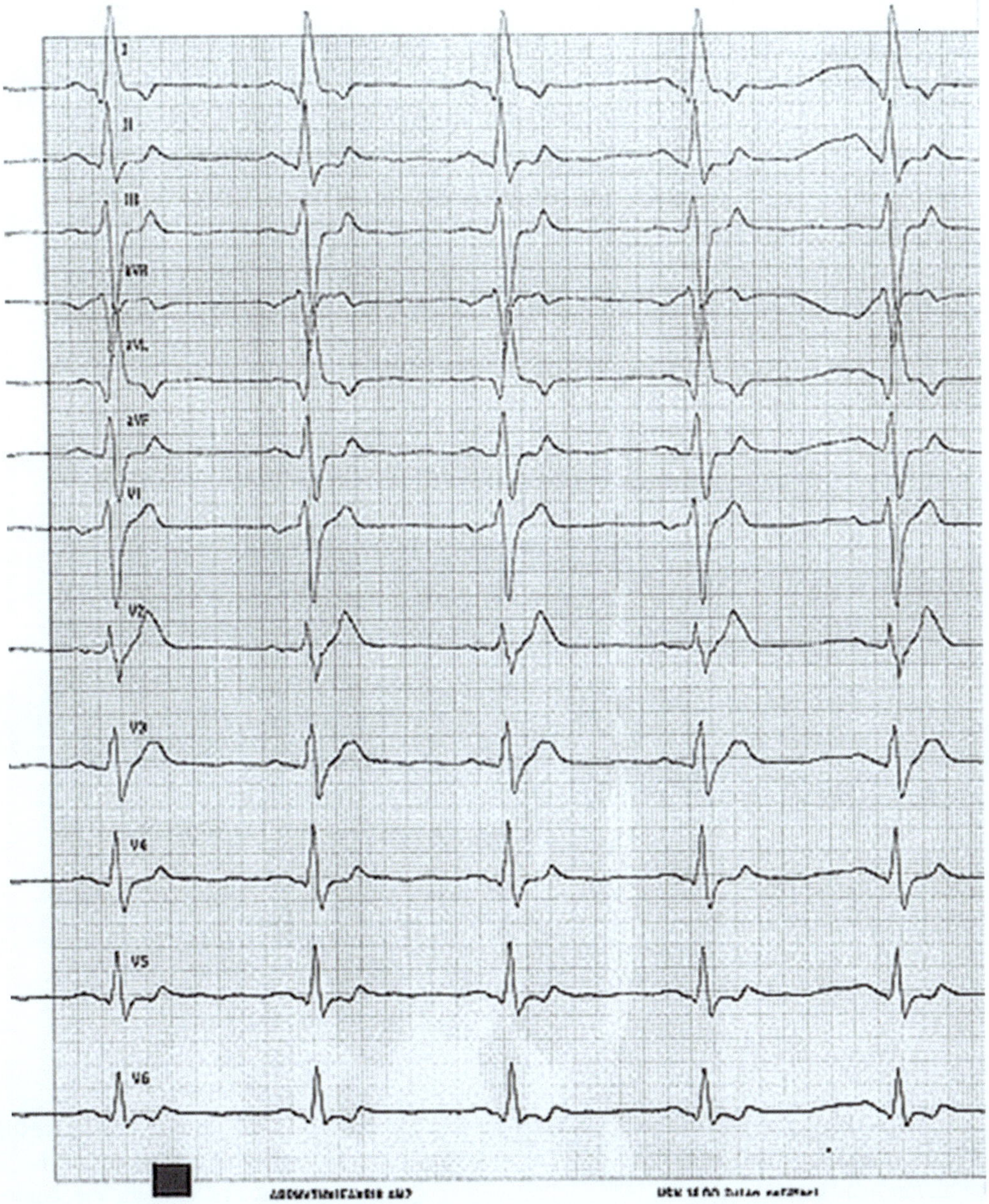

Fig. 13.1 This figure depicts the chest leads of an ECG of a patient with SQT1

Villafane et al. reported the data on paediatric patients with a short QT syndrome. The QTc ranged here from 294 to 355 ms (mean 312 ms) [12, 13].

QT Adaptation to Heart Rate

Another important finding in the initially reported SQT1 patients was the inappropriate adaptation of the QTc interval to heart rate. In the first SQTS patients with a *KCNH2* mutation, the QT interval did not shorten adequately at higher heart rates as compared to controls. Quinidine was able to restore the QTc/heart rate ratio towards the normal range. This lack of adaptation of QT interval with heart rate seemed to be one additional criterion for the diagnosis of SQTS [10, 27].

Giustetto and co-workers further studied the usefulness of exercise testing in the diagnosis of SQTS in the largest series of patients with different mutations in order to see if QT behaviour during exercise helps to differentiate between SQTS patients and individuals with a shorter than normal QT interval. They looked at 21 SQTS patients including the patients from the first report and matched controls. Rest and peak exercise heart rates did not differ between the groups. The baseline QT intervals at resting conditions were 276 vs. 364 ms and at peak exercise 228 ± 27 ms vs. 245 ± 26 ms with a mean variation from rest to peak exercise of 48 ± 14 vs. 120 ± 20 ms. The QT/HR slope never exceeded 0.9 ms/bpm. The mean was −0.53 ms/bpm vs. −1.29 ms/bpm.

Taken together and following the concept of a myocardial repolarization reserve, patients with an SQTS are at the

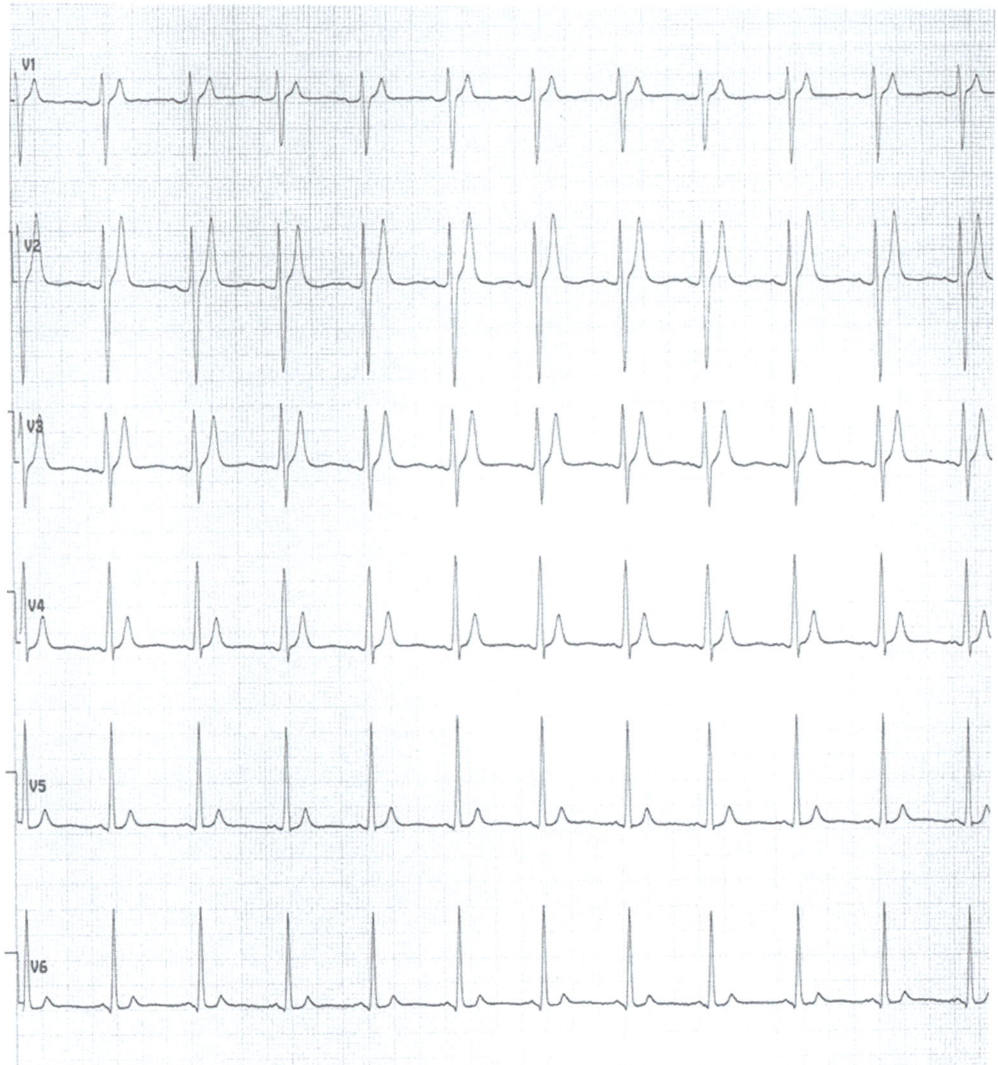

Fig. 13.2 ECG of a patient with SQT syndrome type 1 and a *KCNH2* mutation

lower limit of short repolarization and, subsequently, are not capable to further shorten repolarization as seen in controls at higher heart rates.

Other Cardiac Findings in SQTS Patients

There have been other interesting observations such as PQ-segment depression and echocardiographic findings, which however are not fully understood yet and therefore cannot be considered diagnostic or pathognomonic for SQTS. The first PQ-segment depression was analysed and first described by Tülümen et al. [28]. In their series of patients, the segment between the P wave and the QRS complex was depressed below the isoelectric in 52/64 (81%) of the patients. The authors speculate that a heterogenous abbreviation of atrial repolarization could lead to the PQ-segment depression. They compared the patients with an SQTS to a control group of 117 healthy matched pairs.

Two groups have investigated echocardiographic findings in SQTS patients. The first investigation correlated the surface ECG to the mechanics in SQTS and described a certain electromechanical dissociation of specific phases of relaxation and the time course of repolarization [29]. The second, more recent, report analysed the myocardial performance index, mechanical dispersion and global longitudinal strain. They found that in SQT patients, myocardial function was slightly reduced and the mechanical dispersion was increased [30].

However, these additional observations are only preliminary and have to be confirmed in larger populations.

Invasive Electrophysiological Studies in SQTS

A further diagnostic tool in SQTS patients might be an invasive electrophysiological evaluation. Atrial and ventricular effective refractory periods are significantly shortened, especially in SQT1 (*KCNH2*) [31]. An atrial refractory period of 140 ms and a ventricular effective refractory period of 150 ms or less are highly suspicious criteria of the SQTS. Another finding is the high inducibility of ventricular fibrillation during programmed ventricular stimulation in patients with SQTS1 (Fig. 13.3) [18]. First data from 2003 were confirmed by Rollin and co-workers in 2017, who studied atrial and ventricular effective refractory periods in 16 patients with SQTS. They compared the intervals at 600 and 500 ms basic train cycle length in the RV apex, the RVOT and the right atrium. When using a cut-off of <200 ms, the sensitivity was 86% for the diagnosis of a short QT syndrome, and specificity was 100% compared to controls [32].

The current consensus recommendations and the ESC guidelines [33], however, do not recommend programmed ventricular stimulation for clinical risk stratification in SQTS.

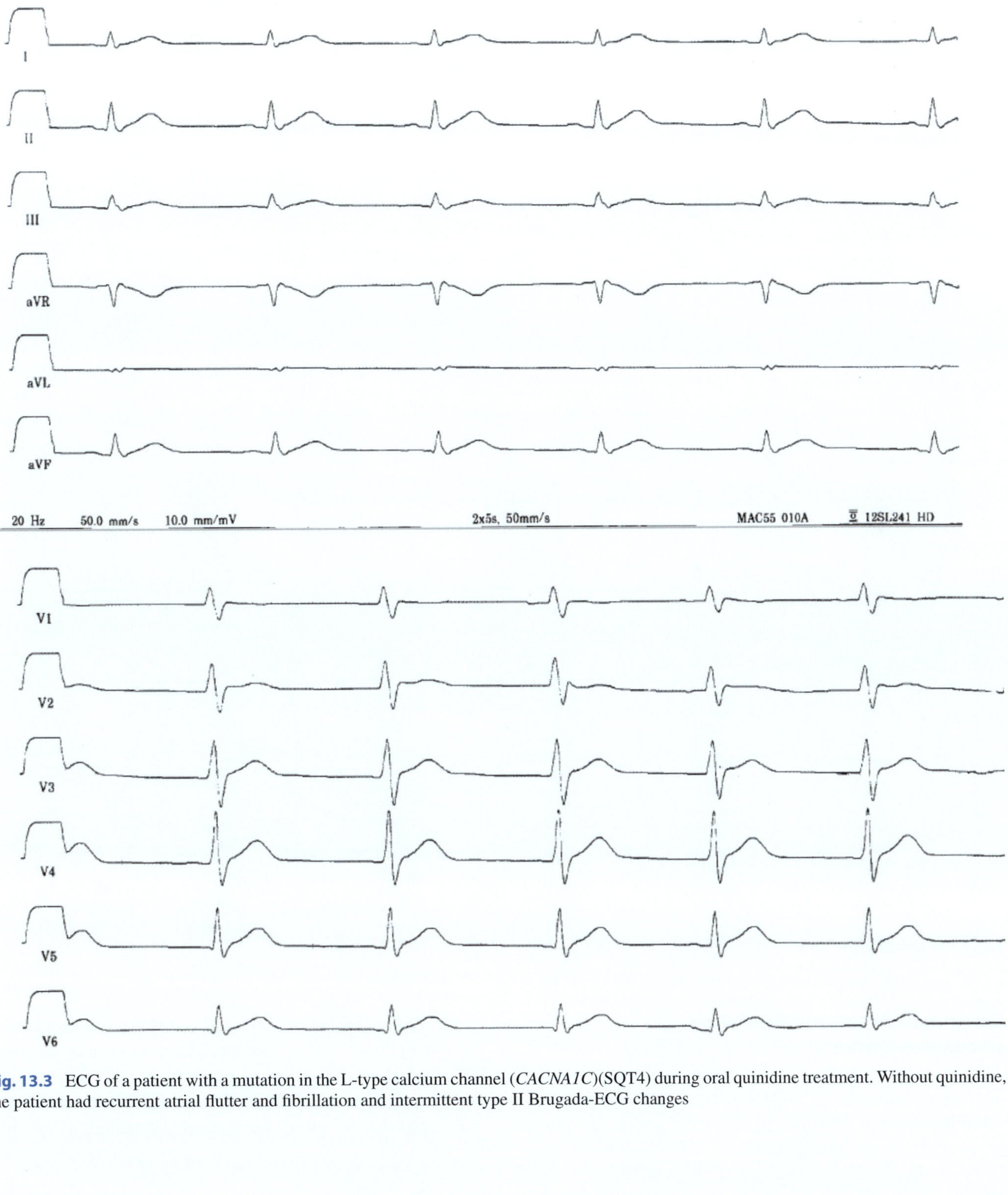

Fig. 13.3 ECG of a patient with a mutation in the L-type calcium channel (*CACNA1C*)(SQT4) during oral quinidine treatment. Without quinidine, the patient had recurrent atrial flutter and fibrillation and intermittent type II Brugada-ECG changes

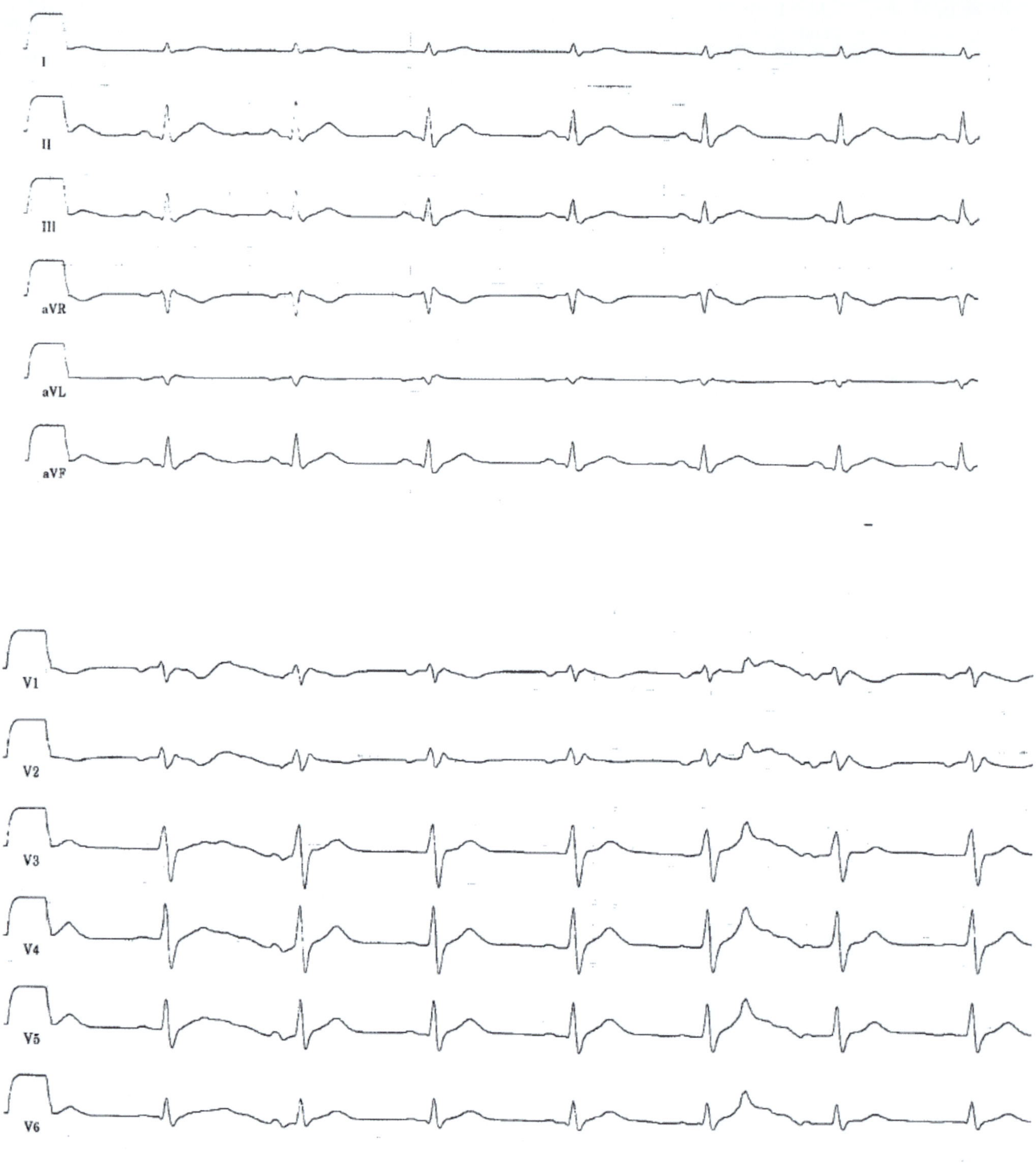

Fig. 13.3 (continued)

Diagnostic Score and Guideline Recommendations

The QTc intervals of SQTS patients are ranging from <360 ms down to <300 ms. In summary, a short QT interval on the 12-lead ECG does not predict risk for life-threatening tachyarrhythmias per se. However, the rare finding of a short QT interval should initiate a diagnostic work-up including family members. In the case of a short QT interval together with episodes of atrial fibrillation, sustained palpitation, unexplained syncope, ventricular fibrillation and/or a positive family history for premature sudden cardiac death, SQTS should be suspected [32, 33].

Gollob et al. proposed a diagnostic criteria score for SQTS analogous to the "Schwartz Score" for long QT syndrome in which a high probability of SQTS was reached when more or equal to 4 points were given; a QTc of <370 ms was 1 point, <350 ms 2 points and <330 ms equal to 3 points [33]. In any case, phenocopying conditions for short QT interval generation in the surface ECG have to be excluded (Table 13.2).

The 2015 ESC guidelines for the management of patients with ventricular arrhythmias and the prevention of sudden cardiac death provide a class I recommendation for a diagnosis of an SQTS when the QTc is <340 ms. It should be considered if the QTc is <360 ms and one or more of the following conditions exists:

(a) A confirmed pathogenic mutation
(b) A family history of SQTS
(c) A family history of sudden death at age < 40 years
(d) Survival from a VT/VF episode in the absence of heart disease

The guidelines emphasize an EP study only as a class III indication ("not recommended") for risk stratification [33].

Genetic Background

So far, around 200 patients with SQTS have been reported, and within this limitation of a small number, not all patients have been systematically investigated through a thorough genetic analysis. Thus, the current mutation detection rate (diagnostic sensitivity) in SQTS is not known, but estimated <25%.

SQTS is a genetically heterogeneous disease similarly as its physiological counterpart, congenital long QT syndrome, and thereby is classified as an ion channel disorder ("ionopathy") with a genetic overlap to LQTS. Currently, more than seven different genes are involved in SQTS indicating not only a moderate degree of genetic heterogeneity but also a lot of unresolved issues on its underlying etiology (Table 13.1). Upon genetic, functional and familial analysis, the majority of SQTS genes appear to be valid, in particular SQT1–SQT3 genes *KCNH2*, *KCNQ1* and *KCNJ2*, the *SLC4A3* and *CACNB2* genes (Table 13.1); for the remaining genes, genetic and in vitro evidence has to be further confirmed by additional studies. So far, the rate of incomplete penetrance (i.e. mutation carriers without any ECG and clinical presentation) is not known for SQTS.

The first gene (*KCNH2*) identified to be causative for the short QT syndrome (SQT1) was a gain-of-function mutation leading to an increase of the rapid component of the delayed rectifier potassium current (I_{Kr}) [7]. Two different nucleotide variants at position 1764 were identified in HERG (*KCNH2*) resulting in the same amino acid change at codon 588 (asparagine is changed into a positively charged lysine (p. Asp588Lys, or N588K). The residue is located in the S5-P loop region of HERG at the outer mouth of the channel and caused a loss of the normal rectification of the current at plateau voltages, which resulted in a significant increase of I_{Kr} during phases 2 and 3 of the action potential leading to an abbreviation of the action potential and both atrial and ventricular refractoriness.

Table 13.1 Genetic subtypes of short QT syndrome (SQTS)

SQTS subform (MIM)	Gene	Protein	Mechanism	Inheritance	Other clinical features
SQT1	*KCNH2*	K_V11.1/hERG (α-subunit of the voltage-dependent K^+ channel)	↑ I_{Kr} Non-synonymous mutations with a gain of function	AD (familial, sporadic)	Atrial fibrillation
SQT2	*KCNQ1*	K_V7.1 (α-subunit of the voltage-dependent K^+ channel)	↑ I_{Ks} Non-synonymous mutations with a gain of function	AD (familial, sporadic)	Atrial fibrillation; sinus bradycardia at birth, junctional bradycardia in infancy
SQT3	*KCNJ2*	Kir2.1 (inward rectifying K+ channel)	↑ I_{K1} Non-synonymous mutations with a gain of function	AD (familial, sporadic)	Atrial fibrillation; autism-epilepsy
	CACNA1C	Ca_V1.2 (α1C-subunit of the voltage-dependent L-type Ca^{2+} channel)	↓ I_{Ca} Non-synonymous mutations with a loss of function	(Sporadic)	Brugada ECG
	CACNB2B	β2-subunit of the voltage-dependent L-type Ca^{2+} channel	↓ I_{Ca}Non-synonymous mutations with a loss of function	AD (familial)	Brugada ECG
	CACNA2D1	α2/δ-subunit of the voltage-dependent L-type Ca^{2+} channel	? ↓I_{Ca} ? Non-synonymous variant with a loss of function	(Case report)	
	SLC4A3	Anion exchanger solute carrier (family 4 member 3, encodes a $Cl^- < >$, HCO_3^- exchanger (AE3)	Decreased $Cl^- < > HCO_3^-$ exchange, increased pH_i non-synonymous mutation with a loss of function	AD (familial)	

The SQT1 subform is the most prevalent (<15%), whereas all other subforms are rare (<1%)

Bellocq et al. shortly after reported on a mutation in a single sporadic case of a 70-year-old patient with SQTS (QTc 302 ms) and sudden cardiac arrest. They identified a gain-of-function mutation (p.Val307Leu) in the *KCNQ1* gene which encodes the slow component of the delayed rectifier potassium channel (I_{Ks}) (SQT2). The mutation caused a −20 mV shift of the half-activation potential and acceleration of the activation kinetics and activation of the mutant channels at more negative potentials. This resulted in a gain of function of I_{Ks} and abbreviation of the action potential. A further missense mutation in the same gene (p.Val141Met) was identified in a baby with bradycardia and atrial fibrillation in utero [6]. The ECG revealed a shortened QT interval and episodes of atrial fibrillation.

Priori and co-workers identified in two relatives without sudden cardiac arrest a gain of function in *KCNJ2* (SQT3) encoding the inward rectifier potassium channel (I_{K1}) causing abbreviation of the QT interval and asymmetrical T waves with a rapid terminal downslope [4]. Deo et al. described also this mutation in *KCNJ2* (p.Ala896Thr (SQT3)) that resulted in a strongly enhanced I_{K1} outward current leading to a phenotype of an extremely abbreviated QT interval and atrial fibrillation [34].

Later, our group together with Antzelevitch and co-workers further described novel mutations of the cardiac L-type calcium channel genes responsible for shortening of the QT interval in families characterized by sudden cardiac death, atrial fibrillation and a Brugada type I ECG pattern. (Fig.13.3) These patients displayed a mixed, overlapping phenotype [5]. Functional analyses revealed loss-of-function missense mutations of the *CACNA1C* (p.Ala39Val and p. Gly490Arg) and *CACNB2b* (p.Ser481Leu) genes encoding the pore forming of $Ca_v1.2$ α1- and β2b-subunits of the cardiac L-type calcium channel. The decreased net current of the cardiac L-type calcium channels led to an abbreviation of the plateau phase of the action potential and thus to a short QT interval. A mutation in the L-type calcium channel gene was recently also reported by Akdis et al. In their study, one family had a non-synonymous variant in *CACNA2D1* causing a loss-of-function effect [35].

There are meanwhile various reports on SQTS patients who had heterozygous mutations in *KCNH2* and *KCNQ1*. A Japanese group identified a novel mutation *KCNH2*-p. Ile560Thr that resulted in a 2.5-fold increase in peak current density in COS-7 cells and a mutation in *KCNH2*-p. Thr618Leu [15]. This identical mutation had already been described by a Chinese group. The Thr618Ile seems to be a mutation hotspot, since Hu et al. described seven families with this particular variant. There was a 100% penetrance with variable clinical expressivity, and the risk of sudden cardiac death was reported as high. Functional studies revealed a significant increase of I_{Kr} tail current density [17]. Others also found a mutation in *KCNQ1*-p.Val141Met.; Moreno et al. presented a male individual with a family history of SCD with a QTc interval of 356 ms who had a mutation in the S5 segment of the KCNQ1 that impaired its association with KCNE1 [9]. Suzuki and co-workers published a case of an asymptomatic 10-year-old boy who displayed a QTc interval of 260 ms who was a carrier of the *KCNH2*-p. Asp588Lys mutation that has been the first one identified in the first two unrelated SQT1 families [36].

A report from a French group presents a family with inherited L-carnitine deficiency, in which a short QT interval was observed in all affected members. After substitution of carnitine, the QT interval was significantly prolonged towards normal range. To confirm the role of carnitine in the evolution of a short QT interval, the authors used a mouse model, in which they could demonstrate that carnitine deficiency induced a short QT interval and a predisposition to inducible ventricular fibrillation [37].

Recently, Thorsen et al. described a loss-of-activity mutation in the cardiac chloride-bicarbonate exchanger AE3 after whole-exome sequencing where the non-synonymous mutation (Arg370His) led to reduced surface expression of AE3 and reduced membrane carbonate transport. The phenotype is a typical SQTS. In one large and a small family, all mutation carriers had a QTc interval of less than 370 ms (340 ± 18 ms) and non-carriers >370 ms (402 ± 24 ms). They expressed the mutation in a zebrafish and found that reduced chloride and higher pH_i lead to an abbreviation of the action potential [38].

So far, the indication for genetic testing of an SQTS proband is a class IIB indication but should be initiated also for scientific reasons. Usually, a multi-gene panel analysis will be performed. In all cases, relatives in the family should be evaluated clinically for a short QT interval, and genetic testing, if successful in the index patient, should be performed in available relatives (class I indication, heterozygosity testing).

Pathophysiological Insights in SQTS

After the identification of the underlying mutations and affected cardiac ion channels, the cellular basis and arrhythmogenesis in experimental SQTS models were examined.

The first experiments in transmural left ventricular wedge preparations and Langendorff heart preparations were performed using pinacidil, an activator of $I_{K,ATP}$ as no specific I_{Kr}, I_{Ks} or I_{K1} agonists were available [39, 40]. Under pinacidil treatment, QT interval was shortened and transmural dispersion of repolarization increased. The action potential was abbreviated heterogeneously among different cell types spanning the ventricular wall and thus opens the window for the genesis for polymorphic ventricular tachycardia (phase-2 re-entry). Transmural dispersion of repolarization was associated with the inducibility of ventricular tachyarrhythmias. Quinidine application was able to reduce monophasic action potential duration and dispersion of repolarization [31].

In the clinical setting, a number of VF or polymorphic VT onsets could be recorded either from monitoring or from ICD data storage. The coupling interval (R-R') of the initiating polymorphic ventricular contraction (PVC) to the previous regular beat was extremely short favouring this hypothesis for arrhythmogenesis in SQTS. Three groups consistently reported on coupling intervals ranging from 190 to 320 ms in humans but predominantly around 230–250 ms [11, 41, 42].

There are some new experiments also on modelling currents in human induced pluripotent stem cell-derived cardiomyocytes (hiPSC-CMs), in which in silico currents are injected to study loss and gain of function of *KCNJ2* mutants. Meijer van Putten et al. nicely demonstrated that effects of specific mutations can be simulated by this new technique [43]. El-Battrawy et al. used hiPSC-CM generated from human skin fibroblasts and reproduced the increased I_{Kr} activity of SQTS-*KCNH2* mutant cells and also the counteracting and therapeutic effect by quinidine to prolong the action potential in this cellular model [44].

Pharmacological Therapy and Follow-up of SQTS

After the identification of the genetic background and the cellular mechanisms of the SQTS, clinical and experimental studies have been conducted with respect to the pharmacological treatment.

Most of the experiences in vitro and in vivo are available for SQT1. Heterogeneous expression studies exhibited that the p.N588K mutation increased the density of I_{Kr} and reduced the affinity of I_{Kr} blockers like d-sotalol 20-fold [7]. Thus, in vitro experiments could prove the failure of d-sotalol restoring QT interval in vivo. McPate et al. could demonstrate that the effect of E-4031, a specific I_{Kr} blocker, was also significantly attenuated by the p.N588K mutation, whereas quinidine was less and disopyramide the least affected by p.N588K-HERG [45]. Cordeiro et al. could nicely show that these findings are based on the +90 mV shift in the voltage dependence of inactivation of the HERG channels. Most I_{Kr} blockers interact with the HERG channels in the inactivated state. Thus, a failure of inactivation of the HERG channel leads to the inefficacy of the specific I_{Kr} blockers [46]. Recently, McPate et al. could demonstrate that besides disopyramide and quinidine also propafenone and amiodarone were only slightly inhibited by the mutant p. N588K [45]. Thus, these drugs may serve as an additional option in the pharmacological treatment of SQT1. For SQT3, El Harchi et al. could identify in vitro that chloroquine is an effective pharmacological inhibitor of the SQT3 p.D172N mutant Kir2.1 [7].

In the clinical setting, several class I and III antiarrhythmic drugs have been tested in patients with the gain-of-function mutation in HERG (SQT1). For class III antiarrhythmics, neither d-sotalol nor ibutilide was able to prolong QT interval in the first SQT1 patients. Flecainide, a Na^+-channel blocker, which has in addition a blocking effect on I_{Kr} and on the transient outward potassium current (I_{to}), led to an increase in ventricular effective refractory periods. However, acute administration of flecainide did cause only a mild prolongation of refractoriness and only a slight prolongation of the QT interval [47]. In contrast, the class I antiarrhythmic agent quinidine was able to normalize the QT interval and to prolong the ventricular effective refractory period in patients with an SQT1 [31]. Additionally, quinidine restored the heart rate dependence of the QT interval towards the normal range and rendered ventricular tachyarrhythmias non-inducible in patients in whom baseline electrophysiological studies demonstrated reproducible inducibility of ventricular fibrillation. Following the positive effects of disopyramide in in vitro experiments, disopyramide has also been shown to be effective in a pilot study in patients with an SQT1.

Another substance that could be of antiarrhythmic effect in patients with SQTS is ranolazine. It has shown to be very effective in experimental models of atrial fibrillation especially when used in conjunction with amiodarone. Ranolazine is mainly inhibiting the late I_{Na} channel. A few studies have looked into the effect of ranolazine [48]. In a Langendorff model of SQTS, in which pinacidil activated the I_{Kr} current, ranolazine reversed the QT shortening, ventricular electrical vulnerability and the ventricular effective refractory periods. The same group tried ivabradine. In the same Langendorff model, they saw that inducibility of VT/VF was reduced following ivabradine. Finally, also the first-generation antihistamine antazoline was investigated [49]. This drug reduced electrical vulnerability in the short QT model. There are, however, no comparable data on off-label use in humans yet.

The most frequently used drug in the past was quinidine. No patient on quinidine therapy suffered from ventricular fibrillation or a recurrence of atrial fibrillation during mid-term follow-up in the SQTS registry. A subset from the SQT1 family published by Bjerregaard et al. treated with propafenone is free of recurrences of atrial fibrillation without prolongation of the QT interval (personal communication). Whether quinidine, propafenone or disopyramide represent an alternative to ICD therapy in prevention of sudden cardiac death cannot be finally answered. Drugs may be an alternative in patients refusing ICD implantation or for those who are not eligible for ICD therapy. In addition, drugs can be given to ICD-bearing patients who experience recurrent electrical shocks. At least, quinidine was shown to prevent life-threatening events in 16 patients reported by Mazzanti and colleagues. In this cohort, after the initiation of quinidine, no further malignant arrhythmias were observed during a relevant follow-up [50].

Whether the electrocardiographic and finally clinical effects of class I or III drugs can be transferred to other SQTS subforms is known to date but seems rationale. However, in a patient with SQT4, quinidine was able to prolong QT interval and suppress paroxysms of atrial fibrillation.

Due to the pathophysiological heterogeneity of the SQTS, any therapy modulating cardiac ion channel function may have very different effects and outcome depending on the type of mutation and the affected cardiac ion channel. Further in vitro, ex vivo and finally in vivo studies are warranted to elucidate the potential long-term benefit of pharmacological treatment.

The 2015 ESC guidelines recommend quinidine or sotalol when patients refuse an ICD or have a contraindication, in asymptomatic patients and in patients having a family history with a class IIb indication. Finally, some drug combinations have been successfully used in patients that are not mentioned in the guidelines, and to some extent, the treatment of this very heterogenous patient population will remain individual.

ICD Therapy in SQTS

The only reliable treatment to prevent sudden cardiac death is the implantation of an implantable cardioverter-defibrillator (ICD). In symptomatic patients with SQTS, the ICD is the therapy of choice for primary or secondary prevention of SCD, while antiarrhythmic drug therapy may represent an adjunct or an alternative therapy in children or in newborns, where ICD implantation is technically challenging and often associated with high morbidity. The risk for inappropriate ICD discharges due to T-wave oversensing is increased in patients with SQTS compared to other conditions with ICD implanted, since intracardiac T waves in general are quite high and closely coupled to the preceding R wave. This issue can be solved by individual ICD programming of the sensing parameters and selection of specific devices. Additionally, quinidine therapy helped to avoid T-wave oversensing by increasing the QT interval and thereby reducing the T-wave amplitude [51]. The urgent need to program the ICD very diligently and carefully select device and leads is underlined by the high reported incidence of inappropriate shocks especially in the paediatric cohort.

Table 13.2 Conditions causing a short QT interval and mimicking short QT syndrome

Hyperkalemia
Hypercalcemia
Digitalis intoxication
Acidosis
Hyperthermia
Drugs

Risk Stratification in SQTS

Risk stratification in SQTS is based on the degree of shortened QTc interval, family history of sudden death <40 years of age in a relative and symptoms. An ICD is indicated following to the 2015 ESC guidelines [33] for survivors of sudden death or patients with a spontaneous documented VT.

Unfortunately, there is no clear statement concerning risk stratification in patients with a history of syncope and a short QTc; this might be evaluated on an individual basis and with regard to the detailed history of syncope and event.

Due to the genetic heterogeneity in SQTS and the low number of patients reported with an indicative genotype, general genotype-phenotype correlations are not established to date. Currently, the yield of genetic testing is still quite low in patients with a clinical short QT syndrome. This suggests that other, unknown genetic (but potentially also non-genetic) mechanisms may be involved. Phenocopying conditions (Table 13.2) for short QT interval generation in the surface ECG have to be excluded. Therefore, clinical risk stratification may rely on the same parameters as noted before.

Summary

The SQTS is one of the primary electrical diseases of the heart with a high incidence of atrial and ventricular fibrillation and thereby sudden cardiac death. Cardiac imaging is unremarkable. The clinical hallmark for the diagnosis is a short QT interval in the baseline ECG, tall T waves and nearly absence of an isoelectric ST segment.

So far, approximately 200 patients are identified worldwide and indicate its role as a rare disease. Due to the limited number of patients and of pathophysiological knowledge and the genetic heterogeneity of the disease, consistent genotype-phenotype relations are not established. Risk stratification is depending on clinical and individual parameters.

Patients with SQTS should be referred for genetic counselling, molecular genetic analysis and initiation of family screening in specialized institutions.

Take Home Message

1. SQTS is a very rare but potentially highly malignant disease.
2. SQTS should be considered in anyone with a QTc < 350 ms without other potential causes.
3. One must always think about SQTS in the following special cases:
   - Aborted cardiac arrest or sudden cardiac death of unknown origin
   - Unexplained atrial fibrillation at young age

References

1. Gussak I, Brugada P, Brugada J, Wright RS, Kopecky SL, Chaitman BR, et al. Idiopathic short QT interval: a new clinical syndrome? Cardiology. 2000;94:99–102.
2. Gaita F, Giustetto C, Bianchi F, Wolpert C, Schimpf R, Riccardi R, et al. Short QT syndrome: a familial cause of sudden death. Circulation. 2003;108:965–70.
3. Bellocq C, van Ginneken AC, Bezzina CR, Alders M, Escande D, Mannens MM, et al. Mutation in the KCNQ1 gene leading to the short QT-interval syndrome. Circulation. 2004;109:2394–7.
4. Priori SG, Pandit SV, Rivolta I, Berenfeld O, Ronchetti E, Dhamoon A, et al. A novel form of short QT syndrome (SQT3) is caused by a mutation in the KCNJ2 gene. Circ Res. 2005;96:800–7.
5. Antzelevitch C, Pollevick GD, Cordeiro JM, Casis O, Sanguinetti MC, Aizawa Y, et al. Loss-of-function mutations in the cardiac calcium channel underlie a new clinical entity characterized by ST-segment elevation, short QT intervals, and sudden cardiac death. Circulation. 2007;115:442–9.
6. Hong K, Piper DR, Diaz-Valdecantos A, Brugada J, Oliva A, Burashnikov E, et al. De novo KCNQ1 mutation responsible for atrial fibrillation and short QT syndrome in utero. Cardiovasc Res. 2005;68:433–40.
7. Brugada R, Hong K, Dumaine R, Cordeiro J, Gaita F, Borggrefe M, et al. Sudden death associated with short-QT syndrome linked to mutations in HERG. Circulation. 2004;109:30–5.
8. El Harchi A, Melgari D, Zhang YH, Zhang H, Hancox C. Action potential clamp and pharmacology of the variant 1 short QT syndrome T618I hERG K+ channel. PLoS One. 2012;7:e52451.
9. Moreno C, Olivera A, de la Cruz A, Bartolucci C, Mun C, Salar E, et al. A new KCNQ1 mutation at the S5 segment that impairs its association with KCNE1 is responsible for short QT syndrome. Cardiovasc Res. 2015;107:613–23.
10. Giustetto C, Di Monte F, Wolpert C, Borggrefe M, Schimpf R, Sbragia P, et al. Short QT syndrome: clinical findings and diagnostic-therapeutic implications. Eur Heart J. 2006;27:2440–7.
11. Mazzanti A, Kanthan A, Monteforte N, Memmi M, Bloise R, Novelli V, et al. Novel insight into the natural history of short QT syndrome. J Am Coll Cardiol. 2014;63:1300–8.
12. Villafane J, Atalla J, Gollob M, Maury P, Wolpert C, Gebauer R, et al. Long-term follow-up of a pediatric cohort with short QT syndrome. J Am Coll Cardiol. 2013;61:1183–91.
13. Villafane J, Fischbach P, Gebauer R. Short QT syndrome manifesting with neonatal atrial fibrillation and bradycardia. Cardiology. 2014;128:236–40.
14. Gollob MH, Redpath CJ, Roberts JD. The short QT syndrome. JACC. 2011;57:802–12.
15. Harrell DT, Ashihara T, Ishikawa T, Tominaga I, Mazzanti A, Takahashi K, et al. Genotype-dependent differences in age of manifestation and arrhythmia complications in short QT syndrome. Int J Cardiol. 2015;190:393–402.
16. Fukuyama M, Ohno S, Wang W, Kimura H, Makivama T, Itoh H, et al. L-type calcium channel mutations in Japanese patients. With inherited arrhythmias. Circ J. 2013;77:1799–806.
17. Hu D, Li Y, Zhang J, Pfeiffer R, Gollob MH, Healey J, et al. The phenotypic spectrum of a mutation hotspot responsible for the short QT syndrome. JACC. 2017;3:727–41.
18. Anttonen O, Junttila MJ, Rissanen H, Reunanen A, Viitasalo M, Huikuri HV. Prevalence and prognostic significance of short QT interval in a middle-aged Finnish population. Circulation. 2007;116:714–20.
19. Funada A, Hayashi K, Ino H, Fujino N, Uchiyama K, Sakata K, et al. Assessment of QT intervals and prevalence of short QT syndrome in Japan. Clin Cardiol. 2008;31:270–4.
20. Gallagher MM, Magliano G, Yap YG, Padula M, Morgia V, Postorino C, et al. Distribution and prognostic significance of QT intervals in the lowest half centile in 12,012 apparently healthy persons. Am J Cardiol. 2006;98:933–5.
21. Kobza R, Roos M, Niggli B, Abacherli R, Lupi GA, Frey F, et al. Prevalence of long and short QT in a young population of 41,767 predominantly male Swiss conscripts. Heart Rhythm. 2009;6:652–7.
22. Viskin S. The QT interval: too long, too short or just right. Heart Rhythm. 2009;6:711–5.
23. Iribarren C, Round AD, Peng J, Lu M, Klatzsky AL, Zaroff JG, et al. Short QT in a cohort of 1.7 million persons: prevalence, correlates, and prognosis. Ann Noninvasive Electrocardiol. 2014;19:490–500.
24. Portugal G, Olivera MM, Cunha P, Ferreira F, Lousinha A, Fiarresga A, et al. Short QT syndrome presenting as syncope: how short is too short? Rev Port Cardiol. 2014;33:649.e1–6.
25. Postema PG, Wilde AMM. The measurement of the QT interval. Curr Cardiol Rev. 2014;10:287–94.
26. Anttonen O, Junttila MJ, Maury P, Schimpf R, Wolpert C, Borggrefe M, et al. Differences in twelve-lead electrocardiogram between symptomatic and asymptomatic subjects with short QT interval. Heart Rhythm. 2009;6:267–71.
27. Giustetto C, Scorocco C, Schimpf R, Maury P, Mazzanti A, Levetto M, et al. Usefulness of exercise test in the diagnosis of short QT syndrome. Europace. 2015;17:628–34.
28. Tülümen E, Giustetto C, Wolpert C, Maury P, Anttonen O, Probst V, et al. PQ segment depression in patients with short QT syndrome: a novel marker for diagnosing short QT syndrome? Heart Rhythm. 2014;11:1024–30.
29. Schimpf R, Antzelevitch C, Haghi D, Giustetto C, Pizzuti A, Gaita F, et al. Electromechanical coupling in patients with the short QT syndrome: further insights into the mechanoelectrical hypothesis of the U wave. Heart Rhythm. 2008;5:241–5.
30. Frea S, Giustetto C, Capriolo M, Scrocco C, Fornengo C, Benedetto S, et al. New echocardiographic insights in short QT syndrome: more than a channelopathy? Heart Rhythm. 2015;12:2096–105.
31. Wolpert C, Schimpf R, Giustetto C, Antzelevitch C, Cordeiro J, Dumaine R, et al. Further insights into the effect of quinidine in short QT syndrome caused by a mutation in HERG. J Cardiovasc Electrophysiol. 2005;16:54–8.
32. Rollin A, Gandjbakhch E, Giustetto C, Scrocco C, Fourcade C, Monteil B. Shortening of the short refractory periods in short QT syndrome. J Am Heart Assoc. 2017;6:e005684.
33. Priori SG, Blomström-Lundqvist C, Mazzanti A, Blom N, Borggrefe M, Camm J, et al. ESC guidelines for the management of patients with ventricular arrhythmias and the prevention of sudden cardiac death. Eur Heart J. 2015;36:2793–867.
34. Deo M, Ruan Y, Pandit SV, Shah K, Berenfeld O, Blaufox A, Cerrone M, et al. KCNJ2 mutation in short QT syndrome 3 results in atrial fibrillation and ventricular proarrhythmia. Proc Natl Acad Sci U S A. 2013;110:4291–6.

35. Akdis D, Saguner AM, Medeiros-Domingo A, Schaller A, Balmer C, Steffel J, et al. Multiple clinical profiles of families with the short QT syndrom. Europace. 2018;20:f113–21.
36. Suzuki H, Hoshina S, Ozawa J, Sato A, Minamino T, Aizawas Y. Short QT syndrome in a boy diagnosed on screening for heart disease. Pediatr Int. 2014;56:775–6.
37. Roussel J, Labarthe F, Thireau J, Ferro F, Farah C, Roy J, et al. Carnitine deficiency induces a short QT syndrome. Heart Rhythm. 2016;13:165–74.
38. Thorsen K, Dam VS, Kjaer-Sorensen K, Pedersen LN, Skeberdis VA, Jurevicius J. Loss-of-activity-mutation in the cardiac chloride-bicarbonate exchanger AE3 causes short QT syndrome. Nat Commun. 2017;1:1696.
39. Extramiana F, Antzelevitch C. Amplified transmural dispersion of repolarization as the basis for arrhythmogenesis in a canine ventricular-wedge model of short-QT syndrome. Circulation. 2004;110:3661–6.
40. Milberg P, Tegelkamp R, Osada N, Schimpf R, Wolpert C, Breithardt G, et al. Reduction of dispersion of repolarization and prolongation of postrepolarization refractoriness explain the antiarrhythmic effects of quinidine in a model of short QT syndrome. J Cardiovasc Electrophysiol. 2007;18:658–64.
41. Schimpf R, Bauersfeld U, Gaita F, Wolpert C. Short QT syndrome: successful prevention of sudden cardiac death in an adolescent by implantable cardioverter-defibrillator treatment for primary prophylaxis. Heart Rhythm. 2005;2:416–7.
42. Giustetto C, Schimpf R, Mazzanti A, Scorocco S, Maury P, Anttonen O, et al. Long-term follow-up of patients with short QT syndrome. JACC. 2011;58:587–95.
43. Meijer van Putten R, Mengarelli I, Guan K, Zegers JG, ACG v G, Verkerk AO. Ion channelopathies in human induced pluripotent stem cell derived cardiomyocytes: a dynamic clamp study with virtual IK1. Frontiers Physiol. 2015;6:1–18.
44. El-Battrawy I, Lan H, Cyganek L, Zhao Z, Li X, Bulubasic F, et al. Modeling short QT syndrome using human-induced pluripotent stem cell-derived cardiomyocytes. J Am Heart Assoc. 2018;7:e007394.
45. McPate MJ, Zhang H, Adeniran I, Cordeiro JM, Witchel HJ, Hancox JC. Comparative effects of the short QT N588K mutation at 37 degrees C on hERG K+ channel current during ventricular, Purkinje fibre and atrial action potentials: an action potential clamp study. J Physiol Pharmacol. 2009;60:23–41.
46. Cordeiro JM, Brugada R, Wu YS, Hong K, Dumaine R. Modulation of I(Kr) inactivation by mutation N588K in KCNH2: a link to arrhythmogenesis in short QT syndrome. Cardiovasc Res. 2005;67:498–509.
47. Gaita F, Giustetto C, Bianchi F, Schimpf R, Haissaguerre M, Calo L, et al. Short QT syndrome: pharmacological treatment. J Am Coll Cardiol. 2004;43:1494–9.
48. Frommeyer G, Weller J, Ellermann C, Kaese S, Kochhaeuser S, Lange PS. Antiarrhythmic properties of ivabradine in an experimental model of short-QT-syndrome. Clin Exp Pharmacol Physiol. 2017;44:941–94.
49. Frommeyer G, Ellermann C, Dechering D, Kochhaeuser S, Boegeholz N, Guener F, et al. Ranolazine and Vernakalant prevent ventricular arrhythmias in an experimental whole-heart model of short-QT-syndrome. J Cardiovasc Electrophysiol. 2016;27:1214–9.
50. Mazzanti A, Maragna R, Vacanti G, Kostopoulou A, Marino M, Monteforte N, et al. Hydroquinidine prevents life-threatening in patient with short QT syndrome. JACC. 2017;24:3010–5.
51. Schimpf R, Wolpert C, Bianchi F, Giustetto C, Gaita F, Bauersfeld U, et al. Congenital short QT syndrome and implantable cardioverter defibrillator treatment: inherent risk for inappropriate shock delivery. J Cardiovasc Electrophysiol. 2003;14:1273–7.

Brugada Syndrome

14

Oscar Campuzano, Georgia Sarquella-Brugada, Ramon Brugada, and Josep Brugada

Introduction

The first manuscript reporting a "*Right bundle branch block, persistent ST segment elevation and sudden cardiac death: A distinct clinical and electrocardiographic syndrome*" was published in 1992 [1]. This report included eight individuals showing mentioned characteristic electrocardiographic (ECG) alterations in a structurally normal heart. All these individuals were resuscitated from sudden cardiac death (SCD) caused by documented ventricular fibrillation (VF). In 1996, a group of Japanese cardiologists proposes the name of Brugada syndrome (BrS) referring to this entity [2]. One year later, BrS was recognized as the same entity that sudden unexplained nocturnal death syndrome (SUNDS) [3] described in the Philippines as *bangungut* [4]. The same disease has been also called *lai tai* in Thailand, *pokkuri death syndrome* in Japan, *dolyeonsa* in Korea, *dream disease* in Hawaii, or *sudden manhood death syndrome* in China. All these entities refer to sudden deaths (SD) in apparently healthy young males that took place at night, during sleep, and an autopsy revealed no pathological evidence to explain the cause of the death. In 1998, the first genetic alteration was identified [5]. In the last 25 years, there has been progressive understanding of the clinical diagnosis, treatment, genetic basis, and cellular electrophysiological mechanisms of BrS. However, several questions remain to be clarified. Here, we will focus on the present knowledge, on clinical, genetic, and molecular features of BrS.

Definition

Nowadays, the diagnosis of BrS is based on a characteristic registry in the ECG: ST-segment elevation with type 1 morphology ≥2 mm in one or more leads among the right precordial leads V_1 and/or V_2 positioned in the second, third, or fourth intercostal space, occurring either spontaneously or after a provocative test with intravenous administration of sodium channel blockers [6]. The presence of all other known causes of ST segment elevation in right precordial leads (known as phenocopies) should be excluded before making the diagnosis of BrS [7].

Disease Burden

The prevalence of BrS is believed to range from 1/5000 to 1/2000 despite significant ethnic, geographic, and gender differences [8]. This rate should be interpreted with caution due to difficulties in determining the real prevalence of

O. Campuzano
Cardiovascular Genetics Centre, University of Girona-IDIBGI, Girona, Spain

Medical Science Department, School of Medicine, University of Girona, Girona, Spain

Centro de Investigación Biomédica en Red de Enfermedades Cardiovasculares (CIBERCV), Madrid, Spain
e-mail: oscar@brugada.org

G. Sarquella-Brugada
Arrhythmia Unit, Hospital Sant Joan de Déu, University of Barcelona, Barcelona, Spain

R. Brugada
Cardiovascular Genetics Centre, University of Girona-IDIBGI, Girona, Spain

Medical Science Department, School of Medicine, University of Girona, Girona, Spain

Centro de Investigación Biomédica en Red de Enfermedades Cardiovasculares (CIBERCV), Madrid, Spain

Familial Cardiomyopathies Unit, Hospital Josep Trueta de Girona, Girona, Spain

J. Brugada (✉)
Centro de Investigación Biomédica en Red de Enfermedades Cardiovasculares (CIBERCV), Madrid, Spain

Arrhythmia Unit, Hospital Sant Joan de Déu, University of Barcelona, Barcelona, Spain

Arrhythmia Section, Cardiovascular Institute, Hospital Clinic, University of Barcelona, Barcelona, Catalonia, Spain
e-mail: jbrugada@clinic.ub.es

H. F. Baars et al. (eds.), *Clinical Cardiogenetics*, https://doi.org/10.1007/978-3-030-45457-9_14

asymptomatic patients and the dynamic variability of the ECG pattern. BrS shows age- and gender-related penetrance, as incomplete penetrance and variable expressivity are hallmarks of this cardiac entity [9]. Therefore, the current prevalence is likely to be underestimated. The incidence of BrS pattern on ECG has ranged from 0.12% to 0.8%, and it has been considered responsible for 4–12% of all SD and up to 20% of SD in patients with structurally normal hearts [10].

Clinical Presentation and Diagnosis

Symptoms

Patients with BrS can present with a wide scale of clinical manifestations, from asymptomatic to syncope, seizures, and nocturnal agonal breathing due to polymorphic VT (PVT) or ventricular fibrillation (VF). If these arrhythmias are sustained, SCD may result [11]. SCD may be the first manifestation of the disease even in asymptomatic patients who never suffered any arrhythmia or syncope. The ECG pattern is now widely recognized, improving the early identification of asymptomatic individuals at risk. A recent study reported nearly 5% of SCD as the first symptom of the disease [12].

Lethal arrhythmias usually occur during sleep or at rest, suggesting an association with bradycardia or vagal events. Febrile episodes have also been commonly associated with symptoms [13]. Symptoms typically first occur during adulthood, average 40 years old, although the onset of first symptoms is also reported in both children and the aged population [8]. Concerning gender differences, male mainly suffer symptoms (3:1). Thus, hormonal influences play a key role in phenotypic manifestation of arrhythmias [14]. However, the pathophysiological mechanisms of these differences remain to clarify. In addition, male predominance among BrS patients does not occur in children under 16 years old, when testosterone levels are low and similar between boys and girls [15]. In a recent study, nearly 30% of preadolescents with a negative pharmacological test showed positive results after puberty [16]. For this reason, negative pharmacological test performed under 16 years old should be repeated after adolescence.

Resting Electrocardiogram

After the first description of BrS, several ambiguities appeared in the characteristic ECG patterns and the specific diagnostic criteria. In 2005, the second BrS Consensus Report stated the current recommendations regarding the diagnostic criteria [8]. Three different ECG patterns have been recognized: Type 1 consists of a coved-type ST-segment elevation greater than 2 mm, followed by a descending negative T wave in at least one right precordial lead (V_1–V_3). It is the only pattern that is diagnostic for BrS. Type 2 and type 3 are saddleback-shaped patterns, with a high initial augmentation followed by an ST elevation of 2 mm for type 2 and less than 2 mm for type 3. Both patterns are suggestive of, but not diagnostic for, BrS (Fig. 14.1). In 2012, an expert consensus was published, establishing two descriptive ECG abnormalities for BrS [17]:

- Type 1 ("coved type"): It is characterized by an ST-segment elevation ≥2 mm in ≥1 right precordial lead (V_1–V_3), followed by an r' wave and a concave or straight ST segment. The descending ST segment crosses the isoelectric line and is followed by a negative and symmetric T wave. This alteration is the only diagnostic pattern for BrS, so far.
- Type 2 ("saddle-back type"): It is characterized by an ST-segment elevation of ≥0.5 mm (generally ≥2 mm in V_2) in ≥1 right precordial lead (V_1–V_3), followed by a convex ST. The r' wave may or may not overlap the J point, but it has a slow downward slope. The ST segment is followed by a positive T wave in V_2 and is of variable morphology in V_1. This ECG anomaly is only suggestive of BrS. To facilitate the differentiation of type 2 ECGs highly indicative of BrS from other Brugada-like patterns, several additional criteria based on the triangle formed by the ascending and descending branch of the r' wave were used:
  - *β angle*: A cutoff value ≥58° provided the best predictive values for conversion to a type 1 BrS pattern (73% positive and 87% negative values) [18].
  - *Length of the base triangle of the r' wave 5 mm below the maximum rise point*: A cutoff value of 4 mm (≥4 mm in patients with BrS) demonstrated 96% specificity and 85% sensitivity (positive predictive value of 95% and negative predictive value 88%) for differentiating the BrS ECG pattern in BrS patients from the ECG pattern of healthy individuals [19].
  - *Other criteria:* The triangle base duration at the isoelectric line (>1.5 mm in patients with BrS) and the relationship between the triangle base at the isoelectric line and its height (>1.3 in BrS patients) may be distinguishing ECG patterns in BrS [20].

Frequent variations in the ECG patterns can occur within a single patient such as the absence of a classic ECG pattern (concealed BrS) [21]. The placement of the right precordial leads in more cranial positions increases sensitivity in some patients due to the variable anatomical correlation between the right ventricular outflow tract and the V_1–V_2 in the standard position [22]. The identification of a spontaneous type 1

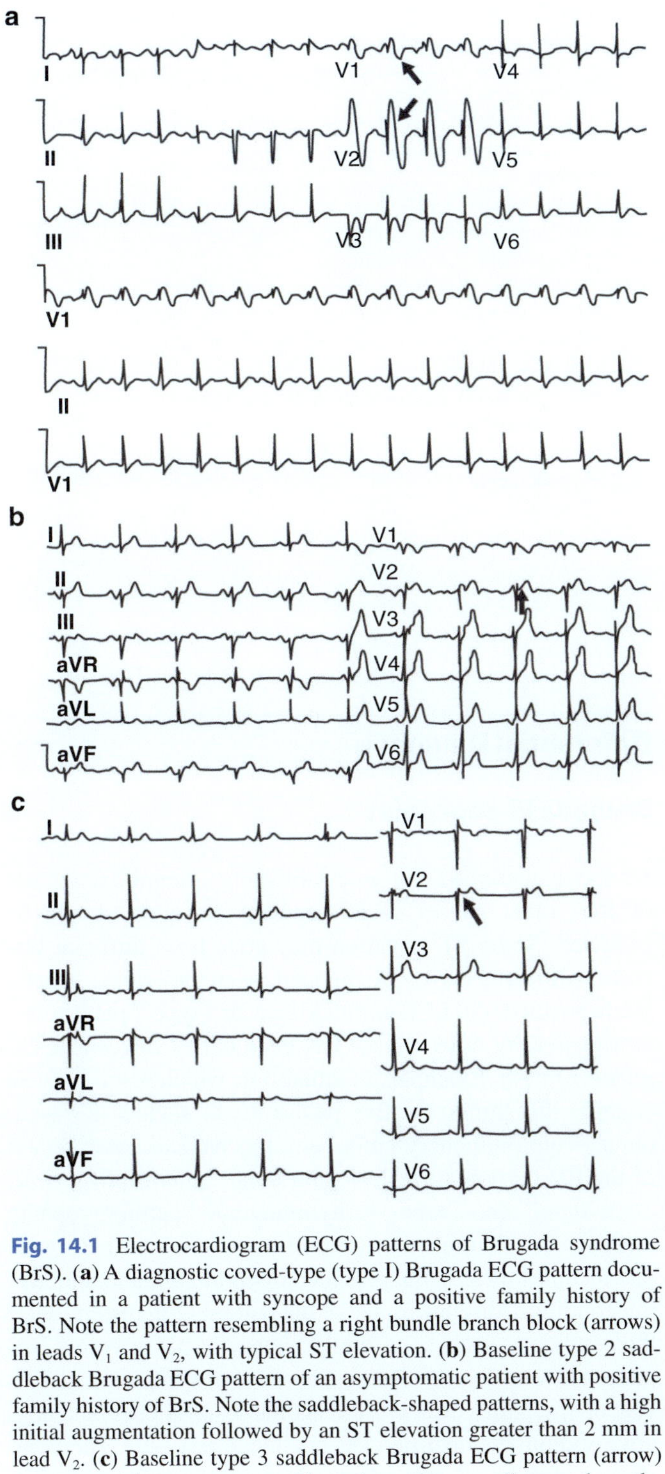

Fig. 14.1 Electrocardiogram (ECG) patterns of Brugada syndrome (BrS). (**a**) A diagnostic coved-type (type I) Brugada ECG pattern documented in a patient with syncope and a positive family history of BrS. Note the pattern resembling a right bundle branch block (arrows) in leads V_1 and V_2, with typical ST elevation. (**b**) Baseline type 2 saddleback Brugada ECG pattern of an asymptomatic patient with positive family history of BrS. Note the saddleback-shaped patterns, with a high initial augmentation followed by an ST elevation greater than 2 mm in lead V_2. (**c**) Baseline type 3 saddleback Brugada ECG pattern (arrow) documented in an asymptomatic patient who was diagnosed on the basis of a positive result on class IC antiarrhythmic drug testing

pattern in the higher intercostal spaces conferred a similar prognosis to individuals with a type 1 pattern in the standard position of V_1–V_2 [23]. Additionally, prolonged ECG monitoring has uncovered spontaneous intermittent type 1 ECG patterns in approximately 30% of patients with only drug-induced type 1 ECG [24, 25]. In addition, prolonged P-wave, PR, or QRS duration is frequently observed, particularly in patients carrying a *SCN5A* pathogenic variant, and sinus node dysfunction may occur [26]. PR prolongation likely represents an HV conduction delay. The QT interval is generally normal, but it can occasionally be slightly prolonged in the right precordial leads [27]. Repolarization abnormalities in the inferior and lateral leads have been reported in up to 11% of patients; these abnormalities are seemingly related to a more severe phenotype. In up to 20% of cases, there may be supraventricular arrhythmias, mainly manifesting as atrial fibrillation, although AV nodal reentry and Wolff-Parkinson-White syndrome have also been described in isolated case reports, probably as coincidental findings rather than genetic association [28, 29].

Pharmacological Tests and Other Diagnostic Tools

The diagnostic pattern of BrS could be documented in approximately 25% of the tracings. Almost every individual with a type 1 ECG will show normalization of the ECG during follow-up. The class IC antiarrhythmic drug test provides a sensitive tool to unmask these concealed forms. A pharmacological test with a sodium channel-blocking agent should be performed to unmask the disease when there is a clinical suspicion without a spontaneous type 1 ECG pattern [30]. Continuous ECG monitoring must be performed during all tests, and it is classified as positive when a type 1 ECG pattern is identified during the infusion. Ventricular arrhythmias can occur during testing; then, widening of the QRS to >130% over the baseline value or the presence of frequent ventricular premature beats should be a warning sign to stop administration (Table 14.1). Nowadays, the most widely used pharmacological test is an intravenous ajmaline and/or flecainide infusion. However, in some countries, procainamide is the only class I iv antiarrhythmic drug available. If not available, oral doses of flecainide or propafenone are used instead [31], but continuous monitoring should be maintained until the ECG reverts to the baseline situation. It is important to remark that nearly 25% of drug-induced tests might be false-negative. A negative flecainide challenge in a patient experiencing aborted SCD is not sufficient to exclude BrS. This should prompt clinicians to ensure long-term ECG follow-up and consider repeating a drug test with another sodium channel blocker [32]. The full stomach test was proposed as an alternative tool in diagnosing BrS [33]. In this test, the ST-segment changes appear to be provoked by an enhanced vagal tone. Adrenergic stimulation decreases the ST-segment elevation, whereas vagal stimulation increases it. Finally, other causes of ST-segment elevation before making the diagnosis of BrS should be excluded.

Table 14.1 Acquired Brugada syndrome (BrS): Differential diagnosis of ST-segment Elevation in electrocardiogram leads V_1 and V_2. RVOT, right ventricular outflow tract

Drugs	Antiarrhythmic drugs	• Class 1C sodium channel blockers (e.g., flecainide, pilsicainide, propafenone) • Class 1A sodium channel blockers (e.g., procainamide, disopyramide, cibenzoline) • Verapamil (L-type calcium channel blocker) • Beta-blockers (inhibit ICa, L)
	Antianginal drugs	• Nitrates • Calcium channel blockers (e.g., nifedipine, diltiazem)
	Psychotropic agents	• Tricyclic antidepressants (e.g., amitriptyline, desipramine, clomipramine, nortriptyline) • Tetracyclic antidepressants (e.g., maprotiline) • Phenothiazines (e.g., perphenazine, cyamemazine) • Selective serotonin uptake inhibitors (e.g., fluoxetine) • Cocaine intoxication
	Antiallergic agents	• Histamine H1 antihistamines. First-generation (dimenhydrinate)
Acute ischemia in RVOT		
Electrolyte disturbances		Hyperkalemia Hypercalcemia
Hyperthermia and hypothermia		
Elevated insulin level		
Mechanical compression of RVOT		

Structural Changes

The clinical phenotype of BrS concomitant with structural changes remains a matter of ongoing scientific investigation [34]. At present, few studies reported the presence of slight structural alterations in both ventricles after microscopic analysis suggesting a plausible structural defect in myocytes [35, 36]. It was supported by the identification in BrS patients of potential pathogenic variants in the *PKP2* gene [37]. This gene encodes the desmosomal protein plakophilin-2, mainly responsible for arrhythmogenic cardiomyopathy (ACM); it is a familial cardiac disease characterized by fibro-fatty substitution of the myocardium in the ventricles of patients. However, all variants reported in *PKP2* as causative for BrS remain to be confirmed [38]. Another study in BrS patients identified tissue- and molecular-level alterations, especially in the right ventricular outflow tract (RVOT) area [39]. In addition, recent studies suggest the pathophysiological mechanism of *PKP2* in BrS, showing no structural alteration, at least at macroscopic and microscopic levels [40, 41]. Taking into account all data published today, the role of structural alterations in BrS is uncertain. Current definition of BrS does not include any structural cardiac alteration. However, usually, this definition concerns to anatomical assessment (postmortem examination or using imaging techniques in alive patients). To date, an exhaustive microscopic or ultramicroscopic study in BrS patients has not been performed.

Differential Diagnosis

Brugada Phenocopies

As abovementioned, before establishing a definite diagnosis of BrS, other causes of ST-segment elevation should be excluded. Some ST elevation may arise from different diseases, while others may be induced by an underlying genetic predisposition. An ECG mimicking a BrS type 1 pattern that is triggered by other causes has been called *Brugada ECG phenocopy* [7]. Examples of situations, which result in ECG changes that mimic the BrS pattern ECG, include RV ischemia, acute pulmonary embolism, mechanical compression of the RV outflow tract, left ventricular hypertrophy, *pectus excavatum*, and even arrhythmogenic cardiomyopathy (ACM). Key findings that support the suspicion of Brugada phenocopies include the presence of an identifiable underlying condition, disappearance of the pattern with resolution of the condition, absence of family history of SD or type 1 BrS pattern in first-degree relatives, absence of symptoms such as syncope, seizures or nocturnal agonal respiration, and a negative sodium channel-blocker challenge test [42]. There are also *modulating factors* that can unmask or exacerbate a typical BrS pattern, which may be due to effects on transmembrane ionic currents [43, 44]. Bradycardia and vagal tone may decrease calcium currents and consequently contribute to ST-segment elevation and pro-arrhythmia [45]. In the case of drugs, one or multiple ionic currents may be affected (decrease in sodium/calcium currents and/or increase in potassium currents). Modulating factors play a major role in the dynamic nature of an ECG and may be responsible for ST-segment elevation in genetically predisposed patients. If any of these modulating factors are present, they should be corrected. Apart from sodium channel blockers, many other drugs have been reported to induce the type 1 BrS ECG pattern, including propofol, tricyclic antidepressants, fluoxetine, lithium, trifluoperazine, antihistamines, and cocaine [46, 47]. This induction is described as an "*acquired form of BrS*." It remains unknown whether acquired BrS is due to individual susceptibility resulting from an increase in latent ion channel dysfunction [48]. For this reason, management during anesthesia and surgery must provide some precautions and drug restrictions [49]. However, the lack of focused studies impedes establishing general rules, and the decision of using each drug must be made after careful consideration of the risks. Their use should always be in controlled conditions and avoiding other factors that are known to have the potential to induce arrhythmias [50]. Premature inactivation of the sodium channel is accentuated at higher temperatures in some *SCN5A* pathogenic variants, suggesting that febrile states may unmask certain BrS patients or temporarily increase the risk of malignant arrhythmias [13], particularly in the pediatric population [51]. Finally, ECG changes compatible with BrS can appear immediately after electrical cardioversion, although it is unknown whether they occur in BrS patients who carry a pathogenic genetic variant [52].

Molecular Diagnosis

The first description of BrS supported a potential inherited disease. Later reports also identified BrS in relatives of different families. This inherited factor was finally demonstrated in 1998, when we identified the first genetic alteration in the *SCN5A* gene [5]. Currently, more than 500 potentially pathogenic variations in more than 20 different genes have been associated with BrS (Table 14.2), supporting an autosomal dominant pattern of inheritance [53]. However, this percentage may be an overestimate as many variants previously classified as pathogenic may be of ambiguous significance following recent guidelines of the American College of Medical Genetics and Genomics (ACMG) [54, 55]. A comprehensive genetic analysis identified the genetic cause in nearly 35% of all cases [56]. Therefore, nearly 70% of families remain without an implicated genetic variant [57].

The *SCN5A* gene is the main gene, responsible for 25% of these cases. This gene encodes the alpha subunit of the car-

Table 14.2 Current genes associated with Brugada syndrome (BrS)

Current	Locus	Gene	Protein	Percentage
Sodium	3p21-p24	*SCN5A*	Nav1.5	<30
	3p22.3	*GPD1-L*	Glycerol-3-P-DH-1	<1
	19q13.1	*SCN1B*	Navβ1	<1
	11q24.1	*SCN3B*	Navβ3	<1
	11q23.3	*SCN2B*	Navβ2	<1
	3p22.2	*SCN10A*	Nav1.8	<2
	6q21	*HEY2*	Hes-related family BHLH transcription	<1
	17p13.1	*RANGRF*	factor YRPW motif 2	<1
	3p14.3	*SLMAP*	RAN-G-release factor (MOG1)	<1
	3q28	*FGF12*	Sarcolemma associated protein	<1
	12p11.21	*PKP2*	Fibroblast growth factor 12	<1
	12q15	*LRRC10*	Plakofilin-2	<1
			Leucine-rich repeat-containing protein 10	
Potassium	12p12.1	*ABCC9*	Adenosine triphosphate (ATP)- sensitive	<1
	11q13-q14	*KCNE3*	MiRP2	<1
	12p12.1	*KCNJ8*	Kv6.1 or Kir6.1	<1
	15q24.1	*HCN4*	Hyperpolarization cyclic nucleotide-gated 4	<1
	7q31.31	*KCND2*	KV4.2	<1
	7q36.1	*KCNH2*	HERG or Kv11.1	<1
	1p13.2	*KCND3*	Kv4.3 or Kir4.3	<1
	7p12.1	*SEMA3A*	Semaphorin III	<1
	Xq22.3	*KCNE5*	Potassium voltage-gated channel subfamily E member 1	<1
Calcium	2p13.3	*CACNA1C*	Cav1.2	<5
	10p12.33	*CACNB2B*	Voltage-dependent β-2	<2
	7q21-q22	*CACNA2D1*	Voltage-dependent α2/δ1	<1
	19q13.33	*TRPM4*	Transient receptor potential M4	<1

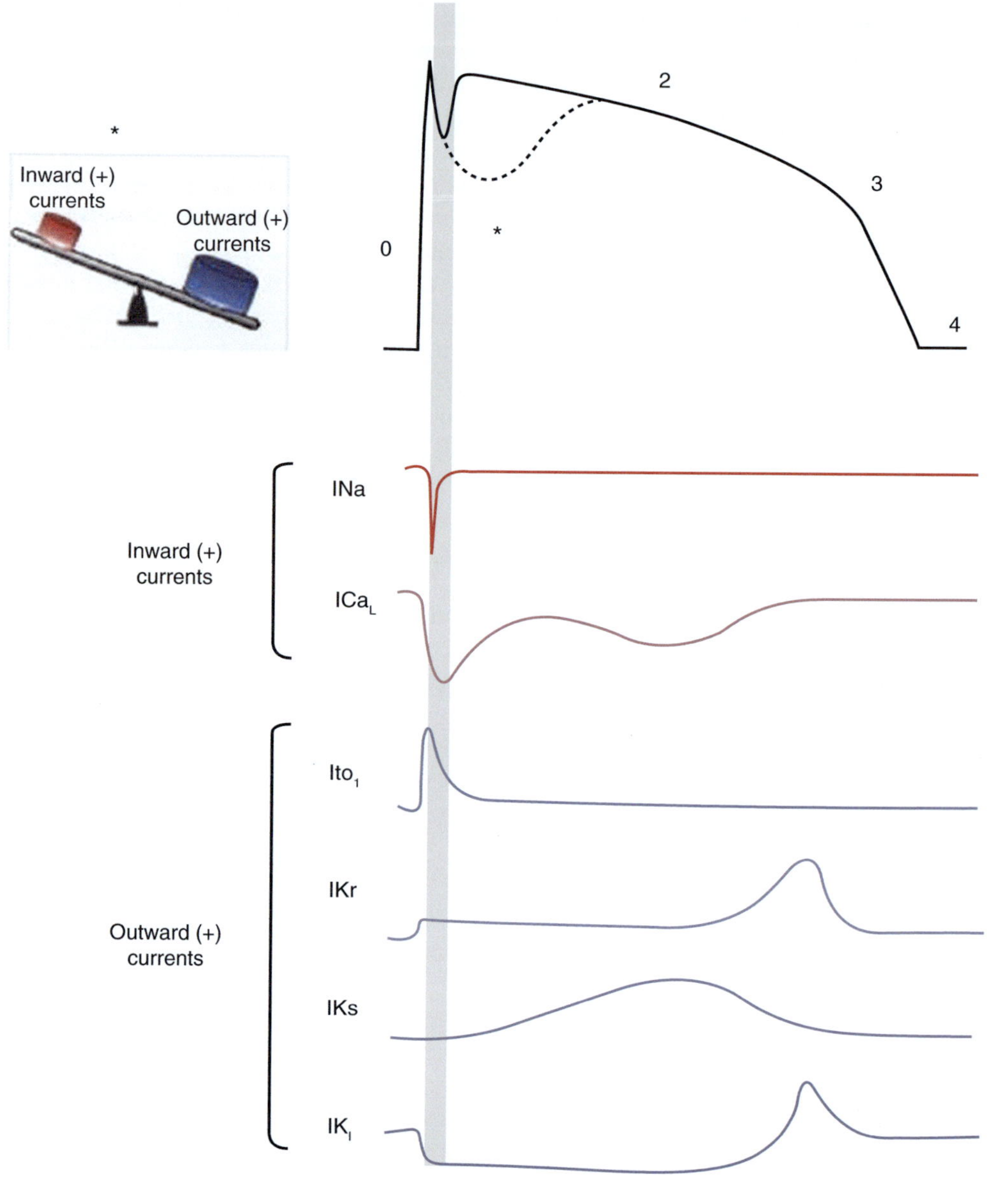

Fig. 14.2 Ventricular myocyte action potential (AP) and main underlying ionic currents. The shaded area highlights phase 1, mostly determined by the balance between INa, ICa, and Ito. When positive inward currents are impaired with respect to positive outward currents (∗), the cell achieves a greater degree of repolarization, and the normal dome of the action potential is lost, leading to the development of a particular notch at the end of phase 1 (dashed line). This is the mechanism that is thought to underlie the Brugada syndrome (BrS). ICa, inward calcium current; INa, inward sodium current; Ito, transient outward potassium current

diac sodium channel Nav1.5. This sodium channel subunit is responsible for phase 0 of the cardiac action potential (Fig. 14.2). In addition to *SCN5A*, a reduced number of pathogenic variants have been identified in other genes (*GPD1L*, *CACNA1C*, *HEY2*, *PKP2*, *RANGRF*, *SCN10A*, *SCN1B*, *SCN2B*, *SCN3B*, *SLMAP*, and *TRPM4*). In recent years, other genes have been also suggested as potential cause of BrS (*ABCC9*, *CACNA2D1*, *CACNB2*, *FGF12*, *HCN4*, *KCND2*, *KCND3*, *KCNE3*, *KCNE5*, *KCNH2*, *KCNJ8*, *LRRC10*, and *SEMA3A*) despite the fact that no comprehensive clinical and cellular studies have confirmed the association, so far. Considering all data, current guidelines recommend a comprehensive genetic analysis of only *SCN5A*. Despite these recent advances, results of genetic screening do not currently influence prognosis or treatment, but merely document the presence of a genetic mutation with either probable or possible cause to explain symptoms in patients with a BrS ECG [9].

Concerning 65% of families diagnosed with BrS but without a conclusive genetic alteration associated with the disease, other genetic alterations have been proposed as responsible for BrS, such as copy number variation (CNV) and alterations in regulatory regions of genes associated with BrS. In a recent study, a comprehensive genetic evaluation of main BrS-susceptibility genes and CNV in a BrS cohort was performed. We identified a low rate for CNVs in the *SCN5A* gene. No CNVs were found in other BrS genes [58]. We reported alterations in GATA transcription factors (GATA5, but especially GATA4) which are main contributors to *SCN5A* gene expression, thus providing a new paradigm of expression regulation that may shed new light on the understanding of BrS [59].

Genetic Interpretation and Clinical Translation

Current guidelines recommend only genetic test of the *SCN5A* gene. However, Next Generation Sequencing (NGS) technology allows a genetic analysis of several genes in a cost-effective way. NGS technology produces extensive genetic data and the current challenge is the interpretation of genetic alterations and their translation into clinical practice. Familial testing helps to clarify the pathogenic role of rare variants identified using NGS technology but also allows the identification of relatives carrying potential genetic variants and, in consequence, at risk of SCD, despite being asymptomatic. Because of controversy on the pathogenic role of variants identified, the ACMG has recently published recommendations focused on classification of genetic variants to clarify their role [54, 55, 57]. Yet, despite these guidelines, most of the BrS genetic variants remain of unknown or ambiguous significance, and translation into clinical practice must be done with caution [60]. The proportion of pathogenic variants associated with BrS should be further analyzed to clarify the real percentage of BrS cases associated with each gene. Family segregation and a comprehensive genotype-phenotype correlation help to interpret genetic variation in BrS; however, incomplete penetrance and variable expressivity exacerbated by the unknown pathophysiological mechanism induced by each genetic variant cloud their definitive roles. Therefore, the main role of *SCN5A* as a cause of pathology has been questioned [61].

Genetic Modulators

The incomplete penetrance of the disease, as well as the variable expression, has brought into question the role of additional genetic factors in the final phenotype. The *SCN5A* polymorphism p.H558R is present in nearly 20% of the population. This polymorphism has been shown to partially restore the sodium current impaired by other co-occurring BrS causing pathogenic variants in the *SCN5A* gene [62]. Thus, this common variant in the population is a genetic modifier of BrS among carriers of a pathogenic variant in *SCN5A*, in whom the presence of this less common allele results in a less severe BrS phenotype [63]. Genetic variants in the *SCN5A* promoter region may also play a pathophysiological role in BrS. One haplotype containing six polymorphisms in the *SCN5A* gene promoter has been identified and functionally linked to a reduced expression of the sodium current in the Japanese population [64]. The *SCN10A* gene (neuronal sodium channel $Na_v1.8$) has been shown to modulate *SCN5A* expression and the electrical function of the heart [65]. In the study, the transcriptional factor HEY2 was also identified as associated with BrS [66]. Other studies have shown the role of double mutations in causing a more severe phenotype [67, 68].

The role of these genetic modifiers in risk stratification has yet to be clearly defined. Recent data proposed the type of genetic pathogenic variant as a tool for risk stratification in BrS. Hence, both patients and relatives who carried a truncated protein showed a more severe phenotype and more severe conduction disorders. Despite the fact that some pathogenic variants appear to confer a worse prognosis, the use of these data in the clinical setting is not yet sufficient to take clinical decisions [69]. In 2015, a study was published that focused on the potential association between BrS and variants in mtDNA. No variants were identified, concluding that a specific mtDNA variation responsible for BrS can be excluded. However, the authors found a high turnover rate in the mtDNA of BrS patients, suggesting this could be an important cofactor for a BrS phenotype modifier [70]. Considering all data published so far, rare pathogenic mutations are responsible for BrS, but other rare and/or common variants may modulate the final phenotype of patients.

Cellular Therapy

In recent years, several advances in unraveling pathophysiological mechanisms associated with BrS have been reported. However, most genetic alterations identified in families suffering from BrS remain without a conclusive role in the disease. The main part of functional studies focused on genetic alterations associated with familial arrhythmogenic disorders has relied on heterologous expression systems in which the mutated ion channel of interest is expressed [71]. However, both electrophysiological and molecular consequences of a potentially pathogenic genetic alteration should be ideally analyzed in the native cardiomyocyte (CM) environment. In 2006, the discovery of somatic cell reprogramming to generate induced pluripotent stem cells (iPSC) [72] created much excitement because of the possibility of producing unique patient- and disease-specific human iPSC (hiPSC) lines as a promising experimental tool for translational heart research and drug development [73, 74]. In 2009, hiPSC were differentiated into functional CMs, making it possible to generate patient-specific human CMs, which are by definition on different genetic backgrounds [75]. These patient-specific hiPSC-CMs are able to incorporate phenotype features of single cells in vitro and allow study of the electrophysiological properties of myocytes that lead to characteristic ECG alterations in BrS [76, 77]. A study using hiPSC-CMs from two BrS patients carrying STOP-codon variants in the *SCN5A* gene did not show rescue of the electrophysiological phenotype by the tested compounds, which initiated a new pharmacological approach in BrS research [78]. Focused on pharmacological effects,

Miller et al. identified ajmaline's mode of action in the hiPSC-CM model and established a simple BrS hiPSC platform to test whether differences in ajmaline response could be determined between BrS patients and controls. Authors concluded that ajmaline can block both depolarization and repolarization of hiPSC-CMs at the cellular level but that a more refined integrated tissue model may be necessary to elicit differences in its effect between BrS patients and controls [79]. In a recent study, we generated hiPSC-CM with a genetic alteration in the *SCN5A* gene. This variant induced a loss of function of sodium channel current typically associated with the disease, leading to pro-arrhythmic changes in channel function not detected using conventional heterologous expression systems [80]. However, hiPSC-CMs usability as a human adult CM model is limited by their functional immaturity; thus, translation of findings from hiPSC-CMs to human disease should be made with great caution. Recently, a mathematical platform focused on quantitative evaluation of hiPSC-CMs was developed, improving the translation from hiPSC-CMs to patients [81]. Despite recent advances, further wide-ranging cellular studies using hiPSC-CM in BrS should be performed to provide insight into the functional effects of the genetic variants as potential therapeutic targets.

Risk Stratification

Risk stratification in BrS remains a challenge not only due to a low rate of cardiac events but also due to SCD as the first manifestation of the disease (Fig. 14.3). Numerous studies have reported that patients who presented arrhythmic events have been initially classified as low risk when following existing guidelines [11, 82]. Clinical studies con-

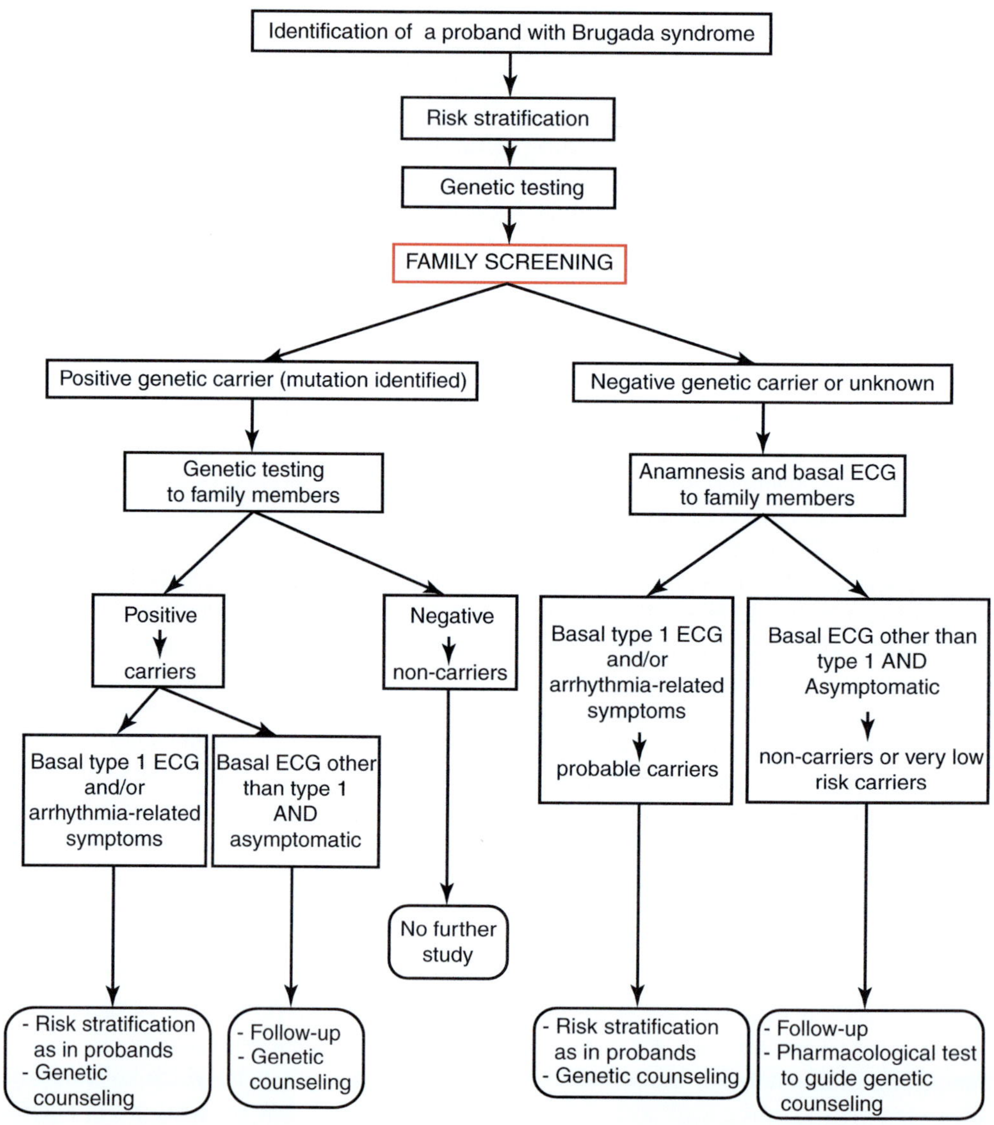

Fig. 14.3 Proposed algorithm for family screening after identification of a patient with a clinically confirmed Brugada syndrome (BrS)

clude that symptomatic patients are at higher risk than asymptomatic ones. In addition, sudden death survivors are at higher risk than patients with syncope. It is also stated that males are at higher risk than females and that patients with type 1 ECG at baseline have a higher risk than those who require class I antiarrhythmics [83, 84]. Identification of asymptomatic patients is the main problem due to SD. No conclusive recommendations have been defined for risk stratification in asymptomatic patients. A study showed a 0.5% annual rate of arrhythmic events in asymptomatic BrS patients [85]. A meta-analysis also recently published showed that asymptomatic subjects with either spontaneous diagnostic ECG pattern or inducible ventricular arrhythmias at programmed ventricular stimulation are at increased risk [86].

Concerning genetics, a family history of SD and the presence of an *SCN5A* pathogenic variant have not been definitively proven risk markers in any of the large studies conducted so far [87, 88]. However, existing data suggest a significantly higher rate of syncope among patients carrying *SCN5A* truncation pathogenic variants and those with *SCN5A* missense pathogenic variants resulting in a decrease of more than 90% of the I_{Na} (nonfunctional Na^+ channels), compared to patients with *SCN5A* missense pathogenic variants that produce a decrease of Na current (≤90%) [69]. In addition, combinations of risk factors with specific genetic mutations may be predictive, such as the combination of a *SCN5A* mutation with a history of SD in young first-degree relatives (<35 years) or in specific mutations such as those that result in a truncated Nav1.5 protein [89, 90]. In 2018, Amin et al. reported that *SCN5A* pathogenic variant is associated with an increased risk of drug-induced ventricular arrhythmia in patients without baseline type 1 ECG. Moreover, the risk for drug-induced arrhythmia depends on the type and topology of the variant in the *SCN5A* gene; in particular, patients with non-missense or missense variants in transmembrane or pore regions of *SCN5A*-encoded channel protein are at high risk of ventricular arrhythmia [91].

In 2016, the last consensus document proposed, for the first time, a multiparametric score system in which a spontaneous appearance of the characteristic ECG would be sufficient for the probable or definite diagnosis of BrS referred to as the Shanghai BrS Score [92]. The score model includes several clinical, echocardiographic, electrocardiographic, and electrophysiological parameters (age, gender, ECG parameters, syncope, and family history) proposed as risk stratifiers. Recently, Kawada et al. published the first report concerning the Shanghai scoring system reporting positive results for the diagnosis of BrS as well as evidence for some potential in the prediction of future events [93]. Despite this fact and in concordance to recent publication [94], further studies are needed for score validation.

Treatment

Implantable Cardioverter Defibrillator

Current guidelines recommend an implantable cardioverter-defibrillator (ICD) as the only proven effective therapeutic strategy for the prevention of SCD in BrS patients (Fig. 14.4) [9]. It should be implanted as primary prophylaxis in patients with BrS who have survived a cardiac arrest suspected to be caused by VT or VF (class IIa) or have documented spontaneous sustained VT (class I). Appropriate shocks were significantly associated with the presence of aborted SCD [95]. In asymptomatic BrS individuals who have inducible sustained VF during programmed ventricular stimulation with two or three extrastimuli at two sites, ICD implantation is controversial and is a class IIb indication. This recommendation is based on the low yearly event rate of 0.5% found in asymptomatic BrS patients [96, 97] coupled with the high complication rate reported for ICDs in BrS [98] and a high rate of complications, mainly consisting of inappropriate shocks [99–102]. A recent study reports that T-wave oversensing is a potential reason for inappropriate shocks in patients with BrS carrying ICDs. In the vast majority, the problem can be solved by reprogramming. However, in some patients, these complications require invasive intervention [103].

Pharmacological Approach

A pharmacological approach to therapy is aimed at rebalancing the ionic currents affected in BrS during the cardiac action potential (AP); drugs that inhibit the transient outward current or increase the Na^+ and Ca^{+2} currents have been tested in BrS (Table 14.1; Fig. 14.2). Hence, drug therapy in BrS has several utilities: first, in the acute management of arrhythmic storm; second, in the prevention of arrhythmic events in patients with implanted ICD who require many shocks; and, third, as an alternative to ICD implantation when the latter is contraindicated, not feasible, unaffordable, or refused by the patient [104].

Quinidine, a class Ia antiarrhythmic drug (AAD) with I_{to} and I_{Kr} blocker effects, is the most extensively studied medication with proven efficacy in successfully controlling and preventing arrhythmic events in BrS. It should be considered as an adjacent therapy to an ICD in high-risk patients and as an alternative to ICD under strict conditions [105]. Unfortunately, the use of quinidine is limited by its availability in many parts of the world and its relatively high incidence of side effects. Available medications effective in the therapy of BrS are isoproterenol, cilostazol, bepridil, denopamine, orciprenaline, and disopyramide and quinine sulfate. Antiarrhythmic medications (amiodarone, beta-blockers, and calcium channel

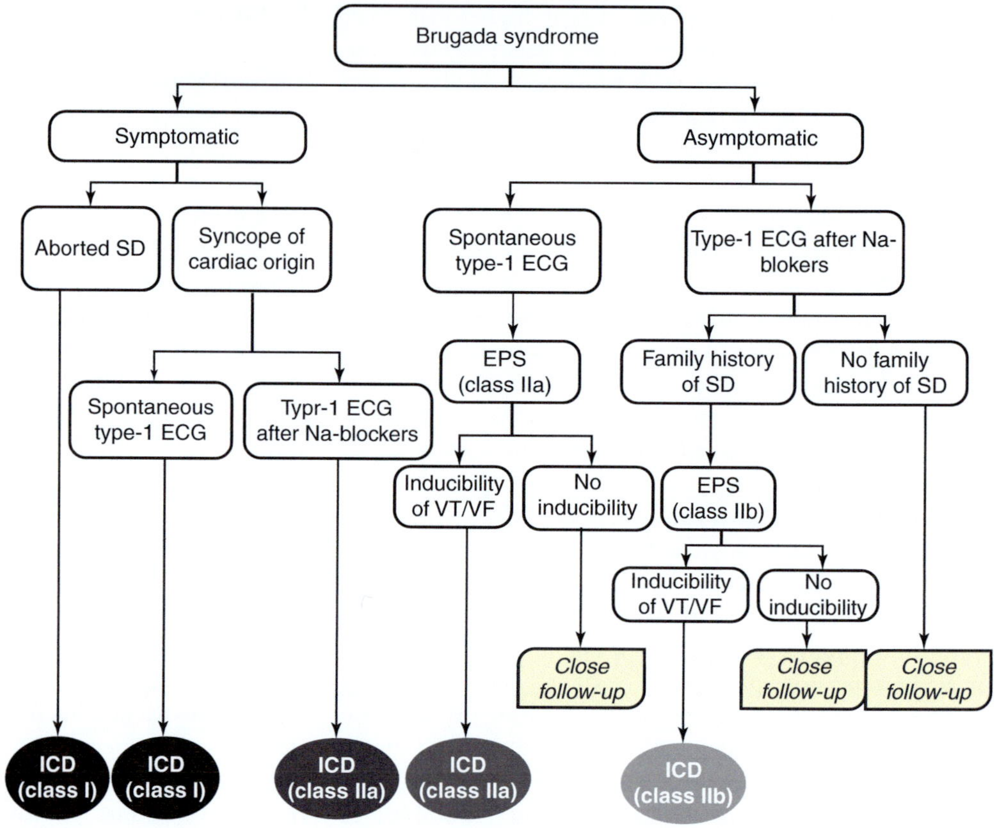

Fig. 14.4 Indications for implantable cardioverter-defibrillator (ICD) implantation in patients with Brugada syndrome. Class I designation indicates clear evidence that the procedure or treatment is useful or effective; Class II, conflicting evidence about usefulness or efficacy; Class IIa, weight of evidence in favor of usefulness or efficacy; Class IIb, usefulness or efficacy less well established

blockers) should be avoided in BrS. In addition, class IA (ajmaline, procainamide) and class IC (flecainide, propafenone, and pilsicainide) sodium channel blockers drugs are known to unmask type 1 ST-segment elevation in the ECG and induce cardiac arrhythmias in BrS. The occurrence of cardiac arrhythmias during sodium channel blocker challenge ranges from 0% to 17.8% [106]. Hence, these drugs are contraindicated in the therapy of BrS.

Radiofrequency Catheter Ablation

Invasive electrophysiology (EP) mapping and radiofrequency catheter ablation (RFCA) have increasingly become the standard of care for many cardiac arrhythmias, including BrS [107]. In 2003, trigger ablation as a viable means of preventing VF in three BrS patients was reported [108]. In 2011, a study including nine symptomatic patients with BrS created three-dimensional electroanatomic map of the endocardial surface of the right ventricle and the epicardial surface [109]. Ablation of the abnormal substrate acutely normalized the ECG pattern in eight of nine patients. After a mean follow-up of 20 months, there was no recurrent VF in all patients. One year later, 10 symptomatic BrS patients were analyzed using three-dimensional electroanatomic map [110]. Ablation was done to target the late activation zone. After endocardial ablation in the group with VF storm, the Brugada ECG was modified in three of four patients. At 30-month follow-up, no patients had recurrence of VF storm. In 2014, a BrS case of an ablation of the epicardial arrhythmogenic substrate in the right ventricular outflow tract was published [111]. In 2015, a BrS case was published in which epicardial ventricular tachycardia ablation was performed and noninducibility of any VT during programmed ventricular stimulation was shown and no recurrences occurred during 9 months of follow-up [112]. Recently, an interesting study focused on epicardial ablation was published. The authors demonstrate that ablation of the arrhythmogenic electrical substrate identified under flecainide can eliminate the BrS phenotype [113]. In 2017, a cohort of 135 symptomatic BrS patients having ICD was analyzed [114]. Arrhythmogenic electrophysiological substrate elimination by radiofrequency ablation results in ECG normalization and VT/VF noninducibility. During a median follow-up of 10 months, the ECG remained normal even after ajmaline in all except two patients who underwent a repeated effective procedure for recurrent VF. Substrate-based ablation is effective in potentially eliminating the arrhythmic consequences of this genetic disease.

With focus on clarifying the pathophysiological mechanism of arrhythmogenesis and its elimination, a recent study in animal models suggests that epicardial RFA exerts its ameliorative effect in the setting of BrS by destroying the cells with the most prominent action potential (AP) notch, thus eliminating sites of abnormal repolarization and the substrate for malignant arrhythmias [115]. Although larger studies with longer follow-up are required, for patients with BrS who have suffered from recurrent VF episodes, epicardial ablation of the BrS substrate should be the treatment of choice [107, 116]. Until we learn more about effectiveness and safety of RF ablation and despite being a life-saving procedure for patients with VF storm, the procedure should be reserved for patients with symptomatic BrS [117].

Pregnancy

The role of hormonal changes during pregnancy as a precipitating factor for arrhythmic events in BrS has been a matter of discussion despite the fact that few articles have been published so far. During pregnancy, autonomic and hemodynamic alterations occur, and estrogen and progesterone blood levels are reduced at peripartum. Some authors stated that elevated hormone levels during pregnancy may increase the risk for arrhythmias in particular cases [118, 119]. However, other authors presented cases with no arrhythmias during pregnancy and postpartum period [120]. Nevertheless, the management of pregnant women affected by BrS should be very strict and multidisciplinary in cooperation with a cardiologist and an anesthesiologist. The largest study of pregnant women with BrS published so far describes a relatively benign course of pregnancy and peripartum period among women with BrS [121]. Additional studies focused on clinical follow-up during the pregnant, postpartum, and peripartum periods should be performed in order to clarify the role of hormones in the risk of malignant arrhythmias.

Children

Despite progress in recent years, little is still known about BrS in the pediatric population. The prevalence, clinical implications, and management of BrS in children and young populations remain to be clarified due to few cases published so far. In large studies of asymptomatic children, BrS ECG pattern was found in 0.01–0.02% [122, 123] suggesting that BrS may exist in children but becomes clinically unmasked with increasing age. Fever is the most important precipitating factor for arrhythmic events, and like adult populations, the risk of arrhythmic events was higher in previously symptomatic patients and in those displaying a spontaneous type 1 ECG [124]. Hence, it is recommended that a 12-lead ECG be performed during febrile episodes, in children with a family history of BrS and in all children with febrile seizures.

Current diagnosis in children is based on ECG patterns [9]. Hence, a spontaneous type 1 ECG pattern in children is considered diagnostic of BrS, as also occurs in adults [125]. Evident disease is rarely reported in children, but malignant conditions such as SCD and syncope due to documented polymorphic VT have been reported [51, 126]. One of the main difficulties of the ECG recording is the optimal positioning of the right precordial leads. Positioning is especially problematic in children due to the different shape of the chest in a growing body. Use of Holter monitors can help identify evident asymptomatic arrhythmias; treadmill exercise test can unmask chronotropic incompetence as a sign of conduction system dysfunction. In addition, the low incidence of BrS in preadolescents suggests the potentially important role of hormones in BrS [127].

Concerning therapy, indications for an ICD in children and adolescents remain challenging, but children presenting with aborted SD, syncope, and a spontaneous type 1 ECG are clearly at high risk for SCD, and an ICD should be considered irrespective of age [51] despite high rates of inappropriate shocks and device-related complications reported [128]. The option of subcutaneous ICD (S-ICD) for young patients with inherited arrhythmic syndromes who do not need pacing therapy is being increasingly considered when feasible despite the lack of conclusive data. A recent study found high rates of sensing screening failure in patients with BrS, due to high T-wave voltages [129]. A recent study suggests a model of risk prediction using four characteristics: SCD or syncope, spontaneous type I ECG, sinus node dysfunction and/or atrial tachycardia, and conduction abnormality [130]. If controversy exists whether performing EPS testing is useful in the adult population, this is even more so in the discussion whether children should undergo programmed extrastimulation techniques to test malignant arrhythmias inducibility [131]. When indicated, the protocol remains the same as in the adult population. Decision-making in children with BrS is challenging and should be individualized according to the specific clinical presentation, family history, and genetic data.

Concerning pharmacological tests, there are limited studies in BrS children. A sodium channel blocker test (ajmaline 1 mg/kg or flecainide 2 mg/kg treatment over 10 min) should be performed after the onset of puberty in patients with a family history of BrS. A drug challenge should be performed if children having an abnormal nondiagnostic ECG or symptoms such as syncope, febrile seizures, or palpitations have appeared. The observation of an age-dependent response to ajmaline challenge is an intriguing recent finding that might have relevant clinical implications [132]. When a patient has had the need of a drug challenge before puberty (symptoms, abnormal ECG), some studies recommend repeating them after puberty. Regarding EPS, if used, the EP protocol is the same as in adults. A pharmacological approach in children at risk using hydroquinidine has been suggested as an alternative to ICD implantation, but little data are available to support this approach [133].

Older Individuals

There are a limited number of studies focused on the older population suffering of BrS. A recent analysis reported a benign prognosis and lower risk of older in comparison to younger patients as older patients presented less ventricular arrhythmias and less family history of SCD [134]. Concerning an ICD, a consensus conference reported that older BrS patients with syncope should undergo ICD implantation if life expectancy is at least 6 months [8]. Recently, another study showed that long-term follow-up of high-risk BrS patients with ICD showed a low incidence of VF in those more than 70 years old and avoidance of ICD implantation or replacement may be considered in elderly BrS patients who remain free from VF until 70 years of age [135]. A study focused on spontaneous Brugada ECG patterns in a Taiwanese population older than 55 years of age showed a higher prevalence of ECG with BrS patterns than the global average [136], mainly due to the endemic expression of this entity in Southeast Asia [137–139]. However, the report also disclosed that the all-cause mortality and cardiac mortality were not significantly different between subjects with or without Brugada ECG patterns. Despite these recent studies, the prevalence and long-term prognosis of individuals with the Brugada ECG pattern in the geriatric population is unknown, and the clinical course and prognosis of BrS in older individuals remains to be clarified. Therefore, decisions in older populations regarding use of drug-induced tests and device-guided management should be made on a case-by-case basis due to sparse data specific to BrS in aged individuals.

Summary

Brugada syndrome is an arrhythmogenic familial entity characterized by a typical ECG (persistent ST-segment elevation in right precordial leads followed by negative T waves), leading to VF and risk of SCD in the absence of structural heart disease. Several pharmacological approaches are currently being used despite the fact that ICD is the only proven effective therapy for patients at high risk so far. Recently, epicardial ablation has been used as a new effective therapy in BrS patients experiencing frequent appropriate ICD shocks. Nowadays, more than 20 genes have been associated with the disease, explaining nearly 35% of cases. However, almost 25% of cases carry a genetic alteration in the *SCN5A* gene. Genetic analysis is helpful in the identification of relatives at risk but for neither risk stratification nor prognosis. Despite recent advances, pathophysiological mechanisms responsible for incomplete penetrance and variable expressivity remain to be elucidated for development of cardio-selective and ion-channel-specific drugs for treatment of BrS. These variables, the asymptomatic and symptomatic presentations, and the unmasking of BrS only in the setting of specific triggers all lead to the present uncertainty and impede a proper clinical diagnosis, risk stratification, and management of patients. Additional studies of large cohorts including clinical and genetic analysis should be done for improving current knowledge of this pathology.

Take Home Message

- The BrS is a rare inherited channelopathy characterized by "*right bundle branch block, ST-segment elevation, and sudden death syndrome*" in the ECG. SCD may be the first symptom of the disease, mainly in men and usually at night during rest.
- The diagnosis of BrS occurs in patients with ECG pattern type 1 and any of the following clinical features: ventricular fibrillation documented polymorphic ventricular tachycardia (PVT), inducibility of PVT with programmed electrical stimulation, family history of SCD less than 45 years, type 1 ECG in family members, unexplained syncope or nocturnal agonal respiration, and no structural heart alterations.
- Ajmaline is the drug with better results unmasking the BrS type 1 pattern. Fever may be also unraveling the diagnostic pattern, especially in children.
- The main gene associated with BrS is *SCN5A*. Family segregation should be performed in order to clarify the real role of genetic alteration identified despite incomplete penetrance, and variable expressivity usually occurs.
- If a certain pathogenic mutation is identified in a family, no further clinical actions should be done in relatives with a negative genetic analysis.
- The main current challenge is the preventive measures in asymptomatic patients who carry a pathogenic genetic alteration and who are at risk of developing symptoms and even SCD.
- The ICD is the most effective strategy for the prevention of SCD in patients suffering from BrS. Recently, radiofrequency catheter ablation has been reported as an effective new treatment.

References

1. Brugada P, Brugada J. Right bundle branch block, persistent ST segment elevation and sudden cardiac death: a distinct clinical and electrocardiographic syndrome. A multicenter report. J Am Coll Cardiol. 1992;20(6):1391–6.
2. Miyazaki T, Mitamura H, Miyoshi S, Soejima K, Aizawa Y, Ogawa S. Autonomic and antiarrhythmic drug modulation of ST segment elevation in patients with Brugada syndrome. J Am Coll Cardiol. 1996;27(5):1061–70.
3. Nademanee K, Veerakul G, Nimmannit S, Chaowakul V, Bhuripanyo K, Likittanasombat K, et al. Arrhythmogenic

marker for the sudden unexplained death syndrome in Thai men. Circulation. 1997;96(8):2595–600.
4. Guazon M. Algunas notas sobre bangungut. Revista Filipina de Medicina Y Farmacia. 1917;8:437–42.
5. Chen Q, Kirsch GE, Zhang D, Brugada R, Brugada J, Brugada P, et al. Genetic basis and molecular mechanism for idiopathic ventricular fibrillation. Nature. 1998;392(6673):293–6.
6. Brugada J, Campuzano O, Arbelo E, Sarquella-Brugada G, Brugada R. Present status of Brugada syndrome: JACC state-of-the-art review. J Am Coll Cardiol. 2018;72(9):1046–59.
7. Baranchuk A, Nguyen T, Ryu MH, Femenia F, Zareba W, Wilde AA, et al. Brugada phenocopy: new terminology and proposed classification. Ann Noninvasive Electrocardiol. 2012;17(4):299–314.
8. Antzelevitch C, Brugada P, Borggrefe M, Brugada J, Brugada R, Corrado D, et al. Brugada syndrome: report of the second consensus conference: endorsed by the Heart Rhythm Society and the European heart rhythm association. Circulation. 2005;111(5):659–70.
9. Priori SG, Blomstrom-Lundqvist C. 2015 European Society of Cardiology Guidelines for the management of patients with ventricular arrhythmias and the prevention of sudden cardiac death summarized by co-chairs. Eur Heart J. 2015;36(41):2757–9.
10. Quan XQ, Li S, Liu R, Zheng K, Wu XF, Tang Q. A meta-analytic review of prevalence for Brugada ECG patterns and the risk for death. Medicine. 2016;95(50):e5643.
11. Milman A, Andorin A, Gourraud JB, Postema PG, Sacher F, Mabo P, et al. Profile of patients with Brugada syndrome presenting with their first documented arrhythmic event: data from the survey on arrhythmic events in BRUgada syndrome (SABRUS). Heart Rhythm. 2018;15(5):716–24.
12. Casado-Arroyo R, Berne P, Rao JY, Rodriguez-Manero M, Levinstein M, Conte G, et al. Long-term trends in newly diagnosed Brugada syndrome: implications for risk stratification. J Am Coll Cardiol. 2016;68(6):614–23.
13. Michowitz Y, Milman A, Sarquella-Brugada G, Andorin A, Champagne J, Postema PG, et al. Fever-related arrhythmic events in the multicenter survey on arrhythmic events in Brugada syndrome (SABRUS). Heart Rhythm. 2018;15(9):1394–401.
14. Sieira J, Dendramis G, Brugada P. Pathogenesis and management of Brugada syndrome. Nat Rev Cardiol. 2016;13(12):744–56.
15. Shimizu W, Matsuo K, Kokubo Y, Satomi K, Kurita T, Noda T, et al. Sex hormone and gender difference--role of testosterone on male predominance in Brugada syndrome. J Cardiovasc Electrophysiol. 2007;18(4):415–21.
16. Conte G, de Asmundis C, Ciconte G, Julia J, Sieira J, Chierchia GB, et al. Follow-up from childhood to adulthood of individuals with family history of Brugada syndrome and normal electrocardiograms. JAMA. 2014;312(19):2039–41.
17. Bayes de Luna A, Brugada J, Baranchuk A, Borggrefe M, Breithardt G, Goldwasser D, et al. Current electrocardiographic criteria for diagnosis of Brugada pattern: a consensus report. J Electrocardiol. 2012;45(5):433–42.
18. Chevallier S, Forclaz A, Tenkorang J, Ahmad Y, Faouzi M, Graf D, et al. New electrocardiographic criteria for discriminating between Brugada types 2 and 3 patterns and incomplete right bundle branch block. J Am Coll Cardiol. 2011;58(22):2290–8.
19. Serra G, Baranchuk A, Bayes-De-Luna A, Brugada J, Goldwasser D, Capulzini L, et al. New electrocardiographic criteria to differentiate the Type-2 Brugada pattern from electrocardiogram of healthy athletes with r'-wave in leads V1/V2. Europace. 2014;16(11):1639–45.
20. Serra G, Baranchuk A, Bayes-De-Luna A, Brugada J, Goldwasser D, Capulzini L, et al. Base of the triangle to determine a Brugada electrocardiogram pattern. Europace. 2015;17(3):505.
21. Richter S, Sarkozy A, Veltmann C, Chierchia GB, Boussy T, Wolpert C, et al. Variability of the diagnostic ECG pattern in an ICD patient population with Brugada syndrome. J Cardiovasc Electrophysiol. 2009;20(1):69–75.
22. Nagase S, Hiramatsu S, Morita H, Nishii N, Murakami M, Nakamura K, et al. Electroanatomical correlation of repolarization abnormalities in Brugada syndrome: detection of type 1 electrocardiogram in the right ventricular outflow tract. J Am Coll Cardiol. 2010;56(25):2143–5.
23. Miyamoto K, Yokokawa M, Tanaka K, Nagai T, Okamura H, Noda T, et al. Diagnostic and prognostic value of a type 1 Brugada electrocardiogram at higher (third or second) V1 to V2 recording in men with Brugada syndrome. Am J Cardiol. 2007;99(1):53–7.
24. Cerrato N, Giustetto C, Gribaudo E, Richiardi E, Barbonaglia L, Scrocco C, et al. Prevalence of type 1 brugada electrocardiographic pattern evaluated by twelve-lead twenty-four-hour holter monitoring. Am J Cardiol. 2015;115(1):52–6.
25. Gray B, Kirby A, Kabunga P, Freedman SB, Yeates L, Kanthan A, et al. Twelve-lead ambulatory electrocardiographic monitoring in Brugada syndrome: potential diagnostic and prognostic implications. Heart Rhythm. 2017;14(6):866–74.
26. Smits JP, Eckardt L, Probst V, Bezzina CR, Schott JJ, Remme CA, et al. Genotype-phenotype relationship in Brugada syndrome: electrocardiographic features differentiate SCN5A-related patients from non-SCN5A-related patients. J Am Coll Cardiol. 2002;40(2):350–6.
27. Pitzalis MV, Anaclerio M, Iacoviello M, Forleo C, Guida P, Troccoli R, et al. QT-interval prolongation in right precordial leads: an additional electrocardiographic hallmark of Brugada syndrome. J Am Coll Cardiol. 2003;42(9):1632–7.
28. Shi S, Liu T, Barajas-Martinez H, Pfeiffer R, Jiang H, Huang C, et al. Atrial fibrillation associated with Wolff-Parkinson-White syndrome in a patient with concomitant Brugada syndrome. Heart Rhythm Case Rep. 2017;3(1):13–7.
29. Kaiser E, Sacilotto L, Darrieux F, Sosa E. Coexistence of Wolff-Parkinson-White and Brugada syndrome: mere curiosity? Ann Noninvasive Electrocardiol. 2014;19(5):504–7.
30. Poli S, Toniolo M, Maiani M, Zanuttini D, Rebellato L, Vendramin I, et al. Management of untreatable ventricular arrhythmias during pharmacologic challenges with sodium channel blockers for suspected Brugada syndrome. Europace. 2018;20(2):234–42.
31. Therasse D, Sacher F, Petit B, Babuty D, Mabo P, Martins R, et al. Sodium-channel blocker challenge in the familial screening of Brugada syndrome: safety and predictors of positivity. Heart Rhythm. 2017;14(10):1442–8.
32. Chauveau S, Le Vavasseur O, Chevalier P. Delayed diagnosis of Brugada syndrome in a patient with aborted sudden cardiac death and initial negative flecainide challenge. Clin Case Rep. 2017;5(12):2022–4.
33. Ikeda T, Abe A, Yusu S, Nakamura K, Ishiguro H, Mera H, et al. The full stomach test as a novel diagnostic technique for identifying patients at risk of Brugada syndrome. J Cardiovasc Electrophysiol. 2006;17(6):602–7.
34. Saffitz JE. Structural heart disease, SCN5A gene mutations, and Brugada syndrome: a complex menage a trois. Circulation. 2005;112(24):3672–4.
35. Frustaci A, Russo MA, Chimenti C. Structural myocardial abnormalities in asymptomatic family members with Brugada syndrome and SCN5A gene mutation. Eur Heart J. 2009;30(14):1763.
36. Catalano O, Antonaci S, Moro G, Mussida M, Frascaroli M, Baldi M, et al. Magnetic resonance investigations in Brugada syndrome reveal unexpectedly high rate of structural abnormalities. Eur Heart J. 2009;30(18):2241–8.
37. Cerrone M, Lin X, Zhang M, Agullo-Pascual E, Pfenniger A, Chkourko Gusky H, et al. Missense mutations in plakophilin-2 cause sodium current deficit and associate with a Brugada syndrome phenotype. Circulation. 2014;129(10):1092–103.

38. Campuzano O, Fernandez-Falgueras A, Iglesias A, Brugada R. Brugada syndrome and PKP2: evidences and uncertainties. Int J Cardiol. 2016;214:403–5.
39. Nademanee K, Raju H, de Noronha SV, Papadakis M, Robinson L, Rothery S, et al. Fibrosis, Connexin-43, and conduction abnormalities in the Brugada syndrome. J Am Coll Cardiol. 2015;66(18):1976–86.
40. Cerrone M, Delmar M. Desmosomes and the sodium channel complex: implications for arrhythmogenic cardiomyopathy and Brugada syndrome. Trends Cardiovasc Med. 2014;24(5):184–90.
41. Moncayo-Arlandi J, Brugada R. Unmasking the molecular link between arrhythmogenic cardiomyopathy and Brugada syndrome. Nat Rev Cardiol. 2017;14(12):744–56.
42. Anselm DD, Baranchuk A. Terminological clarification of Brugada Phenocopy, Brugada Syndrome, and the Brugada ECG pattern: re. early repolarization pattern in patients with provocable Brugada Phenocopy: a marker of additional arrhythmogenic cardiomyopathy. Int J Cardiol. 2014;171(2):288.
43. Postema PG, Neville J, de Jong JS, Romero K, Wilde AA, Woosley RL. Safe drug use in long QT syndrome and Brugada syndrome: comparison of website statistics. Europace. 2013;15(7):1042–9.
44. Dumaine R, Towbin JA, Brugada P, Vatta M, Nesterenko DV, Nesterenko VV, et al. Ionic mechanisms responsible for the electrocardiographic phenotype of the Brugada syndrome are temperature dependent. Circ Res. 1999;85(9):803–9.
45. Yan GX, Antzelevitch C. Cellular basis for the Brugada syndrome and other mechanisms of arrhythmogenesis associated with ST-segment elevation. Circulation. 1999;100(15):1660–6.
46. Junttila MJ, Gonzalez M, Lizotte E, Benito B, Vernooy K, Sarkozy A, et al. Induced Brugada-type electrocardiogram, a sign for imminent malignant arrhythmias. Circulation. 2008;117(14):1890–3.
47. Yap YG, Behr ER, Camm AJ. Drug-induced Brugada syndrome. Europace. 2009;11(8):989–94.
48. Shimizu W. Acquired forms of the Brugada syndrome. J Electrocardiol. 2005;38(4 Suppl):22–5.
49. Duque M, Santos L, Ribeiro S, Catre D. Anesthesia and Brugada syndrome: a 12-year case series. J Clin Anesth. 2017;36:168–73.
50. Dendramis G, Paleologo C, Sgarito G, Giordano U, Verlato R, Baranchuk A, et al. Anesthetic and perioperative Management of Patients with Brugada Syndrome. Am J Cardiol. 2017;120(6):1031–6.
51. Gonzalez Corcia MC, de Asmundis C, Chierchia GB, Brugada P. Brugada syndrome in the paediatric population: a comprehensive approach to clinical manifestations, diagnosis, and management. Cardiol Young. 2016;26(6):1044–55.
52. Gurevitz O, Lipchenca I, Yaacoby E, Segal E, Perel A, Eldar M, et al. ST-segment deviation following implantable cardioverter defibrillator shocks: incidence, timing, and clinical significance. Pacing Clin Electrophysiol. 2002;25(10):1429–32.
53. Sarquella-Brugada G, Campuzano O, Arbelo E, Brugada J, Brugada R. Brugada syndrome: clinical and genetic findings. Genet Med. 2016;18(1):3–12.
54. Richards S, Aziz N, Bale S, Bick D, Das S, Gastier-Foster J, et al. Standards and guidelines for the interpretation of sequence variants: a joint consensus recommendation of the American College of Medical Genetics and Genomics and the Association for Molecular Pathology. Genet Med. 2015;17(5):405–24.
55. Amendola LM, Jarvik GP, Leo MC, McLaughlin HM, Akkari Y, Amaral MD, et al. Performance of ACMG-AMP variant-interpretation guidelines among nine Laboratories in the Clinical Sequencing Exploratory Research Consortium. Am J Hum Genet. 2016;98(6):1067–76.
56. Selga E, Campuzano O, Pinsach-Abuin ML, Perez-Serra A, Mademont-Soler I, Riuro H, et al. Comprehensive genetic characterization of a Spanish Brugada syndrome cohort. PLoS One. 2015;10(7):e0132888.
57. Kapplinger JD, Tester DJ, Alders M, Benito B, Berthet M, Brugada J, et al. An international compendium of mutations in the SCN5A-encoded cardiac sodium channel in patients referred for Brugada syndrome genetic testing. Heart Rhythm. 2010;7(1):33–46.
58. Mademont-Soler I, Pinsach-Abuin ML, Riuro H, Mates J, Perez-Serra A, Coll M, et al. Large genomic imbalances in Brugada syndrome. PLoS One. 2016;11(9):e0163514.
59. Tarradas A, Pinsach-Abuin ML, Mackintosh C, Llora-Batlle O, Perez-Serra A, Batlle M, et al. Transcriptional regulation of the sodium channel gene (SCN5A) by GATA4 in human heart. J Mol Cell Cardiol. 2017;102:74–82.
60. Starita LM, Ahituv N, Dunham MJ, Kitzman JO, Roth FP, Seelig G, et al. Variant interpretation: functional assays to the rescue. Am J Hum Genet. 2017;101(3):315–25.
61. Probst V, Wilde AA, Barc J, Sacher F, Babuty D, Mabo P, et al. SCN5A mutations and the role of genetic background in the pathophysiology of Brugada syndrome. Circ Cardiovasc Genet. 2009;2(6):552–7.
62. Poelzing S, Forleo C, Samodell M, Dudash L, Sorrentino S, Anaclerio M, et al. SCN5A polymorphism restores trafficking of a Brugada syndrome mutation on a separate gene. Circulation. 2006;114(5):368–76.
63. Lizotte E, Junttila MJ, Dube MP, Hong K, Benito B. M DEZ, et al. genetic modulation of brugada syndrome by a common polymorphism. J Cardiovasc Electrophysiol. 2009;20(10):1137–41.
64. Bezzina CR, Shimizu W, Yang P, Koopmann TT, Tanck MW, Miyamoto Y, et al. Common sodium channel promoter haplotype in Asian subjects underlies variability in cardiac conduction. Circulation. 2006;113(3):338–44.
65. Hu D, Barajas-Martinez H, Pfeiffer R, Dezi F, Pfeiffer J, Buch T, et al. Mutations in SCN10A are responsible for a large fraction of cases of Brugada syndrome. J Am Coll Cardiol. 2014;64(1):66–79.
66. Bezzina CR, Barc J, Mizusawa Y, Remme CA, Gourraud JB, Simonet F, et al. Common variants at SCN5A-SCN10A and HEY2 are associated with Brugada syndrome, a rare disease with high risk of sudden cardiac death. Nat Genet. 2013;45(9):1044–9.
67. Makita N, Mochizuki N, Tsutsui H. Absence of a trafficking defect in R1232W/T1620M, a double SCN5A mutant responsible for Brugada syndrome. Circ J. 2008;72(6):1018–9.
68. Cordeiro JM, Barajas-Martinez H, Hong K, Burashnikov E, Pfeiffer R, Orsino AM, et al. Compound heterozygous mutations P336L and I1660V in the human cardiac sodium channel associated with the Brugada syndrome. Circulation. 2006;114(19):2026–33.
69. Meregalli PG, Tan HL, Probst V, Koopmann TT, Tanck MW, Bhuiyan ZA, et al. Type of SCN5A mutation determines clinical severity and degree of conduction slowing in loss-of-function sodium channelopathies. Heart Rhythm. 2009;6(3):341–8.
70. Stocchi L, Polidori E, Potenza L, Rocchi MB, Calcabrini C, Busacca P, et al. Mutational analysis of mitochondrial DNA in Brugada syndrome. Cardiovasc Pathol. 2016;25(1):47–54.
71. Watanabe H, Koopmann TT, Le Scouarnec S, Yang T, Ingram CR, Schott JJ, et al. Sodium channel beta1 subunit mutations associated with Brugada syndrome and cardiac conduction disease in humans. J Clin Invest. 2008;118(6):2260–8.
72. Takahashi K, Yamanaka S. Induction of pluripotent stem cells from mouse embryonic and adult fibroblast cultures by defined factors. Cell. 2006;126(4):663–76.
73. Takahashi K, Tanabe K, Ohnuki M, Narita M, Ichisaka T, Tomoda K, et al. Induction of pluripotent stem cells from adult human fibroblasts by defined factors. Cell. 2007;131(5):861–72.
74. Yu J, Vodyanik MA, Smuga-Otto K, Antosiewicz-Bourget J, Frane JL, Tian S, et al. Induced pluripotent stem cell lines derived from human somatic cells. Science. 2007;318(5858):1917–20.
75. Zhang J, Wilson GF, Soerens AG, Koonce CH, Yu J, Palecek SP, et al. Functional cardiomyocytes derived from human induced pluripotent stem cells. Circ Res. 2009;104(4):e30–41.

76. Veerman CC, Mengarelli I, Guan K, Stauske M, Barc J, Tan HL, et al. hiPSC-derived cardiomyocytes from Brugada Syndrome patients without identified mutations do not exhibit clear cellular electrophysiological abnormalities. Sci Rep. 2016;6:30967.
77. Liang P, Sallam K, Wu H, Li Y, Itzhaki I, Garg P, et al. Patient-specific and genome-edited induced pluripotent stem cell-derived Cardiomyocytes elucidate single-cell phenotype of Brugada syndrome. J Am Coll Cardiol. 2016;68(19):2086–96.
78. Kosmidis G, Veerman CC, Casini S, Verkerk AO, van de Pas S, Bellin M, et al. Readthrough-promoting drugs gentamicin and PTC124 fail to rescue Nav1.5 function of human-induced pluripotent stem cell-derived cardiomyocytes carrying nonsense mutations in the sodium channel gene SCN5A. Circ Arrhythm Electrophysiol. 2016 Nov;9(11):e004227.
79. Miller DC, Harmer SC, Poliandri A, Nobles M, Edwards EC, Ware JS, et al. Ajmaline blocks INa and IKr without eliciting differences between Brugada syndrome patient and control human pluripotent stem cell-derived cardiac clusters. Stem Cell Res. 2017;25:233–44.
80. Selga E, Sendfeld F, Martinez-Moreno R, Medine CN, Tura-Ceide O, Wilmut SI, et al. Sodium channel current loss of function in induced pluripotent stem cell-derived cardiomyocytes from a Brugada syndrome patient. J Mol Cell Cardiol. 2018;114:10–9.
81. Koivumaki JT, Naumenko N, Tuomainen T, Takalo J, Oksanen M, Puttonen KA, et al. Structural immaturity of human iPSC-derived Cardiomyocytes: in Silico investigation of effects on function and disease modeling. Front Physiol. 2018;9:80.
82. Raju H, Papadakis M, Govindan M, Bastiaenen R, Chandra N, O'Sullivan A, et al. Low prevalence of risk markers in cases of sudden death due to Brugada syndrome relevance to risk stratification in Brugada syndrome. J Am Coll Cardiol. 2011;57(23):2340–5.
83. Brugada J, Brugada R, Brugada P. Right bundle-branch block and ST-segment elevation in leads V1 through V3: a marker for sudden death in patients without demonstrable structural heart disease. Circulation. 1998;97(5):457–60.
84. Benito B, Sarkozy A, Mont L, Henkens S, Berruezo A, Tamborero D, et al. Gender differences in clinical manifestations of Brugada syndrome. J Am Coll Cardiol. 2008;52(19):1567–73.
85. Sieira J, Ciconte G, Conte G, Chierchia GB, de Asmundis C, Baltogiannis G, et al. Asymptomatic Brugada syndrome: clinical characterization and long-term prognosis. Circ Arrhythm Electrophysiol. 2015;8(5):1144–50.
86. Letsas KP, Liu T, Shao Q, Korantzopoulos P, Giannopoulos G, Vlachos K, et al. Meta-analysis on risk stratification of asymptomatic individuals with the Brugada phenotype. Am J Cardiol. 2015;116(1):98–103.
87. Sarkozy A, Sorgente A, Boussy T, Casado R, Paparella G, Capulzini L, et al. The value of a family history of sudden death in patients with diagnostic type I Brugada ECG pattern. Eur Heart J. 2011;32(17):2153–60.
88. Gehi AK, Duong TD, Metz LD, Gomes JA, Mehta D. Risk stratification of individuals with the Brugada electrocardiogram: a meta-analysis. J Cardiovasc Electrophysiol. 2006;17(6):577–83.
89. Sommariva E, Pappone C, Martinelli Boneschi F, Di Resta C, Rosaria Carbone M, Salvi E, et al. Genetics can contribute to the prognosis of Brugada syndrome: a pilot model for risk stratification. Eur J Hum Genet. 2013;21(9):911–7.
90. Sieira J, Conte G, Ciconte G, Chierchia GB, Casado-Arroyo R, Baltogiannis G, et al. A score model to predict risk of events in patients with Brugada syndrome. Eur Heart J. 2017;38(22):1756–63.
91. Amin AS, Reckman YJ, Arbelo E, Spanjaart AM, Postema PG, Tadros R, et al. SCN5A mutation type and topology are associated with the risk of ventricular arrhythmia by sodium channel blockers. Int J Cardiol. 2018;266:128–32.
92. Antzelevitch C, Yan GX, Ackerman MJ, Borggrefe M, Corrado D, Guo J, et al. J-wave syndromes expert consensus conference report: emerging concepts and gaps in knowledge. Heart Rhythm. 2016;13(10):e295–324.
93. Kawada S, Morita H, Antzelevitch C, Morimoto Y, Nakagawa K, Watanabe A, et al. Shanghai score system for diagnosis of Brugada syndrome: validation of the score system and system and reclassification of the patients. JACC Clin Electrophysiol. 2018;4(6):724–30.
94. Wilde AAM. The Shanghai score system in Brugada syndrome: using it beyond a diagnostic score. JACC Clin electrophysiol. 2018;4(6):731–2.
95. Conte G, Sieira J, Ciconte G, de Asmundis C, Chierchia GB, Baltogiannis G, et al. Implantable cardioverter-defibrillator therapy in Brugada syndrome: a 20-year single-center experience. J Am Coll Cardiol. 2015;65(9):879–88.
96. Probst V, Veltmann C, Eckardt L, Meregalli PG, Gaita F, Tan HL, et al. Long-term prognosis of patients diagnosed with Brugada syndrome: results from the FINGER Brugada syndrome registry. Circulation. 2010;121(5):635–43.
97. Kamakura S, Ohe T, Nakazawa K, Aizawa Y, Shimizu A, Horie M, et al. Long-term prognosis of probands with Brugada-pattern ST-elevation in leads V1-V3. Circ Arrhythm Electrophysiol. 2009;2(5):495–503.
98. Miyazaki S, Uchiyama T, Komatsu Y, Taniguchi H, Kusa S, Nakamura H, et al. Long-term complications of implantable defibrillator therapy in Brugada syndrome. Am J Cardiol. 2013;111(10):1448–51.
99. Sarkozy A, Boussy T, Kourgiannides G, Chierchia GB, Richter S, De Potter T, et al. Long-term follow-up of primary prophylactic implantable cardioverter-defibrillator therapy in Brugada syndrome. Eur Heart J. 2007;28(3):334–44.
100. Rosso R, Glick A, Glikson M, Wagshal A, Swissa M, Rosenhek S, et al. Outcome after implantation of cardioverter defibrillator [corrected] in patients with Brugada syndrome: a multicenter Israeli study (ISRABRU). Isr Med Assoc J. 2008;10(6):435–9.
101. Zipes DP, Camm AJ, Borggrefe M, Buxton AE, Chaitman B, Fromer M, et al. ACC/AHA/ESC 2006 guidelines for management of patients with ventricular arrhythmias and the prevention of sudden cardiac death--executive summary: A report of the American College of Cardiology/American Heart Association Task Force and the European Society of Cardiology Committee for Practice Guidelines (Writing Committee to Develop Guidelines for Management of Patients with Ventricular Arrhythmias and the Prevention of Sudden Cardiac Death) Developed in collaboration with the European Heart Rhythm Association and the Heart Rhythm Society. Eur Heart J. 2006;27(17):2099–140.
102. Sacher F, Probst V, Maury P, Babuty D, Mansourati J, Komatsu Y, et al. Outcome after implantation of a cardioverter-defibrillator in patients with Brugada syndrome: a multicenter study-part 2. Circulation. 2013;128(16):1739–47.
103. Rodriguez-Manero M, de Asmundis C, Sacher F, Arbelo E, Probst V, Castro-Hevia J, et al. T-wave oversensing in patients with Brugada syndrome: true bipolar versus integrated bipolar implantable cardioverter defibrillator leads: multicenter retrospective study. Circ Arrhythm Electrophysiol. 2015;8(4):792–8.
104. Brodie OT, Michowitz Y, Belhassen B. Pharmacological therapy in Brugada syndrome. Arrhythmia Electrophysiol Rev. 2018;7(2):135–42.
105. Schweizer PA, Becker R, Katus HA, Thomas D. Successful acute and long-term management of electrical storm in Brugada syndrome using orciprenaline and quinine/quinidine. Clin Res Cardiol. 2010;99(7):467–70.
106. Dobbels B, De Cleen D, Ector J. Ventricular arrhythmia during ajmaline challenge for the Brugada syndrome. Europace. 2016;18(10):1501–6.

107. Nademanee K, Hocini M, Haissaguerre M. Epicardial substrate ablation for Brugada syndrome. Heart Rhythm. 2017;14(3):457–61.
108. Haissaguerre M, Extramiana F, Hocini M, Cauchemez B, Jais P, Cabrera JA, et al. Mapping and ablation of ventricular fibrillation associated with long-QT and Brugada syndromes. Circulation. 2003;108(8):925–8.
109. Nademanee K, Veerakul G, Chandanamattha P, Chaothawee L, Ariyachaipanich A, Jirasirirojanakorn K, et al. Prevention of ventricular fibrillation episodes in Brugada syndrome by catheter ablation over the anterior right ventricular outflow tract epicardium. Circulation. 2011;123(12):1270–9.
110. Sunsaneewitayakul B, Yao Y, Thamaree S, Zhang S. Endocardial mapping and catheter ablation for ventricular fibrillation prevention in Brugada syndrome. J Cardiovasc Electrophysiol. 2012;23(Suppl 1):S10–6.
111. Szeplaki G, Ozcan EE, Osztheimer I, Tahin T, Merkely B, Geller L. Ablation of the epicardial substrate in the right ventricular outflow tract in a patient with brugada syndrome refusing implantable cardioverter defibrillator therapy. Can J Cardiol. 2014;30(10):1249e9–e11.
112. Forkmann M, Tomala J, Huo Y, Mayer J, Christoph M, Wunderlich C, et al. Epicardial ventricular tachycardia ablation in a patient with Brugada ECG pattern and mutation of PKP2 and DSP genes. Circ Arrhythm Electrophysiol. 2015;8(2):505–7.
113. Brugada J, Pappone C, Berruezo A, Vicedomini G, Manguso F, Ciconte G, et al. Brugada syndrome phenotype elimination by Epicardial substrate ablation. Circ Arrhythm Electrophysiol. 2015;8(6):1373–81.
114. Pappone C, Brugada J, Vicedomini G, Ciconte G, Manguso F, Saviano M, et al. Electrical substrate elimination in 135 consecutive patients with Brugada syndrome. Circ Arrhythm Electrophysiol. 2017;10(5):e005053.
115. Patocskai B, Yoon N, Antzelevitch C. Mechanisms underlying Epicardial radiofrequency ablation to suppress Arrhythmogenesis in experimental models of Brugada syndrome. JACC Clin Electrophysiol. 2017;3(4):353–63.
116. Fernandes GC, Fernandes A, Cardoso R, Nasi G, Rivera M, Mitrani RD, et al. Ablation strategies for the management of symptomatic Brugada syndrome: a systematic review. Heart Rhythm. 2018;15(8):1140–7.
117. Viskin S. Radiofrequency ablation of asymptomatic Brugada syndrome: Don't go burning my heart. Circulation. 2018;137(18):1883–4.
118. Sharif-Kazemi MB, Emkanjoo Z, Tavoosi A, Kafi M, Kheirkhah J, Alizadeh A, Sadr-Ameli MA, Sharif-Kazemi MB, et al. Electrical storm in Brugada syndrome during pregnancy. Pacing Clin Electrophysiol. 2011 Feb;34(2):e18-21.
119. Prochnau D, Figulla HR, Surber R. First clinical manifestation of Brugada syndrome during pregnancy. Herzschrittmacherther Elektrophysiol. 2013;24(3):194–6.
120. Giambanco L, Incandela D, Maiorana A, Alio W, Alio L. Brugada syndrome and pregnancy: highlights on antenatal and prenatal management. Case Rep Obstet Gynecol. 2014;2014:531648.
121. Rodriguez-Manero M, Casado-Arroyo R, Sarkozy A, Leysen E, Sieira JA, Namdar M, et al. The clinical significance of pregnancy in Brugada syndrome. Rev Esp Cardiol (Engl Ed). 2014;67(3):176–80.
122. Yamakawa Y, Ishikawa T, Uchino K, Mochida Y, Ebina T, Sumita S, et al. Prevalence of right bundle-branch block and right precordial ST-segment elevation (Brugada-type electrocardiogram) in Japanese children. Circ J. 2004;68(4):275–9.
123. Oe H, Takagi M, Tanaka A, Namba M, Nishibori Y, Nishida Y, et al. Prevalence and clinical course of the juveniles with Brugada-type ECG in Japanese population. Pacing Clin Electrophysiol. 2005;28(6):549–54.
124. Probst V, Denjoy I, Meregalli PG, Amirault JC, Sacher F, Mansourati J, et al. Clinical aspects and prognosis of Brugada syndrome in children. Circulation. 2007;115(15):2042–8.
125. Sorgente A, Sarkozy A, De Asmundis C, Chierchia GB, Capulzini L, Paparella G, et al. Ajmaline challenge in young individuals with suspected Brugada syndrome. Pacing Clin Electrophysiol. 2011;34(6):736–41.
126. Gonzalez Corcia MC, Sieira J, Sarkozy A, de Asmundis C, Chierchia GB, Hernandez Ojeda J, et al. Brugada syndrome in the young: an assessment of risk factors predicting future events. Europace. 2016;19(11):1864–73.
127. Brugada R, Campuzano O, Sarquella-Brugada G, Brugada J, Brugada P. Brugada syndrome. Methodist Debakey Cardiovasc J. 2014;10(1):25–8.
128. Gonzalez Corcia MC, Sieira J, Pappaert G, de Asmundis C, Chierchia GB, La Meir M, et al. Implantable Cardioverter-defibrillators in children and adolescents with Brugada syndrome. J Am Coll Cardiol. 2018;71(2):148–57.
129. Conte G, Kawabata M, de Asmundis C, Taravelli E, Petracca F, Ruggiero D, et al. High rate of subcutaneous implantable cardioverter-defibrillator sensing screening failure in patients with Brugada syndrome: a comparison with other inherited primary arrhythmia syndromes. Europace. 2018;20(7):1188–93.
130. Gonzalez Corcia MC, Sieira J, Pappaert G, de Asmundis C, Chierchia GB, Sarkozy A, et al. A clinical score model to predict lethal events in young patients (≤19 years) with the Brugada syndrome. Am J Cardiol. 2017;120(5):797–802.
131. Brugada J, Brugada R, Brugada P. Determinants of sudden cardiac death in individuals with the electrocardiographic pattern of Brugada syndrome and no previous cardiac arrest. Circulation. 2003;108(25):3092–6.
132. Conte G, Brugada P. The challenges of performing ajmaline challenge in children with suspected Brugada syndrome. Open Heart. 2014;1(1):e000031.
133. Probst V, Evain S, Gournay V, Marie A, Schott JJ, Boisseau P, et al. Monomorphic ventricular tachycardia due to Brugada syndrome successfully treated by hydroquinidine therapy in a 3-year-old child. J Cardiovasc Electrophysiol. 2006;17(1):97–100.
134. Conte G. C DEA, Sieira J, Levinstein M, Chierchia GB, G DIG, et al. clinical characteristics, management, and prognosis of elderly patients with Brugada syndrome. J Cardiovasc Electrophysiol. 2014;25(5):514–9.
135. Kamakura T, Wada M, Nakajima I, Ishibashi K, Miyamoto K, Okamura H, et al. Evaluation of the necessity for cardioverter-defibrillator implantation in elderly patients with Brugada syndrome. Circ Arrhythm Electrophysiol. 2015;8(4):785–91.
136. Juang JM, Chen CY, Chen YH, Wu IC, Hsu CC, Chen LN, et al. Prevalence and prognosis of Brugada electrocardiogram patterns in an elderly Han Chinese population: a nation-wide community-based study (HALST cohort). Europace. 2015;17(Suppl 2):ii54–62.
137. Ito H, Yano K, Chen R, He Q, Curb JD. The prevalence and prognosis of a Brugada-type electrocardiogram in a population of middle-aged Japanese-American men with follow-up of three decades. Am J Med Sci. 2006;331(1):25–9.
138. Uhm JS, Hwang IU, Oh YS, Choi MS, Jang SW, Shin WS, et al. Prevalence of electrocardiographic findings suggestive of sudden cardiac death risk in 10,867 apparently healthy young Korean men. Pacing Clin Electrophysiol. 2011;34(6):717–23.
139. Gervacio-Domingo G, Isidro J, Tirona J, Gabriel E, David G, Amarillo ML, et al. The Brugada type 1 electrocardiographic pattern is common among Filipinos. J Clin Epidemiol. 2008;61(10):1067–72.

Catecholaminergic Polymorphic Ventricular

15

Isabelle Denjoy, Alice Maltret, Krystien V. Lieve, Christian van der Werf, and Antoine Leenhardt

Introduction

Catecholaminergic polymorphic ventricular tachycardia (CPVT) is a malignant cardiac channelopathy with polymorphic ventricular tachyarrhythmias during exercise or emotion as its key feature [1]. In some patients, the classic bidirectional ventricular tachycardia, characterized by a beat-to-beat 180-degree alternating QRS axis, can be observed (Fig. 15.1).

The prevalence of CPVT is frequently estimated at 1 in 10,000 in the literature [2, 3], accounting for about 12% of autopsy-negative sudden death and 1.5% of sudden infant death [4, 5]. The first descriptions of patients with clinical characteristics of CPVT were published in 1960 [6] and 1975 [7]. Thereafter, two important case series were published by the Paris group of Philippe Coumel in 1978 [8] and 1995 [9], resulting in the definite recognition of CPVT as a distinct inherited arrhythmia syndrome.

Aetiology

CPVT is secondary to cardiomyocyte calcium imbalance which is the substrate of afterdepolarization. The genetic background of CPVT was discovered in 2001, when mutations in the cardiac ryanodine receptor gene (*RYR2*) [10] and cardiac calsequestrin (*CASQ2*) [11] were found to underlie the common autosomal-dominant and rare autosomal-recessive forms of CPVT, respectively. Since then, several other genes have been identified.

I. Denjoy (✉) · A. Leenhardt
Cardiology Department, APHP, Hopital Bichat, Refering Centre for Cardiac Hereditary Diseases, Paris Sorbonne University Paris, France

A. Maltret
M3C-Necker, Hôpital Universitaire Necker Enfants Malades, Université Paris Descartes, Paris, France

K. V. Lieve · C. van der Werf
Department of Clinical and Experimental Cardiology, Amsterdam Cardiovascular Sciences, Amsterdam UMC, University of Amsterdam, Heart Centre, Amsterdam, The Netherlands

Clinical Presentation

CPVT is considered as a childhood-onset channelopathy since symptoms typically occur within the first two decades [12, 13]. RyR2 mutations are often associated with this juvenal form. Recent studies suggest an adult-onset type of CPVT in which symptoms occur after the third or fourth decade. In the latter, females are more concern and RyR2 is less likely to be involve [14, 15]. Cerebral anoxia secondary to ventricular arrhythmia can mimic seizures and often lead to false diagnosis of epilepsy, causing a mean delay of 2–3 years between initial presentation and diagnosis [16, 17].

Every seizure occurring with exercise or emotional stress has to be considered as CPVT until proven otherwise, especially if the seizure does not respond to antiepileptic medication, if there is a personal or familial history of syncope or sudden death before 30 years [18].

Clinical Diagnosis

A definite clinical diagnosis of CPVT requires the presence of reproducible exercise- or emotion-induced polymorphic or bidirectional ventricular tachycardia in the absence of structural heart disease and resting ECG abnormalities [19, 20]. In individuals over 40 years of age, the exclusion of (significant) coronary artery disease is required [19]. In addition, CPVT is diagnosed in individuals who carry a pathogenic CPVT-associated mutation in *RYR2* or *CASQ2* with or without clinical signs of the disease [19, 20].

According to the HRS/EHRA/APHRS expert consensus recommendations, CPVT can also be diagnosed in patients

H. F. Baars et al. (eds.), *Clinical Cardiogenetics*, https://doi.org/10.1007/978-3-030-45457-9_15

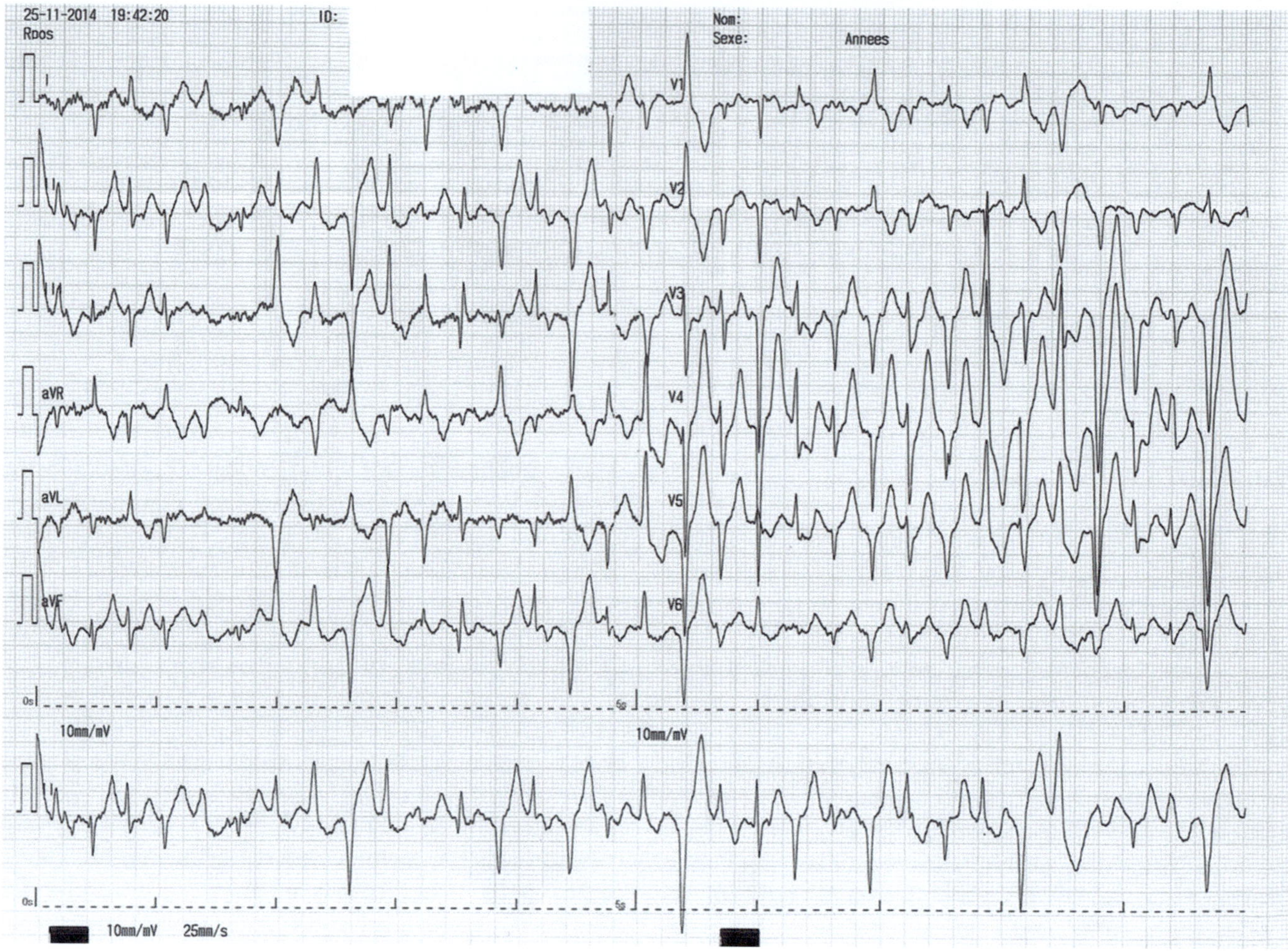

Fig. 15.1 ECG recording during stress test showing bidirectional ventricular premature beats and polymorphic ventricular salvoes typical of CPVT

with adrenergically mediated polymorphic or bidirectional ventricular premature beats, although the minimally required ventricular arrhythmia burden is not further detailed [19, 20]. In patients with possible CPVT, i.e. not meeting the aforementioned clinical diagnostic criteria, genetic testing is critical to make a definite diagnosis of CPVT.

CPVT patients typically have a normal 12-lead resting electrocardiogram, including a normal QTc interval. However, sinus bradycardia and prominent U-waves can be observed [2] as well as supraventricular ectopy or non-sustained supraventricular tachycardia [2, 21–23].

Provocative testing, preferably using exercise testing, is the gold standard to diagnose CPVT. Typically, a gradual increase of ventricular arrhythmia burden and complexity is observed. First, isolated late-coupled ventricular premature beats (VPB) with a predominant left bundle branch inferior axis or right bundle branch block superior axis morphology appear at a heart rate of approximately 110–130 beats per minute [14, 24]. Ventricular arrhythmia threshold heart rate and VPB morphology are usually accurately reproducible in an individual patient, unless important therapeutic modifications are made. Later, bigeminal VPBs and polymorphic couplets or non-sustained ventricular tachycardia, including bidirectional ventricular tachycardia, usually appear. When exercise testing is terminated, the ventricular arrhythmias usually rapidly recede, and VPBs recorded more than one minute into the recovery phase are uncommon [24]. In some patients who reach a high maximum heart rate, the ventricular arrhythmias are paradoxically suppressed at maximum heart rates [25], although the exercise test might be stopped before this point is reached in case of severe ventricular arrhythmias.

Other tests to diagnose CPVT are adrenaline infusion and Holter monitoring (Fig. 15.2). Adrenaline infusion is initiated at a dose of 0.05 μg per kg per minute and then titrated at 4- or 5-minute intervals to a maximum dose of 0.2–0.4 μg per kg per minute. One study which compared the diagnostic accuracy of adrenaline infusion and exercise testing in 36 CPVT patients and 45 unaffected relatives showed a low sensitivity of adrenaline infusion, probably because maximum heart rate achieved upon adrenaline challenge was markedly lower compared with exercise testing [26]. Only seven of 25 CPVT patients with a positive exercise test had a positive

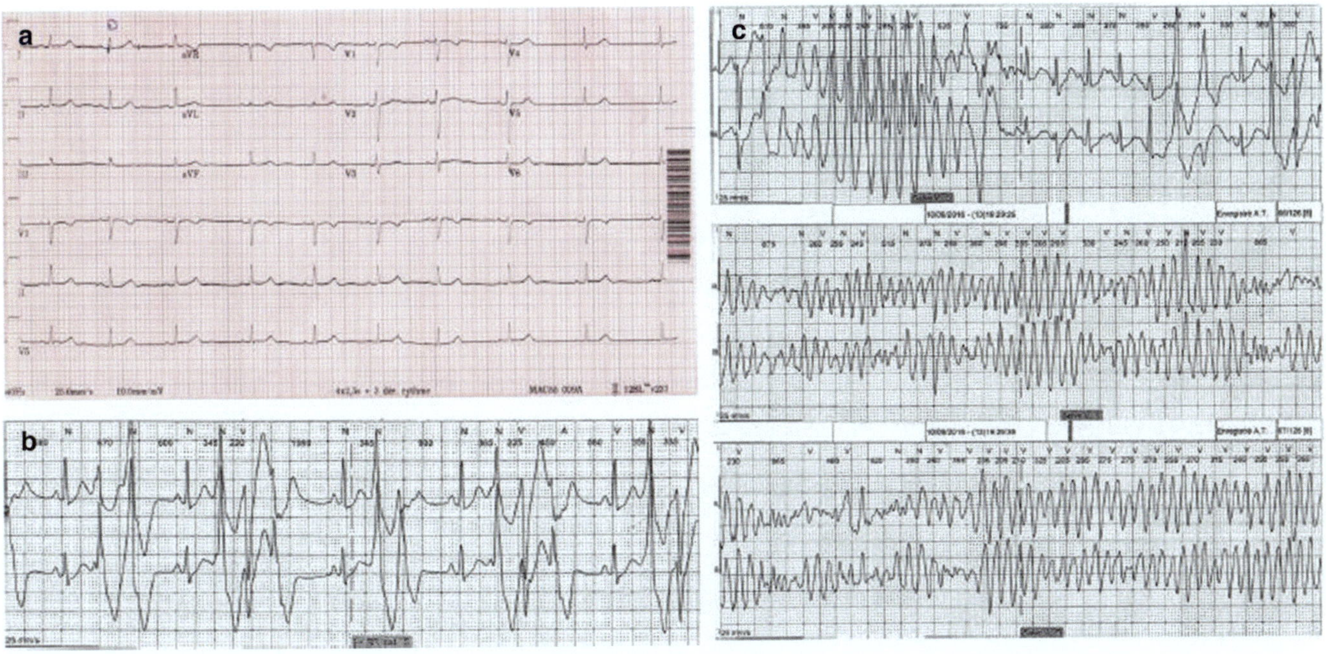

Fig. 15.2 ECG of a 9-year-old girl, referred for syncope while running. Normal ECG at rest (**a**). Bidirectional triplet on the Holter monitoring (**b**) and polymorphic salvoes degenerating into ventricular fibrillation while running (**c**)

adrenaline test, yielding a poor sensitivity of 28%. The specificity of adrenaline infusion was 98%.

Holter monitoring, during which a patient should be encouraged to perform exercise, can be used in selected patients, such as very young or old patients who are unable to undergo exercise testing, but has a lower diagnostic yield as compared with other provocative tests. Holter monitoring may also help to identify supraventricular dysrhythmias (including intermittent ectopic atrial rhythm and tachyarrhythmias), which have been reported in 16–26% of patients with CPVT [2, 14] (Fig. 15.3).

Cardiac imaging is mandatory in every patient suspected of CPVT to rule out structural heart disease. Structural heart disease is, by definition, absent in patients with CPVT. However, mutations in *RYR2* have been linked to fibrofatty myocardial replacement in the right ventricle, mimicking arrhythmogenic cardiomyopathy [27], (left ventricular) non-compaction cardiomyopathy [28] and a complex phenotype including sinoatrial node and atrioventricular node dysfunction, atrial fibrillation, atrial standstill and left ventricular dysfunction and dilatation [29], in addition to the classic CPVT phenotype.

Differential Diagnosis

CPVT manifestation shouldn't be mistaken with epilepsy as described above. The differential diagnosis of CPVT often includes congenital long-QT syndrome, Andersen-Tawil syndrome and concealed structural heart disease.

In patients with a non-diagnostic resting ECG, exercise testing is helpful in distinguishing CPVT and congenital long-QT syndrome. QTc interval prolongation in the recovery phase of the exercise test may unmask congenital long-QT syndrome patients with a normal or borderline QTc interval at rest [30]. The presence of exercise-induced ventricular ectopy beyond isolated VPBs points towards a diagnosis of CPVT [31].

Andersen-Tawil syndrome is characterized by the classic triad of ventricular arrhythmias, periodic paralysis and facial and limb dysmorphism. Mutations in the gene encoding potassium inwardly rectifying channel Kir2.1 (*KCNJ2*) are in approximately 60% of cases. Common cardiac manifestations include mild QTc prolongation, prominent U-waves and ventricular arrhythmias, which include bidirectional or polymorphic ventricular tachycardia. In patients lacking the classic triad of Andersen-Tawil syndrome, the phenotype may very much mimic CPVT. For example, in a series of 24 *KCNJ2* mutation carriers, two individuals (8%) displayed a CPVT phenotype [32]. Genetic testing may distinguish Andersen-Tawil syndrome from CPVT, which is important, because the prognosis in Andersen-Tawil syndrome is more benign.

Initially concealed structural heart disease that may cause exercise-induced ventricular arrhythmias includes arrhythmogenic or hypertrophic cardiomyopathy, mitral valve prolapse or ischemic heart disease. Advanced cardiac imaging and genetic testing may help making a specific diagnosis, although in some cases the underlying condition may reveal only during follow-up.

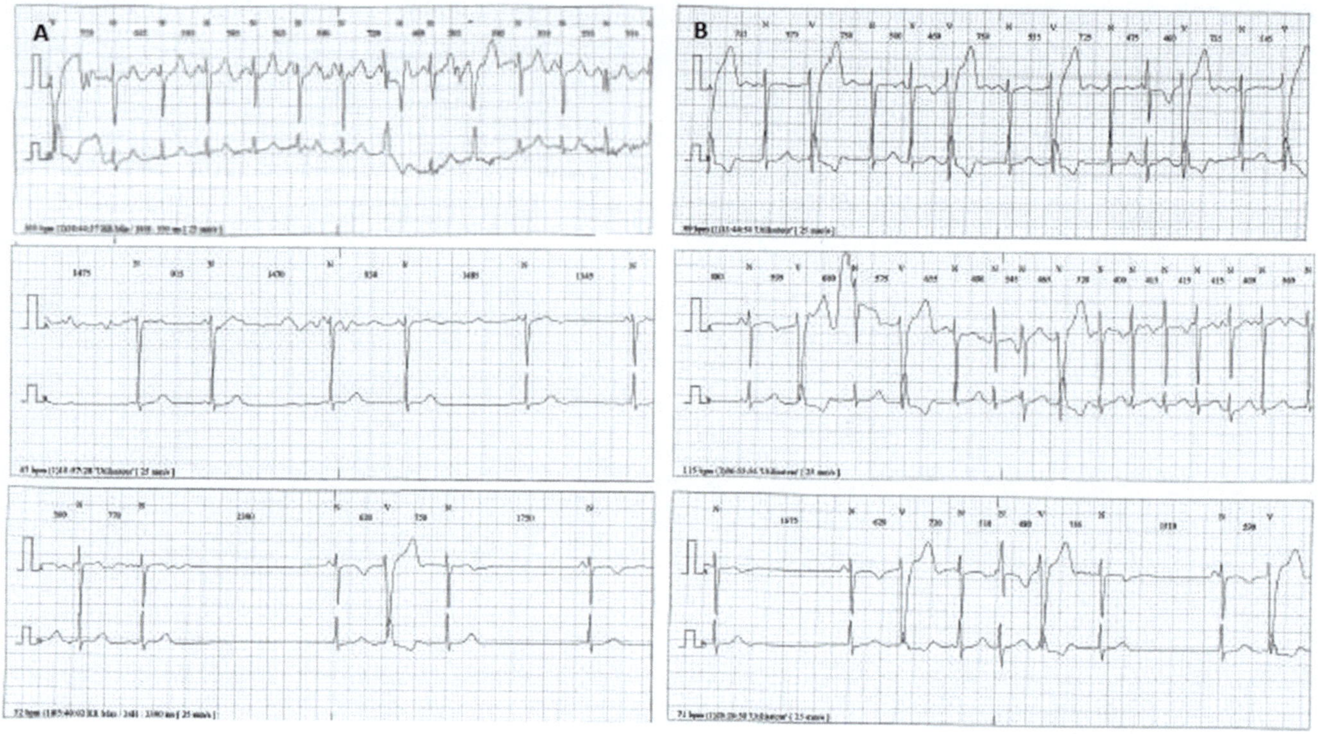

Fig. 15.3 Holter monitoring of a 12-year-old patient treated by nadolol and flecainide for CPVT. Fatigue with beta-blockers. Left panel (**a**) indicates correct beta-blocking during exercise (upper panel) and rest (medium panel), with sinus pause at night (lower panel). Right panel (**b**) shows remaining VPBs (upper panel) and supraventricular arrhythmias (medium and lower panel). Increase dosage of flecainide can be discussed

Molecular Diagnostics

DNA Testing

In CPVT, genetic testing has a diagnostic value. The results of genetic testing may help confirm the diagnosis in patients with a possible clinical diagnosis of CPVT. Current guidelines recommend comprehensive CPVT genetic testing including Ryr2, CASQ2, CALM and TRDN genes in probands with a suspicion for CPVT based on examination of the patient's clinical history, family history and expressed electrocardiographic phenotype during provocative stress testing with cycle, treadmill or catecholamine infusion [33]. In addition, genetic testing may also be considered in cases of adrenergically mediated idiopathic ventricular fibrillation, which may justify genetic testing in such instances [33]. This recommendation is based on several case reports that described patients with idiopathic ventricular fibrillation with no CPVT phenotype in whom *RYR2* mutations were identified [34].

CPVT Genes

Mutation in *RYR2* shows an autosomal dominant inheritance [10] and is identified in approximately 60% of patients with CPVT [35, 36]. RYR2 regulates the release of calcium from the sarcoplasmic reticulum, which initiates cardiac muscle contraction. Today, over 170 unique, mostly missense, mutations in *RYR2* have been identified [37]. Approximately 20% of the *RYR2* mutations are de novo in origin, and in one study, multiple *RYR2* mutations were identified in 5.5% of patients [35]. Mutations in *RYR2* tend to cluster in three hotspots: the N-terminal domain (codons 44–466; ~16% of mutations), the central domain (codons 2246–2534; ~20% of mutations) and the C-terminal channel-forming domain (codons 3778–4959; ~50% of mutations). Several *RYR2* founder mutations have been identified, including the p. G357S mutation in approximately 180 family members from the Canary Islands [38] and the p.R420W mutation in over 60 family members from the Netherlands [39].

In one study, rare missense mutations in *RYR2* were, however, also identified in 3% of control populations [35]. Another study reported a prevalence of previously reported CPVT-associated *RYR2* variants of 6.7% in control subjects, yielding a prevalence of up to 1:150, which is much higher than the estimated prevalence of clinically diagnosed CPVT [37]. It is therefore likely that a proportion of the *RYR2* variants identified is not the major or monogenic cause of CPVT [40]. Therefore, extreme caution needs to be taken before classifying a novel *RYR2* variant as pathogenic, in particular when the variant resides outside of the three regional hotspots, or in case of weak clinical diagnosis.

Mutations in *CASQ2* cause a malignant autosomal recessive inherited form of CPVT [11] and are identified in less than 5% of CPVT index cases. CASQ2 is located within the sarcoplasmic reticulum and also plays an important role in calcium homeostasis. *CASQ2* mutations are typically identified in consanguineous families, but compound heterozygosity in non-consanguineous families has also been observed.

Mutations in the gene encoding triadin (*TRDN*) have been identified in autosomal recessively inherited cases of CPVT [41]. In the first report, three *TRDN* mutations were identified in two out of 97 genotype-negative CPVT probands (2%) [41]. Next, three related children carrying two heterozygous *TRDN* mutations and displaying significant ventricular arrhythmias during isoproterenol infusion testing were reported [42]. A heterozygous missense mutation in *CALM1* (encoding calmodulin) was identified in a large family with a classic CPVT phenotype [43]. Subsequently, another *CALM1* missense mutation was identified in 63 *RYR2* mutation-negative individuals [43]. A mutation in *CALM3* has been associated with CPVT, and both *CALM1* and *CALM3* mutations favour arrhythmogenic Ca disturbances via ryanodine receptor 2 dysregulation [44]. Triadin and calmodulin are also components of the cardiac calcium release complex. Another autosomal recessive form of CPVT was previously mapped to a 25-Mb interval on chromosome 7p14–p22 in a report including four children from an inbred Arabic family [45]. The causal gene, *TECRL*, was recently identified (unpublished data).

CPVT Phenocopies

Patients with mutations in other genes may cause adrenergically mediated ventricular arrhythmias, making these CPVT phenocopies (Table 15.1).

Loss-of-function mutations in the membrane adaptor protein ankyrin-B (*ANK2*) are associated with type 4 congenital long-QT syndrome. However, some patients have exercise-induced ventricular arrhythmias in the absence of QTc interval prolongation [46].

Mutations in *KCNJ2* are generally associated with Andersen-Tawil syndrome but may also cause a CPVT phenocopy including the classic bidirectional VT (see differential diagnosis).

A phenotype with polymorphic ventricular ectopy in carriers of gain-of-function mutations in gene encoding the pore-forming subunit of the cardiac sodium channel Nav 1.5 (*SCN5A*) has been reported [47, 48], including families in which these ventricular arrhythmias were exercise-induced [47].

Table 15.1 Genes associated with CPVT and CPVT phenocopies

Gene	Protein	Prevalence
CPVT		
RYR2	Cardiac ryanodine receptor	60%
CASQ2	Cardiac calsequestrin	<5%
TRDN	Triadin	<1%
CALM1, *CALM3*	Calmodulin	Unknown
TECRL	Trans-2,3-enoyl-CoA reductase-like	Unknown
CPVT phenocopies		
ANK2	Ankyrin-B	Unknown
KCNJ2	Kir 2.1	Unknown
SCN5A	Nav 1.5	Unknown

Therapy (Table 15.2)

β-Blockers

β-Blockers are the mainstay of therapy in CPVT. β-Blockers are recommended in all patients with a clinical diagnosis of CPVT (class I recommendation) and should be considered in genotype-positive-phenotype-negative individuals (class IIa recommendation) [19, 20].

β-Blockers significantly reduce the risk of arrhythmic events, and nadolol seems superior to other β-blockers [12, 49]. β-Blocker should be titrated to the highest tolerable dose. In a meta-analysis on the efficacy of β-blockers including 11 CPVT patient series, the estimated overall 4- and 8-year arrhythmic event rates were 18.0% (95% confidence interval (CI): 7.7–28.9) and 35.9% (95% CI: 15.3–56.5), respectively [50]. Four- and 8-year fatal or near-fatal arrhythmic event rates were 7.2% (95% CI: 3.1–11.3%) and 14.3% (95% CI: 6.1–22.5), respectively.

In a recent large series of 211 children with CPVT, arrhythmic events occurred in 25% of patients on β-blockers [13]. However, nonoptimal dosing and poor adherence contributed to 40% and 48% of all events, respectively. Among 98 *RYR2* mutation-carrying relatives, only two asymptomatic relatives experienced exercise-induced syncope during a median follow-up of 4.7 years (range: 0.3–19 years), while no other arrhythmic events occurred [39].

Thus, β-blocker therapy seems sufficiently protective in the majority of CPVT patients, in particular relatives who are identified through cascade screening and display a mild phenotype. The presence of side effects (reported in approximately a quarter of CPVT patients) [39] should be seriously addressed, as these may hamper medication adherence.

Calcium Channel Blockers

Verapamil along with beta-blockers seems to reduce exercise-induced ventricular arrhythmia in small series [12, 51, 52] especially in CPVT2 patient as demonstrated in mice model

Table 15.2 Therapy

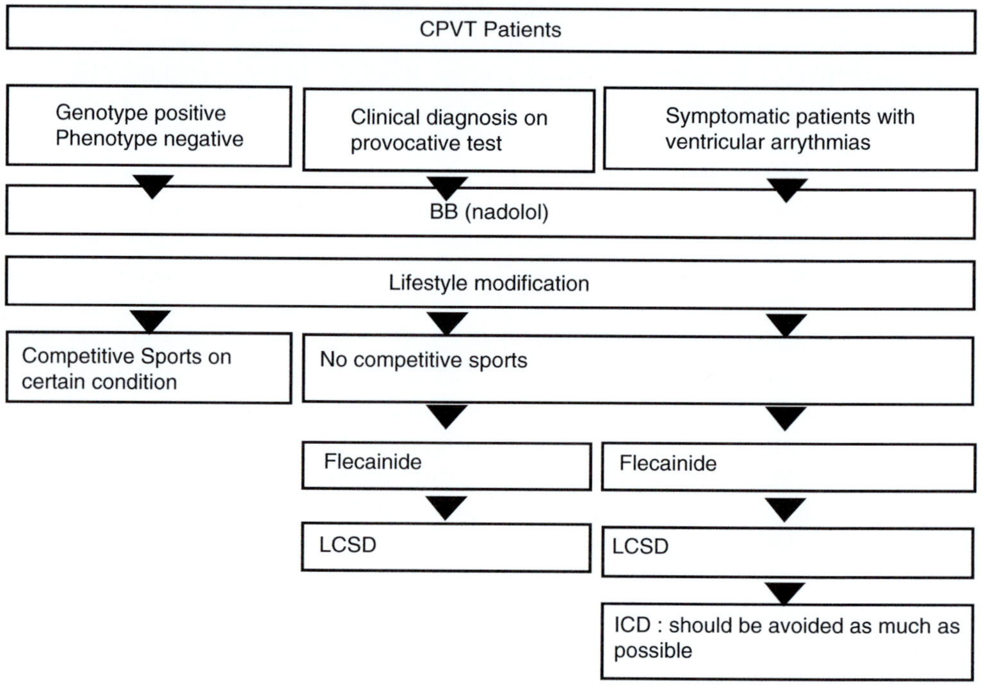

[53]. This drug is not included in the current therapeutic recommendations.

Sodium Channel Blockers

Flecainide (2–3 mg per kg per day) in addition to β-blockers is recommended in patients who experience an arrhythmic event while on β-blockers (class IIa recommendation) [12, 49]. In addition, flecainide should be considered in addition to β-blockers and carriers of an implantable cardioverter-defibrillator (ICD) to reduce the risk of appropriate ICD shocks (class IIa recommendation) [20]. Adding flecainide is effective when patients display couplets or non-sustained ventricular tachycardia during exercise testing while on β-blockers [54].

Flecainide has a possible direct RYR2 blocking effect in a CPVT mouse model [55], although this has been disputed by others [56]. The efficacy of flecainide was shown in a study including 33 severely affected patients, in whom flecainide (1.5–4.5 mg per kg body weight) partially or completely suppressed exercise-induced ventricular arrhythmias in 76% of patients [57]. Arrhythmic events were prevented during a median follow-up of 20 months (range: 12–40), except for one patient who received appropriate ICD shocks after non-adherence. A similar efficacy of flecainide was observed in a series of 12 patients with genotype-negative CPVT [58] and 10 insufficiently controlled CPVT patients carrying *CASQ2* mutations [59]. In 51 children treated with flecainide, eight (16%) experienced an arrhythmic event. However, seven events occurred on a suboptimal dose, and six were probably related to non-adherence. A small case series reported favourable ventricular arrhythmia-suppressing effects of flecainide monotherapy [60], but at present, this is only recommended in patients who are intolerant to β-blocker therapy.

Left Cardiac Sympathetic Denervation

Left cardiac sympathetic denervation (LCSD), usually by use of video-assisted thoracoscopic surgery, may be considered when ventricular arrhythmias cannot be controlled by medication (class IIb recommendation) [12, 49]. During LCSD, the lower half of the left stellate ganglion and thoracic ganglia T2–T4 are removed, thereby inhibiting and largely preventing norepinephrine release in the heart. In the largest series on LCSD in CPVT, the 2-year cumulative event-free survival rate in 63 severely symptomatic patients who underwent LCSD was 81% [61]. Patients with an incomplete LCSD were more likely to experience major arrhythmic events. Quality of life of CPVT patients who underwent LCSD was well, despite minor side effects that were reported by the majority of patients [62, 63].

Lifestyle

All patients with CPVT are advised to limit or avoid competitive sports, strenuous exercise and exposure to stressful environments (class I recommendation) [19, 20]. However, very recent recommendations state that genotype-positive-phenotype-negative athletes may participate in all competitive sports with appropriate precautionary measures, including acquisition of a personal automatic external defibrillator and establishment of an emergency action plan [64].

Importantly, patients should thoroughly be educated about the importance of medication adherence since most of ventricular arrhythmias are secondary to lack of compliance [65, 66].

Risk Stratification

Current guidelines recommend β-blocker therapy in all patients diagnosed with CPVT, including mutation carriers with no ventricular arrhythmias during provocative tests [14, 15]. This is because very little clinical and genetic risk factors for the occurrence of arrhythmic events in CPVT have been identified. In one large CPVT series, a young age at diagnosis and a history of aborted cardiac arrest were associated with future arrhythmic events [8]. Among asymptomatic *RYR2* or *CASQ2* mutation-carrying relatives who are identified by cascade screening, the presence of exercise-induced ventricular arrhythmias seems to increase the risk of arrhythmic events [25]. In one series, relatives with an RYR2 mutation in the C-terminal channel-forming domain had an increased odds of non-sustained ventricular tachycardia compared with those carrying an RYR2 N-terminal mutation [12], but whether this translates into an increased risk of arrhythmic events is unknown. In summary, studies including larger patient populations and longer follow-up durations are needed to develop a more detailed risk stratification model.

Implantable Cardioverter-Defibrillator Indications

ICD implantation is indicated in patients who experienced an aborted cardiac arrest on treatment and in patients with arrhythmic events or polymorphic or bidirectional ventricular tachycardia despite optimal medical therapy (class 1 recommendation) [19, 20].

Two early case reports pointed towards the possible pro-arrhythmic effect of ICD therapy in CPVT by describing patients in whom appropriate or inappropriate ICD shocks and its subsequent catecholamine release initiated fatal ventricular arrhythmia storms [67, 68]. Two recent studies demonstrated that ICD shocks delivered to terminate ventricular tachycardia were often unsuccessful, whereas ventricular fibrillation was frequently terminated [66, 69]. In addition, one study reported induction of more malignant ventricular arrhythmias by ICD therapy in 36% of patients, including electrical storm in 29%, and 8.5% of total shocks [69]. In 94 children with CPVT, appropriate and inappropriate shocks occurred in 46% and 22% of cases, respectively [13]. Electrical storm occurred in 18% and ICD-related complications in 23%. In a meta-analysis on ICD harm in young patients with inherited cardiac diseases, CPVT patients had the highest annual rate of inappropriate shocks (7.6%) and other ICD-related complications (21.2%) [70].

Thus, among patients who did not have an aborted cardiac arrest, ICD implantation should in our opinion be restricted to CPVT patients who do not sufficiently respond to an aggressive therapeutic strategy including β-blockers, flecainide and LCSD. Even in patients with an aborted cardiac arrest, ICD should be avoided as much as possible [71]. If an ICD is implanted, additional therapy with β-blockers, flecainide and sometimes LCSD should be considered to lower the risk of appropriate and inappropriate ICD shocks. Careful ICD programming, i.e. with one ventricular fibrillation zone with a detection interval of 240 beats per minute and (exceptionally) long detection intervals, is crucial.

Recommendations During Pregnancy and Delivery

Unlike other channelopathy (i.e. congenital long-QT syndrome), there is no data showing an increased risk during pregnancy [72–75]. A very recent study among 96 CPVT patients who had 228 pregnancies showed that the pregnancy and postpartum arrhythmic risk was not elevated compared with the nonpregnant period [75]. All patients with events were not taking beta-blockers at the time of the event. In patients under treatment, medication should not be withdrawn as long as potential benefit outweighs potential risk. Beta-blockers can be responsible for foetal bradycardia and hypoglycaemia but also low birth weight. We recommend to continue nadolol or metoprolol treatment during pregnancy. Human data are not available regarding flecainide.

Family Screening

When a (likely) pathogenic mutation is identified in an index patient with CPVT, genetic testing of all first-degree relatives is indicated (Fig. 15.4) [33]. Genetic testing is recommended at a young age, usually after age 2 years, because of the young age of CPVT manifestation [33]. Among *RYR2* mutation-carrying relatives identified by cascade screening, approximately 50% have exercise-induced ventricular arrhythmias [39]. Relatives who are noncarrier of the familial CPVT-causing mutation can be dismissed from further cardiologic evaluation after initial negative clinical investigation.

Fig. 15.4 Family screening in CPVT

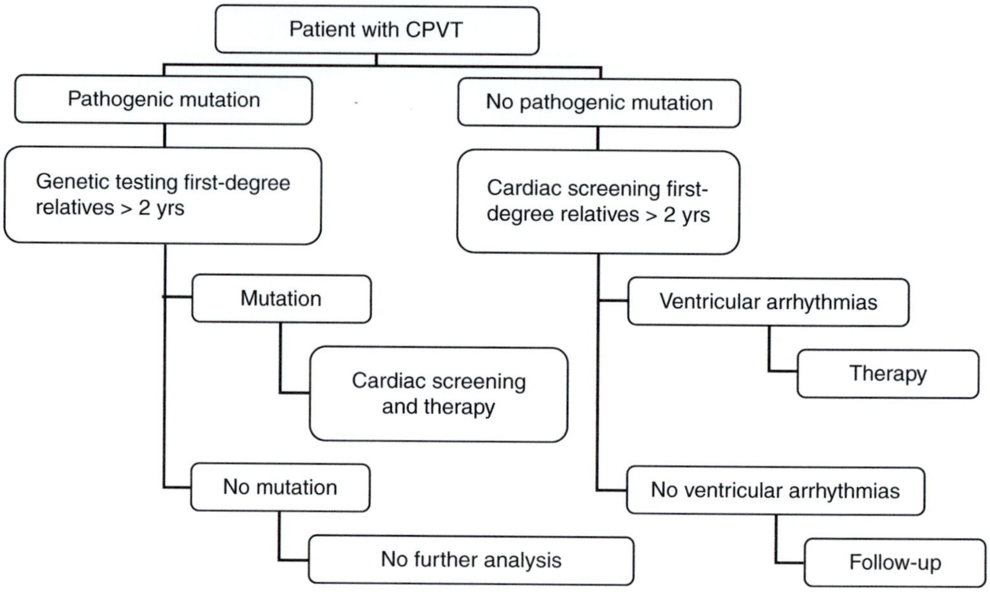

First-degree relatives of a mutation-negative index patient should be screened clinically, starting at age 2 years, in particular with exercise testing, Holter recording or pharmacological challenge (Fig. 15.2). Children and young adults should be followed up regularly, even if the initial clinical screening is normal.

Summary

- CPVT is a rare yet severe inherited arrhythmia syndrome characterized by polymorphic ventricular tachyarrhythmias during exercise or emotion.
- CPVT must be considered in anyone with adrenergically mediated ventricular arrhythmias or cardiac symptoms, such as stress- or emotion-induced syncope or cardiac arrest, or a positive family history for such events.
- CPVT is caused by mutations in genes involved in intracellular calcium cycling, in particular the cardiac ryanodine receptor (*RYR2*) in the majority of cases.
- β-Blockers and lifestyle advices are the cornerstone of therapy, whereas flecainide, LCSD and ICD implantation may be indicated in severely affected patients.

Take-Home Messages

- Stress test ± pharmacological challenge should be performed in stress-induced syncope or unexplained resuscitated sudden cardiac arrest in the young with a normal baseline ECG.
- Cascade family screening is mandatory.

References

1. Leenhardt A, Denjoy I, Guicheney P. Catecholaminergic polymorphic ventricular tachycardia. Circ Arrhythm Electrophysiol. 2012 Oct;5(5):1044–52.
2. van der Werf C, Nederend I, Hofman N, van Geloven N, Ebink C, Frohn-Mulder IME, et al. Familial evaluation in catecholaminergic polymorphic ventricular tachycardia: disease penetrance and expression in cardiac ryanodine receptor mutation-carrying relatives. Circ Arrhythm Electrophysiol. 2012 Aug 1;5(4):748–56.
3. Liu N, Ruan Y, Priori SG. Catecholaminergic polymorphic ventricular tachycardia. Prog Cardiovasc Dis. 2008 Aug;51(1):23–30.
4. Wilders R. Cardiac ion channelopathies and the sudden infant death syndrome. ISRN Cardiol. 2012;2012:846171.
5. Tester DJ, Medeiros-Domingo A, Will ML, Haglund CM, Ackerman MJ. Cardiac channel molecular autopsy: insights from 173 consecutive cases of autopsy-negative sudden unexplained death referred for postmortem genetic testing. Mayo Clin Proc. 2012 Jun;87(6):524–39.
6. Berg K. Multifocal ventricular extrasystoles with Adams-stokes syndrome in children. Am Heart J. 1960;60(6):965–70.
7. Reid DS, Tynan M, Braidwood L, Fitzgerald GR. Bidirectional tachycardia in a child. A study using his bundle electrography. Br Heart J. 1975 Mar;37(3):339–44.
8. Coumel P, Fidelle J, Lucet V, Attuel P, Bouvrain Y. Catecholamine-induced severe ventricular arrhythmias with Adam-Stokes in children: report of four cases. Br Heart J. 1978;40(Supplement):28–37.
9. Leenhardt A, Lucet V, Denjoy I, Grau F, Ngoc DD, Coumel P. Catecholaminergic polymorphic ventricular tachycardia in children. A 7-year follow-up of 21 patients. Circulation. 1995 Mar 1;91(5):1512–9.
10. Priori SG, Napolitano C, Tiso N, Memmi M, Vignati G, Bloise R, et al. Mutations in the cardiac ryanodine receptor gene (hRyR2) underlie catecholaminergic polymorphic ventricular tachycardia. Circulation. 2001 Jan 16;103(2):196–200.
11. Lahat H, Pras E, Olender T, Avidan N, Ben-Asher E, Man O, et al. A missense mutation in a highly conserved region of CASQ2 is associated with autosomal recessive catecholamine-induced

polymorphic ventricular tachycardia in Bedouin families from Israel. Am J Hum Genet. 2001 Dec;69(6):1378–84.
12. Hayashi M, Denjoy I, Extramiana F, Maltret A, Buisson NR, Lupoglazoff J-M, et al. Incidence and risk factors of arrhythmic events in catecholaminergic polymorphic ventricular tachycardia. Circulation. 2009 May 12;119(18):2426–34.
13. Roston TM, Vinocur JM, Maginot KR, Mohammed S, Salerno JC, Etheridge SP, et al. Catecholaminergic polymorphic ventricular tachycardia in children: an analysis of therapeutic strategies and outcomes from an international multicenter registry. Circ Arrhythm Electrophysiol. 2015 Feb 24;8:633–42.
14. Sy RW, Gollob MH, Klein GJ, Yee R, Skanes AC, Gula LJ, et al. Arrhythmia characterization and long-term outcomes in catecholaminergic polymorphic ventricular tachycardia. Heart Rhythm. 2011 Jun;8(6):864–71.
15. Sumitomo N. Are there juvenile and adult types in patients with catecholaminergic polymorphic ventricular tachycardia? Heart Rhythm. 2011 Jun;8(6):872–3.
16. Priori SG, Napolitano C, Memmi M, Colombi B, Drago F, Gasparini M, et al. Clinical and molecular characterization of patients with catecholaminergic polymorphic ventricular tachycardia. Circulation. 2002 Jul 2;106(1):69–74.
17. Kozlovski J, Ingles J, Connell V, Hunt L, McGaughran J, Turner C, et al. Delay to diagnosis amongst patients with catecholaminergic polymorphic ventricular tachycardia. Int J Cardiol. 2014 Oct 20;176(3):1402–4.
18. Hazle MA, Shellhaas RA, Bradley DJ, Dick M, Lapage MJ. Arrhythmogenic channelopathy syndromes presenting as refractory epilepsy. Pediatr Neurol. 2013 Aug;49(2):134–7.
19. Priori SG, Wilde AA, Horie M, Cho Y, Behr ER, Berul C, et al. HRS/EHRA/APHRS expert consensus statement on the diagnosis and management of patients with inherited primary arrhythmia syndromes. Heart Rhythm. 2013 Dec;10(12):1932–63.
20. Authors/Task Force Members, Priori SG, Blomström-Lundqvist C, Mazzanti A, Blom N, Borggrefe M, et al. 2015 ESC Guidelines for the management of patients with ventricular arrhythmias and the prevention of sudden cardiac death: the task force for the management of patients with ventricular arrhythmias and the prevention of sudden cardiac death of the European Society of Cardiology (ESC) Endorsed By: Association For European Paediatric and Congenital Cardiology (AEPC). Eur Heart J. 2015 Aug 29;36(41):2793–867.
21. van der Werf C, Wilde AAM. Catecholaminergic polymorphic ventricular tachycardia: from bench to bedside. Heart Br Card Soc. 2013 Apr;99(7):497–504.
22. Lawrenz W, Krogmann ON, Wieczorek M. Complex atrial arrhythmias as first manifestation of catecholaminergic polymorphic ventricular tachycardia: an unusual course in a patient with a new mutation in ryanodine receptor type 2 gene. Cardiol Young. 2014 Aug;24(4):741–4.
23. Faggioni M, van der Werf C, Knollmann BC. Sinus node dysfunction in catecholaminergic polymorphic ventricular tachycardia: risk factor and potential therapeutic target? Trends Cardiovasc Med. 2014 Oct;24(7):273–8.
24. Blich M, Marai I, Suleiman M, Lorber A, Gepstein L, Boulous M, et al. Electrocardiographic comparison of ventricular premature complexes during exercise test in patients with CPVT and healthy subjects. Pacing Clin Electrophysiol. 2015 Mar;38(3):398–402.
25. Faggioni M, Hwang HS, van der Werf C, Nederend I, Kannankeril PJ, Wilde AAM, et al. Accelerated sinus rhythm prevents catecholaminergic polymorphic ventricular tachycardia in mice and in patients. Circ Res. 2013 Feb 15;112(4):689–97.
26. Marjamaa A, Hiippala A, Arrhenius B, Lahtinen AM, Kontula K, Toivonen L, et al. Intravenous epinephrine infusion test in diagnosis of catecholaminergic polymorphic ventricular tachycardia. J Cardiovasc Electrophysiol. 2012 Feb;23(2):194–9.
27. Tiso N, Stephan DA, Nava A, Bagattin A, Devaney JM, Stanchi F, et al. Identification of mutations in the cardiac ryanodine receptor gene in families affected with arrhythmogenic right ventricular cardiomyopathy type 2 (ARVD2). Hum Mol Genet. 2001 Feb 1;10(3):189–94.
28. Ohno S, Omura M, Kawamura M, Kimura H, Itoh H, Makiyama T, et al. Exon 3 deletion of RYR2 encoding cardiac ryanodine receptor is associated with left ventricular non-compaction. Europace. 2014 Nov;16(11):1646–54.
29. Bhuiyan ZA, van den Berg MP, van Tintelen JP, Bink-Boelkens MTE, Wiesfeld ACP, Alders M, et al. Expanding spectrum of human RYR2-related disease: new electrocardiographic, structural, and genetic features. Circulation. 2007 Oct 2;116(14):1569–76.
30. Sy RW, van der Werf C, Chattha IS, Chockalingam P, Adler A, Healey JS, et al. Derivation and validation of a simple exercise-based algorithm for prediction of genetic testing in relatives of LQTS probands. Circulation. 2011 Nov 15;124(20):2187–94.
31. Horner JM, Ackerman MJ. Ventricular ectopy during treadmill exercise stress testing in the evaluation of long QT syndrome. Heart Rhythm. 2008 Dec;5(12):1690–4.
32. Kimura H, Zhou J, Kawamura M, Itoh H, Mizusawa Y, Ding W-G, et al. Phenotype variability in patients carrying KCNJ2 mutations. Circ Cardiovasc Genet. 2012 Jun;5(3):344–53.
33. Ackerman MJ, Priori SG, Willems S, Berul C, Brugada R, Calkins H, et al. HRS/EHRA expert consensus statement on the state of genetic testing for the channelopathies and cardiomyopathies this document was developed as a partnership between the Heart Rhythm Society (HRS) and the European heart rhythm association (EHRA). Heart Rhythm. 2011 Aug;8(8):1308–39.
34. Paech C, Gebauer RA, Karstedt J, Marschall C, Bollmann A, Husser D. Ryanodine receptor mutations presenting as idiopathic ventricular fibrillation: a report on two novel familial compound mutations, c.6224T>C and c.13781A>G, with the clinical presentation of idiopathic ventricular fibrillation. Pediatr Cardiol. 2014 Dec;35(8):1437–41.
35. Medeiros-Domingo A, Bhuiyan ZA, Tester DJ, Hofman N, Bikker H, van Tintelen JP, et al. The RYR2-encoded ryanodine receptor/calcium release channel in patients diagnosed previously with either catecholaminergic polymorphic ventricular tachycardia or genotype negative, exercise-induced long QT syndrome: a comprehensive open reading frame mutational analysis. J Am Coll Cardiol. 2009 Nov 24;54(22):2065–74.
36. Bai R, Napolitano C, Bloise R, Monteforte N, Priori SG. Yield of genetic screening in inherited cardiac channelopathies: how to prioritize access to genetic testing. Circ Arrhythm Electrophysiol. 2009 Feb;2(1):6–15.
37. Jabbari J, Jabbari R, Nielsen MW, Holst AG, Nielsen JB, Haunsø S, et al. New exome data question the pathogenicity of genetic variants previously associated with catecholaminergic polymorphic ventricular tachycardia. Circ Cardiovasc Genet. 2013 Oct;6(5):481–9.
38. Wangüemert F, Bosch Calero C, Pérez C, Campuzano O, Beltran-Alvarez P, Scornik FS, et al. Clinical and molecular characterization of a cardiac ryanodine receptor founder mutation causing catecholaminergic polymorphic ventricular tachycardia. Heart Rhythm. 2015 Jul;12(7):1636–43.
39. van der Werf C, Nederend I, Hofman N, van Geloven N, Ebink C, Frohn-Mulder IME, et al. Familial evaluation in catecholaminergic polymorphic ventricular tachycardia: disease penetrance and expression in cardiac ryanodine receptor mutation-carrying relatives. Circ Arrhythm Electrophysiol. 2012 Aug 1;5(4):748–56.
40. Kapplinger JD, Pundi KN, Larson NB, Callis TE, Tester DJ, Bikker H, et al. Yield of the RYR2 genetic test in suspected Catecholaminergic polymorphic ventricular tachycardia and implications for test interpretation. Circ Genomic Precis Med. 2018 Feb;11(2):e001424.

41. Roux-Buisson N, Cacheux M, Fourest-Lieuvin A, Fauconnier J, Brocard J, Denjoy I, et al. Absence of triadin, a protein of the calcium release complex, is responsible for cardiac arrhythmia with sudden death in human. Hum Mol Genet. 2012 Jun 15;21(12):2759–67.
42. Rooryck C, Kyndt F, Bozon D, Roux-Buisson N, Sacher F, Probst V, et al. New family with Catecholaminergic polymorphic ventricular tachycardia linked to the Triadin gene. J Cardiovasc Electrophysiol. 2015 Oct;26(10):1146–50.
43. Nyegaard M, Overgaard MT, Søndergaard MT, Vranas M, Behr ER, Hildebrandt LL, et al. Mutations in calmodulin cause ventricular tachycardia and sudden cardiac death. Am J Hum Genet. 2012 Oct 5;91(4):703–12.
44. Gomez-Hurtado N, Boczek NJ, Kryshtal DO, Johnson CN, Sun J, Nitu FR, et al. Novel CPVT-Associated Calmodulin Mutation in CALM3 (CALM3-A103V) Activates Arrhythmogenic Ca Waves and Sparks. Circ Arrhythm Electrophysiol. 2016;9(8):e004161.
45. Bhuiyan ZA, Hamdan MA, Shamsi ETA, Postma AV, Mannens MMAM, Wilde AAM, et al. A novel early onset lethal form of catecholaminergic polymorphic ventricular tachycardia maps to chromosome 7p14-p22. J Cardiovasc Electrophysiol. 2007 Sep;18(10):1060–6.
46. Mohler PJ, Splawski I, Napolitano C, Bottelli G, Sharpe L, Timothy K, et al. A cardiac arrhythmia syndrome caused by loss of ankyrin-B function. Proc Natl Acad Sci U S A. 2004 Jun 15;101(24):9137–42.
47. Swan H, Amarouch MY, Leinonen J, Marjamaa A, Kucera JP, Laitinen-Forsblom PJ, et al. Gain-of-function mutation of the SCN5A gene causes exercise-induced polymorphic ventricular arrhythmias. Circ Cardiovasc Genet. 2014 Dec;7(6):771–81.
48. Laurent G, Saal S, Amarouch MY, Béziau DM, Marsman RFJ, Faivre L, et al. Multifocal ectopic Purkinje-related premature contractions: a new SCN5A-related cardiac channelopathy. J Am Coll Cardiol. 2012 Jul 10;60(2):144–56.
49. Leren IS, Saberniak J, Majid E, Haland TF, Edvardsen T, Haugaa KH. Nadolol decreases the incidence and severity of ventricular arrhythmias during exercise stress testing compared with β1-selective β-blockers in patients with catecholaminergic polymorphic ventricular tachycardia. Heart Rhythm. 2015 Sep 30;13(2):433–40.
50. van der Werf C, Zwinderman AH, Wilde AAM. Therapeutic approach for patients with catecholaminergic polymorphic ventricular tachycardia: state of the art and future developments. Europace. 2012 Feb;14(2):175–83.
51. Swan H, Laitinen P, Kontula K, Toivonen L. Calcium channel antagonism reduces exercise-induced ventricular arrhythmias in catecholaminergic polymorphic ventricular tachycardia patients with RyR2 mutations. J Cardiovasc Electrophysiol. 2005 Feb;16(2):162–6.
52. Rosso R, Kalman JM, Rogowski O, Diamant S, Birger A, Biner S, et al. Calcium channel blockers and beta-blockers versus beta-blockers alone for preventing exercise-induced arrhythmias in catecholaminergic polymorphic ventricular tachycardia. Heart Rhythm. 2007 Sep;4(9):1149–54.
53. Katz G, Khoury A, Kurtzwald E, Hochhauser E, Porat E, Shainberg A, et al. Optimizing catecholaminergic polymorphic ventricular tachycardia therapy in calsequestrin-mutant mice. Heart Rhythm. 2010 Nov;7(11):1676–82.
54. Kannankeril PJ, Moore JP, Cerrone M, Priori SG, Kertesz NJ, Ro PS, et al. Efficacy of flecainide in the treatment of Catecholaminergic polymorphic ventricular tachycardia: a randomized clinical trial. JAMA Cardiol. 2017 Jul 1;2(7):759–66.
55. Watanabe H, Chopra N, Laver D, Hwang HS, Davies SS, Roach DE, et al. Flecainide prevents catecholaminergic polymorphic ventricular tachycardia in mice and humans. Nat Med. 2009 Apr;15(4):380–3.
56. Bannister ML, Thomas NL, Sikkel MB, Mukherjee S, Maxwell C, MacLeod KT, et al. The mechanism of flecainide action in CPVT does not involve a direct effect on RyR2. Circ Res. 2015 Apr 10;116(8):1324–35.
57. van der Werf C, Kannankeril PJ, Sacher F, Krahn AD, Viskin S, Leenhardt A, et al. Flecainide therapy reduces exercise-induced ventricular arrhythmias in patients with catecholaminergic polymorphic ventricular tachycardia. J Am Coll Cardiol. 2011 May 31;57(22):2244–54.
58. Watanabe H, van der Werf C, Roses-Noguer F, Adler A, Sumitomo N, Veltmann C, et al. Effects of flecainide on exercise-induced ventricular arrhythmias and recurrences in genotype-negative patients with catecholaminergic polymorphic ventricular tachycardia. Heart Rhythm. 2013 Apr;10(4):542–7.
59. Khoury A, Marai I, Suleiman M, Blich M, Lorber A, Gepstein L, et al. Flecainide therapy suppresses exercise-induced ventricular arrhythmias in patients with CASQ2-associated catecholaminergic polymorphic ventricular tachycardia. Heart Rhythm. 2013 Nov;10(11):1671–5.
60. Padfield GJ, AlAhmari L, Lieve KVV, AlAhmari T, Roston TM, Wilde AA, et al. Flecainide monotherapy is an option for selected patients with catecholaminergic polymorphic ventricular tachycardia intolerant of β-blockade. Heart Rhythm. 2015 Sep 28;13(2):609–13.
61. De Ferrari GM, Dusi V, Spazzolini C, Bos JM, Abrams DJ, Berul CI, et al. Clinical Management of Catecholaminergic Polymorphic Ventricular Tachycardia: the role of left cardiac sympathetic denervation. Circulation. 2015 Jun 23;131(25):2185–93.
62. Waddell-Smith KE, Ertresvaag KN, Li J, Chaudhuri K, Crawford JR, Hamill JK, et al. Physical and psychological consequences of left cardiac sympathetic denervation in long-QT syndrome and Catecholaminergic polymorphic ventricular tachycardia. Circ Arrhythm Electrophysiol. 2015 Oct;8(5):1151–8.
63. Antiel RM, Bos JM, Joyce DD, Owen HJ, Roskos PL, Moir C, et al. Quality of life after videoscopic left cardiac sympathetic denervation in patients with potentially life-threatening cardiac channelopathies/cardiomyopathies. Heart Rhythm. 2015 Sep 1;13(1):62–9.
64. Ackerman MJ, Zipes DP, Kovacs RJ, Maron BJ. Eligibility and disqualification recommendations for competitive athletes with cardiovascular abnormalities: task force 10: the cardiac Channelopathies: a scientific statement from the American Heart Association and American College of Cardiology. J Am Coll Cardiol. 2015 Oct 27;132(22):e326–9.
65. van der Werf C, Zwinderman AH, Wilde AAM. Therapeutic approach for patients with catecholaminergic polymorphic ventricular tachycardia: state of the art and future developments. Eur Pacing Arrhythm Card Electrophysiol J Work Groups Card Pacing Arrhythm Card Cell Electrophysiol Eur Soc Cardiol. 2012 Feb;14(2):175–83.
66. Miyake CY, Webster G, Czosek RJ, Kantoch MJ, Dubin AM, Avasarala K, et al. Efficacy of implantable cardioverter defibrillators in young patients with catecholaminergic polymorphic ventricular tachycardia: success depends on substrate. Circ Arrhythm Electrophysiol. 2013 Jun;6(3):579–87.
67. Pizzale S, Gollob MH, Gow R, Birnie DH. Sudden death in a young man with catecholaminergic polymorphic ventricular tachycardia and paroxysmal atrial fibrillation. J Cardiovasc Electrophysiol. 2008 Dec;19(12):1319–21.
68. Mohamed U, Gollob MH, Gow RM, Krahn AD. Sudden cardiac death despite an implantable cardioverter-defibrillator in a young female with catecholaminergic ventricular tachycardia. Heart Rhythm. 2006 Dec;3(12):1486–9.
69. Roses-Noguer F, Jarman JWE, Clague JR, Till J. Outcomes of defibrillator therapy in catecholaminergic polymorphic ventricular tachycardia. Heart Rhythm. 2014 Jan;11(1):58–66.
70. Olde Nordkamp LRA, Postema PG, Knops RE, van Dijk N, Limpens J, Wilde AAM, et al. Implantable cardioverter-defibrillator

harm in young patients with inherited arrhythmia syndromes: a systematic review and meta-analysis of inappropriate shocks and complications. Heart Rhythm. 2015 Sep 15;13(2):443–54.

71. Christian van der Werf, Krystien V Lieve, J Martijn Bos, Conor M Lane, Isabelle Denjoy, Ferran Roses-Noguer, et al. (2019) Implantable cardioverter-defibrillators in previously undiagnosed patients with catecholaminergic polymorphic ventricular tachycardia resuscitated from sudden cardiac arrest. European Heart Journal 40 (35):2953–61.
72. Silversides CK, Harris L, Haberer K, Sermer M, Colman JM, Siu SC. Recurrence rates of arrhythmias during pregnancy in women with previous tachyarrhythmia and impact on fetal and neonatal outcomes. Am J Cardiol. 2006 Apr 15;97(8):1206–12.
73. Ekholm EM, Piha SJ, Erkkola RU, Antila KJ. Autonomic cardiovascular reflexes in pregnancy. A longitudinal study. Clin Auton Res Off J Clin Auton Res Soc. 1994 Aug;4(4):161–5.
74. Page RL. Treatment of arrhythmias during pregnancy. Am Heart J. 1995 Oct;130(4):871–6.
75. Cheung CC, Lieve KV, Roston TM, van der Ree MH, Deyell MW, Andrade JG, et al. Pregnancy in catecholaminergic polymorphic ventricular tachycardia. JACC Clin Electrophysiol. 2019 Mar;5(3):387–94.

Idiopathic Ventricular Fibrillation and Early Repolarization Syndrome

16

Tetsuo Sasano and Masayasu Hiraoka

Idiopathic Ventricular Fibrillation

Idiopathic ventricular fibrillation (IVF) is a rare condition in which patients without any major structural heart disease develop VF and often suffer from sudden cardiac death (SCD). While sporadic case reports of VF developing in patients without any pathological condition of the heart have been presented in the literature, collected case studies termed under IVF have appeared as several publications from the late 1980s to early 1990s [1–3]. Several conditions, which are now included in primary electrical diseases developing into VF without any major cardiac structural abnormalities, are generally excluded from IVF as they are a different disease entity due to unique clinical manifestations and special pathogenetic mechanisms. Further, IVF may not be composed of a single entity but may contain multiple forms by clinical manifestations and a possible pathogenetic background.

In this chapter, IVF is described as two groups: (A) early repolarization syndrome (ERS) and (B) IVF, in a narrow sense excluding ERS. An early repolarization (ER) pattern in the ECG is indicated by an elevation of the QRS-ST-segment junction (J-point) and a notch and slur of the terminal portion of the QRS complex. IVF, excluding ERS, does not exhibit an ER pattern on the ECG and can develop into VF events. The clinical presentation in both groups of IVF develops as a sudden onset of VF and/or aborted SCD in subjects without structural heart disease or any known conditions to cause fatal arrhythmic events. In some cases, there is a family history of an ECG sign of an ER pattern and/or SCD. A diagnosis of ERS can be achieved in patients after resuscitation from VF/aborted SCD with the exclusion of any structural heart disease or other reason for fatal arrhythmic events. The ECG during sinus rhythm exhibits an ER pattern in the inferior and/or lateral leads. Prevention of SCD by anti-arrhythmic drugs is not sufficiently achieved, and an ICD implantation is the only available therapy for the prevention of SCD. The mechanism of ERS is assumed to be explained by a repolarization theory based on experimental studies, but the clinical and genetic proof of this concept has not been fully clarified. Other types of IVF include several different types of clinical manifestations, and their diagnostic criteria as well as their mechanisms are mostly unknown. Some forms of IVF have a familial inheritance, and a genetic background has been identified as a possible pathogenic cause in limited cases.

Early Repolarization Syndrome (ERS)

Introduction

Early repolarization syndrome is a type of IVF in which patients with an ER pattern on the ECG develop sudden attacks of VF in the absence of any structural heart disease and without any known causes of fatal arrhythmias. An ER pattern on the ECG has been considered for a long time to be a benign ECG sign except for "Osborn waves" due to hypothermia [4, 5].

In 1992, Brugada and Brugada reported a unique form of IVF, now known as Brugada syndrome (see Chap. 11, in detailed description), where patients with a J-point and ST-segment elevation (ER pattern) in leads V1–V3 without any structural heart disease are prone to develop VF and SCD [6]. The introduction of Brugada syndrome has brought about a strong interest in ER as having a possible correlation to or being a trigger of the development of fatal arrhythmias. Actually, several studies on IVF with an ER pattern excluding Brugada syndrome have been published as reports of a

The authors have no conflicts of interest to declare.

T. Sasano (✉)
Department of Cardiovascular Medicine, Tokyo Medical and Dental University, Bunkyo-ku, Tokyo, Japan
e-mail: Sasano.cvm@tmd.ac.jp

M. Hiraoka
Tokyo Medical and Dental University, Bunkyo-ku, Tokyo, Japan
e-mail: m-hiraoka0401@ivory.plala.or.jp

H. F. Baars et al. (eds.), *Clinical Cardiogenetics*, https://doi.org/10.1007/978-3-030-45457-9_16

single or collected cases, suggesting a possible arrhythmogeneity of ER [7–11]. This hypothesis was supported by an experimental study dealing with canine wedge preparations for a model of ER, which was shown to be capable of developing rapid polymorphic ventricular tachycardias (PVT) [12, 13].

The clinical results supporting this hypothesis were then supported by the seminal work by Haissaguerre et al. who demonstrated the high prevalence of an ER pattern in patients with IVF [14]. In their study, 206 IVF and 412 control cases were explored, and an ER pattern was more frequently observed in IVF patients than the controls (31% vs. 5%, respectively). The odds ratio (OR) for the presence of ER in the IVF patients compared to the control was 10.9 (95% confidence interval 6.3–18.9) after adjusting for the age, sex, race, and level of physical activity. Similar observations were confirmed in IVF patients with case-control studies [15, 16]. The ratio of an ER pattern in patients with IVF was 42–60%, which was significantly higher than that in the controls (3.3–13%, $p < 0.05$). Figure 16.1 presents representative ECGs from IVF patients with and without ER. Subsequently, Tikkanen et al. studied the prognostic significance of an ER pattern in the general population [17]. An ER pattern in the inferior leads was associated with an increased risk of cardiac death in the middle-aged population.

"Early repolarization" (ER) in the 12-lead ECG has been used in cardiology for many years, but its exact definition has varied widely. Because of such variations, the prevalence of ER in the normal population has varied between 2% and 31% [18]. Kambara and Phillips [19] proposed the following definition of ER: (1) end-QRS notching or slurring; (2) elevation of the ST segment; and (3) an upward-sloping ST segment followed by a tall, symmetrical T wave. In clinical practice, many physicians have regarded the presence of a J-point and ST-segment elevation merged with a positive T wave as ER but as a benign ECG sign.

Therefore, the definition of ER, as well as its terminology, has not reached a consensus. Recently, Macfarlene et al. proposed a unified definition of ER to assist future studies [20]. According to their consensus paper, ER is present if all the following criteria are met:

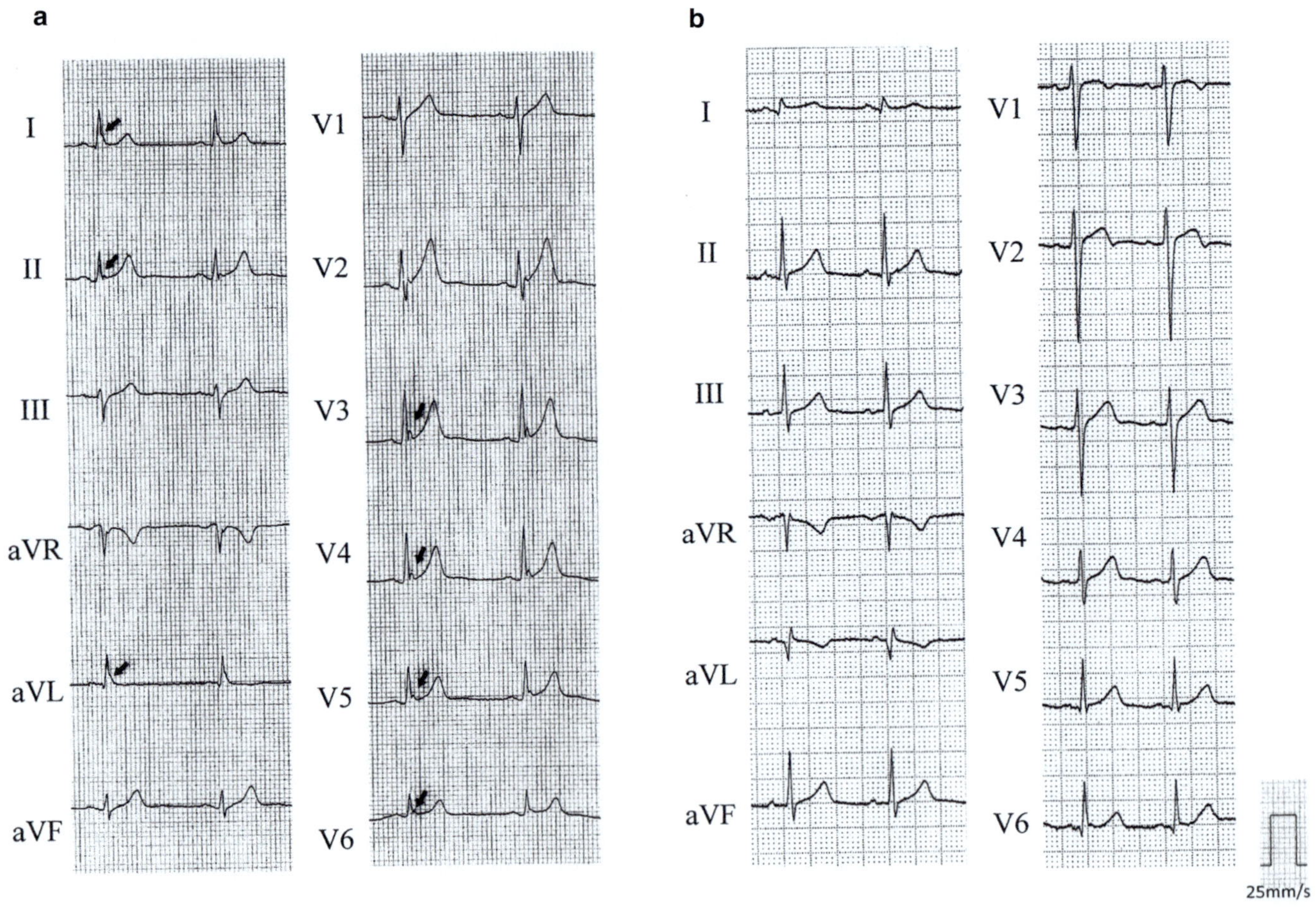

Fig. 16.1 Representative electrocardiograms (ECGs) of the IVF patients with ER (panel A) and without ER (panel B). Panel A: ER was recorded in both the lateral and inferior leads. Panel B: ER was not observed in any lead. (Reproduced by permission from Sekiguchi Y, Hiraoka M, et al. [63])

1. There is an end-QRS notch or slur on the downslope of a prominent R wave. The notch should lie entirely above the baseline. The onset of a slur must also be above the baseline. (The notch and slur should occur during the final 50% of the segment of the QRS complex.)
2. The peak of the J-point should be ≥0.1 mV in two or more contiguous leads of the 12-lead ECG, excluding leads V1–V3.
3. The QRS duration should be <120 ms.

If the ST segment is upward sloping and followed by an upright T wave, the pattern should be described as "ER with an ascending ST segment."

If the ST segment is horizontal or downward sloping, the pattern should be described as "ER with a horizontal or descending ST segment."

Clinical Presentation of ERS

ERS refers to patients with IVF exhibiting an ER pattern on the ECG in the inferior and/or lateral leads. It is important to recognize that ERS and an ER pattern on the ECG should be separated from each other, since an ER pattern itself is mostly a benign ECG sign. A clinical diagnosis of ERS can be made in specific patients who are resuscitated from cardiac arrest due to VF or PVT and with a 12-lead ECG demonstrating an ER pattern during sinus rhythm. At the same time, it is absolutely necessary to exclude any structural heart disease and other primary electrical disorders including long QT syndrome, Brugada syndrome, catecholaminergic polymorphic ventricular tachycardia, and short QT syndrome.

The most difficult diagnostic dilemma is to differentiate malignant ER from benign ER in subjects with this particular ECG sign in the inferior and/or lateral leads. The prevalence of the ER pattern in the inferior and/or lateral leads has been reported to be in a range of 3–24% in the general population [21, 22]. The prevalence varies considerably depending on age, sex, race, and physical activity. Most of these subjects are asymptomatic and without developing VF events. While the clinical implications of an ER pattern in asymptomatic subjects are not clear, it is assumed that the presence of an ER pattern triples the risk of VF. Despite this increase, the overall risk is still negligible because IVF itself is a quite rare disorder. Adler et al. estimated that the risk of developing IVF in an individual younger than 45 years is 3:100,000. The risk increases to 11:100,000 when a J-point elevation is present [23]. A meta-analysis estimated that the absolute difference in subjects with an ER pattern is seven cases of arrhythmic death per 100,000 subjects per year [24]. Although the presence of an ER pattern increases the relative risk of VF, the absolute risk is still very low.

Clinical Diagnosis and Differential Diagnosis

ERS usually develops with a sudden and unexpected onset of syncope and/or aborted SCD due to life-threatening ventricular arrhythmias, VF/PVT. A diagnosis of ERS can be confirmed by resuscitated patients from VF who exhibit an ER pattern in the ECG, and other causes of arrhythmic events are excluded (Figs. 16.2 and 16.3). The HRS/EHRA/APHRS expert consensus statement has provided recommendations for an early repolarization diagnosis [25] (Table 16.1). The diagnostic definition is stated as "ERS is diagnosed in the presence of J-point elevation ≥1 mm in ≥2 contiguous inferior and/or lateral leads of a standard 12-lead ECG in a patient resuscitated from otherwise unexplained VF/PVT." A highly possible case and definition of an ER pattern are also described.

Other features of the clinical manifestations have been presented in various reports on an observational basis with limited numbers of cases. Thus, a definite diagnostic criteria for ERS as well as the risk stratification are lacking at the present time, but physicians should follow the HRS/EHRA/APHRS expert consensus recommendations for the diagnostic decision-making. In addition, following the findings may help diagnose suspected cases of an atypical manifestation in clinical practice.

ERS has a male predominance. The mean age of the first VF episode is between 35–43 years old [14–16, 26, 27]. VF attacks are more likely to develop during sleep than during physical activity [14]. In patients with ERS, the amplitude of the J-point elevation increases with a slow heart rate and after a pause [27] (Fig. 16.4). VF is usually triggered by a short-long-short sequence and a short-coupled extrasystole initiates the arrhythmic events [28]. Circadian variations in the J-point elevation often occur in association with the vagal tone [26]. An increased vagal tone augments and sympathetic stimulation by isoproterenol attenuates the amplitude of the J-point elevation [27]. Sodium channel blockers also attenuate the J-point elevation [27, 29–31]. The amplitude of the ER increases prominently just before VF episodes [11, 14, 16, 28]. An ERS increase is recognized as a hallmark of the disease. A global appearance of a J-point elevation on the 12-lead ECG is suggested to develop within 30 min of VF storms [16]. Such a J-point elevation may completely disappear within weeks after the VF events [27]. A dynamic manifestation of the J-point elevation in malignant cases of ERS might be in contrast to the rather stable expression of an ER pattern in healthy individuals [17, 32, 33]. The magnitude of the J-point elevation may have some prognostic significance. Either a slurred or notched J-point elevation of ≥0.2 mV is relatively rare in the general population and appears to be associated with an increased risk [17]. A horizontal or descending ST segment following the J-point elevation is associated with a worse outcome in the general population [32]. This ECG pattern also provides infor-

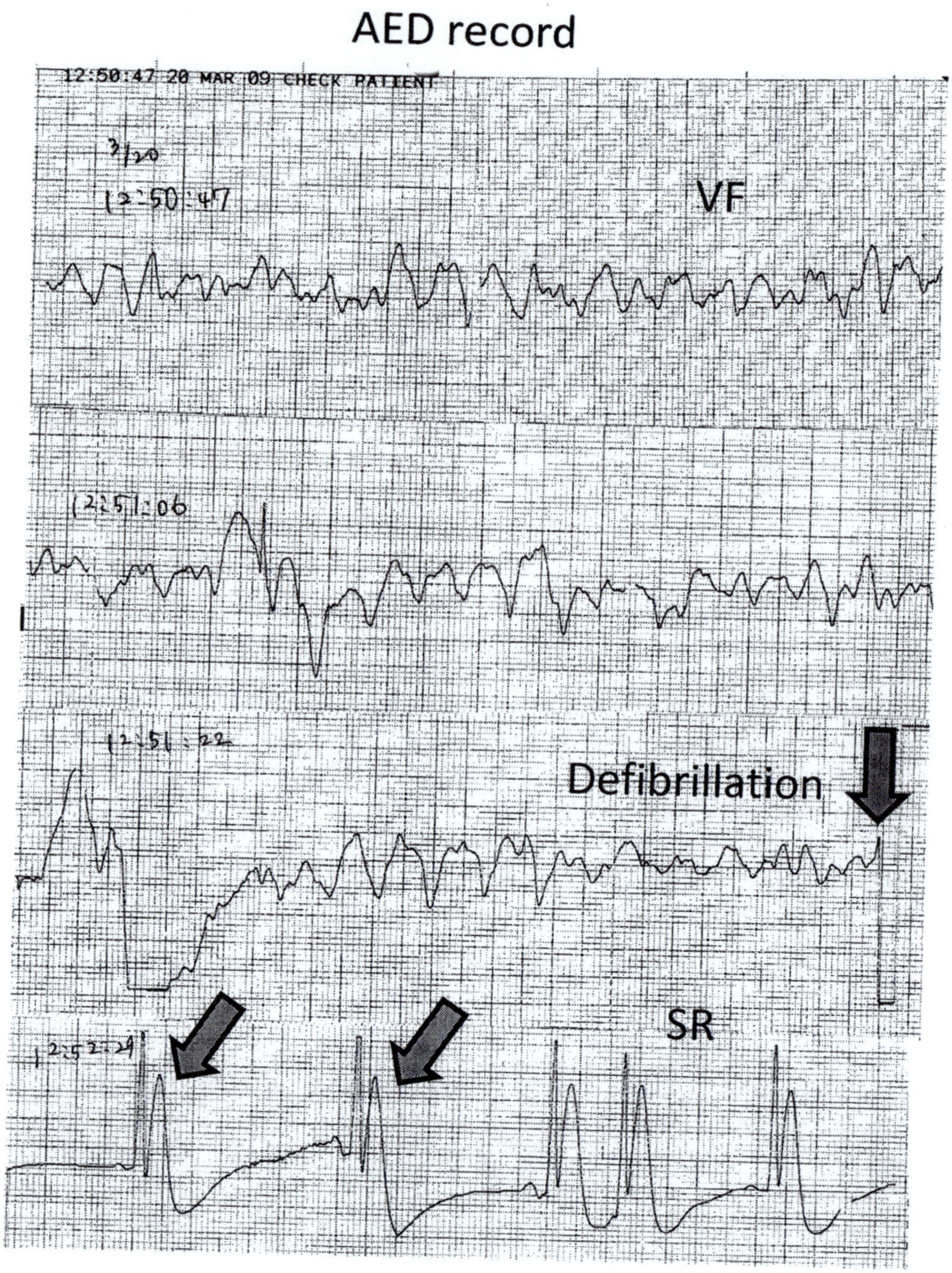

Fig. 16.2 VF and giant J waves in sinus rhythm after defibrillation. Electrocardiograms recorded by an automated external defibrillator (AED) from a 37-year-old man with an aborted sudden cardiac death. The AED detected VF and delivered an electric shock (the right corner of the third row) restoring sinus rhythm with giant J waves (the bottom row). He was shown to have no structural heart disease by various cardiac examinations including echocardiography, coronary angiography, and a pilsicainide provocation test for Brugada syndrome

mation for distinguishing IVF patients from matched controls and probably is a key sign to differentiate a malignant form from a benign ER pattern [33].

The signal-averaged ECG demonstrates that late potentials are frequently positive and concordant with the time of VF events in ERS patients, but no such correlation in IVF cases without ER or controls has been observed [26]. The repolarization parameters (T-wave alternans and QT dispersion) are not different between IVF patients with and without an ER pattern. An electrophysiological study (EPS) is not an effective method to assess the risk of ERS patients. The inducibility of VF is low (34%) in patients with a history of VF and does not differ in IVF patients with or without an ER pattern [14]. The results of a multicenter study to determine the role of an EPS in the risk stratification of ERS patients with a recent history of VF have shown a low (22%) inducibility as well as a low prediction rate (33%) for VF recurrences in EPS-positive cases [34]. Therefore, the current programmed stimulation protocol does not enhance the risk stratification in patients with ERS.

A differential diagnosis is performed to exclude any form of structural heart disease in the development of life-

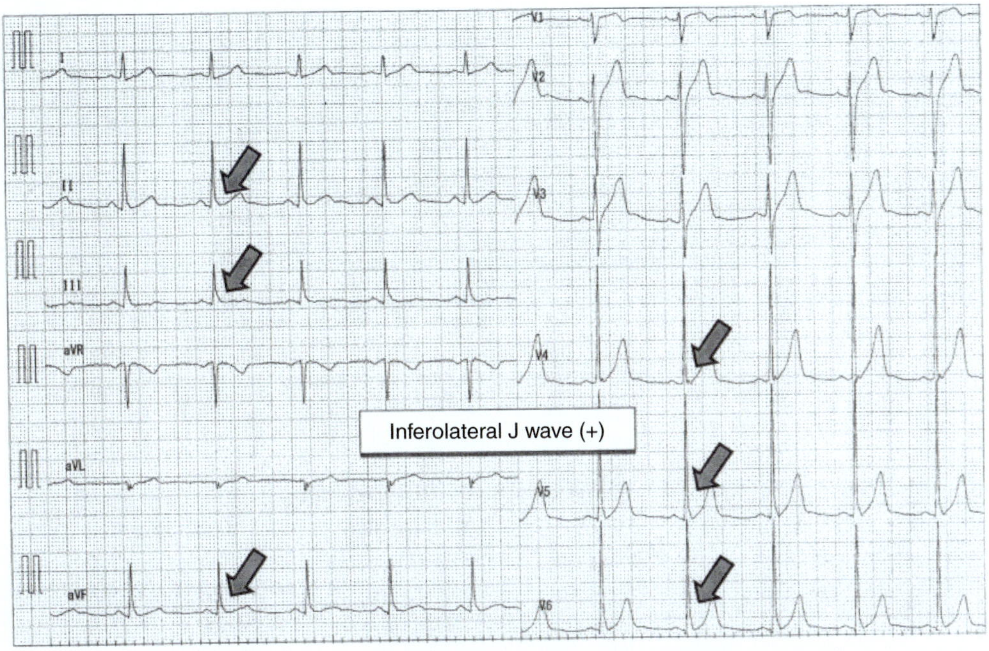

Fig. 16.3 Twelve-lead ECG with infero-lateral ER. An ECG was recorded in the same patient as in Fig. 16.2 on admission. ER (arrows) was observed in the inferior (II, III, and a VF) and lateral (V3–V6) leads

Table 16.1 Early repolarization diagnosis

1. ER syndrome is diagnosed in the presence of a J-point elevation of ≥1 mm in ≥2 contiguous inferior and/or lateral leads of the standard 12-lead ECG in a patient resuscitated from otherwise unexplained VF/polymorphic VT
2. ER syndrome can be diagnosed in an SCD victim with a negative autopsy and medical chart review with a previous ECG demonstrating a J-point elevation of ≥1 mm in ≥2 contiguous inferior and/or lateral leads of the standard 12-lead ECG
3. An ER pattern can be diagnosed in the presence of a J-point elevation of ≥1 mm in ≥2 contiguous inferior and/or lateral leads of the standard 12-lead ECG

ECG electrocardiogram, *ER* early repolarization, *VF* ventricular fibrillation, *SCD* sudden cardiac death (Reproduced by permission from Priori et al. [25])

threatening ventricular arrhythmias and electrolyte imbalance, especially hypokalemia. Primary electrical diseases should be excluded by unique clinical manifestations depending on each disorder and genetic screening. A recent expert consensus report summarized differential diagnosis of ERS and proposed Shanghai Score system for diagnosis of ERS [35].

Clinical Therapy

Table 16.2 presents the therapeutic interventions for ERS patients by the HRS/EHRA/APHRS expert consensus recommendations [25]. The table indicates the medical treatment and indication for an ICD implantation. It also stresses that an ICD implantation is not recommended for asymptomatic patients with an isolated ER pattern on the ECG.

Electrical storms are relatively common after an ICD implantation in patients with ERS. The acute use of isoproterenol has been effective for the suppression of recurrent VF and VF storms. Isoproterenol is typically initiated at 1.0 μg/min, targeting a 20% increase in the heart rate or an absolute heart rate of >90 bpm, and titrated to a hemodynamic response and suppression of recurrent ventricular arrhythmias [25]. Quinidine together with an ICD implantation has been suggested for the long-term suppression of VF recurrences during the chronic phase [16, 29]. A small series in a case study demonstrated that the combination of cilostazol and bepridil suppressed VF recurrences and attenuated the amplitude of the J waves in patients with an ICD implantation [36].

The clinical implications for asymptomatic subjects with an ER pattern on the ECG are not clear. While the presence of an ER pattern is associated with three times the risk of developing VF, the absolute risk is still negligible in the general population [24, 37]. Based on these population studies, as well as clinical observations, middle-aged subjects with an ER pattern on the ECG, especially those with a high amplitude (≥0.2 mV) J-point elevation and horizontal/descending ST segment, should pay attention to carrying out a risk reduction for the long-term basis, especially during acute coronary events in clinical practice [38].

The Mechanism of an ER Pattern and Early Repolarization Syndrome

The genesis of J waves or an ER pattern on the ECG was proposed by the group of Antzelevitch et al. based on animal experiments using canine ventricular wedge preparations

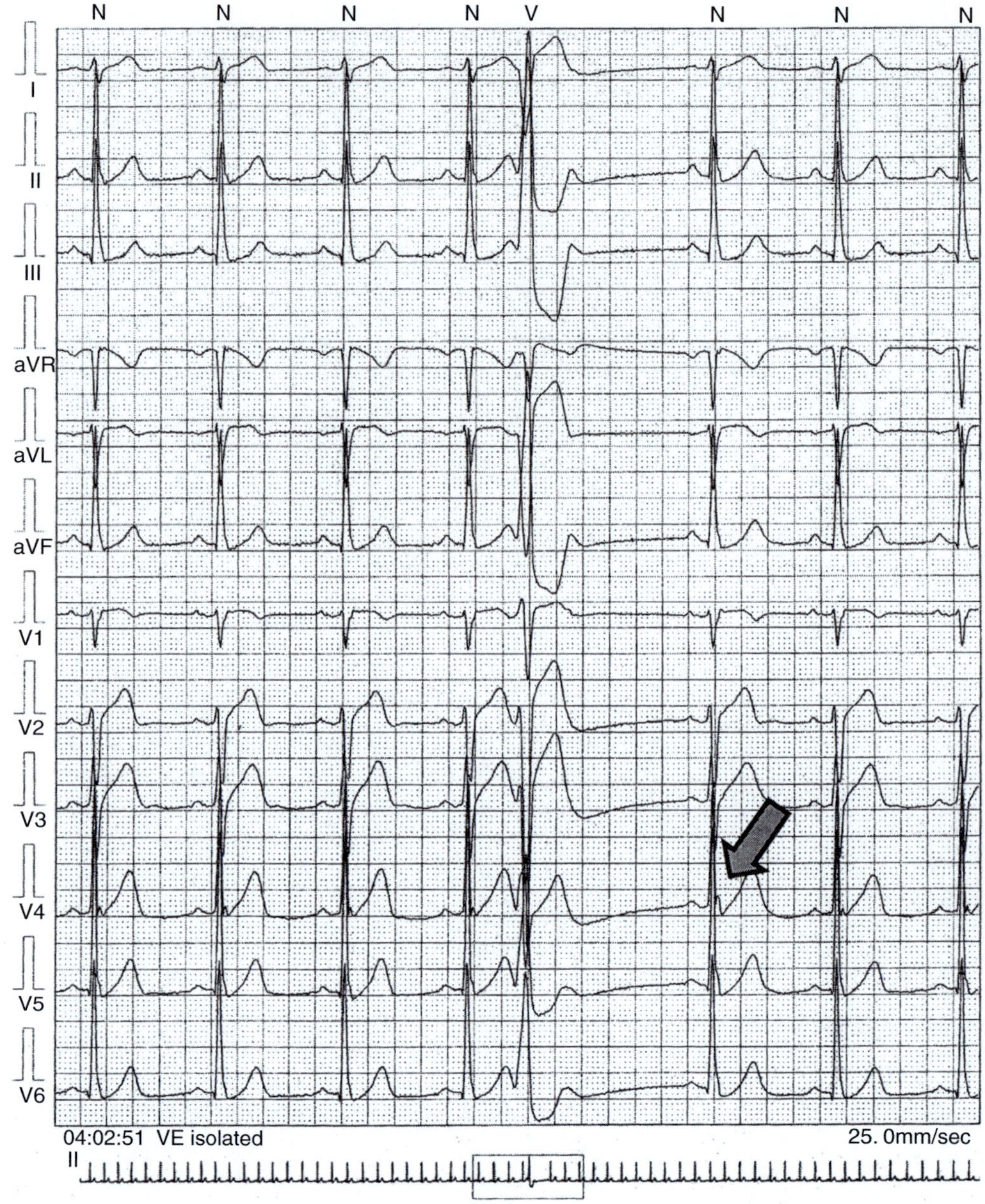

Fig. 16.4 Pause-dependent augmentation of ER. ER was augmented in a beat (arrow) following a long pause after a premature ventricular contraction (recorded from the same patient as shown in Fig. 16.2)

Table 16.2 Early repolarization therapeutic interventions

Class I 1. An ICD implantation is recommended in patients with a diagnosis of ER syndrome who have survived a cardiac arrest
Class IIa 2. An isoproterenol infusion can be useful in suppressing electrical storms in patients with a diagnosis of ER syndrome
3. Quinidine in addition to an ICD can be useful for secondary prevention of VF in patients with a diagnosis of ER syndrome
Class IIb 4. An ICD implantation may be considered in symptomatic family members of ER syndrome patients with a history of syncope in the presence of ST-segment elevation >1 mm in two or more inferior or lateral leads
5. An ICD implantation may be considered in asymptomatic individuals who demonstrate a high-risk ER ECG pattern (high J-wave amplitude, horizontal/descending ST segment) in the presence of a strong family history of juvenile unexplained sudden death with or without pathogenic mutation
Class III 6. An ICD implantation is not recommended in asymptomatic patients with an isolated ER ECG pattern

ICD implantable cardioverter defibrillator (Reproduced by permission from Priori et al. [25]

[12, 13]. The proposed mechanism explains that the genesis of J waves is formed by a transmural voltage gradient during the early repolarization phase due to different action potential configurations between the epicardium and endocardium. The action potential of the epicardial cells exhibits a prominent notch during the early phase of repolarization and that of endocardial cells lacks such a notch. The voltage gradient caused by the presence and absence of the notch between the epicardial and endocardial action potentials produces a J-wave configuration on the ECG. The differences in the action potential configurations are brought about by a membrane current distribution in which the epicardial cells are rich in a transient outward potassium current (I_{to}), while the endocardial cells have a lesser I_{to} current [39]. Conditions that augment or reduce the I_{to} could modify the manifestation of the J waves on the ECG. When the I_{to} is augmented or the current kinetics are changed by exposure to hypothermia, a

slow heart rate, the application of calcium and sodium channel blockers, or I_{to} agonists such as NS5806, the epicardial action potential notch and J waves are augmented. A reduction in the I_{to} by the application of I_{to} blockers such as 4-aminopyridine, quinidine, or premature stimulation causes parallel changes in the decrease in the notch and J waves [12, 40]. With a further increase in the I_{to}-mediated notch, some areas of the epicardial action potential become markedly abbreviated, while those in other areas and the endocardium are not shortened much, which provides the substrate for "phase 2 reentry" and the initiation of PVT/VF.

Antzelevitch and Yan [41] proposed the terminology "J-wave syndrome." This concept is based on several observations suggesting that arrhythmias associated with an ER pattern in the infero-lateral leads, Brugada syndrome, hypothermia, and acute ST-segment elevation myocardial infarctions are mechanistically linked to abnormalities in the manifestation of I_{to}-mediated J waves. Although ERS and Brugada syndrome differ with respect to the lead location and the magnitude of an abnormal J-wave manifestation, they can be considered to represent a continuous spectrum of the phenotypic expression that the authors proposed as "J-wave syndrome." They divided J-wave syndrome into three types: Type 1, displaying an ER pattern predominantly in the lateral leads, is prevalent among healthy male athletes and rarely seen in VF survivors; Type 2, displaying an ER pattern predominantly in the inferior or infero-lateral leads, is associated with a higher level of risk; and Type 3, displaying an ER pattern globally in the inferior, lateral, and right precordial leads, is associated with the highest level of risk for the development of malignant arrhythmias and is often associated with VF storms. This terminology may not be widely accepted since it includes both benign and malignant forms.

The concept of the repolarization theory can explain the experimental results and support some clinical observations. There are, however, several problems left unclarified. For example, contiguous myocardial cells exhibit fairly good electrical coupling among individual cells so that the different action potential configurations are prone to be averaged and a steep voltage gradient is not likely to exist between the epicardium and endocardium or among adjacent cells in the epicardial regions [42]. There may be an additional factor necessary to create the observed conditions in the limited region of the inferior or lateral walls of the ventricle, such as myocardial fibrosis. Second, the I_{to} current is composed of different genetic subunits, which exhibit fast and slow current kinetics: the fast component is formed by *Kv4.2 (KCND2)* + *Kv4.3 (KCND3)* and the slow one by *Kv1.5 (KCNA4)*. Their expression and the combination vary in different cardiac regions and species [43]. It is not known whether the candidate genes for the I_{to} in the human heart, especially, their distribution on the infero-lateral wall, are similar to those in canines or not. Clinically, if the heterogeneity of repolarization caused by I_{to} is the mechanism for developing VF in patients with ERS, it is still difficult to explain why the risk of arrhythmic death is so low (7 cases per 100,000 subjects per year), while an ER pattern in the general population is common (3–24%) [21–24]. Electrophysiological, genetic, and clinical documentations to prove the repolarization theory as an actual mechanism for ERS await further study.

Molecular Diagnostics and Molecular Genetics

A familiar ER pattern on the ECG has been reported to have an autosomal dominant inheritance with incomplete penetrance. Population-based studies also have suggested some degree of inheritance of an ER pattern in the general population [44, 45]. A genetic background of ER has been suggested by observations in subjects of with a common family history of SCD associated with ER and IVF [14, 46], but the inheritance of a malignant ER pattern has not been clearly demonstrated.

Mutations in the L-type Ca channel genes, including *CACNA1C*, *CACNB2B*, and *CACNA2D1* [47], as well as loss-of-function mutations in *SCN5A* [48] have also been reported in patients with ERS, but an inheritance has not been clearly identified. Because of the high prevalence of an ER pattern in the general population, ER may be polygenic and influenced by non-genomic factors as well. A recent genome-wide association meta-analysis in three independent populations of European ancestry found eight loci associated with ER, the strongest association being found with SNPs located at the *KCND3* genes, which encode the I_{to} channel (*Kv4.3*) coding gene [49]. These observations need further confirmation in other populations.

Family Screening and Follow-Up in Relatives

There are currently no recommendations to screen the families of individuals with an asymptomatic ER pattern. No provocation tests are available to diagnose concealed ER in family members of ERS patients. The therapeutic recommendations by the HRS/EHRA/APHRS consensus statement use the term "strong family history" [25]. There is no clear definition of this term, but it is typically chosen when more than one family member is affected, deaths occur at an early age, and a first-degree relative is affected.

Summary

ERS is a specific type of IVF, which is a very rare but highly malignant disease. A diagnosis can be made in resuscitated patients from VF with a J-point elevation in the inferior and/or lateral leads during sinus rhythm, and major structural heart disease and primary electrical disorders are excluded. Treatment should be directed to protect from recurrences of VF and SCD by an implantation of an ICD. An isoproterenol infusion is effective for suppressing VF events during the acute phase and VF storms. Quinidine may be useful in patients with an ICD implantation for preventing recurrent VF events. The mechanism and genetic background of ERS have not been fully clarified.

Take Home Message

- ERS is a very rare but potentially highly malignant disease.
- ERS should be considered in anyone resuscitated from VF with an ER pattern in the inferior and/or lateral leads of the standard 12-lead ECG during sinus rhythm and a strong family history of juvenile unexpected sudden death, without any other potential cause.
- One always must think about ERS in the following cases:
  - Aborted cardiac arrest or SCD of unknown origin
  - The presence of a J-point elevation of ≥1 mm in ≥2 contiguous inferior and/or lateral leads of a standard 12-lead ECG during sinus rhythm
  - A family history of juvenile unexplained sudden death

Idiopathic Ventricular Fibrillation Without an ER Pattern

Idiopathic ventricular fibrillation (IVF) without an ER pattern is characterized by spontaneous VF in the absence of structural heart disease and in the absence of any known electrical disorders. IVF cases are diagnosed and studied only after the resuscitation from cardiac arrest with the exclusion of any structural heart disease and primary electrical disorders. While the incidence of IVF without ER is quite rare, scattered descriptions of small numbers of IVF patients have been presented in the literature without achieving a definite and uniform clarification of the clinical characterization, genetic background, and diagnostic criteria/risk stratification of arrhythmic events. There are several clinical forms of IVF, which may be caused by different pathogenetic mechanisms.

IVF Related to His-Purkinje Conduction Disturbances

Recently, several reports have described that conduction disturbances in the His-Purkinje system are involved in the mechanism of IVF. In the latter part of this chapter, we focus on His-Purkinje conduction disturbances and their involvement in IVF.

Deletion of Irx3 in the Mouse Model

The Iroquois homeobox (Irx) family is an iroquois homeobox transcription factor which contains a highly conserved DNA-binding homeodomain and Iro motif in *Drosophila* and vertebrates. The *Irx* gene family has six subtypes, and they are located forming two clusters (*Irx* 1, 2, and 4 on chromosome 13 and *Irx* 3, 5, and 6 on chromosome 16 in humans) [50]. The *Irx* family genes are expressed in the heart during mouse development [51–53]. Among them, it has been reported that *Irx3* is selectively expressed in the subendocardial layer of the ventricles and plays a critical role in generating the His-Purkinje system. Zhang et al. reported that a genetic deletion of *Irx3* in mice resulted in the disruption of the fast conducting system through the His-Purkinje network [54]. The Purkinje cells express connexin-40 (Cx40) rather than connexin-43 (Cx43), dominantly expressed in working ventricular myocytes. The conductance of Cx40 is larger than that of Cx43, which explains the faster conduction through the Purkinje network. The deletion of *Irx3* results in a reduced expression of Cx40 in the His-Purkinje system.

A study utilizing *Irx3* knockout mice revealed that the deletion of *Irx3* exhibited not only a ventricular conduction disturbance but also ventricular tachyarrhythmias [55]. Ventricular tachyarrhythmias are not seen in the baseline condition, but are evoked by physical exercise, sympathetic activation, or an acute myocardial infarction. An ex vivo electrophysiological study by optical mapping showed that a delayed conduction in the RVOT at baseline and the administration of isoproterenol induced atrioventricular block, followed by non-sustained VT (Fig. 16.5). Those findings suggested that these stimulations increase the discrepancy in the conduction between an impaired His-Purkinje system and the intact myocardium.

IRX3 Mutations Related to IVF

Koizumi et al. further performed genetic screening of *IRX3* in 130 IVF cases including Brugada syndrome, short QT syndrome, and ERS and found two novel point mutations in VF cases (R421P and p485T) [55]. For a functional analysis of these mutations, they generated identical mutations using a murine *Irx3* and transfected a wild-type and mutated *Irx3* into HL-1 murine atrial cells or neonatal mouse ventricular myocytes. Transfection of the wild-type *Irx3* increased the expression of *Cx40* and *SCN5A*, but the transfection of these two mutated *Irx3* genes exhibited a significantly reduced expression of *Cx40* and *SCN5A*. Thus, these mutations contributed to the conduction disturbance in the His-Purkinje system.

The intriguing feature of these cases was that they suffered from VF during physical activity. One case with R421P had a Brugada-type ECG but suffered from syncope while he was ice-skating. Another case had syncope during commuting. These findings indicate that IVF associated with the IRX3 mutation has a different clinical entity than Brugada syndrome. However, the following paper by Kimura et al. described that one of the common variants of

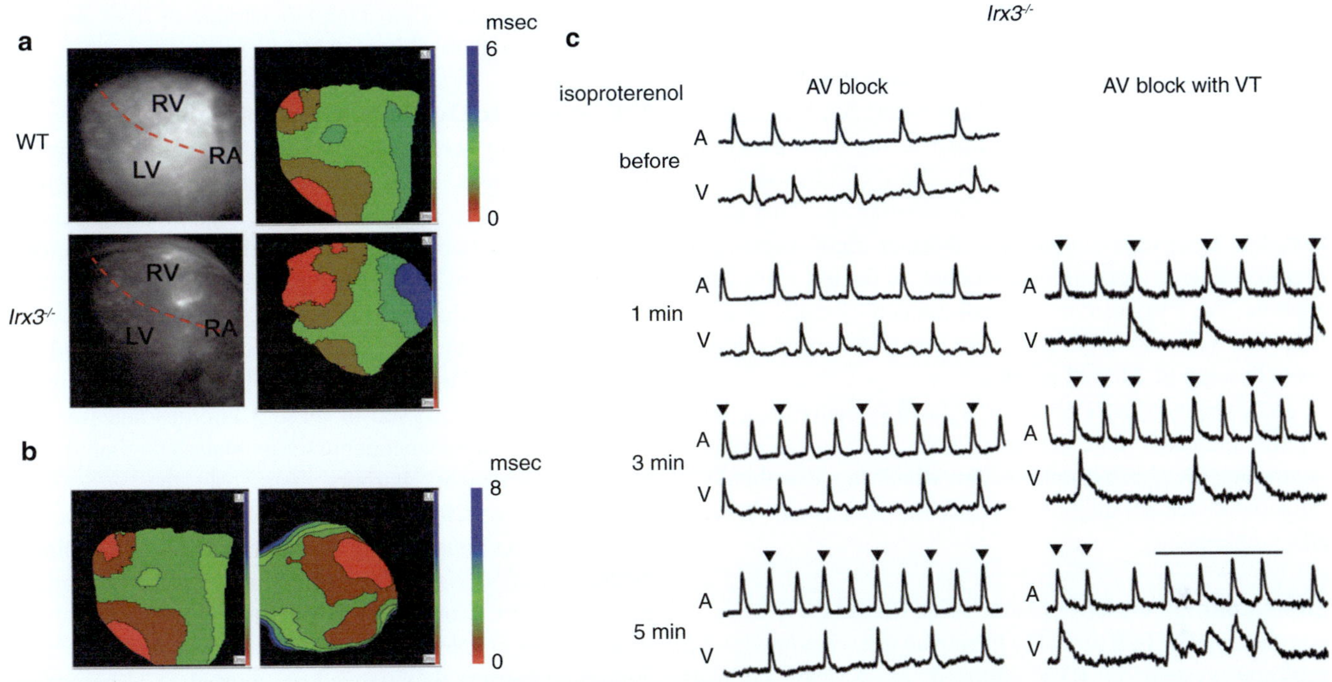

Fig. 16.5 Ex vivo optical epicardial mapping and arrhythmia development in Irx3$^{-/-}$ mice. Panel A: Representative optical epicardial mapping in WT and Irx3$^{-/-}$ mice under basal conditions. Panel B: Representative optical epicardial mapping in WT and Irx3$^{-/-}$ mice after an isoproterenol application. In Irx3$^{-/-}$ mice, an epicardial breakthrough occurs from the base of the right ventricle and propagates to the apex; the propagation of the depolarization became markedly slow. Panel C: AV block and AV block with non-sustained VT occurred after the administration of isoproterenol. Reverse triangles indicate the atrial action potential without a following ventricular action potential. The solid bar indicates non-sustained VT. (Reproduced by permission from Koizumi A, Sasano T, et al. [55])

IRX3 (Q479H) works as a modifier to manifest the electrophysiological phenotype of Brugada syndrome with a polymorphism in SCN5A (A735V), by decreasing the expression of SCN5A [56].

Although the physiological phenotype of *Irx3* knockout mice is evident, the precise molecular mechanism linking Irx3 and a conduction disturbance resulting in IVF has not been fully elucidated. Although the expression of *Cx40* and *SCN5A* is reduced in *Irx3* knockout mice, other factors may be involved in the electrophysiological phenotype. A recent paper described that Irx3 is essential for postnatal morphological maturation of the ventricular conduction system in addition to the regulation of gap junction channels [57]. In addition, two mutations found in IVF cases are not found in the already known functional domains (TALE-homeobox domain and Iro domain). Thus, the mechanism explaining the reduced expression of Cx40 in these two mutations is still under investigation.

Other IVF Related to Conduction Disturbances

The accumulation of several observational studies has indicated an additional possibility of the involvement of the His-Purkinje system in IVF. One phenotype is the association of right bundle branch block (RBBB). Aizawa et al. investigated 87 cases diagnosed with IVF, excluding Brugada syndrome and catecholaminergic polymorphic VT, and found that 10 of 87 patients (11.5%) had complete RBBB and the incidence was much higher than that in the age- and sex-comparable controls (1.37%) [58]. There were no differences in the ECG parameters except for the QRS duration.

The Japanese Idiopathic Ventricular Fibrillation Study (J-IVFS) summarized 64 IVF cases excluding Brugada syndrome [59]. Out of those 64 cases, 24 had an ER pattern in the ECG. In the remaining 40 patients, 9 cases (14%) had an abnormal axis deviation and/or RBBB, indicating a conduction disturbance (CD). They classified the IVF cases into the ER(+) group, ER(−)CD(−) group, and ER(−)CD(+) group. The ER(−)CD(+) group consisted of five males and four females, which was a lower proportion of males than in the ER(+) group. The ER(−)CD(+) group also had a longer PR interval and QRS duration than the ER(−)CD(−) and ER(+) groups. Two studies indicated that about 10% of IVF patients had ventricular conduction disturbances, but no specific ECG parameters were noted in the rest of the IVF cases. VF was initiated with short-coupled premature ventricular contractions (PVCs) in some cases. The inducibility of VF by EPS was low in both types. There were no indications for a familial pattern of IVF with or without RBBB in the two studies. No risk stratification is available; thus, far and drug treatment for the prevention of SCD is not effective. An isoproterenol infusion has been proven to be effective for the treatment of VF storms in some cases. ICD implantations are the only therapeutic option for the prevention of SCD.

Haissaguerre et al. described short-coupled PVCs originating from the distal Purkinje fibers as the main triggering factor for VF in IVF patients [60]. The PVCs had different morphologies and were mapped in several locations of the Purkinje system, including the anterior right ventricular region and large areas of the lower half of the left ventricular septum. The PVC origins were eliminated by catheter ablation, and 89% of the patients were free of VF events during the follow-up of 24 ± 28 months.

In contrast to the IVF cases with *IRX3* mutations, both reports indicated that the prevalence of exercise-induced ventricular tachyarrhythmias is low, which suggests that IVF related with RBBB might have a different mechanism that an *IRX3* deficiency.

Short-Coupled Variant of Torsade de Pointes

Another type of IVF probably having an association with the Purkinje system is PVT initiated by a short-coupled PVT. Leenhardt et al. described a unique form of idiopathic ventricular tachyarrhythmias in young adults and called it a "short-coupled variant of torsade de pointes (TdP)" [61]. The unique feature of this arrhythmia was the development of TdP under a normal QT interval, in contrast to the common association with QT prolongation in congenital and acquired forms of long QT syndrome. The TdP was initiated by PVCs with a short coupling interval (245 ± 28 ms), and one-third of these patients had a family history of sudden death. Approximately 70% of patients with a short-coupled variant of TdP degenerate into VF. In the following year, similar characteristics of patients were reported [62], and the term "short-coupled variant of TdP" was well recognized as a specific form of PVT/VF. This form of arrhythmias is prevalent in females. The initial clinical presentation of the patients is often syncope, and this type of arrhythmia is not inducible by EPS. This arrhythmia can be partially suppressed by verapamil, but the drug cannot prevent SCD and an ICD implantation is the only option for the prevention of SCD. Recently, several studies have been based on treating triggering PVCs from the Purkinje system in patients with PVT/VF by catheter ablation. It has been reported that ablation can achieve freedom from VF recurrences during a follow-up on a short- and long-term basis [60, 63, 64].

The underlying molecular mechanism of the short-coupled variant of TdP has not been elucidated yet. A recent case report, however, indicated that a point mutation in ryanodine receptor 2 (*RyR2*-H29D) is related to PVT [65]. In contrast to the *RyR2* mutation associated with catecholaminergic polymorphic VT, this case has short-coupled PVCs and PVT at rest. The H29D mutation converts *RyR2* to a leaky channel. This may explain some part of or the principal mechanism of the short-coupled variant of TdP, *but this observation may need further clarification.*

IVF Related to Overexpression of DPP6

Studies dealing with a large cohort of familiar IVF in the Netherlands were conducted to clarify the pathogenetic mechanism and risk stratification for asymptomatic patients in the affected family members. Alders et al. performed a genome-wide haplotype-sharing analysis for the identification of a responsible gene in three Dutch families in which multiple individuals died suddenly or were resuscitated at a young age [66]. They identified a haplotype, on chromosome 7q36, that was conserved in these 3 families and was also shared by 7 of 42 independent IVF patients. The shared chromosomal segment harbors part of the *dipeptidyl-aminopeptidase-like protein 6 (DPP6)* gene, which encodes a putative component of I_{to} in the heart [67]. The clinical evaluation of 84 risk-haplotype carriers and 71 noncarriers revealed no ECG or structural parameters indicative of cardiac disease. Penetrance of IVF was high; 50% of risk-haplotype carriers experienced an aborted SCD before the age of 58 years. Their study also demonstrated a 20-fold increase in the *DPP6* mRNA level in the myocardium of carriers as compared to controls. From these results, they proposed *DPP6* as a gene for IVF and an increased *DPP6* expression as the likely pathogenetic mechanism. Despite the finding of an association between familial IVF and a risk haplotype on chromosome 7q36, identification of asymptomatic patients at risk for IVF remains challenging, and no clinical parameters to guide the treatment have been defined [68–70].

Further study by Xiao et al. [71] explored the link between the overexpression of *DPP6* and the pathogenesis of IVF. According to the results, the baseline ECG is normal in *DPP6* risk-haplotype carriers. Ventricular arrhythmias manifest as short-coupled PVCs that sometimes initiate PVT. PVCs consistently display a left bundle branch morphology with a superior/left axis, suggesting a lower RV origin. The short-coupling interval of PVCs under a normal QT interval along with relatively narrow QRS complexes suggested an origin in the Purkinje system, as observed by Haissaguerre et al. [60] in 25% of their IVF patients. In one patient undergoing ablation for repeated VF storms after an ICD implantation, RV pace mapping produced a morphology similar to that of the PVCs. Radiofrequency ablation was applied at a site with early diastolic Purkinje fiber potentials in the anterior lower RV. Neither VF nor a typical morphology of the PVCs recurred during 43 months of follow-up.

While the Ito density is similar in Purkinje fibers and ventricular muscle, the tetraethylammonium (TEA) sensitivity and slow recovery from inactivation are different between the I_{to} in the two tissues [72, 73]. In non-diseased human hearts, the expressions of *DPP6* and *neuronal calcium sensor-1 (NCS-1)* are rich in Purkinje fibers, while *K^+-channel interacting protein type 2 (KChIP2)* is rich in ventricular muscle, which indicates different β-subunit compositions of the I_{to} channels in the two tissues. The heterologous expression of *Kv4.3* in Chinese hamster ovary cells demonstrated that the coexpression of *DPP6* and *NCS-1* (to mimic the Purkinje Ito composition) enhanced the I_{to} as compared to *Kv4.3/NCS-1* alone, and recapitulated the kinetic/pharmacologic properties of the Purkinje I_{to}. Overexpression of *DPP6* enhanced and knockdown of *DPP6* suppressed the native Purkinje fiber I_{to}. A mathematical model of cardiac Purkinje fiber action potentials showed that I_{to} enhancement can greatly accelerate the repolarization of the Purkinje fiber action potential. From these results, the authors suggest that a *DPP6*-mediated Purkinje fiber early repolarization might be a novel molecular mechanism for some forms of IVF. While the suggested mechanism is related to the ER of the Purkinje fibers, further clarification is mandatory as to whether it represents a subset of ERS limited to the conduction system, or other additional mechanisms may be involved in the clinical manifestation of IVF.

Possible Gene Mutations for Other Types of IVF Without an ER Pattern

Genetic screening of Japanese IVF patients disclosed a mutation of the human cardiac sodium channel α-subunit (*SCN5A*) in a symptomatic IVF patient who did not exhibit a typical Brugada ECG and showed a rate-dependent RBBB [74]. A novel *SCN5A* missense mutation, S1710L, was identified, and its channel function studied by a heterologous expression system revealed a markedly reduced current due to an accelerated current decay, negative shift in the steady-state inactivation, and positive shift in the activation (Fig. 16.6). Genetic

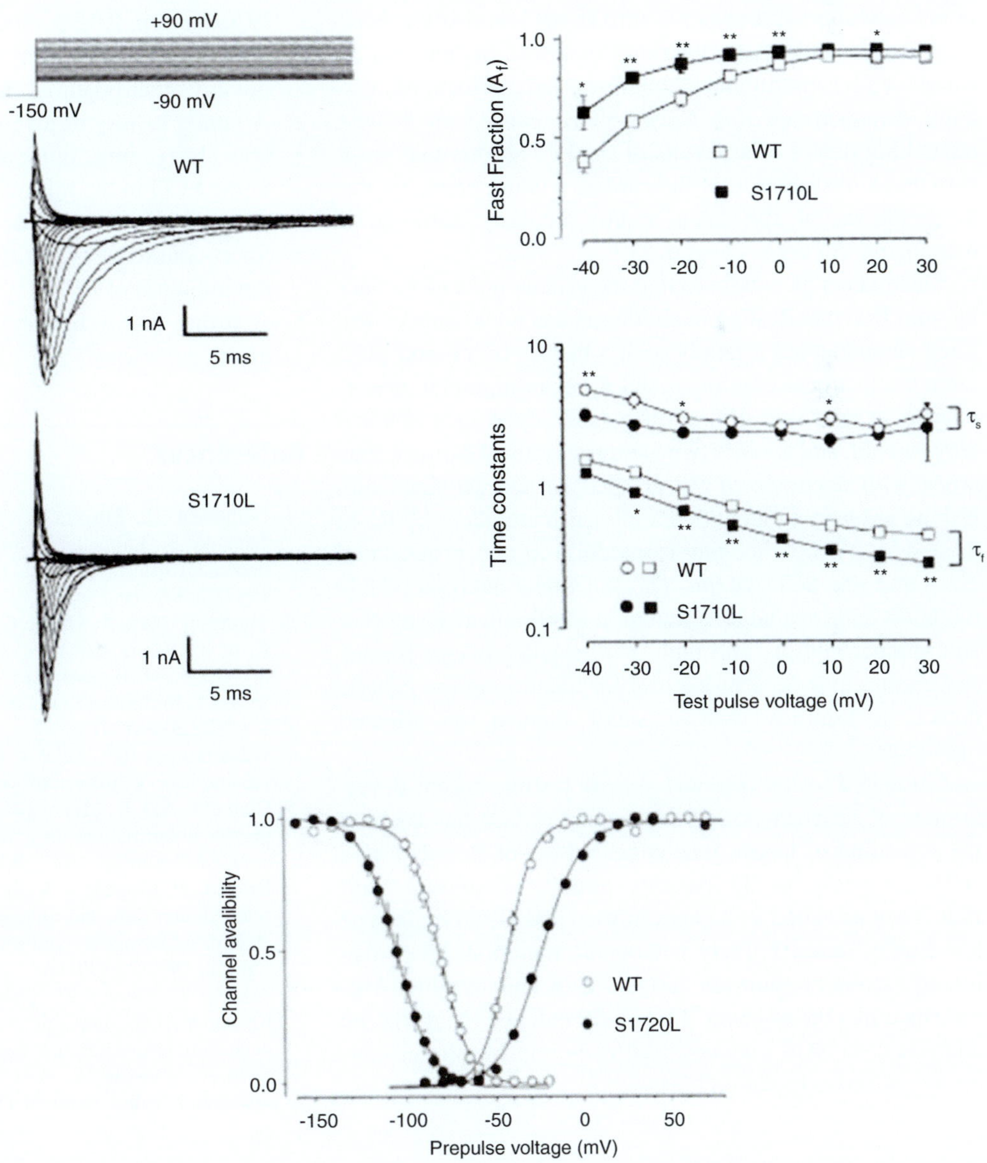

Fig. 16.6 Whole-cell current and its analysis obtained from HEK-hβ1 cells transfected with either WT or S1710L sodium channels. A: Whole-cell current recordings obtained from HEK cells transfected with either WT and S1710L sodium channels. The current was recorded from a holding potential of −150 mV stepped from −90 to +90 mV for 20 ms in 10 mV increments. The current decay is faster in S1710L than WT. B: The time course of the inactivation was fit with a double exponential function. A_f in the upper panel indicates the fraction of the fast inactivation component. τ_f and τ_s in the lower panel indicate the fast and slow time constant of the fast and slow inactivation components, respectively. C: Voltage dependence of the steady-state inactivation and activation. The S1710L current shows a negative shift in the inactivation and a positive shift in the activation compared to WT. (Reproduced by permission from Akai et al. [74])

screening of his family members was not accepted, and a genotype-phenotype co-segregation was not explored.

Valdivia et al. reported a loss-of-function mutation of the *SCN3B*-encoded sodium channel β3 subunit [75]. A 20-year-old healthy male suddenly lost consciousness while playing basketball, and the emergency team found him in VF. After resuscitation from VF, his ECG exhibited epsilon waves in the right precordial leads without inverted T waves. A cardiac examination including echocardiography and cardiac CT scan did not reveal any structural abnormality of the heart, and hence, he was diagnosed with IVF. A mutation analysis disclosed a missense mutation, V54G, in *SCN3B*, which was absent in 800 reference alleles. His mother was an asymptomatic gene-mutation carrier and exhibited a J-point elevation on her ECG. A functional analysis of her HEK293 cells expressing *SCN5A* coexpressed with *Navβ3*-V54G revealed a markedly decreased peak sodium current density, with a positive shift in the activation and negative shift in the inactivation compared to the wild type, resulting in a loss-of-function by *Navβ3*-V54G. Immunocytochemistry and confocal microscopy demonstrated that *Navβ3*-V54G caused an *SCN5A* trafficking defect. The results of the two reports may indicate that a dysfunction of the cardiac sodium channels due to mutations of the main and/or auxiliary subunits is responsible for some cases of IVF.

Marsman et al. sought to find the genetic defect in a family with IVF manifesting in childhood and adolescence [76]. They characterized a family with a history of VF and SCD without electrocardiographic and echocardiographic abnormalities at rest. Two siblings died suddenly at ages of 9 and 10 years old, and another two were resuscitated from cardiac arrest with documented VF at ages 10 and 16 years old. Exome sequencing identified a missense mutation, F90L, in the *CALM1* gene encoding calmodulin in two resuscitated cases and one SCD victim. The functional analysis of this mutation is not available. A mutation was found in the mother and another sibling, and both were asymptomatic. Exome sequencing may be a strong tool for identifying the genetic defect in families with a small number of affected individuals.

Compared to the classical genetic testing, recent development of next-generation sequencing (NGS) has enabled the screening of larger gene panel. Visser et al. performed NGS screening in 33 patients initially diagnosed with IVF. They screened 212 genes in total and DPP6 haplotype and finally found 1 likely pathogenic mutation. NGS also identified one or multiple variants with undetermined significance in 15% of cases. This study indicated that routine analysis with NGS may not drastically improve the discovery of causative mutation [77].

Summary

IVF without an ER pattern in the ECG may include several different types of electrocardiographic and clinical manifestations. They can show either no specific ECG sign, a ventricular conduction disturbance, or a short-coupled variant of TdP with a normal QT interval. The ventricular tachyarrhythmias in most of these cases are initiated by short-coupled PVCs without QT prolongation. A diagnosis of IVF can be made only after resuscitation from VF events excluding structural heart disease and primary electrical disorders. No risk stratification is available at the present time, and an ICD implantation is the only option to prevent SCD.

Take Home Message

- IVF without an ER pattern in the ECG is a very rare but potentially highly malignant disease.
- IVF without an ER pattern in the ECG should be considered in anyone resuscitated from VF showing no specific ECG pattern, RBBB, or short-coupled variant of TdP with a normal QT interval in the standard 12-lead ECG, without any other potential causes.
- A family history of juvenile unexpected sudden death.
- One always must think about IVF without an ER pattern in the ECG in the following cases:
- Aborted cardiac arrest or SCD of an unknown origin
- Short-coupled PVCs with a normal QT interval preceding the initiation of PVT
- A strong family history of juvenile unexplained sudden death

References

1. Belhassen B, Shapira I, Shoshani D, Paredes A, Miller H, Laniado S. Idiopathic ventricular fibrillation: inducibility and beneficial effects of class I antiarrhythmic agents. Circulation. 1987;75:809–16.
2. Martini B, Nava A, Thiene G, Buja GF, Canciani B, Scognamiglio R, et al. Ventricular fibrillation without apparent heart disease: description of six cases. Am Heart J. 1989;118:1203–9.
3. Viskin S, Belhassen B. Idiopathic ventricular fibrillation. Am Heart J. 1990;120:661–71.
4. Wasserburger RH, Alt WJ. The normal RS-T segment elevation variant. Am J Cardiol. 1961;8:184–92.
5. Clements SD Jr, Hurst JW. Diagnostic value of electrocardiographic abnormalities observed in subjects accidentally exposed to cold. Am J Cardiol. 1972;29:729–34.
6. Brugada P, Brugada J. Right bundle branch block, persistent ST segment elevation and sudden cardiac death: a distinct clinical and electrocardiographic syndrome: a multicenter report. J Am Coll Cardiol. 1992;20:1391–6.
7. Aizawa Y, Tamura M, Chinushi M, Naitoh N, Uchiyama H, Kusano Y, et al. Idiopathic ventricular fibrillation and bradycardia-dependent intraventricular block. Am Heart J. 1993;126:1473–4.
8. Garg A, Finneran W, Fred GK. Familiar sudden cardiac death associated with a terminal QRS abnormality on surface 12-lead

electrocardiogram in the index case. J Cardiovasc Electrophysiol. 1998;9:642–7.
9. Takagi M, Aihara N, Takaki H, Taguchi A, Shimizu W, Kurita T, et al. Clinical characteristics of patients with spontaneous or inducible ventricular fibrillation without apparent heart disease presenting with J wave and ST segment elevation in inferior leads. J Cardiovasc Electrophysiol. 2000;11:844–8.
10. Kalla H, Yan GX, Marinchak R. Ventricular fibrillation in a patient with prominent J (Osborn) wave and ST segment elevations in the inferior electrocardiographic leads: a Brugada syndrome variant. J Cardiovasc Electrophysiol. 2000;11:95–8.
11. Shinohara T, Takahashi N, Saikawa T, Yoshimura H. Characterization of J wave in a patient with idiopathic ventricular fibrillation. Heart Rhythm. 2006;3:1082–4.
12. Yan GX, Antzelevitch C. Cellular basis for the electrocardiographic J wave. Circulation. 1996;93:372–9.
13. Gussak I, Antzelevitch C. Early repolarization syndrome: clinical characteristics and possible cellular and ionic mechanisms. J Electrocardiol. 2000;33:299–309.
14. Haissaguerre M, Derval N, Sacher F, et al. Sudden cardiac arrest associated with early repolarization. N Engl J Med. 2008;358:2016–23.
15. Rosso R, Kogan E, Belhassen B, Rozovski U, Sheinman M, et al. J-point elevation in survivors of primary ventricular fibrillation and matched control subjects: incidence and clinical significance. J Am Coll Cardiol. 2008;52:1231–8.
16. Nam GB, Kim YH, Antzelevitch C. Augmentation of J waves and electrical storms in patients with early repolarization. New Eng J Med. 2008;358:2078–9.
17. Tikkanen JT, Anttonen O, Junttila MJ, Aro AL, Kerola T, Rissanen HA, et al. Long-term outcome associated with early repolarization on electrocardiography. New Eng J Med. 2009;361:2529–37.
18. Maury P, Rollin A. Prevalence of early repolarization/J wave pattern in the normal population. J Electrocardiol. 2013;46:411–6.
19. Kambara H, Phillips J. Long-term evaluation of early repolarization syndrome (normal variant RST-T segment elevation). Am J Cardiol. 1976;38:157–61.
20. Macfarlene PW, Antzelevitch C, Haissaguerre M, Huikuri HV, Potse M, Rosso R, et al. The early repolarization. A consensus paper. J Am Coll Cardiol. 2015;66:470–7.
21. Junttila MJ, Sager SJ, Tikkanen JT, Anttonen O, Huikuri HV, Myerburg RJ. Clinical significance of variants of J-points and J-waves: early repolarization patterns and risk. Eur Heart J. 2012;33:2639–43.
22. Huikuri HV, Marcus F, Krahn AD. Early repolarization: an epidemiologist's and a clinician's view. J Electrocardiol. 2013;46:466–9.
23. Adler A, Rosso R, Viskin D, Halkin A, Viskin S. What do we know about the "malignant form" of early repolarization. J Am Coll Cardiol. 2013;62:863–8.
24. Wu S-H, Lin X-X, Cheng Y-J, Qiang C-C, Zhang J. Early repolarization pattern and risk for arrhythmia death. A meta-analysis. J Am Coll Cardiol. 2013;61:645–50.
25. Priori SG, Wilde AA, Horie M, Cho Y, Behr ER, Berul C, et al. HRS/EHRA/APHRS expert consensus statement on the diagnosis and management of patients with inherited primary arrhythmic syndromes. Heart Rhythm. 2013;10:1932–63.
26. Abe A, Ikeda T, Tsukada T, Ishiguro H, Miwa Y, Miyakoshi M, et al. Circadian variation of late potentials in idiopathic ventricular fibrillation associated with J wave: insights into alternative pathophysiology and risk stratification. Heart Rhythm. 2010;7:675–82.
27. Aizawa Y, Sato A, Watanabe H, Chinushi M, Furushima H, Horie M, et al. Dynamicity of the J-wave in idiopathic ventricular fibrillation with a special reference to pause-dependent augmentation of the J-wave. J Am Coll Cardiol. 2012;59:1948–53.
28. Nam GB, Ko KH, Kim J, Park KM, Rhee KS, Choi KJ, Kim YH, Antzelevitch C. Mode of onset of ventricular fibrillation in patients with early repolarization pattern vs. Brugada syndrome. Eur Heart J. 2010;31:330–9.
29. Haissaguerre M, Sacher F, Nogami A, Komiya N, Bernard A, Probst V, et al. Characteristics of recurrent ventricular fibrillation associated with inferolateral early repolarization: role of drug therapy. J Am Coll Cardiol. 2009;53:612–9.
30. Kawata H, Noda T, Yamada Y, Okamura H, Satomi K, Aiba T, et al. Effect of sodium-channel blockade on early repolarization in infero/lateral leads in patients with idiopathic ventricular fibrillation and Brugada syndrome. Heart Rhythm. 2012;9:77–83.
31. Roten L, Derval N, Sacher F, Pascale P, Wilton SB, Scherr D, et al. Ajmaline attenuates electrocardiogram characteristics of inferolateral early repolarization. Heart Rhythm. 2012;9:232–9.
32. Tikkanen JT, Junttila MJ, Anttonen O, , Aro AL, Luttinen S, Kerola T, et al. Early repolarization: electrocardiographic phenotypes associated with favorable long-term outcome. Circulation 2011;123:2666–2673.
33. Rosso R, Glikson E, Belhassen B, Katz A, Halkin A, Steinvil A, et al. Distinguishing "benign" from "malignant early repolarization": the value of the ST-segment morphology. Heart Rhythm. 2012;9:225–9.
34. Mahida S, Derval N, Sacher F, Leenhardt A, Deisenhofer I, Babuty D, et al. Role of electrophysiologic studies in predicting risk of ventricular arrhythmia in early repolarization syndrome. J Am Coll Cardiol. 2015;65:151–9.
35. Antzelevitch C, Yan G-X, Ackerman MJ, Borggrefe M, Corrado D, Guo J, et al. J-wave syndromes expert consensus conference report: emerging concepts and gaps in knowledge. Heart Rhythm. 2016;13:e295–324.
36. Shinohara T, Ebata Y, Ayabe R, Fukui A, Okada N, Yufu K, et al. Combination therapy of cilostazol and bepridil suppresses recurrent ventricular fibrillation related to J-wave syndrome. Heart Rhythm. 2014;11:1441–5.
37. Rosso R, Adler A, Halkin A, Viskin S. Risk of sudden death among young individuals with J wave and early repolarization: putting the evidence into perspective. Heart Rhythm. 2011;8:923–9.
38. Naruse Y, Tada H, Harimura Y, Hayashi M, Noguchi Y, Sato A, et al. Early repolarization is an independent predictor of occurrences of ventricular fibrillation in the very early phase of acute myocardial infarction. Circ Arrhythm Electrophysiol. 2012;5:506–13.
39. Litovsky SH, Antzelevitch C. Transient outward current prominent in canine ventricular epicardium but not endocardium. Circ Res. 1988;62:116–26.
40. Antzelevitch C, Yan GX. J wave syndrome: Brugada and early repolarization syndromes. Heart Rhythm. 2015;12:1852–66.
41. Antzelevitch C, Yan GX. J wave syndrome. Heart Rhythm. 2010;7:549–58.
42. Kleber AG, Rudy Y. Basic mechanisms of cardiac impulse propagation and associated arrhythmia. Physiol Rev. 2004;84:431–88.
43. Niwa N, Nelbonne JM. Molecular determinants of cardiac transient outward potassium current (Ito) expression and regulation. J Mol Cell Cardiol. 2010;48:12–25.
44. Noseworthy PA, Tikkanen JT, Porthan K, Oikarinen L, Pietiila A, Harald K, et al. The early repolarization pattern in the general population: clinical correlates and heritability. J Am Coll Cardiol. 2011;57:2284–9.
45. Reinhard W, Kaess BM, Debiec R, Nelson CP, Stark K, Tobin MD, et al. Heritability of early repolarization: a population-based study. Circulation Cardiovasc Genetics. 2011;4:134–8.
46. Nunn LM, Bhar-Amato J, Lowe MD, Macfarlane PW, Rogers P, McKenna WJ, et al. Prevalence of J-point elevation in sudden arrhythmic death syndrome families. J Am Coll Cardiol. 2011;58:286–90.
47. Burashnikov E, Pfeiffer R, Barajas-Martinez H, Delpon E, Hu D, Desai M, et al. Mutations in the cardiac L-type calcium channel

associated with inherited J-wave syndromes and sudden cardiac death. Heart Rhythm. 2010;7:1872–82.
48. Watanabe H, Nogami A, Ohkubo K, Kawata H, Hayashi Y, Ishikawa T, et al. Electrocardiographic characteristics and SCN5A mutations in idiopathic ventricular fibrillation associated with early repolarization. Circ Arrhythm Electrophysiol. 2011;4:874–81.
49. Sinner MF, Porthan K, Noseworthy PA, Havulinna AS, Tikkanen JT, Muller-Narasyid M, et al. A meta-analysis of genome-wide association studies of the electrocardiographic early repolarization pattern. Heart Rhythm. 2012;9:1627–34.
50. Gómez-Skarmeta JL, Modolell J. Iroquois genes: genomic organization and function in vertebrate neural development. Curr Opin Genet Dev. 2002;12(4):403–8.
51. Bruneau BG, Bao Z-Z, Fatkin D, Xavier-Neto J, Georgakopoulos D, Maguire CT, et al. Cardiomyopathy in Irx4-deficient mice is preceded by abnormal ventricular gene expression. Mol Cell Biol. 2001;21(5):1730–6.
52. Christoffels VM, Keijser AGM, Houweling AC, Clout DEW, Moorman AFM. Patterning the embryonic heart: identification of five mouse Iroquois Homeobox genes in the developing heart. Dev Biol. 2000;224(2):263–74.
53. Costantini DL, Arruda EP, Agarwal P, Kim K-H, Zhu Y, Zhu W, et al. The homeodomain transcription factor Irx5 establishes the mouse cardiac ventricular repolarization gradient. Cell. 2005;123(2):347–58.
54. Zhang S-S, Kim K-H, Rosen A, Smyth JW, Sakuma R, Delgado-Olguín P, et al. Iroquois homeobox gene 3 establishes fast conduction in the cardiac His–Purkinje network. Proc Natl Acad Sci. 2011;108(33):13576–81.
55. Koizumi A, Sasano T, Kimura W, Miyamoto Y, Aiba T, Ishikawa T, et al. Genetic defects in a his-Purkinje system transcription factor, IRX3, cause lethal cardiac arrhythmias. Eur Heart J. 2016;37:1469–75.
56. Kimura Y, Aiba T, Sasano T, Frukawa T, Kusano K, Shimizu W. IRX3 variant as a modifier of Brugada syndrome with frequent ventricular fibrillation. HeartRhythm Case Rep. 2016;2:465–8.
57. Kim K-H, Rosen A, Hussein SMI, Puviindran V, Korogyi AS, Chiarello C, et al. Irx3 is required for postnatal maturation of the mouse ventricular conduction system. Sci Rep. 2016;6:19197.
58. Aizawa Y, Takatsuki S, Kimura T, Nishiyama N, Fukumoto K, Tanimoto Y, et al. Ventricular fibrillation associated with complete right bundle branch block. Heart Rhythm. 2013;10:1028–35.
59. Sekiguchi Y, Aonuma K, Takagi M, Aihara N, Yokoyama Y, Hiraoka M. New clinical and electrocardiographic classification in patients with idiopathic ventricular fibrillation. J Cardiovasc Electrophysiol. 2013;24:902–8.
60. Haissaguerre M, Shoda M, Jais P, Nogami A, Shah DC, Kautzner J, et al. Mapping and ablation of idiopathic ventricular fibrillation. Circulation. 2002;106:962–7.
61. Leenhardt A, Glaser E, Burguera M, Numberg M, Maison-Blanche P, Coumel P. Short-coupled variant of torsade de pointes. A new electrocardiographic entity in the spectrum of idiopathic ventricular tachyarrhythmias. Circulation. 1994;89:206–15.
62. Eisenberg SJ, Scheinman MM, Dullet NK, Finkbeiner WE, Griffin JC, Eldar M, et al. Sudden cardiac death and polymorphous ventricular tachycardia in patients with normal QT intervals and normal systolic function. Am J Cardiol. 1995;75:687–92.
63. Nogami A, Sugiyasu A, Kubota S, Kato K. Mapping and ablation of idiopathic ventricular fibrillation from the Purkinje system. Heart Rhythm. 2004;2:646–9.
64. Knecht S, Sacher F, Wright M, Hocini M, Nogami A, Arentz T, et al. Long-term follow-up of idiopathic ventricular fibrillation ablation: A multicenter study. J Am Coll Cardiol. 2009;54:522–8.
65. Cheung JW, Meli AC, Xie W, Mittal S, Reiken S, Wronska A, et al. Short-coupled polymorphic ventricular tachycardia at rest linked to a novel ryanodine receptor (RyR2) mutation: leaky RyR2 channels under non-stress conditions. Int J Cardiol. 2015;189:228–36.
66. Alders M, Koopmann TT, Christiaan I, Postema PG, Beekman L, Tanck MW, et al. Haplotype-sharing analysis implicates chromosome 7q36 harboring DPP6 in familial idiopathic ventricular fibrillation. Am J Hum Genet. 2009;84:468–76.
67. Radicke S, Cottella D, Graf EM, Ravens U, Wettwer E. Expression and function of dipeptidyl-aminopeptidase-like protein 6 as a putative beta-subunit of human cardiac transient outward current encoded by Kv4.3. J Physiol. 2005;565:751–6.
68. van der Warf C, Hofman N, Tan HL, et al. Diagnostic yield in sudden unexplained death and aborted cardiac arrest in the young: the experience of a tertiary referral center in the Netherlands. Heart Rhythm. 2010;7:1383–9.
69. Postema PG, Christiaans I, Hofman N, Alders M, Koopmann TT, Bezzina CR, et al. Founder mutations in the Netherlands: familial idiopathic ventricular fibrillation and DPP6. Neth Heart J. 2011;19:290–6.
70. ten Sande JN, Postema PG, Boekholdt SM, Tan HL, van der Heijden JF, de Groot NMS, et al. Detailed characterization of familial idiopathic ventricular fibrillation linked to the DPP6 locus. Heart Rhythm. 2016;13:905–12.
71. Xiao L, Koopmann T, Ordog B, Postema PG, Verkerk AO, Iyer V, et al. Unique cardiac Purkinje fiber transient outward current β-subunit composition. A potential molecular link to idiopathic ventricular fibrillation. Circ Res. 2013;112:1310–22.
72. Han W, Wang Z, Nattel SA. A comparison of transient outward currents in cardiac Purkinje cells and ventricular myocytes. Am J Physiol Heart Circ Physiol. 2000;279:H466–74.
73. Han W, Xhang L, Schram G, Nattel SA. Properties of potassium currents in Purkinje cells of failing human hearts. Am J Physiol Heart Circ Physiol. 2002;282:H2495–503.
74. Akai J, Makita N, Sakurada H, Shirai N, Ueda K, Kitabatake A, et al. A novel SCN5A mutation associated with idiopathic ventricular fibrillation without typical ECG findings of Brugada syndrome. FEBS Lett. 2000;479:29–34.
75. Valdivia CR, Medeiros-Domingo A, Ye B, Shen W-K, Algiers TJ, Ackerman MJ, Makielski JC. Loss-of-function mutation of the SCN3B-encoded sodium channel β3 subunit associated with a case of idiopathic ventricular fibrillation. Cardiovasc Res. 2010;86:392–400.
76. Marsman RF, Barc J, Beekman L, Alders M, Dooijes D, van der Wijngaard A, et al. A mutation in CALM1 encoding calmodulin in familiar idiopathic ventricular fibrillation in childhood and adolescence. J Am Coll Cardiol. 2014;63:259–66.
77. Visser M, Dooijes D, van der Smagt JJ, van der Heijden JF, Doevendans PA, Loh P, et al. Next-generation sequencing of a large gene panel in patients initially diagnosed with idiopathic ventricular fibrillation. Heart Rhythm. 2017;14:1035–40.

17 Hereditary Cardiac Conduction Diseases

Rafik Tadros and Julia Cadrin-Tourigny

Introduction

Cardiac conduction disease (CCD) is very common in clinical practice. Its first description dates back to more than a century ago. Although the co-occurrence of fainting episodes and severe bradycardia was reported by Morgagni in the eighteenth century and again later by Stokes and Adams (to whom the term Stokes-Adams attacks was dedicated) [1, 2], the first documentation of atrioventricular block (AVB) on surface electrocardiography was achieved later [3]. Familial CCD have been was? first described in 1901 by Morquio and by many others thereafter [4–7].

Reflecting on its numerous etiologies and electrical manifestations, the definition of CCD is highly variable. We here define it as *any persistent defect in the formation or propagation of the cardiac impulse at any level of the specialized cardiac electrical system in the absence of drug or metabolic disturbance known to affect cardiac conduction.* Unlike most cardiovascular conditions discussed in this book, CCD is primarily caused by non-genetic etiologies (Table 17.1). In many cases, CCD is *secondary* to structural heart disease (e.g., ischemic heart disease, cardiomyopathy), to a cardiac intervention (e.g., aortic valve replacement, arrhythmia ablation), or to auto-immune process (e.g., neonatal lupus syndrome). CCD can also be *primary*, most often in the context of senile degeneration of the conduction system in an elderly patient. Primary CCD in a young patient should raise the suspicion for an inherited etiology, especially if there is a positive family history. The mechanism of CCD is either functional (decreased depolarizing currents or impaired cellular coupling) or associated with premature conduction system degeneration (referred to as Lenègre disease). This chapter is focused on primary CCD in the young, which could have an inherited etiology. We will review the subject in a clinically oriented manner, in a similar fashion as other chapters. A general discussion on the clinical evaluation and management of suspected hereditary CCD will be followed by a review of the molecular genetics of the disease (section "Molecular Genetics") highlighting gene-specific aspects.

R. Tadros (✉)
Cardiovascular Genetics Center, Montreal Heart Institute, Montréal, Canada

Department of Medicine, Université de Montréal, Montréal, Canada

Department of Experimental and Clinical Cardiology, Academic Medical Center, Amsterdam, Netherlands
e-mail: rafik.tadros@umontreal.ca

J. Cadrin-Tourigny
Cardiovascular Genetics Center, Montreal Heart Institute, Montréal, Canada

Department of Medicine, Université de Montréal, Montréal, Canada

Clinical Presentation

Primary CCD is a progressive disease with variable age of onset and clinical course. During early stages, patients are generally asymptomatic, and ECG abnormalities are detected incidentally or during family screening. With the progression of disease, symptoms occur either because of *severe bradycardia* or *chronotropic incompetence* (incapacity to increase heart rate during exercise). In the *former*, patients may present with pre-syncope or syncope occurring during periods of ventricular asystole (typically >4 seconds), due to sinus pauses or high degrees of AVB. In the *latter*, patients could present with exercise intolerance and/or dyspnea. Rarely, patients can be symptomatic in the absence of severe bradycardia and chronotropic incompetence. This may occur because of hemodynamic consequences of electrical dyssynchrony (e.g., excessive PR prolongation causing atrioventricular dyssynchrony) or due to re-entrant arrhythmia secondary to excessively slowed conduction (e.g., bundle branch re-entrant ventricular tachycardia).

Hereditary forms of CCD can be associated with other cardiac electrical or structural diseases as well as neurological disease (Table 17.2). As such, the first manifestation of disease might not be related to CCD but to the associated

H. F. Baars et al. (eds.), *Clinical Cardiogenetics*, https://doi.org/10.1007/978-3-030-45457-9_17

Table 17.1 Etiologies of CCD

Etiology	Definition and suggestive clinical clues
Primary CCD	
Senile progressive CCD	Progressive sinus node dysfunction, atrial arrhythmias, and/or atrioventricular conduction defects typically with fascicular blocks (wide QRS). Late onset (e.g., >50 years old)
Hereditary (see Table 17.2)	As above but with a premature onset (e.g., <50 years old). Family history of CCD, SCD, DCM, and CHD and/or presence of a pathogenic mutation in susceptibility genes
Idiopathic	Unexplained CCD
Secondary CCD	
Ischemic heart disease	Known coronary artery disease or presence of risk factors for atherosclerosis. Presence of Q waves on the ECG and presence of wall motion abnormalities and/or scar on cardiac imaging (typically involving the septum)
Cardiomyopathy	Diagnosed with cardiac imaging. Any cardiomyopathy (most often DCM) can progressively affect the conduction system in proportion with myocardial involvement. When CCD is out of proportion with the severity of cardiomyopathy, a primary CCD should be suspected (e.g., *LMNA* mutations; see Table 17.2)
Cardiac sarcoidosis and myocarditis	Presents with CCD, ventricular arrhythmia, and/or heart failure. Presence of inflammation or scar on cardiac magnetic resonance or positron emission tomography. Diagnosis may require cardiac or extracardiac biopsy. Sarcoidosis should be suspected in all young patients with unexplained severe CCD
Neonatal lupus syndrome	Maternal lupus with transplacental passage of anti-Ro/SSA and anti-La/SSB antibodies resulting in congenital non-progressive AVB at the level of the AV node (narrow QRS). Recurrence in siblings could mimic a hereditary etiology
Congenital heart disease	CCD commonly seen with certain CHD such as ccTGA and partial or complete AVSD. ccTGA can first present with CCD in adult life. AVSD is often associated with Down syndrome. Diagnosis requires cardiac imaging. Co-occurrence of CCD and CHD also observed in certain hereditary conditions (e.g., *NKX2–5* and *TBX5* mutations; see Table 17.2)
Iatrogenic CCD	CCD resulting from a surgical or transcatheter procedure near the conduction system. Typical examples: valvular procedures (most commonly aortic valve replacement), closure of septal defects, arrhythmia ablation, septal reduction therapy in hypertrophic cardiomyopathy
Other rare causes	Infiltrative malignancies and cardiac tumors, trauma, rheumatological disorders
Causes of transient/reversible cardiac conduction defects	
Increased vagal tone	Often seen in well-trained endurance athletes. Can also be triggered by emotion or posture in susceptible individuals (neurocardiogenic/vasovagal syncope). Presents with sinus bradycardia and different degrees of AVB with a narrow QRS
Metabolic disturbances	Examples include hyperkalemia, hypothermia, and thyroid dysfunction
Drugs	Drugs affecting autonomic cardiac modulation or ion channel function. Examples include beta-blockers, calcium channel blockers, sodium channel blockers, digitalis, and amiodarone

AV atrioventricular, *AVB* atrioventricular block, *AVSD* atrioventricular septal defect, *CCD* cardiac conduction disease, *ccTGA* congenitally corrected transposition of the great arteries, *CHD* congenital heart disease, *DCM* dilated cardiomyopathy, *SCD* sudden cardiac death

disease. For instance, patients with loss-of-function mutations in *SCN5A* can have both Brugada syndrome (BS) and CCD. In such cases, the first manifestation of disease can be ventricular arrhythmias in the context of BS. Patients with mutations in *NKX2–5* also present with atrial septal defects, while patients with *LMNA* mutation typically develop CCD in association with dilated cardiomyopathy (DCM) in a later stage of disease development. Other genotype-phenotype correlations are summarized in Table 17.2 and further discussed below. A detailed review of symptoms, physical examination, and cardiac imaging are thus crucial in establishing a correct diagnosis and guide molecular genetic testing.

Systematic longitudinal data on the course and natural history of hereditary CCD are limited. When available, such data will be discussed below along with the specific genetic defects (section "Molecular Genetics"). In contrast, the clinical course and prognosis of conduction defects in the general population without known structural heart disease has been abundantly studied. For instance, unexplained sinus bradycardia (<50 beats/min) in healthy volunteers is not associated with adverse events during a mean follow-up of 5.4 years [8]. In a Finnish populational study of 10,685 individuals aged 30–59 years old and followed for 30 ± 11 years, isolated first-degree AVB (2.1% of patients) was not associated with increased risk of adverse events [9]. Mobitz type I second-degree AVB in individuals without underlying heart disease, as often seen in athletes due to increased vagal tone, is often caused by block in the atrioventricular (AV) node and also has a benign prognosis [10]. In contrast, Mobitz type II second-degree AVB is caused by conduction block below the AV node and is associated with a bad prognosis, with high risk of progression to complete AVB, syncope, and sudden cardiac death (SCD) [11]. The association of right bundle branch block (RBBB) with mortality in the general population is controversial, with a recent meta-analysis showing an increased risk of mortality during follow-up (HR 1.17; 95% confidence interval [CI] 1.03–1.33) [12]. The prognosis of left bundle branch block (LBBB) in asymptomatic healthy individuals appears to be age-dependent. Earlier large cohort studies including patients with a mean age below 55 and mean follow-up less than 10 years do not detect an increased

Table 17.2 Clinical characteristics of the major subtypes of hereditary CCD

Gene/disease (mutation)	Transmission	Relative frequency in CCD	Other arrhythmias	Cardiomyopathy	CHD	Risk of SCD	Typical ECG	Extracardiac features/ diseases	Management particularities
SCN5A (missense and truncating—loss of function)	AD	++	BS, LQTS, AF	+/−(mild)	−	+	Prolonged PR and QRS. Left axis deviation	−	Avoid sodium channel blockers Treat fever
TRPM4 (missense—gain of function)	AD	++	−	−	−	+	RBBB, fascicular blocks	−	Usual CCD management
LMNA (missense, truncating, large deletion)	AD	++ (in CCD with DCM)	Atrial arrhythmias	++	−	++	Low-voltage P wave, prolonged PR, narrow QRS (initially)	Cardio-embolic stroke *LMNA* also linked to muscular dystrophies (EDMD and LGMD) and other diseases	ICD to be considered in presence of left ventricular dysfunction, ventricular arrhythmia, or severe CCD
NKX2–5 (missense, truncating)	AD	+	AF	+/−	++	+	Various degrees of AVB, narrow QRS	−	Usual CCD management
TBX5 (missense, truncating, large deletion)	AD	+/−	AF	−	+	+/−	Various degrees of AVB, narrow QRS	Upper limb skeletal anomalies (HOS)	Usual CCD management
MD (repeat expansions in ***DMPK*** [type I] or ***CNBP*** [type II])	AD	++ (in CCD with muscular dystrophy	Atrial and ventricular arrhythmias	+/−	−	++	Progressive PR prolongation and fascicular blocks	Myotonia, muscle pain, muscle weakness, cataracts, GI complaints. Mild CK elevation	Low threshold for pacemaker or ICD. Consider invasive EPS. Optimal approach yet to be developed
EDMD (***EMD***, ***FHL1***, ***LMNA***)	XR AD AR	+/−	Atrial arrhythmias	+	−	+	Sinus bradycardia, atrial standstill, AVB	Contractures, humeroperoneal muscle weakness, cardio-embolic stroke. Moderate CK elevation	Low threshold for pacemaker and anticoagulation
LGMD type IB (***LMNA***)	AD	+/−	Atrial arrhythmias	+	−	+	Sinus bradycardia, atrial standstill, AVB	Progressive weakness and atrophy of shoulder and pelvic girdle. Overlap with EDMD. Moderate CK elevation	Low threshold for pacemaker? Little available data
DES	AD	+/−	Atrial and ventricular arrhythmias	+	−	+	AVB, fascicular blocks	Proximal and distal muscular weakness. Mild CK elevation	Similar to *LMNA*? Little available data
HCN4 (missense, truncating)	AD	+	AF	LVNC	−	+	Sinus bradycardia	−	Usual CCD management CCD without LVNC has good prognosis

(continued)

Table 17.2 (continued)

Gene/disease (mutation)	Transmission	Relative frequency in CCD	Other arrhythmias	Cardiomyopathy	CHD	Risk of SCD	Typical ECG	Extracardiac features/ diseases	Management particularities
TNNI3K (missense, splice variants)	AD	+/–	Supraventricular tachycardia, atrial and ventricular arrhythmias	+	–	?	Sinus bradycardia, AVB, RBBB, fascicular blocks	–	Usual CCD management? Little available data
PRKAG2 (missense, truncating)	AD	+/–	WPW, AF	HCM	–	+	Ventricular pre-excitation	–	Usual CCD/HCM/WPW management

AD autosomal dominant, *AF* atrial fibrillation, *AR* autosomal recessive, *AVB* atrioventricular block, *BS* Brugada syndrome, *CCD* cardiac conduction disease, *CHD* congenital heart disease, *CK* creatine kinase, *DCM* dilated cardiomyopathy, *EDMD* Emery-Dreifuss muscular dystrophy, *EPS* electrophysiological study, *GI* gastrointestinal, *HCM* hypertrophic cardiomyopathy, *HOS* Holt-Oram syndrome, *ICD* implantable cardioverter-defibrillator, *LGMD* limb-girdle muscular dystrophy, *LQTS* long QT syndrome, *LVNC* left ventricular non-compaction cardiomyopathy, *MD* myotonic dystrophy, *RBBB* right bundle branch block, *SCD* sudden cardiac death, *WPW* Wolff-Parkinson-White syndrome, *XR* X-linked recessive adverse event rate associated with LBBB [13, 14]. In contrast, more recent studies including older patients and longer follow-up show a significant increase in high-degree AVB and cardiovascular as well as total mortality [15–17]. Taken together, these data suggest that conduction defects in the young asymptomatic patient have a good prognosis, with the exception of Mobitz type II second-degree AVB. Whether these data can be extrapolated to hereditary CCD is debatable. Since the mechanism of hereditary CCD is in part an accelerated degeneration of the conduction system, conduction defects in these patients likely occur at a higher rate than in an unselected CCD population.

Diagnosis and Differential Diagnosis

The clinical diagnosis of CCD requires the presence of a conduction abnormality on the ECG, at any single or multiple levels (Fig. 17.1). Secondary causes of CCD should be excluded (Table 17.1). An echocardiogram is indicated in all cases to assess the presence of structural heart disease, either causing or associated with CCD. Other diagnostic tests can be performed depending on patient's age, comorbidities, and clinical findings. Accumulating evidence from independent groups suggests that cardiac sarcoidosis and giant cell myocarditis are common causes of unexplained high-degree AVB in young patients (<55–60 years) [18, 19]. In such patients, advanced cardiac imaging with cardiac magnetic resonance (CMR) or fluorodeoxyglucose (^{18}F) cardiac positron emission tomography should be considered in the diagnostic strategy. In endemic regions, Lyme disease, an infectious disease caused by the spirochete *Borrelia Burgdorferi*, should also be suspected in young patients with unexplained AVB [20]. In the presence of a clinical presentation compatible with the disease, the diagnosis is established by serologic testing. It is important to recognize this etiology in order to start an appropriate antibiotic treatment. Because AVB is most often reversible, permanent pacemaker placement is most often unnecessary.

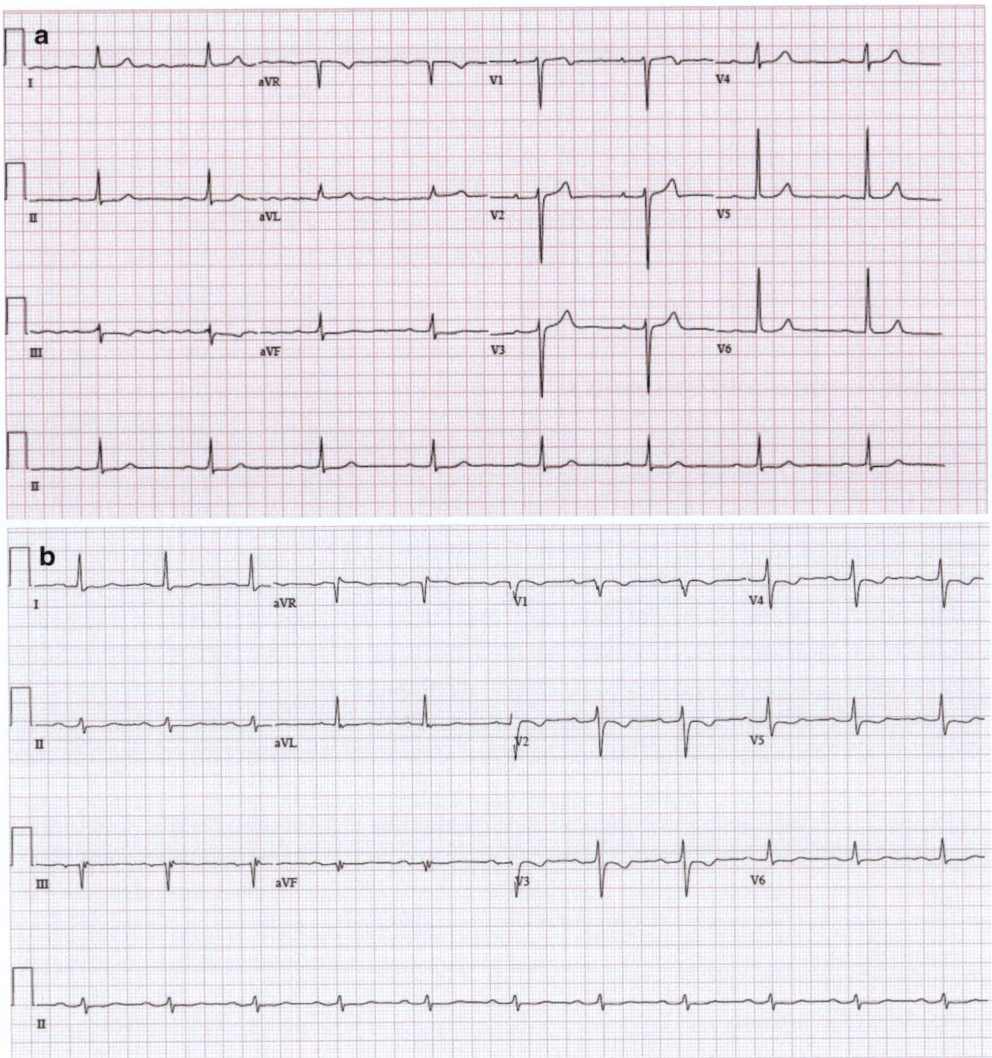

Fig. 17.1 (**a**) ECG obtained from a 50-year-old female with mild dilated cardiomyopathy (left ventricular ejection fraction 52%) and a truncating mutation in *LMNA* (Q410X) mutation. Note the low-voltage P wave, prolonged PR interval, and narrow QRS, typical for *LMNA* disease. (**b**) ECG obtained from a 63-year-old female with structurally normal heart and a truncating mutation in *SCN5A* (R222X). Note the prolonged PR and QRS intervals and left axis deviation, typical for *SCN5A* loss-of-function mutations

A three-generation family history is recommended when evaluating a young patient with an unexplained cardiac conduction defect. Family history taking is detailed in Chap. 2. In the context of CCD, one should specifically assess for the presence of family history of CCD, SCD, arrhythmia, pacemaker or defibrillator implantation, heart failure or cardiomyopathy, cardiac transplantation, congenital heart disease, as well as neuromuscular disease. When assessing the inheritance pattern, one should note that CCD often accompanies many acquired diseases. For instance, ischemic or valvular heart diseases are common causes of CCD. Age is also an important factor in interpreting family history. The prevalence of CCD greatly increases with age. In a prospective cohort study of randomly selected 855 males born in 1913 [21], the prevalence of bundle branch block increased from 1% at the age of 50 to 17% at 80 years old. Likewise, populational studies from the United States and Australia estimate the prevalence of permanent pacemaker therapy to be less than 0.5% in patients below 65 years old but higher than 2% in patients over 75 years old [22, 23]. This age-dependent prevalence is important to keep in mind when assessing the etiology of CCD in family members: In young patients, CCD is rare and more likely to be inherited, while CCD in older patients is common and more likely to be caused by senile degeneration of the conduction system. In sum, a detailed clinical review of family members with suspected CCD, including age at onset and comorbidities, is important to understand the presence and pattern of heritability and identify phenocopies.

Clinical Therapy and Follow-Up

The management of patients with CCD is aimed at alleviating symptoms and preventing SCD. No drug therapy is yet available. Pacemaker implantation is indicated in patients with symptomatic bradycardia as well as those at high risk of complete AVB and SCD. Clinical guidelines on cardiac pacing are periodically updated and published [24]. With the exception of a few locus- and disease-specific management differences (e.g., *LMNA* mutations, muscular dystrophies, discussed below), patients with suspected or established hereditary CCD are treated similarly as patients with other etiologies of CCD.

In the following situations, pacemaker implantation is recommended (Class I indication):

- Sinus node dysfunction with symptoms clearly attributed to bradycardia
- Third-degree or Mobitz type II second-degree AVB, irrespective of symptoms
- Syncope with bundle branch block and demonstration of conduction impairment below the AV node during an invasive electrophysiological study
- Alternating bundle branch block (e.g., RBBB and LBBB), irrespective of symptoms

In the following situations, pacemaker implantation should be considered (Class IIa indication):

- Mobitz type I second-degree AVB, with symptoms or invasive study showing a block below the AV node
- Syncope and demonstration of asymptomatic pauses >6 s

Because of the progressive nature of the disease, a recent expert consensus statement on inherited arrhythmia syndromes also suggests that pacemaker implantation be considered (Class IIa) in presence of bifascicular block with or without first-degree AVB [25].

Patients with manifest CCD as well as carriers of a pathogenic loss-of-function mutation in *SCN5A* should also avoid the use of medication with conduction-slowing properties, such as those listed in http://www.brugadadrugs.org [26, 27].

Since the disease is progressive, patients with CCD should be periodically assessed with ECG and review of symptoms. Longer electrocardiographic recordings such as Holter monitoring and loop recording should be considered in symptomatic patients without ECG criteria for pacemaker implantation, to detect intermittent deterioration of the conduction abnormality. Patients reporting exercise intolerance should undergo exercise testing to detect chronotropic incompetence or exercise-induced AVB. Echocardiography should also be repeated in select patients, periodically in *LMNA*, *DES*, and *SCN5A* mutation carriers and whenever there is clinical suspicion of heart failure. The frequency of follow-up should be individualized, taking into account the severity of conduction anomalies, the rate of disease progression, the presence of symptoms, and the patient's age. Patients with muscular dystrophy and CCD should be monitored more closely. Patients should be advised to consult rapidly if they have a syncopal event, to assess the need for an urgent pacemaker implantation.

Molecular Diagnostics

Genetic testing should be considered in patients with primary CCD developing at a young age (<50 years old) with or without cardiomyopathy or congenital heart disease, especially in the presence of a positive family history [28]. The optimal diagnostic strategy remains unclear. As for other conditions, one should balance the desires for getting a higher yield yet avoiding the detection of variants of unknown significance. In patients with isolated CCD, sequencing of *TRPM4* and *SCN5A* is desirable. For those with associated DCM, sequencing of *LMNA*, *DES*, and *SCN5A* should be undertaken, while patients with CCD associated with congenital heart defects such as atrial septal defects can be screened for mutations in *NKX2–5* and *TBX5*. Mutations in other genes have been identified in few families or isolated cases with CCD, with some supportive functional data. These genes often appear on next-generation sequencing (NGS) "arrhythmia" or "cardiac" panels. Data from the Netherlands suggest the yield of genetic testing in CCD (mostly limited to *SCN5A* sequencing) to be approximately 30%, with a single recurrent *SCN5A* mutation (c.2582_2583delTT) accounting for most of the cases [29]. The yield of targeted genetic testing in large diverse populations and the added value of NGS remain to be explored.

Molecular Genetics

SCN5A

Mutations in *SCN5A* causing CCD were first identified by Schott [30]. The authors reported a large French family with autosomal dominant CCD presenting with first-degree AVB, LBBB, RBBB, or complete AVB requiring pacemaker implantation, in the absence of structural heart disease. Follow-up of the family showed a progressive disease. Using a targeted linkage approach, the authors demonstrated a strong linkage to the 3p21 locus which harbors *SCN5A*. Sequencing revealed a splice site variant predicting skipping of exon 22. The authors also performed sequencing of *SCN5A* in an independent Dutch nuclear family with asymptomatic first-degree AVB, RBBB, and/or nonspecific intraventricular conduction delay and identified a frameshift variant predicting a premature stop codon and co-segregating with the phenotype. In sum, this study was the first to link CCD with *SCN5A*, which was earlier identified as a disease gene in long QT syndrome type III (LQT3) [31] and Brugada syndrome (BS) [32]. Similar to BS, *SCN5A* mutations causing CCD result in loss of function of Nav1.5, the major cardiac sodium channel responsible for cardiomyocyte depolarization. It is thus not uncommon for loss-of-function mutations to result in a mixed phenotype of BS and CCD, either in the same patient or in family members carrying the same variant. In contrast, LQT3 is caused by gain-of-function *SCN5A* mutations which result in impaired inactivation of Nav1.5 with increased late sodium current. Interestingly, mutations resulting in both a decrease in peak sodium current (loss of function) and increase in late current (gain of function) have been identified in families with CCD, BS, and LQT3 [33]. The 1795insD mutation is the best characterized example of such an *overlap syndrome* [26, 27]. *SCN5A* mutations have also been observed in families with sinus node dysfunction, atrial fibrillation, as well as DCM, emphasizing the high heterogeneity of phenotypes associated with *SCN5A* [34]. Highlighting the important role of *SCN5A* and its product Nav1.5 in normal cardiac electrical function, common variants in the *SCN5A-SCN10A* locus have been associated with PR, QRS, and QT intervals as well as BS and ST-T voltages in multiple genome-wide association studies (GWAS) [35–40].

Clinically, CCD associated with *SCN5A* mutations initially presents with a prolonged PR interval, wide QRS, as well as left axis deviation (Fig. 17.1b) which could progress to high-degree AVB. In addition to the general CCD management described in section "Clinical Therapy and Follow-up", patients with a pathogenic mutation in *SCN5A* should be counselled to avoid drugs with sodium channel blocking effects and should suppress fever, a potential trigger of arrhythmic events. Because of the possible overlap with other syndromes causing ventricular tachyarrhythmia, one should be attentive to investigate syncopal events appropriately, as these may sometimes be caused by malignant ventricular arrhythmia. While a standard pacemaker is usually the treatment of choice (when indicated; see above), some patients may benefit from an implantable cardioverter-defibrillator (ICD), especially in overlap syndromes.

TRPM4

In 2009, mutations in *TRPM4* were identified as a cause of CCD [41]. In fact, the story behind this discovery dates back to the 1960s, when Combrink et al. [1] and later Steenkamp et al. [42] described large South African families with autosomal dominant CCD manifesting as RBBB, fascicular blocks, and SCD. Later, a large Lebanese family with a similar phenotype was reported [43]. In 1995, linkage analysis in both the South African and Lebanese families mapped the CCD phenotype to chromosome 19q13.3, which includes *TRPM4* [44, 45]. Sequencing of *TRPM4* identified two different missense mutations in these families, co-segregating with the CCD phenotype [41, 46]. Mutations were also identified in an additional large French family as well as smaller families and sporadic cases with CCD [46–48]. Based on recent data from relatively small cohorts without systematic co-segregation analysis, the estimated yield of TRPM4 testing in progressive CCD is about 15% [47, 48]. Of note, the classic phenotype of *TRPM4*-related CCD is that of RBBB with or without fascicular block which progresses to complete AVB, but rarely isolated LBBB.

TRPM4 encodes a Ca^{2+}-activated non-selective cation channel predominantly expressed in Purkinje fibers. The mechanism of *TRPM4*-related CCD is attenuated deSUMOylation of the protein which results in decreased endocytosis, thus increasing channel density at the cell surface [41]. This increased cation channel density is thought to result in membrane depolarization, thus reducing the availability of Nav1.5, necessary for fast conduction in the specialized cardiac conduction system [49].

LMNA

Mutations in *LMNA* are associated with a wide spectrum of diseases, known as laminopathies. These include Hutchinson-Gilford progeria, autosomal recessive Charcot-Marie-Tooth, Emery-Dreifuss muscular dystrophy, as well as DCM preceded by or accompanied with marked CCD. LMNA-related cardiomyopathy is a progressive disease which initially presents with CCD, typically sinus bradycardia, low-voltage P waves, first-degree AVB, and initially a normal QRS (Fig. 17.1a). The disease is often accompanied by arrhythmia starting at an early stage (premature atrial complexes, atrial tachycardia or fibrillation, premature ventricular complexes, or VT). With disease progression, the patient could present with complete AVB, malignant ventricular arrhythmia or SCD, and eventually DCM with heart failure or embolic stroke. Family data suggest that CCD typically precedes DCM by a median time interval of 7 years [50]. Patients with CCD and an LMNA mutation have a high risk of developing malignant ventricular tachyarrhythmia, even if left ventricular systolic function is preserved [51, 52]. In patients with an indication for pacemaker therapy and an *LMNA* mutation, ICD implantation should thus be considered [25], especially in the presence of additional risk factors such as male sex, non-sustained VT, left ventricular ejection fraction <45%, and the presence of a non-missense mutation [53].

When no mutation is detected in *LMNA* by sequencing in a patient with a typical presentation (CCD, DCM, arrhythmia, and family history), one should consider testing for structural variants, such as a large deletion, using appropriate techniques (e.g., multiplex ligation-dependent probe amplification). Such an approach has been proven useful in some cases [54–56].

CCD Associated with Congenital Heart Defects: *NKX2–5* and *TBX5*

In 1998, Schott identified one missense and two nonsense variants in ***NKX2–5*** in four families affected with an autosomal dominant form of congenital heart defects, mostly (27 of 33 cases) secundum atrial septal defects (ASD) but also a few with other defects with or without ASD [57]. All affected individuals had CCD manifesting as various degrees of AVB. Invasive electrophysiological studies performed in three patients revealed that the site of conduction delay was the AV node, and patients who were later followed show progressive CCD. *NKX2–5* encodes a transcription factor involved in cardiac morphogenesis, specifically in septation during development, and is also important for normal function of the AV node in postnatal life. Other groups also reported mutations in *NKX2–5* in smaller families with a similar phenotype, reproducing the original findings [58].

Holt-Oram syndrome (HOS) is an autosomal dominant disease affecting the heart and hand (heart and hand syndrome) and is caused by mutations in the transcription factor ***TBX5*** in >70% of cases [59, 60]. Virtually all affected individuals have skeletal anomalies involving the radius, carpal, or hand bones, sometimes only seen on radiography. Most patients also have a congenital heart defect, typically a secundum ASD or VSD (ventricular septal defect), but more severe lesions have been reported. Patients with the syndrome are also at risk for severe progressive CCD requiring pacemaker implantation, regardless of the presence of a structural defect. The exact prevalence of CCD in HOS has not been reported. Likewise, the prevalence of pathogenic *TBX5* mutations in suspected hereditary CCD is unknown. Both missense and truncating *TBX5* variants have been associated with HOS. The mutation type and the location of missense variants have been suggested as predicting the phenotype [61]. In presence of a typical HOS and absence of mutation using sequencing, one should also consider testing for large deletions, which have been previously reported [62]. *TBX5* is critical for normal cardiac development in prenatal life, while its control of *SCN5A* expression makes it important in regulating cardiac conduction in postnatal life [63]. In addition to its involvement in HOS, GWAS identified common variations in the *TBX5* locus associated with both PR and QRS durations, again highlighting its role in normal cardiac conduction [37, 39, 64].

CCD Associated with Muscular Dystrophies: An Overview

Muscular dystrophies are a group of clinically and genetically heterogeneous inherited skeletal muscle diseases that often also affect the heart [65]. The prevalence, type, and severity of cardiac involvement depend on the specific muscular dystrophy. In the X-linked recessive *Duchenne and Becker dystrophies* caused by mutations in dystrophin (*DMD*), DCM is the predominant cardiac phenotype, and CCD is infrequent. In contrast, in the autosomal dominant *myotonic dystrophies* caused by repeat expansions in *DMPK* (type I) or *CNBP* (type II), CCD is very common and progressive, while DCM is uncommon. In myotonic dystrophy type I (Steinert's disease), the majority of patients develop

CCD. When CCD is severe (defined as non-sinus rhythm, PR > 240 ms, QRS > 120 ms, or second- or third-degree AVB), it is associated with an increased risk of SCD [66]. Interestingly, the number of CTG repeats in *DMPK* and the severity of the muscular phenotype are predictors of severe CCD. Because SCD is responsible for 30% of mortality and that CCD is thought to play a major role in the mechanism of SCD, the threshold for pacemaker implantation should be low in patients affected with this disease. While the presence of second- or third-degree AVB is a clear indication for pacemaker implantation, the optimal approach for risk stratification and prophylactic device implantation in other patients remains unclear. Some experts suggest the use of an invasive electrophysiological study. A large non-randomized study showed that an invasive electrophysiological study-guided device implant strategy was associated with increased survival, when compared to a conservative noninvasive strategy, after adjusting for baseline differences or matching using propensity scores [67]. Because of a risk of ventricular arrhythmia-mediated SCD, ICD implantation should also be considered instead of a standard pacemaker [68]. *Emery-Dreifuss muscular dystrophy* (EDMD) is a rare disease inherited as either X-linked recessive (caused by mutations in *EMD* or *FHL1*) or autosomal dominant or recessive (mutations in *LMNA*). EDMD is associated with CCD presenting with sinus bradycardia, atrial standstill, and AVB. Patients are also at risk of DCM and atrial arrhythmias with cardioembolic stroke [69]. Patients with both autosomal dominant and X-linked recessive EDMD forms are at risk, but *LMNA* mutation carriers are believed to be at higher risk to have a cardiac involvement [70]. *LMNA* mutations can also cause autosomal dominant *limb-girdle muscular dystrophy* (LGMD) type IB with a high prevalence of cardiac involvement (CCD and DCM). Other autosomal dominant and autosomal recessive subtypes of LGMD can be associated with DCM at various degrees but rarely with CCD. Other types of muscular dystrophies are rarely seen in the context of CCD or DCM.

Myofibrillar myopathy is another genetically heterogeneous neuromuscular disease associated with CCD with or without DCM. Its most common form observed in cardiogenetics is the autosomal dominant desmin-related myopathy. The latter is caused by mutation in *DES* and is characterized by isolated cardiac involvement (25%), isolated neurological involvement (25%), or both (50%) [71]. Cardiac disease consists of cardiomyopathy (mainly DCM), CCD, supraventricular arrhythmias, as well as ventricular arrhythmias including a few cases of SCD despite a pacemaker. Considering the potential risk of SCD from ventricular arrhythmias, some clinicians suggest the use of an ICD in *DES* mutation carriers with a pacemaker indication [71]. Mitochondrial disease caused by mitochondrial DNA deletion can also present with both a neuromuscular defect and CCD with or without cardiomyopathy. The *Kearns-Sayre syndrome* is the classic example, where rapidly progressive AVB is observed.

Management of patients with neuromuscular disease and CCD can be challenging given the limited available literature and the associated muscular morbidity. Given the increased risk of SCD in many of these diseases, clinical practice guidelines suggest a more aggressive approach than with other CCD patients. For instance, permanent pacemaker implantation may be considered for myotonic dystrophy and limb-girdle muscular dystrophy, with any degree of AV block (including first-degree AV block) or bifascicular block, with or without symptoms [72]. Such an aggressive approach based on little clinical data does not make a consensus among experts [24].

Other CCD Genes

Loss-of-function mutations in ***HCN4***, which encodes the major pacemaker channel protein in humans, have been identified in patients and families with sinus node dysfunction, sometimes in association with paroxysmal atrial fibrillation [73, 74]. The severity of the phenotype is highly variable and sometimes benign with isolated asymptomatic sinus bradycardia in a whole family [75]. Recently, loss-of-function mutations were identified in four families with sinus bradycardia in combination with left ventricular non-compaction cardiomyopathy [76] and mild aortic dilatation [77]. Of interest, a gain-of-function mutation in *HCN4* was identified in a familial form of inappropriate sinus tachycardia [78].

The cardiac voltage-gated sodium channel (Nav1.5) is part of a protein complex composed of the α-subunit (encoded by *SCN5A*), as well as β-subunits (e.g., *SCN1B*) and ancillary proteins. Following the association of *SCN5A* with CCD and BS, a candidate gene sequencing study identified mutations in ***SCN1B*** in three small pedigrees affected by CCD with or without BS [79]. The investigators performed functional studies showing that co-expression of *SCN5A* with the mutant *SCN1B* resulted in a decreased sodium current as compared to co-expression of both wild-type proteins. Although these functional data are supportive, the lack of robust human genetic data (three small pedigrees and lack of convincing validation studies) makes one question the role of *SCN1B* in CCD.

The fast propagation of the electrical impulse in the His-Purkinje system depends on the availability of Nav1.5 and also high-conductance gap junctional channels. In a 6-year-old boy with CCD (LBBB and second-degree AVB) who later died suddenly, Makita et al. [80] identified a missense variant in ***GJA5***, which encodes the high-conductance gap junctional channel subunit connexin40. The variant was also present in his mother with documented CCD (LBBB) who later had a SCD, as well as in his 4-year-old sister with a QRS duration at the upper limit of normal. Expression of the mutant proteins showed a reduction in junctional conductance compared to wild-type connexin40. Somatic *GJA5* mutations in left atrial DNA have also been previously identified in patients with atrial fibrillation [81], although this finding was not reproduced in a larger cohort [82] (see Chap. 15 for discussion).

Recently, using linkage analysis and whole-exome sequencing, two groups identified missense variants in ***TNNI3K*** in families with supraventricular tachyarrhythmia and CCD, sometimes associated with DCM [83, 84]. *TNNI3K* encodes for the troponin I-interacting kinase, a cardiac-specific kinase that was previously implicated in atrioventricular conduction in mice [85]. The pathophysiological mechanism implicating *TNNI3K* in arrhythmogenesis is an area of active investigation.

In 2001, Gollob identified missense mutations in ***PRKAG2*** in families with CCD and ventricular pre-excitation with or without cardiac hypertrophy [86, 87]. Multiple families with mutations in *PRKAG2* and an identical phenotype have been identified since then. Sequencing of this gene should be performed in presence of CCD in association with ventricular pre-excitation and/or cardiac hypertrophy. *PRKAG2* encodes the gamma2 regulatory subunit of AMP-activated protein kinase which is part of the AMP-activated protein kinase complex involved in cardiomyocyte metabolism and energetics.

Family Screening

Given the limited long-term data available on familial CCD, it is difficult to recommend a detailed family screening and follow-up algorithm. Instead, the clinician should adapt the follow-up plan to each patient and family. Below are some points for guidance depending on whether a pathogenic variant is identified and whether the disease is familial or sporadic.

When a pathogenic mutation is identified in the proband, cascade screening using mutation analysis in family members is recommended [28]. Mutation carriers should have a complete baseline cardiological evaluation, consisting of a review of symptoms, physical evaluation, ECG, and echocardiography. Exercise testing, Holter monitoring, and loop recoding are suggested if the patient reports any intermittent symptom. Given the progressive nature of the disease, mutation carriers need to be periodically evaluated (e.g., every 1–3 years) depending on age and the extent of ECG abnormalities, if present. Follow-up evaluation should include a review of symptoms and ECG. For patients with *LMNA* mutations, repeating the echocardiogram every 1–2 years is suggested. Patients should be advised to seek urgent medical attention if they present a syncopal event. Family members that do not carry the mutation can be reassured, unless the pathogenicity of the variant is questionable. A baseline ECG is encouraged, while a more extensive evaluation should be performed if symptoms develop.

In genetically elusive unexplained CCD in a young patient without a clear familial disease, a baseline ECG should be performed in first-degree relatives. If the proband also has structural heart disease, an echocardiogram should also be performed in first-degree relatives. If the baseline evaluation is normal, the patient can be discharged from cardiological care and instructed to consult if symptoms develop (e.g., presyncope, syncope, exercise intolerance). If the baseline evaluation is abnormal, the patient should be treated accordingly and periodically followed.

In genetically elusive CCD with a clear familial disease, advanced genetic testing (e.g., whole-exome sequencing, large sequencing gene panel, targeted deletion assays) with appropriate co-segregation analysis should be considered, recognizing that the yield is likely to be low. Clinical screening of first-degree relatives should be performed as above. However, if the baseline evaluation is normal, it is probably prudent to follow up the patients periodically for a long-term, unless the disease onset in affected family members is at a young age.

Summary and Take-Home Messages

- Cardiac conduction disease (CCD) is a clinically heterogeneous disorder involving genetic and non-genetic etiologies.
- A genetic etiology and genetic testing should be considered in presence of a family history of CCD, cardiomyopathy, or congenital heart disease as well as in young patients (<50 years old) with unexplained severe sporadic CCD.
- Isolated CCD can be caused by mutations in *SCN5A* or *TRPM4*.
- CCD in association with dilated cardiomyopathy (DCM) can be caused by *LMNA* and *DES* mutations. Patients with such mutations and severe CCD are also at risk of ventricular arrhythmia. Implantable cardioverter-defibrillator (ICD) therapy should be considered in such cases.
- CCD in association with congenital heart disease can be caused by mutations in *NKX2–5* and *TBX5*. The latter is invariably associated with upper limb skeletal anomalies (Holt-Oram syndrome).
- CCD in association with ventricular pre-excitation or unexplained cardiac hypertrophy is suggestive for mutations in *PRKAG2*.

- *TNNI3K* is a novel CCD gene with heterogeneous phenotypic manifestations including supraventricular and ventricular tachyarrhythmias and cardiomyopathy.
- CCD can accompany some muscular dystrophies (e.g., myotonic dystrophy, Emery-Dreifuss muscular dystrophy, limb-girdle muscular dystrophy type IB). In these cases, aggressive therapy with a pacemaker or ICD can be considered in early stages.
- Device therapy is the only available treatment for hereditary CCD. The decision to implant a device usually follows the same principles as with other causes of CCD, with the exceptions mentioned above.
- Family screening with genetic testing and/or phenotypic testing is recommended in established or suspected hereditary CCD.

References

1. Combrink JM, Davis WH, Snyman HW. Familial bundle branch block. Am Heart J. 1962;64:397–400.
2. Harbison J, Newton JL, Seifer C, Kenny RA. Stokes Adams attacks and cardiovascular syncope. Lancet. 2002;359(9301):158–60.
3. van den Heuvel GCJ. Die ziekte van Stokes-Adams en een geval van aangeboren hartblok 1908.
4. Gourraud JB, Kyndt F, Fouchard S, Rendu E, Jaafar P, Gully C, et al. Identification of a strong genetic background for progressive cardiac conduction defect by epidemiological approach. Heart. 2012;98(17):1305–10.
5. Lynch HT, Mohiuddin S, Sketch MH, Krush AJ, Carter S, Runco V. Hereditary progressive atrioventricular conduction defect. A new syndrome? JAMA. 1973;225(12):1465–70.
6. Lynch RJ, Engle MA. Familial congenital complete heart block. Its occurrence in 2 children with another genetically determined anomaly. Am J Dis Child. 1961;102:210–7.
7. Morquio L. Sur une maladie infantile caractérisée par des modifications permanentes du pouls, des attaques syncopales et épileptiformes. Arch Med Enfants. 1901;4:467–75.
8. Tresch DD, Fleg JL. Unexplained sinus bradycardia: clinical significance and long-term prognosis in apparently healthy persons older than 40 years. Am J Cardiol. 1986;58(10):1009–13.
9. Aro AL, Anttonen O, Kerola T, Junttila MJ, Tikkanen JT, Rissanen HA, et al. Prognostic significance of prolonged PR interval in the general population. Eur Heart J. 2014;35(2):123–9.
10. Strasberg B, Amat YLF, Dhingra RC, Palileo E, Swiryn S, Bauernfeind R, et al. Natural history of chronic second-degree atrioventricular nodal block. Circulation. 1981;63(5):1043–9.
11. Dhingra RC, Denes P, Wu D, Chuquimia R, Rosen KM. The significance of second degree atrioventricular block and bundle branch block. Observations regarding site and type of block. Circulation. 1974;49(4):638–46.
12. Xiong Y, Wang L, Liu W, Hankey GJ, Xu B, Wang S. The prognostic significance of right bundle branch block: a meta-analysis of prospective cohort studies. Clin Cardiol. 2015;38(10):604–13.
13. Fahy GJ, Pinski SL, Miller DP, McCabe N, Pye C, Walsh MJ, et al. Natural history of isolated bundle branch block. Am J Cardiol. 1996;77(14):1185–90.
14. Rotman M, Triebwasser JH. A clinical and follow-up study of right and left bundle branch block. Circulation. 1975;51(3):477–84.
15. Badheka AO, Singh V, Patel NJ, Deshmukh A, Shah N, Chothani A, et al. QRS duration on electrocardiography and cardiovascular mortality (from the National Health and nutrition examination survey-III). Am J Cardiol. 2013;112(5):671–7.
16. Eriksson P, Wilhelmsen L, Rosengren A. Bundle-branch block in middle-aged men: risk of complications and death over 28 years. The primary prevention study in Goteborg, Sweden. Eur Heart J. 2005;26(21):2300–6.
17. Zhang ZM, Rautaharju PM, Soliman EZ, Manson JE, Cain ME, Martin LW, et al. Mortality risk associated with bundle branch blocks and related repolarization abnormalities (from the Women's Health Initiative [WHI]). Am J Cardiol. 2012;110(10):1489–95.
18. Kandolin R, Lehtonen J, Kupari M. Cardiac sarcoidosis and giant cell myocarditis as causes of atrioventricular block in young and middle-aged adults. Circ Arrhythm Electrophysiol. 2011;4(3):303–9.
19. Nery PB, Beanlands RS, Nair GM, Green M, Yang J, McArdle BA, et al. Atrioventricular block as the initial manifestation of cardiac sarcoidosis in middle-aged adults. J Cardiovasc Electrophysiol. 2014;25(8):875–81.
20. Steere AC, Batsford WP, Weinberg M, Alexander J, Berger HJ, Wolfson S, et al. Lyme carditis: cardiac abnormalities of Lyme disease. Ann Intern Med. 1980;93(1):8–16.
21. Eriksson P, Hansson PO, Eriksson H, Dellborg M. Bundle-branch block in a general male population: the study of men born 1913. Circulation. 1998;98(22):2494–500.
22. Bradshaw PJ, Stobie P, Knuiman MW, Briffa TG, Hobbs MS. Trends in the incidence and prevalence of cardiac pacemaker insertions in an ageing population. Open Heart. 2014;1(1):e000177.
23. Silverman BG, Gross TP, Kaczmarek RG, Hamilton P, Hamburger S. The epidemiology of pacemaker implantation in the United States. Public Health Rep. 1995;110(1):42–6.
24. Brignole M, Auricchio A, Baron-Esquivias G, Bordachar P, Boriani G, Breithardt OA, et al. 2013 ESC guidelines on cardiac pacing and cardiac resynchronization therapy: the task force on cardiac pacing and resynchronization therapy of the European Society of Cardiology (ESC). Developed in collaboration with the European heart rhythm association (EHRA). Eur Heart J. 2013;34(29):2281–329.
25. Priori SG, Wilde AA, Horie M, Cho Y, Behr ER, Berul C, et al. Executive summary: HRS/EHRA/APHRS expert consensus statement on the diagnosis and management of patients with inherited primary arrhythmia syndromes. Europace. 2013;15(10):1389–406.
26. Postema PG, Van den Berg M, Van Tintelen JP, Van den Heuvel F, Grundeken M, Hofman N, et al. Founder mutations in the Netherlands: SCN5a 1795insD, the first described arrhythmia overlap syndrome and one of the largest and best characterised families worldwide. Neth Heart J. 2009a;17(11):422–8.
27. Postema PG, Wolpert C, Amin AS, Probst V, Borggrefe M, Roden DM, et al. Drugs and Brugada syndrome patients: review of the literature, recommendations, and an up-to-date website (www.brugadadrugs.org/). Heart Rhythm. 2009b;6(9):1335–41.
28. Ackerman MJ, Priori SG, Willems S, Berul C, Brugada R, Calkins H, et al. HRS/EHRA expert consensus statement on the state of genetic testing for the channelopathies and cardiomyopathies: this document was developed as a partnership between the Heart Rhythm Society (HRS) and the European heart rhythm association (EHRA). Europace. 2011;13(8):1077–109.
29. Hofman N, Tan HL, Alders M, Kolder I, de Haij S, Mannens MM, et al. Yield of molecular and clinical testing for arrhythmia syndromes: report of 15 years' experience. Circulation. 2013;128(14):1513–21.
30. Schott JJ, Alshinawi C, Kyndt F, Probst V, Hoorntje TM, Hulsbeek M, et al. Cardiac conduction defects associate with mutations in SCN5A. Nat Genet. 1999;23(1):20–1.
31. Wang Q, Shen J, Splawski I, Atkinson D, Li Z, Robinson JL, et al. SCN5A mutations associated with an inherited cardiac arrhythmia, long QT syndrome. Cell. 1995;80(5):805–11.

32. Chen Q, Kirsch GE, Zhang D, Brugada R, Brugada J, Brugada P, et al. Genetic basis and molecular mechanism for idiopathic ventricular fibrillation. Nature. 1998;392(6673):293–6.
33. Remme CA, Verkerk AO, Nuyens D, van Ginneken AC, van Brunschot S, Belterman CN, et al. Overlap syndrome of cardiac sodium channel disease in mice carrying the equivalent mutation of human SCN5A-1795insD. Circulation. 2006;114(24):2584–94.
34. Veerman CC, Wilde AA, Lodder EM. The cardiac sodium channel gene SCN5A and its gene product NaV1.5: role in physiology and pathophysiology. Gene. 2015;573(2):177–87.
35. Arking DE, Pulit SL, Crotti L, van der Harst P, Munroe PB, Koopmann TT, et al. Genetic association study of QT interval highlights role for calcium signaling pathways in myocardial repolarization. Nat Genet. 2014;46(8):826–36.
36. Bezzina CR, Barc J, Mizusawa Y, Remme CA, Gourraud JB, Simonet F, et al. Common variants at SCN5A-SCN10A and HEY2 are associated with Brugada syndrome, a rare disease with high risk of sudden cardiac death. Nat Genet. 2013;45(9):1044–9.
37. Holm H, Gudbjartsson DF, Arnar DO, Thorleifsson G, Thorgeirsson G, Stefansdottir H, et al. Several common variants modulate heart rate, PR interval and QRS duration. Nat Genet. 2010;42(2):117–22.
38. Pfeufer A, van Noord C, Marciante KD, Arking DE, Larson MG, Smith AV, et al. Genome-wide association study of PR interval. Nat Genet. 2010;42(2):153–9.
39. Sotoodehnia N, Isaacs A, de Bakker PI, Dorr M, Newton-Cheh C, Nolte IM, et al. Common variants in 22 loci are associated with QRS duration and cardiac ventricular conduction. Nat Genet. 2010;42(12):1068–76.
40. Verweij N, Mateo Leach I, Isaacs A, Arking DE, Bis JC, Pers TH, et al. Twenty-eight genetic loci associated with ST-T wave amplitudes of the electrocardiogram. Hum Mol Genet. 2016;25(10):2093–103.
41. Kruse M, Schulze-Bahr E, Corfield V, Beckmann A, Stallmeyer B, Kurtbay G, et al. Impaired endocytosis of the ion channel TRPM4 is associated with human progressive familial heart block type I. J Clin Invest. 2009;119(9):2737–44.
42. Steenkamp WF. Familial trifascicular block. Am Heart J. 1972;84(6):758–60.
43. Stephan E. Hereditary bundle branch system defect: survey of a family with four affected generations. Am Heart J. 1978;95(1):89–95.
44. Brink PA, Ferreira A, Moolman JC, Weymar HW, van der Merwe PL, Corfield VA. Gene for progressive familial heart block type I maps to chromosome 19q13. Circulation. 1995;91(6):1633–40.
45. de Meeus A, Stephan E, Debrus S, Jean MK, Loiselet J, Weissenbach J, et al. An isolated cardiac conduction disease maps to chromosome 19q. Circ Res. 1995;77(4):735–40.
46. Liu H, El Zein L, Kruse M, Guinamard R, Beckmann A, Bozio A, et al. Gain-of-function mutations in TRPM4 cause autosomal dominant isolated cardiac conduction disease. Circ Cardiovasc Genet. 2010;3(4):374–85.
47. Daumy X, Amarouch MY, Lindenbaum P, Bonnaud S, Charpentier E, Bianchi B, et al. Targeted resequencing identifies TRPM4 as a major gene predisposing to progressive familial heart block type I. Int J Cardiol. 2016;207:349–58.
48. Stallmeyer B, Zumhagen S, Denjoy I, Duthoit G, Hebert JL, Ferrer X, et al. Mutational spectrum in the Ca(2+)--activated cation channel gene TRPM4 in patients with cardiac conductance disturbances. Hum Mutat. 2012;33(1):109–17.
49. Abriel H, Syam N, Sottas V, Amarouch MY, Rougier JS. TRPM4 channels in the cardiovascular system: physiology, pathophysiology, and pharmacology. Biochem Pharmacol. 2012;84(7):873–81.
50. Brodt C, Siegfried JD, Hofmeyer M, Martel J, Rampersaud E, Li D, et al. Temporal relationship of conduction system disease and ventricular dysfunction in LMNA cardiomyopathy. J Card Fail. 2013;19(4):233–9.
51. Anselme F, Moubarak G, Savoure A, Godin B, Borz B, Drouin-Garraud V, et al. Implantable cardioverter-defibrillators in Lamin a/C mutation carriers with cardiac conduction disorders. Heart Rhythm. 2013;10(10):1492–8.
52. Hasselberg NE, Edvardsen T, Petri H, Berge KE, Leren TP, Bundgaard H, et al. Risk prediction of ventricular arrhythmias and myocardial function in Lamin a/C mutation positive subjects. Europace. 2014;16(4):563–71.
53. van Rijsingen IA, Arbustini E, Elliott PM, Mogensen J, Hermans-van Ast JF, van der Kooi AJ, et al. Risk factors for malignant ventricular arrhythmias in Lamin a/c mutation carriers a European cohort study. J Am Coll Cardiol. 2012;59(5):493–500.
54. Gupta P, Bilinska ZT, Sylvius N, Boudreau E, Veinot JP, Labib S, et al. Genetic and ultrastructural studies in dilated cardiomyopathy patients: a large deletion in the Lamin a/C gene is associated with cardiomyocyte nuclear envelope disruption. Basic Res Cardiol. 2010;105(3):365–77.
55. Marsman RF, Bardai A, Postma AV, Res JC, Koopmann TT, Beekman L, et al. A complex double deletion in LMNA underlies progressive cardiac conduction disease, atrial arrhythmias, and sudden death. Circ Cardiovasc Genet. 2011;4(3):280–7.
56. van Tintelen JP, Tio RA, Kerstjens-Frederikse WS, van Berlo JH, Boven LG, et al. Severe myocardial fibrosis caused by a deletion of the 5′ end of the Lamin a/C gene. J Am Coll Cardiol. 2007;49(25):2430–9.
57. Schott JJ, Benson DW, Basson CT, Pease W, Silberbach GM, Moak JP, et al. Congenital heart disease caused by mutations in the transcription factor NKX2-5. Science. 1998;281(5373):108–11.
58. Stallmeyer B, Fenge H, Nowak-Gottl U, Schulze-Bahr E. Mutational spectrum in the cardiac transcription factor gene NKX2.5 (CSX) associated with congenital heart disease. Clin Genet. 2010;78(6):533–40.
59. Basson CT, Bachinsky DR, Lin RC, Levi T, Elkins JA, Soults J, et al. Mutations in human TBX5 [corrected] cause limb and cardiac malformation in Holt-Oram syndrome. Nat Genet. 1997;15(1):30–5.
60. McDermott DA, Fong JC, Basson CT. Holt-oram syndrome. In: Pagon RA, Adam MP, Ardinger HH, Wallace SE, Amemiya A, LJH B, et al., editors. GeneReviews(R). Seattle (WA): University of Washington; 1993.
61. Basson CT, Huang T, Lin RC, Bachinsky DR, Weremowicz S, Vaglio A, et al. Different TBX5 interactions in heart and limb defined by Holt-Oram syndrome mutations. Proc Natl Acad Sci U S A. 1999;96(6):2919–24.
62. Borozdin W, Bravo Ferrer Acosta AM, Bamshad MJ, Botzenhart EM, Froster UG, Lemke J, et al. Expanding the spectrum of TBX5 mutations in Holt-Oram syndrome: detection of two intragenic deletions by quantitative real time PCR, and report of eight novel point mutations. Hum Mutat. 2006;27(9):975–6.
63. Arnolds DE, Liu F, Fahrenbach JP, Kim GH, Schillinger KJ, Smemo S, et al. TBX5 drives Scn5a expression to regulate cardiac conduction system function. J Clin Invest. 2012;122(7):2509–18.
64. den Hoed M, Eijgelsheim M, Esko T, Brundel BJ, Peal DS, Evans DM, et al. Identification of heart rate-associated loci and their effects on cardiac conduction and rhythm disorders. Nat Genet. 2013;45(6):621–31.
65. Groh WJ. Arrhythmias in the muscular dystrophies. Heart Rhythm. 2012;9(11):1890–5.
66. Groh WJ, Groh MR, Saha C, Kincaid JC, Simmons Z, Ciafaloni E, et al. Electrocardiographic abnormalities and sudden death in myotonic dystrophy type 1. N Engl J Med. 2008;358(25):2688–97.
67. Wahbi K, Meune C, Porcher R, Becane HM, Lazarus A, Laforet P, et al. Electrophysiological study with prophylactic pacing and survival in adults with myotonic dystrophy and conduction system disease. JAMA. 2012;307(12):1292–301.
68. Bhakta D, Shen C, Kron J, Epstein AE, Pascuzzi RM, Groh WJ. Pacemaker and implantable cardioverter-defibrillator use

in a US myotonic dystrophy type 1 population. J Cardiovasc Electrophysiol. 2011;22(12):1369–75.
69. Boriani G, Gallina M, Merlini L, Bonne G, Toniolo D, Amati S, et al. Clinical relevance of atrial fibrillation/flutter, stroke, pacemaker implant, and heart failure in Emery-Dreifuss muscular dystrophy: a long-term longitudinal study. Stroke. 2003;34(4):901–8.
70. Bonne G, Leturcq F, Ben YR. Emery-dreifuss muscular dystrophy. In: Pagon RA, Adam MP, Ardinger HH, Wallace SE, Amemiya A, LJH B, et al., editors. GeneReviews(R). Seattle (WA): University of Washington; 1993.
71. van Spaendonck-Zwarts KY, van Hessem L, Jongbloed JD, de Walle HE, Capetanaki Y, van der Kooi AJ, et al. Desmin-related myopathy. Clin Genet. 2011;80(4):354–66.
72. Epstein AE, DiMarco JP, Ellenbogen KA, Estes NA 3rd, Freedman RA, Gettes LS, et al. 2012 ACCF/AHA/HRS focused update incorporated into the ACCF/AHA/HRS 2008 guidelines for device-based therapy of cardiac rhythm abnormalities: a report of the American College of Cardiology Foundation/American Heart Association task force on practice guidelines and the Heart Rhythm Society. J Am Coll Cardiol. 2013;61(3):e6–75.
73. Milanesi R, Baruscotti M, Gnecchi-Ruscone T, DiFrancesco D. Familial sinus bradycardia associated with a mutation in the cardiac pacemaker channel. N Engl J Med. 2006;354(2):151–7.
74. Schulze-Bahr E, Neu A, Friederich P, Kaupp UB, Breithardt G, Pongs O, et al. Pacemaker channel dysfunction in a patient with sinus node disease. J Clin Invest. 2003;111(10):1537–45.
75. Nof E, Luria D, Brass D, Marek D, Lahat H, Reznik-Wolf H, et al. Point mutation in the HCN4 cardiac ion channel pore affecting synthesis, trafficking, and functional expression is associated with familial asymptomatic sinus bradycardia. Circulation. 2007;116(5):463–70.
76. Milano A, Vermeer AM, Lodder EM, Barc J, Verkerk AO, Postma AV, et al. HCN4 mutations in multiple families with bradycardia and left ventricular noncompaction cardiomyopathy. J Am Coll Cardiol. 2014;64(8):745–56.
77. Vermeer AM, Lodder EM, Thomas D, Duijkers FA, Marcelis C, van Gorselen EO, et al. Dilation of the aorta ascendens forms part of the clinical spectrum of HCN4 mutations. J Am Coll Cardiol. 2016;67(19):2313–5.
78. Baruscotti M, Bucchi A, Milanesi R, Paina M, Barbuti A, Gnecchi-Ruscone T, et al. A gain-of-function mutation in the cardiac pacemaker HCN4 channel increasing cAMP sensitivity is associated with familial inappropriate sinus tachycardia. Eur Heart J. 2015;38(4):280–8.
79. Watanabe H, Koopmann TT, Le Scouarnec S, Yang T, Ingram CR, Schott JJ, et al. Sodium channel beta1 subunit mutations associated with Brugada syndrome and cardiac conduction disease in humans. J Clin Invest. 2008;118(6):2260–8.
80. Makita N, Seki A, Sumitomo N, Chkourko H, Fukuhara S, Watanabe H, et al. A connexin40 mutation associated with a malignant variant of progressive familial heart block type I. Circ Arrhythm Electrophysiol. 2012;5(1):163–72.
81. Gollob MH, Jones DL, Krahn AD, Danis L, Gong XQ, Shao Q, et al. Somatic mutations in the connexin 40 gene (GJA5) in atrial fibrillation. N Engl J Med. 2006;354(25):2677–88.
82. Roberts JD, Longoria J, Poon A, Gollob MH, Dewland TA, Kwok PY, et al. Targeted deep sequencing reveals no definitive evidence for somatic mosaicism in atrial fibrillation. Circ Cardiovasc Genet. 2015;8(1):50–7.
83. Theis JL, Zimmermann MT, Larsen BT, Rybakova IN, Long PA, Evans JM, et al. TNNI3K mutation in familial syndrome of conduction system disease, atrial tachyarrhythmia and dilated cardiomyopathy. Hum Mol Genet. 2014;23(21):5793–804.
84. Xi Y, Honeywell C, Zhang D, Schwartzentruber J, Beaulieu CL, Tetreault M, et al. Whole exome sequencing identifies the TNNI3K gene as a cause of familial conduction system disease and congenital junctional ectopic tachycardia. Int J Cardiol. 2015;185:114–6.
85. Lodder EM, Scicluna BP, Milano A, Sun AY, Tang H, Remme CA, et al. Dissection of a quantitative trait locus for PR interval duration identifies Tnni3k as a novel modulator of cardiac conduction. PLoS Genet. 2012;8(12):e1003113.
86. Gollob MH, Green MS, Tang AS, Gollob T, Karibe A, Ali Hassan AS, et al. Identification of a gene responsible for familial Wolff-Parkinson-white syndrome. N Engl J Med. 2001a;344(24):1823–31.
87. Gollob MH, Seger JJ, Gollob TN, Tapscott T, Gonzales O, Bachinski L, et al. Novel PRKAG2 mutation responsible for the genetic syndrome of ventricular preexcitation and conduction system disease with childhood onset and absence of cardiac hypertrophy. Circulation. 2001b;104(25):3030–3.

A Molecular Genetic Perspective on Atrial Fibrillation

18

Jason D. Roberts and Michael H. Gollob

Introduction

Atrial fibrillation (AF), the most common sustained cardiac arrhythmia, is a source of significant morbidity and mortality predominantly through its sequelae of heart failure and stroke. Despite its prevalence and clinical significance, its pathophysiology remains incompletely understood, and treatment strategies remain relatively ineffective. In recent years, the importance of *genetics* in predisposing to AF has been clearly recognized, and in a remarkably short time period, there have been a flurry of landmark discoveries. Insight into the molecular genetics of this condition promises to lead to more effective forms of therapy that will help reduce the burden currently carried by patients and healthcare systems (Table 18.1).

Epidemiology

AF represents the most common cardiac arrhythmia and affects well over two million Americans [1]. Its prevalence increases with age and ranges from less than 0.5% in those aged less than 55 to 9% in octogenarians [2]. Because of the advancing age of Western populations, its incidence is expected to increase over the coming years and has been projected to affect as many as 16 million Americans by 2050 [3]. AF independently increases the risk of mortality with an age-adjusted odds ratio for death of 1.9 in females and 1.5 in males; however, its sequelae of stroke and heart failure represent the greatest sources of morbidity and mortality [4].

J. D. Roberts
Arrhythmia Service, Division of Cardiology, University of Western Ontario, London, ON, Canada
e-mail: jason.roberts@lhsc.on.ca

M. H. Gollob (✉)
Inherited Arrhythmia and Cardiomyopathy Program, Peter Munk Cardiac Centre, Division of Cardiology, Toronto General Hospital, University of Toronto, Toronto, ON, Canada
e-mail: michael.gollob@uhn.ca

Accounting for a large proportion of strokes in the elderly, AF has been estimated to cost the American healthcare system over US $6.5 billion annually [5, 6]. Its burden on the global population, in terms of both health and healthcare dollars, will likely only get worse in the coming years as populations age. This is further exacerbated by the current lack of highly effective therapies for this exceedingly common condition.

In addition to advancing age, structural heart disease also represents a major risk factor for AF [7]. However, approximately 10–20% of cases of AF occur in the absence of known risk factors and have been termed *lone AF* [8]. Without obvious contributing factors, genetics have been hypothesized to play an important role in the development of this form of the arrhythmia. Indeed, a family with lone AF transmitted with an autosomal dominant pattern of inheritance was first documented by Wolff in 1943 [9]. A study of siblings found that brothers and sisters of patients with lone AF have a 70-fold and 34-fold increased risk of developing the arrhythmia relative to the general population, respectively [10]. Further support for AF being a heritable arrhythmia has come from large population-based studies. Analyses from the Framingham Heart Study and Iceland have shown that presence of AF in a first-degree relative is associated with a marked increased risk of developing the arrhythmia and conferred an increased risk for development of the arrhythmia in their offspring (odds ratio of 1.85) [11–13].

Molecular Background

AF reflects a disturbance of the electrical activity within the top chambers of the heart. Transmission of electrical impulses within the heart occurs through *ion channels*, pore-forming proteins present within the plasma membranes of cardiomyocytes [14]. There are a variety of different types of cardiac ion channels, each of which contributes to the cardiac action potential. The two major types of cardiomyocytes within the heart include pacemaker cells and car-

H. F. Baars et al. (eds.), *Clinical Cardiogenetics*, https://doi.org/10.1007/978-3-030-45457-9_18

Table 18.1 The genes associated with atrial fibrillation and the putative mechanisms leading to the arrhythmia

Gene	Study method	Mode of inheritance	Protein and function	Functional effect of mutation	Mechanism for AF
Potassium channels					
KCNQ1	Linkage analysis	Autosomal dominant	α-Subunit of I_{Ks}	Gain of function	Reduced atrial ERP/APD
KCNH2[a]	Candidate gene approach	Autosomal dominant	α-Subunit of I_{Kr}	Gain of function	Reduced atrial ERP/APD
KCNE2	Candidate gene approach	Autosomal dominant	β-Subunit of background potassium current	Gain of function	Reduced atrial ERP/APD
KCNJ2	Candidate gene approach	Autosomal dominant	$K_{ir}2.1$ responsible for I_{K1}	Gain of function	Reduced atrial ERP/APD
KCNA5	Candidate gene approach	Autosomal dominant	$K_v1.5$ responsible for I_{Kur}	Loss of function	Prolonged atrial ERP/APD
Connexins					
GJA5	Candidate gene approach	Sporadic and autosomal dominant	Connexin 40 responsible for cell coupling	Loss of function	Conduction velocity dispersion
Sodium channels					
SCN5A	Candidate gene approach	Autosomal dominant	$Na_v1.5$ responsible for I_{Na}	Loss of function	Prolonged atrial ERP/APD
		Autosomal dominant		Gain of function	Cellular hyperexcitability
Circulating hormones					
NPPA	Linkage analysis	Autosomal dominant	Atrial natriuretic peptide	Unknown	Unknown
Atrial sarcomeric proteins					
MYL4	Exome sequencing	Autosomal dominant	Myosin light chain 4	Loss of function	Atrial myopathy
Unknown loci					
10q22–24	Linkage analysis	Autosomal dominant	Unknown	Unknown	Unknown
6q14–16	Linkage analysis	Autosomal dominant	Unknown	Unknown	Unknown
10p11–q21	Linkage analysis	Autosomal dominant	Unknown	Unknown	Unknown
5p15	Linkage analysis	Autosomal dominant	Unknown	Unknown	Unknown

[a]Identified as a familial cause of atrial fibrillation in the context of short QT syndrome. *ERP* effective refractory period, *APD* action potential duration

diac muscle cells, each with its own distinct *action potential* [14]. The action potential for the cardiac muscle cell is designed to allow for rapid conduction of electrical impulses. In contrast, cardiac pacemaker cells are endowed with a property termed intrinsic automaticity, which allows these cells to function as pacemakers within the heart. The action potential of the cardiac muscle cell will be the main focus of this discussion.

Figure 18.1 depicts the action potential of the cardiac muscle cell, which is divided into five phases. Phase 0 reflects the rapid depolarizing upstroke that occurs secondary to rapid sodium influx into cells and is referred to as I_{Na}. It is mediated by a *voltage-gated sodium channel*, termed $Na_v1.5$, which is the protein product of the *SCN5A* gene [15]. The rapid upstroke, reflective of the rapid flow of current, endows these cells with an ability to transmit electrical impulses with a high conduction velocity. Phase 1 involves a transient current of *repolarization*, termed I_{to}, that occurs secondary to an efflux of potassium ions from the cell. Phase 2, also referred to as the plateau or dome phase, reflects a balance of inward calcium current and outward potassium current [14]. Flow of calcium occurs through voltage-gated L-type calcium channels. The calcium influx during phase 2 not only plays a critical role in the kinetics of the cardiac action potential but is also important in excitation-contraction coupling [16].

Repolarization is mediated by a current that arises secondary to the flow of potassium ions out of the cell. Referred to as the delayed rectifier potassium current, it is divided into three different components on the basis of timing. The first, termed the *ultrarapid component of the delayed rectifier potassium current* (I_{Kur}), is unique to the atria and is felt to be mediated by Kv1.5, a voltage-gated potassium channel encoded by *KCNA5* [18, 19]. Following I_{Kur} is the *rapid component of the delayed rectifier potassium current* (I_{Kr}) that involves the gene products of both *KCNH2* (HERG) and *KCNE2* [20]. Lastly, there is the *slow component of the delayed rectifier potassium current* (I_{Ks}), which involves the gene products of both *KCNQ1* and *KCNE1* [21]. Although I_{Kur} only is exclusive to the atria, I_{Kr} and I_{Ks} are present in both the atria and the ventricles [22].

Phase 4 reflects a resting phase whose properties are in part modulated by the cardiac *inward rectifier potassium current*, or $\boldsymbol{I_{K1}}$, mediated by Kir2.1 and encoded by the *KCNJ2* gene [23]. Although I_{K1} is voltage-gated, its activity differs markedly relative to the previously mentioned voltage-gated potassium channels involved in phase 3. While the delayed rectifier potassium current is triggered by cellular

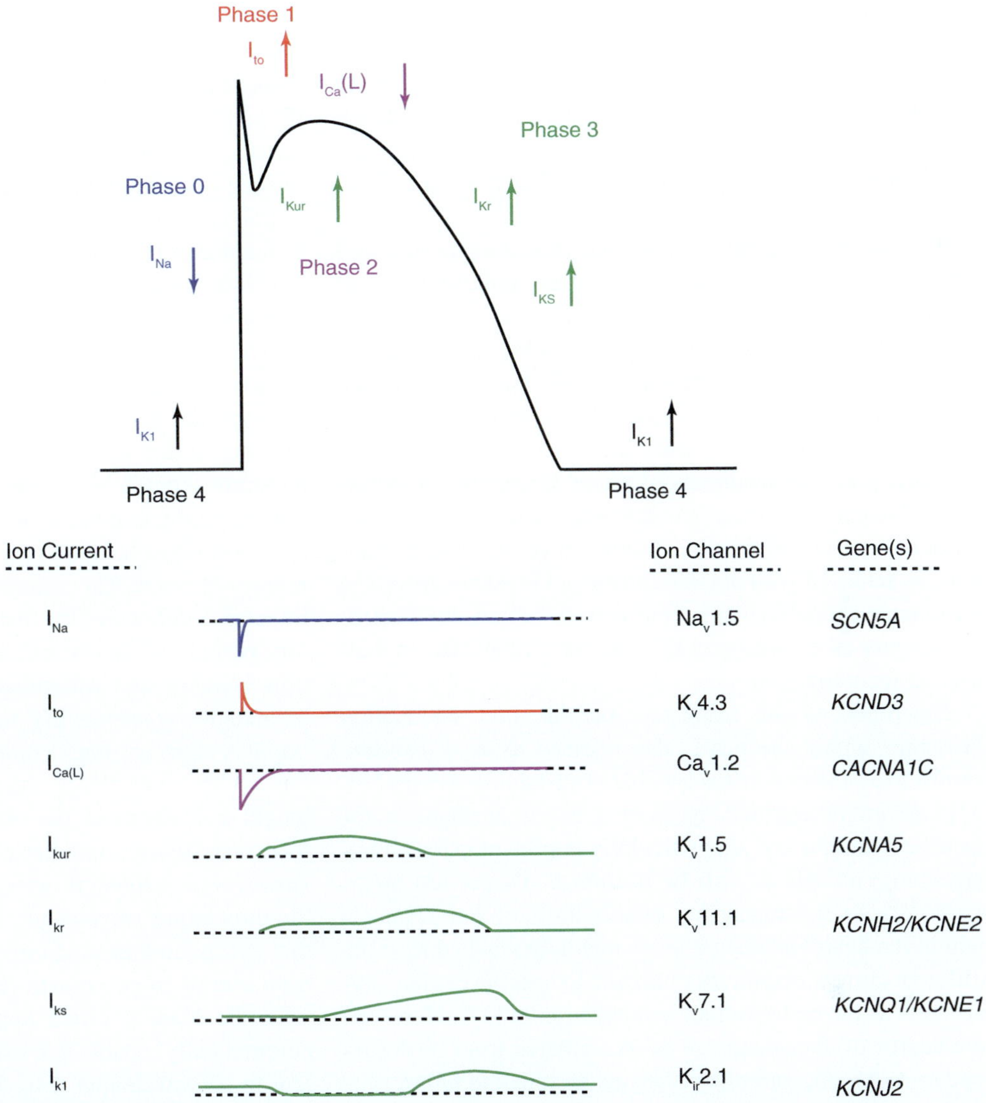

Fig. 18.1 The atrial action potential. The action potential is divided into four phases mediated by distinct ionic currents. These currents are driven by voltage-gated ion channels that allow specific ions to pass across the cardiac sarcolemma. The identity of the currents, the voltage-gated ion channels, and their encoding genes is provided (Adapted from Marban [17])

repolarization, I_{K1} activity predominates when the cell is hyperpolarized or near resting potential [22]. The efflux of potassium ions mediated by I_{K1} during phase 4 serves as an important contributor to the resting membrane potential of the cell and in this context has the potential to influence cellular excitability [24]. Upon depolarization, the magnitude of I_{K1} is dramatically reduced, a property that may be mediated by intracellular magnesium ions and polyamines interfering with the flow of potassium ions through the channel [25]. This reduced current persists until the terminal portion of phase 3 when I_{K1} increases and exerts influence on cellular repolarization and action potential duration [22].

Another important current within cardiac atria is the *muscarinic receptor-activated potassium current*, I_{KACh}, which mediates the flow of potassium ions across the membrane in response to a vagal stimulus [26]. The cardiac muscarinic receptor, M2, is a G-protein-coupled receptor that, upon binding of a cholinergic agonist (acetylcholine), permits the $G_{\beta\gamma}$-subunit to dissociate and subsequently bind and activate I_{KACh} [27]. The constituents of I_{KACh} include Kir3.1 and Kir3.4 encoded by *KCNJ3* and *KCNJ5*, respectively [28]. I_{KACh}, similar to I_{Kur}, is considered to be exclusive to the atria, although mRNA of both subunits has been detected in the ventricles [29]. Activation of I_{KACh} while the cell is depolarized results in a further efflux of potassium ions, which has the potential to shorten the action potential duration and, as will be discussed in subsequent sections, may influence the development of AF [30].

Two major concepts that can be derived from knowledge of the cardiac action potential and its associated currents include the electrical properties of *conduction velocity* and *refractory period*. Conduction velocity reflects the velocity at which an electrical impulse is transmitted through myocardial tissue [14]. Two of the major determinants of conduction velocity include sodium channels and gap junctions. As discussed above, the kinetics of the Na$_v$1.5 channel allow for rapid conduction within the heart [15]. Gap junctions represent intercellular pores that allow electrical current to flow between cells [31]. It is this intercellular coupling, along with the rapid conduction along the cell membrane mediated by $Na_v1.5$, that results in coordinated activity between individual cells of the heart and an ensuing functional electrical syncytium.

The second concept involves the refractory period and refers to the length of time following excitation that a cell requires before it can be re-excited [14]. An electrical impulse that encounters refractory tissue dies out. The length of the refractory period is dependent upon the rate at which a cell is able to repolarize to a potential compatible with re-excitation, and therefore phase 3 of the action potential plays a critical role. The mediators of phase 3, namely, the potassium channels, are therefore important contributors to the refractory period of the cell. Inhibition of potassium channels, as achieved with potassium channel blockers, results in a prolonged repolarization time manifested on the electrocardiogram as a prolonged QT interval in the case of ventricular repolarization.

Heterogeneity of refractory periods and conduction velocities within the heart, also referred to as *dispersion*, results in a substrate that is capable of sustaining *reentry* [32, 33]. Reentrant circuits represent a major mechanism for tachyarrhythmias and are particularly important in the pathophysiology of AF, as will be discussed. Dispersion arises secondary to heterogeneous distributions of ion channels within the heart and occurs in normal individuals due to the different current magnitudes intrinsic to specific cardiac layers such as the endocardium and epicardium [34]. However, the degree of dispersion can be exacerbated from birth secondary to genetic variations altering the function of key protein mediators or can occur over time as a result of asymmetric cardiac electrical and structural remodeling processes. An example of dispersion on the 12-lead ECG is that of QT dispersion reflecting regional heterogeneity of ventricular repolarization.

An understanding of these concepts is necessary in order to properly address the pathophysiology of AF and its associated molecular genetics.

Pathophysiology

AF reflects disorganized and chaotic activity of the atria with impulses firing at a rate of approximately 400–600 times per minute. The mechanisms underlying the development and maintenance of AF remain incompletely understood, and there continues to be a variety of competing theories [35]. The dominant conceptual model of AF over the past 50 years, the *multiple wavelet hypothesis*, is derived from the work of Gordon Moe and involves multiple circuit reentry excitation [36]. In this model, which has been confirmed by high-resolution electrical mapping during AF, irregular atrial activity arises from multiple self-perpetuating micro-reentrant circuits that exhibit spatial and temporal variability [37, 38]. A second model implicates rapidly discharging atrial ectopic foci, a concept that has been strengthened following the recognition that ectopic beats originating from pulmonary veins frequently initiate AF [39–41]. This had led to the use of radiofrequency catheter ablation techniques, in which the pulmonary veins are electrically isolated from the surrounding atria, in order to treat AF [42].

The multiple wavelet hypothesis suggests that increasing numbers of reentrant wavelets within the atria favor the maintenance of AF. A wavelet is a small wave of depolarizing current that may circle back upon itself to form a micro-reentrant circuit. In order to appreciate the conditions governing the number of wavelets that can be established, it is important to have an understanding of the *wavelength of reentry* concept. The wavelength of a circulating electrical impulse is defined as the distance traveled within one refractory period and can be calculated as the product of conduction velocity and refractory period [43]. In contrast, the pathlength represents the distance traveled by an electrical impulse during one complete circuit. As denoted in Fig. 18.2b, a wavelength that is greater in size than its pathlength will result in the circulating impulse encountering refractory tissue, and the circuit will be terminated [43]. However, a pathlength traveled, that is greater in size than the circulating wavelength, will introduce an excitable gap that will permit ensuing circus movement allowing the reentrant circuit to perpetuate (Fig. 18.2c) [44]. In accordance with the leading circle hypothesis, a circulating wavelet automatically establishes itself within a pathlength equivalent to its wavelength (Fig. 18.2a) [43]. On this basis, coupled with wavelength being the product of conduction velocity and refractory period, the number of wavelets that can be supported by atria of a given size is inversely proportional to both conduction velocity and refractory period.

The notion of an increased number of wavelets promoting the maintenance of AF is supported by an increased atrial size serving as a risk factor for the arrhythmia [45]. In a similar fashion, an increase in circulating wavelets through a reduction in refractory period and an ensuing reduction in wavelength theoretically promotes the maintenance of AF. The theory that a shorter wavelength, through a reduced refractory period, predisposes to AF serves as the rationale for using potassium channel blockers to terminate AF. Potassium channel blockers prolong atrial repolarization and result in an increased refractory period, thereby reducing the potential number of circulating wavelets that can be supported by atria of a given size. Of note, the use of sodium channel blockers in AF is not supported by the wavelength of reentry concept. These medications decrease conduction velocity and, given the associated reduction in wavelength, would increase the number of circulating atrial wavelets.

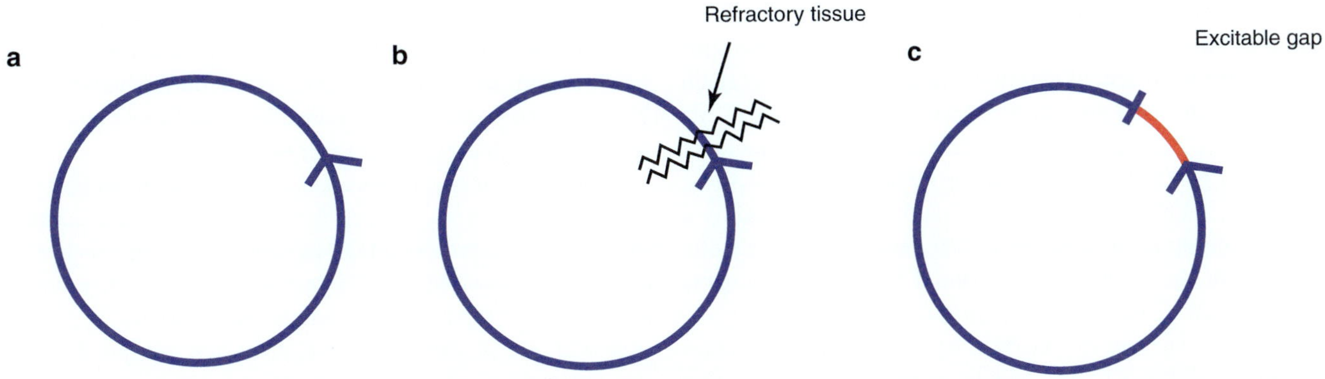

Fig. 18.2 Micro-reentrant circuits in atrial fibrillation. (**a**) A circulating wavelet, whose wavelength is equivalent to its pathlength, exhibiting circus activity. (**b**) An increase in the refractory period of the micro-reentrant circuit has resulted in a wavelength that exceeds the pathlength. The depolarizing current encounters refractory tissue, and the circuit is terminated. (**c**) A reduction in the refractory period of the circulating wavelet from A generates a wavelength that is shorter than the corresponding pathlength resulting in the introduction of an excitable gap (Adapted from Nattel [35])

Their efficacy provides support for mechanistic heterogeneity within AF, a concept that will become evident as the genetic heterogeneity of the arrhythmia is further explored. Sodium channel blockers may be effective in treating a form of AF characterized by focal firing, a concept that will be addressed in the discussion surrounding *gain-of-function* sodium channel mutations.

The aforementioned atrial electrical properties, conduction velocity and refractory period, are often viewed as contributing to the substrate for arrhythmogenesis. The development of a reentry circuit is dependent upon both substrate and trigger, examples being an early afterdepolarization or enhanced automaticity resulting in a premature beat. It is important to note that the physiology responsible for both trigger and substrate is not static but dynamic secondary to modulation by the autonomic nervous system. As such, the *autonomic nervous system* has been recognized as a critical component of arrhythmogenesis. In the setting of lone AF, the sentinel observations of the eminent electrophysiologist Phillipe Coumel implicated the parasympathetic nervous system as the major culprit [46]. He noted that the arrhythmia tended to be triggered during periods of high vagal tone such as sleep and postprandially. The mechanism through which the parasympathetic nervous system mediates lone AF appears to be in part dependent upon I_{KACh} [22]. As previously discussed, activation of I_{KACh} when the cell is depolarized triggers an efflux of potassium ions, shortening the atrial action potential duration and the corresponding refractory period. The heterogeneous vagal innervation of the atria has the potential to result in regional variation of refractory periods [30]. The resultant dispersion in cellular refractoriness throughout the atria has the potential to serve as an ideal substrate for reentry and arrhythmogenesis.

As evidenced by this discussion, there are multiple variables within atrial electrical physiology that can help contribute to the development of AF. The pathophysiological heterogeneity of this disorder is further supported by the varied genetics that characterize the condition. Effective treatment is likely dependent upon targeted therapy that addresses the specific aberrant pathway, which triggers the arrhythmia development in an individual. As a result, a detailed understanding of the molecular mechanisms underlying AF is warranted.

Molecular Genetics

A genetic contribution to AF was supported by informal observations of familial clustering of the arrhythmia; however, the first molecular genetic evidence did not come until 1997 when a genetic locus was found to segregate with the arrhythmia in a Spanish family that suffered from an autosomal dominant form of lone AF [47]. Linkage analysis localized the culprit locus to the long arm of chromosome 10 (10q22–24). Despite isolation of the locus to a relatively small genomic region, a culprit gene could not be identified. Candidate genes in that region included the β-adrenergic receptor (*ADRB1*), the α-adrenergic receptor (*ADRA2*), and a G-protein-coupled receptor kinase (*GPRK5*). Sequencing of these genes, however, did not reveal a mutation that segregated with disease. Over 20 years later, the culprit gene within this locus remains unknown.

Potassium Channels: Gain-of-Function Mutations

KCNQ1

The first causative gene for familial AF was not found until 6 years following identification of the 10q22–24 locus. The discovery came from the study of a four-generation Chinese family exhibiting an autosomal dominant pattern of inheritance of lone AF [48]. Linkage analysis mapped the culprit locus to the short arm of chromosome 11 (11p15.5), a region distinct from that found in the Spanish family. This on its own was a significant finding given that it demonstrated that AF was a genetically heterogeneous disorder that could be caused by more than one gene, a finding corroborated by a separate group in the same year [49]. Review of the genetic contents of the 11p15.5 region found that it contained the *KCNQ1* gene, whose protein product encodes the pore-forming α-subunit of I_{Ks} (*KCNQ1/KCNE1*). *Loss-of-function* mutations within *KCNQ1* had been previously implicated with congenital long QT syndrome type 1, and its previous association with arrhythmia made it an ideal candidate gene [50]. Sequencing of *KCNQ1* found a Ser140Gly mutation that was present in all affected family members and absent from all but one of the unaffected members. The finding that the Ser140Gly mutation appeared to segregate with disease was further strengthened by its absence in 188 healthy control individuals, coupled with it being a highly conserved residue across different species.

Following identification of the putative culprit mutation, functional studies were undertaken in an effort to elucidate the mechanism through which it resulted in a phenotype of AF. Coexpression of mutant *KCNQ1* with *KCNE1* in COS-7 cells resulted in markedly increased current density relative to wild type, consistent with a gain of function. Given that *KCNQ1* contributes to the slow component of the delayed rectifier potassium current (I_{Ks}) and is responsible for repolarization of cardiomyocytes, a gain-of-function mutation could result in more rapid repolarization and reduce the effective refractory period of cells (Fig. 18.3). As discussed previously, this would create a substrate ideal for multiple circuit reentry and promote maintenance of the arrhythmia in a manner consistent with the multiple wavelet hypothesis. This notion is supported by the observation that up to 30% of patients with short QT syndrome, a condition characterized by enhanced ventricular repolarization and malignant ventricular arrhythmias, suffer from AF [51, 52].

Although this theory fits nicely, it is worth noting that 9 of the 16 patients with the Ser140Gly mutation were actually found to have a prolonged QT interval on 12-lead electrocardiography. A prolonged QT interval, being consistent with a slower rate of repolarization within the ventricles, is in contrast with the in vitro functional data. It is conceivable that the mutation may have different effects on the atria and ventricles as a result of the different electrical and structural properties of these chambers. This theory was hypothesized by Lundby et al. who identified a Gln147Arg *KCNQ1* substitution in a patient with lone AF and a prolonged QT interval [53]. When mutant *KCNQ1* was coexpressed with *KCNE1* in *Xenopus laevis* oocytes, a loss of function was observed; however, coexpression with *KCNE2* resulted in a gain of function. Although these findings are intriguing, it is difficult to arrive at firm conclusions as the relative distributions of *KCNE1* and *KCNE2* within the atria and ventricles are largely unknown [53]. An alternative explanation for the seemingly discordant in vitro and electrocardiographic findings may be secondary to single-cell in vitro studies failing to recapitulate the complex physiology of the heart.

KCNE2 and KCNJ2

The discovery that a mutation within a potassium channel gene caused an autosomal dominant form of AF alluded to the possibility that other potassium channel genes may contribute to the arrhythmia. Given that linkage analysis studies

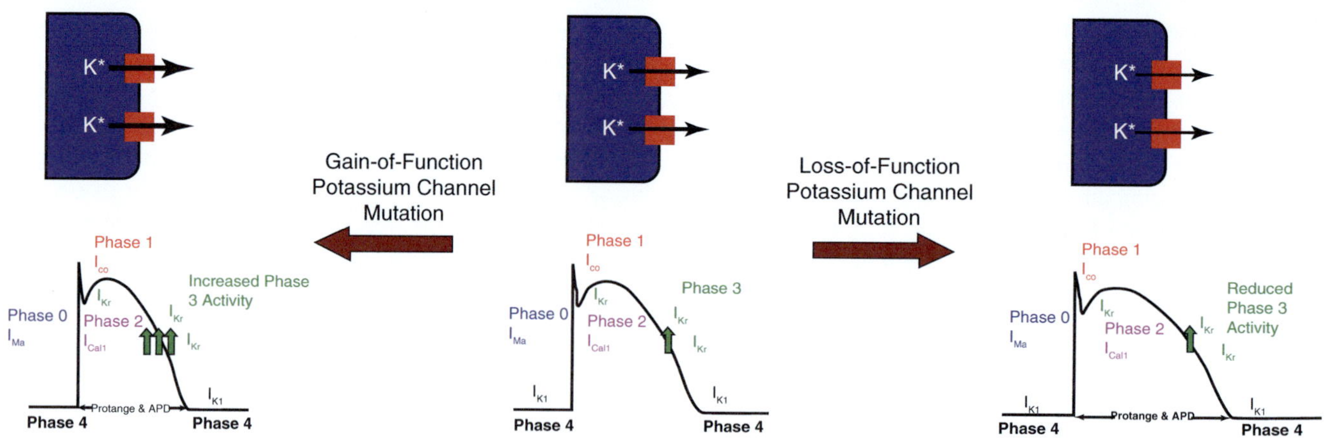

Fig. 18.3 The effect of potassium channel gene mutations on atrial action potential duration. A gain-of-function mutation in a voltage-gated potassium channel increases the efflux of potassium ions during phase 3 resulting in a shortening of the action potential duration. Conversely, the decrease in phase 3 current secondary to a loss-of-function mutation in a voltage-gated potassium channel causes prolongation of the atrial action potential

are frequently limited by small pedigree size, subsequent studies employed a candidate gene approach in which multiple potassium channel genes were screened for mutations in AF families. This approach led to the identification of two additional potassium channel genes, namely, *KCNE2* and *KCNJ2*, as being causal for familial forms of lone AF in two separate studies performed by the same group. A mutation within *KCNE2*, considered to encode the β-subunit of I_{Kr}, was discovered following screening of 28 unrelated Chinese kindreds with familial AF for mutations within 8 different potassium channels genes (*KCNQ1*, *KCNH2*, *KCNE1–5*, and *KCNJ2*) [54]. Two of the 28 probands were found to carry an Arg27Cys mutation that was subsequently found in affected members of the 2 kindreds and was absent in 462 healthy controls. It is important to note that each family only had two affected members, while multiple unaffected members carried the Arg27Cys mutation. This may potentially be accounted for by the mutation carrying a low degree of penetrance and necessitating additional genetic and environmental factors in order for the phenotype of AF to be expressed. Additionally, although *KCNE2* is generally considered to serve as the β-subunit of I_{Kr}, coexpression of Arg27Cys *KCNE2* with *KCNH2* did not result in a change in current relative to wild type. However, there was an increase in current noted when it was coexpressed with *KCNQ1*. Previous work with COS cells has demonstrated that the protein products of *KCNE2* and *KCNQ1* are capable of interacting to generate a background current that is not voltage dependent [55]. It is conceivable that the mutant *KCNE2* may predispose to AF through a background current that may affect cellular repolarization. It should also be noted that recent work in the context of long QT syndrome has questioned if *KCNE2* is sufficient to serve as a monogenic culprit of arrhythmia [56].

KCNJ2 was identified using a similar approach in which 30 Chinese AF kindreds were screened for mutations in 10 ion channel or transporter-related genes (*KCNQ1*, *KCNH2*, *SCN5A*, *ANK-B*, *KCNJ2*, and *KCNE1–5*) [57]. *KCNJ2* encodes Kir2.1, which is responsible for the cardiac inward rectifier potassium current I_{K1}. As discussed, this channel mediates a background potassium current that contributes to the resting membrane potential of the cell and influences cellular excitability and repolarization within the heart. It is also the causative gene for congenital long QT syndrome type 7, also referred to as Andersen-Tawil syndrome [58]. The proband and the other 4 affected family members were all found to carry a Val93Ile mutation within *KCNJ2*, a mutation not found in 420 healthy individuals. In this instance, two unaffected family members were found to carry the mutation; however, their unaffected status may have been secondary to their relatively young ages (33 and 42 years old). Functional analysis of the mutant protein revealed increased current density at potentials ranging from −140 to −80 mV and from −60 to −40 mV consistent with a gain-of-function effect. The putative predisposing mechanism of Val93Ile *KCNJ2* for AF involves enhanced repolarization and a reduction in refractory period, as hypothesized with *KCNQ1*.

KCNH2

The short QT syndrome is a rare inherited arrhythmia syndrome characterized by, as its name suggests, a short QT interval on surface ECG [52, 59]. Affected patients suffer from an increased risk of sudden cardiac death secondary to malignant ventricular arrhythmias, including polymorphic ventricular tachycardia and ventricular fibrillation [51]. In addition to ventricular arrhythmias, short QT syndrome is also characterized by an increased likelihood of developing atrial fibrillation [60]. To date, a total of six genes have been implicated in the condition [61–65]. The first three genes encode voltage-gated potassium channels and have also been identified as culprits in the long QT syndrome. In contrast to the long QT syndrome, which develops secondary to loss-of-function mutations in potassium channels, the pathogenic potassium channel mutations in short QT syndrome result in a gain of function. The first gene identified in short QT syndrome was *KCNH2*, which encodes the pore-forming α-subunit of I_{Kr}. In the original study evaluating for genetic culprits in this condition, investigators identified an identical *KCNH2* N588K mutation among two of the three families evaluated [61]. Both of these families had affected members who suffered from paroxysmal atrial fibrillation. Functional evaluation of the *KCNH2* N588K mutation through its expression in tsA201 cells in the presence and absence of the KCNE2 β-subunit revealed an abbreviation of the cardiac action potential secondary to increased I_{Kr}. These findings were consistent with the short QT interval observed on surface ECG and are likely operative in both the atria and ventricles given the clinical features of patients, coupled with the known expression of *KCNH2* in both chambers. Similar to the aforementioned genetic culprits with gain-of-function mutations, *KCNH2* gain-of-function mutations have been presumed to predispose to a mechanistic sub-phenotype of atrial fibrillation reflective of the multiple wavelet hypothesis. More recently, a mutation within *KCNJ2* (E299V) has also been linked to atrial fibrillation in the setting of short QT syndrome [66].

Potassium Channels: Loss-of-Function Mutations

KCNA5

Up until this point, all of the potassium channel genes implicated in the development of lone AF had been shown to exhibit gain-of-function effects on in vitro functional analysis. As discussed, the purported mechanism involved a reduction in effective refractory period and reentrant wavelength, which in accordance with the multiple wavelet hypothesis would promote and maintain AF. However, was it conceivable that a loss-of-function effect in a potassium channel could result in AF?

Using the candidate gene approach, 154 patients with lone AF were screened for mutations within the *KCNA5* gene, encoding the atrial-specific voltage-gated potassium channel $K_v1.5$ responsible for I_{Kur} [67]. A unique sequence variant was identified in a patient with a family history of the arrhythmia. The patient carried a nonsense mutation (E375X) that resulted in the production of a truncated protein that lacked the S4–S6 voltage sensor, the pore region, and the C-terminus. Because of a lack of available DNA, stringent genetic support for the mutation segregating with the arrhythmia was not possible. Subsequent functional studies revealed that expression of mutant KCNA5-p. E375X within HEK293 cells failed to generate current. This was consistent with a loss-of-function effect and not unexpected given the drastic effect of the nonsense mutation on the mature protein. In addition, when coexpressed with wild-type *KCNA5*, cells exhibited a significant reduction in current density compatible with a dominant-negative effect, which accounted for the autosomal dominant pattern of inheritance in the setting of a loss-of-function mutation.

Given that loss of function within a voltage-gated potassium channel involved in repolarization presumably results in a prolonged refractory period, the mechanism through which mutant KCNA5-p. E375X predisposes to AF would have to be different from the previously described gain-of-function potassium channel mutations (Fig. 18.3). In vitro studies using human atrial myocytes and in vivo studies with a murine model found that administration of 4-aminopyridine, a known blocker of I_{Kur}, dramatically increased the incidence of early afterdepolarizations. The authors hypothesized that increased early afterdepolarizations, in combination with a prolonged atrial action potential duration, could result in disorganized atrial activity akin to that seen in torsades de pointes within the ventricles. Early afterdepolarizations serving as a trigger for AF had previously been suggested in an animal model whereby injection of cesium chloride, a potassium channel blocker, into the sinus node artery of dogs resulted in a polymorphic atrial tachycardia that subsequently degenerated into AF, leading the investigators to coin the term “atrial torsades” [68].

It is important to note that the mechanisms underlying a form of AF caused by a gain-of-function voltage-gated potassium channel appear to be dramatically different and essentially opposing to a form of the arrhythmia driven by a loss of function in a similar channel. The distinct triggers and substrates in these phenotypically identical forms of the arrhythmia serve to emphasize the marked heterogeneity that likely underlies the pathophysiology of AF and may provide insight into the variable efficacies of many therapies.

A Potassium Channel Variant and “Secondary Hit” Hypothesis

Although genetics play an important role in the development of AF, the critical role of the environment is emphasized by the notion that the arrhythmia rarely develops in childhood and becomes increasingly common with advancing age. The interaction of genetics with environmental influences was eloquently illustrated in a family with autosomal dominant AF who also suffered from a high incidence of hypertension [69]. Mutation screening in four genes (*KCNQ1*, *KCNE1–3*) identified a novel missense mutation within *KCNQ1*, namely, Arg14Cys. Analysis of the family pedigree suggested that the mutation segregated with the arrhythmia, while it was absent in 100 control patients. The interesting findings came following in vitro functional studies in which the mutant Arg14Cys *KCNQ1* was coexpressed with *KCNE1* in CHO cells. The mutant potassium channel initially behaved identically to wild type; however, following treatment with a hypotonic solution to simulate the cell swelling and stretching consistent with the atrial milieu in a hypertensive patient, the mutant channels exhibited a marked increase in current and a leftward shift in the voltage dependence of activation consistent with a gain-of-function effect. Wild-type channel properties were unaffected by exposure to the hypotonic media. The authors hypothesized that the inherited ion channel defect represented the “first hit”; however, a “second hit” mediated by environmental factors such as hypertension was necessary for development of the arrhythmia. This phenomenon would help to account for the increasing prevalence of AF with aging.

Are Potassium Channel Mutations Common?

Although many of the genes responsible for familial AF encode potassium channel proteins, an obvious question is whether potassium channel mutations are a common cause of AF. Furthermore, most of the genetic studies discussed involved Chinese kindreds, and it was therefore uncertain if these results were applicable to other ethnicities. In order to address this question, two separate studies from the same group screened over 200 patients of Western European ancestry with lone AF and AF with hypertension for mutations within potassium channel genes (*KCNQ1*, *KCNJ2*, and *KCNE1–5*) [70, 71]. Although a number of common polymorphisms were detected, no disease-causing mutations were discovered. It was, therefore, concluded that potassium channel gene mutations represent a rare cause of AF in patients of Western European descent.

Cardiac Gap Junctions

Gap junctions are specialized channels that directly connect cytoplasmic compartments of adjacent cells, allowing for passage of charged ions and coordinated propagation of cardiac action potentials [31]. The molecular constituents of gap junction channels are connexin proteins, which oligomerize into hexameric structures known as connexons or hemichannels. Adjacent cells each contribute a hemichannel to form a functional gap junction channel (Fig. 18.4) [72]. There are multiple different isoforms of connexin proteins; however, the two most highly expressed isoforms within the heart are *connexin 40* and 43 [73]. Connexin 40 is of particular interest in AF, since it is expressed in atrial myocytes and is absent from ventricular cells [73]. The importance of connexins to AF has been well established in animal studies. In knockout mice lacking the connexin 40 gene, atrial tachyarrhythmias could be induced by burst atrial pacing, whereas this was not possible in wild-type mice [74]. A goat model of persistent AF revealed that connexin 40 distribution within the atria was markedly heterogeneous, a phenomenon also seen in humans with AF [75, 76]. Although the latter finding does not establish causality, it does suggest that heterogeneous distribution of connexins within the heart may form an ideal substrate for AF.

In the light of the atrial-specific expression of Cx40, and the vulnerability of Cx40 knockout mice to AF, our group subsequently screened a group of 15 patients with sporadic, lone AF for mutations within connexin 40 (*GJA5*) and 43 (*GJA1*) [77, 78]. We initially identified a Ala96Ser mutation within the highly conserved transmembrane-spanning domain of the connexin 40 protein. Functional studies of the mutant Cx40 Ala96Ser protein were performed in a gap junction-deficient cell line, N2A cells. Cells expressing the Ala96Ser mutation displayed appropriate trafficking; however, functional electrical cell-to-cell coupling through these channels was significantly reduced. The mutation also demonstrated a dominant-negative effect on wild-type Cx40, as well as a trans-dominant-negative effect on wild-type Cx43. This latter finding provides strong support for the concept of heteromeric interaction of Cx40 and Cx43 in hemichannel formation. Subsequent work has further validated the role of connexin mutations in atrial fibrillation based on findings from multiple patients and families [79–84]. In addition, a dedicated transgenic murine model possessing the Ala96Ser mutation revealed significantly reduced atrial conduction and prolonged episodes of atrial fibrillation following burst atrial pacing [85]. Collectively, these findings provide strong evidence to support a role for connexins in the pathogenesis of atrial fibrillation.

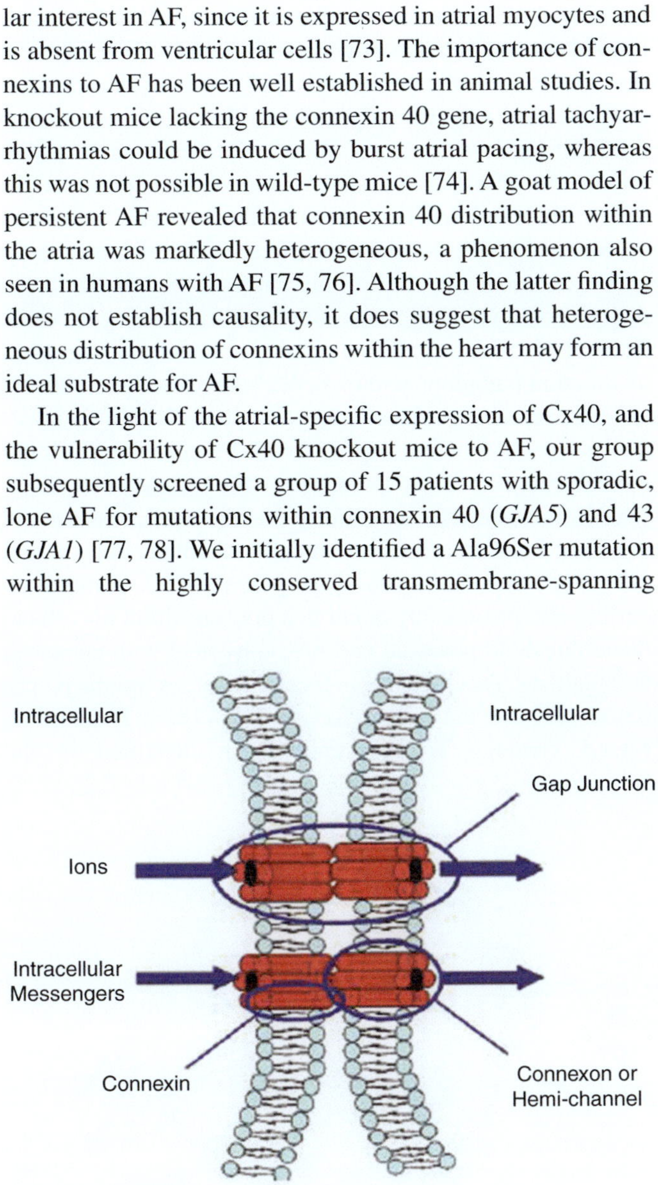

Fig. 18.4 Gap junctions form intercellular pores that permit passage of ions and intracellular messengers between the cytoplasm of adjacent cells. A gap junction is composed of two adjoining connexons or hemichannels, whose molecular constituents are termed connexins

Sodium Channels: Loss-of-Function Mutations

SCN5A encodes the sodium channel, $Na_v1.5$, responsible for the rapid depolarization upstroke of the cardiac action potential. It has been associated with numerous arrhythmic disorders including the Brugada syndrome, congenital long QT syndrome type 3, sick sinus syndrome, and bundle branch reentrant ventricular tachycardia [86–89]. Given its obvious importance with the electrical properties of the heart, multiple groups employed a candidate gene approach screening patients with AF for mutations within *SCN5A*. The first study involved 157 patients with lone AF; screening did not identify any novel mutations felt to be causative for AF [90]. The H558R single nucleotide polymorphism (SNP), of which approximately one third of the population are heterozygous, was also examined in these patients along with 314 matched controls. The R558 allele, which had previously been shown to alter $Na_v1.5$ function by reducing depolarizing sodium current, was found to confer an increased risk of developing AF (odds ratio 1.6) [90, 91]. However, the sample size in this study was rather small, and the data has yet to be duplicated in larger cohorts.

A second study involving 375 patients with AF (118 had lone AF, while 257 had AF associated with heart disease) and 360 well-matched controls identified 8 novel mutations in 10 separate AF patients [92]. None of the variants were found in controls, and all involved highly conserved residues within $Na_v1.5$. Six of the patients appeared to represent familial cases, and in each case, the variant appeared to segregate with the disease. Functional studies were not performed, and therefore the mechanism through which these variants cause

AF is unknown. These findings suggest, in contrast to the previous study, that mutations within *SCN5A* represent a relatively common cause of AF in patients with and without heart disease.

A third group screened *SCN5A* in 57 patients with lone AF or AF with hypertension and a confirmed family history of the arrhythmia [93]. A single novel mutation was found, Asn1986Lys, which was not found in 300 ethnically matched controls. The father of the proband, who also suffered from AF, was found to be a carrier of the mutation, while the unaffected mother did not have any sequence variants within *SCN5A*. Unfortunately, further genetic profiling of the family was not possible due to unwillingness to participate in the study. Expression of the mutant gene within *Xenopus laevis* oocytes suggested a loss-of-function effect as evidenced by a significant hyperpolarizing shift in the midpoint of steady-state inactivation. This alteration was predicted to prolong the atrial action potential duration, and, therefore, Asn1986Lys-SCN5A presumably triggers AF through a manner akin to the aforementioned atrial torsade. These findings, which confirmed the association of *SCN5A* with AF, however, suggested that it is not a frequent cause of the condition.

Sodium Channels: Gain-of-Function Mutations

Although previous studies had implicated loss-of-function *SCN5A* mutations in association with AF, subsequent work indicated that gain-of-function mutations within *SCN5A* are also part of the genetic spectrum responsible for AF. Prior to these studies, the only disease related to an *SCN5A* gain-of-function effect was long QT syndrome type 3, which is mediated by a persistent late sodium current [87].

In a four-generation Japanese family with an autosomal dominant form of AF, a novel Met1875Thr mutation was identified within *SCN5A* [94]. The proband was reported to have increased right atrial excitability during radiofrequency catheter ablation for AF. All affected family members were found to carry the mutation, while the mutation was absent in all unaffected family members and 210 ethnically matched controls. Functional analysis of Met1875Thr revealed a pronounced depolarizing shift in the midpoint of steady-state inactivation consistent with a gain-of-function effect. No persistent sodium current was observed, consistent with the observation that affected individuals had QT intervals within the normal range.

A second study from our group involving a mother and son with lone AF identified a Lys1493Arg mutation involving a highly conserved residue within the DIII-IV linker located six amino acids downstream from the fast inactivation motif of sodium channels [95]. Biophysical studies demonstrated a significant positive shift in the voltage dependence of inactivation and a large ramp current near resting membrane potential, consistent with a gain of function. When expressed in HL-1 atrial cardiomyocytes, enhanced cellular excitability was observed in the form of spontaneous action potential depolarizations and a lower threshold for action potential firing as compared to wild-type cells. Collectively, these studies suggest that both gain- and loss-of-function mutations within *SCN5A* are associated with AF.

The existing evidence suggests that *SCN5A* gain-of-function mutations predispose to AF by enhancing cellular hyperexcitability. The depolarizing shift in steady-state inactivation increases the probability that the channel will be in the open conformation and capable of conducting current [95]. This alteration in the gating of the Na_v1–5-mediated current will presumably result in a predisposition for cells to reach threshold potential and fire, consistent with enhanced automaticity. This increase in focal discharges has the potential to serve as the trigger for AF (Fig. 18.5). In addition, $Na_v1.5$ channels have recently been identified in the

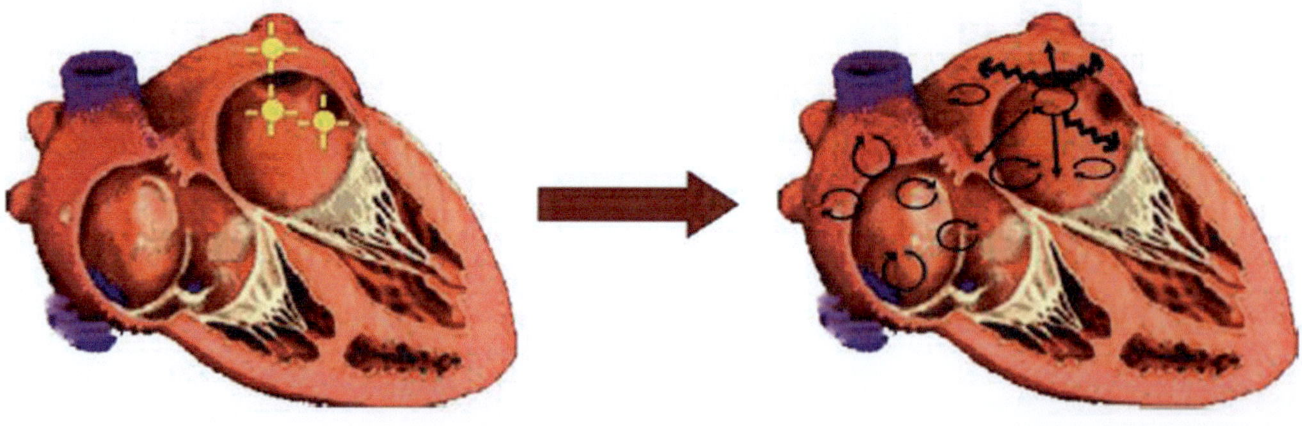

Fig. 18.5 Cellular hyperexcitability triggering atrial fibrillation. Ectopic foci originating from the pulmonary veins contribute to the development of a self-perpetuating micro-reentrant circuit. Rapid, heterogeneous conduction from the reentrant circuit to the surrounding atria results in electrical activity consistent with atrial fibrillation

autonomic ganglia that surround the pulmonary veins [96]. Mutations within *SCN5A* may therefore result in neuronal hyperexcitability that may trigger AF through a parasympathetic pathway and contribute to the rapidly firing ectopic foci observed in the region of the pulmonary veins in some patients with the arrhythmia.

Atrial Natriuretic Peptide

In contrast to the previous culprits, which all involved cardiac ion channels, the subsequent genetic culprit implicated in the arrhythmia was a circulating hormone, the *atrial natriuretic peptide* (ANP). Although known to be important in cardiac physiology, ANP had been largely viewed as cardioprotective in the setting of heart failure [97]. It was known, however, to be capable of modulating the electrical activities of the heart, and there were reports of its effects on specific ion channels [98–100]. However, little work had been done on ANP in the context of AF, and previous studies that had examined for a possible relationship had been negative [101].

Linkage analysis of a Caucasian family of Northern European ancestry with autosomal dominant AF mapped the causative locus to the small arm of chromosome 1 (1p36–35) [102]. Review of the genes within this region revealed the presence of *NPPA*, the gene encoding ANP, and subsequent sequencing revealed a two-base-pair deletion in exon 3 that resulted in a frameshift associated with loss of the stop codon. Extension of the reading frame results in an elongated peptide that is 40 amino acids in length relative to the 28 amino acid length of the wild type. The deletion was present in all of the affected family members and absent in unaffected family members and 560 control patients. Functional studies involving an isolated rat whole-heart model suggested that the mutant ANP resulted in a reduced effective refractory period; however, the mechanism was not entirely clear. ANP mediates its effects on cells through binding to natriuretic peptide receptors that possess intracellular guanylate cyclase activity [103]. Previous work has suggested that ANP molecules with an elongated C-terminus may be more resistant to degradation and therefore may circulate at higher levels [104]. Therefore, the authors hypothesized that increased circulating ANP may produce increased intracellular levels of cGMP that may in turn, through an unknown mechanism, reduce the effective refractory period.

Atrial Myosin Light Chain 4

Individuals that suffer from genetic forms of ventricular cardiomyopathies, including familial dilated cardiomyopathy and hypertrophic cardiomyopathy, have markedly increased risks of developing atrial fibrillation. The presumed mechanism for this association has generally been assumed to be increased atrial pressure arising secondary to ventricular systolic and/or diastolic dysfunction. Notably, the genetic culprits responsible for these forms of ventricular cardiomyopathy are also expressed within the atria giving rise to the possibility that atrial fibrillation in these conditions may actually occur secondary to a concomitant atrial myopathy [105].

Our group identified a family with an autosomal dominant form of atrial fibrillation characterized by an early age of onset in the setting of normal biventricular function [106]. Affected family members derived minimal benefit from both antiarrhythmic drugs and catheter ablation for maintenance of sinus rhythm. Notably, while in sinus rhythm, affected individuals had low amplitude p-waves on surface ECG and on echocardiography had markedly dilated atria and severely reduced atrial function. Collectively, these findings, coupled with evidence of large regions of electrical silence observed at the time of catheter ablation, were suggestive of a sub-phenotype of atrial fibrillation that developed secondary to an atrial myopathy.

In an effort to identify a genetic culprit, we performed exome sequencing on affected and unaffected family members and identified an *MYL4* missense mutation, Glu11Lys, that tracked with the affected phenotype. The *MYL4* gene encodes the atrial-specific myosin light chain, a sarcomeric constituent whose expression is restricted to the atrium. This differential cardiac chamber expression was felt to account for the phenotype in our family consisting of a myopathy restricted to the atria. Subsequent functional work using a transgenic zebrafish model revealed that fish carrying the mutation had markedly dilated atria and prolonged p-wave durations reflective of slow intra-atrial conduction. Electron microscopy revealed evidence of sarcomeric disarray by abnormal organization of H-zones and Z-discs (Fig. 18.6). Collectively, these findings were consistent with an atrial myopathy and mirrored the clinical phenotype exhibited by affected family members. In addition to introducing a novel genetic culprit for atrial fibrillation, our findings serve to validate a novel sub-phenotype of atrial fibrillation characterized by an underlying atrial myopathy. Additional studies from other groups have supported a role for *MYL4* in AF pathogenesis [107, 108].

Unknown Loci

Finally, in addition to 10q22–24, there are multiple other loci that have been identified through linkage analysis in kindreds with autosomal dominant forms of lone AF. These loci include 6q14–16, 10p11–q21, and 5p15; the specific causative genes remain unknown [109–111].

Wild-Type

Tg(myh6:cmlc1^{E17K})

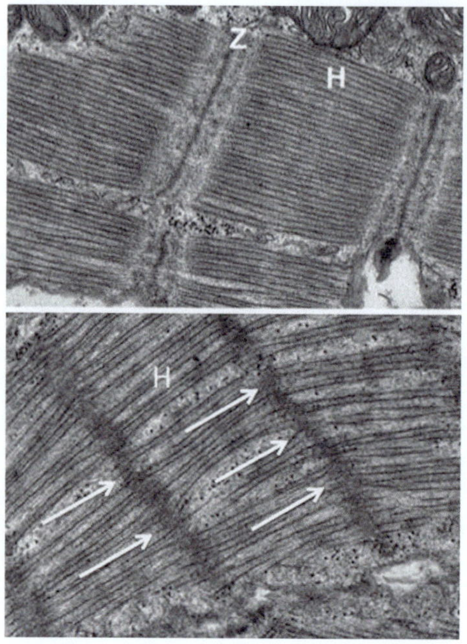

Fig. 18.6 Atrial sarcomeric structure in wild-type and transgenic Glu17Lys zebrafish. Electron microscopy reveals normal H-zones and Z-discs in wild type, but absent Z-discs (arrows) in the transgenic atrium. *H* H-zone, *Z* Z-disc

Genome-Wide Association Studies

The availability of DNA microarrays containing hundreds of thousands of *single nucleotide polymorphisms* (SNPs) has resulted in the opportunity to screen the entire genome for regions that may confer an increased risk for disease. This robust mechanism is proving to be an invaluable tool in unraveling the complex genetics underlying many common diseases including coronary artery disease and AF.

A *genome-wide association study* using a DNA microarray containing 316,515 SNPs was performed on 550 patients with AF or flutter in combination with 4476 control patients from Iceland [112]. They discovered a strong association with SNPs on chromosome 4q25, the most significant being rs2200733 with an odds ratio of 1.84 (95% confidence intervals 1.54–2.21). Replication studies using additional samples from Iceland (2251 cases and 13,238 controls), Sweden (143 cases and 738 controls), the USA (636 cases and 804 controls), and China (333 cases and 2836 controls) further reinforced the association with rs2200733. The odds ratio for the combined European population was 1.72 (95% confidence interval 1.59–1.86), while that for the Chinese cohort was 1.42 (95% confidence interval 1.16–1.73) The haplotype block corresponding to the associated SNPs does not contain a known gene, and, therefore, the mechanism for this association is currently unknown. Candidate genes present within the adjacent haplotype block include *PITX2*, which encodes a protein involved in cardiac development, and *ENPEP*, whose protein product is involved in angiotensin II breakdown [90, 91]. Research to delineate the genetic factors at the 4q25 locus responsible for the increased risk for the development of AF is ongoing, and insights are gradually being gleaned [113–115].

Following identification of the 4q25 locus, two subsequent genome-wide association studies were performed with larger numbers of cases and controls in order to improve power and identify previously undetected loci associated with AF. Both groups independently identified two separate SNPs, rs7193343 and rs2106261, which localized to an intronic region within the *ZFHX3* gene on chromosome 16q22 [116, 117]. *ZFHX3* encodes a transcription factor, AT motif-binding factor 1, whose function in the heart is currently unclear. The *ZFHX3* gene has recently been implicated in a vasculitis involving the coronary arteries (Kawasaki disease) [118]. The association of 16q22 with AF was not as strong as for 4q25, with an odds ratio in the range of 1.2 in most European populations. Furthermore, it was not significantly associated with AF in the Chinese population [117]. Lastly, it is important to note that although the 16q22 SNPs did localize to a gene, it does not necessarily implicate *ZFHX3* in the pathogenesis of AF. These SNPs may appear to associate with AF due to linkage disequilibrium with the true causal variants in surrounding regions. As with the 4q25 locus, further work is necessary in order to better appreciate the apparent relationship between 16q22 and AF.

Subsequent genome-wide association studies with steadily increasing sizes have now identified upward of 140 common genetic variants that exhibit statistically significant associations with atrial fibrillation at genome-wide levels of significance [119–125]. The precise mechanism through which each of these SNPs predisposes to the arrhythmia remains unclear, although details are gradually emerging [113, 126, 127]. Experts have hypothesized that these SNPs reside in enhancer or repressor regions and influence expression of nearby genes; however further work will be necessary to definitively clarify their role in the development of the arrhythmia. Pathway analysis of the collection of SNPs implicated in AF has begun to suggest that genetic susceptibility to the arrhythmia may be secondary to the development of an underlying atrial cardiomyopathy [125]. Although the precise biological roles of these AF-risk SNPs remain unclear, their collective use in the form of polygenic risk scores to predict the risk of developing AF has begun to show promise, and experts have started to argue for transitioning their use into the clinical setting [128, 129].

The Autonomic Nervous System

Clinical observations suggest that the autonomic nervous system plays a critical role in the pathogenesis of AF, and this has been supported in different animal models. AF can be readily triggered in structurally normal hearts through exposure to a cholinergic agonist such as carbachol followed by burst pacing. In a canine model, atrial vagal denervation through radiofrequency catheter ablation prevented subsequent induction of the arrhythmia through burst pacing and vagal stimulation [107]. In an effort to investigate the molecular mechanisms underlying this phenomenon, knockout mice that lacked Kir3.4 (previously referred to as GIRK4) were developed [29]. As discussed previously, Kir3.1 and Kir3.4 encode the protein products responsible for I_{KACh}, and the absence of either results in the complete loss of I_{KACh}. Unlike wild-type mice, burst pacing in the presence of carbachol was unable to induce AF in the I_{KACh}-deficient knockout mice. This data serves to implicate I_{KACh} in the pathogenesis of AF and suggests that blockers of I_{KACh} may potentially serve as an effective treatment for the arrhythmia. This is an especially attractive treatment option given that I_{KACh}, like I_{Kur}, appears to be localized predominantly to the atria.

Although there is relatively robust data supporting the involvement of the cholinergic system in the pathogenesis of AF, genetic mutations in genes encoding the molecular mediators of the cholinergic response in the heart have not been reported.

Clinical Aspects: Genetic Diagnosis and Targeted Therapy

Our understanding of the genetic contributions to AF remains in its infancy, and genetics have yet to be incorporated into routine clinical practice for management of the arrhythmia [130]. The current status of clinical genetics in AF is in contrast to other known inherited arrhythmia diseases, such as long QT syndrome and arrhythmogenic cardiomyopathy. In these conditions, a majority of the genetic causes are considered to be known, and the yield of clinical genetic testing is above 50%. In contrast, the yield of genetic testing in most AF patients is anticipated to be less than 10%. The reasons for the lower yield are multifactorial and related to development of AF being polygenic, likely dependent on both rare and common variants, coupled with additional critical contributions from conventional clinical and environmental factors.

A detailed understanding of the genetics contributing to the pathophysiology of AF may allow for the development of pharmacogenomic strategies associated with improved treatment efficacy and reduced adverse events [131]. AF is likely a heterogeneous disorder, a concept that has been nicely illustrated by genetic findings. In one instance, it may arise secondary to a gain-of-function effect within a potassium channel, whereas in another case, it may result from a loss-of-function effect in the same channel. Although phenotypically they may be indistinguishable on electrocardiography, the most efficacious treatment choice may be markedly different in the light of differing electrophysiologic triggers. Given their identical phenotype, genetic characterization will likely be necessary in order to identify the particular AF subtype. In the first example given above, the arrhythmia has likely developed secondary to a shortened atrial refractory period, which has resulted in an ideal substrate for multiple reentrant wavelets within the atria. Effective treatment with a potassium channel blocker that restores the atrial effective refractory period to its normal length, thereby disrupting the reentrant wavelets, may be the optimal agent to restore and maintain sinus rhythm. However, the same treatment in the second case would likely exacerbate the arrhythmia, given that it is secondary to a prolonged atrial refractory period, which may have resulted in "atrial torsade." The genetic and pathophysiologic heterogeneity underlying the arrhythmia is likely responsible for the variable treatment response observed in cases of lone AF [131].

In addition to the above example with potassium channel mutations, a similar approach can be extended to the other genes that have been implicated in AF. For example, forms of AF that develop secondary to cellular hyperexcitability as a result of gain-of-function mutations within sodium channels may benefit from sodium channel blockers. In the context of an AF subtype characterized by conduction velocity heterogeneity that arose secondary to a loss-of-function connexin mutation, such a patient may benefit from a form of therapy that keeps gap junctions in their open state. Although not currently available, there are emerging gap junction pharmacophores that may serve this purpose [108]. Targeted therapy, consistent with a pharmacogenomic approach, should be a goal that is strived for in the coming years. Along with being more efficacious, this strategy should also reduce the unwanted proarrhythmic effects seen with antiarrhythmic drugs.

Beyond personalized forms of targeted therapy for AF, genetics also holds promise for facilitating recognition of individuals most susceptible to arrhythmia development. Recent work has shown that use of polygenic risk scores comprised of over 1000 and even millions of SNPs enables identification of large proportions of the general population at significantly increased risk of AF [128, 129]. In this fashion, genetics may allow for more aggressive risk factor modification of those at risk, including blood pressure control and weight loss, which may help reduce the rapidly expanding prevalence of the condition. Beyond disease prevention, polygenic risk scores may also serve to facilitate identification of AF as a culprit of stroke and enable initiation of effective preventive therapy through oral anticoagulation [132].

Summary

An understanding of the genetic factors that lead to the development of AF holds great promise for the development of effective therapies against this exceedingly common arrhythmia. The ability to identify the specific electrophysiologic mechanisms, on the basis of genetic discovery, may lead to more effective forms of targeted therapy that carry less risk. This era of pharmacogenomics has yet to arrive for AF; however, it may be gradually inching closer. In the more immediate future, the use of polygenic risk scores may improve our ability to predict the risk of AF within the general population, which may allow for more aggressive risk factor modification among individuals at greatest risk for developing the arrhythmia. Improved insight into the factors governing the arrhythmia and identification of those at risk may help curb the rapidly expanding prevalence of AF and reduce its burden on patients and healthcare systems.

At present, the use of genetic testing for AF remains within the research domain and is currently not recommended for clinical use [130]. Prior to transitioning genetic testing to the clinical setting, a more thorough understanding of the genetic architecture underlying the arrhythmia is desirable. Unlike classic inherited arrhythmia syndromes, such as long QT syndrome and catecholaminergic polymorphic ventricular tachycardia, which are most often secondary to a single genetic culprit, the development of AF in the majority of cases is likely dependent on polygenic mechanisms with contributions from both rare and common variants. It is hoped that improved insight into the anticipated existence of genetic sub-phenotypes may yield clinically actionable treatment strategies. That said, given that environmental factors likely play a prominent role in the majority of cases, it is probable that genetic testing for AF will be most useful for cases of the arrhythmia with an early age of onset and also develop in the absence of clinical risk factors.

References

1. Feinberg WM, Blackshear JL, Laupacis A, Kronmal R, Hart RG. Prevalence, age distribution, and gender of patients with atrial fibrillation. Analysis and implications. Arch Intern Med. 1995;155:469–73.
2. Go AS, Hylek EM, Phillips KA, Chang Y, Henault LE, Selby JV, Singer DE. Prevalence of diagnosed atrial fibrillation in adults: national implications for rhythm management and stroke prevention: the AnTicoagulation and risk factors in atrial fibrillation (ATRIA) study. JAMA. 2001;285:2370–5.
3. Miyasaka Y, Barnes ME, Gersh BJ, Cha SS, Bailey KR, Abhayaratna WP, Seward JB, Tsang TSM. Secular trends in incidence of atrial fibrillation in Olmsted County, Minnesota, 1980 to 2000, and implications on the projections for future prevalence. Circulation. 2006;114:119–25.
4. Benjamin EJ, Wolf PA, D'Agostino RB, Silbershatz H, Kannel WB, Levy D. Impact of atrial fibrillation on the risk of death: the Framingham heart study. Circulation. 1998;98:946–52.
5. Coyne KS, Paramore C, Grandy S, Mercader M, Reynolds M, Zimetbaum P. Assessing the direct costs of treating nonvalvular atrial fibrillation in the United States. Value Health. 2006;9:348–56.
6. Wolf PA, Abbott RD, Kannel WB. Atrial fibrillation: a major contributor to stroke in the elderly. The Framingham Study. Arch Intern Med. 1987;147:1561–4.
7. Benjamin EJ, Levy D, Vaziri SM, D'Agostino RB, Belanger AJ, Wolf PA. Independent risk factors for atrial fibrillation in a population-based cohort. The Framingham Heart Study. JAMA. 1994;271:840–4.
8. Kopecky SL, Gersh BJ, McGoon MD, Whisnant JP, Holmes DR, Ilstrup DM, Frye RL. The natural history of lone atrial fibrillation. A population-based study over three decades. N Engl J Med. 1987;317:669–74.
9. Wolff L. Familial Auricular Fibrillation. N Engl J Med. 1943;229:396–8.
10. Ellinor PT, Yoerger DM, Ruskin JN, MacRae CA. Familial aggregation in lone atrial fibrillation. Hum Genet. 2005;118:179–84.
11. Fox CS, Parise H, D'Agostino RB, Lloyd-Jones DM, Vasan RS, Wang TJ, Levy D, Wolf PA, Benjamin EJ. Parental atrial fibrillation as a risk factor for atrial fibrillation in offspring. JAMA. 2004;291:2851–5.
12. Arnar DO, Thorvaldsson S, Manolio TA, Thorgeirsson G, Kristjansson K, Hakonarson H, Stefansson K. Familial aggregation of atrial fibrillation in Iceland. Eur Heart J. 2006;27:708–12.
13. Lubitz SA, Yin X, Fontes JD, Magnani JW, Rienstra M, Pai M, Villalon ML, Vasan RS, Pencina MJ, Levy D, Larson MG, Ellinor PT, Benjamin EJ. Association between familial atrial fibrillation and risk of new-onset atrial fibrillation. JAMA. 2010;304:2263–9.
14. Katz AM. Cardiac ion channels. N Engl J Med. 1993;328:1244–51.
15. Abriel H. Cardiac sodium channel Nav1.5 and its associated proteins. Arch Mal Coeur Vaiss. 2007;100:787–93.
16. Bers DM. Cardiac excitation-contraction coupling. Nature. 2002;415:198–205.
17. Marbán E. Cardiac channelopathies. Nature. 2002;415:213–8.
18. Tamkun MM, Knoth KM, Walbridge JA, Kroemer H, Roden DM, Glover DM. Molecular cloning and characterization of two voltage-gated K+ channel cDNAs from human ventricle. FASEB J Off Publ Fed Am Soc Exp Biol. 1991;5:331–7.
19. Wang Z, Fermini B, Nattel S. Sustained depolarization-induced outward current in human atrial myocytes. Evidence for a novel delayed rectifier K+ current similar to Kv1.5 cloned channel currents. Circ Res. 1993;73:1061–76.
20. Abbott GW, Sesti F, Splawski I, Buck ME, Lehmann MH, Timothy KW, Keating MT, Goldstein SA. MiRP1 forms IKr potassium channels with HERG and is associated with cardiac arrhythmia. Cell. 1999;97:175–87.
21. Sanguinetti MC, Curran ME, Zou A, Shen J, Spector PS, Atkinson DL, Keating MT. Coassembly of K(V)LQT1 and minK (IsK) proteins to form cardiac I(Ks) potassium channel. Nature. 1996;384:80–3.
22. Tamargo J, Caballero R, Gómez R, Valenzuela C, Delpón E. Pharmacology of cardiac potassium channels. Cardiovasc Res. 2004;62:9–33.
23. Kubo Y, Baldwin TJ, Jan YN, Jan LY. Primary structure and functional expression of a mouse inward rectifier potassium channel. Nature. 1993;362:127–33.
24. Dhamoon AS, Jalife J. The inward rectifier current (IK1) controls cardiac excitability and is involved in arrhythmogenesis. Heart Rhythm Off J Heart Rhythm Soc. 2005;2:316–24.
25. Lu Z. Mechanism of rectification in inward-rectifier K+ channels. Annu Rev Physiol. 2004;66:103–29.
26. Sakmann B, Noma A, Trautwein W. Acetylcholine activation of single muscarinic K+ channels in isolated pacemaker cells of the mammalian heart. Nature. 1983;303:250–3.
27. Pfaffinger PJ, Martin JM, Hunter DD, Nathanson NM, Hille B. GTP-binding proteins couple cardiac muscarinic receptors to a K channel. Nature. 1985;317:536–8.

28. Corey S, Krapivinsky G, Krapivinsky L, Clapham DE. Number and stoichiometry of subunits in the native atrial G-protein-gated K+ channel, IKACh. J Biol Chem. 1998;273:5271–8.
29. Kovoor P, Wickman K, Maguire CT, Pu W, Gehrmann J, Berul CI, Clapham DE. Evaluation of the role of I(KACh) in atrial fibrillation using a mouse knockout model. J Am Coll Cardiol. 2001;37:2136–43.
30. Liu L, Nattel S. Differing sympathetic and vagal effects on atrial fibrillation in dogs: role of refractoriness heterogeneity. Am J Phys. 1997;273:H805–16.
31. Rohr S. Role of gap junctions in the propagation of the cardiac action potential. Cardiovasc Res. 2004;62:309–22.
32. Brachmann J, Karolyi L, Kübler W. Atrial dispersion of refractoriness. J Cardiovasc Electrophysiol. 1998;9:S35–9.
33. Weiss JN, Qu Z, Chen P-S, Lin S-F, Karagueuzian HS, Hayashi H, Garfinkel A, Karma A. The dynamics of cardiac fibrillation. Circulation. 2005;112:1232–40.
34. Antzelevitch C. Modulation of transmural repolarization. Ann N Y Acad Sci. 2005;1047:314–23.
35. Nattel S. New ideas about atrial fibrillation 50 years on. Nature. 2002;415:219–26.
36. Moe GK, Rheinboldt WC, Abildskov JA. A computer model of atrial fibrillation. Am Heart J. 1964;67:200–20.
37. Konings KT, Kirchhof CJ, Smeets JR, Wellens HJ, Penn OC, Allessie MA. High-density mapping of electrically induced atrial fibrillation in humans. Circulation. 1994;89:1665–80.
38. Cox JL, Canavan TE, Schuessler RB, Cain ME, Lindsay BD, Stone C, Smith PK, Corr PB, Boineau JP. The surgical treatment of atrial fibrillation. II. Intraoperative electrophysiologic mapping and description of the electrophysiologic basis of atrial flutter and atrial fibrillation. J Thorac Cardiovasc Surg. 1991;101:406–26.
39. Mandapati R, Skanes A, Chen J, Berenfeld O, Jalife J. Stable microreentrant sources as a mechanism of atrial fibrillation in the isolated sheep heart. Circulation. 2000;101:194–9.
40. Jalife J, Berenfeld O, Mansour M. Mother rotors and fibrillatory conduction: a mechanism of atrial fibrillation. Cardiovasc Res. 2002;54:204–16.
41. Haïssaguerre M, Jaïs P, Shah DC, Takahashi A, Hocini M, Quiniou G, Garrigue S, Le Mouroux A, Le Métayer P, Clémenty J. Spontaneous initiation of atrial fibrillation by ectopic beats originating in the pulmonary veins. N Engl J Med. 1998;339:659–66.
42. Pappone C, Rosanio S, Oreto G, Tocchi M, Gugliotta F, Vicedomini G, Salvati A, Dicandia C, Mazzone P, Santinelli V, Gulletta S, Chierchia S. Circumferential radiofrequency ablation of pulmonary vein ostia: a new anatomic approach for curing atrial fibrillation. Circulation. 2000;102:2619–28.
43. Allessie MA, Bonke FI, Schopman FJ. Circus movement in rabbit atrial muscle as a mechanism of tachycardia. III. The "leading circle" concept: a new model of circus movement in cardiac tissue without the involvement of an anatomical obstacle. Circ Res. 1977;41:9–18.
44. Rensma PL, Allessie MA, Lammers WJ, Bonke FI, Schalij MJ. Length of excitation wave and susceptibility to reentrant atrial arrhythmias in normal conscious dogs. Circ Res. 1988;62:395–410.
45. Psaty BM, Manolio TA, Kuller LH, Kronmal RA, Cushman M, Fried LP, White R, Furberg CD, Rautaharju PM. Incidence of and risk factors for atrial fibrillation in older adults. Circulation. 1997;96:2455–61.
46. Coumel P, Attuel P, Lavallée J, Flammang D, Leclercq JF, Slama R. The atrial arrhythmia syndrome of vagal origin. Arch Mal Coeur Vaiss. 1978;71:645–56.
47. Brugada R, Tapscott T, Czernuszewicz GZ, Marian AJ, Iglesias A, Mont L, Brugada J, Girona J, Domingo A, Bachinski LL, Roberts R. Identification of a genetic locus for familial atrial fibrillation. N Engl J Med. 1997;336:905–11.
48. Chen Y-H, Xu S-J, Bendahhou S, Wang X-L, Wang Y, Xu W-Y, Jin H-W, Sun H, Su X-Y, Zhuang Q-N, Yang Y-Q, Li Y-B, Liu Y, Xu H-J, Li X-F, Ma N, Mou C-P, Chen Z, Barhanin J, Huang W. KCNQ1 gain-of-function mutation in familial atrial fibrillation. Science. 2003;299:251–4.
49. Darbar D, Herron KJ, Ballew JD, Jahangir A, Gersh BJ, Shen W-K, Hammill SC, Packer DL, Olson TM. Familial atrial fibrillation is a genetically heterogeneous disorder. J Am Coll Cardiol. 2003;41:2185–92.
50. Wang Q, Curran ME, Splawski I, Burn TC, Millholland JM, VanRaay TJ, Shen J, Timothy KW, Vincent GM, de Jager T, Schwartz PJ, Toubin JA, Moss AJ, Atkinson DL, Landes GM, Connors TD, Keating MT. Positional cloning of a novel potassium channel gene: KVLQT1 mutations cause cardiac arrhythmias. Nat Genet. 1996;12:17–23.
51. Giustetto C, Di Monte F, Wolpert C, Borggrefe M, Schimpf R, Sbragia P, Leone G, Maury P, Anttonen O, Haissaguerre M, Gaita F. Short QT syndrome: clinical findings and diagnostic-therapeutic implications. Eur Heart J. 2006;27:2440–7.
52. Gollob MH, Redpath CJ, Roberts JD. The short QT syndrome: proposed diagnostic criteria. J Am Coll Cardiol. 2011;57:802–12.
53. Lundby A, Ravn LS, Svendsen JH, Olesen S-P, Schmitt N. KCNQ1 mutation Q147R is associated with atrial fibrillation and prolonged QT interval. Heart Rhythm. 2007;4:1532–41.
54. Yang Y, Xia M, Jin Q, Bendahhou S, Shi J, Chen Y, Liang B, Lin J, Liu Y, Liu B, Zhou Q, Zhang D, Wang R, Ma N, Su X, Niu K, Pei Y, Xu W, Chen Z, Wan H, Cui J, Barhanin J, Chen Y. Identification of a KCNE2 gain-of-function mutation in patients with familial atrial fibrillation. Am J Hum Genet. 2004;75:899–905.
55. Tinel N, Diochot S, Borsotto M, Lazdunski M, Barhanin J. KCNE2 confers background current characteristics to the cardiac KCNQ1 potassium channel. EMBO J. 2000;19:6326–30.
56. Roberts JD, Krahn AD, Ackerman MJ, Rohatgi RK, Moss AJ, Nazer B, Tadros R, Gerull B, Sanatani S, Wijeyeratne YD, Baruteau A-E, Muir AR, Pang B, Cadrin-Tourigny J, Talajic M, Rivard L, Tester DJ, Liu T, Whitman IR, Wojciak J, Conacher S, Gula LJ, Leong-Sit P, Manlucu J, Green MS, Hamilton R, Healey JS, Lopes CM, Behr ER, Wilde AA, Gollob MH, Scheinman MM. Loss-of-function KCNE2 variants: true monogenic culprits of long-QT syndrome or proarrhythmic variants requiring secondary provocation? Circ Arrhythm Electrophysiol. 2017;10:e005282. https://doi.org/10.1161/CIRCEP.117.005282.
57. Xia M, Jin Q, Bendahhou S, He Y, Larroque M-M, Chen Y, Zhou Q, Yang Y, Liu Y, Liu B, Zhu Q, Zhou Y, Lin J, Liang B, Li L, Dong X, Pan Z, Wang R, Wan H, Qiu W, Xu W, Eurlings P, Barhanin J, Chen Y. A Kir2.1 gain-of-function mutation underlies familial atrial fibrillation. Biochem Biophys Res Commun. 2005;332:1012–9.
58. Plaster NM, Tawil R, Tristani-Firouzi M, Canún S, Bendahhou S, Tsunoda A, Donaldson MR, Iannaccone ST, Brunt E, Barohn R, Clark J, Deymeer F, George AL, Fish FA, Hahn A, Nitu A, Ozdemir C, Serdaroglu P, Subramony SH, Wolfe G, Fu YH, Ptácek LJ. Mutations in Kir2.1 cause the developmental and episodic electrical phenotypes of Andersen's syndrome. Cell. 2001;105:511–9.
59. Gaita F, Giustetto C, Bianchi F, Wolpert C, Schimpf R, Riccardi R, Grossi S, Richiardi E, Borggrefe M. Short QT syndrome a familial cause of sudden death. Circulation. 2003;108:965–70.
60. Hong K, Bjerregaard P, Gussak I, Brugada R. Short QT syndrome and atrial fibrillation caused by mutation in KCNH2. J Cardiovasc Electrophysiol. 2005;16:394–6.
61. Brugada R, Hong K, Dumaine R, Cordeiro J, Gaita F, Borggrefe M, Menendez TM, Brugada J, Pollevick GD, Wolpert C, Burashnikov E, Matsuo K, Wu YS, Guerchicoff A, Bianchi F, Giustetto C, Schimpf R, Brugada P, Antzelevitch C. Sudden

death associated with short-QT syndrome linked to mutations in HERG. Circulation. 2004;109:30–5.
62. Bellocq C, van Ginneken ACG, Bezzina CR, Alders M, Escande D, Mannens MMAM, Baró I, Wilde AAM. Mutation in the KCNQ1 gene leading to the short QT-interval syndrome. Circulation. 2004;109:2394–7.
63. Priori SG, Pandit SV, Rivolta I, Berenfeld O, Ronchetti E, Dhamoon A, Napolitano C, Anumonwo J, di Barletta MR, Gudapakkam S, Bosi G, Stramba-Badiale M, Jalife J. A novel form of short QT syndrome (SQT3) is caused by a mutation in the KCNJ2 gene. Circ Res. 2005;96:800–7.
64. Antzelevitch C, Pollevick GD, Cordeiro JM, Casis O, Sanguinetti MC, Aizawa Y, Guerchicoff A, Pfeiffer R, Oliva A, Wollnik B, Gelber P, Bonaros EP, Burashnikov E, Wu Y, Sargent JD, Schickel S, Oberheiden R, Bhatia A, Hsu L-F, Haïssaguerre M, Schimpf R, Borggrefe M, Wolpert C. Loss-of-function mutations in the cardiac calcium channel underlie a new clinical entity characterized by ST-segment elevation, short QT intervals, and sudden cardiac death. Circulation. 2007;115:442–9.
65. Templin C, Ghadri J-R, Rougier J-S, Baumer A, Kaplan V, Albesa M, Sticht H, Rauch A, Puleo C, Hu D, Barajas-Martinez H, Antzelevitch C, Lüscher TF, Abriel H, Duru F. Identification of a novel loss-of-function calcium channel gene mutation in short QT syndrome (SQTS6). Eur Heart J. 2011;32:1077–88.
66. Deo M, Ruan Y, Pandit SV, Shah K, Berenfeld O, Blaufox A, Cerrone M, Noujaim SF, Denegri M, Jalife J, Priori SG. KCNJ2 mutation in short QT syndrome 3 results in atrial fibrillation and ventricular proarrhythmia. Proc Natl Acad Sci U S A. 2013;110:4291–6.
67. Olson TM, Alekseev AE, Liu XK, Park S, Zingman LV, Bienengraeber M, Sattiraju S, Ballew JD, Jahangir A, Terzic A. Kv1.5 channelopathy due to KCNA5 loss-of-function mutation causes human atrial fibrillation. Hum Mol Genet. 2006;15:2185–91.
68. Satoh T, Zipes DP. Cesium-induced atrial tachycardia degenerating into atrial fibrillation in dogs: atrial torsades de pointes? J Cardiovasc Electrophysiol. 1998;9:970–5.
69. Otway R, Vandenberg JI, Guo G, Varghese A, Castro ML, Liu J, Zhao J, Bursill JA, Wyse KR, Crotty H, Baddeley O, Walker B, Kuchar D, Thorburn C, Fatkin D. Stretch-sensitive KCNQ1 mutation a link between genetic and environmental factors in the pathogenesis of atrial fibrillation? J Am Coll Cardiol. 2007;49:578–86.
70. Ellinor PT, Moore RK, Patton KK, Ruskin JN, Pollak MR, Macrae CA. Mutations in the long QT gene, KCNQ1, are an uncommon cause of atrial fibrillation. Heart Br Card Soc. 2004;90:1487–8.
71. Ellinor PT, Petrov-Kondratov VI, Zakharova E, Nam EG, MacRae CA. Potassium channel gene mutations rarely cause atrial fibrillation. BMC Med Genet. 2006;7:70.
72. Hervé J-C, Bourmeyster N, Sarrouilhe D, Duffy HS. Gap junctional complexes: from partners to functions. Prog Biophys Mol Biol. 2007;94:29–65.
73. Vozzi C, Dupont E, Coppen SR, Yeh HI, Severs NJ. Chamber-related differences in connexin expression in the human heart. J Mol Cell Cardiol. 1999;31:991–1003.
74. Hagendorff A, Schumacher B, Kirchhoff S, Lüderitz B, Willecke K. Conduction disturbances and increased atrial vulnerability in Connexin40-deficient mice analyzed by transesophageal stimulation. Circulation. 1999;99:1508–15.
75. van der Velden HM, Ausma J, Rook MB, Hellemons AJ, van Veen TA, Allessie MA, Jongsma HJ. Gap junctional remodeling in relation to stabilization of atrial fibrillation in the goat. Cardiovasc Res. 2000;46:476–86.
76. Wilhelm M, Kirste W, Kuly S, Amann K, Neuhuber W, Weyand M, Daniel WG, Garlichs C. Atrial distribution of connexin 40 and 43 in patients with intermittent, persistent, and postoperative atrial fibrillation. Heart Lung Circ. 2006;15:30–7.
77. Gollob MH, Jones DL, Krahn AD, Danis L, Gong X-Q, Shao Q, Liu X, Veinot JP, Tang ASL, Stewart AFR, Tesson F, Klein GJ, Yee R, Skanes AC, Guiraudon GM, Ebihara L, Bai D. Somatic mutations in the connexin 40 gene (GJA5) in atrial fibrillation. N Engl J Med. 2006;354:2677–88.
78. Thibodeau IL, Xu J, Li Q, Liu G, Lam K, Veinot JP, Birnie DH, Jones DL, Krahn AD, Lemery R, Nicholson BJ, Gollob MH. Paradigm of genetic mosaicism and lone atrial fibrillation: physiological characterization of a connexin 43-deletion mutant identified from atrial tissue. Circulation. 2010;122:236–44.
79. Yang Y-Q, Liu X, Zhang X-L, Wang X-H, Tan H-W, Shi H-F, Jiang W-F, Fang W-Y. Novel connexin40 missense mutations in patients with familial atrial fibrillation. Europace. 2010;12:1421–7.
80. Yang Y-Q, Zhang X-L, Wang X-H, Tan H-W, Shi H-F, Jiang W-F, Fang W-Y, Liu X. Connexin40 nonsense mutation in familial atrial fibrillation. Int J Mol Med. 2010;26:605–10.
81. Christophersen IE, Holmegard HN, Jabbari J, Sajadieh A, Haunsø S, Tveit A, Svendsen JH, Olesen MS. Rare variants in GJA5 are associated with early-onset lone atrial fibrillation. Can J Cardiol. 2013;29:111–6.
82. Shi H-F, Yang J-F, Wang Q, Li R-G, Xu Y-J, Qu X-K, Fang W-Y, Liu X, Yang Y-Q. Prevalence and spectrum of GJA5 mutations associated with lone atrial fibrillation. Mol Med Rep. 2013;7:767–74.
83. Sun Y, Yang Y-Q, Gong X-Q, Wang X-H, Li R-G, Tan H-W, Liu X, Fang W-Y, Bai D. Novel germline GJA5/connexin40 mutations associated with lone atrial fibrillation impair gap junctional intercellular communication. Hum Mutat. 2013;34:603–9.
84. Sun Y, Tong X, Chen H, Huang T, Shao Q, Huang W, Laird DW, Bai D. An atrial-fibrillation-linked connexin40 mutant is retained in the endoplasmic reticulum and impairs the function of atrial gap-junction channels. Dis Model Mech. 2014;7:561–9.
85. Lübkemeier I, Andrié R, Lickfett L, Bosen F, Stöckigt F, Dobrowolski R, Draffehn AM, Fregeac J, Schultze JL, Bukauskas FF, Schrickel JW, Willecke K. The Connexin40A96S mutation from a patient with atrial fibrillation causes decreased atrial conduction velocities and sustained episodes of induced atrial fibrillation in mice. J Mol Cell Cardiol. 2013;65:19–32.
86. Chen Q, Kirsch GE, Zhang D, Brugada R, Brugada J, Brugada P, Potenza D, Moya A, Borggrefe M, Breithardt G, Ortiz-Lopez R, Wang Z, Antzelevitch C, O'Brien RE, Schulze-Bahr E, Keating MT, Towbin JA, Wang Q. Genetic basis and molecular mechanism for idiopathic ventricular fibrillation. Nature. 1998;392:293–6.
87. Wang Q, Shen J, Splawski I, Atkinson D, Li Z, Robinson JL, Moss AJ, Towbin JA, Keating MT. SCN5A mutations associated with an inherited cardiac arrhythmia, long QT syndrome. Cell. 1995;80:805–11.
88. Benson DW, Wang DW, Dyment M, Knilans TK, Fish FA, Strieper MJ, Rhodes TH, George AL. Congenital sick sinus syndrome caused by recessive mutations in the cardiac sodium channel gene (SCN5A). J Clin Invest. 2003;112:1019–28.
89. Roberts JD, Gollob MH, Young C, Connors SP, Gray C, Wilton SB, Green MS, Zhu DW, Hodgkinson KA, Poon A, Li Q, Orr N, Tang AS, Klein GJ, Wojciak J, Campagna J, Olgin JE, Badhwar N, Vedantham V, Marcus GM, Kwok P-Y, Deo RC, Scheinman MM. Bundle branch re-entrant ventricular tachycardia: novel genetic mechanisms in a life-threatening arrhythmia. JACC Clin Electrophysiol. 2017;3:276–88.
90. Chen LY, Ballew JD, Herron KJ, Rodeheffer RJ, Olson TM. A common polymorphism in SCN5A is associated with lone atrial fibrillation. Clin Pharmacol Ther. 2007;81:35–41.
91. Makielski JC, Ye B, Valdivia CR, Pagel MD, Pu J, Tester DJ, Ackerman MJ. A ubiquitous splice variant and a common polymorphism affect heterologous expression of recombinant human SCN5A heart sodium channels. Circ Res. 2003;93:821–8.

92. Darbar D, Kannankeril PJ, Donahue BS, Kucera G, Stubblefield T, Haines JL, George AL, Roden DM. Cardiac sodium channel (SCN5A) variants associated with atrial fibrillation. Circulation. 2008;117:1927–35.
93. Ellinor PT, Nam EG, Shea MA, Milan DJ, Ruskin JN, MacRae CA. Cardiac sodium channel mutation in atrial fibrillation. Heart Rhythm. 2008;5:99–105.
94. Makiyama T, Akao M, Shizuta S, Doi T, Nishiyama K, Oka Y, Ohno S, Nishio Y, Tsuji K, Itoh H, Kimura T, Kita T, Horie M. A novel SCN5A gain-of-function mutation M1875T associated with familial atrial fibrillation. J Am Coll Cardiol. 2008;52:1326–34.
95. Li Q, Huang H, Liu G, Lam K, Rutberg J, Green MS, Birnie DH, Lemery R, Chahine M, Gollob MH. Gain-of-function mutation of Nav1.5 in atrial fibrillation enhances cellular excitability and lowers the threshold for action potential firing. Biochem Biophys Res Commun. 2009;380:132–7.
96. Scornik FS, Desai M, Brugada R, Guerchicoff A, Pollevick GD, Antzelevitch C, Pérez GJ. Functional expression of "cardiac-type" Nav1.5 sodium channel in canine intracardiac ganglia. Heart Rhythm. 2006;3:842–50.
97. Rubattu S, Sciarretta S, Valenti V, Stanzione R, Volpe M. Natriuretic peptides: an update on bioactivity, potential therapeutic use, and implication in cardiovascular diseases. Am J Hypertens. 2008;21:733–41.
98. Crozier I, Richards AM, Foy SG, Ikram H. Electrophysiological effects of atrial natriuretic peptide on the cardiac conduction system in man. Pacing Clin Electrophysiol PACE. 1993;16:738–42.
99. Sorbera LA, Morad M. Atrionatriuretic peptide transforms cardiac sodium channels into calcium-conducting channels. Science. 1990;247:969–73.
100. Le Grand B, Deroubaix E, Couétil JP, Coraboeuf E. Effects of atrionatriuretic factor on Ca2+ current and Cai-independent transient outward K+ current in human atrial cells. Pflüg Arch Eur J Physiol. 1992;421:486–91.
101. Ellinor PT, Low AF, Patton KK, Shea MA, Macrae CA. Discordant atrial natriuretic peptide and brain natriuretic peptide levels in lone atrial fibrillation. J Am Coll Cardiol. 2005;45:82–6.
102. Hodgson-Zingman DM, Karst ML, Zingman LV, Heublein DM, Darbar D, Herron KJ, Ballew JD, de Andrade M, Burnett JC, Olson TM. Atrial natriuretic peptide frameshift mutation in familial atrial fibrillation. N Engl J Med. 2008;359:158–65.
103. Levin ER, Gardner DG, Samson WK. Natriuretic peptides. N Engl J Med. 1998;339:321–8.
104. Chen HH, Lainchbury JG, Burnett JC. Natriuretic peptide receptors and neutral endopeptidase in mediating the renal actions of a new therapeutic synthetic natriuretic peptide dendroaspis natriuretic peptide. J Am Coll Cardiol. 2002;40:1186–91.
105. McNally EM, Barefield DY, Puckelwartz MJ. The genetic landscape of cardiomyopathy and its role in heart failure. Cell Metab. 2015;21:174–82.
106. Orr N, Arnaout R, Gula LJ, Spears DA, Leong-Sit P, Li Q, Tarhuni W, Reischauer S, Chauhan VS, Borkovich M, Uppal S, Adler A, Coughlin SR, Stainier DYR, Gollob MH. A mutation in the atrial-specific myosin light chain gene (MYL4) causes familial atrial fibrillation. Nat Commun. 2016;7:11303.
107. Gudbjartsson DF, Holm H, Sulem P, Masson G, Oddsson A, Magnusson OT, Saemundsdottir J, Helgadottir HT, Helgason H, Johannsdottir H, Gretarsdottir S, Gudjonsson SA, Njølstad I, Løchen M-L, Baum L, Ma RCW, Sigfusson G, Kong A, Thorgeirsson G, Sverrisson JT, Thorsteinsdottir U, Stefansson K, Arnar DO. A frameshift deletion in the sarcomere gene MYL4 causes early-onset familial atrial fibrillation. Eur Heart J. 2017;38:27–34.
108. Peng W, Li M, Li H, Tang K, Zhuang J, Zhang J, Xiao J, Jiang H, Li D, Yu Y, Sham PC, Nattel S, Xu Y. Dysfunction of myosin light-chain 4 (MYL4) leads to heritable atrial cardiomyopathy with electrical, contractile, and structural components: evidence from genetically-engineered rats. J Am Heart Assoc. 2017;6:007030.
109. Ellinor PT, Shin JT, Moore RK, Yoerger DM, MacRae CA. Locus for atrial fibrillation maps to chromosome 6q14-16. Circulation. 2003;107:2880–3.
110. Volders PGA, Zhu Q, Timmermans C, Eurlings PMH, Su X, Arens YH, Li L, Jongbloed RJ, Xia M, Rodriguez L-M, Chen YH. Mapping a novel locus for familial atrial fibrillation on chromosome 10p11-q21. Heart Rhythm. 2007;4:469–75.
111. Darbar D, Hardy A, Haines JL, Roden DM. Prolonged signal-averaged P-wave duration as an intermediate phenotype for familial atrial fibrillation. J Am Coll Cardiol. 2008;51:1083–9.
112. Gudbjartsson DF, Arnar DO, Helgadottir A, Gretarsdottir S, Holm H, Sigurdsson A, Jonasdottir A, Baker A, Thorleifsson G, Kristjansson K, Palsson A, Blondal T, Sulem P, Backman VM, Hardarson GA, Palsdottir E, Helgason A, Sigurjonsdottir R, Sverrisson JT, Kostulas K, Ng MCY, Baum L, So WY, Wong KS, Chan JCN, Furie KL, Greenberg SM, Sale M, Kelly P, MacRae CA, Smith EE, Rosand J, Hillert J, Ma RCW, Ellinor PT, Thorgeirsson G, Gulcher JR, Kong A, Thorsteinsdottir U, Stefansson K. Variants conferring risk of atrial fibrillation on chromosome 4q25. Nature. 2007;448:353–7.
113. Ye J, Tucker NR, Weng L-C, Clauss S, Lubitz SA, Ellinor PT. A functional variant associated with atrial fibrillation regulates PITX2c expression through TFAP2a. Am J Hum Genet. 2016;99:1281–91.
114. Wang J, Klysik E, Sood S, Johnson RL, Wehrens XHT, Martin JF. Pitx2 prevents susceptibility to atrial arrhythmias by inhibiting left-sided pacemaker specification. Proc Natl Acad Sci U S A. 2010;107:9753–8.
115. Kirchhof P, Kahr PC, Kaese S, Piccini I, Vokshi I, Scheld H-H, Rotering H, Fortmueller L, Laakmann S, Verheule S, Schotten U, Fabritz L, Brown NA. PITX2c is expressed in the adult left atrium, and reducing Pitx2c expression promotes atrial fibrillation inducibility and complex changes in gene expression. Circ Cardiovasc Genet. 2011;4:123–33.
116. Benjamin EJ, Rice KM, Arking DE, Pfeufer A, van Noord C, Smith AV, Schnabel RB, Bis JC, Boerwinkle E, Sinner MF, Dehghan A, Lubitz SA, D'Agostino RB, Lumley T, Ehret GB, Heeringa J, Aspelund T, Newton-Cheh C, Larson MG, Marciante KD, Soliman EZ, Rivadeneira F, Wang TJ, Eiríksdottir G, Levy D, Psaty BM, Li M, Chamberlain AM, Hofman A, Vasan RS, Harris TB, Rotter JI, WHL K, Agarwal SK, BHC S, Wang K, Launer LJ, Smith NL, Chakravarti A, Uitterlinden AG, Wolf PA, Sotoodehnia N, Köttgen A, van Duijn CM, Meitinger T, Mueller M, Perz S, Steinbeck G, Wichmann H-E, Lunetta KL, Heckbert SR, Gudnason V, Alonso A, Kääb S, Ellinor PT, JCM W. Variants in ZFHX3 are associated with atrial fibrillation in individuals of European ancestry. Nat Genet. 2009;41:879–81.
117. Gudbjartsson DF, Holm H, Gretarsdottir S, Thorleifsson G, Walters GB, Thorgeirsson G, Gulcher J, Mathiesen EB, Njølstad I, Nyrnes A, Wilsgaard T, Hald EM, Hveem K, Stoltenberg C, Kucera G, Stubblefield T, Carter S, Roden D, Ng MCY, Baum L, So WY, Wong KS, Chan JCN, Gieger C, Wichmann H-E, Gschwendtner A, Dichgans M, Kuhlenbäumer G, Berger K, Ringelstein EB, Bevan S, Markus HS, Kostulas K, Hillert J, Sveinbjörnsdóttir S, Valdimarsson EM, Løchen M-L, Ma RCW, Darbar D, Kong A, Arnar DO, Thorsteinsdottir U, Stefansson K. A sequence variant in ZFHX3 on 16q22 associates with atrial fibrillation and ischemic stroke. Nat Genet. 2009;41:876–8.
118. Burgner D, Davila S, Breunis WB, Ng SB, Li Y, Bonnard C, Ling L, Wright VJ, Thalamuthu A, Odam M, Shimizu C, Burns JC, Levin M, Kuijpers TW, Hibberd ML. International Kawasaki Disease Genetics Consortium. A genome-wide association study identifies novel and functionally related susceptibility Loci for Kawasaki disease. PLoS Genet. 2009;5:e1000319.

119. Ellinor PT, Lunetta KL, Glazer NL, Pfeufer A, Alonso A, Chung MK, Sinner MF, de Bakker PIW, Mueller M, Lubitz SA, Fox E, Darbar D, Smith NL, Smith JD, Schnabel RB, Soliman EZ, Rice KM, Van Wagoner DR, Beckmann B-M, van Noord C, Wang K, Ehret GB, Rotter JI, Hazen SL, Steinbeck G, Smith AV, Launer LJ, Harris TB, Makino S, Nelis M, Milan DJ, Perz S, Esko T, Köttgen A, Moebus S, Newton-Cheh C, Li M, Möhlenkamp S, Wang TJ, Kao WHL, Vasan RS, Nöthen MM, MacRae CA, Stricker BHC, Hofman A, Uitterlinden AG, Levy D, Boerwinkle E, Metspalu A, Topol EJ, Chakravarti A, Gudnason V, Psaty BM, Roden DM, Meitinger T, Wichmann H-E, Witteman JCM, Barnard J, Arking DE, Benjamin EJ, Heckbert SR, Kääb S. Common variants in KCNN3 are associated with lone atrial fibrillation. Nat Genet. 2010;42:240–4.
120. Ellinor PT, Lunetta KL, Albert CM, Glazer NL, Ritchie MD, Smith AV, Arking DE, Müller-Nurasyid M, Krijthe BP, Lubitz SA, Bis JC, Chung MK, Dörr M, Ozaki K, Roberts JD, Smith JG, Pfeufer A, Sinner MF, Lohman K, Ding J, Smith NL, Smith JD, Rienstra M, Rice KM, Van Wagoner DR, Magnani JW, Wakili R, Clauss S, Rotter JI, Steinbeck G, Launer LJ, Davies RW, Borkovich M, Harris TB, Lin H, Völker U, Völzke H, Milan DJ, Hofman A, Boerwinkle E, Chen LY, Soliman EZ, Voight BF, Li G, Chakravarti A, Kubo M, Tedrow UB, Rose LM, Ridker PM, Conen D, Tsunoda T, Furukawa T, Sotoodehnia N, Xu S, Kamatani N, Levy D, Nakamura Y, Parvez B, Mahida S, Furie KL, Rosand J, Muhammad R, Psaty BM, Meitinger T, Perz S, Wichmann H-E, Witteman JCM, Kao WHL, Kathiresan S, Roden DM, Uitterlinden AG, Rivadeneira F, McKnight B, Sjögren M, Newman AB, Liu Y, Gollob MH, Melander O, Tanaka T, Stricker BHC, Felix SB, Alonso A, Darbar D, Barnard J, Chasman DI, Heckbert SR, Benjamin EJ, Gudnason V, Kääb S. Meta-analysis identifies six new susceptibility loci for atrial fibrillation. Nat Genet. 2012;44:670–5.
121. Sinner MF, Tucker NR, Lunetta KL, Ozaki K, Smith JG, Trompet S, Bis JC, Lin H, Chung MK, Nielsen JB, Lubitz SA, Krijthe BP, Magnani JW, Ye J, Gollob MH, Tsunoda T, Müller-Nurasyid M, Lichtner P, Peters A, Dolmatova E, Kubo M, Smith JD, Psaty BM, Smith NL, Jukema JW, Chasman DI, Albert CM, Ebana Y, Furukawa T, Macfarlane PW, Harris TB, Darbar D, Dörr M, Holst AG, Svendsen JH, Hofman A, Uitterlinden AG, Gudnason V, Isobe M, Malik R, Dichgans M, Rosand J, Van Wagoner DR, METASTROKE Consortium, AFGen Consortium, Benjamin EJ, Milan DJ, Melander O, Heckbert SR, Ford I, Liu Y, Barnard J, Olesen MS, Stricker BHC, Tanaka T, Kääb S, Ellinor PT. Integrating genetic, transcriptional, and functional analyses to identify 5 novel genes for atrial fibrillation. Circulation. 2014;130:1225–35.
122. Low S-K, Takahashi A, Ebana Y, Ozaki K, Christophersen IE, Ellinor PT, AFGen Consortium, Ogishima S, Yamamoto M, Satoh M, Sasaki M, Yamaji T, Iwasaki M, Tsugane S, Tanaka K, Naito M, Wakai K, Tanaka H, Furukawa T, Kubo M, Ito K, Kamatani Y, Tanaka T. Identification of six new genetic loci associated with atrial fibrillation in the Japanese population. Nat Genet. 2017 [cited 2017 May 18];advance online publication. Available from: http://www.nature.com/ng/journal/vaop/ncurrent/full/ng.3842.html?WT.feed_name=subjects_biological-sciences
123. Christophersen IE, Rienstra M, Roselli C, Yin X, Geelhoed B, Barnard J, Lin H, Arking DE, Smith AV, Albert CM, Chaffin M, Tucker NR, Li M, Klarin D, Bihlmeyer NA, Low S-K, Weeke PE, Müller-Nurasyid M, Smith JG, Brody JA, Niemeijer MN, Dörr M, Trompet S, Huffman J, Gustafsson S, Schurmann C, Kleber ME, Lyytikäinen L-P, Seppälä I, Malik R, Horimoto ARVR, Perez M, Sinisalo J, Aeschbacher S, Thériault S, Yao J, Radmanesh F, Weiss S, Teumer A, Choi SH, Weng L-C, Clauss S, Deo R, Rader DJ, Shah SH, Sun A, Hopewell JC, Debette S, Chauhan G, Yang Q, Worrall BB, Paré G, Kamatani Y, Hagemeijer YP, Verweij N, Siland JE, Kubo M, Smith JD, Van Wagoner DR, Bis JC, Perz S, Psaty BM, Ridker PM, Magnani JW, Harris TB, Launer LJ, Shoemaker MB, Padmanabhan S, Haessler J, Bartz TM, Waldenberger M, Lichtner P, Arendt M, Krieger JE, Kähönen M, Risch L, Mansur AJ, Peters A, Smith BH, Lind L, Scott SA, Lu Y, Bottinger EB, Hernesniemi J, Lindgren CM, Wong JA, Huang J, Eskola M, Morris AP, Ford I, Reiner AP, Delgado G, Chen LY, Chen YDI, Sandhu RK, Li M, Boerwinkle E, Eisele L, et al. Large-scale analyses of common and rare variants identify 12 new loci associated with atrial fibrillation. Nat Genet. 2017;49:946–52.
124. Roselli C, Chaffin MD, Weng L-C, Aeschbacher S, Ahlberg G, Albert CM, Almgren P, Alonso A, Anderson CD, Aragam KG, Arking DE, Barnard J, Bartz TM, Benjamin EJ, Bihlmeyer NA, Bis JC, Bloom HL, Boerwinkle E, Bottinger EB, Brody JA, Calkins H, Campbell A, Cappola TP, Carlquist J, Chasman DI, Chen LY, YDI C, Choi E-K, Choi SH, Christophersen IE, Chung MK, Cole JW, Conen D, Cook J, Crijns HJ, Cutler MJ, Damrauer SM, Daniels BR, Darbar D, Delgado G, Denny JC, Dichgans M, Dörr M, Dudink EA, Dudley SC, Esa N, Esko T, Eskola M, Fatkin D, Felix SB, Ford I, Franco OH, Geelhoed B, Grewal RP, Gudnason V, Guo X, Gupta N, Gustafsson S, Gutmann R, Hamsten A, Harris TB, Hayward C, Heckbert SR, Hernesniemi J, Hocking LJ, Hofman A, ARVR H, Huang J, Huang PL, Huffman J, Ingelsson E, Ipek EG, Ito K, Jimenez-Conde J, Johnson R, Jukema JW, Kääb S, Kähönen M, Kamatani Y, Kane JP, Kastrati A, Kathiresan S, Katschnig-Winter P, Kavousi M, Kessler T, Kietselaer BL, Kirchhof P, Kleber ME, Knight S, Krieger JE, Kubo M, Launer LJ, Laurikka J, Lehtimäki T, Leineweber K, Lemaitre RN, Li M, Lim HE, et al. Multi-ethnic genome-wide association study for atrial fibrillation. Nat Genet. 2018;50:1225–33.
125. Nielsen JB, Thorolfsdottir RB, Fritsche LG, Zhou W, Skov MW, Graham SE, Herron TJ, Mc Carthy S, Schmidt EM, Sveinbjornsson G, Surakka I, Mathis MR, Yamazaki M, Crawford RD, Gabrielsen ME, Skogholt AH, Holmen OL, Lin M, Wolford BN, Dey R, Dalen H, Sulem P, Chung JH, Backman JD, Arnar DO, Thorsteinsdottir U, Baras A, O'Dushlaine C, Holst AG, Wen X, Hornsby W, Dewey FE, Boehnke M, Kheterpal S, Mukherjee B, Lee S, Kang HM, Holm H, Kitzman J, Shavit JA, Jalife J, Brummett CM, Teslovich TM, Carey DJ, Gudbjartsson DF, Stefansson K, Abecasis GR, Hveem K, Willer CJ. Biobank-driven genomic discovery yields new insight into atrial fibrillation biology. Nat Genet. 2018;50:1234–9.
126. Hsu J, Gore-Panter S, Tchou G, Castel L, Lovano B, Moravec CS, Pettersson GB, Roselli EE, Gillinov AM, McCurry KR, Smedira NG, Barnard J, Van Wagoner DR, Chung MK, Smith JD. Genetic control of left atrial gene expression yields insights into the genetic susceptibility for atrial fibrillation. Circ Genomic Precis Med. 2018;11:e002107.
127. Roberts JD. Noncoding genetic variation and gene expression: deciphering the molecular drivers of genome-wide association study signals in atrial fibrillation. Circ Genomic Precis Med. 2018;11:e002109.
128. Weng L-C, Preis SR, Hulme OL, Larson MG, Choi SH, Wang B, Trinquart L, McManus DD, Staerk L, Lin H, Lunetta KL, Ellinor PT, Benjamin EJ, Lubitz SA. Genetic predisposition, clinical risk factor burden, and lifetime risk of atrial fibrillation. Circulation. 2017;137(10):1027–38.
129. Khera AV, Chaffin M, Aragam KG, Haas ME, Roselli C, Choi SH, Natarajan P, Lander ES, Lubitz SA, Ellinor PT, Kathiresan S. Genome-wide polygenic scores for common diseases identify individuals with risk equivalent to monogenic mutations. Nat Genet. 2018;50:1219–24.
130. Ackerman MJ, Priori SG, Willems S, Berul C, Brugada R, Calkins H, Camm AJ, Ellinor PT, Gollob M, Hamilton R, Hershberger RE, Judge DP, Le Marec H, McKenna WJ, Schulze-Bahr E, Semsarian C, Towbin JA, Watkins H, Wilde A, Wolpert C, Zipes DP. HRS/

EHRA expert consensus statement on the state of genetic testing for the channelopathies and cardiomyopathies this document was developed as a partnership between the Heart Rhythm Society (HRS) and the European Heart Rhythm Association (EHRA). Heart Rhythm. 2011;8:1308–39.
131. Roberts JD, Gollob MH. Impact of genetic discoveries on the classification of lone atrial fibrillation. J Am Coll Cardiol. 2010;55:705–12.
132. Lubitz SA, Parsons OE, Anderson CD, Benjamin EJ, Malik R, Weng L-C, Dichgans M, Sudlow CL, Rothwell PM, Rosand J, Ellinor PT, Markus HS, Traylor M, WTCCC2, International Stroke Genetics Consortium, and AFGen Consortia. Atrial fibrillation genetic risk and ischemic stroke mechanisms. Stroke. 2017;48:1451–6.

Part IV

Hereditary Thoracic Aortic Diseases

Heritable Thoracic Aortic Diseases: Syndromal and Isolated (F)TAAD

19

Barbara J. M. Mulder, Ingrid M. B. H. van de Laar, and Julie De Backer

Introduction

Heritable thoracic aortic disease (H-TAD) comprises a heterogeneous group of disorders with as a common denominator aortic aneurysm or dissection on one or several levels from the aortic root till the diaphragm. Aneurysms and dissections in more distal parts of the aorta and/or other vessels may co-occur in some H-TAD entities. Depending on the presence or absence of manifestations in other organ systems, H-TAD can be further subdivided into syndromic and nonsyndromic H-TAD. For both clinical entities, multiple underlying gene defects have been identified, although we must recognize that in a substantial number of patients and families, especially in the nonsyndromic group, no causal variant is identifiable, defining them as "heritable" but strictly speaking not (yet) as "genetic."

Currently known causal genes that have been identified in H-TAD can be grouped into those affecting structure (i.e., genes encoding extracellular matrix (ECM) components (e.g., *FBN1*, *COL3A1*, *MFAP5*, *FBN2*, *BGN*, *LOX*)) and those that affect the ability to modify structure in response to changes in mechanical load imposed on the aortic wall. The latter group can be divided into genes encoding various proteins involved in TGFβ signaling (e.g., *TGFBR1*, *TGFBR2*, *TGFB2*, *TGFB3*, *SMAD2*, *SMAD3, SMAD4*) and genes encoding proteins involved in vascular smooth muscle cell contractility (e.g., *ACTA2*, *MYH11*, *MYLK*, *PRKG1*). Table 19.1 provides a schematic overview of the currently known genes and their associated clinical entities.

In this chapter, we will cover the clinical and molecular aspects of four relevant syndromic H-TAD entities, Marfan syndrome, vascular Ehlers-Danlos syndrome, Loeys-Dietz syndrome, and multisystemic smooth muscle cell dysfunction syndrome, as well as the current knowledge on nonsyndromic H-TAD.

Clinical Presentation

Marfan Syndrome

Marfan syndrome (MFS, ORPHA 558, OMIM #154700) is a common yet under-recognized autosomal dominant systemic disorder of connective tissue, caused by heterozygous mutations in the *FBN1* gene at 15q21.1, which encodes the extracellular matrix protein fibrillin-1. The disorder shows characteristic but highly variable manifestations mainly in the cardiovascular, ocular, and musculoskeletal systems. It was first reported in 1896, when Antoine Bernard-Jean Marfan described a young girl with unusual musculoskeletal features [37]. It was not until the mid-1950s that cardiovascular involvement in Marfan syndrome was well recognized and described in Victor McKusick's monograph [38]. The age of onset of clinical manifestations is highly variable, ranging from severe cardiovascular involvement at birth in the neonatal form to patients developing manifestations only in midlife. The estimated prevalence of Marfan syndrome is 1 in 3,000–5,000 individuals, with no ethnic or gender predilection. About 25% of patients represent new mutations. Prognosis is mainly determined by progressive dilation of the aorta, which may lead to aortic dissection and death at a young age. Mean survival of untreated patients is about 40 years. Fortunately, improved management and ongoing research have led to a significant increase in life expectancy of at least 30 years [39, 40] which does not imply that life

B. J. M. Mulder
Department of Cardiology, Academic Medical Centre, Amsterdam, The Netherlands
e-mail: b.j.mulder@amc.uva.nl

Ingrid M. B. H. van de Laar (✉)
Department of Clinical Genetics, Erasmus Medical Center, Rotterdam, The Netherlands
e-mail: i.vandelaar@erasmusmc.nl

J. De Backer
Department of Cardiology and Center for Medical Genetics, Ghent University Hospital, Ghent, Belgium
e-mail: Julie.debacker@ugent.be

H. F. Baars et al. (eds.), *Clinical Cardiogenetics*, https://doi.org/10.1007/978-3-030-45457-9_19

Table 19.1 Schematic overview of heritable thoracic aortic disease (H-TAD) entities, according to the underlying gene defects and according to the degree of manifestations outside the aorta (syndromic gradient, from left to right). Two major groups of gene mutations associated with H-TAD can be distinguished, namely, those affecting structure (i.e., the ECM) and those that affect the ability to modify structure in response to changes in mechanical load imposed on the aortic wall (i.e., cell signaling pathways and the contractile apparatus)

Gene name	Clinical entities associated with the gene—from highly syndromic on the left to nonsyndromic on the right		
H-TAD related to genes encoding components of the extracellular matrix			
FBN1	Neonatal MFS [1, 2]	Classic MFS/MFS features [2]	Isolated/nonsyndromic H-TAD [3]
COL3A1	vEDS [4]		Isolated/nonsyndromic H-TAD [5]
MFAP5		MFS features [6]	Isolated/nonsyndromic H-TAD [6]
BGN	Meester-Loeys syndrome		
LOX			Isolated/nonsyndromic H-TAD [7]
H-TAD related to genes encoding components of the TGFβ pathway			
TGFBR1	LDS; vEDS [8, 9]	Classic MFS/MFS features [10, 11]	Isolated/nonsyndromic H-TAD [10, 11]
TGFBR2	LDS; vEDS [8, 9]	Classic MFS/MFS features [11–13]	Isolated/nonsyndromic H-TAD [14, 15]
SMAD2		Marfanoid features	Isolated/nonsyndromic H-TAD [16]
SMAD3	LDS [17, 18]	AOS, classic MFS/MFS features [19]	Isolated/nonsyndromic H-TAD [5, 20]
SMAD4	Juvenile polyposis syndrome HHT Myhre syndrome		Isolated/nonsyndromic H-TAD [21]
TGFβ2	LDS [17, 22]	Classic MFS/MFS features [23]	Isolated/nonsyndromic H-TAD [24]
TGFβ3	LDS, syndrome presenting at birth with distal arthrogryposis, hypotonia, bifid uvula, a failure of normal postnatal muscle development [25]	MFS features [26, 27]	
H-TAD related to genes encoding proteins involved in the contractile apparatus of vascular smooth muscle cells			
ACTA2	Multisystemic SMC dysfunction syndrome [28–30]	H-TAD with mild associated skin/ocular/vascular lesions [31]	Isolated/nonsyndromic H-TAD [32]
MYLK			Isolated/nonsyndromic H-TAD [33]
PRKG1			Isolated/nonsyndromic H-TAD [34]
MYH11		H-TAD with patent ductus arteriosus [35, 36]	Isolated/nonsyndromic H-TAD [32]

AOS aneurysm-osteoarthritis syndrome, *HHT* hereditary hemorrhagic telangiectasia, *H-TAD* heritable thoracic aortic disease, *MFS* Marfan syndrome, *LDS* Loeys-Dietz syndrome, *SMC* smooth muscle cell, *vEDS* vascular Ehlers-Danlos syndrome

expectancy in MFS is normal—a recent population study demonstrated a median age at death in MFS patients of 50 years, which is 8–13 years lower than in the general population [41]. A key factor in improving prognosis is early identification of patients with Marfan syndrome. Precipitating factors reported to accelerate progressive dilatation or dissection include increased blood pressure, intense physical exercise, and pregnancy [42–45].

Loeys-Dietz Syndrome

In 2005, Loeys-Dietz syndrome (LDS, ORPHA 60030, OMIM # 609192, 610380, 610168, 608967, 615582) was recognized as a new disease entity. Currently five types of Loeys-Dietz syndrome are described, labeled types 1 through 5, which are distinguished by their genetic cause. Regardless of the type, signs and symptoms of Loeys-Dietz syndrome can become apparent anytime ranging from early childhood to late adulthood, and the severity is variable. The prevalence of all types of LDS is currently unknown.

LDS is mainly characterized by aneurysms and/or dissections of the aortic root, although 50% of LDS patients have aneurysms/dissections in other arteries, including cerebral, thoracic, and abdominal arteries. In most patients, arterial tortuosity of head and neck arteries is present. Fatal aortic events can occur at a young age, and fatal aortic dissection and rupture in the aortic root can occur with diameters smaller than 45 mm. In addition to the cardiovascular abnormalities, skeletal (pectus, scoliosis, joint laxity, osteoarthritis, arachnodactyly, talipes equinovarus), craniofacial (hypertelorism, bifid uvula/cleft palate, craniosynostosis), and cutaneous (translucent skin, easy bruising, dystrophic scars) abnormalities can occur in varying severity among the different types of LDS.

The initial reports in LDS types 1 and 2 described a poor prognosis for LDS patients with a mean age at death of 26 years due to aortic dissection and cerebral hemorrhage as major causes of death. This figure may be somewhat biased by the clinical severity of individuals initially ascertained as having LDS. Also there is a large inter- and intrafamilial variation [14, 46]. More recent reports indeed indicate a wide spectrum of clinical severity in LDS with mean aortic root growth rates being not significantly different from MFS [47]. The extent of craniofacial/skeletal features appears as an indicator for aortic disease severity, especially in small-sized women with *TGFBR2* mutations [47, 48].

Vascular Ehlers-Danlos Syndrome

Ehlers-Danlos syndrome (EDS) is an inherited heterogeneous group of connective tissue disorders, comprising several different clinical subtypes. The prevalence is estimated at 1 in 10.000 to 1 in 25.000 for all types. Classification of Ehlers-Danlos syndromes has recently been updated, now including the identification of an underlying genetic defect as a requirement for the diagnosis [49]. The vascular subtype of Ehlers-Danlos syndrome (vEDS, ORPHA 286, *OMIM* #130050), formerly known as EDS type 4, is an autosomal dominant connective tissue disorder caused by mutations in the *COL3A1* gene. vEDS is clinically characterized by vascular, intestinal, and uterine fragility. The prevalence of vEDS has been estimated at 1/50.000 to 1/150.000 [50]. Actually, the true rate is unknown, and estimates based on ascertained cases might significantly underestimate the true prevalence in the population. Studies of natural history in vEDS indicated that life span is significantly decreased, almost always related to arterial rupture. The largest (retrospective) series reporting on clinical events and survival mentions a median survival of 48 years. The age at death ranged from 6 to 73 years [4]. Mean age at first complication was 23.5+/−11.1 years. Overall, complications are rare in childhood, but 25% of patients have a first complication by the age of 20 years, and more than 80% have suffered from at least one complication by the age of 40 years. There are no gender differences. Bowel rupture affects about a quarter of affected individuals and in some is the first indication of a connective tissue abnormality. Mortality related to intestinal rupture—which is more often amenable to surgical treatment—is significantly lower than mortality related to arterial complications (estimated at 3%) [4]. A more recent smaller-scale study on 31 patients treated for vascular events showed slightly better survival rates with 68% of patients surviving at the age of 50 years [51].

Pregnancy complications that included both intrapartum and peripartum vascular ruptures could lead to death although recent data could not confirm pregnancy as a trigger for adverse outcome [52].

Multisystemic Smooth Muscle Dysfunction Syndrome

Multisystemic smooth muscle dysfunction syndrome (MSMD syndrome, ORPHA 404463, OMIM #613834) caused by specific de novo mutations in the *ACTA2* gene (R179H) is a rare disorder characterized by widespread SMC dysfunction manifesting in the iris, bladder, gastrointestinal (GI) tract, and vasculature [28, 53]. Median age at diagnosis with molecular genetic testing is 11 years [54]. All patients present in early infancy with congenital cardiovascular lesions including patent ductus arteriosus (91%), aortic arch hypoplasia, aortic coarctation, or aortopulmonary window (9%) requiring surgery [54, 55].

Nonsyndromic H-TAD

The majority of TAD patients will not present additional clinical features, related to an underlying syndromic entity. TAD can result from diverse etiologies, including infectious agents and hemodynamic forces. The vast majority of descending thoracic aneurysms are associated with atherosclerosis, and the risk factors for aneurysm formation are the same as those for atherosclerosis (e.g., hypertension, hypercholesterolemia, smoking) [56]. Atherosclerosis is an infrequent cause of ascending thoracic aortic aneurysms, however [56], and the underlying heritable forms should always be considered. It has been recognized for many years that up to 20% of patients presenting with an aortic aneurysm/dissection have an affected first-degree relative, in which case the term nonsyndromic heritable thoracic aortic disease applies (NS H-TAD, ORPHA 91387, OMIM #132900; 607086; 607087; 609192; 610168; 611788; 613780; 614816; 615436; 615582; 616166). The younger the proband, the greater the chance of having affected relatives. We now know that simply asking about aortic disease is insufficient. One needs to query about intracerebral arterial disease, precocious coronary artery disease, congenital heart disease (specifically coarctation and patent ductus), and bicuspid aortic valve [57].

Aortic dilation progresses more rapidly in patients with familial aortopathy with a greater risk of aortic complications [58, 59].

Gene panels available for testing patients with NS H-TAD vary widely. In selecting how many—and which—genes need to be included on such panels, one needs to carefully make a balance between smaller panels, potentially lacking some genes, and larger panels, concurring a higher risk of finding variants of unknown significance (VUSs). Gene-disease validity needs to be well established for genes to be included on these panels. Within the framework of ClinGen, tools have been provided for this purpose [60]. Using this semiquantitative method, we have analyzed a set of 53 genes and identified a set of 12 genes strongly linked to NS H-TAD [61].

The selection of patients in whom genetic testing is recommended has changed over time and is driven by costs on

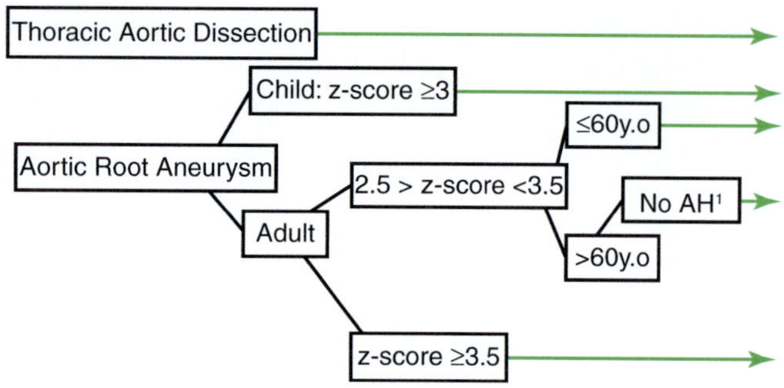

Fig. 19.1 Flowchart illustrating the indications for clinical genetic evaluation and testing in patients with aortic aneurysms/dissections. Z-scores should be calculated based on appropriate formulas, taking into account the age and BSA (body surface area) of the patient. *AHT* arterial hypertension (adjusted from the pathway developed for VASCERN—www.vascern.eu)

Table 19.2 The revised Ghent criteria for diagnosis of Marfan syndrome

Family history	Aortic dilation ($Z \geq 2$) or dissection	Ectopia lentis	Systemic score (≥7 of 20)	Pathogenic *FBN1* mutation
	X	X		
	X		X	
	X			X
		X		X
X	X			
X		X		
X			X	

Each line represents a possible combination leading to Marfan syndrome. *Xao FBN1* mutation associated with aortic pathology

the one hand and actionability on the other hand. Technical advances have led to a significant reduction in costs over the last decade, and recent data indicate that gene-based management is important. We therefore suggest to apply a low threshold for additional genetic testing in patients presenting with H-TAD. A flowchart based on patients' age and aortic Z-score is provided in Fig. 19.1. Recent studies assessing the mutation uptake rate in these patients show figures varying between 15 and 30% [5, 62]. In addition to pathogenic variants, found in 9%, patients with early-onset sporadic thoracic aortic dissection also appear to carry a higher number of VUSs in H-TAD genes (in up to 28% of cases). These data not only support genetic testing in individuals with dissections <56 years of age but also emphasize how critical it is to classify these variants as disrupting protein function and predisposing to dissection or as completely benign [63].

The risk of aortic complications in nonsyndromic H-TAD patients is influenced by the underlying genetic defect, as has already been shown for a small number of genes and is confirmed in unpublished data from the Montalcino Aortic Consortium [64]. Evident additional patient-related factors for developing aortic complications include smoking, hypertension, and strenuous physical exercise as well as anatomical factors such as the presence of a bicuspid aortic valve.

Clinical Diagnosis and Differential Diagnosis

Clinical Diagnosis

Marfan Syndrome

Early identification and establishment of the diagnosis in patients with Marfan syndrome is of considerable importance because prophylactic surgery can prevent aortic dissection and rupture. Elucidation of the molecular mechanisms behind Marfan syndrome will allow improvement in diagnostic testing, but so far, the diagnosis of Marfan syndrome has to be made on clinical grounds, following the revised Ghent criteria (Table 19.2) [1].

The diagnosis of Marfan syndrome requires the coexistence of aortic root aneurysm or aortic dissection together with either a pathogenic *FBN1* mutation, ectopia lentis, or a positive family history. The remaining cardinal manifestations of Marfan syndrome are incorporated in a systemic score, where a systemic score > 7 also contributes to the diagnosis (Table 19.3) [1].

Marfan syndrome shows a high penetrance but marked inter- and intrafamilial variability. The disorder should be regarded as a spectrum of diverse and highly variable manifestations in the different organs, and not all patients display the classic habitus. Most of the manifestations have an age-dependent penetrance. Moreover, many of the physical findings are also encountered in the general population or in other syndromic H-TAD entities, such as Loeys-Dietz syndrome and Ehlers-Danlos syndrome. The variability in clinical expression, with manifestations that emerge from childhood onwards, the presence of *FBN1* mutations in the different fibrillinopathies, and the high rate of de novo mutations can pose difficulties in establishing the diagnosis in some patients, particularly in younger individuals with few symptoms [2]. Some patients need follow-up before a definitive judgment can be made. A multidisciplinary approach, including clinical genetics, cardiology, ophthalmology, and radiology, is essential in establishing the diagnosis, treatment, and follow-up. When the diagnosis has been established in an individual, first-degree relatives should be screened for the disorder as well.

Cardiovascular System

The major sources of morbidity and mortality in Marfan syndrome are due to manifestations in the cardiovascular system, of which aortic aneurysm and dissection are the most life-threatening. Dilatation of the sinus of Valsalva is found in up to 80% of adults with Marfan syndrome

Table 19.3 Scoring of the systemic features

Feature	Score
Wrist and thumb sign	3 (wrist or thumb: 1)
Pectus carinatum deformity	2 (pectus excavatum or chest asymmetry: 1)
Hindfoot deformity	2 (plain pes planus: 1)
Pneumothorax	2
Dural ectasia	2
Protrusio acetabuli	2
Reduced upper segment/lower segment ratio AND increased arm/height WITHOUT severe scoliosis	1
Scoliosis or thoracolumbar kyphosis	1
Reduced elbow extension	1
Facial features (3/5): dolichocephaly, enophthalmos, downslanting palpebral fissures, malar hypoplasia, retrognathia	1
Skin striae	1
Myopia >3 diopters	1
Mitral valve prolapse (all types)	1

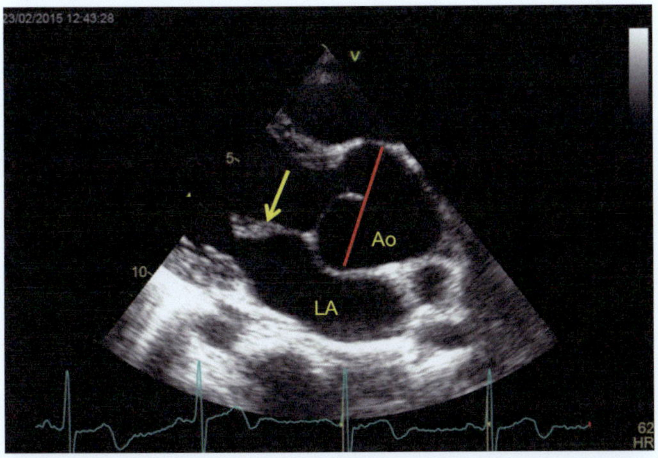

Fig. 19.2 Transthoracic echocardiography image of an aortic sinus of Valsalva aneurysm in a 15-year-old boy with Marfan syndrome. Note the pear-shaped aortic root and the thickened mitral valve leaflets (arrow). *Ao* aorta, *LA* left atrium

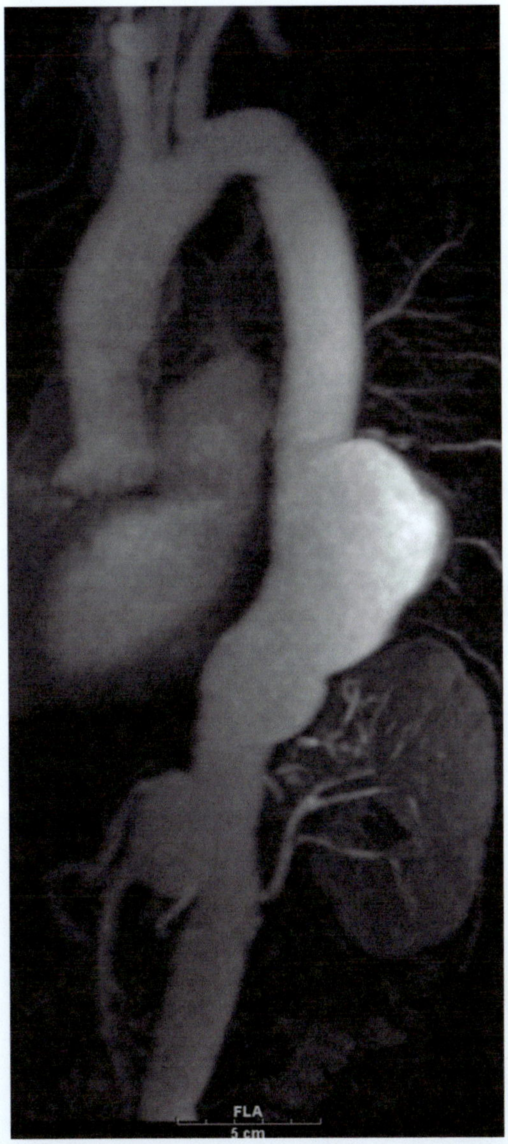

Fig. 19.3 MR image of an aneurysm at the level of the descending thoracic aorta in a 52-year-old lady with Marfan syndrome who underwent previous replacement of the proximal descending and abdominal aorta

(Fig. 19.2), resulting in a typical pear shape of the aortic root. Aortic root aneurysm/dissection is a major criterion for the diagnosis of Marfan syndrome (Table 19.2). The onset and progression of aortic dilatation is highly variable, in rare cases beginning in utero, while other individuals never develop dilatation to critical diameters. Normal aortic dimensions are dependent on body surface area, sex, and age, and therefore, the dimensions measured—especially in pediatric patients—have to be compared with age-dependent nomograms using the same measurement methods [52, 53, 65]. In adults, aortic roots ≥40 mm diameter can generally be considered dilated [66].

Without preventive surgery, dissections in Marfan syndrome mostly constitute type A aortic dissections involving the aortic root, in many cases propagating along the descending aorta. The risk of type A dissection clearly increases with increasing aortic root diameter, but dissection may occasionally occur in patients with no or only mild aortic dilatation. Other risk factors for dissection include rate of aortic growth and a family history of aortic dissection. MFS is associated with a HR of 200 of having aortic disease [41].

As Marfan patients currently survive longer after surgical replacement of the aortic root, an increasing amount of patients develop aneurysms and/or dissections elsewhere in the arterial tree (Fig. 19.3, [67–69]). Apart from increasing diameters, the aorta also elongates, which forces the anatomically fixed aorta to curve and become tortuous. By means of magnetic resonance imaging (MRI), the aortic and vertebral tortuosity index can be measured [70, 71], both of which correlate well with aortic outcome. Apart from aortic diameters and tortuosity index, MRI may be useful to determine aortic elasticity in the distal aorta. A decreased local distensibility and increased flow wave velocity as an expression of decreased aortic elasticity can be found in many but not all unoperated patients with Marfan syndrome. Patients with Marfan syndrome with prior prophylactic aortic surgery are at substantial risk for type B aortic dissection, even when the descending aorta is only slightly dilated. In about 17% of patients, the aorta distal from the root is the first site of complications [68]. Predictors for aortic growth and adverse events in the distal aorta include a larger aortic diameter, lower aortic distensibility, higher aortic tortuosity index, and previous aortic root replacement [72–74].

Eight to 15% of Marfan patients require initial surgery in the descending aorta [67, 75]. Patients with initial type B aortic dissection are at a significantly higher risk for re-intervention (86% for previous type B dissection versus 42% for previous type A dissection). The majority of re-interventions are required in patients with previous dissection (48% versus 11% re-intervention in the patients presenting with aortic aneurysm) [75]. A large contemporary series of 96 thoraco-abdominal aortic aneurysm repairs in patients with MFS shows an excellent survival rate of 97% [76]. Recommendations are slightly different from the ones applied for the aortic root (see below): repair at the level of the thoraco-abdominal aorta in MFS is recommended when the aneurysm diameter exceeds 5.5 cm [77]. However, the high risk of surgical intervention at this level should be weighed against the risk of type B dissection, which may occur at substantially smaller aortic diameters.

Dilatation of the main pulmonary artery is a frequent finding in patients with Marfan syndrome [78, 79] but with limited clinical consequences.

Within the heart, the atrioventricular valves are most often involved, with thickening and prolapse of mitral and/or tricuspid valves and subsequent regurgitation [80] (Fig. 19.4). Mitral valve prolapse accounts for one point in the systemic score. Aortic valve regurgitation usually arises in the context of stretching of the aortic annulus due to a dilated aortic root.

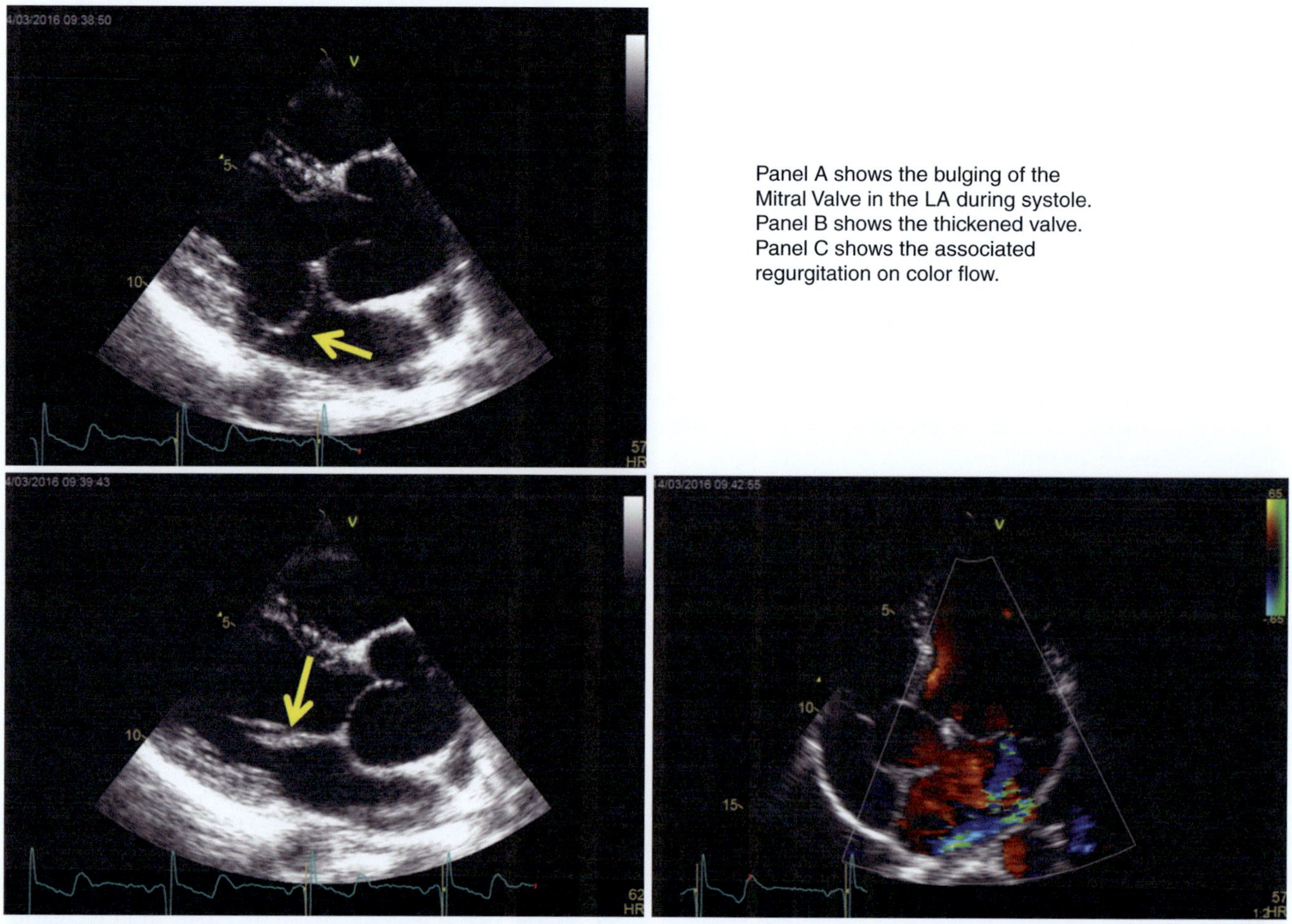

Fig. 19.4 Transthoracic echocardiographic images of mitral valve prolapse in a 15-year-old Marfan boy. Panel A shows the bulging of the mitral valve in the LA during systole. Panel B shows the thickened valve. Panel C shows the associated regurgitation on color flow

Severe aortic valve regurgitation may lead to left ventricular failure. Although not included in the diagnostic criteria for Marfan syndrome, it has been speculated that a fibrillin-1 defect in the myocardium may predispose MFS patients to left ventricular dilation and reduced left ventricular function. In several studies, evidence has been found for mild but significant impairment of left ventricular systolic and diastolic function in Marfan patients, not related to valvular heart disease [81–83]. These findings have also been corroborated in different mouse models of MFS. Possibly related to left ventricular dysfunction, arrhythmias and even sudden cardiac death occur with a higher frequency in Marfan syndrome indicating the need for careful evaluation in patients with palpitations [84].

Patients with a dilated aorta are usually asymptomatic. The presence of significant aortic, tricuspid, or mitral regurgitation may lead to symptoms of ventricular volume overload. Patients with Marfan syndrome tend to feel fatigued, which may, at least partly, be explained by orthostatic hypotension. The combination of increased height and a structural abnormality of the blood vessels may cause impaired orthostatic tolerance. In Marfan patients, fatigue and low orthostatic tolerance have been correlated [85]. Patients can be educated in physical counterpressure maneuvers, such as leg crossing and muscle tensing, to counteract orthostatic drops in blood pressure.

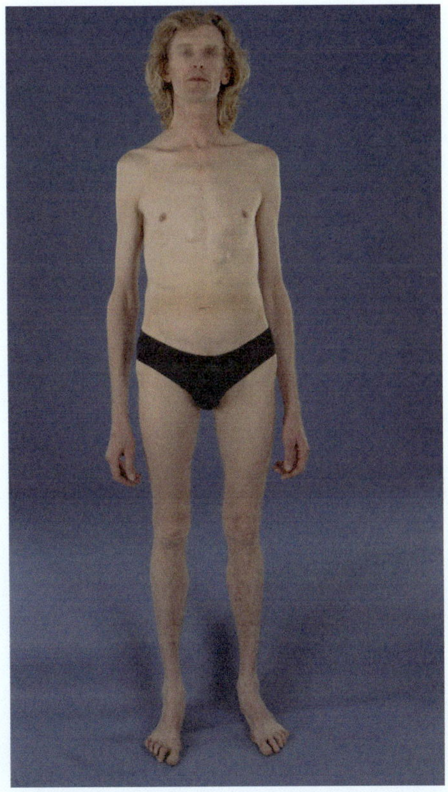

Fig. 19.5 Patient with a typical habitus of Marfan syndrome with overgrowth of long bones and hypoplasia of skeletal muscle and adipose tissue

Ocular System

Ocular lens dislocation (ectopia lentis), often bilateral and symmetric and mostly upward, is considered a major criterion and occurs in about 60% of patients with Marfan syndrome [86]. When dislocation of a lens is detected in the absence of a traumatic event (the most common cause), Marfan syndrome should always be considered. Subluxation usually develops in childhood but may first appear later in life. A slit-lamp examination is an essential part of the diagnostic examination. Myopia, often rapidly progressing during childhood, is the most common ocular finding in patients with Marfan syndrome. It is associated with an increased length of the globe and an increased risk of retinal detachment [87]. The cornea can be flat and the iris or ciliary muscle may be hypoplastic [88]. A predisposition of cataracts and glaucoma exists. The lens dislocation, retinal detachment, cataract, and glaucoma may cause significant visual impairment.

Skeletal System

The most striking skeletal manifestation is the overgrowth of the long bones, leading to the characteristic appearance of patients with MFS. The extremities are disproportionately long for the size of the trunk (dolichostenomelia), which leads to an increased arm span-to-height and upper-lower segment ratio (Fig. 19.5): the fingers and toes are long and thin (arachnodactyly), and in combination with hypermobility of the joints, this leads to the characteristic wrist (Walker-Murdoch)—and thumb (Steinberg)—sign. Individuals with MFS are taller than predicted based on their non-affected relatives; however, they are not necessarily tall compared to the general population (Fig. 19.6). Overgrowth of the rib cartilage can lead to pectus excavatum or pectus carinatum. Scoliosis, affecting around 60% of patients, may lead to deformity, pain, and even respiratory problems. Additional skeletal manifestations include pes planus and an abnormally deep acetabulum (protrusion acetabuli) with accelerated erosion, which can be confirmed on radiographs. Typical facial features of MFS are a long and narrow face with underdeveloped cheekbones (malar hypoplasia), downward slanting palpebral fissures, enophthalmos, and retro- or micrognathia. A highly arched and narrow palate and tooth crowding are often present as well. Skeletal abnormalities in Marfan syndrome emerge and may progress during childhood and adolescence, typically during periods of rapid growth. The most specific skeletal manifestations are incorporated in the systemic score (Table 19.3).

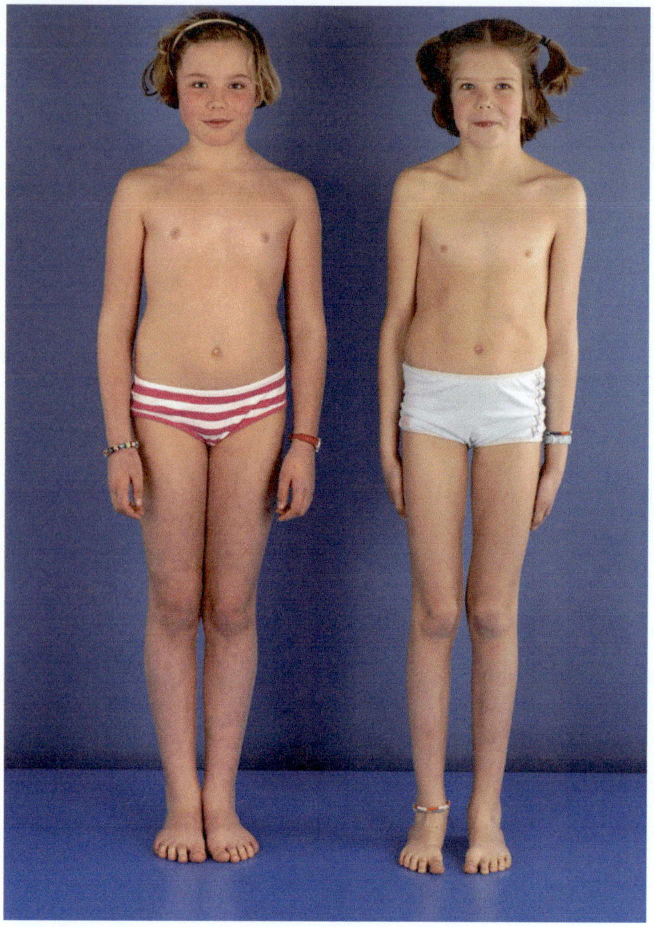

Fig. 19.6 The 8-year-old girl on the right has Marfan syndrome. She is 2 years younger than her sister on the left, though the girls have the same height

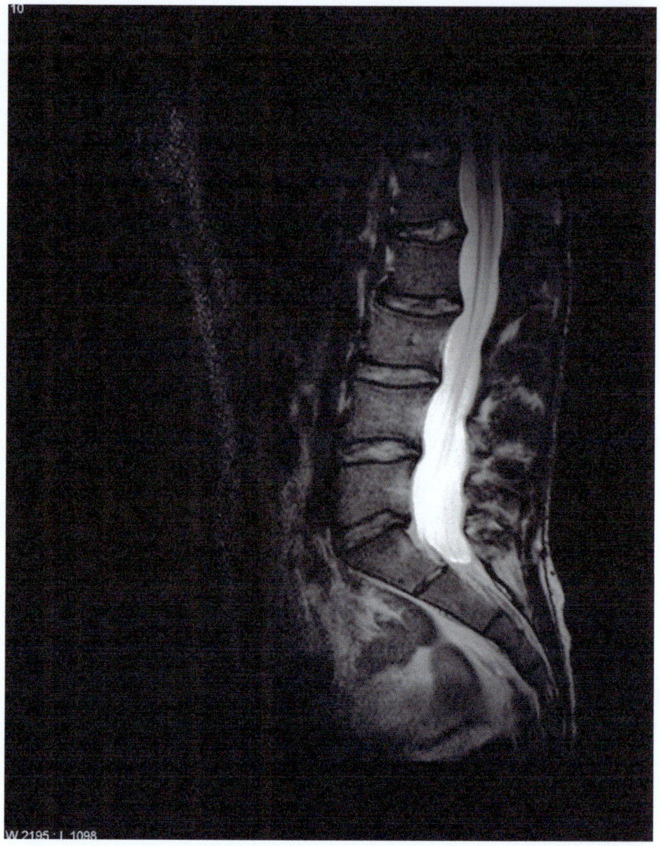

Fig. 19.7 Magnetic resonance imaging showing lumbar and sacral dural ectasia in a patient with Marfan syndrome

Pulmonary System

In the lungs, widening of distal airspaces and lung bullae or blebs may be present, particularly in the upper lobes, which can predispose to spontaneous pneumothorax [89]. In addition, pectus deformities and scoliosis may lead to significantly reduced lung capacity. The prevalence of obstructive sleep apnea syndrome is increased in MFS (almost one in three patients present at least mild sleep apnea) [90] and was related to aortic events in one study [91].

Dural Sac

Stretching and ballooning of the dural sac (dural ectasia) in the lumbosacral region is seen in about two-thirds of patients with Marfan syndrome. It can be assessed by lumbosacral imaging with MRI or CT (Fig. 19.7, [92]). The presence of dural ectasia accounts for two points in the systemic score. Dural ectasia can also be present in other connective tissue disorders [93, 94] and in healthy individuals. Possible symptoms include back pain and weakness, pain, and numbness in the proximal legs [95], although it is often asymptomatic. Bone erosion and nerve entrapment may occur.

Skin and Integuments

In contrast to many other connective tissue disorders, most patients with Marfan syndrome have a normal skin texture and elasticity, although in some people, the skin is unusually thin or elastic. A common feature in Marfan syndrome is the presence of stretch marks (striae distensae) that are not associated with rapid weight gain and at sites that are not typically stretched, such as the lumbar area and the anterior and posterior sides of the shoulders (Fig. 19.8). Inguinal and umbilical hernias, congenital or acquired, are also common. Only striae distensae are included in the systemic score.

Others

Hypoplasia of the skeletal muscle and adipose tissue, often present in Marfan syndrome, contributes to the slender and asthenic appearance of some patients (Fig. 19.5).

Loeys-Dietz Syndrome

There are no specific clinical criteria for the diagnosis of LDS. Patients with mutations in *TGFBR1*, *TGFBR2*,

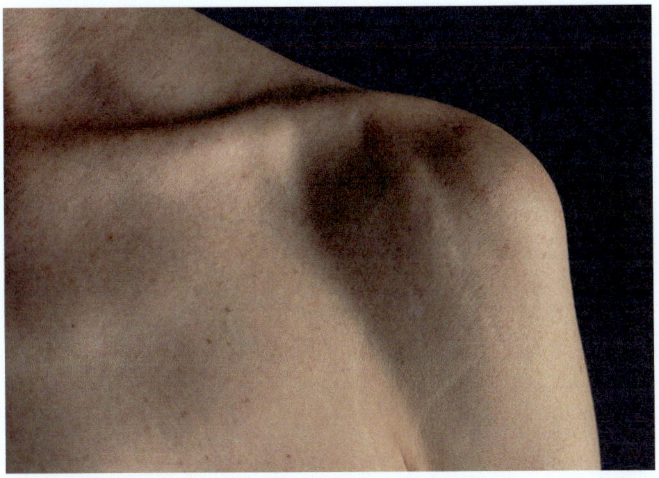

Fig. 19.8 Typical striae atrophicae on the anterior side of the shoulder of an adult patient with Marfan syndrome

Table 19.4 LDS subtypes and associated clinical entities

LDS type (OMIM #)	ORPHA code	Gene (OMIM #)	Chromosome	Other disorders reported
LDS type 1 (609192)	60030	*TGFBR1* (190181)	9q22.33	Furlong syndrome, nonsyndromic H-TAD
LDS type 2 (610168)	60030	*TGFBR2* (190182)	3p24.1	Nonsyndromic H-TAD, MFS2
LDS type 3 (613795)	284984	*SMAD3* (603109)	15q22.33	Aneurysm-osteoarthritis syndrome (AOS), nonsyndromic H-TAD
LDS type 4 (614816)	91387	*TGFB2* (190220)	1q41	MFS, nonsyndromic H-TAD
LDS type 5 (615582)	91387	*TGFB3* (190230)	14q24.3	Rienhoff syndrome, nonsyndromic H-TAD

SMAD3, *TGFB2*, or *TGFB3* gene in combination with documented aneurysm or dissection or a family history of documented LDS is sufficient to establish the diagnosis of LDS [17]. The clinical LDS continuum is subdivided into multiple disease classes named LDS types 1 to 5. Initially Loeys et al. described mutations in TGFBR1 and TGFBR2 in syndromic H-TAD patients which are now considered to have LDS types 1 and 2, respectively [9, 17]. *SMAD3* mutations are identified in patients with aneurysm-osteoarthritis syndrome (AOS) [19]. Since the phenotype of individuals with *SMAD3* mutations shows significant overlap with the findings in patients with LDS, AOS is also indicated as LDS type 3. LDS 4 and 5 have now been allocated to mutations in the ligands of the TGFB receptors, *TGFB2* and *TGFB3*, respectively [22, 23, 96]. Also mutations in the *SMAD2* gene were identified in syndromic aneurysm patients, but no LDS type has been assigned to this gene yet [97, 98] (Table 19.4).

Cardiovascular System

All subtypes of LDS are characterized by variable degrees of aortic and arterial aneurysm and dissection, which range from aggressive and early-onset presentations to milder forms, closely resembling cardiovascular features in Marfan syndrome [47, 48]. A type A aortic dissection has been reported in individuals as young as 3 months of age [99]. Aneurysms are mainly present in the aortic root, at the level of the sinuses of Valsalva, and less commonly involve the descending or abdominal aorta. Arterial aneurysm can also be present in other arteries throughout the body and most commonly occur in the major arteries that arise from the aorta in the thorax and abdomen and those that supply the head and neck.

Dissections occur at aortic dimensions that are not considered hazardous in other connective tissue disorders such as Marfan syndrome, i.e., ≤ 45 mm, or without prior dilatation. In LDS type 5, no examples of early arterial dissection or dissection at small aortic dimension are reported so far.

Arterial tortuosity is most commonly observed in the vertebral and carotid arteries (Fig. 19.9) but can also be seen in the aorta or other arteries throughout the body. Tortuosity of the vertebral arteries is also present in MFS, but its prevalence is much higher in LDS patients [100]. The severity of the arterial tortuosity is a poor prognostic factor and correlates with the degree of aortic dilation and younger age at dissection, cardiac surgery, and death [101]. Thus far no arterial tortuosity is observed in LDS type 5 patients [25, 27, 96, 102].

Mitral valve prolapse and/or insufficiency appears less common in LDS than in MFS but can be seen in all types of LDS and ranges from mild-to-severe mitral valve disease. Congenital heart disease is more prevalent in LDS than in the general population and includes atrial septal defect (ASD), patent ductus arteriosus (PDA), and bicuspid aortic valve (BAV). In LDS type 3, atrial fibrillation (24%) and left ventricular hypertrophy (18%) have been reported. Impaired left ventricular systolic function has been reported in LDS type 1 [103].

For the more recently identified LDS genes, *TGFB2* and *TGFB3*, the aortic/arterial phenotypes seem less severe than LDS types 1, 2, and 3, and a higher degree of non-penetrance is reported [104]. However, these observations are based on limited data, and detailed genotypic and phenotypic data have yet to emerge.

TGFBR1, *TGFBR2*, *SMAD3*, and *TGFB2* mutations have not only been associated with syndromic H-TAD presentations; rare mutations have also been described in nonsyndromic H-TAD patients [5, 14, 20, 62].

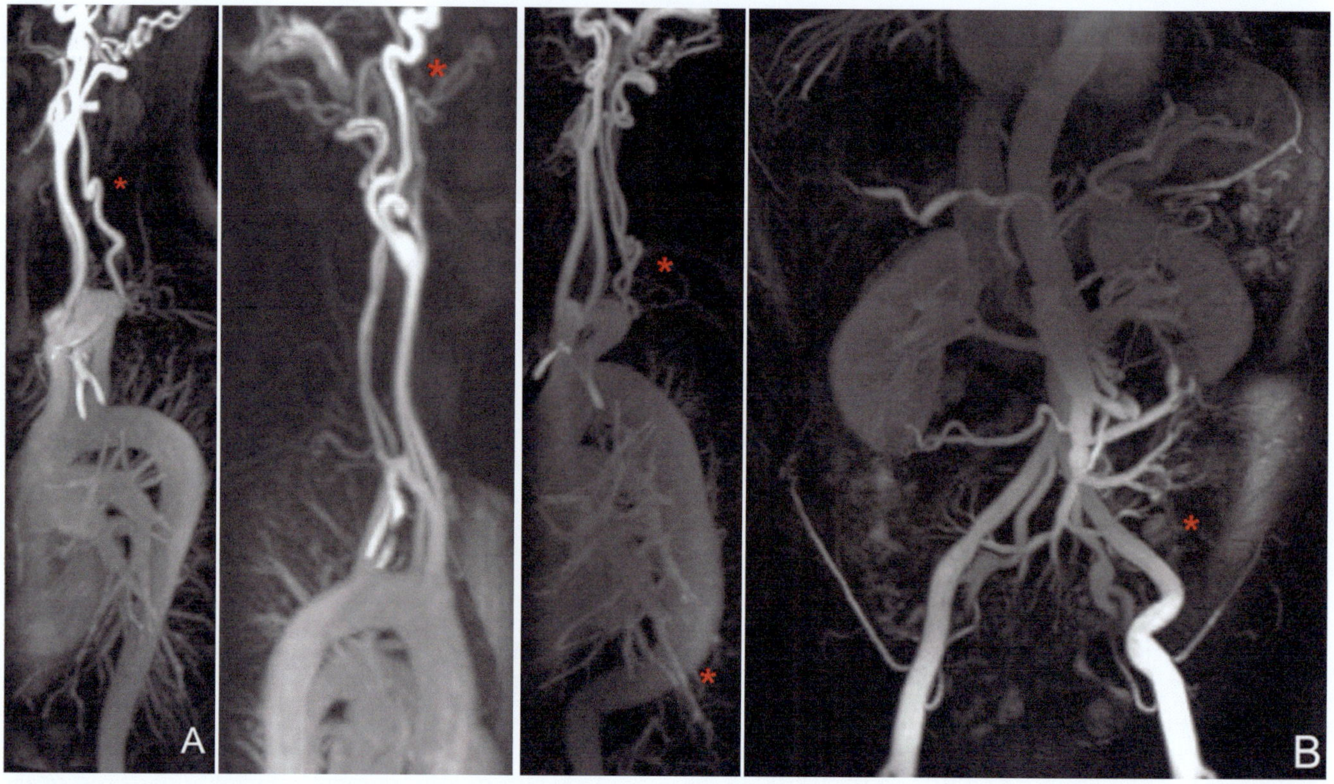

Fig. 19.9 MRI images of the head and neck vessels in two sisters with a TGFBR2 mutation (panel A) and of the upper thoracic aorta and head and neck vessels as well as the lower abdominal aorta and iliac arteries in a patient with a TGFBR1 mutation (panel B). Note the marked tortuosity of the marked vessels

Skeletal Anomalies
Skeletal manifestations that overlap with MFS include pectus deformity, scoliosis, flat feet, and arachnodactyly. Craniosynostosis occurs in LDS but rarely in MFS. Joint hypermobility is also common, including congenital hip dislocation and recurrent or multiple joint subluxations. Paradoxically, contractures of extremities like clubfoot, camptodactyly, and contractures of other joints are also described in LDS. In LDS types 1 and 2, cervical spine abnormalities, like subluxations or instability, have been reported in 51% of patients in the series reported by MacCarrick [17]. Spondylolisthesis and scoliosis can be mild or severe and progressive.

Osteoarthritis is particularly present in LDS type 3. In the initial report of LDS3, it was noted that almost all *SMAD3* mutation carriers developed early-onset joint abnormalities including osteoarthritis and osteochondritis dissecans, meniscal lesions, and intervertebral disc degeneration [105]. Osteoarthritis mainly affects the spine, hands and/or wrists, and knees, but it is also reported in all other joints. These abnormalities may be present at a young age and may be the patient's presenting symptom. They seem to be discriminating clinical features in LDS type 3.

However, in recent years, several studies have reported individuals with pathogenic *SMAD3* mutations without osteoarticular manifestations indicating that this finding is not mandatory but can be an important diagnostic clue [20, 106–113].

Joint anomalies like osteoarthritis, osteochondritis dissecans, and meniscal lesions are rarely described in LDS due to *TGFBR1*, *TGFBR2*, *TGFB2*, and *TGFB3* mutations and Marfan syndrome, but no systematic joint studies in these patients are reported. Further studies to establish the frequency of osteoarthritis and osteochondritis dissecans in these related syndromes are warranted [114, 115].

Craniofacial Abnormalities
The facial features in LDS patients include hypertelorism and cleft palate. Uvula anomalies (ranging from bifid to broad) can be seen as the mildest form of cleft palate. It may be an easy diagnostic clue, as it only occurs in Loeys-Dietz syndrome, but not in other syndromic or nonsyndromic forms of H-TAD.

There is a marked inter- and intrafamilial variability in facial features. In many cases, no craniofacial features are described. This might indicate that craniofacial anomalies are less frequent or milder than initially reported.

Skin and Integuments

Some features that are common in connective tissue disorders are also frequent in LDS like inguinal, umbilical, and hiatal hernia and thin translucent skin with a tendency to poor wound healing and atrophic scars. Some patients with *TGFBR1/2* mutations show significant clinical overlap with vascular Ehlers-Danlos syndrome and have initially been designated as LDS type 2 [8].

Others

Apart from joint, skeletal, craniofacial, and cutaneous abnormalities, pulmonary manifestations including spontaneous pneumothorax, restrictive lung disease, and obstructive sleep apnea are more frequent in LDS. Also immunological features like allergic manifestations, especially asthma, food allergy, eczema, and allergic rhinitis, occur at a higher prevalence in LDS [116]. Autoimmune features, such as Sjogren's disease, rheumatoid arthritis, and Hashimoto's disease, have been described. Gastrointestinal disease including eosinophilic esophagitis and inflammatory bowel disease like ulcerative colitis and Crohn disease are frequently seen in LDS [17, 110]. Infants and children with LDS often present with failure to thrive and constipation which might persist throughout life [17, 116]. Dural ectasia occurs with similar frequency and severity as in MFS [117]. In LDS type 3, neurological features such as muscle cramps, paresthesia, hypoesthesia, or gait disturbance have been described [110].

Other features, such as hydrocephalus, hypotonia, and headaches, are also part of the syndrome. Arnold-Chiari type 1 malformation, developmental delay, defective tooth enamel, and osteoporosis have been rarely described in LDS types 1 and 2.

Vascular Ehlers-Danlos Syndrome

The clinical diagnosis of the vascular type of Ehlers-Danlos syndrome is usually suspected on the basis of family history or a clinical history of arterial rupture, dissection or aneurysm, rupture of the large intestine, or pregnancy complications at young ages. Because of clinical overlap with some forms of Loeys-Dietz syndrome, Marfan syndrome, and familial arterial aneurysm and dissection syndromes, the diagnosis should be confirmed by identification of pathogenic variants in COL3A1 [118].

Cardiovascular System

In many vEDS patients, the diagnosis is made only after a catastrophic vascular complication or at postmortem examination. vEDS patients are at risk for aneurysms and rupture or dissection, especially of medium-sized arteries [4, 51]. Multiple locations (synchronous) or recurring ruptures or dissections in different anatomical regions in medium-sized arteries in individuals under the age of 40 should raise this diagnostic consideration. The proximal and distal branches of the aortic arch, the descending thoracic aorta, and abdominal aorta are often affected, as well as vertebral and carotid arteries. Dissection and rupture often occur without preceding aneurysm formation, rendering management very challenging. In a recent literature review, Berqvist et al. reported arterial rupture without underlying aneurysm in 33% of patients with a serious hemorrhagic complication [119]. Aneurysm and arterial-venous fistula in the cavernous portion of the carotid (often referred to as a carotid-cavernous sinus fistula (CCSF)) are rare conditions with a higher than expected prevalence in people with vEDS.

Mitral valve prolapse has been reported in several cases of vEDS [120, 121], but subsequent larger studies could not confirm this finding [122] indicating that mitral valve prolapse is an aspecific finding in vEDS.

Skin and Facial Characteristics

Distinctive facial features—although present in less than 30% of the patients [123]—consist of an "old-looking" face, with prominent cheekbones, sunken or bulging eyes, a thin and pinched nose, as well as thin lips (Fig. 19.10). The skin on the extremities, especially the hands, appears aged (acrogeria) (Fig. 19.11). Unlike other types of EDS, affected individuals often have inelastic, thin, translucent skin [124]. Easy bruising may be prominent, especially in children.

Skeletal System

Hypermobility of small joints can be present (Fig. 19.12), while hypermobility of large joints, characteristic of the more common forms of Ehlers-Danlos syndrome, is unusual in the vascular type. Clubfeet and congenital hip dislocations are more prevalent in vEDS patients [4].

Gastrointestinal System

Rupture of the gastrointestinal tract is another serious complication, occurring in about 25% of affected individuals and being lethal in 3% of cases [4]. It mostly occurs in the sigmoid colon, but the small intestine and stomach can also be affected.

Pulmonary System

Spontaneous pneumothorax is seen in 12% of individuals, often as a first manifestation. Rupture of pulmonary blebs is probably the major cause of pneumothorax [118].

Pregnancy

Pregnancy was initially considered as a potential trigger for uterine and vascular rupture, and historical data reported pregnancy-related complications in 12% [4]. Recent observations in a larger study however reported slightly lower percentages of pregnancy-related deaths in 5.3% of pregnancies and found no difference in survival between parous and nul-

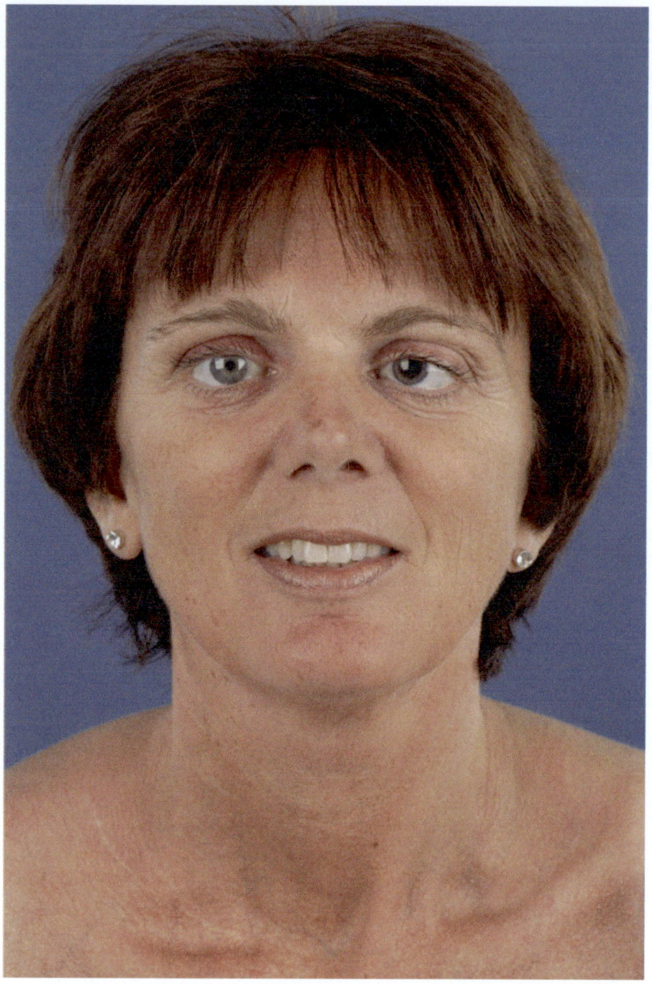

Fig. 19.10 A 43-year-old with vascular Ehlers-Danlos syndrome. Typical facial features including protruding eyes and a thin and pinched nose. The left pupil is wide and unresponsive to light, resulting from a vascular complication and surgery

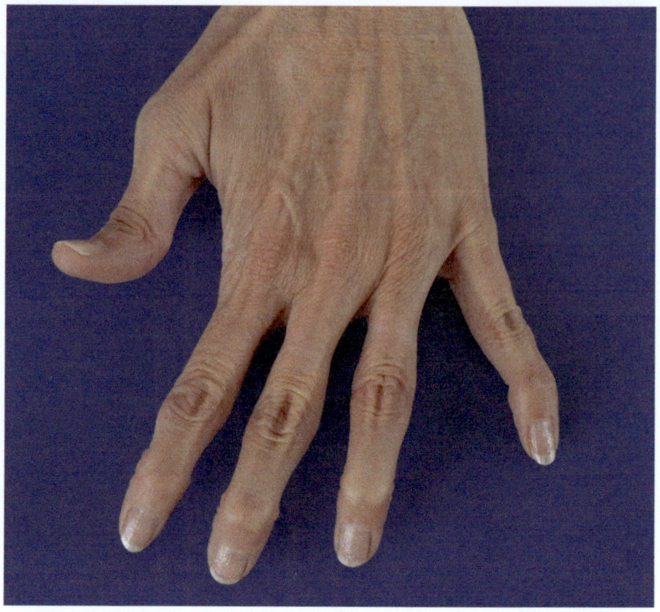

Fig. 19.11 Hand of the a 43-year-old woman with vascular Ehlers-Danlos syndrome showing acrogeria

liparous women, suggesting that age is the main risk factor and not pregnancy itself [52]. The most common pregnancy-related complications in this study were third-/fourth-degree lacerations (20%), arterial dissection/rupture (9.2%), uterine rupture (2.6%), and surgical complications (2.6%). Preterm delivery (occurring in up to 19% of cases) occurs more frequently in the setting of an affected fetus, owing to increased fragility of the membranes [125].

Multisystemic Smooth Muscle Dysfunction Syndrome

Specific missense de novo mutations, R179 in *ACTA2*, cause a syndrome characterized by dysfunction of SMCs throughout the body, with widespread manifestations [28].

Cardiovascular System

Patients reported so far invariable presented with a hemodynamically significant patent ductus arteriosus (PDA) or aortopulmonary window requiring intervention in the neonatal period. Ascending aortic aneurysms develop during childhood, and a majority of patients need surgery at a young age (<15 years). One 14-year-old boy reported by Ades developed a type A dissection at the age of 14 years [126].

Patients go on to develop fusiform ascending aortic aneurysms extending to the arch during childhood, also necessitating surgical repair. By the age of 25 years, aortic disease is fully penetrant [54].

Cerebrovascular lesions include small vessel disease (hyperintense periventricular white matter lesions, 95%), intracranial artery stenosis (77%), ischemic strokes (27%), and seizures (18%). Hemiparesis in a 10 year old and global neurodevelopmental delay have been reported [29, 54].

The prevalence of the disease is unknown but presumably very low with about 40 patients reported in literature worldwide. The outcome in these patients is poor—most known cases do not survive beyond the third decade of life and die from aortic complications or obstructive cerebro-or cardiovascular lesions.

Cerebrovascular abnormalities have been encountered on imaging studies in all patients, including fusiform dilatation of the internal carotids and stenoses at the more terminal portions of these same vessels, reminiscent but not entirely similar to what is seen in moyamoya disease [29, 127] (Fig. 19.13). All patients for whom imaging was reported had bilateral periventricular white matter hyperintensities suggesting concurrent angiographically occult small vessel disease [29]. Clinically, one young child has been reported with hemiparesis, and global developmental delay has been reported in 2/13 patients in one series [29].

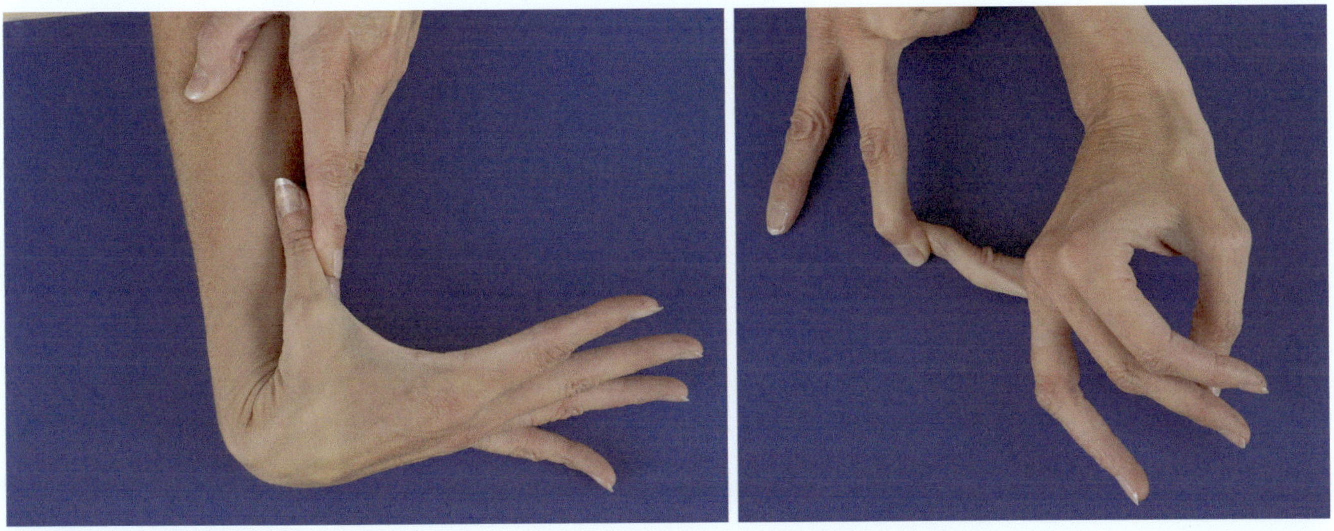

Fig. 19.12 Hypermobility of the wrist and fingers in vascular Ehlers-Danlos syndrome

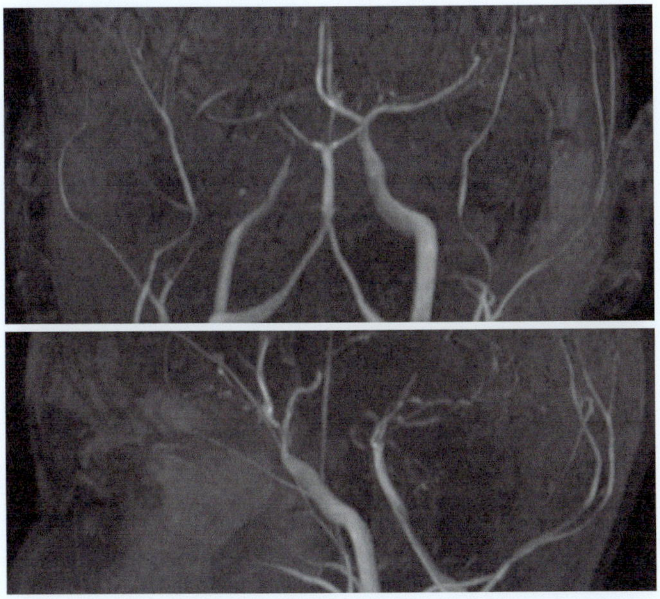

Fig. 19.13 MR angiography of the brain in a 17-year-old girl with multisystemic smooth muscle cell dysplasia syndrome. Note the dilated left internal carotid artery to the terminal portion, occlusive disease of distal intracranial circulation, an abnormally straight course of intracranial arteries, and absence of "moyamoya" collaterals

Other Organ System Manifestations

Congenital mydriasis or fixed dilated pupils is a feature shared by all patients with the R179 mutation [28, 128]. Other reported manifestations indicating SMC dysfunction include hypotonic bladder and malrotation and hyperperistalsis of the GI tract.

Pulmonary manifestations include asthma, cystic lung disease in infancy, and primary pulmonary hypertension necessitating bilateral lung transplantation at the age of 18 months in one case [28, 30, 53].

Nonsyndromic H-TAD

About 20% of individuals with a thoracic aortic aneurysm or a type A aortic dissection without a history of connective tissue disorder have an affected first-degree relative and therefore may have a genetic predisposition [59, 129]. Nonsyndromic H-TAD (NS H-TAD) is diagnosed in the presence of familial dilatation and/or dissection of the thoracic aorta; in the absence of MFS, LDS, vEDS, or other syndromic features; and in the absence of other underlying factors for aortic disease such as atherosclerosis. NS H-TAD is inherited in an autosomal dominant manner with decreased penetrance and variable expression.

The genetic background of NS H-TAD is heterogeneous, and mutations in nearly all genes reported in the setting of syndromic H-TAD entities may give rise to NS H-TAD. A comprehensive list of genes with a confirmed strong gene-disease validity for H-TAD has been published recently [61] and shown in Fig. 19.14:

Mutations in the *ACTA2* gene (actin, α-2, smooth muscle, aorta; OMIM #102620) are most frequently encountered in the setting of NS H-TAD and responsible for 12%–21% of cases [31, 32, 130]. Mutations in genes encoding other proteins involved in smooth muscle cell contraction also cause an inherited predisposition to thoracic aortic disease, including *MYH11*, *MYLK*, *PRKG1*, and *MFAP5* [6, 33, 35, 36, 131]. Mutations in genes encoding components of the ECM can give rise to NS H-TAD as has been illustrated by the identification of *FBN1* mutations in 3% of a large cohort of NS H-TAD patients [132] [6].

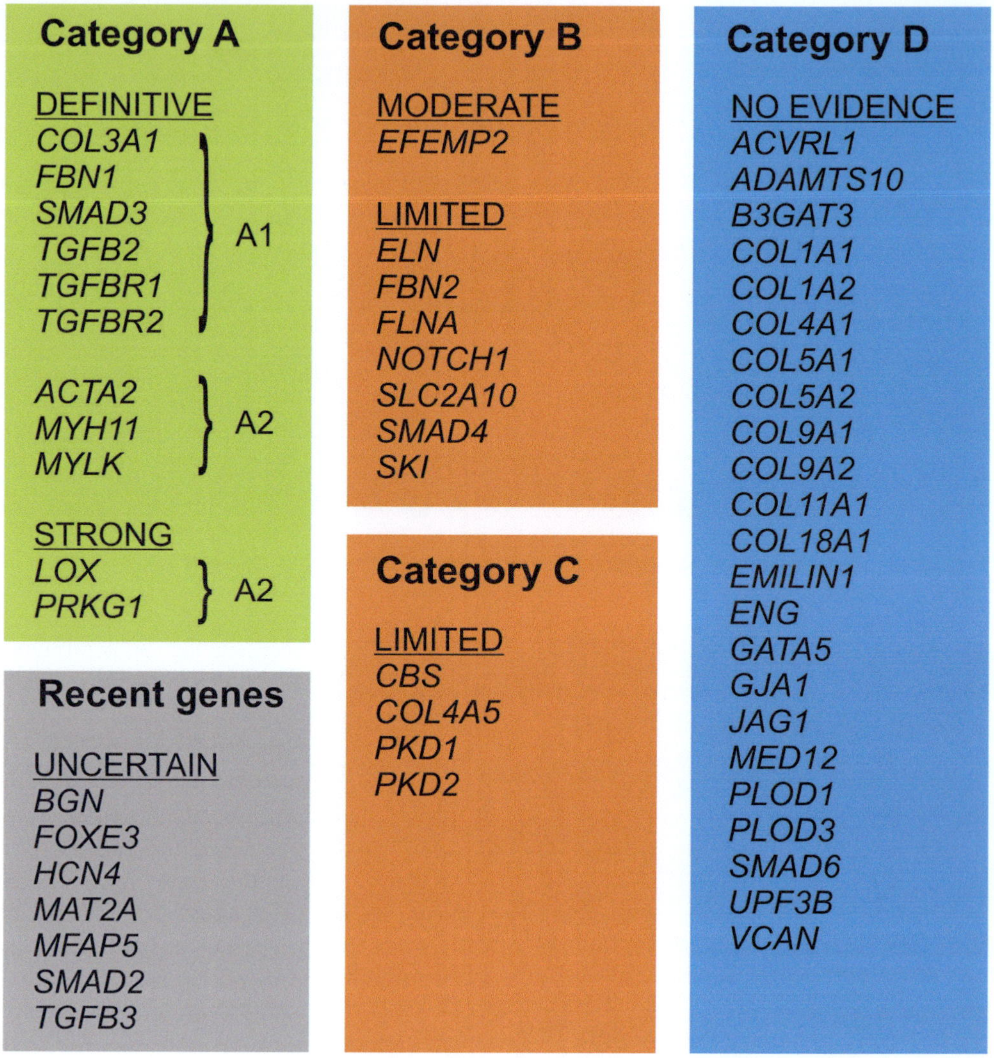

Fig. 19.14 Schematic overview of genes involved in HTAD categorized according to the strength of the gene-disease validity using the framework developed by ClinGen - reprinted from Renard et al. [61] with permission

Cardiovascular System

Affected individuals have progressive aortic dilatation of the sinuses of Valsalva and/or ascending aorta and aortic dissection. In the majority of individuals with NS H-TAD, enlargement of the aorta precedes dissection although the extent of dilatation may be much lower than conventional thresholds for treatment [64, 133]. In NS H-TAD, the onset and rate of progression of aortic dilatation are highly variable, with some individuals developing dilatation in childhood, while others reach high age without aneurysms. A higher growth rate was observed in one study comparing familial to sporadic cases of TAD [58]. Individuals with familial H-TAD have a younger mean age at presentation than individuals with non-familial thoracic aortic aneurysms, but older than individuals with Marfan syndrome [59]. Aortic dissection in childhood is rare.

A recent study describing aortic features in a large series of patients with *ACTA2* mutations indicated that aortic events occurred in 48% of individuals, with the vast majority presenting with thoracic aortic dissections (88%) associated with 25% mortality. Type A dissections were more common than type B dissections (54% versus 21%), but the median age of onset of type B dissections was significantly younger than type A dissections (27 years versus 36 years). In this extensive series, the lifetime risk for an aortic event was 76%, suggesting that additional environmental or genetic factors play a role in expression of aortic disease in individuals with *ACTA2* mutations. Mutations disrupting p.R179 and p.R258 were associated with significantly increased risk for aortic events, whereas p.R185Q and p.R118Q mutations showed significantly lower risk of aortic events compared with other mutations [130]. Mitral valve prolapse in *ACTA2* mutation patients is reported in only 3% of cases which is in contrast to Marfan syndrome and Loeys-Dietz syndrome and approaches the prevalence in the general population [14, 130, 134].

Patients harboring specific *ACTA2* mutations also show an increased risk for early-onset stroke or coronary artery

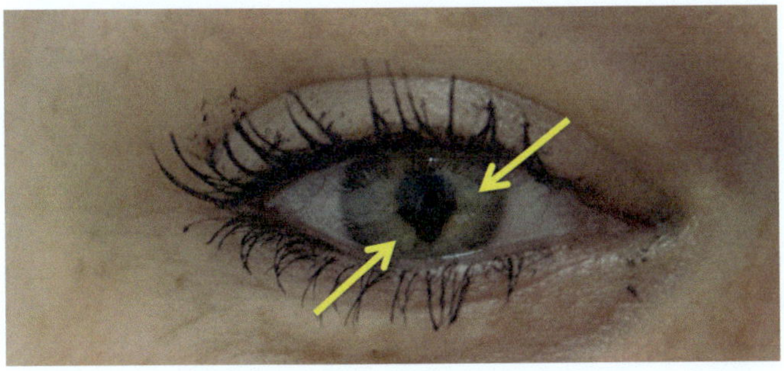

Fig. 19.15 Illustration of iris flocculi in a patient harboring a pathogenic variant on the ACTA2 gene

disease [130]. Other features associated with *ACTA2* mutations include livedo reticularis and iris flocculi (Fig. 19.15).

Patients with *MFAP5* mutations present with aortic root dilatation, mostly occurring at middle age and associated with various and very mild syndromic features in some individuals (pectus deformities, mitral valve prolapse). Interestingly several patients also presented lone atrial fibrillation.

Sixty-three percent of the 31 patients reported with mutations in the *PRKG1* gene presented with aortic dissection, commonly at a young age (mean 31 years) [34].

Patients with *MAT2A* mutations have a predisposition for thoracic aortic aneurysms/dissections. Bicuspid aortic valves are seen more frequently [135].

The majority of patients with a mutation in the *MYH11* gene also present a patent ductus arteriosus [32, 35, 36, 131]. Aortic stiffness in mutation carriers is increased even in those without significant aortic dilatation [131].

Differential Diagnosis

All entities described above show significant clinical and genetic overlap and should therefore always be considered in their respective differential diagnosis.

Genetic testing is important in the differential diagnosis, and for some entities, very characteristic clinical features can give the clue to the diagnosis as is, for example, the case for lens luxation, which is a feature unique to Marfan syndrome. Diagnostic distinctions have prognostic value and may affect the clinical management and lifestyle of patients and are therefore of great importance.

Data collected within the International Montalcino Aortic Consortium indicate that there are clear gene-specific differences in aortic outcome. Patients with *SMAD3* mutations have the latest onset of aortic events, whereas *PRKG1* carriers have youngest age of onset of aortic events (D. Milewicz, personal communication).

Table 19.5 provides an overview of the clinical and genetic findings of the most relevant differential diagnoses to be taken into account in H-TAD. The entities not already mentioned above are briefly listed below.

In an individual with Marfan-like skeletal manifestations, several disorders have to be considered. There is extensive overlap in clinical features between Loeys-Dietz syndrome and Marfan syndrome, such as aortic root aneurysm and dissection, scoliosis, pectus deformity, and arachnodactyly. The main distinguishing features between Loeys-Dietz syndrome and Marfan syndrome are the presence of the typical triad of hypertelorism, cleft palate/bifid uvula, and arterial tortuosity. Moreover, patients with Loeys-Dietz syndrome do not have ectopia lentis, and the majority do not have the typical overgrowth of long bones as seen in Marfan syndrome.

Mitral valve prolapse syndrome (MVPS) and MASS phenotype (MASS) are Marfan-like syndromes that exhibit aortic dilatation and mitral valve prolapse. Differentiating between MFS on the one hand and MVPS or MASS on the other hand can be particularly challenging in children and adolescents because of the age-dependent penetrance of many features in Marfan syndrome. Unlike in MFS, the presence of ectopia lentis and aortic aneurysm precludes the diagnosis of MVPS and MASS. A recent study demonstrated that aortic dilatation in these clinical entities is mild and does not progress over time, as opposed to what is observed in MFS [142].

Arterial tortuosity syndrome, an autosomal recessive disorder, is characterized by generalized tortuosity of arteries but can also present with other connective tissue findings such as cutis laxa, joint hypermobility, or skin hyperextensibility. Arterial stenoses may occur in the systemic as well as in the pulmonic vascular bed, and mild aortic root dilatation has occasionally been reported. So far, no vascular ruptures have been reported in patients with this syndrome [143, 144].

Shprintzen-Goldberg syndrome is a rare craniosynostosis syndrome characterized by Marfanoid skeletal manifestations, exophthalmos, hypertelorism, downslanting palpebral fissures and other dysmorphic features, and developmental delay. The majority of patients do not show vascular involvement. Although a mutation in *FBN1* has been reported in two cases in the past presenting Marfanoid features with craniosynostosis [145], the actual underlying gene defect has recently been identified as heterozygous mutations in exon 1 of the *SKI* gene [137, 138]. The dysmorphic features in patients harboring *SKI* mutations are strikingly more severe than in those harboring *FBN1* mutations.

Congenital contractural arachnodactyly is a condition primarily affecting the skeleton with contractures of digits, elbows, and knees evident at birth, elongated long bones, and kyphoscoliosis. In addition, the pinna of the

Table 19.5 Overview of clinical entities to be taken into account in the differential diagnosis of H-TAD (both syndromic and nonsyndromic)

Disorder	Gene(s)	Main cardiovascular features	Additional clinical features
Syndromic H-TAD			
Marfan	*FBN1* [136], *TGFBR1* and 2 [5, 12], *SMAD3* [5], *TGFB2* [23]	**Sinus of Valsalva aneurysm**, aortic dissection, mitral valve prolapse, main pulmonary artery dilatation, left ventricular dysfunction	**Lens luxation**, skeletal features (arachnodactyly, pectus deformity, scoliosis, flat feet, increased arm span, dolichocephaly), dural ectasia, striae
Loeys-Dietz	*TGFBR1* and *2* [8, 9], *SMAD3*, *TGFB2* [22], *TGFB3*	**Sinus of Valsalva aneurysm**, aortic dissection, arterial aneurysms and dissections, **arterial tortuosity**, patent ductus arteriosus, atrial septal defect, bicuspid aortic valve	**Bifid uvula/cleft palate, hypertelorism**, pectus abnormalities, scoliosis, clubfeet
Vascular Ehlers-Danlos	*COL3A1*	**Arterial rupture and dissection without preceding dilatation/aneurysm**	**Gastrointestinal rupture, thin and translucent skin**, dystrophic scars, facial characteristics (Madonna face, thin lips, deep set eyes), clubfeet, uterine rupture
Multisystemic smooth muscle dysfunction syndrome	ACTA2 [28]	**Ascending aortic aneurysm**, aortic dissection, **patent ductus arteriosus**, aortic coarctation, aortopulmonary window, pulmonary arterial hypertension	**Congenital mydriasis**, malrotation of the gut, moyamoya disease, periventricular white matter hyperintensities
Shprintzen-Goldberg syndrome	*SKI* [137, 138]	**Mild aortic root dilatation**, mitral valve prolapse	**Craniosynostosis**, distinctive craniofacial features, skeletal changes, neurologic abnormalities, mild-to-moderate intellectual disability
Arterial tortuosity syndrome	*SLC2A10* [139]	**Arterial tortuosity**, arterial stenoses and aneurysms, mild aortic root dilatation	Hyperlax skin and joints, beaked nose, elongated face, micrognathia
Cutis laxa syndromes (autosomal dominant and recessive)	*ELN* [140], *FBLN4* [141], *FBLN5*	Mild aortic dilatation and tortuosity	Skin hyperlaxity, emphysema, downslanting palpebral fissures, inguinal hernia
Nonsyndromic TAAD			
	ACTA2 (10–21%)	Thoracic aortic aneurysm/dissection, cerebrovascular disease, coronary artery disease	Lack of Marfanoid skeletal features, **livedo reticularis, iris flocculi, coronary artery/cerebrovascular disease**
	TGFBR1/2 (3–5%)	Thoracic aortic aneurysm/dissection	Lack of syndromal features
	FBN1 (3%)	Sinus of Valsalva aneurysms	**Lack of syndromal features**
	MYLK	Thoracic aortic aneurysm/dissections often at low aortic diameters	
	SMAD3 (2%)	Intracranial and other arterial aneurysms	
	TGFB2	**Mitral valve prolapse**	
	NOTCH1	**Highly calcified bicuspid aortic valve**	
	MYH11	**Patent ductus arteriosus**	
	PRKG1	**Aortic dissection at young age**	
	MAT2A	**Bicuspid aortic valve**	
	MFAP5	**Lone atrial fibrillation**	

Distinctive cardiovascular and other clinical features are indicated in bold

ear is typically crumpled. Mitral valve prolapse and aortic root dilatation have been reported, with unknown frequency and generally in a milder degree than in MFS. Mutations in the *FBN2* gene account for about half of cases [146, 147].

Homocystinuria is a disorder caused by a deficiency of the cystathionine β-synthase (CBS) enzyme. Clinical features are variable and include developmental delay, ectopia lentis, severe myopia, skeletal abnormalities (excessive height and long bone overgrowth), and thromboembolism. Homocystinuria is inherited in an autosomal recessive manner, the causative gene being the *CBS* gene, with mutations identified in over 95% of patients [148, 149].

Clinical Therapy

Many aspects of treatment and medical management in H-TAD are based on the large body of knowledge obtained in Marfan syndrome. This will therefore be discussed in more detail—only specific aspects related to treatment and management for the other entities will be mentioned below.

Marfan Syndrome

Medical Treatment

In patients with Marfan syndrome, and especially in patients with aortic dissection, rigorous antihypertensive medical treatment is important, aiming at a systolic blood pressure less than 120 mm Hg. The most commonly prescribed drugs are β-adrenergic blockers, which reduce the aortic dilation rate in patients with Marfan syndrome, due to its effects in reducing the blood pressure and the force of the left ventricular ejection [150, 151]. Losartan, an angiotensin II receptor 1 blocker, might be an alternative or complementary therapy to β-blockers, since losartan reduces arterial pressure and potentially interferes with the pathophysiology of Marfan syndrome by TGFβ antagonism. After evidence for effectiveness of losartan in a mouse model of Marfan syndrome [152], a small pilot study in children and adults demonstrated a beneficial effect of losartan combined with β-blockers (n = 15) on aortic dilation rate compared with β-blockers alone (n = 13) after 35 months of echocardiographic follow-up [153]. Subsequently, eight randomized clinical trials were initiated to test losartan effectiveness; so far four studies have been published [154]. The COMPARE trial confirmed these results in a larger cohort (n = 145) as measured by MRI and additionally demonstrated the beneficial effect of losartan on the distal part of the aorta after aortic root surgery [155]. The Marfan Sartan trial evaluated the benefit of adding losartan to a high dose of β-blockers. Remarkably, in this cohort of 292 children and adults, aortic dilation rate was similar for the losartan- and placebo-treated group after 3.5 years of echocardiographic follow-up [156]. The Pediatric Heart Network Study demonstrated that both losartan and atenolol were equally effective in reducing aortic dilatation rate in a large, blinded trial including 608 children during 3 years by echocardiography [157]. The last published trial so far demonstrated in 140 Marfan patients aged 5 to 60 years that losartan was not inferior in respect of atenolol and tended to be more favorable in the losartan monotherapy group when corrected for BSA or Z-score measured by MRI over 3 years of follow-up [158]. The discrepancies in outcome between the studies may be explained by the different study designs [154, 159]. With the available data, we can conclude that losartan does not seem to be more effective in reducing the aortic dilation rate than a high dosage of β-blockers but that losartan can safely be administered as an alternative or as an additive to β-blocker therapy, especially in patients with intolerance or side effects of β-blockers [154].

Surgical Treatment

The threshold diameter for aortic surgery is 50 mm for any level of the aorta or 45 mm for the aortic root in combination with either a family history of dissection, progressive dilation of more than 2 mm/year, or severe aortic or mitral valve regurgitation or if pregnancy is desired. Lower thresholds for intervention may be considered according to body surface area (BSA) in patients of small stature or according to patient's preference [160]. On average, women have a smaller aorta (by 5 mm), which is only partly explained by a smaller BSA [161]. An indexed aortic diameter (adjusted for BSA) could be useful for operative decision-making [162], and surgery then would be indicated at an aortic diameter of 4.5 cm in patients with a BSA of 1.65 m^2, 5.0 cm at a BSA of 1.8 m^2, and 5.5 cm at a BSA of 2 m^2.

Over the past 30 years, the composite replacement of the aortic valve and ascending aorta ("Bentall procedure") (Fig. 19.16) has been a low-risk and very durable operation for aortic root aneurysm in Marfan patients. In a series of 675 Marfan patients undergoing aortic root surgery, the operative mortality rate was 1.5% for elective operations and 11.7% for emergency operations [163]. However, in patients with initially normal aortic valves, valve-sparing operations with root replacement by a Dacron prosthesis and reimplantation of the coronary arteries into the prosthesis (the David procedure) have now become the preferred choice of surgery. Either type of aortic root replacement appears to be safe, reproducible, and associated with excellent 5- to 10-year results. Freedom from reoperation of the aortic valve after the David procedure was 94.8%, with a slow progressive deterioration of aortic valve function after long-term follow-

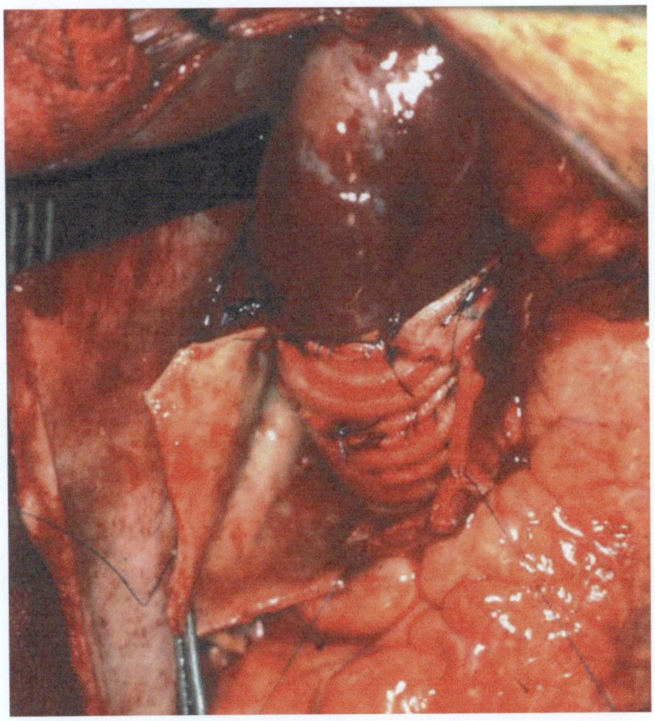

Fig. 19.16 Bentall procedure: the graft and mechanical valve have been incorporated and the coronary arteries have been reimplanted

up [164]. A homograft or bioprosthetic valve may also be considered to avoid anticoagulant therapy.

Endovascular stenting is a minimally invasive surgical procedure with some advantages as compared to open repair in patients with abdominal aortic aneurysms [165]. Less information concerning the outcomes of endovascular stenting in Marfan patients is available. In ten Marfan patients treated with an endovascular stent procedure, the technical success rates were excellent. However, in Marfan patients with aortic dissection, the use of endovascular stenting should be considered in life-threatening emergencies only, as a bridge to definite therapy, since these aortas dilate progressively, resulting in high endoleak rates, a 12% mortality rate, and a 14–18% need of a new surgical procedure [166–168].

Personalized external aortic root support (PEARS) is a novel surgical approach, stabilizing the aortic root and decreasing the risk of aortic dissection in patients with Marfan syndrome. Although long-term follow-up data is currently lacking, PEARS seems effective in stabilizing the aortic root and preventing its dilatation. It is a viable alternative for prevention of aortic root dissection in Marfan patients [169].

Follow-Up

Optimal long-term outcome demands lifelong follow-up with imaging of the aortic root by means of echocardiography and the entire aorta by means of MRI at regular intervals. This is particularly true if a dissection has occurred and its stability is being monitored. Patients with mitral valve prolapse and moderate or severe mitral regurgitation should also be followed with yearly echocardiography. Antihypertensive medical treatment, aiming at a systolic blood pressure less than 120 mm Hg, is important in all patients with Marfan syndrome. After aortic dissection, systolic blood pressure should not exceed 110 mm Hg. Lifelong and regular follow-up of these patients requires involvement of trained specialists with ample expertise in a tertiary referral center.

Regular imaging of the aortic root and all other parts of the aorta is crucial in the follow-up of patients with Marfan syndrome (Table 19.6).

Echocardiography in the parasternal long-axis view is mostly used for measurement of the aortic root (Fig. 19.2). By means of Doppler echocardiography, the presence and hemodynamic consequences of aortic regurgitation, mitral valve prolapse, mitral regurgitation, and occasionally tricuspid valve prolapse can be assessed. MRI is particularly useful for imaging of the entire aorta, for patients with deformation of the chest wall and asymmetrical aortic roots (Fig. 19.17, [170]). Imaging of the entire aorta should be performed in every patient. When parts of the aorta are dilated, regular follow-up should be performed at least once every year. Even when the aorta shows no abnormalities, imaging should be repeated within 5 years. Computed tomography (CT) may be used when MRI cannot be performed because of contraindications or unavailability. With MRI, aortic elasticity can be measured and is often reduced. Aortic elasticity of the thoracic descending aorta appeared to be an independent predictor for progressive descending aortic dilation [171]. Holter monitoring should be performed in symptomatic patients, because ventricular arrhythmias, conduction disturbances, and sudden cardiac death may occasionally occur.

Lifestyle Advice

Patients should be advised to avoid both physical and emotional situations that increase blood pressure and heart rate dramatically. Furthermore, patients should be advised to avoid exertion at maximal capacity, competitive sports, contact sports, and isometric sports.

Endocarditis Prophylaxis

Endocarditis prophylaxis is recommended only in patients with a prosthetic valve and in patients with previous endocarditis and in patients with complete repair using prosthetic material (surgical or percutaneous) for up to 6 months after the procedure (until endothelializa-

Table 19.6 Different imaging modalities

	Transthoracic echocardiography	Transesophageal echocardiography	Magnetic resonance imaging or computed tomography
Aortic root dilation	X		X
Presence and severity of aortic regurgitation	X	X	
Presence and severity of mitral regurgitation	X	X	
Reparability of mitral and aortic valves		X	
Dilation of the pulmonary trunk	X		X
Evidence of endocarditis	X	X	X
Presence of ascending aortic dissection	X	X	X
Intraoperative evaluation of aortic and mitral valve surgery		X	
Dimensions of major branches and arteries			X
Presence of lumbosacral dural ectasia			X
Aortic elasticity and tortuosity			X

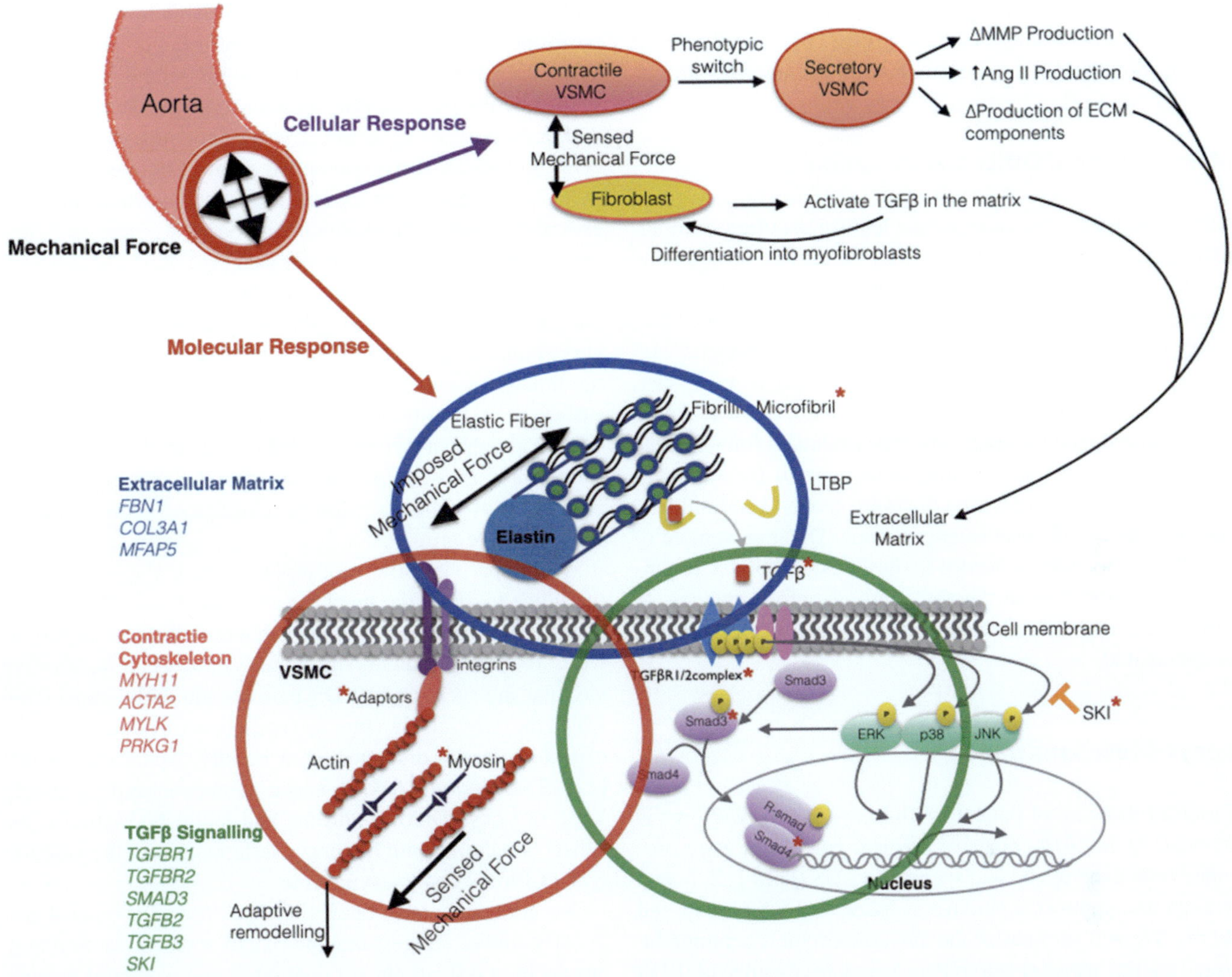

Fig. 19.17 Concept of mechanobiology underlying homeostasis in the thoracic aorta. Alterations, either due to higher imposed forces (hypertension) or due to (genetic) alterations in the various components required for proper sensing and/or transduction of the signal may lead to aneurysms/dissections. Mutations in the various components may affect the mechanical properties of the microfibrils or the signaling pathways, leading to an altered mechanotransduction signal and initiation of cellular response mechanisms including increased TGFβ signaling

tion) and ongoing only when a residual defect persists at the site of prosthetic material [172].

Pregnancy

For women with Marfan syndrome, pregnancy presents a twofold problem: a 50% chance that the child will be affected and an increased risk of aortic dissection during or (especially) shortly after pregnancy. Women with an aortic diameter above 45 mm are strongly discouraged to become pregnant before surgical repair. An aortic diameter below 40 mm rarely presents a problem, although a completely safe diameter does not exist. With an aorta between 40 and 45 mm, recent aortic growth and a family history of aortic events are important for advising pregnancy with or without preconception aortic repair [44]. A study on 55 pregnancies in 35 women with Marfan syndrome showed an increased aortic growth rate of 0.3 mm/month, which decreased after delivery, but remained higher than the pre-pregnancy growth rate [45]. Two other smaller studies have reported no difference between the baseline and the pregnancy aortic dilation rate [173, 174]. Pregnancy, however, did influence long-term growth rate in Marfan women with an aortic root diameter above 40 mm (0.36 mm/year vs 0.14 mm/year in the childless Marfan women) [44].

In addition to cardiovascular complications, pregnancy in women with Marfan syndrome is associated with a high rate of premature deliveries, premature rupture of membranes, and increased mortality in the offspring [173]. Especially the use of β-blockers is associated with intrauterine growth retardation [175].

Management of Other Manifestations

Periodic ophthalmic review is appropriate in childhood and early adolescence because ectopia lentis most often becomes evident in preschool years and may be slowly progressive. Adult patients should have ophthalmic screening at low frequency, because of the risk of glaucoma and cataracts. Most often, the myopia and lens dislocation can be managed with eyeglasses. Sometimes surgical intervention is necessary, including the implantation of artificial lenses. Growth should be monitored, and the spine has to be evaluated for scoliosis. Surgical interventions are sometimes needed for stabilization of the spine or correction of severe pectus abnormalities, for medical as well as cosmetic reasons. The involvement of a skilled orthopedist is needed in these severe cases. Growth-reducing sex hormone therapy, starting before puberty, to limit adult height may be considered when an extreme height is anticipated.

Loeys-Dietz Syndrome

Careful follow-up of patients with Loeys-Dietz syndrome is mandatory. In 2014 extensive medical guidelines were provided both generalized and specific to LDS types 1, 2, 3, and 4, even though most experience is based on LDS types 1 and 2 [17]. We will summarize the most important recommendations on the medical surveillance and treatments of LDS patients.

Cardiovascular Management

Many of the measures recommended for patients with Marfan syndrome also apply to patients with Loeys-Dietz syndrome. Avoidance of isometric exercise, contact sports, competitive sports, and exercising to the point of exhaustion are indicated. Blood pressure-lowering medication is advised in order to reduce hemodynamic stress. Beta-blockers are the standard-of-care treatment for individuals with syndromic aneurysmal disease, but angiotensin receptor blockers can be considered due to their effects on the TGF-beta signaling cascade. Also angiotensin-converting enzyme inhibitors have been used in some institutions. All patients with LDS require at least yearly echocardiography to monitor the aortic root, ascending aorta, and heart valves. Congenital heart defects, arrhythmias, and heart failure should be managed by according protocols. Because the vascular pathology can be seen throughout the entire arterial tree, baseline surveillance includes imaging of the arterial tree from head through pelvis by magnetic resonance or computed tomography angiography. Initially these diagnostic investigations should be performed annually to determine the rate of progression. Thereafter, frequency of head to pelvis imaging should be guided by progression rate, location, and size of aneurysm.

For LDS types 1, 2, and 3, aortic root surgery in adolescents and adults is recommended at lower diameters than in other aortic aneurysm syndromes, that is, when maximal ascending aortic dimensions approach 4.5 cm or when expanding more than 0.5 cm per year [17]. Surgical intervention at smaller dimensions may be indicated, based upon family history or personal risk assessments. In children, surgery should be considered when the maximal ascending aortic dimension exceeds the 99th percentile for age and body surface area (in patients with severe craniofacial features) or 4.0 cm (in the presence of mild craniofacial features) and should preferably be performed when the size of the aortic annulus allows the insertion of a sufficiently sized graft to accommodate growth.

Valve-sparing aortic root replacement is the intervention of choice to avoid the need for anticoagulation. Aneurysms distant from the aortic root are often amenable to surgery as well. To prevent aneurysm rupture or dissection, elective vascular intervention in LDS patients should be considered when the arterial diameter exceeds two to three times the expected arterial diameter or in rapidly expanding arteries [17]. The reported risk of aortic surgery is approximately 1.7% in Loeys-Dietz syndrome and might be higher in the subset of patients with features overlapping with the vascular type of Ehlers-Danlos syndrome.

No guidelines have been suggested for LDS types 4 and 5; early studies suggest that the risk of aortic dissection may not occur at 4.0 cm but surgical intervention should be considered at 4.5 cm, depending on family history and/or adult aortic dimension. More phenotypic data are needed on these types of LDS in order to provide guidelines.

Management of Other Manifestations

In order to assess cervical spine instability, flexion-extension X-rays of the cervical spine should be performed at diagnosis. It is recommended to repeat imaging every 3–5 years during growth. Management of scoliosis and pectus deformities should be performed as for Marfan patient. McCarrick et al. also provided extensive guidelines for management of allergies; gastroenterologic and nutritional, craniofacial, cutaneous, ophthalmologic, and pulmonary manifestations; and the psychosocial implications of the diagnosis on a patient and its family.

Vascular Ehlers-Danlos Syndrome

Management of patients with vascular Ehlers-Danlos syndrome is difficult due to the unpredictability of the events.

The same rules with regard to blood pressure control and lifestyle recommendations as mentioned for MFS apply here. Given the known tissue and especially vascular fragility, it is sensible to limit exposure to vigorous contact sports. Because of significant risks of arterial pathology and fragility, any sudden onset of unusual pain needs prompt and meticulous investigation, by both clinical examination and appropriate noninvasive imaging.

Antiplatelets and anticoagulants should be used only after careful consideration of the risks and benefits. This also applies to the use of NSAIDs. A medical alert bracelet or the carrying of a note with essential medical information, which briefly notifies attending physicians of potential EDS vascular-type complications, is recommended. Some general guidelines for anesthesia and surgery have been suggested [176]. These include crossmatching of adequate amounts of blood for transfusion, avoiding intramuscular premedication, establishing adequate peripheral venous access, and avoiding arterial lines and central venous lines whenever possible.

In general, the management of a vascular dissection or rupture should be conservative, whenever possible. Special surgical preventive measures need to be taken into account, and surgery is more likely to be successful if the surgeon is well-informed about the condition [51]. More recently developed techniques for endovascular repair have been used successfully in the right hands in small series [177]. The outcome of surgical management in such highly specialized centers is better than the average natural evolution but remains associated with high morbidity as demonstrated by complication in 46% in a series of 31 patients from the Mayo Clinic and in 33% in 9 patients from the Johns Hopkins Hospital [51, 177]. Mortality of open surgery and endovascular procedures in a recent retrospective analysis was 30% and 24%, respectively, and the overall mortality was 39% [119]. As with all retrospective analyses, and especially in the case of rare disorders, selection bias cannot be excluded.

The pros and cons of serial vascular imaging are elusive but are probably at least potentially beneficial. One should balance the risk of causing anxiety [119] against the potential benefits of detecting previously unknown aneurysms or progressive dilatations that are potentially treatable and potentially life-saving [51]. So far, the reduction of mortality or morbidity by serial imaging capable of predicting potential early signs of arterial wall weakness has not been systematically explored in vEDS.

The only drug with a proven beneficial effect in vEDS is the selective B1 receptor blocker with B2 mimetic properties, celiprolol. A multicenter randomized open-label controlled trial with celiprolol in 53 patients was ended prematurely due to treatment benefit with a 36% reduction in vascular events in the treated group as compared to the untreated group [178]. It needs to be acknowledged though that the occurrence rate of vascular events remained high at 20% in the treated patient group.

Multisystemic Smooth Muscle Dysfunction Syndrome

Recently recommendations for surveillance and management of MSMD syndrome have been published [54]. Surgical repair of the PDA should be considered in infants with MSMD, since delaying this surgery has the risk to escalate the pulmonary arterial hypertension. Evaluation of the entire aorta at the time of diagnosis is recommended. Follow-up imaging should be performed by echocardiography or cardiac MRI/MRA. Surveillance of the descending thoracic and abdominal aorta should be started at 10 years of age or earlier if abnormalities were noted on the initial scan. When possible, elective aortic root repair should be delayed in children until the annulus can accommodate an adult-sized graft. Valve-sparing elective surgical repair of aneurysms of the ascending aorta should be discussed when the aortic diameter reaches 45 mm. Asymptomatic peripheral artery aneurysm should be monitored annually by ultrasound. Surgical repair of symptomatic, thrombotic, or large aneurysms (>20 mm in diameter) should be considered. No drug treatments have been specifically tested in individuals with *ACTA2* mutations. Extensive recommendations on the neurologic, pulmonary, gastrointestinal, urogenital, ocular, and reproductive complications are available [54].

Nonsyndromic H-TAD

When a patient is diagnosed with a thoracic aortic aneurysm, clinical evaluation including family history, physical examination, and ocular assessment is recommended to exclude underlying syndromic entities.

In contrast to patients with syndromic H-TAD entities who may come to medical attention through associated clinical manifestations, patients with nonsyndromic forms are often diagnosed on presentation with aortic events, which are overwhelmingly acute aortic dissections. In patients with *ACTA2* mutations, (complex) type B dissections appeared to be more common than type A aortic dissection, leading the authors to conclude that anyone presenting with an acute aortic dissection without syndromic features and with a family history of the disease, along with young people with aortic dissections, especially type B aortic dissections, should raise a suspicion for an underlying *ACTA2* mutation. Because these individuals present with complicated dissections often requiring surgical intervention, transfer to a tertiary care center should be considered [130]. Since aortic disease in *ACTA2* mutation carriers often extends to the distal thoracic aorta, more extensive imaging with CT/MRI in these patients is recommended. In patients with *ACTA2* mutations, more extensive involvement of the aortic root, ascending aorta, and aortic arch should be taken into account when planning thoracic aortic repair, and consideration should be given to repairing all these regions even if a specific location is not yet enlarged [130].

Medications that reduce hemodynamic stress, such as β-adrenergic blockers, are recommended for individuals with H-TAD. Careful follow-up is warranted. In nonsyndromic H-TAD with confirmed genetic defect and/or familial occurrence, aortic surgery is recommended at ascending aortic diameters similar to Marfan syndrome and should be individualized for each patient, taking into account family history, rate of aortic growth, underlying gene defect, etc.

The threshold for surgical intervention may be guided by the aortic size at which other family members have had aortic complications, if known. If not known, then a size threshold of 4.5–5.0 cm for the ascending aorta and 5.5–6.0 cm for the descending thoracic aorta is reasonable because of the high complication rate of thoraco-abdominal aortic surgery at this level [179]. The current guidelines of the American College of Cardiology [77] recommend prophylactic surgery based on different scenarios according to the underlying gene as different clinical courses are expected in patients with different gene mutations. The more recent ESC guidelines on management of aortic disease have not adopted these rules [160]. Recent studies indicate that the course of aortic disease related to mutations in the *TGFBR* genes appears to be less aggressive in at least a subset of patients [14, 46]. Studies are ongoing to assess whether clinical or biochemical parameters could help us to better estimate the risk in an individual patient.

Molecular Diagnostics

Molecular confirmation of the correct diagnosis is increasingly important for gene-tailored patient management in H-TAD patients. Traditional genetic testing involved Sanger sequencing of a number of genes in a step-wise manner to try to identify the causal mutation. Currently, many genetic laboratories have introduced next-generation sequencing (NGS) into diagnostics, which changed the whole field of genetics. With NGS, or massive parallel sequencing, millions of small DNA fragments can be sequenced at the same time, creating a massive pool of data. Bioinformatic analyses are used to piece together these fragments by mapping the individual reads to the human reference genome providing accurate data on DNA variation. NGS can be used to sequence all 22,000 coding genes (whole exome) or targeted to small numbers of individual genes (panels).

Several studies have shown that the NGS approach including all syndromic and nonsyndromic genes for H-TAD is by far less time-consuming than consecutive Sanger sequencing of each TAD gene, and as a consequence, the labor costs also diminished proportionally.

Marfan Syndrome

The mutation detection rate for the *FBN1* gene in patients fulfilling the diagnostic criteria for Marfan syndrome is about 90% [180]. In the remaining 10% of patients, no causal mutation or deletion in *FBN1* can be identified. In those cases, the causative mutation in *FBN1* might not be detectable with conventional techniques, or these patients may harbor a mutation in another (unknown) gene.

In a few *FBN1*-negative patients fulfilling the criteria of Marfan syndrome, as well as in patients with "incomplete" Marfan syndrome, mutations in genes involved in the transforming growth factor β pathway have been identified. A discriminative feature with MFS caused by *FBN1* mutations is ectopia lentis, which seems to be an exclusive feature for patients with *FBN1* mutations.

From a practical standpoint, single-gene mutation screening of the *FBN1* gene may be considered in patients fulfilling the diagnostic criteria for MFS including ectopia lentis. In all others, more extensive NGS panel sequencing or targeted exome sequencing, including the *FBN1* gene, may be more appropriate.

Loeys-Dietz Syndrome

In rare cases, careful work-up by an experienced clinical geneticist or cardiologist can help to make the correct clinical diagnosis and predict the molecular cause. However, LDS genes frequently lead to a range of phenotypes, and in a majority of cases, the features are less obvious or are evolving in children or young adults. Moreover, several LDS genes have been implicated in the pathogenesis of nonsyndromic H-TAD.

In order to overcome these hurdles, targeted NGS panel of genes involved in H-TAD or whole exome sequencing (WES) with a filter for the known H-TAD genes is advised in LDS patients.

Vascular Ehlers-Danlos Syndrome

As is the case with the other syndromes, isolated screening of the *COL3A1* gene may be considered in those cases with a very typical phenotype, for example, in those cases presenting with gastrointestinal rupture or extensive ruptures/

dissections in different arterial beds. In all other cases, extended genetic screening using NGS panels of targeted exome sequencing seems more appropriate.

Multisystemic Smooth Muscle Dysfunction Syndrome

In patients with this distinct phenotype, specific mutational analysis of the *ACTA2* R179 mutation is indicated as a first step and if negative to be complemented with more extensive screening.

Nonsyndromic H-TAD

In several countries, targeted NGS of a panel of genes involved in H-TAD or whole exome sequencing (WES) with a filter of the known H-TAD genes is available. Deleterious mutations in cohorts of both syndromic and nonsyndromic H-TAD adults are identified in 4–27% of patients using a targeted NGS panels with different numbers of TAAD genes [5, 62, 181] [182]. The addition of copy number variation analysis was shown to significantly increase the diagnostic yield [183].

Lists of "core genes" and "additional genes" to be tested in the setting of H-TAD are provided in Arslan-Kirchner et al. [184].

The downside of more extended genetic screening is that many variants of unknown significance (around 20%) are identified and it is challenging to assign causality with certainty to the found variants [62, 182]. Collaborative international networks including the ClinGen initiative are currently being installed with the aim to improve strategies for variant curation [185].

Molecular Genetics and Specific Consequences of the Genotype

Marfan Syndrome

Molecular Genetics

FBN1 is a large gene with 65 exons coding for fibrillin-1 [186, 187], a 320 kDa glycoprotein consisting of 2871 amino acids. Fibrillins are large (~350,000 MW) structural macromolecules that contribute to the integrity and function of all connective tissues. They are considered to be "structural macromolecules" because, like the collagens, the fibrillins form fibers that are visible in transmission electron micrographs.

Fibrillin-1 is highly conserved among different species. The polypeptide comprises 47 repeated cysteine-rich motifs resembling epidermal growth factor (EGF-like) and an 8-cysteine motif (TB/8-cys). Forty-three of the 47 motifs contain a consensus sequence for calcium binding and are termed calcium-binding EGF-like (cbEGF-like) motifs (Fig. 19.1) [188, 189].

Fibrillin molecules polymerize to form the microfibrils, a constituent of the extracellular matrix. Microfibrils can associate with elastin to form elastic fibers. The microfibrils and elastic fibers have a widespread distribution in connective tissue throughout the body, including the skin, vascular wall, tendons, fascia, alveolar wall, and ciliary zonules that suspend the ocular lens, where they provide force-bearing structural support needed by these individual organ systems. Fibrillin microfibrils are organized to best suit the functional integrity of the tissue: for example, in tendons, elastic fibers run parallel to the long axis, whereas in muscular arteries, elastic fibers encircle the lumen [190].

In addition, it has become increasingly clear that fibrillin-rich microfibrils have functions that are not directly related to structural integrity but rather have to do with homeostasis of the elastic matrix, matrix-cell attachments, and regulation of cytokines [188, 189].

To date, about 2000 different mutations have been reported in *FBN1.* Most of the reported mutations are missense mutations affecting the conserved cysteine residues or residues of the consensus sequence of the cbEGF-like motifs. Nonsense mutations, mutations of splice sites associated with exon skipping, and, more rarely, small deletions are also found. The majority of mutations are private mutations that are unique to a family or an individual patient. Approximately 25% of cases of Marfan syndrome are caused by de novo mutations. Most of the infants with a severe form of Marfan syndrome are isolated (de novo) cases, which reflects the low likelihood of these patients to survive to reproductive age.

Many mutations in *FBN1* are believed to adversely affect the normal, wild-type gene product, i.e., they are thought to have a dominant-negative effect. However, Marfan syndrome and related disorders can also be caused by mutations that prevent or reduce the expression of the mutant allele. Haploinsufficiency may therefore also contribute to the pathogenesis [191].

Pathophysiology

The current knowledge of the role of fibrillin-1 in the pathogenesis of aortic aneurysm formation is at least threefold: [1] structural role in elastic fiber composition, [2] regulator of TGFβ signaling, and [3] role in mechanotransduction.

Early theories of disease pathogenesis in Marfan syndrome assumed that the manifestations of the disease were caused by the loss of structural integrity of affected tissues, due to mutant fibrillin-1 in the microfibrils. It was thought that this resulted in weak tissue that could not withstand enduring stress over time. Some features of Marfan syndrome could indeed be explained by these models, such as aortic aneurysms, ectopia lentis, and dural ectasia. However, other features, including bone overgrowth, craniofacial features, and myxomatous changes of the mitral valve, did not seem compatible with these theories. It has become increasingly clear that other mechanisms indeed contribute to the pathogenesis of Marfan syndrome.

Animal studies have shown that fibrillin-rich microfibrils have an essential role in homeostasis of the elastic matrix during postnatal life [192]. Elastic fibers have intimate connections with adjacent vascular endothelial cells and smooth muscle cells, mediated by fibrillin-1. As a result of defective fibrillin-1, these connections may be absent or inadequate. In mice, this resulted in abortive matrix remodeling, characterized by overproduction of multiple structural components and matrix-degrading enzymes, including metalloproteinases 2 and 9. Subsequent events are infiltration of inflammatory cells, intimal hyperplasia, elastic fiber calcification, and structural collapse of the vessel wall leading to aneurysm formation [192]. These manifestations have also been observed in pathologic specimens from patients with Marfan syndrome [193].

In addition to their structural function, fibrillin-rich microfibrils also play a significant role in the regulation of cytokines. Transforming growth factors β (TGFβs) are multifunctional cytokines that can induce many cellular events including proliferation, differentiation, cell cycle arrest, programmed cell death, and matrix deposition [194]. The activation of TGFβ is limited by fibrillin-1. It was therefore hypothesized that abnormal fibrillin-1 or reduced levels of fibrillin-1 result in excessive amounts of active TGFβ [195]. Subsequently, an increased output of TGFβ-responsive genes, such as collagen and connective tissue growth factor (CTGF), and altered cellular events lead to the phenotypic manifestations of Marfan syndrome. TGFβ is a multifunctional peptide that controls proliferation, differentiation, and other functions in many cell types. Fibrillin-1 is homologous to the family of latent TGFβ-binding proteins (LTBPs), which serve to hold TGFβ in an inactive complex in various tissues, including the extracellular matrix [196]. Indeed, fibrillin-1 was shown to bind TGFβ and LTBPs [197, 198]. Hence, it was hypothesized that mutations in fibrillin-1 could lead to perturbed sequestration of the inactive TGFβ complex [195]. Indeed, increased TGFβ signaling has been demonstrated in several tissues in MFS patients and murine models for MFS.

Surprisingly, more recent studies demonstrated that a *Fbn1* mouse in which the LTBP binding site was deleted (*Fbn1*$^{H1\Delta}$) did not present features of MFS [199]. This observation refuted the importance of TGFβ sequestration by fibrillin-1, and an alternative hypothesis was proposed whereby mutant microfibrils influence TGFβ activation in a different way. Increased TGFβ signaling is now considered as the result of a final common pathway in the disease process. The role of the TGFβ signaling pathway may also vary during the dynamic transition from aortic aneurysm predisposition to end-stage disease, such as dissection [200].

Moreover, fibrillins do not only contribute to cell signaling in the vessel wall through regulation of growth factor bioavailability, but these microfibrils are also important in *mechanotransduction* from the endothelium and extracellular matrix to the vascular smooth muscle cells. The process of mechanotransduction is critical to maintain homeostasis within the aortic wall by regulating aortic remodeling in response to hemodynamic stress. Mutations in fibrillin-1 may perturb this mechanism [201, 202]. Hence, a recent hypothesis states that the mechanical state of the matrix is sensed by cells in the vessel wall, which consequently send a signal through integrins and the cytoskeleton, resulting in inappropriate remodeling and aneurysm formation and this is via a common pathway of inappropriate TGFβ signaling. A schematic overview of the pathogenesis is provided in Fig. 19.17.

Genotype-Phenotype Correlation

No definitive genotype-phenotype correlations seem to be present in Marfan syndrome [203, 204]. Therefore, the identification of a particular mutation in a patient has little prognostic value and cannot determine individual management. However, some generalizations in genotype-phenotype correlations can be made—an overview is provided in Table 19.7. Mutations causing in-frame loss or gain of central coding sequence due to deletions, insertions, or splicing errors are associated with more severe disease. In contrast, mutations that create a premature termination codon leading to rapid degradation of the transcript can be associated with mild manifestations that may not fulfill the criteria for Marfan syndrome [212–214]. The mutations that have been found in patients with a neonatal presentation of severe and rapidly progressive Marfan syndrome, the so-called neonatal Marfan syndrome, are located in the central portion of the *FBN1* gene between exons 24 and 32, although many other patients with mutations in this region have a classic or mild phenotype [215].

A recent study of *FBN1* mutations in patients with MFS indicated that MFS patients with a haploinsufficient mutation are at increased risk for cardiovascular death and aortic dissection compared to patients with a dominant-negative effect mutation [211].

Loeys-Dietz Syndrome

Molecular Genetics

Loeys-Dietz syndrome types 1 and 2 are caused by mutations in the transforming growth factor β receptor type 1 (*TGFBR1*) gene and transforming growth factor β receptor

Table 19.7 Main genotype-phenotype correlations in Marfan syndrome caused by *FBN1* mutations

Type of *FBN1* mutation	Phenotype
Cysteine substitutions in EGF-like domains [205]	High incidence of ectopia lentis; severe early onset in exons 26–32
Premature termination codons (PTC) [206]	Low incidence of ectopia lentis; high incidence of large joint hypermobility; high incidence of skin striae; higher incidence of aortic dissection?
First 15 exons; arginine to cysteine mutations [207]	Predominant ectopia lentis
All mutation types [208]	Cysteine mutations correlate strongly with ectopia lentis; PTC mutations are associated with severe skeletal and skin phenotypes; mutations in exons 24–32 are associated with severe disease
Pediatric cohort; 33% of mutations occurred in exons 24–32; incidence of PTCs was smaller than in adult cohort [2]	Lethal neonatal Marfan syndrome is a genuine clinical entity; clinical manifestations increase with age
All mutation types [209]	"Incomplete" or mild Marfan syndrome was associated with mutations in exons 59–65; mutations at the ends (in exons 1–15 and 59–65) may be milder than mutations in between
All mutation types [210]	Truncating and splicing mutations were associated with aortic events
Dominant-negative (DN) vs haploinsufficient (HI) *FBN1* mutations [211]	Marfan syndrome patients with an HI mutation are at increased risk for cardiovascular death and aortic dissection compared to patients with a DN mutation

type 2 (*TGFBR2*) gene. Several hundreds of inactivating mutations have been identified in *TGFBR1* or *TGFBR2*. These are mostly missense substitutions of evolutionary conserved residues that encode the intracellular serine-threonine kinase domain of the receptors. No differences exist in clinical manifestation of patients with mutations in either gene. Mutations in *TGFBR1* and *TGFBR2* have also been reported in patients with familial thoracic aortic aneurysm and dissection (TAAD), without the other features of the Loeys-Dietz syndrome [15], as well as in patients fulfilling the criteria for Marfan syndrome [12]. There are no apparent differences in the type of mutations in these disorders as opposed to those found in Loeys-Dietz syndrome.

There is considerable intrafamilial variability in phenotype in Loeys-Dietz syndrome, and multiple cases of apparent non-penetrance have been reported [8, 10]. Most cases of severe Loeys-Dietz syndrome are due to de novo mutations.

LDS type 3 is caused by mutations in the SMAD family member 3 (*SMAD3*). The *SMAD3* gene contains three main functional domains, namely, the MH1 and MH2 domain and the linker region, and mutations occur throughout the entire 9 exon-containing gene. The mutation spectrum encompasses both truncating and missense mutations, with the latter clustering within the MH2 protein domain [19, 104]. The most likely effect of these mutations is a loss of function, with TGFβ signals not being propagated via SMAD3. Until now, no clear genotype-phenotype correlation has been established.

LDS types 4 and 5 are caused by mutations in the TGFβ binding ligands *TGFB2* and *TGFB3*. Various *TGFB2/3* mutation types, i.e., missense, frameshift, nonsense, and splice site mutations, have been reported, most likely leading to loss of function of the respective protein [104].

For all types of LDS, it is unknown why some mutations cause a severe LDS phenotype, while others account for the mild end of the disease spectrum.

In a minority of cases, LDS results from a new gene mutation (de novo) and occurs in people with no history of the disorder in their family. More frequently, an affected person inherits the mutation from one affected parent.

Pathophysiology

All LDS genes are essential in TGF-beta signaling. At the aortic tissue level, a recurrent pattern of enhanced TGFβ signaling is observed despite a loss of function at the molecular level. Histology and immunohistochemistry of aorta fragments of LDS cases show upregulation of both upstream ligands and downstream targets of the TGFβ pathway. This observation is similar to patients with other syndromic and nonsyndromic aneurysms like Marfan syndrome, arterial tortuosity syndrome, aneurysms associated with bicuspid aortic valve, and degenerative aneurismal aortic disease. This clearly indicates the existence of common (TGFβ-related) pathogenic mechanisms leading to arterial wall disease.

The precise mechanisms underlying the attenuation of TGFβ signaling remain elusive and a matter of debate. Several mechanisms that could explain this TGFβ paradox have been proposed but need experimental validation. These theories include altered receptor trafficking, impaired autoregulation of TGFβ signaling, alternative signaling cascades, or non-autonomous cellular events.

Vascular Ehlers-Danlos Syndrome

COL3A1 located on chromosome 2q24.3-q31 encodes type 3 collagen. There are N- and C-terminal propeptides coded, respectively, by 5 exons for the N propeptide and 4 exons for the C propeptide and in between an uninterrupted perfect triple helix coding for Gly-X-Y triplets, in which X or Y are frequently lysine (4%) or proline (10%). Mutations of the triple helix are generally caused by missense point mutations converting glycine to a larger amino acid. Such errors distort the dimensions of the triple helix, interrupting helical winding and leading to incorporation of mutant alpha chains into mature triple helices. This leads to diminished collagen secretion and assembly, resulting in weakened tissues containing the mutant molecules. Similar effects arise from exon skips in which shortened triple helices are similarly disruptive. In the case of stop codon mutations or large deletions, dosage effects are exerted, by mechanisms of haploinsufficiency. An extensive list of *COL3A1* mutations and polymorphisms can be found at https://eds.gene.le.ac.uk/home.php?select_db=COL3A1.

Pathophysiology

Despite the fact that vEDS and its underlying genetic defect have been known since the early 1990s, there has been limited progress on understanding the disease mechanism beyond that of connective tissue weakness due to structural defects or reduced amounts of type 3 procollagen. Based on the recent established role of the altered TGFβ signaling in Marfan syndrome and related thoracic aortic aneurysm disorders, the role of this mechanism was studied by Morissette and colleagues. They observed that mutations in *COL3A1* do not seem to alter the TGFβ signaling pathway in dermal fibroblasts from vEDS patients [216]; data regarding TGFβ signaling in arterial tissue are unfortunately not yet available.

Genotype/Phenotype Correlation

Two recent studies [217, 218] indicated that individuals with missense mutations substituting glycine and splice site or in-frame insertions-deletions have a more severe and earlier onset of the disease than *COL3A1* null mutations, non-glycine mutations, or mutations in the N- or C-terminal part of *COL3A1*. The latter groups also had less digestive complications. Within the glycine substituting group, substitutions for serine and arginine seem to have a better outcome than those for valine and aspartic acid [218] (Pepin et al).

COL3A1 mutations are occasionally encountered in patients presenting with NS H-TAD [5, 219].

Multisystemic Smooth Muscle Dysfunction Syndrome

In patients presenting the characteristic phenotype of neonatal PDA, fixed congenital mydriasis, moyamoya-like cerebrovascular disease, and TAA, targeted mutation analysis of the *ACTA2* R179 mutation may be considered. The R179 mutation is located close to a key protein-protein interaction site on the macromolecular surface of α-actin, leading to the assumption that the mutation may disrupt critical interaction and disrupt downstream signaling events necessary for smooth muscle cell function. Analysis of the nucleotide sequence around the mutation failed to identify a mutable motif to explain the increased frequency of this mutation. Therefore, the recurrent identification of this mutation may be due to a recruitment bias resulting from the unique phenotype in these patients [28].

Nonsyndromic H-TAD

Molecular Genetics

As already mentioned and as indicated in Table 19.1, the genetic background of NS H-TAD is heterogeneous. In the majority of patients and families, the underlying genetic basis is not found. Mutations in *FBN1*, *COL3A1*, *TGFBR1*, *TGFBR2*, *SMAD3*, and *TGFB2* have been reported in small proportions of patients with NS H-TAD [[5, 10, 20, 132].

Pathophysiology

The identification and characterization of these genes suggests that altered ECM function and increased TGFβ signaling play a role in pathogenesis. Another mechanism underlying NS H-TAD is through interaction with the vascular smooth muscle contractile apparatus. Several hypotheses exist to explain the link between H-TAD and impaired vascular SMC contractility. Mutations in genes involved in the smooth muscle cell apparatus (*MYLK*, *MYH11*, *ACTA2*, *PRKAG1*) may lead to upregulation of stress and repair pathways. In the vascular wall of patients harboring a *MYH11* mutation, angiotensin-converting enzyme (ACE) and insulin-like growth factor 1 (IGF-1) are upregulated [36]. Upregulation of ACE and IGF-1 activates the angiotensin II, phosphoinositide-3 kinase (PI3K), and canonical and non-canonical TGFβ pathways (SMAD2/3 and ERK, respectively), subsequently leading to increased smooth muscle cell contractility and proliferation and upregulation of TGFβ [36, 220]. TGFβ can in itself induce a contractile phenotype of vascular SMCs, since it regulates transcription of contractile genes [221–223]. TGFβ upregulation has been demonstrated in the aortic wall of patients with missense mutations in *ACTA2* and *MYH11* [32]. However, Pannu and colleagues did not find increased CTGF staining or increased expression of CTGF and TGFβ1 in aortic tissue and smooth muscle cells of patients harboring *MYH11* mutations [15]. For *MYLK*, *FLNA*, and *PRKG1*, no data have been reported so far on a possible association with TGFβ signaling.

The cytoskeleton also plays a role in maintaining the ECM integrity. The cytoskeleton is involved in the assembly of fibronectin fibrils via integrin receptors [224]. A stable fibronectin fibrillar matrix is in turn indispensable for C-terminal association of fibrillin-1 monomers into bead-like structures and their linear assembly into microfibrils [225]. The inability of the contractile apparatus to exert its function can consequently affect the integrity of the extracellular matrix, and this may thus indirectly trigger cellular response mechanisms, including increased TGFβ signaling.

Mutations leading to perturbed contractility of vascular SMCs may also impair mechanical homeostasis and lead to maladaptive remodeling, since mechanosensing requires intact load-bearing structures [202].

Genotype/Phenotype Correlations

In the era of personalized medicine, it is very tempting to say that the genotype may guide us in predicting the phenotype. Great caution is however warranted, especially since no large series of any of these diseases are currently available. An example to illustrate this is found in the identification of mutations in the *TGFBR1/2* genes. Initial reports of patients harboring these mutations indicated that the aortic phenotype was markedly more aggressive than the one common phenotype observed in Marfan syndrome [8]. Subsequent observations could however not confirm these findings [14, 46], indicating that the phenotype in patients with *TGFBR* mutations may vary widely from severe syndromic presentations as in Loeys-Dietz syndrome to milder nonsyndromic phenotypes. Currently, efforts are undertaken to collect data on a larger scale in order to obtain data from representative cohorts of patients.

Within each H-TAD gene, genotype-specific phenotypes have been reported as, for example, in the *ACTA2* gene with the severe phenotype associated with the R179 mutation [28]. Similarly, more severe phenotypes have been reported for other substitutions at that position and for the R258 mutations [130].

Family Screening and Follow-Up in Relatives

A molecular diagnosis provides the opportunity of carrier testing in asymptomatic family members. However, genetic testing can have potential negative ethical, legal, and social implications. During pretest genetic counseling, the potential risks, benefits, and limitations of genetic testing need to be discussed, facilitating autonomous decision-making. Predictive genetic testing of minors is generally accepted for childhood-onset conditions if preventative or therapeutic measurements are available to reduce morbidity or mortality. Accordingly, predictive testing seems justified in asymptomatic children at risk for MFS, LDS, and other H-TAD entities. Although clinical expression of these conditions is highly variable and age-dependent, severe cardiovascular manifestations have been observed in early childhood, and children may benefit from early prophylactic treatment. Early knowledge of the diagnosis may also be useful for the timely treatment of skeletal and ocular manifestations in these disorders.

Testing in children for adult-onset disorders including vascular EDS is more controversial and needs to be decided on an individual basis. Patients (and their parents) should be informed of the fact that 12%–24% of individuals have a major complication by age 20 years [217] and that preventive treatment with celiprolol may be considered before the age of 18 years. Other potential benefits of testing for vEDS in minors include [1] elimination of concern for those children who do not have the familial *COL3A1* pathogenic variant, [2] awareness of and preparedness for potential complications, and (3) restriction of high-impact sports and high-risk activities for those with the pathogenic variant [226]. Given the opportunity to consider testing for children at 50% risk of having inherited the pathogenic variant, parents usually do not wait until a complication arises or until the child reaches adulthood for a test to be performed [226].

In nonsyndromic H-TAD, the medical benefit for genetic testing in children is less obvious, and genetic testing is usually postponed until adulthood to protect the child's future autonomy. We strongly recommend that testing of children always involves psychosocial support.

In the many families without an identified causal mutation, it is not possible to determine which individuals are at risk of developing aneurysms and dissection. Therefore, all first-degree relatives (children, siblings, and parents) of H-TAD patients are advised to undergo regular aortic imaging, as recommended by the ESC and ACC guidelines [77, 160]. The timing of screening depends on the family history.

In case of familial TAD, we suggest to start screening at the age of 25 years or 10 years below the youngest case in the family, if the latter ends up below 25 years. We assume that clinically relevant disease will rarely be detected in children or young adults below these age limits, while the psychological impact of screening should not be underestimated. If the initial screening reveals no abnormalities, we recommend to continue screening every 5 years. If the aortic diameters are very small or remain stable over time, 10-year intervals seem reasonable. We suggest to discontinue screening by age 65 years. However, if the first screening takes place after the age of 60 years, we recommend at least one follow-up. In case the screening reveals an abnormality, follow-up should be adjusted accordingly [227] (Fig. 19.18).

In sporadic TAD patients (aneurysm ≥45 mm or dissection) either aged <50 years or between 50 and 60 years without hypertension or syndromic features, we believe a single screening will suffice. However, if this screening takes place before the age of 40 years, a second screening might be considered at older age (above 50 years) [227] (Fig. 19.18).

Transthoracic echocardiography (TTE) is the primary imaging tool for screening of family members. We recommend to perform CT or MRI at initial evaluation, to exclude the presence of aneurysms at areas poorly visualized by TTE [227] (Fig. 19.18). Furthermore, we encourage routine screening of the abdominal aorta. If there is a family history of aneurysms, dissections, or tortuosity outside the thoracic

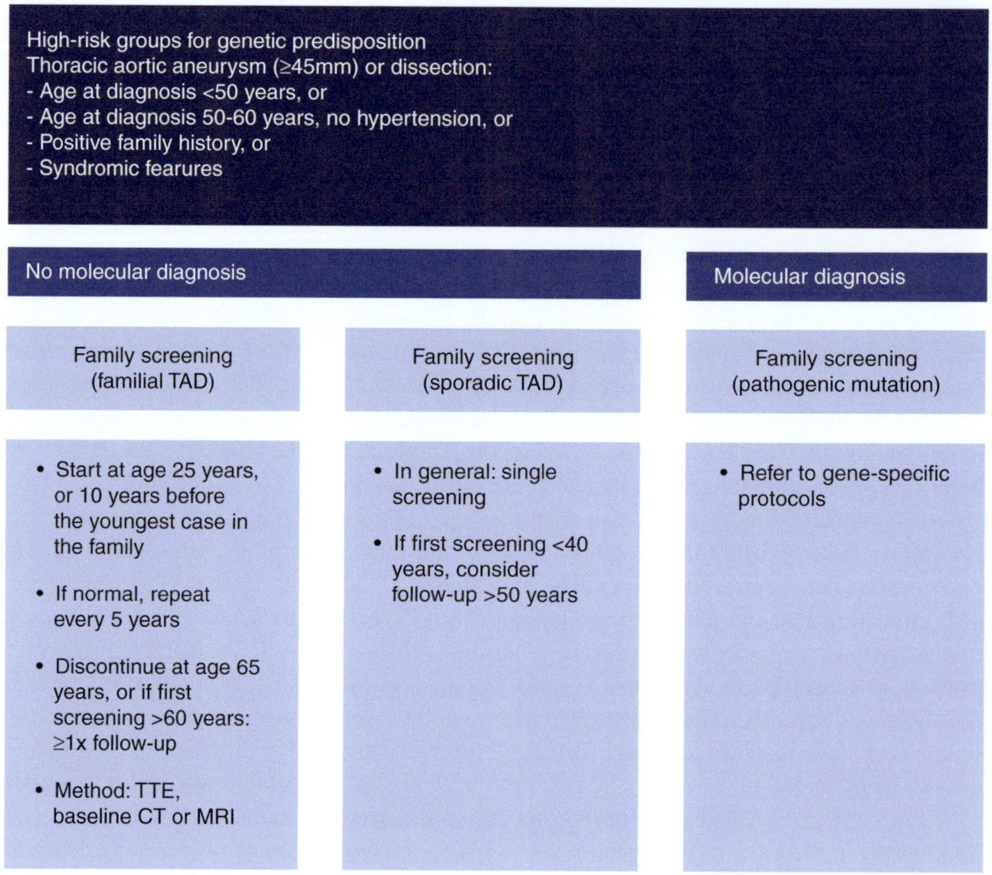

Fig. 19.18 Summary of recommendations for family screening

aorta, more extensive screening should be considered. Screening for intracranial aneurysms is usually recommended in families with at least two affected [228].

Prenatal diagnosis (PND) and preimplantation diagnosis (PGD) can be offered to those H-TAD patients with a known mutation in most countries. A French study in MFS patients indicated that a majority of patients (74%) was in favor of prenatal testing. The opinion of caregivers varied, but most of them agreed that these issues should be addressed in a multidisciplinary team [65].

Summary/Take-Home Message

Heritable thoracic aortic disease (H-TAD) comprise a heterogeneous group of disease entities with significant clinical and genetic overlap. Both syndromic and nonsyndromic forms are recognized. Identification of the underlying genetic defect is important for confirmation of the diagnosis and may help in risk stratification and guidance of management. A substantial proportion of (mainly nonsyndromic) families with H-TAD remains in whom the underlying gene defect has not been identified yet, and in these cases, clinical imaging of patients and relatives is the mainstay of follow-up.

Next-generation sequencing techniques have significantly improved the diagnostic yield in patients with H-TAD, and NGS panel sequencing and/or targeted exome sequencing is the method of choice for mutation screening.

Life expectancy in H-TAD patients is determined by the risk for aortic dissection and depends at least partly on the underlying molecular diagnosis. Timely diagnosis and treatment is crucial and should be performed in a multidisciplinary setting. Prophylactic aortic surgery is beyond doubt the most life-saving treatment modality, and more research is needed to better define the optimal thresholds for—especially descending—aortic surgery in the individual patient.

Take-Home Messages

- At least 20% of patients presenting with thoracic aortic disease have an affected relative, and a detailed family history with clinical evaluation of first-degree relatives is an essential component of the evaluation.
- Both syndromic and nonsyndromic entities of H-TAD are recognized with significant clinical and genetic overlap. Careful clinical assessment of all patients is required to exclude syndromic entities. Clinical molecular testing is appropriate after pretest genetic counseling.

- Over 15 genes have been identified so far that can cause Mendelian forms of thoracic aortic disease when mutated. These encode for components of the extracellular matrix, the TGFβ signaling pathway, or the smooth muscle cell contractile apparatus.
- Mutations lead to altered structural and functional properties in the aortic wall through interaction with mechanobiology.

References

1. Loeys BL, Dietz HC, Braverman AC, Callewaert BL, De Backer J, Devereux RB, et al. The revised Ghent nosology for the Marfan syndrome. J Med Genet. 2010 Jun 30;47(7):476–85.
2. Faivre L, Masurel-Paulet A, Collod-Beroud G, Callewaert BL, Child AH, Stheneur C, et al. Clinical and molecular study of 320 children with Marfan syndrome and related type I fibrillinopathies in a series of 1009 probands with pathogenic FBN1 mutations. Pediatrics. 2009 Jan;123(1):391–8. Available from: http://eutils.ncbi.nlm.nih.gov/entrez/eutils/elink.fcgi?dbfrom=pubmed&id=19117906&retmode=ref&cmd=prlinks
3. Milewicz DM, Michael K, Fisher N, Coselli JS, Markello T, Biddinger A. Fibrillin-1 (FBN1) mutations in patients with thoracic aortic aneurysms. Circulation. 1996 Dec 1;94(11):2708–11.
4. Pepin M, Schwarze U, Superti-Furga A, Byers PH. Clinical and genetic features of Ehlers-Danlos syndrome type IV, the vascular type. N Engl J Med. 2000 Mar 9;342(10):673–80.
5. Campens L, Callewaert B, Muiño Mosquera L, Renard M, Symoens S, de Paepe A, et al. Gene panel sequencing in heritable thoracic aortic disorders and related entities – results of comprehensive testing in a cohort of 264 patients. Orphanet J Rare Dis. 2015;10(1):9.
6. Barbier M, Gross M-S, Aubart M, Hanna N, Kessler K, Guo D-C, et al. MFAP5 loss-of-function mutations underscore the involvement of matrix alteration in the pathogenesis of familial thoracic aortic aneurysms and dissections. Am J Hum Genet. 2014 Dec 4;95(6):736–43.
7. Guo DC, Regalado ES, Gong L, Duan X, Santos-Cortez RL, Arnaud P, et al. LOX mutations predispose to thoracic aortic aneurysms and dissections. Circ Res. 2016 Mar 18;118(6):928–34.
8. Loeys BL, Schwarze U, Holm T, Callewaert BL, Thomas GH, Pannu H, et al. Aneurysm syndromes caused by mutations in the TGF-beta receptor. N Engl J Med. 2006 Aug 24;355(8):788–98.
9. Loeys BL, Chen J, Neptune ER, Judge DP, Podowski M, Holm T, et al. A syndrome of altered cardiovascular, craniofacial, neurocognitive and skeletal development caused by mutations in TGFBR1 or TGFBR2. Nat Genet. 2005 Jan 30;37(3):275–81.
10. Stheneur C, Collod-Beroud G, Faivre L, Gouya L, Sultan G, Le Parc J-M, et al. Identification of 23 TGFBR2 and 6 TGFBR1 gene mutations and genotype-phenotype investigations in 457 patients with Marfan syndrome type I and II, Loeys-Dietz syndrome and related disorders. Hum Mutat. 2008 Nov;29(11):E284–95.
11. Singh KK, Rommel K, Mishra A, Karck M, Haverich A, Schmidtke J, et al. TGFBR1 and TGFBR2 mutations in patients with features of Marfan syndrome and Loeys-Dietz syndrome. Hum Mutat. 2006 Aug;27(8):770–7.
12. Mizuguchi T, Collod-Beroud G, Akiyama T, Abifadel M, Harada N, Morisaki T, et al. Heterozygous TGFBR2 mutations in Marfan syndrome. Nat Genet. 2004 Aug 4;36(8):855–60.
13. Disabella E, Grasso M, Marziliano N, Ansaldi S, Lucchelli C, Porcu E, et al. Two novel and one known mutation of the TGFBR2 gene in Marfan syndrome not associated with FBN1 gene defects. Eur J Hum Genet. 2006 Jan;14(1):34–8.
14. Attias D, Stheneur C, Roy C, Collod-Beroud G, Detaint D, Faivre L, et al. Comparison of clinical presentations and outcomes between patients with TGFBR2 and FBN1 mutations in Marfan syndrome and related disorders. Circulation. 2009 Dec 22;120(25):2541–9.
15. Pannu H. Mutations in transforming growth factor- receptor type II cause familial thoracic aortic aneurysms and dissections. Circulation. 2005 Jul 18;112(4):513–20.
16. Micha D, Guo DC, Hilhorst-Hofstee Y, van Kooten F, Atmaja D, Overwater E, et al. SMAD2 mutations are associated with arterial aneurysms and dissections. Hum Mutat. 2015 Dec;36(12):1145–9.
17. MacCarrick G, Black JH, Bowdin S, El-Hamamsy I, Frischmeyer-Guerrerio PA, Guerrerio AL, et al. Loeys-Dietz syndrome: a primer for diagnosis and management. Genet Med. 2014;27:576–87.
18. van der Linde D, van de Laar IMBH, Bertoli-Avella AM, Oldenburg RA, Bekkers JA, Mattace-Raso FUS, et al. Aggressive cardiovascular phenotype of aneurysms-osteoarthritis syndrome caused by pathogenic SMAD3 variants. J Am Coll Cardiol. 2012 Jul 31;60(5):397–403. Available from: http://eutils.ncbi.nlm.nih.gov/entrez/eutils/elink.fcgi?dbfrom=pubmed&id=22633655&retmode=ref&cmd=prlinks
19. van de Laar IMBH, Oldenburg RA, Pals G, Roos-Hesselink JW, de Graaf BM, Verhagen JMA, et al. Mutations in SMAD3 cause a syndromic form of aortic aneurysms and dissections with early-onset osteoarthritis. Nat Genet. 2011 Feb 1;43(2):121–6.
20. Regalado ES, Guo D-C, Villamizar C, Avidan N, Gilchrist D, McGillivray B, et al. Exome sequencing identifies SMAD3 mutations as a cause of familial thoracic aortic aneurysm and dissection with intracranial and other arterial aneurysms. Circ Res. 2011 Sep 2;109(6):680–6.
21. Wang Y, Huang HY, Bian GL, Yu YS, Ye WX, Hua F, et al. A functional variant of SMAD4 enhances thoracic aortic aneurysm and dissection risk through promoting smooth muscle cell apoptosis and proteoglycan degradation. EBioMedicine. 2017 Jul;21:197–205.
22. Lindsay ME, Schepers D, Bolar NA, Doyle JJ, Gallo E, Fert-Bober J, et al. Loss-of-function mutations in TGFB2 cause a syndromic presentation of thoracic aortic aneurysm. Nat Genet. 2012 Jul;8:1–7. https://doi.org/10.1038/ng.2349.
23. Guo D-C, Hanna N, Regalado ES, Detaint D, Gong L, Varret M, et al. TGFB2 mutations cause familial thoracic aortic aneurysms and dissections associated with mild systemic features of Marfan syndrome. Nat Genet. 2012;8:1–8.
24. Renard M, Callewaert B, Malfait F, Campens L, Sharif S, Del Campo M, et al. Thoracic aortic-aneurysm and dissection in association with significant mitral valve disease caused by mutations in TGFB2. Int J Cardiol. 2012 Oct 22;165(3):584–7. Available from: http://eutils.ncbi.nlm.nih.gov/entrez/eutils/elink.fcgi?dbfrom=pubmed&id=23102774&retmode=ref&cmd=prlinks
25. Rienhoff HY, Yeo C-Y, Morissette R, Khrebtukova I, Melnick J, Luo S, et al. A mutation in TGFB3 associated with a syndrome of low muscle mass, growth retardation, distal arthrogryposis and clinical features overlapping with marfan and loeys-dietz syndrome. Am J Med Genet A. 2013 Jul;3:2040–6.
26. Morisaki H, Akiko Y, Itaru Y, Razia S, Tatsuya O, Hiroshu T. Pathogenic mutations found in 3 Japanese families with MFS/LDS-like disorder. Paris.
27. Matyas G, Naef P, Oexle K. De novo TGFB3 mutation in a patient with overgrowth and Loeys-Dietz Syndrome features. Paris.
28. Milewicz DM, Ostergaard JR, Ala-Kokko LM, Khan N, Grange DK, Mendoza-Londono R, et al. De novo ACTA2 mutation causes a novel syndrome of multisystemic smooth muscle dysfunction. Am J Med Genet A. 2010 Oct;152A(10):2437–43.

29. Munot P, Saunders DE, Milewicz DM, Regalado ES, Ostergaard JR, Braun KP, et al. A novel distinctive cerebrovascular phenotype is associated with heterozygous Arg179 ACTA2 mutations. Brain. 2012 Aug;135(Pt 8):2506–14.
30. Meuwissen MEC, Lequin MH, Bindels-de Heus K, Bruggenwirth HT, Knapen MFCM, Dalinghaus M, et al. ACTA2 mutation with childhood cardiovascular, autonomic and brain anomalies and severe outcome. Am J Med Genet A. 2013 Jun;161A(6):1376–80.
31. Guo D-C, Pannu H, Tran-Fadulu V, Papke CL, Yu RK, Avidan N, et al. Mutations in smooth muscle α-actin (ACTA2) lead to thoracic aortic aneurysms and dissections. Nat Genet. 2007 Nov 11;39(12):1488–93.
32. Renard M, Callewaert B, Baetens M, Campens L, Macdermot K, Fryns J-P, et al. Novel MYH11 and ACTA2 mutations reveal a role for enhanced TGFbeta signaling in FTAAD. Int J Cardiol. 2011 Sep 19;165(2):314–21. Available from: http://eutils.ncbi.nlm.nih.gov/entrez/eutils/elink.fcgi?dbfrom=pubmed&id=21937134&retmode=ref&cmd=prlinks
33. Wang L, Guo D-C, Cao J, Gong L, Kamm KE, Regalado E, et al. Mutations in myosin light chain kinase cause familial aortic dissections. Am J Hum Genet. 2010 Nov 12;87(5):701–7.
34. Guo D-C, Regalado E, Casteel DE, Santos-Cortez RL, Gong L, Kim JJ, et al. Recurrent gain-of-function mutation in PRKG1 causes thoracic aortic aneurysms and acute aortic dissections. Am J Hum Genet. 2013 Aug 8;93(2):398–404.
35. Zhu L, Vranckx R, van Kien PK, Lalande A, Boisset N, Mathieu F, et al. Mutations in myosin heavy chain 11 cause a syndrome associating thoracic aortic aneurysm/aortic dissection and patent ductus arteriosus. Nat Genet. 2006 Jan 29;38(3):343–9.
36. Pannu H, Tran-Fadulu V, Papke CL, Scherer S, Liu Y, Presley C, et al. MYH11 mutations result in a distinct vascular pathology driven by insulin-like growth factor 1 and angiotensin II. Hum Mol Genet. 2007 Apr 5;16(20):2453–62.
37. Marfan AB. Un cas de déformation congénitale des quatres membres, plus prononcée aux extrémités, caractérisée par l"allongement des avec un certain degré d"amincissement. Bull Mem Soc Med Hop Paris. 1896 Jan 1;13:220–6.
38. VA MK, editor. Heritable disorders of connective tissue. St Louis: Mosby CA; 1956.
39. Pyeritz RE. Marfan syndrome: 30 years of research equals 30 years of additional life expectancy. Heart. 2008 Nov 25;95(3):173–5.
40. Silverman DI, Burton KJ, Gray J, Bosner MS, Kouchoukos NT, Roman MJ, et al. Life expectancy in the Marfan syndrome. Am J Cardiol. 1995 Jan 15;75(2):157–60.
41. Groth KA, Stochholm K, Hove H, Andersen NH, Gravholt CH. Causes of mortality in the Marfan syndrome (from a Nationwide Register Study). Am J Cardiol. 2018 Oct 1;122(7):1231–5.
42. Braverman AC, Harris KM, Kovacs RJ, Maron BJ. Eligibility and disqualification recommendations for competitive athletes with cardiovascular abnormalities: task force 7: aortic diseases, including Marfan syndrome: a scientific statement from the American Heart Association and American College of Cardiology. Circulation. 2015;132:e303–9.
43. Jondeau G, Detaint D, Tubach F, Arnoult F, Milleron O, Raoux F, et al. Aortic event rate in the Marfan population: a cohort study. Circulation. 2012 Jan 17;125(2):226–32.
44. Meijboom LJ. Pregnancy and aortic root growth in the Marfan syndrome: a prospective study. Eur Heart J. 2005 Mar 21;26(9):914–20.
45. Donnelly RT, Pinto NM, Kocolas I, Yetman AT. The immediate and long-term impact of pregnancy on aortic growth rate and mortality in women with Marfan syndrome. J Am Coll Cardiol. 2012 Jul 17;60(3):224–9.
46. Teixido-Tura G, Franken R, Galuppo V, Gutiérrez García-Moreno L, Borregan M, BJM M, et al. Heterogeneity of aortic disease severity in patients with Loeys-Dietz syndrome. Heart. 2016 Feb 4;102(8):626–32.
47. Teixidó-Tura G, Franken R, Galuppo V, Gutiérrez García-Moreno L, Borregan M, Mulder BJ, et al. Heterogeneity of aortic disease severity in patients with Loeys-Dietz syndrome. Heart. 2016 Apr;102(8):626–32.
48. Jondeau G, Ropers J, Regalado E, Braverman A, Evangelista A, Teixedo G, et al. International registry of patients carrying TGFBR1 or TGFBR2 mutations: results of the MAC (Montalcino Aortic Consortium). Circ Cardiovasc Genet. 2016 Dec;9(6):548–58.
49. Malfait F, Francomano C, Byers P, Belmont J, Berglund B, Black J, et al. The 2017 international classification of the Ehlers-Danlos syndromes. Am J Med Genet C Semin Med Genet. 2017 Mar;175(1):8–26.
50. Byers PH. Ehlers-Danlos syndrome: recent advances and current understanding of the clinical and genetic heterogeneity. J Invest Dermatol. 1994 Nov;103(5 Suppl):47S–52S.
51. Oderich GS, Panneton JM, Bower TC, Lindor NM, Cherry KJ, Noel AA, et al. The spectrum, management and clinical outcome of Ehlers-Danlos syndrome type IV: a 30-year experience. J Vasc Surg. 2005 Jul;42(1):98–106.
52. Murray ML, Pepin M, Peterson S, Byers PH. Pregnancy-related deaths and complications in women with vascular Ehlers-Danlos syndrome. Genet Med. 2014 Dec;16(12):874–80.
53. Lemire BD, Buncic JR, Kennedy SJ, Dyack SJ, Teebi AS. Congenital mydriasis, patent ductus arteriosus, and congenital cystic lung disease: new syndromic spectrum? Am J Med Genet A. 2004 Dec 15;131(3):318–9.
54. Regalado ES, Mellor-Crummey L, De Backer J, Braverman AC, Ades L, Benedict S, et al. Clinical history and management recommendations of the smooth muscle dysfunction syndrome due to ACTA2 arginine 179 alterations. Genet Med. 2018 Oct;20(10):1206–15.
55. Logeswaran T, Friedburg C, Hofmann K, Akintuerk H, Biskup S, Graef M, et al. Two patients with the heterozygous R189H mutation in ACTA2 and Complex congenital heart defects expands the cardiac phenotype of multisystemic smooth muscle dysfunction syndrome. Am J Med Genet A. 2017 Apr;173(4):959–65.
56. Isselbacher EM. Thoracic and abdominal aortic aneurysms. Circulation. 2005 Feb 15;111(6):816–28.
57. Pyeritz RE. Heritable thoracic aortic disorders. Curr Opin Cardiol. 2014 Jan;29(1):97–102.
58. Albornoz G, Coady M, Roberts M, Davies R, Tranquilli M, Rizzo J, et al. Familial thoracic aortic aneurysms and dissections—incidence, modes of inheritance, and phenotypic patterns. Ann Thorac Surg. 2006 Oct;82(4):1400–5.
59. Coady MA, Rizzo JA, Goldstein LJ, Elefteriades JA. Natural history, pathogenesis, and etiology of thoracic aortic aneurysms and dissections. Cardiol Clin. 1999 Nov;17(4):615–35.
60. Strande NT, Riggs ER, Buchanan AH, Ceyhan-Birsoy O, DiStefano M, Dwight SS, et al. Evaluating the clinical validity of gene-disease associations: an evidence-based framework developed by the clinical genome resource. Am J Hum Genet. 2017 Jun 1;100(6):895–906.
61. Renard M, Francis C, Ghosh R, Scott AF, Witmer PD, Adès LC, et al. Clinical validity of genes for heritable thoracic aortic aneurysm and dissection. J Am Coll Cardiol. 2018 Aug 7;72(6):605–15.
62. Wooderchak-Donahue W, VanSant-Webb C, Tvrdik T, Plant P, Lewis T, Stocks J, et al. Clinical utility of a next generation sequencing panel assay for Marfan and Marfan-like syndromes featuring aortopathy. Am J Med Genet A. 2015 May 5;167A(8):1747–57.

63. Guo DC, Hostetler EM, Fan Y, Kulmacz RJ, Zhang D. GenTAC Investigators et al. Heritable thoracic aortic disease genes in sporadic aortic dissection. J Am Coll Cardiol. 2017 Nov 28;70(21):2728–30.
64. Regalado ES, Guo DC, Prakash S, Bensend TA, Flynn K, Estrera A, et al. Aortic disease presentation and outcome associated with ACTA2 mutations. Circ Cardiovasc Genet. 2015 Jun;8(3):457–64.
65. Coron F, Rousseau T, Jondeau G, Gautier E, Binquet C, Gouya L, et al. What do French patients and geneticists think about prenatal and preimplantation diagnoses in Marfan syndrome? Prenat Diagn. 2012 Dec;32(13):1318–23.
66. Radonic T, de Witte P, Groenink M, de Bruin-Bon RACM, Timmermans J, Scholte AJH, et al. Critical appraisal of the revised Ghent criteria for diagnosis of Marfan syndrome. Clin Genet. 2011 Oct;80(4):346–53.
67. Finkbohner R, Johnston D, Crawford ES, Coselli J, Milewicz DM. Marfan syndrome. Long-term survival and complications after aortic aneurysm repair. Circulation. 1995 Feb 1;91(3):728–33.
68. Engelfriet PM. Beyond the root: dilatation of the distal aorta in Marfan's syndrome. Heart. 2006 Jul 19;92(9):1238–43.
69. Mulder BJM. The distal aorta in the Marfan syndrome. Neth Heart J. 2008 Nov;16(11):382–6.
70. Franken R, El Morabit A, de Waard V, Timmermans J, Scholte AJ, van den Berg MP, et al. Increased aortic tortuosity indicates a more severe aortic phenotype in adults with Marfan syndrome. Int J Cardiol. 2015 Sep 1;194:7–12.
71. Morris SA. Arterial tortuosity in genetic arteriopathies. Curr Opin Cardiol. 2015 Nov;30(6):587–93.
72. den AW H, Franken R, Zwinderman AH, Timmermans J, Scholte AJ, van den Berg MP, et al. The risk for type B aortic dissection in marfan syndrome. J Am Coll Cardiol. 2015 Jan;65(3):246–54.
73. Nollen GJ, Groenink M, Tijssen JGP, Van Der Wall EE, Mulder BJM. Aortic stiffness and diameter predict progressive aortic dilatation in patients with Marfan syndrome. Eur Heart J. 2004 Jul;25(13):1146–52.
74. Franken R, Morabit El A, de Waard V, Timmermans J, Scholte AJ, van den Berg MP, et al. Increased aortic tortuosity indicates a more severe aortic phenotype in adults with Marfan syndrome. Int J Cardiol. 2015 May 15;194:7–12.
75. Schoenhoff FS, Jungi S, Czerny M, Roost E, Reineke D, Mátyás G, et al. Acute aortic dissection determines the fate of initially untreated aortic segments in Marfan syndrome. Circulation. 2013 Apr 16;127(15):1569–75.
76. Lemaire SA, de La Cruz KI, Coselli JS. The thoracoabdominal aorta in Marfan syndrome. London: Springer London; 2014. p. 423–34.
77. Hiratzka LF, Bakris GL, Beckman JA, Bersin RM, Carr VF, Casey DE, et al. ACCF/AHA/AATS/ACR/ASA/SCA/SCAI/SIR/STS/SVM guidelines for the diagnosis and management of patients with thoracic aortic disease: a report of the American College of Cardiology Foundation/American Heart Association Task Force on Practice Guidelines, American Association for Thoracic Surgery, American College of Radiology, American Stroke Association, Society of Cardiovascular Anesthesiologists, Society for Cardiovascular Angiography and Interventions, Society of Interventional Radiology, Society of Thoracic Surgeons, and Society for Vascular Medicine. Circulation. 2010;121:e266–369.
78. Sheikhzadeh S, De Backer J, Gorgan N, Rybczynski M, Hillebrand M, Schüler H, et al. The main pulmonary artery in adults: a controlled multicenter study with assessment of echocardiographic reference values, and the frequency of dilatation and aneurysm in Marfan syndrome. Orphanet J Rare Dis. 2014 Dec 10;9(1):203.
79. Nollen GJ, van Schijndel KE, Timmermans J, Groenink M, Barentsz JO, van der Wall EE, et al. Pulmonary artery root dilatation in Marfan syndrome: quantitative assessment of an unknown criterion. Heart. 2002 May;87(5):470–1.
80. De Backer J, Loeys B, Devos D, Dietz H, de Sutter J, de Paepe A. A critical analysis of minor cardiovascular criteria in the diagnostic evaluation of patients with Marfan syndrome. Genet Med 2006 Jul;8(7):401–8. Available from: http://eutils.ncbi.nlm.nih.gov/entrez/eutils/elink.fcgi?dbfrom=pubmed&id=16845272&retmode=ref&cmd=prlinks
81. de Backer JF, Devos D, Segers P, Matthys D, François K, Gillebert TC, et al. Primary impairment of left ventricular function in Marfan syndrome☆. Int J Cardiol 2006 Oct 10;112(3):353–8. Available from: http://eutils.ncbi.nlm.nih.gov/entrez/eutils/elink.fcgi?dbfrom=pubmed&id=16316698&retmode=ref&cmd=prlinks
82. Meijboom LJ, Timmermans J, van Tintelen JP, Nollen GJ, De Backer J, van den Berg MP, et al. Evaluation of left ventricular dimensions and function in Marfan's syndrome without significant valvular regurgitation. Am J Cardiol. 2005 Mar 15;95(6):795–7.
83. Campens L, Renard M, Trachet B, Segers P, Muiño Mosquera L, de Sutter J, et al. Intrinsic cardiomyopathy in Marfan syndrome: results from in-vivo and ex-vivo studies of the Fbn1(C1039G/+) model and longitudinal findings in humans. Pediatr Res. 2015 Jun;78(3):256–63.
84. Schaeffer BN, Rybczynski M, Sheikhzadeh S, Akbulak RÖ, Moser J, Jularic M, et al. Heart rate turbulence and deceleration capacity for risk prediction of serious arrhythmic events in Marfan syndrome. Clin Res Cardiol. 2015 Dec;104(12):1054–63.
85. van Dijk N, Boer MC, Mulder BJM, van Montfrans GA, Wieling W. Is fatigue in Marfan syndrome related to orthostatic intolerance? Clin Auton Res. 2008 Aug;18(4):187–93.
86. Maumenee IH. The eye in the Marfan syndrome. Trans Am Ophthalmol Soc. 1981;79:684–733.
87. Dotrelova D, Karel I, Clupkova E. Retinal detachment in Marfan's syndrome. Characteristics and surgical results. Retina. 1997;17(5):390–6.
88. Maumenee IH. The eye in the Marfan syndrome. Birth Defects Orig Artic Ser. 1982;18(6):515–24.
89. Wood JR, Bellamy D, Child AH, Citron KM. Pulmonary disease in patients with Marfan syndrome. Thorax. 1984 Oct;39(10):780–4.
90. Rybczynski M, Koschyk D, Karmeier A, Gessler N, Sheikhzadeh S, Bernhardt AMJ, et al. Frequency of sleep apnea in adults with the Marfan syndrome. Am J Cardiol. 2010 Jun 15;105(12):1836–41. Available from: http://eutils.ncbi.nlm.nih.gov/entrez/eutils/elink.fcgi?dbfrom=pubmed&id=20538140&retmode=ref&cmd=prlinks
91. Kohler M, Pitcher A, Blair E, Risby P, Senn O, Forfar C, et al. The impact of obstructive sleep apnea on aortic disease in Marfan's syndrome. Respiration. 2013;86(1):39–44.
92. Oosterhof T, Groenink M, Hulsmans FJ, Mulder BJ, van der Wall EE, Smit R, et al. Quantitative assessment of dural ectasia as a marker for Marfan syndrome. Radiology. 2001 Aug;220(2):514–8.
93. Villeirs GM, Van Tongerloo AJ, Verstraete KL, Kunnen MF, de Paepe AM. Widening of the spinal canal and dural ectasia in Marfan's syndrome: assessment by CT. Neuroradiology. 1999 Nov;41(11):850–4.
94. Sheikhzadeh S, Brockstaedt L, Habermann CR, Sondermann C, Bannas P, Mir TS, et al. Dural ectasia in Loeys-Dietz syndrome: comprehensive study of 30 patients with a TGFBR1 or TGFBR2 mutation. Clin Genet. 2014 Dec;86(6):545–51.
95. Foran JRH, Pyeritz RE, Dietz HC, Sponseller PD. Characterization of the symptoms associated with dural ectasia in the Marfan patient. Am J Med Genet A. 2005 Apr 1;134A(1):58–65.
96. Bertoli-Avella AM, Gillis E, Morisaki H, Verhagen JMA, de Graaf BM, van de Beek G, et al. Mutations in a TGF-β ligand, TGFB3,

cause syndromic aortic aneurysms and dissections. J Am Coll Cardiol. 2015 Apr 7;65(13):1324–36.
97. Micha D, Guo D-C, Hilhorst-Hofstee Y, van Kooten F, Atmaja D, Overwater E, et al. SMAD2 mutations are associated with arterial aneurysms and dissections. Hum Mutat. 2015 Aug;6:1145–9.
98. Cannaerts E, Kempers M, Maugeri A, Marcelis C, Gardeitchik T, Richer J, et al. Novel pathogenic SMAD2 variants in five families with arterial aneurysm and dissection: further delineation of the phenotype. J Med Genet. 2019 Apr;56(4):220–7.
99. Gupta-Malhotra M, Devereux RB, Dave A, Bell C, Portman R, Milewicz D. Aortic dilatation in children with systemic hypertension. J Am Soc Hypertens. 2014 Jan;9:239–45.
100. Kono AK, Higashi M, Morisaki H, Morisaki T, Tsutsumi Y, Akutsu K, et al. High prevalence of vertebral artery tortuosity of Loeys-Dietz syndrome in comparison with Marfan syndrome. Jpn J Radiol. 2010 May;28(4):273–7.
101. Morris SA, Orbach DB, Geva T, Singh MN, Gauvreau K, Lacro RV. Increased vertebral artery tortuosity index is associated with adverse outcomes in children and young adults with connective tissue disorders. Circulation. 2011 Jul 25;124(4):388–96.
102. Kuechler A, Altmüller J, Nürnberg P, Kotthoff S, Kubisch C, Borck G. Exome sequencing identifies a novel heterozygous TGFB3 mutation in a disorder overlapping with Marfan and Loeys-Dietz syndrome. Mol Cell Probes. 2015 Oct;29(5):330–4.
103. Eckman PM, Hsich E, Rodriguez ER, Gonzalez-Stawinski GV, Moran R, Taylor DO. Impaired systolic function in Loeys-Dietz syndrome: a novel cardiomyopathy? Circ Heart Fail. 2009 Nov;2(6):707–8.
104. Schepers D, Tortora G, Morisaki H, MacCarrick G, Lindsay M, Liang D, et al. A mutation update on the LDS-associated genes TGFB2/3 and SMAD2/3. Hum Mutat. 2018 May;39(5):621–34.
105. van de Laar IMBH, van der Linde D, Oei EHG, Bos PK, Bessems JH, Bierma-Zeinstra SM, et al. Phenotypic spectrum of the SMAD3-related aneurysms-osteoarthritis syndrome. J Med Genet. 2011 Dec 13;49(1):47–57. Available from: http://eutils.ncbi.nlm.nih.gov/entrez/eutils/elink.fcgi?dbfrom=pubmed&id=22167769&retmode=ref&cmd=prlinks
106. Wischmeijer A, Van Laer L, Tortora G, Bolar NA, Van Camp G, Fransen E, et al. Thoracic aortic aneurysm in infancy in aneurysms-osteoarthritis syndrome due to a novel SMAD3 mutation: further delineation of the phenotype. Am J Med Genet A. 2013 Mar 29;161A(5):1028–35.
107. Hilhorst-Hofstee Y, Scholte AJHA, Rijlaarsdam MEB, van Haeringen A, Kroft LJ, Reijnierse M, et al. An unanticipated copy number variant of chromosome 15 disrupting SMAD3 reveals a three-generation family at serious risk for aortic dissection. Clin Genet. 2013 Apr;83(4):337–44.
108. Fitzgerald-Butt SM, Klima J, Kelleher K, Chisolm D, McBride KL. Genetic knowledge and attitudes of parents of children with congenital heart defects. Am J Med Genet A. 2014 Sep;164A(12):3069–75.
109. Martens T, Van Herzeele I, De Ryck F, Renard M, de Paepe A, François K, et al. Multiple aneurysms in a patient with aneurysms-osteoarthritis syndrome. Ann Thorac Surg; 2013 Jan 1;95(1):332–5. Available from: http://eutils.ncbi.nlm.nih.gov/entrez/eutils/elink.fcgi?dbfrom=pubmed&id=23272854&retmode=ref&cmd=prlinks
110. Aubart M, Gobert D, Aubart-Cohen F, Detaint D, Hanna N, d'Indya H, et al. Early-onset osteoarthritis, Charcot-Marie-tooth like neuropathy, autoimmune features, multiple arterial aneurysms and dissections: an unrecognized and life threatening condition. PLoS One. 2014;9(5):e96387.
111. Panesi P, Foffa I, Sabina S, Ait Alì L, Andreassi MG. Novel TGFBR2 and known missense SMAD3 mutations: two case reports of thoracic aortic aneurysms. Ann Thorac Surg. 2015 Jan;99(1):303–5.
112. Berthet E, Hanna N, Giraud C, Soubrier M. A case of rheumatoid arthritis associated with SMAD3 gene mutation: a new clinical entity? J Rheumatol. 2015 Mar;42(3):556.
113. Courtois A, Coppieters W, Bours V, Defraigne JO, Colige A, Sakalihasan N. A novel SMAD3 mutation caused multiple aneurysms in a patient without osteoarthritis symptoms. Eur J Med Genet. 2017 Apr;60(4):228–31.
114. Grahame R, Pyeritz RE. The Marfan syndrome: joint and skin manifestations are prevalent and correlated. Br J Rheumatol. 1995 Feb;34(2):126–31.
115. Law C, Bunyan D, Castle B, Day L, Simpson I, Westwood G, et al. Clinical features in a family with an R460H mutation in transforming growth factor beta receptor 2 gene. J Med Genet. 2006 Dec;43(12):908–16.
116. Frischmeyer-Guerrerio PA, Guerrerio AL, Oswald G, Chichester K, Myers L, Halushka MK, et al. TGFβ receptor mutations impose a strong predisposition for human allergic disease. Sci Transl Med. 2013 Jul 24;5(195):195ra94.
117. Sheikhzadeh S, Sondermann C, Rybczynski M, Habermann CR, Brockstaedt L, Keyser B, et al. Comprehensive analysis of dural ectasia in 150 patients with a causative FBN1 mutation. Clin Genet. 2013 Aug;86(3):238–45.
118. Byers PH, Belmont J, Black J, De Backer J, Frank M, Jeunemaitre X, et al. Diagnosis, natural history, and management in vascular Ehlers-Danlos syndrome. Am J Med Genet C Semin Med Genet. 2017 Mar;175(1):40–7.
119. Bergqvist D, Björck M, Wanhainen A. Treatment of vascular Ehlers-danlos syndrome: a systematic review. Ann Surg. 2013 Aug;258(2):257–61.
120. Watanabe S, Ishimitsu T, Inoue K, Tomizawa T, Noguchi Y, Sugishita Y, et al. Type IV Ehlers-Danlos syndrome associated with mitral valve prolapse: a case report. J Cardiol Suppl. 1988;18:97–105–discussion106.
121. Jaffe AS, Geltman EM, Rodey GE, Uitto J. Mitral valve prolapse: a consistent manifestation of type IV Ehlers-Danlos syndrome. The pathogenetic role of the abnormal production of type III collagen. Circulation. 1981 Jul;64(1):121–5.
122. Dolan AL, Mishra MB, Chambers JB, Grahame R. Clinical and echocardiographic survey of the Ehlers-Danlos syndrome. Br J Rheumatol. 1997 Apr;36(4):459–62.
123. Zilocchi M, Macedo TA, Oderich GS, Vrtiska TJ, Biondetti PR, Stanson AW. Vascular Ehlers-Danlos syndrome: imaging findings. AJR Am J Roentgenol. 2007 Sep;189(3):712–9.
124. Heidbreder AE, Ringelstein EB, Dittrich R, Nabavi D, Metze D, Kuhlenbäumer G. Assessment of skin extensibility and joint hypermobility in patients with spontaneous cervical artery dissection and Ehlers-Danlos syndrome. J Clin Neurosci. 2008 Jun;15(6):650–3.
125. Lind J, Wallenburg HCS. Pregnancy and the Ehlers-Danlos syndrome: a retrospective study in a Dutch population. Acta Obstet Gynecol Scand. 2002 Apr;81(4):293–300.
126. Adès LC, DAVIES R, Haan EA, Holman KJ, Watson KC, Sreetharan D, et al. Aortic dissection, patent ductus arteriosus, iris hypoplasia and brachytelephalangy in a male adolescent. Clin Dysmorphol. 1999 Oct;8(4):269–76.
127. Khan N, Schinzel A, Shuknecht B, Baumann F, Ostergaard JR, Yonekawa Y. Moyamoya angiopathy with dolichoectatic internal carotid arteries, patent ductus arteriosus and pupillary dysfunction: a new genetic syndrome? Eur Neurol. 2004;51(2):72–7.
128. Roulez FMJ, Faes F, Delbeke P, Van Bogaert P, Rodesch G, De Zaeytijd J, et al. Congenital fixed dilated pupils due to ACTA2- multisystemic smooth muscle dysfunction syndrome. J Neuroophthalmol. 2014 Jun;34(2):137–43.
129. Biddinger A, Rocklin M, Coselli J, Milewicz DM. Familial thoracic aortic dilatations and dissections: a case control study. J Vasc Surg. 1997 Mar;25(3):506–11.

130. Regalado ES, Guo D, Prakash S, Bensend TA, Flynn K, Estrera A, et al. Aortic disease presentation and outcome associated with ACTA2 mutations. Circ Cardiovasc Genet. 2015 Mar 10;8(3):457–64.
131. van Kien PK. Mapping of familial thoracic aortic aneurysm/dissection with patent Ductus Arteriosus to 16p12.2-p13.13. Circulation. 2005 Jul 12;112(2):200–6. Available from: http://circ.ahajournals.org/cgi/doi/10.1161/CIRCULATIONAHA.104.506345
132. Regalado ES, Guo D-C, Santos-Cortez RLP, Hostetler E, Bensend TA, Pannu H, et al. Pathogenic FBN1 variants in familial thoracic aortic aneurysms and dissections. Clin Genet. 2015 Dec; 89 (6), 719–23. Available from: http://eutils.ncbi.nlm.nih.gov/entrez/eutils/elink.fcgi?dbfrom=pubmed&id=26621581&retmode=ref&cmd=prlinks
133. Milewicz DM, Chen H, Park ES, Petty EM, Zaghi H, Shashidhar G, et al. Reduced penetrance and variable expressivity of familial thoracic aortic aneurysms/dissections. Am J Cardiol. 1998 Aug 15;82(4):474–9.
134. Freed LA, Levy D, Levine RA, Larson MG, Evans JC, Fuller DL, et al. Prevalence and clinical outcome of mitral-valve prolapse. N Engl J Med. 1999 Jul 1;341(1):1–7.
135. Guo D-C, Gong L, Regalado ES, Santos-Cortez RL, Zhao R, Cai B, et al. MAT2A mutations predispose individuals to thoracic aortic aneurysms. Am J Hum Genet. 2015 Jan 8;96(1):170–7.
136. Dietz HC, Cutting GR, Pyeritz RE, Maslen CL, Sakai LY, Corson GM, et al. Marfan syndrome caused by a recurrent de novo missense mutation in the fibrillin gene. Nature. 1991 Jul 25;352(6333):337–9.
137. Carmignac V, Thevenon J, Adès L, Callewaert B, Julia S, Thauvin-Robinet C, et al. In-frame mutations in exon 1 of SKI cause dominant Shprintzen-Goldberg syndrome. Am J Hum Genet; 2012 Nov 2;91(5):950–7. Available from: http://eutils.ncbi.nlm.nih.gov/entrez/eutils/elink.fcgi?dbfrom=pubmed&id=23103230&retmode=ref&cmd=prlinks
138. Doyle AJ, Doyle JJ, Bessling SL, Maragh S, Lindsay ME, Schepers D, et al. Mutations in the TGF-β repressor SKI cause Shprintzen-Goldberg syndrome with aortic aneurysm. Nat Genet. 2012 Nov;44(11):1249–54.
139. Coucke PJ. Homozygosity mapping of a gene for arterial tortuosity syndrome to chromosome 20q13. J Med Genet. 2003 Oct 1;40(10):747–51.
140. Callewaert B, Renard M, Hucthagowder V, Albrecht B, Hausser I, Blair E, et al. New insights into the pathogenesis of autosomal-dominant cutis laxa with report of five ELN mutations. Hum Mutat. 2011 Apr;32(4):445–55.
141. Renard M, Holm T, Veith R, Callewaert BL, Adès LC, Baspinar O, et al. Altered TGFbeta; signaling and cardiovascular manifestations in patients with autosomal recessive cutis laxa type I caused by fibulin-4 deficiency. Eur J Hum Genet. 2010 Apr 14;18(8):895–901.
142. Rippe M, De Backer J, Kutsche K, Mosquera LM, Schüler H, Rybczynski M, et al. Mitral valve prolapse syndrome and MASS phenotype: stability of aortic dilatation but progression of mitral valve prolapse. Int J Cardiol Heart Vasc. 2016 Mar 1;10:39–46.
143. Coucke PJ, Willaert A, Wessels MW, Callewaert B, Zoppi N, De Backer J, et al. Mutations in the facilitative glucose transporter GLUT10 alter angiogenesis and cause arterial tortuosity syndrome. Nat Genet. 2006 Mar 19;38(4):452–7.
144. Callewaert BL, Willaert A, Kerstjens-Frederikse WS, de Backer J, Devriendt K, Albrecht B, et al. Arterial tortuosity syndrome: clinical and molecular findings in 12 newly identified families. Hum Mutat. 2008 Jan;29(1):150–8.
145. Kosaki K, Takahashi D, Udaka T, Kosaki R, Matsumoto M, Ibe S, et al. Molecular pathology of Shprintzen-Goldberg syndrome. Am J Med Genet A. 2006 Jan 1;140(1):104–8–authorreply109–10.
146. Gupta PA, Wallis DD, Chin TO, Northrup H, Tran-Fadulu VT, Towbin JA, et al. FBN2 mutation associated with manifestations of Marfan syndrome and congenital contractural arachnodactyly. J Med Genet. 2004 May;41(5):e56.
147. Nishimura A, Sakai H, Ikegawa S, Kitoh H, Haga N, Ishikiriyama S, et al. FBN2, FBN1, TGFBR1, and TGFBR2 analyses in congenital contractural arachnodactyly. Am J Med Genet A. 2007 Apr 1;143A(7):694–8.
148. Kruger WD, Wang L, Jhee KH, Singh RH, Elsas LJ. Cystathionine beta-synthase deficiency in Georgia (USA): correlation of clinical and biochemical phenotype with genotype. Hum Mutat. 2003 Dec;22(6):434–41.
149. De Lucca M, Casique L. Characterization of cystathionine beta-synthase gene mutations in homocystinuric Venezuelan patients: identification of one novel mutation in exon 6. Mol Genet Metab. 2004 Mar;81(3):209–15.
150. Shores J, Berger KR, Murphy EA, Pyeritz RE. Progression of aortic dilatation and the benefit of long-term beta-adrenergic blockade in Marfan's syndrome. N Engl J Med. 1994 May 12;330(19):1335–41.
151. Engelfriet P, Mulder B. Is there benefit of beta-blocking agents in the treatment of patients with the Marfan syndrome? Int J Cardiol. 2007 Jan 18;114(3):300–2.
152. Habashi JP, Judge DP, Holm TM, Cohn RD, Loeys BL, Cooper TK, et al. Losartan, an AT1 antagonist, prevents aortic aneurysm in a mouse model of Marfan syndrome. Science. 2006 Apr 7;312(5770):117–21.
153. Chiu H-H, Wu M-H, Wang J-K, Lu C-W, Chiu S-N, Chen C-A, et al. Losartan added to β-blockade therapy for aortic root dilation in Marfan syndrome: a randomized, open-label pilot study. Mayo Clin Proc. 2013 Mar;88(3):271–6.
154. Franken R, Mulder BJM. Aortic disease: Losartan versus atenolol in the Marfan aorta-how to treat? Nat Rev Cardiol. 2015 Jun 16;12(8):447–8.
155. Groenink M, den AW H, Franken R, Radonic T, de Waard V, Timmermans J, et al. Losartan reduces aortic dilatation rate in adults with Marfan syndrome: a randomized controlled trial. Eur Heart J. 2013 Sep 2;34(45):3491–500.
156. Milleron O, Arnoult F, Ropers J, Aegerter P, Detaint D, Delorme G, et al. Marfan Sartan: a randomized, double-blind, placebo-controlled trial. Eur Heart J. 2015 Aug 21;36(32):2160–6.
157. Lacro RV, Dietz HC, Sleeper LA, Yetman AT, Bradley TJ, Colan SD, et al. Atenolol versus Losartan in children and young adults with Marfan's syndrome. N Engl J Med. 2014 Nov 27;371(22):2061–71.
158. Forteza A, Evangelista A, Sánchez V, Teixido-Tura G, Sanz P, Gutiérrez L, et al. Efficacy of losartan vs. atenolol for the prevention of aortic dilation in Marfan syndrome: a randomized clinical trial. Eur Heart J. 2015 Oct 29;37(12):978–85.
159. De Backer J. Marfan and Sartans: time to wake up! Eur Heart J. 2015 Jun 1;36(32):2131–3.
160. Erbel R, Aboyans V, Boileau C, Bossone E, Di Bartolomeo R, Authors/Task Force Members, et al. ESC guidelines on the diagnosis and treatment of aortic diseases. Eur Heart J. 2014;35(41):2873–926.
161. Meijboom LJ, Timmermans J, Zwinderman AH, Engelfriet PM, Mulder BJM. Aortic root growth in men and women with the Marfan's syndrome. Am J Cardiol. 2005 Nov 15;96(10):1441–4.
162. Davies RR, Gallo A, Coady MA, Tellides G, Botta DM, Burke B, et al. Novel measurement of relative aortic size predicts rupture of thoracic aortic aneurysms. Ann Thorac Surg. 2006 Jan;81(1):169–77.
163. Gott VL, Greene PS, Alejo DE, Cameron DE, Naftel DC, Miller DC, et al. Replacement of the aortic root in patients with Marfan's syndrome. N Engl J Med. 1999 Apr 29;340(17):1307–13.

164. David TE, Feindel CM, David CM, Manlhiot C. A quarter of a century of experience with aortic valve-sparing operations. J Thorac Cardiovasc Surg. 2014 Sep;148(3):872–9–discussion879–80.
165. Lederle FA, Freischlag JA, Kyriakides TC, Matsumura JS, Padberg FT, Kohler TR, et al. Long-term comparison of endovascular and open repair of abdominal aortic aneurysm. N Engl J Med. 2012 Nov 22;367(21):1988–97.
166. Preventza O, Mohammed S, Cheong BY, Gonzalez L, Ouzounian M, Livesay JJ, et al. Endovascular therapy in patients with genetically triggered thoracic aortic disease: applications and short- and mid-term outcomes. Eur J Cardiothorac Surg. 2014 Aug;46(2):248–53–discussion 253.
167. Pacini D, Parolari A, Berretta P, Di Bartolomeo R, Alamanni F, Bavaria J. Endovascular treatment for type B dissection in Marfan syndrome: is it worthwhile? Ann Thorac Surg. 2013 Feb;95(2):737–49.
168. Nordon IM, Hinchliffe RJ, Holt PJ, Morgan R, Jahangiri M, Loftus IM, et al. Endovascular management of chronic aortic dissection in patients with Marfan syndrome. J Vasc Surg. 2009 Nov;50(5):987–91.
169. Izgi C, Newsome S, Alpendurada F, Nyktari E, Boutsikou M, Pepper J, Treasure T, Mohiaddin R. External aortic root support to prevent aortic dilatation in patients with Marfan syndrome. J Am Coll Cardiol. 2018;72:1095–105.
170. Meijboom LJ, Groenink M, van der Wall EE, Romkes H, Stoker J, Mulder BJ. Aortic root asymmetry in marfan patients; evaluation by magnetic resonance imaging and comparison with standard echocardiography. Int J Card Imaging. 2000 Jun;16(3):161–8.
171. Nollen GJ. Aortic pressure-area relation in Marfan patients with and without blocking agents: a new non-invasive approach. Heart. 2004 Mar 1;90(3):314–8. https://doi.org/10.1136/hrt.2003.010702.
172. Nishimura RA, Otto CM, Bonow RO, Carabello BA, Erwin JP, Guyton RA, et al. 2014 AHA/ACC guideline for the management of patients with valvular heart disease: a report of the American College of Cardiology/American Heart Association Task Force on practice guidelines. J Am Coll Cardiol. 2014 Jul;148(1):e1–e132.
173. Meijboom LJ, Drenthen W, Pieper PG, Groenink M, van der Post JAM, Timmermans J, et al. Obstetric complications in Marfan syndrome. Int J Cardiol. 2006 Jun 7;110(1):53–9.
174. Rossiter JP, Repke JT, Morales AJ, Murphy EA, Pyeritz RE. A prospective longitudinal evaluation of pregnancy in the Marfan syndrome. Am J Obstet Gynecol. 1995 Nov;173(5):1599–606.
175. Ersbøll AS, Hedegaard M, Sondergaard L, Ersbøll M, Johansen M. Treatment with oral beta-blockers during pregnancy complicated by maternal heart disease increases the risk of fetal growth restriction. BJOG. 2014 Apr;121(5):618–26.
176. Dolan P, Sisko F, Riley E. Anesthetic considerations for Ehlers-Danlos syndrome. Anesthesiology. 1980 Mar;52(3):266–9.
177. Brooke BS, Arnaoutakis G, McDonnell NB, Black JH. Contemporary management of vascular complications associated with Ehlers-Danlos syndrome. J Vasc Surg. 2010 Jan 1;51(1):131–9.
178. Ong K-T, Perdu J, De Backer J, Bozec E, Collignon P, Emmerich J, et al. Effect of celiprolol on prevention of cardiovascular events in vascular Ehlers-Danlos syndrome: a prospective randomised, open, blinded-endpoints trial. Lancet. 2010 Oct 30;376(9751):1476–84.
179. Boodhwani M, Andelfinger G, Leipsic J, Lindsay T, MS MM, Therrien J, et al. Canadian Cardiovascular Society position statement on the management of thoracic aortic disease. Can J Cardiol. 2014;30:577–89.
180. Loeys B, de Backer J, van Acker P, Wettinck K, Pals G, Nuytinck L, et al. Comprehensive molecular screening of the FBN1 gene favors locus homogeneity of classical Marfan syndrome. Hum Mutat. 2004 Aug;24(2):140–6.
181. Proost D, Vandeweyer G, Meester JAN, Salemink S, Kempers M, Ingram C, et al. Performant mutation identification using targeted next generation sequencing of fourteen thoracic aortic aneurysm genes. Hum Mutat. 2015 Apr; 36 (8), 808–814. Available from: http://eutils.ncbi.nlm.nih.gov/entrez/eutils/elink.fcgi?dbfrom=pubmed&id=25907466&retmode=ref&cmd=prlinks
182. Ziganshin BA, Bailey AE, Coons C, Dykas D, Charilaou P, Tanriverdi LH, et al. Routine genetic testing for thoracic aortic aneurysm and dissection in a clinical setting. Ann Thorac Surg. 2015 Nov;100(5):1604–11.
183. Eline Overwater, Luisa Marsili, Marieke J.H. Baars, Annette F. Baas, Irma van de Beek, Eelco Dulfer, et al. Results of next-generation sequencing gene panel diagnostics including copy-number variation analysis in 810 patients suspected of heritable thoracic aortic disorders. Hum Mutat. 2018 Sep; 39(9):1173–1192. https://doi.org/10.1002/humu.23565. Epub 2018 Jul 12.
184. Arslan-Kirchner M, Arbustini E, Boileau C, Charron P, Child AH, Collod-Beroud G, et al. Clinical utility gene card for: hereditary thoracic aortic aneurysm and dissection including next-generation sequencing-based approaches. Eur J Hum Genet. 2015 Oct;28:146–50.
185. Rehm HL, Berg JS, Brooks LD, Bustamante CD, Evans JP, Landrum MJ, et al. ClinGenDOUBLEHYPHENthe clinical genome resource. N Engl J Med. 2015 Jun 4;372(23):2235–42.
186. Corson GM, Chalberg SC, Dietz HC, Charbonneau NL, Sakai LY. Fibrillin binds calcium and is coded by cDNAs that reveal a multidomain structure and alternatively spliced exons at the 5′ end. Genomics. 1993 Aug;17(2):476–84.
187. Biery NJ, Eldadah ZA, Moore CS, Stetten G, Spencer F, Dietz HC. Revised genomic organization of FBN1 and significance for regulated gene expression. Genomics. 1999 Feb 15;56(1):70–7.
188. Sengle G, Sakai LY. The fibrillin microfibril scaffold: a niche for growth factors and mechanosensation? Matrix Biol. 2015 May 7;47:3–12.
189. Hubmacher D, Tiedemann K, Reinhardt DP. Fibrillins: from biogenesis of microfibrils to signaling functions. Curr Top Dev Biol. 2006;75:93–123.
190. Sakai LY, Keene DR, Renard M, De Backer J. FBN1: the disease-causing gene for Marfan syndrome and other genetic disorders. Gene. 2016;591(1):279–91.
191. Judge DP, Biery NJ, Keene DR, Geubtner J, Myers L, Huso DL, et al. Evidence for a critical contribution of haploinsufficiency in the complex pathogenesis of Marfan syndrome. J Clin Investig. 2004 Jul 15;114(2):172–81.
192. Pereira L, Lee SY, Gayraud B, Andrikopoulos K, Shapiro SD, Bunton T, et al. Pathogenetic sequence for aneurysm revealed in mice underexpressing fibrillin-1. Proc Natl Acad Sci U S A. 1999 Mar 30;96(7):3819–23.
193. Bunton TE, Biery NJ, Myers L, Gayraud B, Ramirez F, Dietz HC. Phenotypic alteration of vascular smooth muscle cells precedes elastolysis in a mouse model of Marfan syndrome. Circ Res. 2001 Jan 19;88(1):37–43.
194. Massagué J. The TGF-beta family of growth and differentiation factors. Cell. 1987 May 22;49(4):437–8.
195. Neptune ER, Frischmeyer PA, Arking DE, Myers L, Bunton TE, Gayraud B, et al. Dysregulation of TGF-beta activation contributes to pathogenesis in Marfan syndrome. Nat Genet. 2003 Mar;33(3):407–11.
196. Isogai Z, Ono RN, Ushiro S, Keene DR, Chen Y, Mazzieri R, et al. Latent transforming growth factor beta-binding protein 1 interacts with fibrillin and is a microfibril-associated protein. J Biol Chem. 2003 Jan 24;278(4):2750–7.

197. Dallas SL, Miyazono K, Skerry TM, Mundy GR, Bonewald LF. Dual role for the latent transforming growth factor-beta binding protein in storage of latent TGF-beta in the extracellular matrix and as a structural matrix protein. J Cell Biol. 1995 Oct;131(2):539–49.
198. Saharinen J, Hyytiäinen M, Taipale J, Keski-Oja J. Latent transforming growth factor-beta binding proteins (LTBPs) DOUBLEHYPHENstructural extracellular matrix proteins for targeting TGF-beta action. Cytokine Growth Factor Rev. 1999 Jun;10(2):99–117.
199. Charbonneau NL, Carlson EJ, Tufa S, Sengle G, Manalo EC, Carlberg VM, et al. In vivo studies of mutant fibrillin-1 microfibrils. J Biol Chem. 2010 Aug 6;285(32):24943–55.
200. Dietz H. A healthy tension in translational research. J Clin Invest. 2014 Apr 1;124(4):1425–9.
201. Jeremy RW, Robertson E, Lu Y, Hambly BD. Perturbations of mechanotransduction and aneurysm formation in heritable aortopathies. Int J Cardiol. 2013 Oct 25;169(1):7–16.
202. Humphrey JD, Milewicz DM, Tellides G, Schwartz MA. Cell biology. Dysfunctional mechanosensing in aneurysms. Science. 2014 May 2;344(6183):477–9.
203. Loeys B, Nuytinck L, Delvaux I, De Bie S, de Paepe A. Genotype and phenotype analysis of 171 patients referred for molecular study of the fibrillin-1 gene FBN1 because of suspected Marfan syndrome. Arch Intern Med. 2001 Nov 12;161(20):2447–54.
204. de Backer J, Nollen GJ, Devos D, Pals G, Coucke P, Verstraete K, et al. Variability of aortic stiffness is not associated with the fibrillin 1 genotype in patients with Marfan's syndrome. Heart. 2006 Jul;92(7):977–8.
205. Schrijver I, Liu W, Brenn T, Furthmayr H, Francke U. Cysteine substitutions in epidermal growth factor-like domains of fibrillin-1: distinct effects on biochemical and clinical phenotypes. Am J Hum Genet. 1999 Oct;65(4):1007–20.
206. Schrijver I, Liu W, Odom R, Brenn T, Oefner P, Furthmayr H, et al. Premature termination mutations in FBN1: distinct effects on differential allelic expression and on protein and clinical phenotypes. Am J Hum Genet. 2002 Aug;71(2):223–37.
207. Comeglio P, Evans AL, Brice G, Cooling RJ, Child AH. Identification of FBN1 gene mutations in patients with ectopia lentis and marfanoid habitus. Br J Ophthalmol. 2002 Dec;86(12):1359–62.
208. Faivre L, Collod-Beroud G, Loeys BL, Child A, Binquet C, Gautier E, et al. Effect of mutation type and location on clinical outcome in 1,013 probands with Marfan syndrome or related phenotypes and FBN1 mutations: an international study. Am J Hum Genet. 2007 Sep;81(3):454–66.
209. Comeglio P, Johnson P, Arno G, Brice G, Evans A, Aragon-Martin J, et al. The importance of mutation detection in Marfan syndrome and Marfan-related disorders: report of 193 FBN1 mutations. Hum Mutat. 2007 Sep;28(9):928.
210. Baudhuin LM, Kotzer KE, Lagerstedt SA. Increased frequency of FBN1 truncating and splicing variants in Marfan syndrome patients with aortic events. Genet Med. 2015 Mar;17(3):177–87.
211. Franken R, Groenink M, de Waard V, HMA F, Scholte AJ, van den Berg MP, et al. Genotype impacts survival in Marfan syndrome. Eur Heart J. 2016 Jan 18;37:3285–90.
212. Nijbroek G, Sood S, McIntosh I, Francomano CA, Bull E, Pereira L, et al. Fifteen novel FBN1 mutations causing Marfan syndrome detected by heteroduplex analysis of genomic amplicons. Am J Hum Genet. 1995 Jul;57(1):8–21.
213. Tynan K, Comeau K, Pearson M, Wilgenbus P, Levitt D, Gasner C, et al. Mutation screening of complete fibrillin-1 coding sequence: report of five new mutations, including two in 8-cysteine domains. Hum Mol Genet. 1993 Nov;2(11):1813–21.
214. Dietz HC, McIntosh I, Sakai LY, Corson GM, Chalberg SC, Pyeritz RE, et al. Four novel FBN1 mutations: significance for mutant transcript level and EGF-like domain calcium binding in the pathogenesis of Marfan syndrome. Genomics. 1993 Aug;17(2):468–75.
215. Faivre L, Collod-Beroud G, Callewaert B, Child A, Binquet C, Gautier E, et al. Clinical and mutation-type analysis from an international series of 198 probands with a pathogenic FBN1 exons 24-32 mutation. Eur J Hum Genet. 2009 Apr;17(4):491–501.
216. Morissette R, Schoenhoff F, Xu Z, Shilane DA, Griswold BF, Chen W, et al. Transforming growth factor-β (TGF-β) and inflammation in vascular (Type IV) Ehlers Danlos syndrome. Circ Cardiovasc Genet. 2014 Jan 6;7(1):80–8. https://doi.org/10.1161/CIRCGENETICS.113.000280.
217. Frank M, Albuisson J, Ranque B, Golmard L, Mazzella J-M, Bal-Theoleyre L, et al. The type of variants at the COL3A1 gene associates with the phenotype and severity of vascular Ehlers-Danlos syndrome. Eur J Hum Genet. 2015 Mar 11;23(12):1657–64.
218. Pepin MG, Schwarze U, Rice KM, Liu M, Leistritz D, Byers PH. Survival is affected by mutation type and molecular mechanism in vascular Ehlers-Danlos syndrome (EDS type IV). Genet Med. 2014 Dec;16(12):881–8.
219. Tromp G, Kuivaniemi H, Stolle C, Pope FM, Prockop DJ. Single base mutation in the type III procollagen gene that converts the codon for glycine 883 to aspartate in a mild variant of Ehlers-Danlos syndrome IV. J Biol Chem. 1989 Nov 15;264(32):19313–7.
220. Rodriguez-Vita J, Angiotensin II. Activates the Smad pathway in vascular smooth muscle cells by a transforming growth factor- -independent mechanism. Circulation. 2005 May 2;111(19):2509–17.
221. Guo X, Chen S-Y. Transforming growth factor-β and smooth muscle differentiation. World J Biol Chem. 2012 Mar 26;3(3):41–52.
222. Wynne BM, Chiao C-W, Webb RC. Vascular smooth muscle cell signaling mechanisms for contraction to Angiotensin II and Endothelin-1. J Am Soc Hypertens. 2009 Mar;3(2):84–95.
223. Inamoto S, Kwartler CS, Lafont AL, Liang YY, Fadulu VT, Duraisamy S, et al. TGFBR2 mutations alter smooth muscle cell phenotype and predispose to thoracic aortic aneurysms and dissections. Cardiovasc Res. 2010 Dec 1;88(3):520–9.
224. Singh P, Carraher C, Schwarzbauer JE. Assembly of fibronectin extracellular matrix. Annu Rev Cell Dev Biol. 2010;26:397–419.
225. Sabatier L, Chen D, Fagotto-Kaufmann C, Hubmacher D, McKee MD, Annis DS, et al. Fibrillin assembly requires fibronectin. Mol Biol Cell. 2009 Feb;20(3):846–58.
226. Pepin MG, Murray ML, Byers PH. Vascular Ehlers-Danlos syndrome. In: Adam MP, Ardinger HH, Pagon RA, Wallace SE, LJH B, Stephens K, Amemiya A, editors. Gene reviews. Seattle: University of Washington; 1999. www.ncbi.nlm.nih.gov–books–NBK1494.
227. Verhagen JMA, Kempers M, Cozijnsen L, Bouma BJ, Duijnhouwer AL, Post JG, et al. Expert consensus recommendations on the cardiogenetic care for patients with thoracic aortic disease and their first-degree relatives. Int J Cardiol. 2018 May 1;258:243–8.
228. Schievink WI, Schaid DJ, Rogers HM, Piepgras DG, Michels VV. On the inheritance of intracranial aneurysms. Stroke. 1994 Oct;25(10):2028–37.

Bicuspid Aortic Valve

20

Aline Verstraeten, Jolien Roos-Hesselink, and Bart Loeys

Introduction

Cardiac valves act as one-way doors, ensuring blood to flow in a single direction through the heart. The heart's left ventricle is separated from the aorta by the aortic valve, a tricuspid valve which normally consists of three crescent-shaped leaflets, named after their orientation relative to the left and right coronary artery: the left coronary cusp (LCC), the right coronary cusp (RCC), and the non-coronary cusp (NCC). About 500 years ago, Leonardo da Vinci first described individuals with an aortic valve with only two, unequally sized leaflets, which is termed a bicuspid aortic valve (BAV) [1]. With a prevalence of 0.5–2% in the general population, BAV is considered the most common congenital cardiac malformation. Considerably more men are affected than women [1, 2], and significant familial clustering (~47–89% heritability) has been observed [2, 3]. Although being intrinsically asymptomatic, BAV associates with severe cardiovascular complications. In earlier years, these manifestations accounted for a higher mortality and morbidity than all other congenital heart defects combined [4]. Nowadays, significant advances in perioperative management have succeeded in roughly equaling the survival rates between BAV individuals without significant valvular complications and tricuspid aortic valve (TAV) individuals [5, 6]. Further improvement of the management of the comorbidities of BAV and development of accurate biomarkers are still necessary though. Numerous investigative efforts into the condition's pathomechanisms have been instigated, which although insightful have increasingly exposed knowledge gaps and, hence, areas where further research is warranted. In this chapter, a comprehensive overview on the clinical and the so far unraveled molecular characteristics of BAV will be provided.

A. Verstraeten (✉)
Center of Medical Genetics, Faculty of Medicine and Health Sciences, University of Antwerp and Antwerp University Hospital, Antwerp, Belgium
e-mail: Aline.verstraeten@uantwerpen.be

J. Roos-Hesselink
Department of Cardiology, Erasmus Medical Centre, Rotterdam, The Netherlands
e-mail: j.roos@erasmusmc.nl

B. Loeys
Center of Medical Genetics, Faculty of Medicine and Health Sciences, University of Antwerp and Antwerp University Hospital, Antwerp, Belgium

Department of Human Genetics, Radboud University Nijmegen Medical Center, Nijmegen, The Netherlands
e-mail: Bart.loeys@uantwerpen.be

Pathophysiology

BAV is believed to result from abnormal embryological fusion of two adjacent cusps or abnormal septation of a primordial cusp. Pertaining to the orientation of the fused cusps, multiple classification systems have been put forward to accurately discriminate between different morphological BAV patterns. The Sievers classification is, by far, the most commonly used one [7]. It takes into account the number of raphes (none, one, or two, i.e., thin ridges of tissue located at the valvular regions where undeveloped cusps form a malformed commissure) and the spatial position of the fused cusps. Most patients have a BAV with one raphe (88%), either stemming from fusion of the RCC and LCC (R-L, 71%) or the RCC and NCC (R-N, 14%) (Fig. 20.1) [7]. Animal studies on their etiology have suggested that the R-N subtype results from defective epithelial-to-mesenchymal transformation (EMT) in the outflow tract (OFT) during aortic cushion formation, whereas the R-L subtype is caused by defective OFT septation due to abnormal activity of neural crest cells [8].

Clinical Presentation

The clinical presentation of BAV is exceedingly heterogeneous. While most BAV patients remain asymptomatic, approximately one third of patients develop cardiovascular

H. F. Baars et al. (eds.), *Clinical Cardiogenetics*, https://doi.org/10.1007/978-3-030-45457-9_20

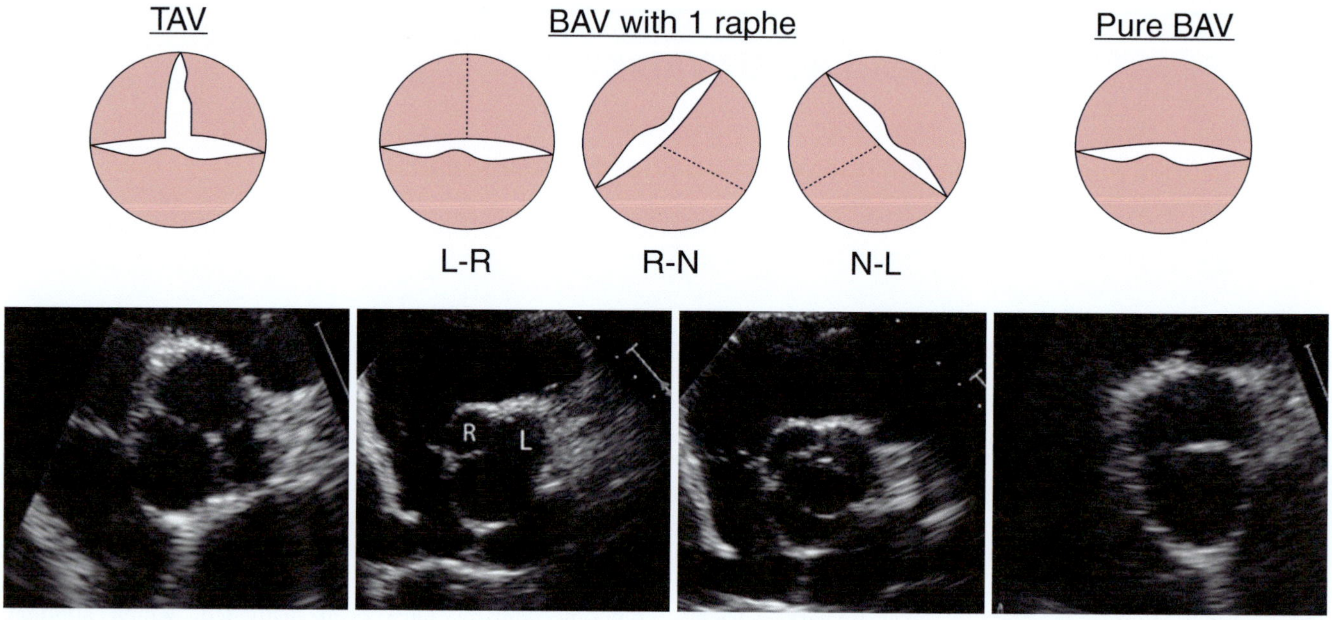

Fig. 20.1 Illustrations and transthoracic echocardiographies of tricuspid and bicuspid aortic valves

complications due to the BAV itself or associated anomalies [4]. Aortic coarctation (±10%) as well as aneurysms (≤50% in BAV patients with normal valve function) and dissections of the distal ascending aorta are considered the most frequent associated lesions, but also ventricular septal defect (VSD), atrial septal defect (ASD), and patent ductus arteriosus are more commonly observed in BAV patients or their relatives [5, 9, 10]. Obviously, auxiliary valve dysfunction results from valve tightening (aortic valve stenosis (AS)), leakiness (aortic regurgitation (AR)), or infective endocarditis. BAV and its associated cardiovascular anomalies can present at any age, from prenatal stages to adulthood. About one half of the patients that undergo aortic valve surgery before age 70 have BAV. Over the past couple of years, a handful of studies suggested associations between the morphological patterns of BAV and the occurrence of valvular complications. Based on a large international multicenter registry comprising more than 2100 BAV patients, the presence of a raphe was found to significantly increase the risk for both AS and AR [11, 12]. Zooming in to patients with a single raphe, those with the R-N fusion subtype were more likely to suffer from AS compared to the others, whereas no difference was observed as regards AR frequencies [12, 13]. The findings of this large-scale study are contradicting prior studies though, warranting replication [14, 15]. Besides valve morphology, gender was also reported to impact on the prevalence of valvular complications in BAV patients, with males being described to be more susceptible to AR and females to AS [6, 12, 16–18]. Also here, further proof is necessary.

Of all established BAV-related complications, thoracic aortic aneurysm (TAA) and particularly the resulting dissections when they are left untreated pose the most serious threat. The R-L fusion subtype comes with the highest TAA risk [12, 18]. In clinical series and autopsy reports of patients with aortic dissection, BAV is reported in 4–9% of the patients [19]. Among the young aortic dissection patients (<40 years), 9–28% of the cases present with BAV. Overall, it is believed that BAV patients have an eight- to ninefold increased risk of deadly dissections compared to TAV individuals, occurring at considerably younger ages [9, 20]. As TAA generally remain unnoticed, careful cardiovascular monitoring of BAV patients is mandatory to prevent sudden cardiac death (SCD) because of aortic dissections or ruptures.

Clinical Diagnosis

Diagnosing BAV

Presently, BAV is being diagnosed at all ages, in very discrete clinical settings, and often even accidentally. Early detection, however, is critical to enable timely surveillance and recognition of the condition's concomitant cardiovascular complications. Based on auscultation and/or an individual's minor complaints (e.g., fatigue, dyspnea, palpitation) alone, BAV cannot reliably be diagnosed [4]. Nonetheless, perception of a mid-systolic ejection click at the apex frequently (in 60–70% of the BAV cases) prompts clinicians to thoroughly inspect valve morphology through alternative, more rigorous techniques [21]. Echocardiography serves already more than 40 years as the first-line test because of its high accuracy and availability at relatively low cost [22]. Whereas systolic long-axis views showing an eccentric leaflet closure plane and leaflet doming hint toward BAV, short-axis views are essential to firmly determine the number of valve leaflets, the fusion subtype, and the presence of a raphe (Fig. 20.1) [23]. In recent years, particularly transesophageal echocardiography (TEE) has proven accurate, reaching sensitivities and specificities up to, respectively, 92% and 96% [24, 25]. Although TEE undeniably outperforms standard transthoracic echocardiography (TTE), it is invasive and may require sedation [26]. Hence, when improved diagnostic precision is warranted, the use of three-dimensional TTE is commonly preferred over TEE.

In patients with moderate-to-severe stenosis and/or calcification of the aortic valve, echocardiography-based differentiation between TAV and BAV is sometimes difficult (~70% accuracy) [21]. In such instances, cardiovascular magnetic resonance (CMR) imaging has been reported to be more sensitive, yet less specific, than echocardiography (>90% accuracy) [21, 27, 28].

Diagnosing BAV-Related Cardiovascular Manifestations

Apart from evaluating their valve morphology, it is warranted to check presumed BAV patients for the presence of TAA as well as AS, AR, ASD, VSD, and coarctation. Although careful echocardiographic studies usually allow to assess pathophysiological aortic root or aorta ascendens dimensions (>40 mm) (Fig. 20.2) [21, 29], computed tomography (CT) and CMR provide a (more) reliable impression of the full spectrum of BAV's associated complications. This has urged the European Society of Cardiology (ESC), the European and American Associations for Thoracic Surgery (EACTS/AATS), and the American College of Cardiology/American Heart Association (ACC/AHA) to recommend them as complementary diagnostic tools [30–33]. Owing to the recent improvements in CT with respect to radiation exposure, it is often the imaging method of choice. In children, however, CMR might still be preferred over CT.

Differential Diagnosis

Several reports on incidental BAV recognition in clinically and pathogenetically diverse disease entities exist, e.g., in chr22q11.2 deletion syndrome [34], familial left ventricular noncompaction (*MYH7*) [35], non-syndromic TAA (*ACTA2*) [36], Joubert syndrome (a case with an unknown genetic defect) [37], and joint dislocation associated with congenital heart disease (*B3GAT3*) [38]. Whether BAV truly belongs to the phenotypic spectrum of these disorders is yet surrounded by uncertainty. More established is the markedly increased prevalence of BAV in Loeys-Dietz syndrome and Turner syndrome. Whereas the majority of the underlying genetic disease causes of these syndromes have been identified, the precise mechanisms with respect to increased BAV susceptibility in these patients remain largely elusive.

Molecular Diagnosis

Molecular Genetics

BAV may occur both sporadically and familially, but its relatively high heritability (47–89%) indicates that disease determination is largely genetic [2, 3]. In rare extended families, an autosomal dominant inheritance pattern with reduced penetrance and variable expressivity has been observed [39,

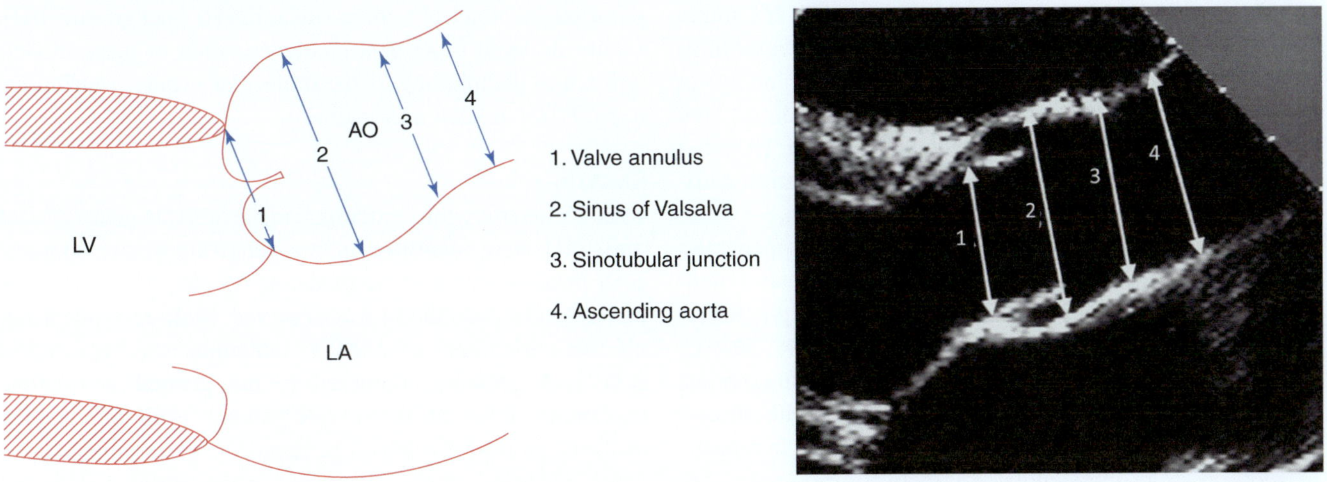

Fig. 20.2 Where to measure aortic dimensions in BAV patients by means of transthoracic echocardiography. Abbreviations – *LV* left ventricle, *LA* left atrium, *Ao* aorta

40]. Also high genetic heterogeneity has been established, further complicating the etiology of BAV [41].

Historically aberrant post-valvular hemodynamics was thought to be the sole trigger for TAA development in BAV patients. Over the last decade, however, increasing evidence for the existence of common genetic defects causing BAV and TAA has emerged [42]. Arguments in favor of this hypothesis include identification of several pedigrees in which BAV and TAA either co-occur or manifest as a single disease entity [43], progression of aneurysm formation after valve replacement [1], and shared embryonic origin of the aortic valve as well as the ascending aorta [44]. Most likely, the etiology of BAV/TAA is complex in nature, with genetic predisposing factors working in combination with abnormal flow patterns [45].

Pertaining to genetics, BAV likely is a consequence of mutations in diverse genes encoding transcription factors, extracellular matrix components, or proteins acting in signaling pathways that regulate cell proliferation, differentiation, adhesion, or apoptosis [46]. The high clinical and genetic heterogeneity of BAV and its accompanying complications, however, have significantly burdened gene identification. As an example, family-based linkage studies have successfully pinpointed BAV loci (chr18q, 5q, and 13q) almost 10 years ago [46]. Nonetheless, the major underlying BAV culprits have still not been identified. Even the recent advent of next-generation sequencing did not (yet) prominently move the BAV genetics field forward. In the following sections, we report on the genetic breakthroughs so far.

BAV Genes in Humans

NOTCH1

To date, *NOTCH1* (OMIM *190198) is considered the only firmly established BAV gene. In 2005, dominantly inherited loss-of-function mutations were first described in two unrelated BAV families suffering from early-onset aortic valve calcification [47]. Meanwhile, additional *NOTCH1* mutations (i.e., missense, splice site, nonsense, and frameshift) have been identified in up to 13% of the familial and 4% of the sporadic BAV, AS, or BAV/AS cases [48]. Reduced penetrance (~16%) has been documented. Although TAA has repeatedly been reported in a fraction of the mutation carriers, *NOTCH1* mutations are not considered as a major cause of non-calcified, non-stenotic BAV with highly penetrant TAA [49]. Occasionally, *NOTCH1* mutations cause non-BAV/AS left-sided cardiovascular pathologies, e.g., (BAV/) coarctation and hypoplastic left heart syndrome [48, 50, 51].

NOTCH1 encodes a 300 kDa single-pass transmembrane receptor consisting of an extracellular domain with 36 epidermal growth factor (EGF)-like and 3 NOTCH/Lin repeats, in addition to an intracellular transactivating domain containing 6 ankyrin repeats. Upon binding of its ligands (i.e., DLL1, DLL3, DLL4, JAG1, and JAG2), NOTCH1 gets cleaved by ADAM metalloproteases and converts into a transcriptional coactivator [52]. Influencing embryonic cell fate decisions, proper NOTCH signaling is crucial for multiple developmental processes, including cardiovascular development [53, 54]. Experimental evidence increasingly converges on abnormal endothelial-to-mesenchymal transition (EMT) as the key culprit for aortic valve malformations in *NOTCH1* mutation carriers. Constitutional Notch1-null mice die early due to severe cardiac defects attributed to abnormal EMT [55]. Furthermore, in aortic endothelial cells of *NOTCH1* mutation carriers, ligand-to-NOTCH binding cannot activate EMT [56]. Excessive mesenchyme proliferation has also been observed in cardiac-specific *Notch1* mutant mice that present with valve dysmorphology (e.g., BAV) [57]. It has been suggested that whereas Dll4-Notch1 signaling mediates EMT, Jag1-Notch1 signaling restricts post-EMT valve mesenchyme proliferation. Interestingly, besides the single mechanisms as such, also crosstalk between both signaling cascades might be affected in *NOTCH1*-related congenital heart disease. Further investigation with respect to these assumptions, however, is warranted.

Scientists have also succeeded in shedding light on the molecular mechanisms underlying aortic valve calcification in *NOTCH1* mutation carriers. Under normal physiological circumstances, NOTCH1 suppresses valve calcification by inducing the expression of *HEY1/2*. In turn, they act through BMP2 to suppress activation of Runx2, a transcriptional activator of osteoblast development [58–62]. Obviously, loss of NOTCH1 disables its protective capacity relating to vascular/valvular calcification, which fits the pathological hallmarks of *NOTCH1* patients.

TAA-related phenotypes have been demonstrated in only recently developed transgenic *NOTCH1* cell and animal models. *NOTCH1*$^{-/-}$-induced pluripotent stem cells showed impaired differentiation to mature smooth muscle cells [63], whereas aortic root dilatation in the absence of BAV was reported in Notch1$^{+/-}$ mice on a 129S6 background [64]. Future in-depth functional characterization of these models will aid in deciphering of the molecular events contributing to *NOTCH1*-related aortopathy.

SMAD6

In 2012, heterozygous mutations in the *SMAD6* gene (OMIM *602931) were identified in two relatively young sporadic BAV patients with mild-to-moderate AS [65]. In one of these patients, also coarctation was observed. More recently, a significant enrichment of *SMAD6* mutations was reported in BAV/TAA patients compared to the general population, explaining 2.5% of BAV/TAA patients [66]. Segregation analysis confirmed reduced penetrance and variable expressivity. *SMAD6* is highly expressed in the cardiac valves and OFT of the human embryonic heart. Its encoded protein consists of two large domains, MH1 and MH2. Whereas the

MH1 domain serves as a DNA-binding module, the MH2 domain interacts with bone morphogenetic protein (BMP) type I receptors to inhibit BMP signaling [67]. A loss-of-function mechanism is suspected, with most of the BAV/TAA- and BAV/AS-causing mutations either being predicted to lead to haplo-insufficiency or affecting these functionally crucial MH protein domains. For the two *SMAD6* missense mutations described in 2012, deficient inhibition of BMPR1A-mediated signaling when compared to wild type has been shown, providing further evidence that *SMAD6* mutations cause BAV through a loss-of-function mechanism [65]. Constitutive loss of murine Smad6 results in incompletely penetrant embryonic and postnatal lethality, likely due to embryonic vessel hemorrhage because of endothelial cell-cell junction destabilization [68, 69]. In surviving animals, thickening of the cardiac valves and OFT septation defects have been observed. Of note, BMP signaling has been documented to cross talk with NOTCH as well as canonical and non-canonical TGF-β signaling, highlighting the emergence of convergent pathomechanisms for BAV [70].

GATA Transcription Factors

GATA4, *GATA5*, and *GATA6* encode transcription factors with a key role in cardiovascular development.

Rare *GATA4* mutations (OMIM ∗600576) have mostly been found in patients with ASD and VSD rather than BAV [71, 72]. However, a recent BAV genome-wide association study pinpointed common protein-coding and regulatory genetic variability in *GATA4* as important disease contributor [73]. Subsequent disruption of *GATA4* in human-induced pluripotent stem cell-derived endothelial cells revealed significantly impaired EMT, a critical process for aortic valve formation. In mice, Gata4 has previously been shown to have a key role in heart formation and endocardial cushion development [74–76]. Gata4$^{-/-}$ mice are embryonically lethal and lack a primitive heart tube [75].

The search for rare *GATA5* sequence variants in humans with BAV was instigated by the discovery of hypoplastic hearts and partially penetrant R-N BAV (~25%) in endocardial cell-specific Gata5$^{-/-}$ mice [77]. Several rare heterozygous mutations in *GATA5* (OMIM ∗611496) have been described in BAV patients [78–81]. No prominent clustering in specific protein domains was observed, yet nearly all mutations were shown to drastically reduce the protein's transcriptional potency. Comparable *GATA5* mutations have also been identified in other strikingly dissimilar cardiovascular disorders: isolated VSD [82], dilated cardiomyopathy [83], lone atrial fibrillation [84], and tetralogy of Fallot [85]. The GATA5 zinc finger transcription factor is exclusively expressed in the endocardial cells and cushions of both the atrioventricular canal and the OFT [86]. In embryonic mice, loss of Gata5 reduces Jag1 expression while increasing Rbpj-κ expression, respectively, a ligand and repressor of Notch, cumulatively resulting in ~20–30% downregulation of the Notch signaling pathway [77]. In contrast to what has been observed in Notch1 knockout mice, EMT was not altered. This might be explained by (partial) compensation for loss of Gata5 by closely related cardiac Gata transcription factors [77]. Besides Notch-related genes, also *Nos3* and *Tbx20* were suggested to be downstream targets of Gata5. Interestingly, mutations in *TBX20* have been linked with valve and septal defects in humans [87], including BAV (unpublished data), and Nos3$^{-/-}$ mice display partially penetrant R-N BAV (see Section "BAV in Animal Models") [88].

GATA6 is closely related to *GATA4* and *GATA5* but has a somewhat different expression pattern. Besides in the fetal heart, it is also highly expressed in the embryonic pancreas. In concordance with this profile, de novo *GATA6* (OMIM ∗601656) mutations have been identified in patients with pancreatic agenesis and, in the majority of the cases (92%), congenital heart defects, including ASD, VSD, tetralogy of Fallot, patent ductus arteriosus, or double outlet right ventricle [89]. Although one of the parents of a patient with a *GATA6*-related ASD was found to have BAV [90] and partially BAV has been observed in Gata6$^{+/-}$ mice [91], the evidence for a role of heterozygous *GATA6* mutations in humans with BAV is limited. Only one rare *GATA6* BAV-causing mutation (p.E386∗) has been reported so far [92]. In addition, common *GATA6* variants reaching nominal significance for an association with BAV have recently been described, but none of them survived multiple testing correction [93]. While constitutive Gata6$^{-/-}$ mice are embryonically lethal, myocyte-, smooth muscle-, or neural crest cell-specific loss leads to cardiac defects such as VSD, interrupted aortic arch, persistent truncus arteriosus, and hypertrophy [94, 95]. No gross anomalies were reported in Gata6$^{+/-}$ mice apart from BAV, which was suggested to (at least partially) result from abnormal valve remodeling due to altered extracellular matrix degradation and cell apoptosis [93].

Clearly, pronounced variability in the phenotypes attributed to loss-of-function mutations in the cardiac GATA transcription factors has been observed, both in humans and mice. This remains to be explained, but one likely hypothesis states that other genetic determinants and/or environmental risk factors influence an individual's ultimate phenotypic outcome.

ROBO4

Based on exome sequencing in a large family with BAV/TAA, a splice site mutation in *ROBO4* was found to segregate with BAV and/or TAA [96]. Subsequent resequencing of *ROBO4* in a large cohort of 441 patients identified enrichment for rare variants in BAV/TAA probands compared to controls. Targeted silencing of *ROBO4* or expression of mutant *ROBO4* in endothelial cell lines imposes relevant functional deficits, including impaired barrier function and a synthetic cell repertoire highly suggestive of increased EMT. Concordant findings are observed in patients and animal models (zebrafish and mouse) with BAV/TAA-associated phenotypes and ROBO4 deficiency. These data highlight the role of dysfunctional endothelial cell biology in the etiology of BAV and/or TAA.

Occasional Findings in NKX2.5 and MATR3

NKX2.5 has been considered a plausible candidate gene for BAV because of multiple reasons: it encodes an important transcription regulator involved in cardiac morphogenesis, BAV has been reported in 11% of the Nkx2.5$^{+/-}$ mice [97], and finally, the human *NKX2.5* gene maps to chr5q34, a linked but yet unexplained locus for BAV. Whereas more than 50 mutations spread over the various functional domains of NKX2.5 (OMIM ∗600584) have been identified in patients with ASD, VSD, hypoplastic left heart syndrome, or tetralogy of Fallot [98], only 2 have been reported in BAV patients. A heterozygous missense mutation (p.Arg25Cys) that had previously been identified in a non-BAV individual with cardiac disease was found in a Down syndrome patient with aneurysm of the membranous septum, aortic coarctation, and BAV [99]. The other mutation (p.Lys192∗) segregated in a three-generational autosomal dominant BAV family [100]. Functional analyses of the latter genetic defect revealed almost complete depletion of transcriptional activity compared to wild-type NKX2.5 as well as loss of the synergistic transcriptional activation of NKX2.5 and GATA5, supporting variant pathogenicity. Yet, owing to the very few *NKX2.5* mutations that have been reported in BAV patients to date, *NKX2.5* is currently not unambiguously recognized as a human BAV gene.

A direct relationship between genetic variability in *MATR3* and BAV development was put forward with the identification of a de novo translocation disrupting the 5' UTR of *AHDC1* and the 3′ UTR of *MATR3* (OMIM ∗164015) in an individual with BAV, coarctation of the aorta, and patent ductus arteriosus in addition to pervasive developmental delay [101]. Whereas *AHDC1* loss of function most probably accounts for the observed developmental impairment [102], subtle perturbations in the level and/or function of the nuclear matrix protein MATR3 have been proposed to explain the cardiovascular manifestations [101]. Arguments in favor for this assumption include strong expression of *Matr3* in the developing mouse heart and the presence of BAV in 15% of heterozygous Matr3 3′ truncated transgenic mice. Missense *MATR3* mutations in humans, however, cause a slowly progressive form of amyotrophic lateral sclerosis, a devastating neuromuscular disorder [103]. Taken together, more supportive evidence is needed, e.g., through the identification of additional BAV patients with *MATR3* mutations, to truly establish an association between BAV and genetic variability in *MATR3*.

BAV in Syndromic Aortopathy

Although some studies have suggested that BAV presents in up to 5% of the MFS cases [104], this finding has not been observed in large observational MFS studies. With MFS being caused by mutations in fibrillin-1 encoded by the *FBN1* gene (OMIM ∗134797), resulting in dysregulation of the TGF-β signaling pathway and impaired extracellular matrix integrity [105, 106], some studies aimed at unraveling the link between *FBN1* and BAV, thus far with inconclusive results. On one hand, decreased fibrillin-1 levels have been observed in the aorta and pulmonary artery of patients with BAV [107], and rare BAV/TAA patients (in whom a clinical MFS diagnosis was excluded) with *FBN1* missense mutations have been reported [108]. The latter *FBN1* missense mutations seem rather mild variants with few other MFS outward features, but in association with a BAV they might be sufficient to cause aortic aneurysm. On the other hand, a significant association between SNPs in or spanning the *FBN1* gene and BAV could not be established [109, 110], whereas genetic *FBN1* variability did associate with increased TAA risk [110]. Fewer studies have investigated the link between BAV and Loeys-Dietz syndrome, a connective tissue disorder that clinically resembles MFS but presents with additional features such as hypertelorism, craniosynostosis, bifid uvula, cleft palate, and arterial tortuosity. The incidence of BAV in Loeys-Dietz patients exceeds that seen in the general population by five times [111]. To date, mutations in six genes (i.e., *TGFBR1*, *TGFBR2*, *SMAD2*, *SMAD3*, *TGFB2*, and *TGFB3*) causing Loeys-Dietz syndrome have been reported, all resulting in a pathological increase in TGF-β signaling [106]. Mutation analysis of *TGFBR1* and *TGFBR2* in BAV cohorts only yielded a single hit (p.Val387Met) of unknown significance [50, 112, 113]. *SMAD2*, *SMAD3*, *TGFB2*, and *TGFB3* have not yet systematically been screened in BAV cohorts as far as we know, but LDS patients with mutations in those genes occasionally present BAV.

BAV (±30%), as well as TAA and aortic coarctation, is remarkably frequent in Turner syndrome, which is caused by either partial or complete absence of one X-chromosome [114]. Apart from the aforementioned cardiovascular defects, affected females generally present with a webbed neck, low-set ears, short stature, diabetes, and low thyroid hormone levels. It is expected that the complex phenotype of Turner syndrome results from loss of function of multiple X-linked genes, including at least one yet to be identified gene that explains the cardiovascular manifestations [115]. A remarkably higher prevalence of BAV in subjects missing only the short arm of the X-chromosome (Xp) has been observed, suggesting Xp location of such gene(s) [116]. Of note, existence of an X-linked BAV gene might, at least partially, explain the prominent male predominance of BAV.

BAV in Animal Models

Besides the above described ones, several more mouse genes have been linked to partially penetrant BAV in mouse knockout models. Additionally, concurrent targeting of multiple genes belonging to the Robo-Slit signaling pathway was shown to cause BAV as well.

The $Nos3^{-/-}$ mouse was one of the first discovered BAV animal models [88]. *Nos3* is highly expressed in the endothelial cells of the aortic valve. It encodes endothelial nitric oxide synthase (eNOS), which is a downstream target of Gata5 and Notch1 [77, 117]. Approximately 27% of the eNos knockout mice develop BAV [118], possibly due to abnormal distribution of neural crest and second heart field cells in the parietal OFT cushion [119]. Backcrossing $Notch1^{+/-}$ into a Nos3-null background yielded a significantly higher penetrance of BAV (~73%), further underlining genetic interaction between the eNos and Notch1 signaling pathways [118]. Interestingly, adult compound $Nos3^{-/-}$;$Notch1^{+/-}$ mice have also been found to develop dilation of the aortic sinus, independent of BAV-related hemodynamic disturbances [120]. Consistent with the mouse findings, decreased protein expression of eNOS was observed in aortic endothelial cells of patients with BAV [121]. Moreover, in BAV patients, a significant inverse correlation between eNOS expression and aortic diameters was observed [121]. Nevertheless, no BAV-causing *NOS3* mutations have been identified so far in humans.

BAV also frequently (~78%) presents in mice lacking *Alk2* in the endocardial cushion mesenchyme [122], though not in neural crest-specific knockouts [123], highlighting a cell autonomous origin of *Alk2*-related BAV development. *Alk2* encodes the activin receptor type I (AcvrI), which has a key role in the BMP signaling pathway. To be exact, AcvrI activation has been shown to stimulate EMT in the aortic valve cushions [124]. In humans, a gain-of-function *ALK2* mutation causes a very rare connective tissue disorder characterized by progressive ectopic ossification of skeletal muscles, fascia, tendons, and ligaments [125]. BAV has not been reported in these patients.

Mice depleted for *Hoxa1*, coding for another essential cardiovascular transcription factor, show a variety of heart defects, including partially penetrant BAV (25%) [126]. During early embryogenesis, *Hoxa1* is expressed in precursors of the cardiac neural crest cells, where it acts upstream of genes driving neural crest specification and maturation [126]. In humans, recessive *HOXA1* mutations cause a complex phenotype characterized by horizontal gaze abnormalities, deafness, facial weakness, hypoventilation, malformations of the internal carotid arteries and OFT, mental retardation, and autism [127]. BAV did not present in *HOXA1* cases, nor have *HOXA1* mutations been observed in BAV patients.

BAV has been observed in 27% of mice completely lacking expression of Krox20 [128]. Neural crest- or endothelium-specific Krox20 deletion, however, only leads to BAV in 10% of animals. This suggests that the aortic valve phenotype attributed to depletion of endothelial or neural crest Krox20 can partially be compensated by other neighboring Krox20-expressing cells. *Krox20* encodes a zinc finger transcription factor that is expressed in the semilunar and atrioventricular valve primordia and drives *Col1a1* and *Col3a1* expression during valve development [129, 130]. Mutations in the human orthologue of *Krox20*, i.e., *EGR2*, cause peripheral neuropathies [131]. BAV has not been documented in any of the *EGR2* mutation carriers.

Mouse embryos lacking endocardial Brg1 show thickened cardiac valves that frequently (~35%) are bicuspid [132]. Brg1 almost entirely makes up the core ATPase subunit of the Brg1-associated factor chromatin remodeling complex, which facilitates activation and repression of genes through ATP-dependent alteration of the chromatin structure. In the cardiovascular system, Brg1 has particularly been shown to be pivotal in regulating proliferation, differentiation, and apoptosis of neural crest cells as well as EMT [132, 133]. Gain- and loss-of-function mutations in the human orthologue of *Brg1*, *SMARCA4*, respectively, cause syndromic mental retardation or rhabdoid tumor predisposition syndrome [134, 135]. BAV does not belong to the phenotypic spectrum of either one of both.

Finally, BAV has been observed in mice depleted for *Robo* and/or *Slit* genes [136]. Whereas BAV presents in all compound Robo1;Robo2 mutants, the aortic valves in single Robo1 or Robo2 mutant mice appear normal, suggesting functional Robo1/2 redundancy in the heart. Of note, BAV was also observed in Slit2 knockout mice, yet with significantly reduced penetrance. The exact mechanisms that interconnect Robo-Slit dysfunction and BAV formation remain to be elucidated. Crosstalk between Robo-Slit and Notch signaling might be part of the explanation, as Robo1 deficiency was shown to impact on *Notch1/2* expression levels [136]. Furthermore, genes relating to the Notch or Robo-Slit pathways show strikingly similar expression patterns in the developing heart. To date, no human disorders have firmly been linked to mutations in *ROBO1*, *ROBO2*, or *SLIT2*.

Molecular Diagnostic Testing

Molecular diagnostic testing encompasses systematic screening of patients and their relatives for the presence of pathogenic variants in known causal genes, enabling early disease management stratification by discriminating between at-risk individuals and those likely to be unaffected.

As discussed in the sections above, the genetic etiology of BAV is considered exceedingly heterogeneous and is, based on the large number of genetically unexplained familial cases, far from solved. Moreover, rare genetic defects in the most established BAV culprits (i.e., *NOTCH1*, *SMAD6*, *ROBO4*, and *GATA5*) are uncommon and hardly ever fully penetrant and associate with exceedingly diverse phenotypes, making interpretation of their pathogenic nature and genetic counseling challenging. Establishment of variant recurrence among multiple families, mutation clustering in certain protein domains, and genotype-phenotype correlations would facilitate the latter process. Routine testing of the known BAV genes in a molecular diagnostic setting, which is still in its infancy, therefore serves a dual purpose, i.e., risk stratification and expansion and validation of the mutational and phenotypic spectrum of the known BAV genes.

In genetically heterogeneous disorders such as BAV, molecular diagnostic testing by means of gene panel sequencing has proven most proficient [137]. However, as presently only a small number of BAV genes have to be screened and their mutation frequencies are low, the approach is of too little yield to be cost-efficient. Consequently, BAV genes are presently being included in large next-generation sequencing panels encompassing genes causal for a variety of congenital heart disorders and/or aortopathies. With the declining cost of exome sequencing, it will likely also replace gene panel sequencing in a diagnostic setting in the near future. Molecular tests to identify patients at risk for specific BAV-related complications, such as AS, AR, or TAA, will require considerably more time and research because their underlying genetic determinants are even more enigmatic. Until the genetic etiology of BAV and its associated complications has been considerably further elucidated, careful cardiovascular surveillance will likely remain an important clinical strategy in the majority of BAV families (see Section "Patient Management").

Patient Management

Despite the fact that the risk for aortic dissection in BAV patients is clearly lower than in MFS, aortic dilatations and aneurysms entail a significant risk for acute aortic dissection and/or rupture, which –despite surgical progress – still associate with poor outcomes. Hitherto, the current medical therapies cannot prevent the progression of aortic dilatation or aneurysm formation in TAA patients in general, nor in BAV cases. As a result, much emphasis has been placed on cardiovascular monitoring and preventive surgery. Recent population-based studies revealed that in BAV patients with minimal valve dysfunction, the mortality rates have become similar to those in the general population [5, 6]. Given the high prevalence of BAV, universal application of imaging-based surveillance as well as preventive aortic surgery represents a costly endeavor for our society.

Medical Therapy

Due to histological similarities between aortic specimens of BAV and Marfan syndrome (MFS) patients [138], the current medical therapies for BAV-related TAA resulted from extrapolating those for MFS. Noteworthy, efficacy of these therapeutic strategies has not yet been demonstrated in large BAV cohorts and is even under debate in the MFS field [106]. Consequently, many efforts are in progress to acquire more evidence regarding the disease-modifying capacities of the currently available drugs and to develop alternative MFS and/or BAV therapies.

The mainstay of current therapeutic approach in MFS-related aortopathy is the administration of β-adrenergic receptor antagonists (β-blockers). Their role in BAV-related aortopathy remains controversial. Prophylactic β-blockers have been suggested to impact on aneurysm progression by reducing the mean arterial pressure and the systolic heart rate [139]. In spite of the established use of β-blockers in TAA management, clinical trials in MFS patients revealed variable outcomes [140–142]. Additionally, in a 4D flow imaging study, aortic blood flows were not shown to be significantly altered in β-blocker-treated BAV patients compared to their untreated counterparts [143]. To allow more powerful estimates of the protective effects of β-blockers on BAV-related aortopathy, larger cohorts that are stratified for dosage in addition to treatment duration should be tested for β-blocker beneficence.

Administration of angiotensin II receptor blockers (ARBs) embodies the second therapeutic approach in patients with aortic dilatation. Angiotensin II binds and exerts its function through two G-protein coupled receptors: AT1 and AT2. Via activation of AT1, the transforming growth factor (TGF-β) pathway becomes stimulated, initiating fibrosis [144]. In 2006, upregulated TGF-β signaling was pinpointed the key culprit in the pathogenesis of MFS-related aortopathy, urging development of TGF-β-neutralizing therapies [145]. The AT1 blocker losartan had already proven capable of attenuating TGF-β signaling in certain animal models and was routinely used to treat hypertension, which rendered it the number one drug to test [146, 147]. While small studies in humans seemed promising [148–150], recent findings did not confirm efficacy of losartan as to MFS-related TAA management [151–154]. A meta-analysis combining all individual trials (±2300 patients) is being conducted at the time of writing [155]. In BAV patients, there is no trial-based evidence yet for beneficence of ARBs, nor for preferred use of ARBs over β-blockers or vice versa.

A randomized multicenter trial addressing efficacy of both β-blocker and ARB treatment in BAV patients has been completed, but the study results remain to be published (https://clinicaltrials.gov/ct2/show/NCT01202721).

The third potential therapeutic strategy involves administration of angiotensin-converting enzyme inhibitors (ACEi), which block the processing of biologically inactive angiotensin I to its active form, i.e., angiotensin II, which after binding to AT1 receptors leads to vasoconstriction. Consequently, ACEi decrease blood pressure by preventing the contraction of blood vessels. In MFS, they are mostly prescribed to patients who are intolerant of β-blockers [156]. Beneficence is under debate though, because ACEi also block the beneficial downstream AT2 pathway. As to BAV-related TAA, a recent study has revealed lack of significant ACEi efficacy [157]. Larger studies are necessary to shed a better light on the added value of ACEi therapy in BAV/TAA patients though.

Surgical Intervention

In the young, implantation of prosthetic valves yields suboptimal clinical outcomes because of the patients' enduring growth. In addition, the anticoagulant therapy, warranted in patients with a mechanical valve, may prohibit sports participation or other activities. Hence, in BAV children and young adults with isolated AS, balloon valvuloplasty (i.e., widening of the stenotic aortic valve by inserting a balloon catheter) or Ross surgery are designated the optimal treatment options [158]. In adults, aortic valve replacement is the preferred management strategy due to superior durability. To treat AR in the absence of AS, valve sparing repair methods avoiding the anticoagulation-related risks that come with mechanical valve implantation have emerged. Their success, however, heavily depends on leaflet tissue quality, that is, the degree of fibrosis and calcification [159]. Other options are bioprosthesis, human tissue valves, and the Ross procedure (especially in children). As to surgical intervention for TAA, the precise timing is mostly being determined by pragmatically established but systematically revised aortic diameter thresholds. In asymptomatic individuals, the current guidelines recommend elective aortic repair when proximal aortic diameters exceed 55 mm [160]. BAV patients in whom additional risk factors have been identified, including a positive family history for SCD due to dissections or ruptures, systemic hypertension, and aortic enlargement at an extremely rapid pace (≥5 mm/year), should undergo surgical intervention if the aortic dimensions are ≥50 mm. A cutoff of 45 mm is advisable if aortic valve repair is anyway being performed because of severe AS or AR.

Taken together, surgical procedures for BAV and/or TAA should be tailored to the presence and degree of valvular dysfunction and aneurysmal disease as well as the desired anticoagulation status. In the early 1970s, the so-called Bentall and De Bono surgical procedures, which replace the aortic root, ascending aorta, and/or aortic valve with, respectively, a Dacron prosthesis and/or mechanical valve, represented the golden standard [161, 162]. More recently, valve sparing techniques such as David's or Yacoub's surgery are becoming increasingly popular, eliminating the need for life-long anticoagulation therapy [163]. Their mid-term results have proven excellent, with at least 90% of the patients being free from reoperation on the aortic valve 10–15 years after surgery, but long-term results have yet to be evaluated [164].

Cardiovascular Management in Pregnancy

Pregnant women with BAV, and particularly those with severe AS, are at increased risk for cardiac and neonatal complications [165]. Hence, female patients should be thoroughly monitored and counseled regarding potential threats and treatment options prior to, during, and after pregnancy. Recent guidelines recommend BAV females to undergo advanced imaging of the valve and thoracic aorta (CT or CMR) before pregnancy [166, 167]. Upon observation of aortic diameters above 50 mm or symptomatic AS and AR, pre-pregnancy surgery should be considered, or pregnancy should be avoided. Nevertheless, in rare instances, highly progressive symptoms may still develop during pregnancy, requiring balloon valvuloplasty or valve/aorta surgery. Only in case of positive, well-substantiated benefit/risk ratios, their execution is justified.

Of note, BAV in pregnancy might not cause major problems in the vast majority of patients. The latter cases are generally not reported in literature as they do not require specific interventions, possibly biasing estimated complication frequencies [168].

Sports Recommendations

In about 5–8% of the athletes below 40 years, SCD during sports is caused by AS and/or ruptured TAA, which are commonly associated with BAV [169, 170]. As such, once athletes have been diagnosed with BAV, specific guidelines on exercise should be followed to prevent SCD. According to the 2015 ACC/AHA guidelines, BAV athletes, without valve problems and with aortic dimensions ≤40 mm, can participate in all competitive sports [171]. For those with a mildly to moderately dilated aorta (40–45 mm), participation in low-intensity competitive sports with a low likelihood of bodily contact may be considered. Intense weight training has to be avoided. Finally, athletes with a markedly dilated aorta (>45 mm) should not participate in any competitive sports.

They can participate safely to recreational golfing or billiards, for example, though. In BAV athletes with asymptomatic or mild aortic valve complications but normal aortic diameters, exercise testing is recommended to decide on the tolerable level and intensity of physical activity [32]. Importantly, it has to be stressed that sports participation has major health benefits over a sedentary lifestyle and that therefore some form of exercise is advisable in most BAV cases.

Patient Follow-Up

To meticulously follow disease progression, serial echocardiography, when necessary complemented with CMR or CT, should be performed. The aortic growth rate is highly variable between BAV patients. It generally ranges from 0.2 to 0.9 mm per year [172–175], which is about fivefold higher than what is observed in TAV individuals [176]. In accordance with the law of Laplace, patients with larger aortas show faster expansion rates [177]. The current ESC and ACC/AHA guidelines advocate yearly cardiac imaging in BAV patients with an aortic root or ascending aortic diameter of ≥45 mm and a negative family history for aortic dissections or considerably increasing interval changes in aortic dimensions [30, 31]. In those with smaller diameters, cardiac imaging every 2–3 years should be sufficient.

Family Screening

Family screening is in practice still predominantly based on expert opinion. Most commonly, family screening is recommended in first-degree relatives of probands with BAV/TAA, young BAV patients with severe cardiovascular complications, or patients with a positive family history for BAV, TAA, or unexplained SCD.

Cascade Clinical Screening

Current ESC guidelines recommend echocardiographic evaluation of all first-degree relatives of patients with BAV (Class 2aC) in search of aortic dilation and/or BAV [139]. However, little is known of the cost-effectiveness of such an approach. A study of Hales and Mahle assessed the cost-effectiveness of family imaging, revealing a per life-year saved cost of $74,884 (2012) [178]. Depending on the available local health system resources (e.g., accessibility to conventional echocardiography, waiting lists), focus echocardiography in first-degree relatives of either all BAV patients or those located at the most severe end of the phenotypic spectrum (e.g., severe valve dysfunction or TAA) should be considered. Whether cardiovascular monitoring should start as soon as possible or from 18 years onward is still under debate. Once BAV has been diagnosed, standard surveillance and management guidelines should be followed (see Section "Patient Follow-Up"). As to TAA monitoring following TAV establishment, no formal recommendations have been drafted. As aortopathy can take years to develop and a recent study revealed TAA in about 10% of TAV first-degree relatives, regular (i.e., every 3–5 years) interval follow-up is advisable though [2].

Cascade Molecular Screening

Molecular diagnostic testing of the yet known congenital heart disease and/or TAA genes is recommended in all BAV/TAA probands below age 60 and BAV index patients with a positive familial history for BAV, TAA, and/or unexplained sudden cardiac death. Upon identification of a pathogenic (Class 5) or likely pathogenic (Class 4) variant, cascade molecular screening should be performed. For variants of unknown significance (VUSs), cascade screening is not advisable. Whenever possible, segregation analysis might be considered to gain extra evidence for or refute variant pathogenicity though.

Conclusions

Due to the high prevalence of BAV, and the life-threatening cardiovascular complications that associate with it, BAV represents a major public health problem. Over the past couple of years, extensive efforts aiming at unraveling the disorder's etiology have revealed valuable insights, typically pinpointing EMT malfunction or distortion of the normal cardiac neural crest cell activity as the key disease culprits. Yet, the pathogenetic picture is still far from complete, hampering development of novel therapies. These are definitely needed, as major uncertainty surrounds the usefulness of the current medical therapies for BAV. Investigations into the basic genetic defects as well as dysfunctional cellular mechanisms and signaling pathways underlying BAV will definitely continue in the upcoming years. Their adequate design necessitates acknowledgment of the factors underlying the current inscrutability of BAV genetics. Some hypotheses can already be put forward. As extended families segregating BAV in a Mendelian manner are rare, gene identification approaches in groups of unrelated BAV patients, commonly taking advantage of the advent of next-generation sequencing technologies, have increasingly gained momentum. In the latter studies, genetic heterogeneity might jeopardize success. Recent findings suggest that distinct BAV subtypes result from different pathomechanisms [8]. Moreover, occurrence of particular cardiovascular complications might correlate with the underlying genetic BAV cause. Considering BAV as a single disease entity can thus unnecessarily compromise homogeneity of patients under study. To increase the probability of finding multiple cases with pathogenic mutations in the same gene in future gene identification studies, it could be advantageous to stratify patient populations for well-defined endophenotypes as to valve morphology and coexisting morbidity. Additionally, one might consider to select cases with a positive family history who have been confronted with prominent valve dysfunction or aortopathy early in life. These individuals are situated at the severest end of the phenotypic BAV spectrum, rendering a major contribution of genetic factors to the disease etiology very likely. A second hypothesis states that oligogenic inheritance accounts for a substantial fraction of the genetic etiology of BAV, implying that one single patient should carry rare mutations in multiple genes, whether or not belonging to one biological pathway. Supportive evidence encompasses low penetrance of BAV in the so far described single gene knockout mice, whereas compound knockouts are more consistently affected [118, 136]. Furthermore, oligogenic inheritance in other left ventricular outflow tract malformations has already been demonstrated [179]. Consequently, future BAV analysis strategies should also be tailored toward non-Mendelian inheritance patterns.

Take-Home Message

Bicuspid aortic valve:

- Is the most common congenital heart defect.
- Is associated with a variety of severe cardiovascular complications.
- Is currently managed by means of:
  - Interval cardiovascular monitoring to diagnose concomitant cardiovascular features
  - Medical therapy (although efficacy remains to be proven)
  - Preventive surgical intervention
- Has a high heritability, which is indicative of a role for genetic factors.
- Is genetically far from explained but seems complex and exceedingly heterogeneous.
- Likely results from defective endothelial-to-mesenchymal transition and/or cardiac neural crest cell activity.
- Imaging-based first-degree relative screening is recommended upon establishment of BAV in an individual, especially if the proband presents with severe valve dysfunction or pronounced TAA.
- Patients with pronounced aortopathy below age 60 or with a positive family history for BAV, TAA, and/or unexplained sudden cardiac death are recommended to be tested for mutations in the currently known congenital heart disease and/or TAA genes.

References

1. Braverman AC, Guven H, Beardslee MA, Makan M, Kates AM, Moon MR. The bicuspid aortic valve. Curr Probl Cardiol. 2005;30(9):470–522.
2. Galian-Gay L, Carro Hevia A, Teixido-Tura G, Rodriguez Palomares J, Gutierrez-Moreno L, Maldonado G, et al. Familial clustering of bicuspid aortic valve and its relationship with aortic dilation in first-degree relatives. Heart. 2018;105(8):603–8.
3. Cripe L, Andelfinger G, Martin LJ, Shooner K, Benson DW. Bicuspid aortic valve is heritable. J Am Coll Cardiol. 2004;44(1):138–43.
4. Ward C. Clinical significance of the bicuspid aortic valve. Heart. 2000;83(1):81–5.
5. Tzemos N, Therrien J, Yip J, Thanassoulis G, Tremblay S, Jamorski MT, et al. Outcomes in adults with bicuspid aortic valves. JAMA. 2008;300(11):1317–25.
6. Michelena HI, Desjardins VA, Avierinos JF, Russo A, Nkomo VT, Sundt TM, et al. Natural history of asymptomatic patients with normally functioning or minimally dysfunctional bicuspid aortic valve in the community. Circulation. 2008;117(21):2776–84.
7. Sievers HH, Schmidtke C. A classification system for the bicuspid aortic valve from 304 surgical specimens. J Thorac Cardiovasc Surg. 2007;133(5):1226–33.
8. Fernandez B, Duran AC, Fernandez-Gallego T, Fernandez MC, Such M, Arque JM, et al. Bicuspid aortic valves with different spatial orientations of the leaflets are distinct etiological entities. J Am Coll Cardiol. 2009;54(24):2312–8.
9. Michelena HI, Khanna AD, Mahoney D, Margaryan E, Topilsky Y, Suri RM, et al. Incidence of aortic complications in patients with bicuspid aortic valves. JAMA. 2011;306(10):1104–12.
10. Fedak PW, Verma S, David TE, Leask RL, Weisel RD, Butany J. Clinical and pathophysiological implications of a bicuspid aortic valve. Circulation. 2002;106(8):900–4.
11. Kong WK, Delgado V, Poh KK, Regeer MV, Ng AC, McCormack L, et al. Prognostic implications of raphe in bicuspid aortic valve anatomy. JAMA Cardiol. 2017;2(3):285–92.
12. Ng ACT, Delgado V, Kong WKF, Bax JJ. Lessons from an international bicuspid aortic valve disease registry: the raphe and beyond. Heart Lung Circ. 2018;27(7):782–4.
13. Ward RM, Marsh JM, Gossett JM, Rettiganti MR, Collins RT 2nd. Impact of bicuspid aortic valve morphology on aortic valve disease and aortic dilation in pediatric patients. Pediatr Cardiol. 2018;39(3):509–17.
14. Kang JW, Song HG, Yang DH, Baek S, Kim DH, Song JM, et al. Association between bicuspid aortic valve phenotype and patterns of valvular dysfunction and bicuspid aortopathy: comprehensive evaluation using MDCT and echocardiography. JACC Cardiovasc Imaging. 2013;6(2):150–61.
15. Kim JS, Ko SM, Chee HK, Shin JK, Song MG, Shin HJ. Relationship between bicuspid aortic valve phenotype, valvular function, and ascending aortic dimensions. J Heart Valve Dis. 2014;23(4):406–13.
16. Kong WK, Regeer MV, Ng AC, McCormack L, Poh KK, Yeo TC, et al. Sex differences in phenotypes of bicuspid aortic valve and aortopathy: insights from a large multicenter, international registry. Circ Cardiovasc Imaging. 2017;10(3):e005155. https://doi.org/10.1161/CIRCIMAGING.116.005155.
17. Andrei AC, Yadlapati A, Malaisrie SC, Puthumana JJ, Li Z, Rigolin VH, et al. Comparison of outcomes and presentation in men-versus-women with bicuspid aortic valves undergoing aortic valve replacement. Am J Cardiol. 2015;116(2):250–5.
18. Roman MJ, Pugh NL, Devereux RB, Eagle KA, Holmes K, LeMaire SA, et al. Aortic dilatation associated with bicuspid aortic valve: relation to sex, hemodynamics, and valve morphology (the National Heart Lung and Blood Institute-sponsored national

registry of genetically triggered thoracic aortic aneurysms and cardiovascular conditions). Am J Cardiol. 2017;120(7):1171–5.
19. Braverman AC. Aortic involvement in patients with a bicuspid aortic valve. Heart. 2011;97(6):506–13.
20. Edwards WD, Leaf DS, Edwards JE. Dissecting aortic aneurysm associated with congenital bicuspid aortic valve. Circulation. 1978;57(5):1022–5.
21. Michelena HI, Prakash SK, Della Corte A, Bissell MM, Anavekar N, Mathieu P, et al. Bicuspid aortic valve: identifying knowledge gaps and rising to the challenge from the international bicuspid aortic valve consortium (BAVCon). Circulation. 2014;129(25):2691–704.
22. Nanda NC, Gramiak R, Manning J, Mahoney EB, Lipchik EO, DeWeese JA. Echocardiographic recognition of the congenital bicuspid aortic valve. Circulation. 1974;49(5):870–5.
23. Freeman RV, Otto CM. Bicuspid aortic valve and aortopathy: see the first, then look at the second. JACC Cardiovasc Imaging. 2013;6(2):162–4.
24. Yousry M, Rickenlund A, Petrini J, Jenner J, Liska J, Eriksson P, et al. Aortic valve type and calcification as assessed by transthoracic and transoesophageal echocardiography. Clin Physiol Funct Imaging. 2015;35(4):306–13.
25. Takeda H, Muro T, Saito T, Hyodo E, Ehara S, Hanatani A, et al. Diagnostic accuracy of transthoracic and transesophageal echocardiography for the diagnosis of bicuspid aortic valve: comparison with operative findings. Osaka City Med J. 2013;59(2):69–78.
26. Cote G, Denault A. Transesophageal echocardiography-related complications. Can J Anaesth. 2008;55(9):622–47.
27. Joziasse IC, Vink A, Cramer MJ, van Oosterhout MF, van Herwerden LA, Heijmen R, et al. Bicuspid stenotic aortic valves: clinical characteristics and morphological assessment using MRI and echocardiography. Neth Hear J. 2011;19(3):119–25.
28. van der Wall EE. Bicuspid aortic valve; optimal diagnosis and latest interventional treatment. Neth Hear J. 2015;23(3):149–50.
29. Mordi I, Tzemos N. Bicuspid aortic valve disease: a comprehensive review. Cardiol Res Pract. 2012;2012:196037.
30. Nishimura RA, Otto CM, Bonow RO, Carabello BA, Erwin JP 3rd, Guyton RA, et al. 2014 AHA/ACC guideline for the Management of Patients with Valvular Heart Disease: executive summary: a report of the American College of Cardiology/American Heart Association Task Force on practice guidelines. Circulation. 2014;129(23):2440–92.
31. Vahanian A, Alfieri O, Andreotti F, Antunes MJ, Baron-Esquivias G, Baumgartner H, et al. Guidelines on the management of valvular heart disease (version 2012). Eur Heart J. 2012;33(19):2451–96.
32. Baumgartner H, Falk V, Bax JJ, De Bonis M, Hamm C, Holm PJ, et al. 2017 ESC/EACTS guidelines for the management of valvular heart disease. Eur Heart J. 2017;38(36):2739–91.
33. Borger MA, Fedak PWM, Stephens EH, Gleason TG, Girdauskas E, Ikonomidis JS, et al. The American Association for Thoracic Surgery consensus guidelines on bicuspid aortic valve-related aortopathy: executive summary. J Thorac Cardiovasc Surg. 2018;156(2):473–80.
34. Ben-Shachar S, Ou Z, Shaw CA, Belmont JW, Patel MS, Hummel M, et al. 22q11.2 distal deletion: a recurrent genomic disorder distinct from DiGeorge syndrome and velocardiofacial syndrome. Am J Hum Genet. 2008;82(1):214–21.
35. Basu R, Hazra S, Shanks M, Paterson DI, Oudit GY. Novel mutation in exon 14 of the sarcomere gene MYH7 in familial left ventricular noncompaction with bicuspid aortic valve. Circ Heart Fail. 2014;7(6):1059–62.
36. Guo DC, Papke CL, Tran-Fadulu V, Regalado ES, Avidan N, Johnson RJ, et al. Mutations in smooth muscle alpha-actin (ACTA2) cause coronary artery disease, stroke, and Moyamoya disease, along with thoracic aortic disease. Am J Hum Genet. 2009;84(5):617–27.
37. Karp N, Grosse-Wortmann L, Bowdin S. Severe aortic stenosis, bicuspid aortic valve and atrial septal defect in a child with Joubert Syndrome and Related Disorders (JSRD) - a case report and review of congenital heart defects reported in the human ciliopathies. Eur J Med Genet. 2012;55(11):605–10.
38. Baasanjav S, Al-Gazali L, Hashiguchi T, Mizumoto S, Fischer B, Horn D, et al. Faulty initiation of proteoglycan synthesis causes cardiac and joint defects. Am J Hum Genet. 2011;89(1):15–27.
39. Huntington K, Hunter AG, Chan KL. A prospective study to assess the frequency of familial clustering of congenital bicuspid aortic valve. J Am Coll Cardiol. 1997;30(7):1809–12.
40. Clementi M, Notari L, Borghi A, Tenconi R. Familial congenital bicuspid aortic valve: a disorder of uncertain inheritance. Am J Med Genet. 1996;62(4):336–8.
41. Ellison JW, Yagubyan M, Majumdar R, Sarkar G, Bolander ME, Atkinson EJ, et al. Evidence of genetic locus heterogeneity for familial bicuspid aortic valve. J Surg Res. 2007;142(1):28–31.
42. Hinton RB. Bicuspid aortic valve and thoracic aortic aneurysm: three patient populations, two disease phenotypes, and one shared genotype. Cardiol Res Pract. 2012;2012:926975.
43. Loscalzo ML, Goh DL, Loeys B, Kent KC, Spevak PJ, Dietz HC. Familial thoracic aortic dilation and bicommissural aortic valve: a prospective analysis of natural history and inheritance. Am J Med Genet A. 2007;143A(17):1960–7.
44. Jain R, Engleka KA, Rentschler SL, Manderfield LJ, Li L, Yuan L, et al. Cardiac neural crest orchestrates remodeling and functional maturation of mouse semilunar valves. J Clin Invest. 2011;121(1):422–30.
45. Rossi A, van der Linde D, Yap SC, Lapinskas T, Kirschbaum S, Springeling T, et al. Ascending aorta dilatation in patients with bicuspid aortic valve stenosis: a prospective CMR study. Eur Radiol. 2013;23(3):642–9.
46. Martin LJ, Ramachandran V, Cripe LH, Hinton RB, Andelfinger G, Tabangin M, et al. Evidence in favor of linkage to human chromosomal regions 18q, 5q and 13q for bicuspid aortic valve and associated cardiovascular malformations. Hum Genet. 2007;121(2):275–84.
47. Garg V, Muth AN, Ransom JF, Schluterman MK, Barnes R, King IN, et al. Mutations in NOTCH1 cause aortic valve disease. Nature. 2005;437(7056):270–4.
48. Kerstjens-Frederikse WS, van de Laar IM, Vos YJ, Verhagen JM, Berger RM, Lichtenbelt KD, et al. Cardiovascular malformations caused by NOTCH1 mutations do not keep left: data on 428 probands with left-sided CHD and their families. Genet Med. 2016;18(9):914–23.
49. Kent KC, Crenshaw ML, Goh DL, Dietz HC. Genotype-phenotype correlation in patients with bicuspid aortic valve and aneurysm. J Thorac Cardiovasc Surg. 2013;146(1):158–65 e1.
50. Foffa I, Ait Ali L, Panesi P, Mariani M, Festa P, Botto N, et al. Sequencing of NOTCH1, GATA5, TGFBR1 and TGFBR2 genes in familial cases of bicuspid aortic valve. BMC Med Genet. 2013;14:44.
51. McBride KL, Riley MF, Zender GA, Fitzgerald-Butt SM, Towbin JA, Belmont JW, et al. NOTCH1 mutations in individuals with left ventricular outflow tract malformations reduce ligand-induced signaling. Hum Mol Genet. 2008;17(18):2886–93.
52. Andersson ER, Sandberg R, Lendahl U. Notch signaling: simplicity in design, versatility in function. Development. 2011;138(17):3593–612.
53. Artavanis-Tsakonas S, Rand MD, Lake RJ. Notch signaling: cell fate control and signal integration in development. Science. 1999;284(5415):770–6.
54. High FA, Epstein JA. The multifaceted role of Notch in cardiac development and disease. Nat Rev Genet. 2008;9(1):49–61.
55. Timmerman LA, Grego-Bessa J, Raya A, Bertran E, Perez-Pomares JM, Diez J, et al. Notch promotes epithelial-mesenchymal

transition during cardiac development and oncogenic transformation. Genes Dev. 2004;18(1):99–115.
56. Kostina AS, Uspensky VE, Irtyuga OB, Ignatieva EV, Freylikhman O, Gavriliuk ND, et al. Notch-dependent EMT is attenuated in patients with aortic aneurysm and bicuspid aortic valve. Biochim Biophys Acta. 2016;1862(4):733–40.
57. MacGrogan D, D'Amato G, Travisano S, Martinez-Poveda B, de Luxan G, Del Monte-Nieto G, et al. Sequential ligand-dependent notch signaling activation regulates valve primordium formation and morphogenesis. Circ Res. 2016;118(10):1480–97.
58. Ducy P, Zhang R, Geoffroy V, Ridall AL, Karsenty G. Osf2/Cbfa1: a transcriptional activator of osteoblast differentiation. Cell. 1997;89(5):747–54.
59. Kaden JJ, Bickelhaupt S, Grobholz R, Vahl CF, Hagl S, Brueckmann M, et al. Expression of bone sialoprotein and bone morphogenetic protein-2 in calcific aortic stenosis. J Heart Valve Dis. 2004;13(4):560–6.
60. Mohler ER 3rd, Gannon F, Reynolds C, Zimmerman R, Keane MG, Kaplan FS. Bone formation and inflammation in cardiac valves. Circulation. 2001;103(11):1522–8.
61. Acharya A, Hans CP, Koenig SN, Nichols HA, Galindo CL, Garner HR, et al. Inhibitory role of Notch1 in calcific aortic valve disease. PLoS One. 2011;6(11):e27743.
62. Nigam V, Srivastava D. Notch1 represses osteogenic pathways in aortic valve cells. J Mol Cell Cardiol. 2009;47(6):828–34.
63. Jiao J, Tian W, Qiu P, Norton EL, Wang MM, Chen YE, et al. Induced pluripotent stem cells with NOTCH1 gene mutation show impaired differentiation into smooth muscle and endothelial cells: implications for bicuspid aortic valve-related aortopathy. J Thorac Cardiovasc Surg. 2018;156(2):515–22 e1.
64. Koenig SN, La Haye S, Feller JD, Rowland P, Hor KN, Trask AJ, et al. Notch1 haploinsufficiency causes ascending aortic aneurysms in mice. JCI Insight. 2017;2(21):e91353. https://doi.org/10.1172/jci.insight.91353.
65. Tan HL, Glen E, Topf A, Hall D, O'Sullivan JJ, Sneddon L, et al. Nonsynonymous variants in the SMAD6 gene predispose to congenital cardiovascular malformation. Hum Mutat. 2012;33(4):720–7.
66. Gillis E, Kumar AA, Luyckx I, Preuss C, Cannaerts E, van de Beek G, et al. Candidate gene Resequencing in a large bicuspid aortic valve-associated thoracic aortic aneurysm cohort: SMAD6 as an important contributor. Front Physiol. 2017;8:400.
67. Hanyu A, Ishidou Y, Ebisawa T, Shimanuki T, Imamura T, Miyazono K. The N domain of Smad7 is essential for specific inhibition of transforming growth factor-beta signaling. J Cell Biol. 2001;155(6):1017–27.
68. Wylie LA, Mouillesseaux KP, Chong DC, Bautch VL. Developmental SMAD6 loss leads to blood vessel hemorrhage and disrupted endothelial cell junctions. Dev Biol. 2018;442(2):199–209.
69. Galvin KM, Donovan MJ, Lynch CA, Meyer RI, Paul RJ, Lorenz JN, et al. A role for smad6 in development and homeostasis of the cardiovascular system. Nat Genet. 2000;24(2):171–4.
70. Chen G, Deng C, Li YP. TGF-beta and BMP signaling in osteoblast differentiation and bone formation. Int J Biol Sci. 2012;8(2):272–88.
71. Garg V, Kathiriya IS, Barnes R, Schluterman MK, King IN, Butler CA, et al. GATA4 mutations cause human congenital heart defects and reveal an interaction with TBX5. Nature. 2003;424(6947):443–7.
72. Li RG, Xu YJ, Wang J, Liu XY, Yuan F, Huang RT, et al. GATA4 loss-of-function mutation and the congenitally bicuspid aortic valve. Am J Cardiol. 2018;121(4):469–74.
73. Yang B, Zhou W, Jiao J, Nielsen JB, Mathis MR, Heydarpour M, et al. Protein-altering and regulatory genetic variants near GATA4 implicated in bicuspid aortic valve. Nat Commun. 2017;8:15481.
74. Rivera-Feliciano J, Lee KH, Kong SW, Rajagopal S, Ma Q, Springer Z, et al. Development of heart valves requires Gata4 expression in endothelial-derived cells. Development. 2006;133(18):3607–18.
75. Molkentin JD, Lin Q, Duncan SA, Olson EN. Requirement of the transcription factor GATA4 for heart tube formation and ventral morphogenesis. Genes Dev. 1997;11(8):1061–72.
76. Kuo CT, Morrisey EE, Anandappa R, Sigrist K, Lu MM, Parmacek MS, et al. GATA4 transcription factor is required for ventral morphogenesis and heart tube formation. Genes Dev. 1997;11(8):1048–60.
77. Laforest B, Andelfinger G, Nemer M. Loss of Gata5 in mice leads to bicuspid aortic valve. J Clin Invest. 2011;121(7):2876–87.
78. Padang R, Bagnall RD, Richmond DR, Bannon PG, Semsarian C. Rare non-synonymous variations in the transcriptional activation domains of GATA5 in bicuspid aortic valve disease. J Mol Cell Cardiol. 2012;53(2):277–81.
79. Bonachea EM, Chang SW, Zender G, LaHaye S, Fitzgerald-Butt S, McBride KL, et al. Rare GATA5 sequence variants identified in individuals with bicuspid aortic valve. Pediatr Res. 2014;76(2):211–6.
80. Shi LM, Tao JW, Qiu XB, Wang J, Yuan F, Xu L, et al. GATA5 loss-of-function mutations associated with congenital bicuspid aortic valve. Int J Mol Med. 2014;33(5):1219–26.
81. Martin M, Alonso-Montes C, Florez JP, Pichel IA, Rozado J, Andia JB, et al. Bicuspid aortic valve syndrome: a heterogeneous and still unknown condition. Int J Cardiol. 2014;177(3):1105.
82. Wei D, Bao H, Zhou N, Zheng GF, Liu XY, Yang YQ. GATA5 loss-of-function mutation responsible for the congenital ventriculoseptal defect. Pediatr Cardiol. 2013;34(3):504–11.
83. Zhang XL, Dai N, Tang K, Chen YQ, Chen W, Wang J, et al. GATA5 loss-of-function mutation in familial dilated cardiomyopathy. Int J Mol Med. 2015;35(3):763–70.
84. Wang XH, Huang CX, Wang Q, Li RG, Xu YJ, Liu X, et al. A novel GATA5 loss-of-function mutation underlies lone atrial fibrillation. Int J Mol Med. 2013;31(1):43–50.
85. Wei D, Bao H, Liu XY, Zhou N, Wang Q, Li RG, et al. GATA5 loss-of-function mutations underlie tetralogy of fallot. Int J Med Sci. 2013;10(1):34–42.
86. Nemer G, Nemer M. Cooperative interaction between GATA5 and NF-ATc regulates endothelial-endocardial differentiation of cardiogenic cells. Development. 2002;129(17):4045–55.
87. Kirk EP, Sunde M, Costa MW, Rankin SA, Wolstein O, Castro ML, et al. Mutations in cardiac T-box factor gene TBX20 are associated with diverse cardiac pathologies, including defects of septation and valvulogenesis and cardiomyopathy. Am J Hum Genet. 2007;81(2):280–91.
88. Lee TC, Zhao YD, Courtman DW, Stewart DJ. Abnormal aortic valve development in mice lacking endothelial nitric oxide synthase. Circulation. 2000;101(20):2345–8.
89. Chao CS, McKnight KD, Cox KL, Chang AL, Kim SK, Feldman BJ. Novel GATA6 mutations in patients with pancreatic agenesis and congenital heart malformations. PLoS One. 2015;10(2):e0118449.
90. Lin X, Huo Z, Liu X, Zhang Y, Li L, Zhao H, et al. A novel GATA6 mutation in patients with tetralogy of Fallot or atrial septal defect. J Hum Genet. 2010;55(10):662–7.
91. Laforest B, Nemer M. Genetic insights into bicuspid aortic valve formation. Cardiol Res Pract. 2012;2012:180297.
92. Xu YJ, Di RM, Qiao Q, Li XM, Huang RT, Xue S, et al. GATA6 loss-of-function mutation contributes to congenital bicuspid aortic valve. Gene. 2018;663:115–20.
93. Gharibeh L, Komati H, Bosse Y, Boodhwani M, Heydarpour M, Fortier M, et al. GATA6 regulates aortic valve remodeling and its Haploinsufficiency leads to RL-type bicuspid aortic valve. Circulation. 2018;138(10):1025–38.

94. Lepore JJ, Mericko PA, Cheng L, Lu MM, Morrisey EE, Parmacek MS. GATA-6 regulates semaphorin 3C and is required in cardiac neural crest for cardiovascular morphogenesis. J Clin Invest. 2006;116(4):929–39.
95. van Berlo JH, Elrod JW, van den Hoogenhof MM, York AJ, Aronow BJ, Duncan SA, et al. The transcription factor GATA-6 regulates pathological cardiac hypertrophy. Circ Res. 2010;107(8):1032–40.
96. Gould RA, Aziz H, Woods CE, Seman-Senderos MA, Sparks E, Preuss C, et al. ROBO4 variants predispose individuals to bicuspid aortic valve and thoracic aortic aneurysm. Nat Genet. 2018;51(1):42–50.
97. Biben C, Weber R, Kesteven S, Stanley E, McDonald L, Elliott DA, et al. Cardiac septal and valvular dysmorphogenesis in mice heterozygous for mutations in the homeobox gene Nkx2-5. Circ Res. 2000;87(10):888–95.
98. Chung IM, Rajakumar G. Genetics of congenital heart defects: the NKX2-5 gene, a key player. Genes. 2016;7(2):6. https://doi.org/10.3390/genes7020006.
99. Beffagna G, Cecchetto A, Dal Bianco L, Lorenzon A, Angelini A, Padalino M, et al. R25C mutation in the NKX2.5 gene in Italian patients affected with non-syndromic and syndromic congenital heart disease. J Cardiovasc Med. 2013;14(8):582–6.
100. Qu XK, Qiu XB, Yuan F, Wang J, Zhao CM, Liu XY, et al. A novel NKX2.5 loss-of-function mutation associated with congenital bicuspid aortic valve. Am J Cardiol. 2014;114(12):1891–5.
101. Quintero-Rivera F, Xi QJ, Keppler-Noreuil KM, Lee JH, Higgins AW, Anchan RM, et al. MATR3 disruption in human and mouse associated with bicuspid aortic valve, aortic coarctation and patent ductus arteriosus. Hum Mol Genet. 2015;24(8):2375–89.
102. Xia F, Bainbridge MN, Tan TY, Wangler MF, Scheuerle AE, Zackai EH, et al. De novo truncating mutations in AHDC1 in individuals with syndromic expressive language delay, hypotonia, and sleep apnea. Am J Hum Genet. 2014;94(5):784–9.
103. Johnson JO, Pioro EP, Boehringer A, Chia R, Feit H, Renton AE, et al. Mutations in the Matrin 3 gene cause familial amyotrophic lateral sclerosis. Nat Neurosci. 2014;17(5):664–6.
104. Nistri S, Porciani MC, Attanasio M, Abbate R, Gensini GF, Pepe G. Association of Marfan syndrome and bicuspid aortic valve: frequency and outcome. Int J Cardiol. 2012;155(2):324–5.
105. Dietz HC, Cutting GR, Pyeritz RE, Maslen CL, Sakai LY, Corson GM, et al. Marfan syndrome caused by a recurrent de novo missense mutation in the fibrillin gene. Nature. 1991;352(6333):337–9.
106. Verstraeten A, Alaerts M, Van Laer L, Loeys B. Marfan syndrome and related disorders: 25 years of gene discovery. Hum Mutat. 2016;37(6):524–31.
107. Fedak PW, de Sa MP, Verma S, Nili N, Kazemian P, Butany J, et al. Vascular matrix remodeling in patients with bicuspid aortic valve malformations: implications for aortic dilatation. J Thorac Cardiovasc Surg. 2003;126(3):797–806.
108. Pepe G, Nistri S, Giusti B, Sticchi E, Attanasio M, Porciani C, et al. Identification of fibrillin 1 gene mutations in patients with bicuspid aortic valve (BAV) without Marfan syndrome. BMC Med Genet. 2014;15:23.
109. Lesauskaite V, Sepetiene R, Jariene G, Patamsyte V, Zukovas G, Grabauskyte I, et al. FBN1 polymorphisms in patients with the dilatative pathology of the ascending thoracic aorta. Eur J Cardiothorac Surg. 2015;47(4):e124–30.
110. Lemaire SA, McDonald ML, Guo DC, Russell L, Miller CC 3rd, Johnson RJ, et al. Genome-wide association study identifies a susceptibility locus for thoracic aortic aneurysms and aortic dissections spanning FBN1 at 15q21.1. Nat Genet. 2011;43(10):996–1000.
111. Loeys BL, Dietz HC. Loeys-Dietz Syndrome. In: Pagon RA, Adam MP, Ardinger HH, Wallace SE, Amemiya A, LJH B, et al., editors. GeneReviews(R). Seattle, WA: University of Washington; 2008.
112. Arrington CB, Sower CT, Chuckwuk N, Stevens J, Leppert MF, Yetman AT, et al. Absence of TGFBR1 and TGFBR2 mutations in patients with bicuspid aortic valve and aortic dilation. Am J Cardiol. 2008;102(5):629–31.
113. Girdauskas E, Schulz S, Borger MA, Mierzwa M, Kuntze T. Transforming growth factor-beta receptor type II mutation in a patient with bicuspid aortic valve disease and intraoperative aortic dissection. Ann Thorac Surg. 2011;91(5):e70–1.
114. Olivieri LJ, Baba RY, Arai AE, Bandettini WP, Rosing DR, Bakalov V, et al. Spectrum of aortic valve abnormalities associated with aortic dilation across age groups in turner syndrome. Circ Cardiovasc Imaging. 2013;6(6):1018–23.
115. Mortensen KH, Andersen NH, Gravholt CH. Cardiovascular phenotype in turner syndrome--integrating cardiology, genetics, and endocrinology. Endocr Rev. 2012;33(5):677–714.
116. Bondy C, Bakalov VK, Cheng C, Olivieri L, Rosing DR, Arai AE. Bicuspid aortic valve and aortic coarctation are linked to deletion of the X chromosome short arm in turner syndrome. J Med Genet. 2013;50(10):662–5.
117. Chang AC, Fu Y, Garside VC, Niessen K, Chang L, Fuller M, et al. Notch initiates the endothelial-to-mesenchymal transition in the atrioventricular canal through autocrine activation of soluble guanylyl cyclase. Dev Cell. 2011;21(2):288–300.
118. Bosse K, Hans CP, Zhao N, Koenig SN, Huang N, Guggilam A, et al. Endothelial nitric oxide signaling regulates Notch1 in aortic valve disease. J Mol Cell Cardiol. 2013;60:27–35.
119. Peterson JC, Chughtai M, Wisse LJ, Gittenberger-de Groot AC, Feng Q, Goumans MTH, et al. Nos3 mutation leads to abnormal neural crest cell and second heart field lineage patterning in bicuspid aortic valve formation. Dis Model Mech. 2018;11(10) https://doi.org/10.1242/dmm.034637.
120. Koenig SN, Bosse KM, Nadorlik HA, Lilly B, Garg V. Evidence of Aortopathy in mice with Haploinsufficiency of in -null background. J Cardiovasc Dev Dis. 2015;2(1):17–30.
121. Aicher D, Urbich C, Zeiher A, Dimmeler S, Schafers HJ. Endothelial nitric oxide synthase in bicuspid aortic valve disease. Ann Thorac Surg. 2007;83(4):1290–4.
122. Thomas PS, Sridurongrit S, Ruiz-Lozano P, Kaartinen V. Deficient signaling via Alk2 (Acvr1) leads to bicuspid aortic valve development. PLoS One. 2012;7(4):e35539.
123. Kaartinen V, Dudas M, Nagy A, Sridurongrit S, Lu MM, Epstein JA. Cardiac outflow tract defects in mice lacking ALK2 in neural crest cells. Development. 2004;131(14):3481–90.
124. Wang J, Sridurongrit S, Dudas M, Thomas P, Nagy A, Schneider MD, et al. Atrioventricular cushion transformation is mediated by ALK2 in the developing mouse heart. Dev Biol. 2005;286(1):299–310.
125. Shore EM, Xu M, Feldman GJ, Fenstermacher DA, Cho TJ, Choi IH, et al. A recurrent mutation in the BMP type I receptor ACVR1 causes inherited and sporadic fibrodysplasia ossificans progressiva. Nature Genet. 2006;38(5):525–7.
126. Makki N, Capecchi MR. Cardiovascular defects in a mouse model of HOXA1 syndrome. Hum Mol Genet. 2012;21(1):26–31.
127. Tischfield MA, Bosley TM, Salih MA, Alorainy IA, Sener EC, Nester MJ, et al. Homozygous HOXA1 mutations disrupt human brainstem, inner ear, cardiovascular and cognitive development. Nat Genet. 2005;37(10):1035–7.
128. Odelin G, Faure E, Coulpier F, Di Bonito M, Bajolle F, Studer M, et al. Krox20 defines a subpopulation of cardiac neural crest cells contributing to arterial valves and bicuspid aortic valve. Development. 2018;145(1) https://doi.org/10.1242/dev.151944.
129. Odelin G, Faure E, Kober F, Maurel-Zaffran C, Theron A, Coulpier F, et al. Loss of Krox20 results in aortic valve regurgitation and impaired transcriptional activation of fibrillar collagen genes. Cardiovasc Res. 2014;104(3):443–55.

130. Theron A, Odelin G, Faure E, Avierinos JF, Zaffran S. Krox20 heterozygous mice: a model of aortic regurgitation associated with decreased expression of fibrillar collagen genes. Arch Cardiovasc Dis. 2016;109(3):188–98.
131. Warner LE, Mancias P, Butler IJ, McDonald CM, Keppen L, Koob KG, et al. Mutations in the early growth response 2 (EGR2) gene are associated with hereditary myelinopathies. Nat Genet. 1998;18(4):382–4.
132. Akerberg BN, Sarangam ML, Stankunas K. Endocardial Brg1 disruption illustrates the developmental origins of semilunar valve disease. Dev Biol. 2015;407(1):158–72.
133. Li W, Xiong Y, Shang C, Twu KY, Hang CT, Yang J, et al. Brg1 governs distinct pathways to direct multiple aspects of mammalian neural crest cell development. Proc Natl Acad Sci U S A. 2013;110(5):1738–43.
134. Schneppenheim R, Fruhwald MC, Gesk S, Hasselblatt M, Jeibmann A, Kordes U, et al. Germline nonsense mutation and somatic inactivation of SMARCA4/BRG1 in a family with rhabdoid tumor predisposition syndrome. Am J Hum Genet. 2010;86(2):279–84.
135. Tsurusaki Y, Okamoto N, Ohashi H, Kosho T, Imai Y, Hibi-Ko Y, et al. Mutations affecting components of the SWI/SNF complex cause coffin-Siris syndrome. Nat Genet. 2012;44(4):376–8.
136. Mommersteeg MT, Yeh ML, Parnavelas JG, Andrews WD. Disrupted slit-Robo signalling results in membranous ventricular septum defects and bicuspid aortic valves. Cardiovasc Res. 2015;106(1):55–66.
137. Xue Y, Ankala A, Wilcox WR, Hegde MR. Solving the molecular diagnostic testing conundrum for Mendelian disorders in the era of next-generation sequencing: single-gene, gene panel, or exome/genome sequencing. Genet Med. 2015;17(6):444–51.
138. Niwa K, Perloff JK, Bhuta SM, Laks H, Drinkwater DC, Child JS, et al. Structural abnormalities of great arterial walls in congenital heart disease: light and electron microscopic analyses. Circulation. 2001;103(3):393–400.
139. Hiratzka LF, Bakris GL, Beckman JA, Bersin RM, Carr VF, Casey DE Jr, et al. ACCF/AHA/AATS/ACR/ASA/SCA/SCAI/SIR/STS/SVM guidelines for the diagnosis and management of patients with thoracic aortic disease: a report of the American College of Cardiology Foundation/American Heart Association Task Force on practice guidelines, American Association for Thoracic Surgery, American College of Radiology, American Stroke Association, Society of Cardiovascular Anesthesiologists, Society for Cardiovascular Angiography and Interventions, Society of Interventional Radiology, Society of Thoracic Surgeons, and Society for vascular medicine. Circulation. 2010;121(13):e266–369.
140. Gersony DR, McClaughlin MA, Jin Z, Gersony WM. The effect of beta-blocker therapy on clinical outcome in patients with Marfan's syndrome: a meta-analysis. Int J Cardiol. 2007;114(3):303–8.
141. Plein A, Calmont A, Fantin A, Denti L, Anderson NA, Scambler PJ, et al. Neural crest-derived SEMA3C activates endothelial NRP1 for cardiac outflow tract septation. J Clin Invest. 2015;125(7):2661–76.
142. Kioussi C, Briata P, Baek SH, Rose DW, Hamblet NS, Herman T, et al. Identification of a Wnt/Dvl/beta-catenin --> Pitx2 pathway mediating cell-type-specific proliferation during development. Cell. 2002;111(5):673–85.
143. Allen BD, Markl M, Barker AJ, van Ooij P, Carr JC, Malaisrie SC, et al. Influence of beta-blocker therapy on aortic blood flow in patients with bicuspid aortic valve. Int J Cardiovasc Imaging. 2016;32(4):621–8.
144. Habashi JP, Doyle JJ, Holm TM, Aziz H, Schoenhoff F, Bedja D, et al. Angiotensin II type 2 receptor signaling attenuates aortic aneurysm in mice through ERK antagonism. Science. 2011;332(6027):361–5.
145. Habashi JP, Judge DP, Holm TM, Cohn RD, Loeys BL, Cooper TK, et al. Losartan, an AT1 antagonist, prevents aortic aneurysm in a mouse model of Marfan syndrome. Science. 2006;312(5770):117–21.
146. Lim DS, Lutucuta S, Bachireddy P, Youker K, Evans A, Entman M, et al. Angiotensin II blockade reverses myocardial fibrosis in a transgenic mouse model of human hypertrophic cardiomyopathy. Circulation. 2001;103(6):789–91.
147. Martin B, Brenneman R, Becker KG, Gucek M, Cole RN, Maudsley S. iTRAQ analysis of complex proteome alterations in 3xTgAD Alzheimer's mice: understanding the interface between physiology and disease. PLoS One. 2008;3(7):e2750.
148. Brooke BS, Habashi JP, Judge DP, Patel N, Loeys B, Dietz HC 3rd. Angiotensin II blockade and aortic-root dilation in Marfan's syndrome. N Engl J Med. 2008;358(26):2787–95.
149. Chiu HH, Wu MH, Wang JK, Lu CW, Chiu SN, Chen CA, et al. Losartan added to beta-blockade therapy for aortic root dilation in Marfan syndrome: a randomized, open-label pilot study. Mayo Clin Proc. 2013;88(3):271–6.
150. Pees C, Laccone F, Hagl M, Debrauwer V, Moser E, Michel-Behnke I. Usefulness of losartan on the size of the ascending aorta in an unselected cohort of children, adolescents, and young adults with Marfan syndrome. Am J Cardiol. 2013;112(9):1477–83.
151. Bhatt AB, Buck JS, Zuflacht JP, Milian J, Kadivar S, Gauvreau K, et al. Distinct effects of losartan and atenolol on vascular stiffness in Marfan syndrome. Vasc Med. 2015;20(4):317–25.
152. Forteza A, Evangelista A, Sanchez V, Teixido-Tura G, Sanz P, Gutierrez L, et al. Efficacy of losartan vs. atenolol for the prevention of aortic dilation in Marfan syndrome: a randomized clinical trial. Eur Heart J. 2015;37(12):978–85.
153. Milleron O, Arnoult F, Ropers J, Aegerter P, Detaint D, Delorme G, et al. Marfan Sartan: a randomized, double-blind, placebo-controlled trial. Eur Heart J. 2015;36(32):2160–6.
154. Lacro RV, Dietz HC, Sleeper LA, Yetman AT, Bradley TJ, Colan SD, et al. Atenolol versus losartan in children and young adults with Marfan's syndrome. N Engl J Med. 2014;371(22):2061–71.
155. Pitcher A, Emberson J, Lacro RV, Sleeper LA, Stylianou M, Mahony L, et al. Design and rationale of a prospective, collaborative meta-analysis of all randomized controlled trials of angiotensin receptor antagonists in Marfan syndrome, based on individual patient data: a report from the Marfan treatment Trialists' collaboration. Am Heart J. 2015;169(5):605–12.
156. Feiner L, Webber AL, Brown CB, Lu MM, Jia L, Feinstein P, et al. Targeted disruption of semaphorin 3C leads to persistent truncus arteriosus and aortic arch interruption. Development. 2001;128(16):3061–70.
157. Ohnemus D, Oster ME, Gatlin S, Jokhadar M, Mahle WT. The effect of angiotensin-converting enzyme inhibitors on the rate of ascending aorta dilation in patients with bicuspid aortic valve. Congenit Heart Dis. 2015;10(1):E1–5.
158. Siu SC, Silversides CK. Bicuspid aortic valve disease. J Am Coll Cardiol. 2010;55(25):2789–800.
159. Della Corte A, Body SC, Booher AM, Schaefers HJ, Milewski RK, Michelena HI, et al. Surgical treatment of bicuspid aortic valve disease: knowledge gaps and research perspectives. J Thorac Cardiovasc Surg. 2014;147(6):1749–57.
160. Accf/Aha/Aats/Acr/Asa/Sca/Scai/Sir/Sts/Svm Guidelines For The D, Management Of Patients With Thoracic Aortic Disease Representative Members, Hiratzka LF, Creager MA, Isselbacher EM, Svensson LG, et al. Surgery for aortic dilatation in patients with bicuspid aortic valves: a statement of clarification from the American College of Cardiology/American Heart Association Task Force on clinical practice guidelines. Circulation. 2016;133(7):680–6.
161. Bentall H, De Bono A. A technique for complete replacement of the ascending aorta. Thorax. 1968;23(4):338–9.

162. Gott VL, Greene PS, Alejo DE, Cameron DE, Naftel DC, Miller DC, et al. Replacement of the aortic root in patients with Marfan's syndrome. N Engl J Med. 1999;340(17):1307–13.
163. Benedetto U, Melina G, Takkenberg JJ, Roscitano A, Angeloni E, Sinatra R. Surgical management of aortic root disease in Marfan syndrome: a systematic review and meta-analysis. Heart. 2011;97(12):955–8.
164. David TE. Aortic valve sparing operations: outcomes at 20 years. Ann Cardiothorac Surg. 2013;2(1):24–9.
165. Orwat S, Diller GP, van Hagen IM, Schmidt R, Tobler D, Greutmann M, et al. Risk of pregnancy in moderate and severe aortic stenosis: from the multinational ROPAC registry. J Am Coll Cardiol. 2016;68(16):1727–37.
166. European Society of Gynecology (ESG), the Association for European Paediatric Cardiology (AEPC), and the German Society for GenderMedicine (DGesGM), Regitz-Zagrosek V, Blomstrom Lundqvist C, Borghi C, et al. ESC guidelines on the management of cardiovascular diseases during pregnancy: the Task Force on the Management of Cardiovascular Diseases during pregnancy of the European Society of Cardiology (ESC). Eur Heart J. 2011;32(24):3147–97.
167. Regitz-Zagrosek V, Roos-Hesselink JW, Bauersachs J, Blomstrom-Lundqvist C, Cifkova R, De Bonis M, et al. 2018 ESC guidelines for the management of cardiovascular diseases during pregnancy. Eur Heart J. 2018;39(34):3165–241.
168. Lésniak-Sobelga A, Kostklewicz M, Wisniowska-Smialek S, Rubis P, Podolec P. Outcome of pregnancy in patients with bicuspid aortic valve – a study of 89 patients. Journal of Rare Cardiovascular Diseases. 2014;2(1):9–14.
169. Maron BJ, Pelliccia A. The heart of trained athletes: cardiac remodeling and the risks of sports, including sudden death. Circulation. 2006;114(15):1633–44.
170. Maron BJ, Zipes DP, Kovacs RJ, American Heart Association E, Arrhythmias Committee of Council on Clinical Cardiology CoCDiYCoC, Stroke Nursing CoFG, et al. Eligibility and disqualification recommendations for competitive athletes with cardiovascular abnormalities: preamble, principles, and general considerations: a scientific statement from the American Heart Association and American College of Cardiology. Circulation. 2015;132(22):e256–61.
171. Braverman AC, Harris KM, Kovacs RJ, Maron BJ. Eligibility and disqualification recommendations for competitive athletes with cardiovascular abnormalities: task force 7: aortic diseases, including Marfan syndrome: a scientific statement from the American Heart Association and American College of Cardiology. J Am Coll Cardiol. 2015;66(21):2398–405.
172. Ferencik M, Pape LA. Changes in size of ascending aorta and aortic valve function with time in patients with congenitally bicuspid aortic valves. Am J Cardiol. 2003;92(1):43–6.
173. Dore A, Brochu MC, Baril JF, Guertin MC, Mercier LA. Progressive dilation of the diameter of the aortic root in adults with a bicuspid aortic valve. Cardiol Young. 2003;13(6):526–31.
174. Detaint D, Michelena HI, Nkomo VT, Vahanian A, Jondeau G, Sarano ME. Aortic dilatation patterns and rates in adults with bicuspid aortic valves: a comparative study with Marfan syndrome and degenerative aortopathy. Heart. 2014;100(2):126–34.
175. Yap SC, Kouwenhoven GC, Takkenberg JJ, Galema TW, Meijboom FJ, van Domburg R, et al. Congenital aortic stenosis in adults: rate of progression and predictors of clinical outcome. Int J Cardiol. 2007;122(3):224–31.
176. Etz CD, Zoli S, Brenner R, Roder F, Bischoff M, Bodian CA, et al. When to operate on the bicuspid valve patient with a modestly dilated ascending aorta. Ann Thorac Surg. 2010;90(6):1884–90. discussion 91-2
177. Shimada I, Rooney SJ, Pagano D, Farneti PA, Davies P, Guest PJ, et al. Prediction of thoracic aortic aneurysm expansion: validation of formulae describing growth. Ann Thorac Surg. 1999;67(6):1968–70. discussion 79–80
178. Hales AR, Mahle WT. Echocardiography screening of siblings of children with bicuspid aortic valve. Pediatrics. 2014;133(5):e1212–7.
179. McBride KL, Pignatelli R, Lewin M, Ho T, Fernbach S, Menesses A, et al. Inheritance analysis of congenital left ventricular outflow tract obstruction malformations: segregation, multiplex relative risk, and heritability. Am J Med Genet A. 2005;134A(2):180–6.

Part V

Miscellaneous

Sudden Cardiac Death in the Young: Post-mortem Investigation and Cardiogenetic Evaluation of Victims and Their Relatives

21

Lennart J. Blom, Annette F. Baas, Aryan Vink, and Rutger J. Hassink

Introduction

Sudden cardiac death (SCD) was recently defined as "Sudden and unexpected death occurring within an hour of the onset of symptoms, or occurring in patients found dead within 24 h of being asymptomatic and presumably due to a cardiac arrhythmia or hemodynamic catastrophe" [1]. Population studies show that over two-thirds of sudden death cases are of suspected cardiac origin and classified as SCD [2].

The incidence of SCD in persons aged 1–40 years varies depending on the population studied and methodology used. The incidence for children is 1.3 per 100,000 person-years and increases to 8.5 per 100,000 in adults up to 40 years of age [3].

The underlying causes identified in autopsy series suggest that in people under 35 years of age, 24–31% of deaths are due to coronary artery disease; 17–37% are associated with cardiomyopathy, predominantly hypertrophic cardiomyopathy, idiopathic left ventricular hypertrophy, and arrhythmogenic cardiomyopathy (depending on the investigated region [4]); and in 31–35%, no cause is found by gross and histological examination, and the death is presumed to be arrhythmic [5, 6]. Due to the probability of inherited disease in these cases, up to 50% in SCD victims without structural heart disease [7], post-mortem diagnosis in the victim is crucial for appropriate management of the victim's family members.

In practice, not all causes of SCD in a young victim are established. Usually, the victim was asymptomatic, and the event is the first presentation of the disease, or the victim suffered from non-specific symptoms, which often are not formally evaluated. The deaths are frequently unwitnessed, and circumstances at the time of death have to be retrieved from ambulance and police reports [3].

When autopsy cannot identify a cause, which happens in up to 30% [6], these cases are referred to as *sudden arrhythmic death syndrome* (SADS). Despite the absence of an apparent underlying cause, the possibility of an underlying inherited cardiac disease remains, and family members should be considered for cardiogenetic consultation and cardiac evaluation.

After the Event

A dedicated and focused post-mortem investigation is essential in detecting potential inherited cardiac diseases in sudden death victims. This involves gathering as much information about the deceased as possible. The investigation should include obtaining a premorbid medical history, occurrence of syncope, exertional symptoms, prior illness, recently prescribed medication, and any previous ECGs or other diagnostic tests performed. Circumstances of SCD often rely on obtaining information from available ambulance and police reports. When no further investigations are performed, these cases are referred to as *sudden unexplained death* (SUD).

Family history is another important part of the post-mortem investigation and should contain a comprehensive three-generation family pedigree focused on identifying a family history of cardiac disease and premature sudden unexplained death. Examples of suspicious symptoms or deaths in family members are *sudden infant death syndrome* (SIDS), epilepsy, recurrent fainting, drowning of experienced swimmers in (shallow) waters, or one-sided vehicle accidents [3, 8].

The recommended steps to be taken after the event are presented in Fig. 21.1.

L. J. Blom (✉) · R. J. Hassink
Department of Cardiology, University Medical Center Utrecht, Utrecht, The Netherlands
e-mail: L.J.Blom-2@umcutrecht.nl

A. F. Baas
Department of Clinical Genetics, University Medical Center Utrecht, Utrecht, The Netherlands

A. Vink
Department of Pathology, University Medical Center Utrecht, Utrecht, The Netherlands

H. F. Baars et al. (eds.), *Clinical Cardiogenetics*, https://doi.org/10.1007/978-3-030-45457-9_21

Fig. 21.1 Flowchart of recommended actions and investigations after a sudden death in the young suspected of inherited heart disease, including the multidisciplinary specialists involved. *SCD* sudden cardiac death

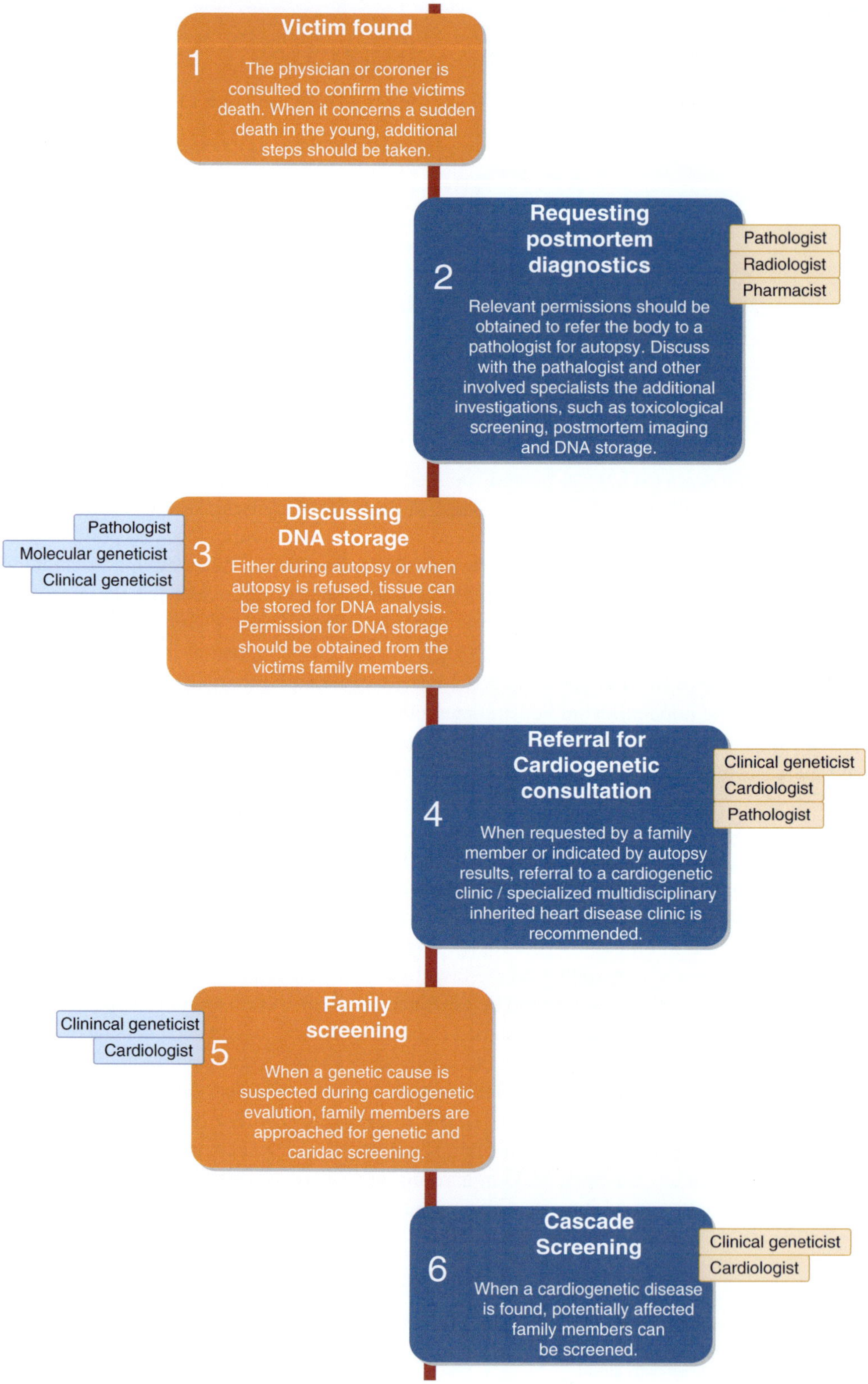

Autopsy and Toxicological Screening

A full post-mortem examination is strongly recommended in all cases of sudden death in the young (between 1 and 40 years old), as this represents the first, and only, opportunity to establish and register an *accurate* cause of death. The international guideline for post-mortem investigation and autopsy in SCD/SUD provides a minimum standard that is required in the routine autopsy practice for the adequate investigation of SCD [9]. If little experience with cardiac examination is available, referral of the heart (tissue) to a cardiac expert pathologist is recommended. In the report of the autopsy, the pathologist should state the certainty to which the findings of the autopsy could have led to the sudden death, since findings of uncertain significance might lead to erroneous interpretation and, e.g., may mask underlying disease [10]. During the autopsy, appropriate material for toxicology, microbiology, biochemistry, and molecular investigation should be obtained. A toxicological examination for drugs (e.g., opiates, amphetamine), alcohol, and medication may be considered necessary in cases with no structural abnormalities at autopsy, although the presence of drugs does not rule out an underlying genetic disease [11, 12]. Over 70% of SCD autopsies yield an underlying diagnosis and are thereby the most effective post-mortem investigation in young SCD victims [2, 5, 6]. Post-mortem diagnosis may give psychological closure for the family [13]. In case a potential inherited disorder was found, this may give rise to cascade screening of family members and preventive management. Autopsy findings that indicate involvement of other inherited disease, such as premature coronary artery disease in familial hypercholesterolemia or genetically vulnerable myocardium which may predispose for myocarditis, should also be considered. When no diagnosis could be made, autopsy findings can be used to guide screening and management of family members [10].

Post-mortem Imaging

Noninvasive imaging modalities may aid in improving diagnostic accuracy when autopsy is not performed. Post-mortem imaging alone, also known as "virtual" or "minimally invasive" autopsy, is as of now insufficient as a substitute for conventional autopsy but can be an alternative when conventional autopsy is, e.g., refused by the victim's relatives [14]. Both post-mortem *computer tomography* (CT) and *cardiac magnetic resonance* (CMR) *imaging* can be performed within a few hours after death. Post-mortem CT usually consists of a scan of the head and neck, thorax, and abdomen and should be interpreted by a radiologist with experience regarding post-mortem imaging techniques. Post-mortem MR imaging is generally dedicated to the heart and brain to detect more subtle abnormalities that could have been the cause of death.

The utility and yield of post-mortem imaging in SCD is still unclear. An Australian investigation compared the outcome of regular post-mortem investigation with post-mortem MRI and CT in 17 SCD victims and showed that MRI had a high sensitivity and positive predictive value compared to traditional autopsy for arrhythmogenic cardiomyopathy, ischemic heart disease, pulmonary embolism, or aortic dissection and could be used as a rule-out when autopsy is not possible [15]. Another issue is cost assessment, which is complicated as mortuary service and post-mortem imaging costs vary considerably between and within countries. A recent report estimated post-mortem imaging could increase costs for post-mortem investigation by >30% and propose a national service for cost-effective implementation [16]. In general, costs of post-mortem investigation are paid by the initiator. When post-mortem investigation is required by law, for example, in unnatural death, the state will refund the costs. When the death occurs in hospital, the post-mortem investigations may be financed by the hospital. Post-mortem investigation of out-of-hospital deaths is usually funded by the family of the deceased. Sudden death of a young individual is a reason for further investigation, which in many countries is still funded by the family when the death occurs out of hospital. In the UK, it is legally required to perform post-mortem investigations in these cases, and therefore, the costs are paid by the state. To improve the rate of post-mortem investigation of young SCD victims in other countries, funding by state or health insurance companies should be considered.

Molecular Autopsy

In SCD victims, post-mortem investigation allows tissue to be collected and stored in the way it is recommended by pathology guidelines. When a hereditary cause of death is suspected, the pathologist can recommend referral of first-degree family members to a cardiogenetic clinic and store DNA of the deceased for potential genetic testing [9]. Even when autopsy is refused, a minimal amount of tissue can be collected from the victim for storage. This tissue can be used for genetic testing. The types of tissue that are usually collected during autopsy are ethylenediaminetetraacetic acid (EDTA) blood and/or frozen (cardiac) muscle, liver, or spleen [17, 18]. A skin biopsy can be taken when no autopsy is performed (with permission from the victim's relatives). Prior to the biopsy, the skin needs to be disinfected with alcohol. The obtained tissue can be temporarily stored in a sterile vial with physiological isotonic saline before sending it to a DNA laboratory [19].

Storage of the victim's DNA enables genetic testing when relatives consult a cardiologist or geneticist for cardiogenetic evaluation. The yield of post-mortem genetic testing in SCD victims is modest (13% in Lahrouchi et al. [20], 27% in Tan et al. [21], and 32% in Kumar et al. [22]); however when combined with clinical evaluation of relatives, the diagnostic yield increases to approximately 40% [21, 23]. The recommended number of genes in molecular autopsy panels is under debate, as the ratio of rare *variants of uncertain significance* (VUS) to pathogenic or likely pathogenic variants is unfavorable. Therefore, pretest counselling of the relatives is essential. The HRS/EHRA consensus states that comprehensive or targeted (KCNQ1, KCNH2, SCN5A, and RyR2) gene testing may be considered in unexplained sudden death cases, where they account for 35% of pathologic mutations found [8, 19]. Further genetic testing should be guided but not limited by phenotypic findings in the deceased, as even in autopsy-negative SADS patients, pathogenic variants are found in cardiomyopathy-associated genes [10].

Together with the clinical evaluation of the family, post-mortem genetic testing (i.e., a molecular autopsy) could uncover the cause of death in the deceased. When a genetic cause is found, cascade screening of at-risk family members can be initiated.

Cardiogenetic Evaluation of First-Degree Relatives of Young SCD Victims

Phenotypic Screening

In most cases of SCD, phenotypic screening of relatives is indicated. The extent of this screening is dependent on the findings in the deceased. These findings can then be used for targeted genetic testing in the victim (if the victim's DNA is available) or in the clinically affected relative (with cardiac abnormalities).

When there are no clues available for a specific diagnosis, in SADS cases, for example, phenotypic screening is important to reveal inherited disease in the family. First-degree relatives, obligate carriers, and symptomatic relatives should be evaluated.

A cardiac examination of the relatives should follow a standard approach and is based largely on the HRS/EHRA consensus document for inherited heart diseases [8]. Examination should include the following aspects: (1) medical and family history; (2) physical examination; (3) standard resting 12-lead electrocardiogram, 12-lead electrocardiogram after brisk standing [24], and 12-lead electrocardiogram with specific right precordial positioning of the leads (leads—V1, V2, 1V1, and 1V2) [25]; (4) exercise testing; and (5) echocardiography. If the initial examination raises the possibility of a specific genetic disorder, further investigations may be indicated, which may include provocation testing (e.g., ajmaline challenging in suspected Brugada syndrome patients), cardiac MRI, Holter recording, or signal-averaged ECG [3, 8].

Mutation-Positive SCD Victim

When a genetic mutation is found in the stored DNA of the SCD victim, as assessed after a first-degree relative has requested cardiogenetic screening, the pathogenicity of the particular mutation must be assessed. In case of a pathogenic (disease-causing) mutation, the presence of the mutation is enough to diagnose inherited disease. Confirmation or exclusion of the presence of a disease-causing mutation in presymptomatic family members of the sudden death victim by cascade screening will guide risk stratification and management [8, 13]. Because most inherited heart diseases show an *autosomal dominant* pattern of inheritance, first-degree relatives (parents, siblings, and children) of SCD victims with genetic disease have a 50% risk of being a carrier of the same disease [26]. This is not the case if a mutation occurred de novo in the victim (is absent in the parents). However, due to the low probability of a germline mosaicism, siblings are still eligible for genetic screening in case of a de novo mutation.

Cascade screening starts with genetic testing of the (genetically) first-degree relatives of an affected individual or second-degree relatives when a first-degree relative has deceased. Subsequently, the screening can be extended to the connecting branch of the pedigree [27]. The absence of the mutation rules out the presence of the disease, and no further testing of the connecting pedigree is needed. In case a causative mutation is present in a relative, cardiologic evaluation and/or diagnostic follow-up is usually indicated.

In case there is uncertainty about the significance of the discovered mutation (classes 2–4), the results should be interpreted together with the outcome of phenotypic screening of relatives to determine the probability of inherited disease in the family members.

Mutation-Negative SCD Victim

Evaluation of family members of SCD victims in whom no genetic diagnosis is established is complex and should preferably involve a multidisciplinary team of specialists. Therefore, cardiogenetic evaluation is best performed in the context of referral of family members to a cardiogenetic clinic [3, 8]. Cascade screening should only be performed together with clinical evaluation of the family and preferably guided by post-mortem findings in the deceased.

The yield of genetic screening in family members varies depending on the phenotypic screening performed and the results of post-mortem investigation in the SCD victim. If these provide clues for cardiac disease, in more than 5% of first-degree relatives, a disease-causing mutation is found. Because of incomplete penetrance and variable expression, the subsequent management and follow-up of relatives differ between diagnoses. The genetic test results must be interpreted cautiously and incorporated in results of clinical evaluation [8]. If no diagnosis is made after comprehensive evaluation, then asymptomatic relatives are generally followed up till age 40 years [3].

Yield of Cardiogenetic Evaluation

With thorough clinical assessment of first-degree *relatives* of SUD victims, a cause of death can be established in up to 50% of selected and comprehensively evaluated families [21, 23, 28]. A Dutch investigation of 43 families of *SUD* victims, of whom 22 were autopsied, found an inherited cardiac disease in 17 of the 43 families that explained the sudden death of the victims [21]. Furthermore, a study executed in the UK revealed an inherited disease in 53% of the 57 families of SADS victims aged 4–64 years [23].

Discovery of inherited disease in an (asymptomatic) relative of a SCD victim does not necessarily have prognostic consequences. Nor does the absence of abnormalities on cardiac evaluation automatically rule out the presence of an inherited disease.

This complicates the management of relatives and requires a disease-specific approach. In some diseases, symptoms develop only at older age (e.g., *HCM*, *DCM,* and *ARVD/C*), which may mandate follow-up in these individuals. In others, an extensive cardiogenetic evaluation is sufficient for diagnosis or exclusion (e.g., *LQTS*, *BrS*, and *CPVT*). However, it should be realized that a relative carrying the mutation of an inherited cardiac disease will not necessarily develop signs or symptoms of the clinical syndrome that is associated with the mutation.

Conclusion

Sudden cardiac death in the young is a devastating event that deserves thorough investigation and care for the benefit of the victim's family members. Many specialized clinical disciplines need to collaborate to perform these investigations, and outcome is dependent on the coordinated efforts of all those involved. A comprehensive overview of the different clinical scenarios and recommended management options is presented in the flowchart in Fig. 21.2.

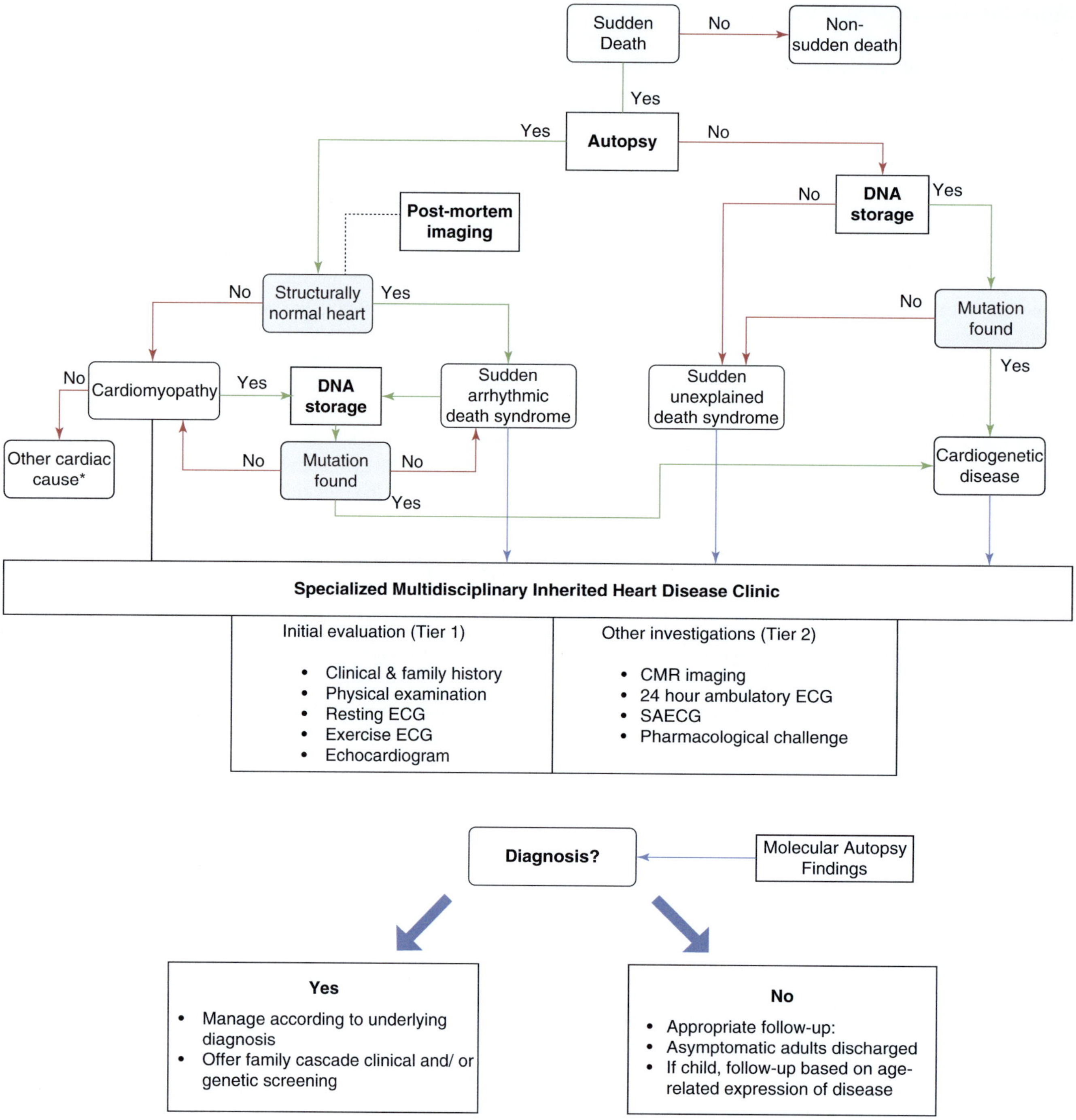

Fig. 21.2 Flowchart of diagnosis and management of inherited heart disease in families of a young sudden death victim. Note: DNA testing of stored DNA sample is initiated only after the relatives visit the outpatient clinic and request on DNA testing. ∗Inherited disease may be suspected; see paragraph "Autopsy and Toxicological Screening." *ECG* electrocardiogram, *CMR* cardiac magnetic resonance imaging, *SAECG* signal-averaged electrocardiogram. Adapted from Semsarian et al. [3]

References

1. Al-Khatib SM, Stevenson WG, Ackerman MJ, et al. 2017 AHA/ACC/HRS guideline for management of patients with ventricular arrhythmias and the prevention of sudden cardiac death: executive summary. Heart Rhythm. 2017;15(10):e190–252. https://doi.org/10.1016/j.hrthm.2017.10.035.
2. Winkel BG, Holst AG, Theilade J, Kristensen IB, Thomsen JL, Ottesen GL, Bundgaard H, Svendsen JH, Haunsø S, Tfelt-Hansen J. Nationwide study of sudden cardiac death in persons aged 1-35 years. Eur Heart J. 2011;32:983–90.
3. Semsarian C, Ingles J, Wilde AAM. Sudden cardiac death in the young: the molecular autopsy and a practical approach to surviving relatives. Eur Heart J. 2015;36:1290–6.
4. Sheppard MN. Aetiology of sudden cardiac death in sport: a histopathologist's perspective. Br J Sports Med. 2012;46:15–21.
5. Eckart RE, Shry EA, Burke AP, et al. Sudden death in young adults: an autopsy-based series of a population undergoing active surveillance. J Am Coll Cardiol. 2011;58:1254–61.
6. Doolan A, Langlois N, Semsarian C. Causes of sudden cardiac death in young Australians. Med J Aust. 2004;180:110–2.
7. Ranthe MF, Winkel BG, Andersen EW, Risgaard B, Wohlfahrt J, Bundgaard H, Haunsø S, Melbye M, Tfelt-Hansen J, Boyd HA. Risk of cardiovascular disease in family members of young sudden cardiac death victims. Eur Heart J. 2013;34:503–11.
8. Ackerman MJ, Priori SG, Willems S, et al. HRS/EHRA expert consensus statement on the state of genetic testing for the Channelopathies and cardiomyopathies. Heart Rhythm. 2011;8:1308–39.
9. Basso C, Aguilera B, Banner J, et al. Guidelines for autopsy investigation of sudden cardiac death: 2017 update from the Association for European Cardiovascular Pathology. Virchows Arch. 2017;471:691–705.
10. Papadakis M, Raju H, Behr ER, De Noronha SV, Spath N, Kouloubinis A, Sheppard MN, Sharma S. Sudden cardiac death with autopsy findings of uncertain significance: potential for erroneous interpretation. Circ Arrhythm Electrophysiol. 2013;6:588–96.
11. Tominaga M, Michiue T, Inamori-Kawamoto O, Hishmat AM, Oritani S, Takama M, Ishikawa T, Maeda H. Efficacy of drug screening in forensic autopsy: retrospective investigation of routine toxicological findings. Legal Med. 2015;17:172–6.
12. Bjune T, Risgaard B, Kruckow L, Glinge C, Ingemann-Hansen O, Leth PM, Linnet K, Banner J, Winkel BG, Tfelt-Hansen J. Post-mortem toxicology in young sudden cardiac death victims: a nationwide cohort study. Europace. 2018;20:614–21.
13. Tester DJ, Ackerman MJ. Evaluating the survivor or the relatives of those who do not survive: the role of genetic testing. Cardiol Young. 2017;27:S19–24.
14. Sonnemans LJP, Kubat B, Prokop M, Klein WM. Can virtual autopsy with postmortem CT improve clinical diagnosis of cause of death? A retrospective observational cohort study in a Dutch tertiary referral Centre. BMJ Open. 2018;8:e018834.
15. Puranik R, Gray B, Lackey H, Yeates L, Parker G, Duflou J, Semsarian C. Comparison of conventional autopsy and magnetic resonance imaging in determining the cause of sudden death in the young. J Cardiovasc Magn Reson. 2014;16:1–11.
16. Karalis J, Denton E. Forensic and post-mortem imaging in England: a national perspective. J Forensic Radiol Imaging. 2016;4:17–9.
17. Priori SG, Blomström-Lundqvist C, Mazzanti A, et al. 2015 ESC guidelines for the management of patients with ventricular arrhythmias and the prevention of sudden cardiac death. Eur Heart J. 2015;36:2793–867.
18. Carturan E, Tester DJ, Brost BC, Basso C, Thiene G, Ackerman MJ. Postmortem genetic testing for conventional autopsy–negative sudden unexplained death. Am J Clin Pathol. 2008;129:391–7.
19. Semsarian C, Hamilton RM. Key role of the molecular autopsy in sudden unexpected death. Heart Rhythm. 2012;9:145–50.
20. Lahrouchi N, Raju H, Lodder EM, et al. Utility of post-mortem genetic testing in cases of sudden arrhythmic death syndrome. J Am Coll Cardiol. 2017;69:2134–45.
21. Tan HL, Hofman N, Van Langen IM, Van Der Wal AC, Wilde AAM. Sudden unexplained death: heritability and diagnostic yield of cardiological and genetic examination in surviving relatives. Circulation. 2005;112:207–13.
22. Kumar S, Peters S, Thompson T, Morgan N, Maccicoca I, Trainer A, Zentner D, Kalman JM, Winship I, Vohra JK. Familial cardiological and targeted genetic evaluation: low yield in sudden unexplained death and high yield in unexplained cardiac arrest syndromes. Heart Rhythm. 2013;10:1653–60.
23. Behr ER, Dalageorgou C, Christiansen M, Syrris P, Hughes S, Tome Esteban MT, Rowland E, Jeffery S, McKenna WJ. Sudden arrhythmic death syndrome: familial evaluation identifies inheritable heart disease in the majority of families. Eur Heart J. 2008;29:1670–80.
24. Adler A, van der Werf C, Postema PG, et al. The phenomenon of "QT stunning": the abnormal QT prolongation provoked by standing persists even as the heart rate returns to normal in patients with long QT syndrome. Heart Rhythm. 2012;9:901–8.
25. Sangwatanaroj S, Prechawat S, Sunsaneewitayakul B, Sitthisook S, Tosukhowong P, Tungsanga K. New electrocardiographic leads and the procainamide test for the detection of the Brugada sign in sudden unexplained death syndrome survivors and their relatives. Eur Heart J. 2001;22:2290–6.
26. Priori SG, Wilde AA, Horie M, et al. HRS/EHRA/APHRS expert consensus statement on the diagnosis and Management of Patients with inherited primary arrhythmia syndromes. Heart Rhythm. 2013;10:1932–63.
27. Heart Rhythm UK Familial Sudden Death Syndromes Statement Development Group. Clinical indications for genetic testing in familial sudden cardiac death syndromes: an HRUK position statement. Heart. 2008;94:502–7.
28. Behr E, Wood DA, Wright M, Syrris P, Sheppard MN, Casey A, Davies MJ, McKenna W. Cardiological assessment of first-degree relatives in sudden arrhythmic death syndrome. Lancet. 2003;362:1457–9.

Hereditary Neuromuscular Diseases and Cardiac Involvement

22

S. M. Schade van Westrum, K. Wahbi, G. Bonne, and A. J. van der Kooi

Introduction

This chapter focuses on the primary cardiac involvement in hereditary neuromuscular diseases, i.e. the primary cardiac changes which are caused by the same genetic anomalies that damage skeletal muscle or nerves. Cardiac involvement can manifest itself as impulse generation or conduction defects; focal or diffuse myocardial thickening; dilation of the cardiac cavities; relaxation abnormality; hypertrophic, dilated, non-compaction or restrictive cardiomyopathy; Takotsubo phenomenon; secondary valve insufficiency; intra-cardiac thrombus formation; or heart failure with systolic or diastolic dysfunction [1]. Secondary cardiac involvement in neuromuscular disorders ultimately manifesting with cor pulmonale is not addressed in detail. Chest wall disorders (e.g. in spinal muscular atrophy type 2 or congenital myopathies/dystrophies) or respiratory muscle weakness (e.g. in *Pompe*'s disease) reduces the pulmonary vascular bed and causes pulmonary hypertension, chronic hypoxia and hypercapnia. Respiratory muscle weakness is confirmed by pulmonary function tests that show a significant reduction of maximal respiratory pressures and vital capacity (VC) consistent with a restrictive ventilatory defect. In such cases, nocturnal ventilatory support is indicated.

This chapter reviews the probability and severity of cardiac disease in each type of hereditary neuromuscular disease and provides recommendations for management.

S. M. S. van Westrum · A. J. van der Kooi (✉)
Amsterdam UMC, Academic Medical Center (AMC), Neuroscience Institute, University of Amsterdam, Amsterdam, The Netherlands
e-mail: a.j.kooi@amc.uva.nl

K. Wahbi
APHP, Cochin Hospital, Cardiology Department, FILNEMUS, Paris-Descartes, Sorbonne Paris Cité University, Paris, France

G. Bonne
Center of Research in Myology, Sorbonne Université, INSERM UMRS 974, Paris, France

Institut de Myologie, Paris, France

Muscle Disorders

Muscular Dystrophies

Muscular dystrophies represent a clinically and genetically heterogeneous group of disorders, characterised by muscle wasting and weakness of variable distribution and severity and dystrophic changes in skeletal muscle. They can be caused by mutations in genes encoding sarcolemma-associated proteins, such as dystrophin and the dystrophin-associated glycoprotein complex, and genes encoding proteins of the nuclear envelope.

Sarcolemma-Associated Proteins/Structural Proteins

Dystrophinopathic Cardiomyopathy

Dystrophinopathic cardiomyopathy is caused by a defect in the *dystrophin* gene on the X-chromosome encoding for the protein dystrophin. Dystrophin is expressed in the heart, skeletal muscle, neural tissues and smooth muscle, but progressive tissue damage is confined to the heart and skeletal muscle. Dystrophin, together with other cytoskeletal proteins, provides mechanical support for the sarcolemma. A change in the amount, size or function of dystrophin causes a structurally weak sarcolemma, which ruptures under mechanical stress, allowing uncontrolled focal ingress of extracellular fluid components, especially calcium, into the muscle fibre interior [2, 3]. Mutations of the dystrophin gene can result in different disorders manifesting with skeletal muscle involvement and/or cardiomyopathy: *Duchenne* muscular dystrophy (DMD, complete absence of dystrophin), *Becker* muscular dystrophy (BMD, qualitative and/or quantitative abnormalities of dystrophin), *X-linked dilated cardiomyopathy* (dystrophin abnormalities confined to the myocardium) and symptomatic carrier (DMD/BMD) manifesting with cardiomyopathy. The lack of dystrophin in cardiac muscle leads to progressive cardiomyocyte degeneration and fibrosis. The posterior basal segment of the left ventricle is consistently the first site in which hypokinesis is detected

H. F. Baars et al. (eds.), *Clinical Cardiogenetics*, https://doi.org/10.1007/978-3-030-45457-9_22

on echocardiography. The characteristic electrocardiographic (ECG) alterations consist of tall right precordial R waves (R/S ratio greater than 1 in V1) and deep Q waves (greater than 3 mm) in the left precordial and limb leads. A progressive, global hypokinesia with ventricular dilatation then evolves. The right side of the heart is rarely affected, and in particular, the right atrium rarely demonstrates any echocardiographic abnormality. The most frequent cardiac abnormality in DMD is sinus tachycardia, occurring in childhood and persisting through life. Another rhythm abnormality frequently found is atrial premature beats. The incidence of cardiac conduction defects remained 6–13% throughout life [4]. AV blocks are only rarely found. Ventricular arrhythmias are infrequent at the early stages, but their incidence increases with the progression of the disease.

Duchenne Muscular Dystrophy

Duchenne muscular dystrophy is caused by frameshift mutations in the dystrophin gene, causing complete absence of the dystrophin protein. DMD has an incidence of 1 in 2500 to 3500 live male births [5]. Predominantly boys are affected in this X-linked disorder. The onset of disease is usually between 2 and 5 years of age with progressive symmetrical proximal weakness, legs more than arms, a characteristic hypertrophic appearance of the calves and marked elevation of serum creatine kinase (CK) activity. Wheelchair dependency occurs around the age of 10–12 years; corticosteroid treatment delays this to a median of 14.5 years [6]. The introduction of ventilatory support led to a considerable extension of the life expectancy, from a mean age of death of 14.4 years in the 1960s to 25.3 years for those who were ventilated since 1990 [7]. From a clinical perspective, a progressive dilated cardiomyopathy eventually occurs in all boys with DMD. Symptoms of overt cardiac failure are rare, probably because boys typically have a severely restricted physical ability. Left untreated, cardiomyopathy makes a significant contribution to early mortality [7]. Sudden cardiac death events and significant Holter findings are rare in DMD patients with an left ventricle ejection fraction (LVEF) >35% [8].

Management. The management of cardiac involvement in DMD falls apart in two parts: follow-up and investigation on one side and treatment or prevention on the other side.

Cardiac assessment once a year is generally advocated in guidelines [9–11]. In patients with symptoms or with abnormalities on investigations, it is advised to monitor more frequently. The method of investigation is dependent on the age of the patient and availability, but noninvasive techniques are advocated. In younger patients, until the age of 7, cardiac investigation with ECG and echocardiography is the method of choice. Conventional 2D echocardiography can be extended with techniques as tissue Doppler- and strain-based methods. Speckle tracking echocardiography is a more recent advancement in strain analysis and is increasingly used. With speckle tracking echocardiography, it is possible to identify small regions of abnormal mobility of the cardiac wall and may show abnormalities even when there is no reduction of the ejection fraction yet [12]. Above the age of 7 years, cardiac MRI, when available, is preferred because of the high sensitivity of cardiac changes with better reproducibility and reliability because it is independent of deformation of the thorax. Cardiac MRI detects in DMD twice as much patients with fraction shortening as with echocardiography [13, 14]. Early fibrotic changes in the myocardium are shown with late gadolinium-enhanced cardiac MRI. The cardiomyopathy patients aside from Duchenne patients can suffer from rhythm disorders requiring treatment. Irrespective of age, these abnormalities are detected with ECG and 24-h ECG.

When considering pharmacological treatment, angiotensin-converting enzymes (ACE) or angiotensin receptor blocker (ARB) is considered a first-line therapy with beta-blockers added when myocardial dilatation evolves. A systematic review concludes that evidence is limited but survival is improved (a) in patients on ACE inhibitors when still having a normal ejection fraction and (b) in patients on ACE or ARB combined with beta-blockers with an abnormal ejection fraction whether symptomatic or asymptomatic. The dosages are variable and generally left to the discretion of the treating cardiologist [11]. The age of starting treatment in patients with no abnormalities is debatable, but 10 years is advised [10]. Glucocorticoids are often used in Duchenne muscular dystrophy. Eplerenone has shown in a randomised trial to diminish the rate of decline in ventricular systolic function when given in combination with ACE or ARBs [15]. Other corticosteroids like deflazacort, prednisolone or prednisone may also delay the development of cardiomyopathy [16].

As heart failure develops, the incidence of arrhythmias also increases. Although generally known and screened, knowledge about optimal treatment is sparse as the National Heart, Lung and Blood Institute expert group stated [10]. They advised to follow the published general adult heart failure guidelines when considering pharmacologic treatment and the placement of implantable cardiac defibrillators. The DMD Care Considerations Working Group has the same expert-based advice. The use of anticoagulation in cardiomyopathy is not clear in DMD, although it is advised according to the same general heart failure guidelines. Since ischaemic strokes might be more prevalent in DMD patients with cardiomyopathy but without atrial fibrillation, the prescription of anticoagulants is sensible [17].

Becker Muscular Dystrophy

Becker muscular dystrophy is caused by in-frame mutations in the dystrophin gene which lead to reduced or otherwise altered dystrophin protein expression. The incidence of BMD is one third of that of DMD, a much higher figure than was previously thought, implying that BMD has been under-diagnosed in the past [18]. The clinical picture is characterised by later age of onset and slower rate of progression as compared to DMD. However, the spectrum of BMD encompasses a variety of phenotypes, including an intermediate form between BMD and DMD ('outliers'), a 'quadriceps-only' form and a very mild form in which BMD may manifest itself with myalgias and muscle cramps, exercise intolerance and myoglobinuria or asymptomatic elevation of the serum CK activity. In most cases, the first symptoms were noticed between the 6th and 18th year of life with a mean age of onset of 11.1 years [19]. The age of loss of ambulation varies from 10 to 78 years (mean age is in the fourth decade). Becker cardiomyopathy evolves in the same manner as DMD cardiomyopathy. In BMD, the severity of cardiac disease does not correlate with that of skeletal muscle weakness [20]. Certain dystrophin mutations are known to predispose to earlier cardiac involvement [21]. A severe dilated cardiomyopathy can occur in patients with BMD with relatively preserved muscle function.

Management. Patients with BMD should have cardiac evaluation (ECG and echocardiography) at diagnosis [22] Subsequent 5-yearly and preferably 2-yearly screening is recommended [9]. If ECG or structural cardiac evaluation (e.g. echocardiography) has abnormal results, or if the patient has episodes of syncope, near-syncope or palpitations, clinicians should order rhythm evaluation (e.g. Holter or event monitor) [22]. When progressive abnormality is found, they should be seen more regularly and treated with ACE inhibitors and/or beta-blockers [23] Cardiac transplantation may be a viable treatment option in this group of patients [24].

X-Linked Dilated Cardiomyopathy

There are descriptions of male patients who present with early-onset dilated cardiomyopathy and do not develop or have only mild skeletal muscle weakness [25, 26]. Many but not all affected patients have an increased serum CK activity [27]. The disease is being referred to as X-linked dilated cardiomyopathy (XL-LDC). X-LDC may be caused by the presence of a single point mutation at the first exon-intron boundary or a nonsense mutation in exon 29, by a rearrangement downstream from the 5′ end of intron 11 or by a deletion in the mid-rod domain of the dystrophin gene. What all these mutations have in common is that they show a different pattern of expression in cardiac as compared to skeletal muscle [28].

Management. Patients should have cardiac evaluation (ECG and echocardiography) at diagnosis. Subsequent 5-yearly and preferably 2-yearly screening is recommended. When progressive abnormality is found, they should be seen more regularly and treated with ACE inhibitors and, if indicated, beta-blockers. Cardiac transplantation may be a viable treatment in this group of patients.

Female Carriers of Duchenne and Becker Muscular Dystrophy

Carriers of DMD and BMD are at risk of developing dilated cardiomyopathy. The cumulative risk of cardiomyopathy is estimated to be between 7% and 10% [29–31]. Dilated cardiomyopathy (DCM) is more frequently found in carriers who have symptomatic weakness. Cardiac abnormalities in DMD/BMD carriers are progressive, as in patients with DMD/BMD [32].

Management. Echocardiography and ECG are recommended in carriers of DMD and BMD at diagnosis and at least every 5 years thereafter, or more frequently, in patients with abnormalities on investigation. There is no indication to test them presymptomatically before the age of 16 years [9]. Clinical geneticists should refer women for cardiac evaluation when carriership is diagnosed. Carriers manifesting severe skeletal muscle symptoms or cardiac symptoms require more frequent investigation. Once significant abnormalities are detected, patients may benefit from treatment with ACE inhibitors and beta-blockers, if indicated. Ultimately cardiac transplantation may be appropriate [9, 33].

Dystrophin-Associated Glycoprotein Complex Cardiomyopathies

Sarcoglycanopathies (limb-girdle muscular dystrophy *(LGMD) types 2C, D, E and F*) constitute about 25% of the LGMD group and are inherited in an autosomal recessive manner. Limb-girdle muscular dystrophies constitute a heterogeneous group of disorders characterised by progressive weakness of the limb-girdle muscles, i.e. the muscles of hip region and upper leg, and shoulder region and proximal arm. LGMD2C-F are caused by defects in alpha, beta, gamma and delta sarcoglycan, which are part of the sarcoglycan transmembrane component of the dystrophin-associated glycoprotein complex. All types of sarcoglycanopathies can be associated with cardiomyopathy. The clinical course is comparable to that of patients with DMD or severe BMD. The frequency of DCM is around 20%, and DCM is progressive over time [34]. There were no significant differences in median age or severity of disease between patients with or without DCM.

Management. It is recommended to investigate sarcoglycanopathy patients with the same frequency as patients with DMD/BMD (see above) [9]. Present perception is that the incidence of tachy- or bradyarrhythmias in sarcoglycanopathies is low, but the issue has not been fully resolved. Arrhythmia surveillance with Holter ECG or other ambulatory ECG registrations is justified. Standard therapy should be effective in these patients with evidence of cardiomyopathy, but trial-based evidence of efficacy is lacking.

Other Plasma Membrane Proteins

Caveolinopathies. Caveolins are the structural proteins that are necessary for the formation of caveolae membrane domains. Caveolae are vesicular organelles (50–100 nm in diameter) that are particularly abundant in cells of the cardiovascular system. In these cell types, caveolae function both in protein trafficking and signal transduction [35]. The gene encoding for caveolin-3, the muscle-specific form of the caveolin family, is located on chromosome 3. Cardiac myocytes and skeletal muscle fibres express caveolin-3. In skeletal muscle, caveolin-3 is partly associated with the complex of dystrophin-associated proteins. Caveolin-3 mutations, predominantly autosomal dominant but occasionally autosomal recessive, may cause a variety of phenotypes, including LGMD1C, distal myopathy, rippling muscle disease, myoglobinuria and asymptomatic hyper-CKemia. The incidence is unknown. There seems to be no evidence to suggest that cardiac surveillance is indicated routinely in LGMD1C [9, 36]. However, several recent observations of familial hypertrophic cardiomyopathy [36]; sudden death, possibly due to arrhythmia [37]; and long QT syndrome [38] associated with caveolin-3 mutations suggest that cardiac involvement is a feature of caveolin-3 deficiency, and careful cardiac assessment of these patients seems reasonable [39].

Proteins with Enzymatic Activity

LGMD2I/MDC1C

LGMD2I, caused by mutations in the *fukutin-related protein* (FKRP) gene, is an autosomal recessive disorder. The *FKRP* gene is a homologue of the fukutin gene encoding for the fukutin-related protein. FKRP is a putative glycosyltransferase, and the precise function is uncertain. It has been localised in the Golgi apparatus and is involved in the glycosylation processing of α-dystroglycan, an indispensable molecule for binding laminin alpha 2. FKRP is ubiquitously expressed. Mutations in the fukutin-related protein gene (*FKRP*) located on chromosome 19q13 give rise to a spectrum of phenotypes including a form of *congenital muscular dystrophy (MDC1C)*, *Walker-Warburg* phenotype and a relatively mild form of limb-girdle muscular dystrophy (LGMD2I). The most common mutation is the c.826C > A mutation. Patients with a homozygous C826A mutation generally exhibit milder and late-onset muscular dystrophy, whereas the compound heterozygous mutations are associated with more severe and early-onset type of muscular dystrophy phenotypically related to DMD [40, 41]. There are considerable regional differences. In the Netherlands, for example, LGMD2I was diagnosed in only 8% of all LGMD families, whereas in the United Kingdom and Denmark, LGMD2I is considered the most frequent cause of LGMD [41–43].

Left ventricular hypokinesis, dilated cardiomyopathy and heart failure have been reported in 30–80% of LGMD2I patients, regardless of the gene mutation and the severity of the muscular disease, suggesting that all patients should be referred for cardiac evaluation [44, 45].

Management. It is recommended to subject all patients with LGMD2I to evaluation for cardiac involvement (ECG and echocardiography) at diagnosis. After that, 2-year screening seems reasonable [9].

Fukuyama Congenital Muscular Dystrophy

Fukuyama congenital muscular dystrophy (FCMD) is an autosomal recessive disorder, caused by mutations in the fukutin gene on chromosome 9q31 [46]. Its protein product, fukutin, has sequence homologies with bacterial glycosyltransferase, but its precise function is unknown. FCMD also belongs to the group of disorders associated with glycosylation defects of α-dystroglycan, the so-called Walker-Warburg syndromes. The disorder is particularly frequent in Japan where its incidence is 40% of that of DMD, while it is rare in Western countries [47]. FCMD is clinically characterised by a triad of mental retardation, brain deformities and congenital muscular dystrophy.

Typically, patients are able to sit but never attain independent ambulation. Most patients with FCMD develop left ventricular dysfunction by 10 years of age, with progressive deterioration in cardiac function [48]. In contrast, the mildest fukutin-related phenotype, *LGMD2M*, presents with minimal muscle weakness, DCM and normal intelligence [49]. Congenital onset FCMD patients should have yearly cardiac investigations especially after the age of 10 [48]. Late-onset LGMD patients with mutations in the fukutin protein should be evaluated with ECG and echocardiography at diagnosis. After that, 2-year screening seems reasonable.

Inner Nuclear Membrane Proteins

Emery-Dreifuss muscular dystrophy (EDMD) can present as an X-linked (EDMD1), autosomal dominant (EDMD2) and, rarely, autosomal recessive disorder (EDMD3). The disease is characterised by early contractures and a humeroperoneal distribution of muscle weakness. Both emerin and lamin A/C, the causative genes in X-linked and autosomal inherited EDMD, respectively, are nuclear lamina genes. Defects in these genes cause conduction disorders and cardiomyopathy. In case of more prominent limb-girdle muscle weakness in the presence of a lamin A/C mutation, the disorder is called LGMD1B.

X-Linked Emery-Dreifuss Muscular Dystrophy

The gene locus for this entity is located at Xq28, and the *gene* (*EMD* previously named *STA*), which is 2100 bp in length and consists of 6 exons encoding a 254-amino acid serine-rich protein, is called emerin [50]. Emerin mutations identified to date include a few missense mutations, and the majority are nonsense, splice site or small deletions/insertions that ultimately result in premature translation termination and complete absence of emerin expression on both Western blotting and immunohistochemistry. The function of the *emerin* protein which is ubiquitously expressed in all tissues [51] and in all vertebrates remains to be fully elucidated.

Clinically, the disorder is characterised by early contractures of the Achilles tendons, elbows and posterior cervical muscles, often before there is any significant weakness. Subsequently, limitation of neck flexion develops, but later forward flexion of the entire spine becomes limited [52]. Muscle wasting and weakness with a distinctive humeroperoneal distribution early in the course of the disease is slowly progressive. Weakness later extends to the proximal limb-girdle musculature, but is rarely profound. Onset in the first few years of life is not exceptional [53, 54]. The variability of the clinical severity in individual members of the same family appears to be much greater as compared to other forms of muscular dystrophy (even compared to Becker muscular dystrophy). Only very rarely, ambulation is lost as a result of muscle weakness or contractures [53]. Very rare cases seem to be completely asymptomatic still in the fourth decade of life [53].

Cardiac features usually occur in patients' (early) teens or 20s, but a boy as young as 5 years, in whom the heart was involved, has been reported [53]. Cardiac involvement is characterised by cardiac conduction defects, ranging from sinus bradycardia, to prolongation of the PR interval on electrocardiography to complete heart block. Atrial paralysis is almost pathognomonic of EDMD. The finding of a dilated right atrium on echocardiography and isolated atrial paralysis with absent 'P' waves on electrocardiography should always prompt the exclusion of EDMD [55]. The severity of heart disease does not correlate with the degree of skeletal muscle involvement, and cardiac involvement can be very prominent [56]. EDMD affects the atria, and right heart involvement predominates. There is progressive replacement of the normal myocardium by fibrous and adipose tissue, which results in the loss of atrial contractility (atrial paralysis) and atrial dilatation. Evidence of left ventricular dysfunction (in addition to the invariable involvement of the conduction system) was reported by some groups but not by others [53].

As with DMD, there may be some female carriers of this X-linked disease who manifest cardiac disease, in particular, atrial paralysis, albeit usually at a later age than male subjects [56]. No association with any sign of muscle weakness, wasting or contractures appears to be present [53]. Published cases of manifesting carriers may have been diluted by cases of dominant disease.

Management. Cardiological evaluation at diagnosis and annually thereafter using 12-lead ECG (preferably at 50 mm/s) requires expert assessment as ECG changes may be subtle and difficult to interpret [9]. Holter monitoring should be recommended annually for tachy- or bradyarrhythmias. Echocardiography can be done on a less regular basis. Permanent pacemaker implantation is justified, even in asymptomatic patients [9] when ECG begins to show abnormalities of sinus node or AV node disease. However, nocturnal AV-Wenckebach may be a normal finding in young people. In the presence of sino-atrial or AV nodal conduction abnormalities on surface ECG, invasive electrophysiology testing probably adds little to the decision to or timing of pacemaker implantation. However, such testing may have a role in determining the optimum mode of and sites for pacing [9]. Whether implantable defibrillators may be a more appropriate form of management than pacemakers when anti-bradycardia pacing is indicated for these patients is as yet unclear [57].

Anticoagulation is indicated in all patients with emerinopathy who develop sustained supraventricular arrhythmia, regardless of their CHADS-VASc score and even for paroxysmal arrhythmias [58].

It is recommended to establish the carrier status in females at risk and to offer them periodic ECG surveillance including 24-h ambulatory Holter monitoring to detect atrial or AV nodal conduction disease [9]. There is a need for more systematic study of the natural history of cardiac involvement in X-linked EDMD carriers.

Autosomal Inherited EDMD/LGMD1B/L-CMD

Mutations in the *LMNA* gene on chromosome 1q11-q23 [59] encoding *lamins A and C* by alternative splicing cause primary laminopathies, inherited predominantly autosomal dominant, including various types of lipodystrophies, muscular dystrophies (EDMD2 and EDMD3, LGMD1B, L-CMD) and *progeroid syndromes*, *mandibulo-acral dysplasia*, dilated cardiomyopathies, *neuropathy*, restrictive *dermopathy* and *arthropathy* with tendinous calcifications. When looking at *LMNA*-related muscular dystrophies, most cases will have an EDMD phenotype, but in some instances, a limb-girdle phenotype, referred to as LGMD1B, is found as well as congenital forms of muscular dystrophy.

Lamins are nuclear intermediate filaments that form the *nuclear lamina*, which lines the inner nuclear membrane. Lamin proteins have been shown to bind to chromatin and to several inner nuclear membrane proteins.

The pattern and severity of cardiac disease is thought to be more severe in the autosomal dominant form as compared to the X-linked EDMD. Among patients with AD-EDMD, 35% will develop a progressive and potentially life-limiting dilated cardiomyopathy by middle age. Ventricular dysrhythmias are also significant in laminopathy patients and are an important cause of sudden death, despite pacing suggesting that implantation of an ICD is warranted when there is an indication for device implantation [60].

Management. ECG at diagnosis and yearly thereafter. Holter monitoring for tachy- or bradyarrhythmias and echocardiography annually. Prevention of sudden death which is mostly caused by ventricular tacharrhythmia is complex and should be based on implantable defibrillators rather than pacemakers despite the greater risk for complications [61]. These patients should be managed in specialised centres and their data collated to contribute to further evidence in the future. In the meantime, there is a strong indication for defibrillator implantation to be considered when anti-bradycardia pacing is indicated or left ventricular function is severely impaired or in patients with sustained ventricular tachycardia. Four risk factors for malignant ventricular tachyarrhythmias have been identified and can help in selecting patients for prophylactic implantations of cardiac defibrillators: (non-)sustained ventricular tachycardia, male gender, non-missense mutations and mild ventricular dysfunction (left ventricular ejection fraction <45%) [62]. ICD therapy is recommended in primary prevention for patients with two or more risk factors. These recommendations need to be validated over time through the collection of high-quality prospective data [9].

Nucleotide Repeat Disorders with Myotonia

Myotonic Dystrophy

Myotonic dystrophy type 1 (*DM1*, also known as *dystrophia myotonica* or *Steinert's* disease) is an autosomal dominant multisystem disorder and the most common myopathy presenting in adults (incidence 1 in 8000 live births; prevalence is approximately 5 per 100,000 in most American and European populations).

DM1 is caused by an aberrantly expanded CTG repeat in the 3′-untranslated region of the DM protein kinase (DMPK) gene on chromosome 19q13.3. The mutated *DMPK* gene is presumed to have a dominant-negative effect on mRNA and aberrant expression of neighbouring genes due to abnormal number of polynucleotide repeats. The CTG repeat expansion can lead to abnormal splicing of several distantly located genes, including chloride channel, cardiac troponin T and insulin receptor genes. The severity of the disease is related to the repeat length, which can expand from generation to generation (anticipation), and varies from very severe often lethal congenital DM to late-onset mild muscle weakness, myotonia and cataract. Patients with adolescent-onset DM1 characteristically manifest with myotonia (delayed muscle relaxation after contraction); progressive weakness and atrophy of the skeletal muscles, with predominant distal weakness; and facial involvement with involvement of systems other than skeletal muscle, such as the heart, endocrine glands, central nervous system and smooth muscle.

Myocardial fibrosis and degeneration of the cardiac conduction system occur in the majority of patients. Approximately, 90% show ECG abnormalities, commonly prolongation of the PR interval and QRS duration. Arrhythmias can occur, including sinus node dysfunction, progressive heart block, atrial tachycardia, flutter or fibrillation and ventricular tachycardia or fibrillation [63]. Patients with adult DM1 are at high risk for arrhythmias and sudden death, even when a pacemaker was implanted [64, 65]. A rhythm other than sinus, PR interval of 240 msec or more, QRS duration of 120 msec or more or second-degree or third-degree atrioventricular block and a diagnosis of atrial tachyarrhythmia (sustained atrial tachycardia, flutter or fibrillation) predict sudden death [64]. Cardiomyopathy and congestive heart failure occur far less frequently than conduction disturbances. The most prevalent echocardiographic changes are mitral valve prolapse and septal and myocardial fibrosis.

Management. Cardiac evaluation includes annual ECG and Holter monitoring if annual ECG shows increasing PR or QRS intervals or other evidence of increased risk of bradycardia. Echocardiogram should be performed at diagnosis in myotonic dystrophy. Invasive measurement of the HV interval may help decide the need for pacing in borderline cases. If atrial tachyarrhythmias (atrial flutter, fibrillation) become symptomatic, anti-arrhythmic treatment may be justified [9]. However, anti-arrhythmic drugs may aggravate any pre-existing tendency to bradycardia or ventricular tachyarrhythmias. Prophylactic pacing remains the first-line treatment for the prevention of sudden death, which is mainly related to conduction defects in the disease. A strategy based on invasive electrophysiological study in patients with mild conduction defects on their ECG has been associated with an improvement of overall long-term survival related to major reduction of sudden death [66]. A subset of patients remains however exposed to sudden death despite permanent pacing, particularly those with non-sustained tachycardia or severe ventricular dysfunction for whom implantable cardiac defibrillators should be considered.

Myotonic Dystrophy Type 2

Myotonic dystrophy type 2 (DM2), also called *proximal myotonic myopathy (PROMM)*, is present in a large number of families of Northern European ancestry. In Germany, it has the same prevalence as DM1. DM2 is caused by an expanded CCTG tetra-nucleotide repeat in the first intron of the zinc finger protein 9 (ZNF9) gene on chromosome 3q21.

DM2 shares many features with DM1, but the patients have less symptomatic distal, facial and bulbar weakness and less pronounced clinical myotonia. Important other differences include the absence of a congenital form of DM2, no mental retardation in juvenile cases and less evident excessive daytime sleepiness.

The heart involvement is comparable to that in DM1 in its characteristics, though less frequent and delayed in the course of the disease [67]. Complete atrioventricular block occurs in most cases during the seventh decade. The risk for sudden death in DM2 appears to be lower than in DM1. A higher proportion of patients develop left ventricular dysfunction and thromboembolic complications associated with atrial fibrillation. Patients with DM2 should benefit from the same approach for risk stratification and preventive treatments for sudden death as for patients with DM1.

Ion Channel Disorder Associated with Periodic Paralysis and Heart Involvement

Andersen Syndrome

Andersen syndrome is a very rare disease and characterised by the clinical triad of dyskalaemic paralytic attack, ventricular ectopy and potential dysmorphic features. It is inherited as an autosomal dominant trait. Mutations in the potassium channel gene *KCNJ2*, which encodes for the Kir2.1 potassium channel generating the I_{K1} current, have been found. Cardiac disturbances may comprise the long QT syndrome (type 7), ventricular extra-systoles or tachycardia [68]. Tachydysrhythmia may cause syncopal attacks and sudden death. The cardiac symptoms are provoked or worsened by hypokalaemia and digitalis. The *paralytic attacks* may be hyperkalaemic or hypokalaemic, and therefore the response to oral potassium is unpredictable.

Myofibrillar Myopathies

The term *myofibrillar myopathies (MFM)* was proposed as a noncommittal designation for a group of chronic neuromuscular diseases associated with common morphologic features, consisting of a distinct pathologic pattern of myofibrillar disorganisation that begins at the Z-disk and is followed by accumulation of myofibrillar degradation products and ectopic expression of diverse proteins. These disorders are transmitted mainly by autosomal dominant inheritance, and typically manifest as distal myopathies, but may also affect proximal muscles [69]. Mutations in the genes encoding desmin, αB-crystallin, myotilin, ZASP, filamin C, FHL1 and BAG3 have been identified in about half of the patients. Median age of onset is 55 years (range 7–77). Serum CK activity is normal or slightly elevated. Cardiomyopathy, often of the arrhythmogenic type, is a frequent associated feature, particularly for patients with mutations in the *DES* gene who develop in a majority of cases complete atrioventricular blocks and ventricular tachyarrhythmias [70]. Cardiomyopathy has been more often reported in childhood-onset myofibrillar myopathy and can manifest as DCM (*DES*, *FHL1*) and HCM (αB-crystallin, *BAG3*, *FHL1*). Mutations in myotilin cause LGMD1A, and *FHL1* mutations may present with an Emery-Dreifuss phenotype (EDMD6). Cardiac involvement in desminopathies resembles cardiac involvement in laminopathies, and the same guidelines for follow-up and management seem to be appropriate, with a strong indication for prophylactic implantation of a defibrillator.

Congenital Myopathies

Central Core Disease

The core myopathies central core disease (CCD) and multiminicore disease are heterogeneous congenital myopathies. They are most frequently caused by mutations in the *ryanodin receptor (RYR1)* or mutations encoding *selenoprotein (SEPN1)*. Mutations in the skeletal muscle alpha-actinin 1 (*ACTA1*) and titin (*TTN*) can also result in core myopathies [71]. CCD can present with hypotonia and weakness in the neonatal period and a non-progressive course but also with milder phenotypes [71]. It is inherited in an autosomal dominant or autosomal recessive pattern. Dysmorphic features may develop secondary to muscle weakness. An association with the potentially fatal malignant hyperthermia syndrome is well known. Serum CK activity is usually normal. Muscle biopsies reveal well-demarcated cores within most muscle fibres. Cardiac involvement in *RYR1*, *SEPN1* and *ACTA1*-related CCD is rare.

Titin is the largest known protein in nature. It is involved in the intrasarcomeric cytoskeleton, providing tension properties to myofilaments and ensuring the diastolic relaxation of the heart. It has been implicated in several neuromuscular disorders such as autosomal dominant myopathy with proximal muscle weakness and early respiratory failure (HMERF), LGMD2J, congenital or early-onset myopathy with fatal cardiomyopathy, multiminicore disease with heart disease and tibial muscular dystrophy (Udd myopathy) [72]. Among patients with congenital titinopathies, cardiac involvement has been reported in approximately 50% of cases. Dilated cardiomyopathy and left ventricular systolic dysfunction represented the most common pattern and were present at birth in approximately one third of the patients, potentially leading to terminal heart failure. Patients with TTN cardiomyopathy do not show any specific risk for arrhythmic complications compared to patients with other cardiomyopathies. Cardiac follow-up is warranted at diagnosis and thereafter on an annual basis and should include ECG and echocardiogram [73].

Nemaline Rod Myopathy

Defects in 11 thin filament protein genes, including skeletal α-actin *(ACTA1)*, nebulin *(NEB)*, α-tropomyosin *(TPM3)*, β-tropomyosin *(TPM2)*, troponin T *(TNNT1)* and cofilin-2 *(CFL2)*, *KBTBD13, KLHL40* and *41*, *LMOD3* and *MYPN*, have so far been shown to result in nemaline myopathy [71]. Inheritance can be autosomal recessive or dominant. Nemaline myopathy is characterised by the presence of rod-shaped structures in the muscle fibres.

The clinical spectrum of nemaline myopathies is wide, ranging from severe often fatal conditions with prenatal onset to early childhood-onset conditions of varying severity. Disproportionately severe axial and respiratory muscle involvement is common in all variants and is often the long-term prognostic determinant. The condition is otherwise essentially stable, though in a few patients with mutations in

ACTA1, severe progression of weakness in late childhood has been noticed.

Primary cardiac involvement is probably not as rare as presumed. Several cases with nemaline myopathy and dilated or hypertrophic cardiomyopathy leading to heart failure and sudden cardiac death have been described [74, 75].

Myosin Storage Myopathy

Mutations in the myosin heavy-chain gene, *MYH7*, cause autosomal dominant myosin storage myopathy and also Laing distal myopathy. Scapuloperoneal and limb-girdle muscle weakness, congenital fibre-type disproportion and multiminicore disease were also reported in connection of *MYH7*. Mutations in *MYH7* is the most frequent cause of hypertrophic cardiomyopathy. Cardiomyopathy has been described in combination with myosin storage myopathy [76, 77].

Centronuclear Myopathy with Cardiomyopathy

Centronuclear myopathies (CNMs) are characterised by muscle weakness and increased numbers of central nuclei within myofibres. It is a very rare disorder, which can present with diverse phenotypes. Striated muscle preferentially expressed protein kinase (*SPEG*), the product of SPEG complex locus, was identified as an MTM1-interacting protein. *SPEG* is present in cardiac muscle, where it plays a critical role. Recently recessively inherited *SPEG* mutations were demonstrated in centronuclear myopathy with cardiomyopathy [78]. In addition, mutations in titin have been found [71].

Metabolic Disorders Affecting Muscle

Lysosomal Glycogenosis

Pompe's Disease or Glycogen Storage Disease Type 2

Pompe's disease is a rare autosomal recessive disorder caused by mutations in the gene that encodes for *α-glucosidase*. Alpha-glucosidase deficiency causes glycogen to accumulate in various tissues and disrupt function of skeletal and cardiac muscle in particular. Presentation in infancy is associated with respiratory failure, cardiomyopathy and severe muscle weakness. Juvenile- or adult-onset cases typically present with proximal muscle weakness and often develop respiratory insufficiency or exertional dyspnoea due to diaphragmatic involvement [79]. Cardiac involvement in glycogenosis type 2 comprises cardiomyopathy, arrhythmias and cardiac decompensation. The cardiac involvement depends on the residual acid alpha-glucosidase activity and the age at symptom onset. In the late-onset forms, cardiac involvement is rare [80].

Management. Until recently, treatment was focused on supportive measures, and infants diagnosed with classical Pompe's disease usually died within the first year of life. The introduction of enzyme replacement therapy (ERT) with recombinant α-glucosidase has dramatically improved the life expectancy of infantile-onset disease with anecdotal improvements in respiratory and motor function observed in juvenile- or adult-onset cases [81]. Cardiac assessment in infants with glycogenosis type 2 should involve an echocardiogram at diagnosis, followed by check-ups at quarterly intervals during the first 2 years of treatment with ERT and then at 6-monthly intervals. For adult patients, it is advocated to perform an ECG at least once in routine clinical follow-up. Additional echocardiography seems indicated only in those patients with abnormal ECG findings, a history of cardiac disease or evident cardiac symptoms [82].

Danon Disease

Danon disease is caused by a primary deficiency of a major lysosomal membrane glycoprotein, *LAMP2 (lysosome-associated membrane protein 2)*. This is a rare X-linked dominant disorder, characterised by hypertrophic cardiomyopathy, skeletal myopathy and variable degree of mental retardation, with autophagic vacuoles in skeletal and cardiac muscle. Males are more affected than females. In probands, cardiac symptoms, such as exertional dyspnoea, start in teenage years. The association of hypertrophic cardiomyopathy and cardiac arrhythmia is common, and patients typically die of cardiac failure or cardiac arrest in their fourth decade. Problems with the electrical activity in the heart can occur, presenting as 'Wolff-Parkinson-White' syndrome. The myopathy is usually mild. Serum CK activities are 5–10 times elevated [83]. Milder variants of the disease have been described [84].

Management. Patients should have a cardiac investigation, including ECG and echocardiography, at diagnosis. Cardiac investigations should be performed every 1–2 years or more frequently, if an abnormal echocardiogram is identified. Heart transplantation is the reliable treatment once heart failure occurs [85].

Mitochondrial Disorders

Primary Disorders of Mitochondrial Function

These are caused by mutations in both mitochondrial and nuclear genes encoding mitochondrial proteins. They are an increasingly recognised cause of multisystem diseases that have disorders of the central nervous system and skeletal muscle as their predominant manifestations. Because of its dependence on oxidative metabolism, the heart is also frequently involved in *mitochondrial* disease (see Chap. 24). Several mitochondrial syndromes that involve the heart include *Kearns-Sayre syndrome*, *MELAS* (mitochondrial myopathy, encephalopathy, lactic acidosis and stroke-like episodes) and *MERFF* (myoclonic epilepsy with ragged red fibres). Several types of cardiac abnormality including hypertrophic cardiomyopathy, DCM (dilated cardiomyopathy), *Wolff-Parkinson-White syndrome* and cardiac arrhythmia have been described [86]. Conduction disturbances may be an important cause of mortality in patients with Kearns-Sayre syndrome. Terminal heart failure is a common cause of death in patients with any type of mutation and is particularly frequent in patients with m.3243A > G mutation in *MT-TL1*. The following parameters have proven their ability to stratify the long-term risk for cardiac life-threatening complications in any adult patient with mitochondrial disease: left ventricular hypertrophy, ventricular premature contractions, diabetes and intraventricular conduction blocks [87].

Management. Patients should have cardiac evaluation (ECG, echocardiography and Holter) at diagnosis. After that, they should be screened for the development of cardiomyopathy and electrical complications with time intervals that depend on initial evaluation, at least yearly for patients with *Kearns-Sayre syndrome* or *MELAS* with hypertrophic cardiomyopathy. Timely placement of a pacemaker can be life-saving in the presence of conduction block. In patients with isolated cardiomyopathy, cardiac transplantation may be required [88].

Carnitine Deficiency

Carnitine plays an essential role in the transfer of long-chain fatty acids across the inner mitochondrial membrane. This transfer requires enzymes and transporters that accumulate carnitine within the cell (*OCTN2 carnitine transporter*), conjugate it with long-chain fatty acids (*carnitine palmitoyltransferase 1* (*CPT1*)), transfer the acylcarnitine across the inner plasma membrane (*carnitine-acylcarnitine translocase* (*CACT*)) and conjugate the fatty acid back to coenzyme A for subsequent beta-oxidation (*carnitine palmitoyltransferase 2* (*CPT2*)). Deficiency of the OCTN2 carnitine transporter causes primary carnitine deficiency, characterised by increased loss of carnitine in the urine and decreased carnitine accumulation in tissues. Patients can present with hypoketotic hypoglycaemia and hepatic encephalopathy or with muscle weakness and cardiomyopathy. This disease responds to carnitine supplementation [89].

CACT deficiency presents in most cases in the neonatal period with hypoglycaemia, hyperammonaemia and cardiomyopathy with arrhythmia leading to cardiac arrest. Plasma carnitine levels are extremely low.

In CPT1 deficiency, the skeletal muscle and heart are usually unaffected. In adults with deficiency of CPT2, rhabdomyolysis triggered by prolonged exercise may occur. More severe variants of CPT2 deficiency present in the neonatal period similar to CACT deficiency. Treatment for deficiency of CPT2 and CACT consists of a low-fat diet supplemented with medium-chain triglycerides that can be metabolised by mitochondria.

Friedreich's Ataxia

Friedreich's ataxia (FRDA) is an autosomal recessive disorder, in most cases caused by a homozygous expanded GAA repeat (55–1700, normal 7–33) localised in the intron of the frataxin gene on chromosome 9q13. There is an inverse correlation between the length of the GAA repeat and onset of the disease, progression and occurrence of cardiomyopathy [90]. The *frataxin gene* encodes for the frataxin protein located at the inner mitochondrial membrane, the function of which remains to be elucidated.

The estimated prevalence is 2–3 per 100,000 inhabitants. Onset of the disease is usually between 5 and 25 years. Progressive gait ataxia and ataxia of the legs are the first manifestations of the disease. Subsequently, cerebellar dysarthria, ataxia of the arms, oculomotor disturbances, pyramidal features and sensory abnormalities due to involvement of the posterior columns and the peripheral nerves occur. Hypertrophic cardiomyopathy is observed in 60–70% and can even precede cerebellar ataxia. In later stages, DCM may develop. Most patients are wheelchair-bound after a disease duration of 8–15 years. There is a great range in age of death (30–70 years), dependent on the occurrence of cardiac involvement [91].

Management. A 2014 consensus statement for the care of patients with FRDA recommended that an ECG and echocardiogram should be performed at the time of initial diagnosis and then at least annually. A Holter and/or loop monitor assessment should be performed if an individual with FRDA has palpitations [92].

Barth Syndrome

Barth syndrome is an extremely rare X-linked cardioskeletal myopathy caused by a deficiency in tafazzin. *Tafazzin*, a phospholipid acyltransferase, is involved in acyl-specific remodelling of cardiolipin, which promotes structural uniformity and molecular symmetry among the cardiolipin molecular species. Inhibition of this pathway leads to changes in mitochondrial architecture and function [93]. Patients have variable clinical findings, often including heart failure, myopathy, cyclic neutropenia, growth retardation and organic aciduria. Female carriers are not affected. Affected boys usually die of heart failure in infancy or early childhood, but there may be relative improvement in those who survive to later childhood [94].

Management. Patients should have a cardiac investigation, including ECG and echocardiography, at diagnosis and thereafter every 1–2 years, or more frequently, if an abnormal echocardiogram is identified.

Neuropathies

Familial Amyloid Polyneuropathy (TTR Amyloidosis)

Familial amyloid polyneuropathy designates a group of dominantly inherited neuropathies, with extracellular deposition of amyloid substance in various tissues. The disease is characterised by the accumulation of misfolded transthyretin protein (TTR) and is therefore now called TTR amyloidosis. TTR-associated neuropathies are by far the most frequent type with a severe sensorimotor and autonomic neuropathy as the hallmark of the disease, most often associated with cardiac manifestations. First described in Portugal, the disorder was subsequently reported across the world, although Portugal, Japan and Sweden are the three main areas of prevalence. In the past years, an increasing number of mutations have been identified in the TTR gene, along with a larger clinical spectrum than initially thought. Variable age of onset and penetrance are also reported with unclear phenotypic-genotypic correlations. Cardiac involvement consists of failure of the right side, conduction blocks or supraventricular arrhythmias. Over the last 15 years, liver transplantation has enabled improved prognosis of this devastating condition. However, in some patients with substantial cardiac involvement prior to liver transplantation, the cardiac condition continues to worsen, as measured by left ventricular wall thickness and ejection fraction [95]. These findings have led to a very small number of combined liver and heart transplantations in cases of hereditary amyloidosis with cardiac involvement. Recently, new therapeutic strategies have emerged, which stabilise TTR or to silence the TTR gene [96].

Management. Patients should undergo cardiac evaluations including ECG, echocardiography and when possible cardiac MRI at diagnosis and at least on a yearly basis during follow-up. Besides etiological treatment of cardiomyopathy, the treatment of heart failure symptoms includes loop diuretics and spironolactone with a close surveillance of blood pressure and blood ionogram since those patients are prone to hypotension and renal failure in combination with angiotensin-converting enzyme inhibitors. Beta-blockers are not recommended since they are often poorly tolerated as they blunt compensatory tachycardia drive and induce greater negative inotropic effects in amyloid-infiltrated hearts [97]. Prophylactic pacing is generally recommended in patients with conduction defect on their ECG regarding the high risk of progression to complete atrioventricular blocks and sudden death [98].

Charcot-Marie-Tooth Disease Type 2 Caused by Lamin A/C Mutations

Charcot-Marie-Tooth (CMT) disease comprises a group of clinically and genetically heterogeneous hereditary motor and sensory neuropathies, which are clinically characterised by distal muscle weakness and wasting, sensory disturbances and foot and hand deformities. An axonal subtype, CMT2, is defined by (near-)normal nerve conduction velocities in combination with the loss of large myelinated fibres and axonal degeneration on nerve biopsy. CMT2 phenotypes are characterised by a large genetic heterogeneity. In one autosomal recessive subtype of CMT2, mutations in the lamin A/C gene have been found. Mutations in this gene also cause AD-EDMD, LGMD1B and DCM with conduction defects, and therefore, similar cardiac involvement may be anticipated, although, as yet, it has not been described.

Refsum's Disease

This is a rare autosomal recessive peroxisomal disorder. The classic triad encompasses ataxia, retinitis pigmentosa and polyneuropathy. Refsum's disease is caused by an inborn error in the metabolism of a fatty acid, called phytanic acid. All patients have markedly increased serum concentrations of phytanic acid. Cardiomyopathy can occur in the course of the disease, mostly at an advanced stage of the disease. Chronic dietary treatment by restricting the exogenous sources of phytanic acid and its precursor phytol results in clinical improvement.

Summary

A fair proportion of the neuromuscular disorders have a genetic cause. Molecular genetic evaluation can reveal a pathogenic mutation in many cases. Heart involvement is either the direct or indirect cause of death in many of these diseases. It is also of importance to consider the presence of cardiac abnormalities in patients with inherited neuromuscular disease who are to be given a general anaesthetic, because arrhythmias and conduction abnormalities may be precipitated perioperatively.

Cardiac involvement related to the primary skeletal muscle disorder can manifest itself as impulse generation or conduction defects or cardiomyopathy.

Patients with neuromuscular disorders, known to be associated with cardiac pathology, should be referred to a cardiologist for extensive evaluation of ventricular function, impulse formation and conduction diseases. Vice versa, patients presenting with dilated cardiomyopathies due to a gene defect related to a neuromuscular disorder or without a detected genetic cause should always be investigated for subclinical neuromuscular disease (Table 22.1).

Table 22.1 Frequency, type and implications of cardiac involvement in different neuromuscular disorders

Disease (gene/proteins)	Cardiac involvement	% of patients with cardiac involvement	Age at onset	Morbidity/ mortality	Evaluation	Management
Duchenne muscular dystrophy (dystrophin)	ECG abnormalities; DCM	Abnormal ECG > 90%; abnormal echocardiography >90%	Detectable from the age of 6 years onwards	Cardiac death 30–40%	ECG and echocardiography at diagnosis, 2-yearly before 10 years, annually thereafter	ACE inhibitors, beta-blockers
Becker muscular dystrophy (dystrophin)	ECG abnormalities; myocardial hypertrophy and DCM	ECG abnormal, 90%; echocardiography abnormal, 65%	Variable, may be disproportionate to skeletal involvement	Cardiac death in up to 50%	ECG and echocardiography every 2–5 years	ACE inhibitors, beta-blockers, heart transplantation in end-stage DCM in patients with relatively preserved skeletal muscle function
DMD/BMD carriers (dystrophin)	ECG abnormalities; DCM	7–10% dilated cardiomyopathy, ECG abnormalities 20–90%	Variable, may be disproportionate to skeletal muscle involvement		Echo and ECG at diagnosis or after the age of 16 years and at least every 5 years thereafter	ACE inhibitors, beta-blockers, cardiac transplantation in end-stage DCM
X-DCM (dystrophin)	ECG abnormalities; DCM	100% by definition	No evident muscle weakness	Cardiac transplantation sometimes necessary	ECG and echocardiography every 2–5 years	ACE inhibitors, beta-blockers. Cardiac transplantation in end-stage DCM
Sarcoglycanopathies (LGMD2C-F) (sarcoglycans)	ECG abnormalities; DCM	20–25%	Variable	Cardiac transplantation sometimes necessary	ECG and echocardiography every 2–5 years	ACE inhibitors, beta-blockers. Cardiac transplantation in end-stage DCM
LGMD1C (caveolin-3)	HCM, long QT	Case reports				
LGMD2I/MDC1C (FKRP)	ECG abnormalities DCM	1/3 of adult-onset cases	Possibly related to severity of overall disease		ECG and echocardiography at diagnosis, every 2 years thereafter	ACE inhibitors, beta-blockers
Fukutin congenital muscular dystrophy/LGMD2M (fukutin)	DCM	Case reports			Late-onset cases: ECG and echocardiography at at diagnosis	ACE inhibitors, beta-blockers, diagnosis, every 2 years thereafter
X-EDMD (emerin)	AV block, atrial paralysis, atrial flutter and fibrillation	>95% by the age of 30 years	10–39	SCD common in non-paced and to a lower extent in paced individuals	ECG and Holter at diagnosis and annually thereafter	Pacemaker or cardiac defibrillator
AD-EDMD/LGMD1B/myofibrillar myopathies (lamin A/C, desmin, alpha-B-crystallin, myotilin, FHL1)	AV block, atrial flutter and fibrillation; HCM; DCM	Rhythm and conduction disturbances >95% by the age of 30 years, DCM 35%		SCD despite pacing, heart failure	ECG and Holter at diagnosis and annually thereafter	ICD, ACE inhibitors, beta-blockers, cardiac transplantation in end-stage DCM
Titinopathies – congenital and early childhood myopathy	DCM	> 50%	Congenital and childhood	Terminal heart failure	ECG and echocardiogram at diagnosis and annually thereafter	Conventional heart failure therapy

(continued)

Table 22.1 (continued)

Disease (gene/proteins)	Cardiac involvement	% of patients with cardiac involvement	Age at onset	Morbidity/ mortality	Evaluation	Management
DM1/DM2 (DMPK)	AV conduction disturbances, atrial flutter and fibrillation, ventricular tachyarrhythmias	90% ECG abnormalities		SCD 30%	ECG and Holter at diagnosis and annually thereafter, echocardiogram	Pacemaker
Andersen syndrome (KCNJ2)	Long QT syndrome, ventricular extra-systoles or tachycardia			Syncopal attacks sudden death; provoked by hypokalaemia and digitalis		
RYR1, SEPN1, TTN	Cardiomyopathy	Reports				
Pompe's disease (alpha-glucosidase)	Cardiomyopathy in neonatal/childhood cases	Rare in adult-onset cases			In infants echocardiography with 3–6-month interval; ECG at least once in adult-onset cases	Enzyme replacement therapy
Danon disease (LAMP2)	HCM			Cardiac failure or cardiac arrest in fourth decade	ECG and echocardiography at diagnosis. Every 1–2 years thereafter	Cardiac transplantation in end-stage HCM
Mitochondrial	HCM, DCM, Wolff-Parkinson-White syndrome and cardiac arrhythmia, conduction disturbances				ECG, Holter ECG and echocardiography at diagnosis and during follow-up according to initial risk stratification	Pacemaker, cardiac transplantation in end-stage DCM
Carnitine deficiency	Cardiomyopathy, arrhythmia					Dietary treatment
Barth syndrome (tafazzin)	DCM, HCM			Heart failure in infancy or early childhood	ECG and echocardiography at diagnosis and thereafter every 1–2 years	
Familial amyloid neuropathy (TTR, apolipoprotein A1, gelsolin)	HCM, DCM					Liver (+heart) transplantation
Refsum's disease	HCM, DCM		Later stages of the disease			Dietary treatment
Friedreich's ataxia (frataxin)	HCM, DCM	60–70%		Cardiac involvement determines age of death	ECG and echocardiography at diagnosis, re-screening every 3–5 years	Idebenone

DCM denotes dilated cardiomyopathy, *HCM* denotes hypertrophic cardiomyopathy, *ACE* denotes angiotensin-converting enzyme, *SCD* denotes sudden cardiac death, *AV* denotes atrioventricular, *X* denotes X-linked, *AD* denotes autosomal dominant, *DM1* denotes myotonic dystrophy type 1, *DM2* denotes myotonic dystrophy type 2

References

1. Finsterer J, Stollberger C. Cardiac involvement in primary myopathies. Cardiology. 2000;94(1):1–11.
2. Mokri B, Engel AG. Duchenne dystrophy: electron microscopic findings pointing to a basic or early abnormality in the plasma membrane of the muscle fiber. Neurology. 1975 Dec;25(12):1111–20.
3. Head SI, Williams DA, Stephenson DG. Abnormalities in structure and function of limb skeletal muscle fibres of dystrophic mdx mice. Proc Biol Sci. 1992 May 22;248(1322):163–9.
4. Nigro G, Comi LI, Politano L, Bain RJI. The incidence and evolution of cardiomyopathy in Duchenne muscular dystrophy. Int J Cardiol. 1990;26:271–7.
5. van Essen AJ, Busch HF, te Meerman GJ, ten Kate LP. Birth and population prevalence of Duchenne muscular dystrophy in the Netherlands. Hum Genet. 1992;88(3):258–66.
6. Ricotti V, Ridout DA, Scott E, Quinlivan R, Robb SA, Manzur AY, Muntoni F, North Star Clinical Network. Long-term benefits and adverse effects of intermittent versus daily glucocorticoids in boys with Duchenne muscular dystrophy. J Neurol Neurosurg Psychiatry. 2013;84(6):698–705.
7. Eagle M, Baudouin SV, Chandler C, Giddings DR, Bullock R, Bushby K. Survival in Duchenne muscular dystrophy: improvements in life expectancy since 1967 and the impact of home nocturnal ventilation. Neuromuscul Disord. 2002 Dec;12(10):926–9.
8. Villa CR, Czosek RJ, Ahmed H, Khoury PR, Anderson JB, Knilans TK, Jefferies JL, Wong B, Spar DS. Ambulatory monitoring and arrhythmic outcomes in pediatric and adolescent patients with Duchenne muscular dystrophy. J Am Heart Assoc. 2015 Dec 31;5(1) https://doi.org/10.1161/JAHA.115.002620.
9. Bushby K, Muntoni F, Bourke JP. 107th ENMC international workshop: the management of cardiac involvement in muscular dystrophy and myotonic dystrophy. 7th-9th June 2002, Naarden, the Netherlands. Neuromuscul Disord. 2003 Feb;13(2):166–72.
10. McNally EM, Kaltman JR, Benson DW, Working Group of the National Heart, Lung, and Blood Institute; Parent Project Muscular Dystrophy, et al. Contemporary cardiac issues in Duchenne muscular dystrophy. Working Group of the National Heart, Lung, and Blood Institute in collaboration with Parent Project Muscular Dystrophy. Circulation. 2015 May 5;131(18):1590–8.
11. Birnkrant DJ, Bushby KMD, Bann CM, et al. Diagnosis and management of Duchenne muscular dystrophy part 2: respiratory, cardiac, bone health and orthopaedic management. Lancet Neurol. 2018;17(4):347–61.
12. Power LC, O'Grady GL, Hornung TS, et al. Imaging the heart to detect cardiomyopathy in Duchenne muscular dystrophy: a review. Neuromuscul Disord. 2018 Sep;28(9):717–30.
13. Buddhe S, Lewin M, Olson A, Ferguson M, Soriano BD. Comparison of left ventricular function assessment between echocardiography and MRI in Duchenne muscular dystrophy. Pediatr Radiol. 2016 Sep;46(10):1399–408.
14. Brunklaus A, Parish E, Muntoni F, et al. The value of cardiac MRI versus echocardiography in the pre-operative assessment of patients with Duchenne muscular dystrophy. Eur J Paediatr Neurol. 2015;19:395–401.
15. Raman SV, Hor KN, Mazur W, et al. Eplerenone for early cardiomyopathy in Duchenne muscular dystrophy: a randomized, double-blind, placebo-controlled trial. Lancet Neurol. 2015 Feb;14(2):153–61.
16. Barber BJ, Andrews JG, Lu Z, et al. Oral corticosteriods and onset of cardiomyopathy in Duchenne muscular dystrophy. J Pediatr. 2013 Oct;163(4):1080–4.
17. Winterholler M, Holländer C, Kerling F, et al. Stroke in Duchenne muscular dystrophy: a retrospective longitudinal study in 54 patients. Stroke. 2016 Aug;47(8):2123–6.
18. Iodice F, Testa G, Averardi M, Brancaccio G, Amodeo A, Cogo P. Implantation of a left ventricular assist device as a destination therapy in Duchenne muscular dystrophy patients with end stage cardiac failure: management and lessons learned. Neuromuscul Disord. 2015 Jan;25(1):19–23.
19. Bushby KM, Thambyayah M, Gardner-Medwin D. Prevalence and incidence of Becker muscular dystrophy. Lancet. 1991;337(8748):1022–4.
20. Emery AE, Skinner R. Clinical studies in benign (Becker type) X-linked muscular dystrophy. Clin Genet. 1976;10(4):189–201.
21. Casazza F, Brambilla G, Salvato A, Morandi L, Gronda E, Bonacina E. Dilated cardiomyopathy and successful cardiac transplantation in Becker's muscular dystrophy. Follow-up after two years. G Ital Cardiol. 1988;18(9):753–7.
22. Narayanaswami P, Weiss M, Selcen D, et al. Evidence-based guideline summary: diagnosis and treatment of limb-girdle and distal dystrophies. Neurology. 2014;83:1453–63.
23. Kwon HW, Kwon BS, Kim GB, et al. The effect of Enalapril and Carvedilol on left ventricular dysfunction in middle childhood an adolescent patients with muscular dystrophy. Korean Circ J. 2012 Mar;42(3):184–91.
24. Hoogerwaard EM, De Voogt WG, Wilde AAM, et al. Evolution of cardiac abnormalities in Becker muscular dystrophy over a 13-year period. J Neurol. 1997;244:657–63.
25. Muntoni F, Cau M, Ganau A, et al. Deletion of the dystrophin muscle-promotor region associated with X-linked dilated cardiomyopathy. N Engl J Med. 1993;329:921–5.
26. Towbin JA, Fielding Hejtmancik J, Brink P, et al. X-linked dilated cardiomyopathy. Circulation. 1993;87:1854–65.
27. Muntoni F, Di LA, Porcu M, et al. Dystrophin gene abnormalities in two patients with idiopathic dilated cardiomyopathy. Heart. 1997 Dec;78(6):608–12.
28. Ferlini A, Galié N, Merlini L, Sewry C, Branzi A, Muntoni F. A novel Alu-like element rearranged in the dystrophin gene causes a splicing mutation in a family with X-linked dilated cardiomyopathy. Am J Hum Genet. 1998 Aug;63(2):436–46.
29. Hoogerwaard EM, van der Wouw PA, Wilde AAM, et al. Cardiac involvement in carriers of Duchenne and Becker muscular dystrophy. Neuromuscul Disord. 1999;9:347–51.
30. Politano L, Nigro V, Nigro G, et al. Development of cardiomyopathy in female carriers of Duchenne and Becker muscular dystrophy. JAMA. 1996;275:1335–8.
31. Grain L, Cortina-Borja M, Forfar C, Hilton-Jones D, Hopkin J, Burch M. Cardiac abnormalities and skeletal muscle weakness in carriers of Duchenne and Becker muscular dystrophies and controls. Neuromuscul Disord. 2001 Mar;11(2):186–91.
32. Schade van Westrum SM, Hoogerwaard EM, Dekker L, et al. Cardiac abnormalities in a follow-up study on carriers of Duchenne and Becker muscular dystrophy. Neurology. 2011 Jul 5;77(1):62–6.
33. Rees W, Schuler S, Hummel M, Hetzer R. Heart transplantation in patients with muscular dystrophy associated with end-stage cardiomyopathy. J Heart Lung Transplant. 1993 Sep;12(5):804–7.
34. Schade van Westrum SM, Dekker LR, de Voogt WG, Wilde AA, Ginjaar IB, de Visser M, van der Kooi AJ. Cardiac involvement in Dutch patients with sarcoglycanopathy: a cross-sectional cohort and follow-up study. Muscle Nerve. 2014 Dec;50(6):909–13.
35. Williams TM, Lisanti MP. The Caveolin genes: from cell biology to medicine. Ann Med. 2004;36(8):584–95.
36. Hayashi T, Arimura T, Ueda K, et al. Identification and functional analysis of a caveolin-3 mutation associated with familial hypertrophic cardiomyopathy. Biochem Biophys Res Commun. 2004 Jan 2;313(1):178–84.
37. Cronk LB, Ye B, Kaku T, et al. Novel mechanism for sudden infant death syndrome: persistent late sodium current secondary to mutations in caveolin-3. Heart Rhythm. 2007 Feb;4(2):161–6.

38. Vatta M, Ackerman MJ, Ye B, et al. Mutant caveolin-3 induces persistent late sodium current and is associated with long-QT syndrome. Circulation. 2006 Nov 14;114(20):2104–12.
39. Goodwin FC, Muntoni F. Cardiac involvement in muscular dystrophies: molecular mechanisms. Muscle Nerve. 2005 Jun 2;32(5):577–88.
40. Brockington M, Yuva Y, Prandini P, et al. Mutations in the fukutin-related protein gene (FKRP) identify limb girdle muscular dystrophy 2I as a milder allelic variant of congenital muscular dystrophy MDC1C. Hum Mol Genet. 2001 Dec 1;10(25):2851–9.
41. Poppe M, Cree L, Bourke J, et al. The phenotype of limb-girdle muscular dystrophy type 2I. Neurology. 2003 Apr 22;60(8):1246–51.
42. van der Kooi AJ, Frankhuizen WS, Barth PG, et al. Limb-girdle muscular dystrophy in the Netherlands: gene defect identified in half the families. Neurology. 2007 Jun 12;68(24):2125–8.
43. Sveen ML, Schwartz M, Vissing J. High prevalence and phenotype-genotype correlations of limb girdle muscular dystrophy type 2I in Denmark. Ann Neurol. 2006 May;59(5):808–15.
44. Wahbi K, Meune C, Hamouda EH, et al. Cardiac assessment of limb-girdle muscular dystrophy 2I patients: an echography, Holter ECG and magnetic resonance imaging study. Neuromuscul Disord. 2008 Aug;18(8):650–5.
45. Petri H, Sveen ML, Thune JJ, Vissing C, Dahlqvist JR, Witting N, Bundgaard H, Køber L, Vissing J. Progression of cardiac involvement in patients with limb-girdle type 2 and Becker muscular dystrophies: a 9-year follow-up study. Int J Cardiol. 2015 Mar 1;182:403–11.
46. Kobayashi K, Nakahori Y, Miyake M, et al. An ancient retrotransposal insertion causes Fukuyama-type congenital muscular dystrophy. Nature. 1998 Jul 23;394(6691):388–92.
47. Toda T, Kobayashi K, Kondo-Iida E, Sasaki J, Nakamura Y. The Fukuyama congenital muscular dystrophy story. Neuromuscul Disord. 2000 Mar;10(3):153–9.
48. Murakami T, Hayashi YK, Noguchi S, et al. Fukutin gene mutations cause dilated cardiomyopathy with minimal muscle weakness. Ann Neurol. 2006 Nov;60(5):597–602.
49. Nakanishi T, Sakauchi M, Kaneda Y, et al. Cardiac involvement in Fukuyama-type congenital muscular dystrophy. Pediatrics. 2006;117(6):e1187–92.
50. Bione S, Maestrini E, Rivella S, et al. Identification of a novel X-linked gene responsible for Emery-Dreifuss muscular dystrophy. Nat Genet. 1994;8:323–7.
51. Manilal S, Nguyen TM, Sewry CA, Morris GE. The Emery-Dreifuss muscular dystrophy protein, emerin, is a nuclear membrane protein. Hum Mol Genet. 1996 Jun;5(6):801–8.
52. Emery AE. Emery-Dreifuss muscular dystrophy – a 40 year retrospective. Neuromuscul Disord. 2000 Jun;10(4–5):228–32.
53. Wehnert M, Muntoni F. 60th ENMC international workshop: non X-linked Emery-Dreifuss muscular dystrophy 5–7 June 1998, Naarden, The Netherlands. Neuromuscul Disord. 1999 Mar;9(2):115–21.
54. Talkop UA, Talvik I, Sonajalg M, et al. Early onset of cardiomyopathy in two brothers with X-linked Emery-Dreifuss muscular dystrophy. Neuromuscul Disord. 2002 Nov;12(9):878–81.
55. Buckley AE, Dean J, Mahy IR. Cardiac involvement in Emery Dreifuss muscular dystrophy: a case series. Heart. 1999 Jul;82(1):105–8.
56. Sakata K, Shimizu M, Ino H, et al. High incidence of sudden cardiac death with conduction disturbances and atrial cardiomyopathy caused by a nonsense mutation in the STA gene. Circulation. 2005 Jun 28;111(25):3352–8.
57. Nigro G, Russo V, Ventriglia VA, et al. Early onset of cardiomyopathy and primary prevention of sudden death in X-linked Emery–Dreifuss muscular dystrophy. Neuromuscul Disord. 2010;20:174–7.
58. Silvestri NJ, Ismail H, Zimetbaum P, Raynor EM. Cardiac involvement in the muscular dystrophies. Muscle Nerve. 2018 May;57(5):707–15.
59. Bonne G, Di Barletta MR, Varnous S, et al. Mutations in the gene encoding Lamin A/C cause autosomal dominant Emery-Dreifuss muscular dystrophy. Nat Genet. 1999 Mar;21(3):285–8.
60. van Berlo JH, de Voogt WG, van der Kooi AJ, et al. Meta-analysis of clinical characteristics of 299 carriers of LMNA gene mutations: do Lamin A/C mutations portend a high risk of sudden death? J Mol Med. 2005 Jan;83(1):79–83.
61. Curtis JP, Luebbert JJ, Wang Y, et al. Association of physician certification and outcomes among patients receiving an implantable cardioverter-defibrillator. JAMA. 2009 Apr 22;301(16):1661–70.
62. Van Rijsingen IA, Arbustini E, Elliott PM, et al. Risk factors for malignant ventricular arrhythmias in Lamin a/c mutation carriers: a European cohort study. J Am Coll Cardiol. 2012 Jan 31;59(5):493–500.
63. Sovari AA, Bodine CK, Farokhi F. Cardiovascular manifestations of myotonic dystrophy-1. Cardiol Rev. 2007 Jul;15(4):191–4.
64. Groh WJ, Groh MR, Saha C, et al. Electrocardiographic abnormalities and sudden death in myotonic dystrophy type 1. N Engl J Med. 2008 Jun 19;358(25):2688–97.
65. Hermans MC, Faber CG, Pinto YM. Sudden death in myotonic dystrophy. N Engl J Med. 2008 Oct 9;359(15):1626–8.
66. Wahbi K, Babuty D, Probst V, et al. Incidence and predictors of sudden death, major conduction defects and sustained ventricular tachyarrhythmias in 1388 patients with myotonic dystrophy type 1. Eur Heart J. 2017;38(10):751–8.
67. Wahbi K, Christophe Meune C, Henri Marc Becane HM, et al. left ventricular arrhythmias are frequent in type 2 myotonic dystrophy: a case control study. Elsevier. Neuromuscul Disord. 2009;19:468–72.
68. Sansone V, Griggs RC, Meola G, et al. Andersen's syndrome: a distinct periodic paralysis. Ann Neurol. 1997 Sep;42(3):305–12.
69. Selcen D. Myofibrillar myopathies. Curr Opin Neurol. 2008 Oct;21(5):585–9.
70. Wahbi K, Béhin A, Charron P, Dunand M, Richard P, Meune C, Vicart P, Laforêt P, Stojkovic T, Bécane HM, Kuntzer T, Duboc D. High cardiovascular morbidity and mortality in myofibrillar myopathies due to DES gene mutations: a 10-year longitudinal study. Neuromuscul Disord. 2012 Mar 22;22(3):211–8.
71. Mah JK, Joseph JT. An overview of congenital myopathies. Continuum. 2016;22(6):1932–53.
72. Savarese M, Sarparanta J, Vihola A, et al. Increasing role of Titin mutations in neuromuscular disorders. Journal of Neuromuscular Diseases. 2016;3:293–308.
73. Oates EC, Jones KJ, Donkervoort S, et al. Congenital Titinopathy: comprehensive characterization and pathogenic insights. Ann Neurol. 2018;83(6):1105–24.
74. Feng JJ, Marston S. Genotype-phenotype correlations in ACTA1 mutations that cause congenital myopathies. Neuromuscul Disord. 2009 Jan;19(1):6–16.
75. Finsterer J, Stollberger C. Review of cardiac disease in Nemaline myopathy. Pediatr Neurol. 2015;53:473–7.
76. Tajsharghi H, Oldfors A, Macleod DP, Swash M. Homozygous mutation in MYH7 in myosin storage myopathy and cardiomyopathy. Neurology. 2007 Mar 20;68(12):962.
77. Uro-Coste E, Arne-Bes MC, Pellissier JF, et al. Striking phenotypic variability in two familial cases of myosin storage myopathy with a MYH7 Leu1793pro mutation. Neuromuscul Disord. 2009 Feb;19(2):163–6.
78. Agrawal PB, Pierson CR, Joshi M, Liu X, Ravenscroft G, Moghadaszadeh B, Talabere T, Viola M, Swanson LC, Haliloğlu G, Talim B, Yau KS, Allcock RJ, Laing NG, Perrella MA, Beggs AH. SPEG interacts with myotubularin, and its deficiency causes

centronuclear myopathy with dilated cardiomyopathy. Am J Hum Genet. 2014 Aug 7;95(2):218–26.
79. Hagemans ML, Hop WJ, Van Doorn PA, Reuser AJ, Van der Ploeg AT. Course of disability and respiratory function in untreated late-onset Pompe disease. Neurology. 2006 Feb 28;66(4):581–3.
80. Sacconi S, Wahbi K, Theodore G, Garcia J, Salviati L, Bouhour F, Vial C, Duboc D, Laforêt P, Desnuelle C. Atrio-ventricular block requiring pacemaker in patients with late onset Pompe disease. Neuromuscul Disord. 2014 Jul;24(7):648–50.
81. Van der Beek NA, Hagemans ML, Van der Ploeg AT, Reuser AJ, Van Doorn PA. Pompe disease (glycogen storage disease type II): clinical features and enzyme replacement therapy. Acta Neurol Belg. 2006 Jun;106(2):82–6.
82. Van der Beek NA, Soliman OI, van Capelle CI, et al. Cardiac evaluation in children and adults with Pompe disease sharing the common c.-32–13T>G genotype rarely reveals abnormalities. J Neurol Sci. 2008 Dec 15;275(1–2):46–50.
83. Danon MJ, Oh SJ, DiMauro S, et al. Lysosomal glycogen storage disease with normal acid maltase. Neurology. 1981 Jan;31(1):51–7.
84. van der Kooi AJ, van Langen IM, Aronica E, et al. Extension of the clinical spectrum of Danon disease. Neurology. 2008 Apr 15;70(16):1358–9.
85. Cheng Z, Fang Q. Danon disease: focusing on heart. J Hum Genet. 2012;57:407–10.
86. Ozawa T, Tanaka M, Sugiyama S, Hattori K, Ito T, Ohno K, Takahashi A, Sato W, Takada G, Mayumi B, et al. Multiple mitochondrial DNA deletions exist in cardiomyocytes of patients with hypertrophic or dilated cardiomyopathy. Biochem Biophys Res Commun. 1990 Jul 31;170(2):830–6.
87. Wahbi K, Bougouin W, Béhin A, et al. Long-term cardiac prognosis and risk stratification in 260 adults presenting with mitochondrial diseases. Eur Heart J. 2015 Nov;36(42):2886–93.
88. Tranchant C, Mousson B, Mohr M, et al. Cardiac transplantation in an incomplete Kearns-Sayre syndrome with mitochondrial DNA deletion. Neuromuscul Disord. 1993 Sep;3(5–6):561–6.
89. Fu L, Huang M, Chen S. Primary Carnitine deficiency and cardiomyopathy. Korean Circulation Journal. 2013 Dec;43(12):785–92.
90. Bit-Avragim N, Perrot A, Schols L, et al. The GAA repeat expansion in intron 1 of the frataxin gene is related to the severity of cardiac manifestation in patients with Friedreich's ataxia. J Mol Med. 2001;78(11):626–32.
91. Weidemann F, Stork S, Liu D, et al. Cardiomyopathy of Friedreich Ataxia. J Neurochem. 2013;126:88–93.
92. Corben LA, Lynch D, Pandolfo M, Schulz JB, Delatycki MB. Clinical Management Guidelines Writing Group Consensus clinical management guidelines for Friedreich ataxia. Orphanet J Rare Dis. 2014 Nov 30;9:184.
93. Barth PG, Valianpour F, Bowen VM, et al. X-linked cardioskeletal myopathy and neutropenia (Barth syndrome): an update. Am J Med Genet A. 2004 May 1;126A(4):349–54.
94. Barth PG, Wanders RJ, Vreken P. X-linked cardioskeletal myopathy and neutropenia (Barth syndrome)-MIM 302060. J Pediatr. 1999 Sep;135(3):273–6.
95. Stangou AJ, Hawkins PN, Heaton ND, et al. Progressive cardiac amyloidosis following liver transplantation for familial amyloid polyneuropathy: implications for amyloid fibrillogenesis. Transplantation. 1998 Jul 27;66(2):229–33.
96. Maurer MS, Schwartz JH, Gundapaneni B, et al. Tafamidis treatment for patients with Transthyretin amyloid cardiomyopathy. N J Med. 2018 Sep 13;379(11):1007–16.
97. Ruberg FL, Berk JL. Transthyretin (TTR) cardiac amyloidosis. Circulation. 2012 Sep 4;126(10):1286–300.
98. Algalarrondo V, Dinanian S, Juin C, Chemla D, Bennani SL, Sebag C, Planté V, Le Guludec D, Samuel D, Adams D, Slama MS. Prophylactic pacemaker implantation in familial amyloid polyneuropathy. Heart Rhythm. 2012 Jul;9(7):1069–75.

Genetic Disorders of Lipoprotein Metabolism: Diagnosis and Management

23

A. J. Cupido, R. M. Stoekenbroek, and J. J. P. Kastelein

Abbreviations

ANGPTL3	angiopoietin-like 3
ABC	Adenosine triphosphate (ATP) binding cassette
ACAT	Acyl-coenzyme A: Cholesterol O-acyltransferase
Apo-A1	Apolipoprotein A1
ASO	Antisense oligonucleotide
BASs	Bile acid sequestrants
CAD	Coronary artery disease
CE	Cholesterylester
CETP	Cholesterylester transfer protein
CHD	Coronary heart disease
cIMT	Carotid intima media thickness
CVD	Cardiovascular disease
EMA	European Medicines Agency
FCH	Familial combined hyperlipidemia
FD	Familial dysbetalipoproteinemia
FDA	Food and Drug Administration
FDB	Familial defective apolipoprotein B
FH	Familial hypercholesterolemia
FHTG	Familial hypertriglyceridemia
HDL-C	High-density lipoprotein cholesterol
HL	Hepatic lipase
HMG-CoA	3-Hydroxyl-3-methylglutaryl coenzyme A
IDL	Intermediate-density lipoprotein
LCAT	Lecithin:cholesteryl acyltransferase
LDL-C	Low-density lipoprotein cholesterol
LDL-R	Low-density lipoprotein receptor
LDLRAP	LDL-receptor-adapting protein
LIPC	Gene-encoding hepatic lipase
LIPG	Gene-encoding endothelial lipase
LPL	Lipoprotein lipase
NPC1L1	Niemann-Pick C1 like 1
PCSK9	Proprotein convertase subtilisin/kexin type 9
PLTP	Phospholipid transfer protein
RCT	Reverse cholesterol transport
SNP	Single nucleotide polymorphism
SR-B1	Scavenger receptor B1
TC	Total cholesterol
VLDL	Very low-density lipoprotein

A. J. Cupido · R. M. Stoekenbroek · J. J. P. Kastelein (✉)
Department of Vascular Medicine, Amsterdam University Medical Centers - location AMC, University of Amsterdam, Amsterdam, The Netherlands
e-mail: a.j.cupido@amsterdamumc.nl
j.j.kastelein@amsterdamumc.nl; j.s.jansen@amc.nl

Introduction

Atherosclerosis, leading to ischemic manifestations in different vascular beds, is the leading cause of morbidity and mortality worldwide. It is a multifactorial disease, driven by a combination of genetic, environmental, and behavioral factors. The process of atherosclerosis accelerates in the presence of classical risk factors such as *dyslipidemia,* hypertension, diabetes mellitus, obesity, and smoking. Dyslipidemia is one of the major contributors to atherosclerosis and includes both elevated low-density lipoprotein cholesterol (*LDL-C*) and remnant cholesterol levels, as well as decreased high-density lipoprotein cholesterol (*HDL-C*) levels [1]. The crucial role of increased plasma LDL-C levels in the pathogenesis of atherosclerosis has been well established. This also applies to the pharmacological reduction of plasma LDL-C levels accomplished by 3-hydroxyl-3-methylglutaryl coenzyme A (HMG-CoA) reductase inhibitors or *statins.* A large prospective meta-analysis including over 90,000 individuals demonstrated that an LDL-C reduction of 1 mmol/L is associated with a 21% reduction in major cardiovascular events [2]. In addition, decreased plasma HDL-C levels are an independent predictor of cardiovascular disease (CVD), as has been unequivocally established by numerous epidemiological studies. Almost 40% of patients with premature coronary artery disease (CAD) have low HDL-C levels, either alone or in conjunction with hypertriglyceridemia or combined hyperlipidemia [3]. However, whether raising HDL-C by pharmacological means

H. F. Baars et al. (eds.), *Clinical Cardiogenetics*, https://doi.org/10.1007/978-3-030-45457-9_23

will result in cardiovascular benefit is questionable. A meta-regression analysis of 108 randomized controlled trials, including more than 300,000 patients using several lipid-modifying interventions, did not show a relationship between treatment-induced increases in HDL-C and a decrease in coronary heart disease events or deaths when corrected for concurrent LDL-C reductions [4]. Nevertheless, this study does not prove that increasing HDL-C in selected patients with low HDL-C levels has no value [5]. In addition, these studies evaluated only HDL-C concentrations and did not address HDL functionality.

Finally, *hypertriglyceridemia* also influences CVD risk. Several epidemiological and genetic studies have indicated elevated plasma triglyceride levels as an independent risk factor for CVD [6–12]. This also applies to remnant cholesterol [10]. For individuals with high triglycerides in the general population, the risks for myocardial infarction, ischemic heart disease, ischemic stroke, and all-cause mortality are significantly increased [10]. In addition, Mendelian randomization studies also established triglycerides as a causal factor for CVD [13].

Although dyslipidemia has a largely polygenic background, a number of *monogenetic disorders* have been identified. Timely identification and diagnosis of monogenic (or sometimes polygenic) lipid disorders is important, as the causal effect of lipid disturbances on the risk of disease seem additive over a lifetime [14]. For example, it has been shown that patients with a monogenic FH mutation (reviewed below) are at higher risk for CVD compared to patients with a polygenic cause or patients from the general population with similarly high LDL-C levels [15]. This chapter provides an overview of genetic causes underlying disturbances in lipid and lipoprotein metabolism, in which the focus will be primarily on these monogenetic disorders. The chapter starts with a global overview of lipid and lipoprotein metabolism, followed by the genetic background of disturbances in LDL-C and HDL-C levels, respectively. Finally, genetic causes of disorders in triglyceride metabolism are also discussed. For each of these categories, genetics, clinical phenotype, diagnosis, and management will be addressed.

Structure of Lipids and Lipoproteins

Cholesterol and *triglycerides* exert essential functions in body cell membranes and in hormone and energy homeostasis. Due to their hydrophobic properties, cholesterol and triglycerides are transported in large macromolecular complexes, the so-called lipoproteins. *Lipoproteins* contain a core of hydrophobic lipids surrounded by hydrophilic molecules such as phospholipids, unesterified cholesterol, and *apolipoproteins*. The latter are proteins that provide structural integrity to the lipoprotein and serve as ligands for binding to specific receptors. Based on their relative density, lipoproteins can be categorized into five major classes: chylomicrons, very low-density lipoproteins (*VLDL*), intermediate-density lipoproteins (*IDL*), *LDL*, and *HDL*. The first two categories are large, buoyant triglyceride-rich particles, whereas the latter three are dense, cholesterol-rich particles. When fasting, plasma cholesterol levels are usually a reflection of the amount of LDL in the plasma, whereas plasma triglyceride levels reflect the amount of VLDL. A special type of lipoprotein that is currently being investigated for its link with CVD is lipoprotein (a) [Lp(a)]. Lp(a) is structurally similar to LDL-C, but holds an apolipoprotein (a) tail, which varies in length and form. The length and form of this tail is genetically determined by so-called kringle-repeats. In general, the concentration of Lp(a) is inversely associated with the amount of kringle repeats [16].

Lipid and Lipoprotein Metabolism

The liver and the intestine are the most important sources of lipoproteins. Their transport and metabolism are generally divided into three systems: absorption of exogenous and endogenous lipids and lipoproteins, endogenous synthesis of lipids and lipoproteins, and *reverse cholesterol transport* (*RCT*). These processes are depicted in Fig. 23.1.

Absorption of Exogenous and Endogenous Lipids

The average Western diet consists of a daily intake of approximately 100 g of fat and 500 mg of cholesterol. Phospholipids and bile acids, present in hepatic bile, emulsify lipids from food to form micelles within the intestinal lumen. Hepatic bile also delivers significant amounts of unesterified cholesterol to these micelles.

Pancreatic lipases secreted into the intestinal lumen digest dietary lipids to chemical entities that can be absorbed by enterocytes. Fatty acids and monoacylglycerides are almost entirely absorbed through both passive diffusion and carrier-mediated processes [17]. By contrast, *cholesterol absorption* is an active process, mediated by several transporter proteins which are located at the intestinal brush-border membrane. Cholesterol and sterols derived from plants are taken up by the enterocyte through the recently identified Niemann-Pick C Like 1 (NPC1L1) transporter [18], whereas the ATP-binding cassette transporters (ABC) G5 and G8 actively secrete plant sterols, and to a lesser extent cholesterol, back into the intestinal lumen [19]. Of note, NPC1L1 and ABCG5 and G8 are also located in the liver, where they are involved in hepatic cholesterol trafficking to the bile [19, 20]. Intestinal cholesterol absorption exhibits on average about 50% efficiency, with large

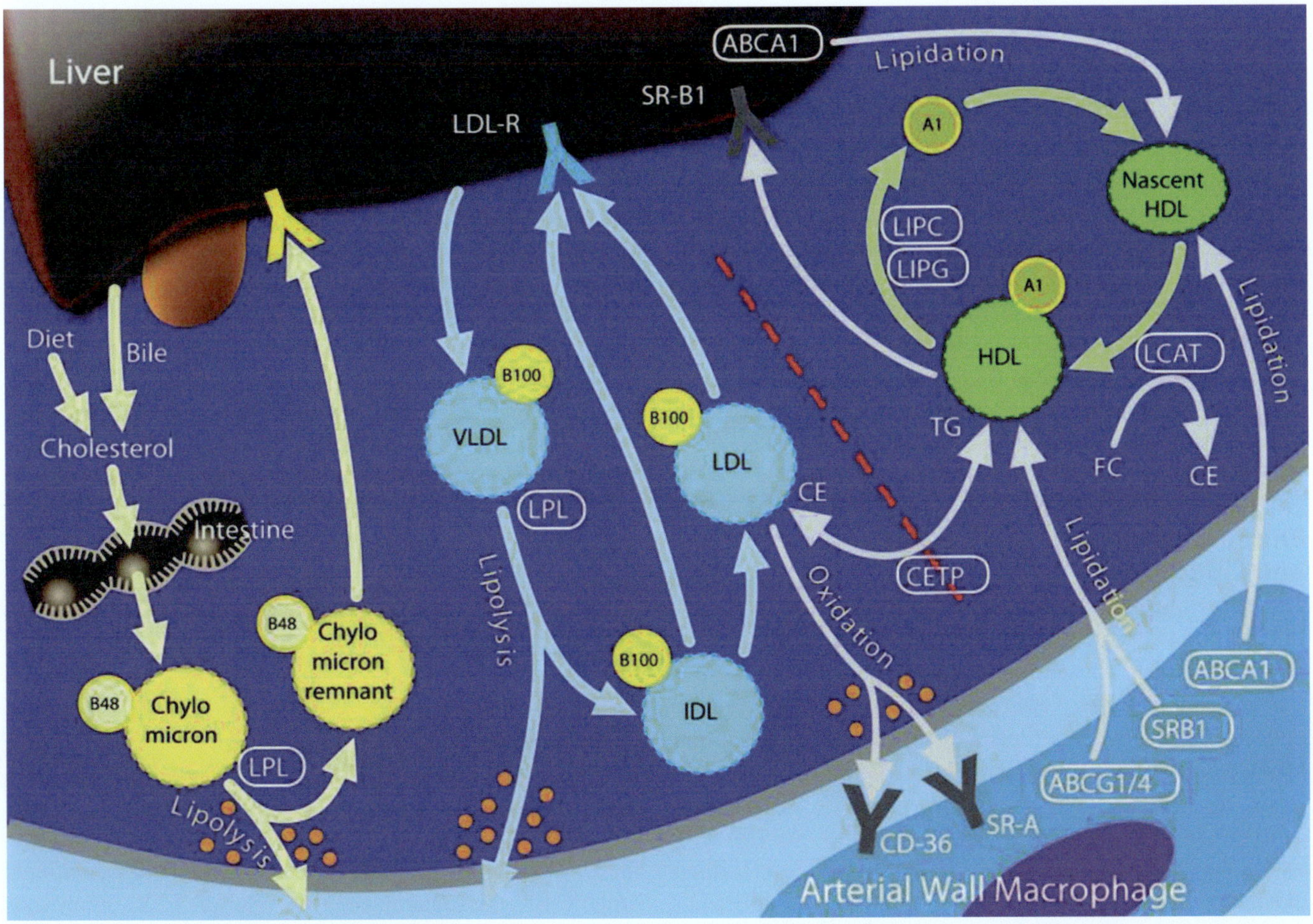

Fig. 23.1 Overview of lipoprotein metabolism. Dietary lipids and cholesterol from the hepatic bile are absorbed in the intestine, packaged into chylomicrons, and secreted into the lymph, which drains into the systemic circulation. In the bloodstream, the triglyceride-rich (*TG*) chylomicrons are hydrolyzed through the action of lipoprotein lipase (*LPL*) and the removed TGs and free fatty acids are taken up by extrahepatic tissues such as the liver and muscles. The chylomicrons remnants are taken up by the liver for further processing. In the fasting state, the liver assembles TG-rich very low-density lipoprotein (*VLDL*). Also VLDL are hydrolyzed by LPL and thereby transformed to smaller VLDL remnants, IDL. Half of the IDL are directly taken up by the liver through binding of the LDL-R, whereas the other half is converted to cholesterol-rich LDL. Most of the plasma LDL-C is cleared from the circulation by binding to the LDL-R of the liver. Of the remaining LDL, some subfractions are especially prone to oxidative modification and then taken up by scavenger receptors (CD-36) of arterial wall macrophages resulting in foam cells and atherosclerotic plaques. High-density lipoprotein (*HDL*) is responsible for the RCT from extrahepatic tissues to the liver. Nascent HDL is formed from lipid-poor Apo-A1, which is secreted by the liver and intestine and which is lipidated through interaction with ABCA1. Nascent HDL is also generated from surface components shed during lipolysis of TG-rich lipoproteins by LPL (not depicted). After lipidation, LCAT esterifies free cholesterol (*FC*) to cholesterylesters (*CE*) which migrates into the core of the HDL making them larger spherical particles. These larger HDL particles acquire additional lipids from extrahepatic tissues, including arterial wall macrophages, by receptor-mediated pathways such as ABCG1, ABCG4, and SR-B1, as well as from lipolysis of TG-rich lipoproteins and passive diffusion (not depicted). The HDL particles can be metabolized in several ways. First, they can deliver CE to the liver by binding to SR-B1 on the hepatocyte surface. In the liver, the cholesterol can be processed and eliminated. Alternatively, CE in HDL can be exchanged for TG in apo-B-containing lipoproteins, by the action of CETP. The TG-enriched HDL is hydrolyzed by LIPC and LIPG to smaller HDL and lipid-poor Apo-A1 particles. These can be either recycled to acquire cholesterol or excreted from the body through the kidneys

interindividual variation, ranging from 20% to 80% [21]. Free cholesterol that has entered the enterocyte is either reesterified intracellularly by Acylcoenzyme A:cholesterol acyltransferase (ACAT) 2 and then packaged into chylomicrons, or trafficked toward the baso-laterally located ATP-binding cassette transport protein A1 (ABCA1) protein for HDL formation.

Chylomicrons consist for approximately 80–95% of triglycerides and apolipoprotein B48 (apo-B48) as their structural surface protein. They are secreted into the lymph, which drains directly into the systemic circulation. In the bloodstream, chylomicrons are hydrolyzed, that is, triglycerides and free fatty acids (FFAs) are removed from the core of the chylomicrons, by *lipoprotein lipase* (*LPL*), thereby generating remnant particles. LPL is anchored to the endothelial surface by proteoglycans and/or by the anchoring protein GPIHBP1 (glycosylphosphatidylinositol-anchored high-density lipoprotein-binding protein 1) [22]. LPL requires apolipoprotein CII as a cofactor for adequate hydrolysis. The removed triglycerides and FFAs are taken up by the liver and muscle, whereas the chylomicrons remnants are taken up by the liver for further processing, as described below. Chylomicrons have a short half-life in the circulation, averaging approximately 10–20 min, provided that clearance is undisturbed. Hence, chylomicrons are not present in the bloodstream in the fasting state. However, when postprandial levels of chylomicrons and their remnants remain high, due to intestinal overproduction or delayed clearance, this can promote delivery of chylomicrons and their remnants to the arterial endothelium, with subsequent generation of *foam cells* and fatty streaks and eventually *atherosclerotic plaque formation*.

Endogenous Synthesis of Lipids and Lipoproteins

In the fasting state, the liver assembles VLDL-C by combining triglycerides, phospholipids, apolipoprotein B100 (apo-B100), and cholesterylesters (CEs). The latter originate either from de novo synthesis and subsequent esterification by ACAT2 or from remnant particles that have been taken up from the circulation. Like chylomicrons, VLDLs are triglyceride-rich particles secreted into the bloodstream, where they are hydrolyzed by LPL and thereby transformed to smaller and denser VLDL remnants, IDL, and finally LDL particles. In general, half of the VLDL remnants are directly taken up by the liver through binding to the *LDL receptor* (LDL-R), whereas the other half is converted to LDL.

LDL is the most abundant cholesterol-carrying particle in humans and accounts for more than 75% of plasma cholesterol. Mediated by *apo-B100*, most of plasma LDL is cleared from the circulation by the LDL-R, which is located at the surface of hepatocytes and internalized entirely (lipoprotein + receptor) upon binding of LDL. The remaining LDL particles are delivered to peripheral tissues such as the adrenals and gonads for the synthesis of steroid and sex hormones. In hepatic endosomes, LDL is degraded to amino acids and free cholesterol, whereas the LDL-R is scavenged back to the cell surface for the uptake of additional LDL particles. Approximately, 70–80% of the LDL catabolism takes place via the LDL-R. The remaining part is cleared via nonspecific routes.

The proprotein convertase subtilisin/kexin type 9 (*PCSK9*) protein plays a pivotal role in LDL metabolism by promoting degradation of LDL-R instead of recycling it back to the cell surface, thereby reducing the number of available LDL receptors at the surface of hepatocytes [23]. It primarily does so by acting on the LDL receptor as a secreted factor and the expression is—similar to LDL-R—modulated by intracellular cholesterol levels. Because of this effect of cholesterol at the transcriptional level, statins increase *PCSK9* expression, thereby partially counteracting their effect in terms of upregulating LDL receptor expression. Therefore, inhibiting PCSK9 could lower LDL-C levels by increasing the available pool of LDL receptors and work synergistically with statins. PCSK9 inhibitors have emerged as the prime candidate to further reduce CVD risk, as will be discussed in section, "Management."

Finally, LDL is not a homogeneous lipoprotein fraction, as it consists of several subfractions with varying mass and density. *Small-dense LDL* is particularly associated with atherosclerotic disease. This subfraction is mostly prevalent in subjects with elevated triglyceride levels. Small-dense LDL particles are prone to oxidative modification, resulting in uptake by scavenger receptors of arterial macrophages, which express a strong affinity for these so-called ox-LDL particles. Since a negative feedback system for these scavenger receptors is lacking, unlimited amounts of ox-LDL can be taken up by these macrophages, which transform into foam cells and atherosclerotic plaques.

HDL Metabolism and RCT

HDL is a highly heterogeneous class of lipoprotein particles that differ in protein component and lipid composition, size, shape, density, and charge. In addition to the observational support for the atheroprotective role of HDL, numerous in vitro and in vivo animal studies have demonstrated various mechanisms through which HDL exerts its beneficial effects on the arterial wall. The most widely acknowledged mechanism is its role in *RCT*. This involves the ability of HDL to stimulate efflux of cholesterol from peripheral tissues, transport in the plasma, and uptake by the liver, followed by biliary excretion and elimination via the feces. Specifically, the efflux of cholesterol from macrophage foam cells in the artery wall is thought to be central to the antiatherogenic properties of HDL. In addition, putative atheroprotective properties of HDL include its ability to improve endothelial function, inhibit LDL oxidation, and induce several antiapoptotic, anti-inflammatory, and antithrombotic effects. However, pharmacotherapeutic interventions aimed to raise HDL-C levels have thus far not resulted in a clinically meaningful benefit in patients [24].

The process of RCT starts by lipidation of *apolipoprotein A1* (Apo-A1) through interaction with the ABCA1 protein. Apo-AI is the most important structural protein of HDL and comprises approximately 70% of the proteins in HDL-C. It is synthesized by the liver and intestine and released into the circulation either in a free non-lipidated form or incorporated in small discoid particles, rich in phospholipids and poor in cholesterol, the so-called nascent or pre-β-HDL. Nascent HDL is also generated from redundant surface components shed during lipolysis of triglyceride-rich lipoproteins such as chylomicrons and VLDL by LPL. The *ABCA1 transporter* resides at the cellular membrane and facilitates the transfer of free cholesterol and phospholipids from intracellular lipid pools to apo-A1. New insights suggest that, in contrast to previous opinion, hepatic ABCA1 appears to be critical for the initial lipidation of lipid-poor apo-A1, protecting it from rapid degradation and allowing it to go on to form mature HDL. Conversely, macrophage ABCA1 appears to contribute little to bulk lipidation of HDL and therefore to plasma HDL-C levels, but does seem to be important for protection against atherosclerosis [25]. After lipidation, lecithin: cholesteryl acyltransferase (*LCAT*) subsequently esterifies the externalized free cholesterol to cholesterylesters on the surface of HDL on activation by its cofactor apo-A1. The esterified cholesterol then migrates into the core of the HDL and as larger amounts of cholesterylesters become incorporated, HDL becomes a larger spherical particle. These larger so-called HDL-3 and HDL-2 particles acquire additional free cholesterol and phospholipids from extrahepatic tissues, including macrophage foam cells, by means of passive diffusion or receptor-mediated pathways, such as ABCG1, ABCG4, and scavenger receptor B1 (SR-B1), as well as from lipolysis of triglyceride-rich lipoproteins [26]. The HDL-3 and HDL-2 particles can be metabolized in several ways. First, they can directly deliver cholesterylesters to the liver by binding to *SR-B1* on the hepatocyte surface. In the liver, the cholesterol can be processed and eliminated as bile or converted to cholesterol-containing steroids. Once the HDL particle is delipidated, it dissociates from SR-B1 and can then reinitiate another cycle of RCT. Alternatively, cholesterylesters in HDL can be exchanged for triglycerides in apo-B-containing lipoproteins such as LDL, by the action of *cholesterylester transfer protein* (*CETP*), after which these cholesterylesters are available for hepatic clearance via the LDL receptor. However, if a population of apo-B-containing lipoproteins enriched with cholesterylesters by CETP interacts with macrophages in arterial walls and promotes net cholesterol uptake, this process is potentially atherogenic. Whether the sum effect of CETP activity in humans is pro- or antiatherogenic is not clear. Most experimental evidence in animal and genetic studies favors a pro-atherogenic role for CETP. The triglyceride-enriched HDL is a substrate for hydrolysis by *hepatic lipase* (LIPC) while phospholipids are mainly hydrolyzed by *endothelial lipase* (LIPG). In this way, HDL is remodeled to lipid poor Apo-A1 and smaller HDL particles which can either be recycled to acquire cholesterol from extrahepatic tissues or dissociated apo-A1 is excreted from the body through the kidneys. *Phospholipid transfer protein* (*PLTP*) also plays a major role in HDL metabolism in various ways. PLTP facilitates the transfer of phospholipids from triglyceride-rich lipoproteins during lipolysis and evidence has accumulated over the years that PLTP can also remodel HDL particles [27].

Genetic Causes of Elevated LDL-C Levels

Mutations in genes involved in LDL metabolism can result in increased plasma LDL-C concentrations. Three genes have been characterized: the *LDLR* gene, the *ApoB* gene, and most recently the *PCSK9* gene [28]. These genes are involved in *autosomal dominant hypercholesterolemia*. The single known *autosomal recessive* form of *hypercholesterolemia* (ARH) is caused by failing internalization of the LDL-R/LDL particle complex in the hepatocytes and is caused by a mutation in the *LDLRAP1* gene [29, 30].

Familial Hypercholesterolemia

Familial hypercholesterolemia (FH) is the most common autosomal dominant inherited disorder of metabolism. Approximately 1:300 people are affected worldwide, although data from most countries is still missing [31]. In some populations, this prevalence is higher due to a founder effect [32]. Homozygosity is rare, with an average of one per 160,000–300,000, with higher frequencies in populations where a founder effect or high rates of consanguinity are present [33]. FH subjects are characterized by plasma LDL-C levels above the 95th percentile for age and gender, due to impaired internalization of LDL particles caused by functional alterations in the LDL receptor [34]. Moreover, the decrease in the hepatic cholesterol pool stimulates cholesterol synthesis, resulting in increased production of VLDL, which further increases LDL-C levels.

Genetics

The molecular defect underlying FH most often consists of a mutation in the *LDLR gene*, located on chromosome 19p13 [34]. At present, over 3500 different mutations in the LDL-R or promoter region leading to an FH phenotype have been described, all of which are publicly available at the University College London low-density lipoprotein receptor gene varaiant database [35].

In addition, mutations in the *PCSK9 gene* on chromosome 1 are a rare cause of the FH phenotype, accounting for 2% of cases [36]. To date, 28 pathogenic mutations in *PCSK9* have been reported. These "gain-of-function" mutations cause hypercholesterolemia due to PCSK9-induced enhanced degradation of LDL receptors, thereby decreasing the available pool of hepatic LDL receptors. Finally, mutations in the LDL-R-binding domain of apo-B100 can result in a phenotype which resembles FH, approximately in 5% of FH cases [36]. This is outlined in the next paragraph on familial defective apolipoprotein B (FDB).

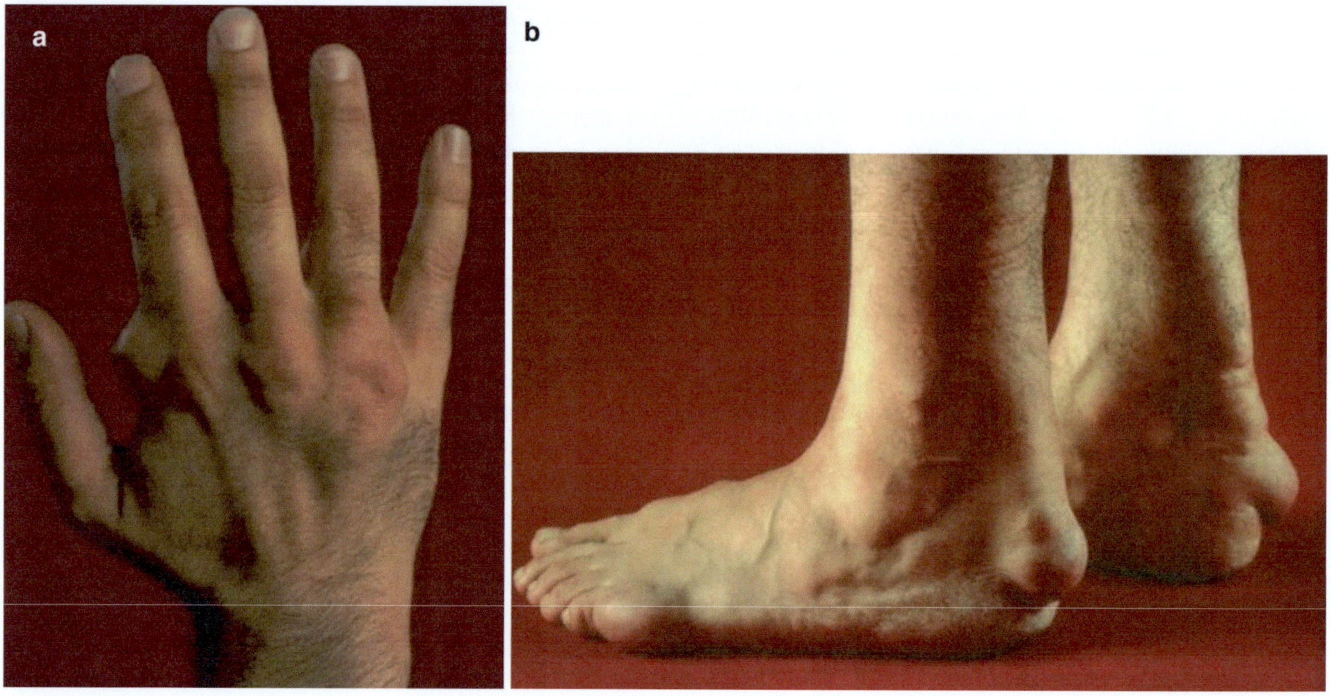

Fig. 23.2 Skin xanthomas (**a**) Xanthomas of the hand and (**b**) Achilles tendon xanthomas

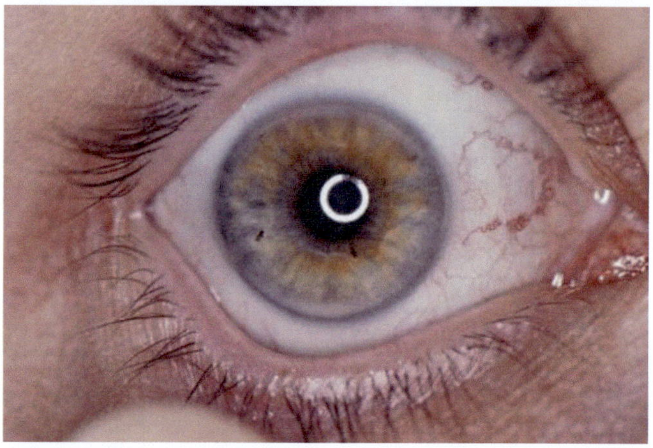

Fig. 23.3 Arcus lipoides

Clinical Characteristics

A hallmark of FH is plasma LDL-C levels above the 95th percentile for age and gender. This induces accelerated deposition of cholesterol in arterial walls and other tissues, resulting in the clinical hallmarks of FH: premature atherosclerosis, *tendon xanthomas*, *xanthelasma*, and corneal arcus [34]. However, these clinical characteristics (Figs. 23.2 and 23.3) are not exclusively associated with or may not be present in every patient with FH. Moreover, the age of appearance of these symptoms varies depending on the severity of the phenotype. If untreated, approximately 50% of male and 30% of female heterozygous FH patients will develop symptomatic CVD before the age of 50 years [37]. However, the onset and progression of atherosclerotic disease varies considerably between FH individuals and within families. It was shown that event-free survival depends more on actual LDL-C levels caused by the mutation, rather than the type of mutation itself [38].

Patients with homozygous FH have plasma cholesterol levels >13 mmol/L. If untreated, patients suffer from CVD before 20 years of age and generally do not survive past 30 years of age [33].

Although cardiovascular events are rare in children heterozygous for FH, affected children were already shown to have an impaired endothelial function [37], as well as an increased *carotid intima-media thickness* (*cIMT*) [39], when compared to their unaffected siblings, which is indicative for an early onset of subclinical atherosclerosis. Based on these findings, current guidelines advise early pharmacological cholesterol-lowering in children with FH, as discussed below.

Diagnosis

FH is usually diagnosed on the basis of clinical features. Several clinical tools have been developed, with different diagnostic criteria, some of which combined with DNA analysis (reviewed in Reference [40]). In the Netherlands, the algorithm of the Dutch Lipid Network is used, as shown in Table. 23.1. The primary clinical diagnostic criteria are elevated LDL-C levels above the 95th percentile for age and gender, the presence of tendon xanthomata in the patient or a first-degree rela-

Table 23.1 Diagnostic algorithm for familial hypercholesterolemia

Family history*	1
I first-degree relative with CVD <55 (men) / 60 (women) years of age II first-degree relative with plasma LDL-cholesterol levels >95th percentile	
III first-degree relative with a corneal arcus <45 years and/or tendon xanthomas IV children <18 years of age with plasma LDL-cholesterol levels >95th percentile	2
Personal medical history	
I CHD <55 (men) / 60 (women) years of age	2
II Cerebro-vascular event or peripheral arterial disease <55 (men) / 60 (women) years of age	1
Physical examination	
I presence of tendon xanthomas	6
II presence of corneal arcus <45 years of age	4
Laboratory parameters	
I LDL-cholesterol >8.5 mmol/l	8
II LDL-cholesterol 6.5–8.4 mmol/l	5
III LDL-cholesterol 5.0–6.4 mmol/l	3
IV LDL-cholesterol 4.0–4.9 mmol/l	1
DNA analysis	
Functional mutation in the *LDLR*, *APOB* or *PCSK9* gene	8
Diagnosis	
Definite FH > 8	
Probable FH 6–8	
Possible FH 3–5	
Unlikely FH <3	
Additional DNA testing is advised if the score > 6	

*In this category, only the highest applicable number should be scored; the highest score for family history is 2

tive, and a pattern of autosomal dominant inheritance of premature coronary heart disease or hypercholesterolemia. The diagnosis can be confirmed through genetic testing of the *LDLR, APO-B, and PCSK9* genes. However, careful selection of patients is important given the costs of genetic analysis. Although the current yield is relatively low (between 54% and 70%), tools to aid physicians in the decision for referral are currently being developed [41].

Early diagnosis—preferably during childhood—of FH is important to enable prompt treatment. Nationally organized genetic cascade-screening programs have been implemented in the Netherlands, Spain, and Wales, in addition to initiatives on a smaller scale in various other countries [42].

Management

Treatment with *high-dose statins* is currently the most effective strategy to reduce CVD risk in FH patients [43]. Lowering LDL-c levels remains the primary target for therapy. Recent studies have confirmed that the inverse relationship between LDL-c and CVD risk persists even at very low LDL-c levels, without apparent adverse effects. In response, updated clinical guidelines argue for treatment with high-intensity statins from the start of therapy and even lower LDL-C treatment targets depending on the patient's combined risk [44–46]. In addition, patients are treated in combination with lifestyle modifications aimed to reduce the risk of other atherogenic factors. Finally, several new pharmacological agents have been developed to optimize cholesterol-lowering treatment in those who do not reach acceptable LDL-C levels or who are unable to tolerate high doses of statins.

Ezetimibe is a cholesterol absorption-inhibiting compound, which acts by blocking the intestinal NPC1L1 protein. Ezetimibe was the first nonstatin drug which has been shown to improve clinical outcomes when added to statins in clinical trials [47]. These results were somewhat surprising, given that earlier studies, using surrogate end points by ultrasound (ENHANCE), did not find a benefit in terms of primary end points [48].

PCSK9 inhibition represents the latest advancement in cholesterol-lowering drugs [49]. Several approaches to PCSK9 inhibition are currently being developed and evaluated in clinical studies, and monoclonal antibodies were the first to be approved by regulating bodies. By virtue of their ability to prevent lysosomal degradation of the LDL receptor, PCSK9 inhibitors increase the available pool of hepatic LDL receptors. Recent meta-analyses [50, 51] of clinical trials comprising >10,000 individuals have unequivocally demonstrated the efficacy of PCSK9 inhibitors in improving lipid profiles: mean LDL reductions were observed of 50%, whereas HDL increased by 6% and Lp(a) decreased by 26%. A recent meta-analysis of all randomized outcome trials showed a 17% reduction in CV events when compared to placebo, with most notably myocardial infarction and stroke reductions [52]. Importantly, PCSK9 inhibitors have shown to be generally safe and well tolerated. Based on these promising results, both the Food and Drug Administration (FDA) and European Medicines Agency (EMA) have approved alirocumab and evolocumab for several categories of patients including hetero- and homozygous FH patients who fail to meet LDL goals as well as statin-intolerant patients. An entirely new approach to PCSK9 inhibition is through the siRNA agent Inclisiran, which lowers PCSK9 levels by interfering with the expression of *PCSK9* [53]. The antisense strand of Inclisiran binds to the RNA Induced Silencing Complex, which in turn binds and degrades PCSK9 mRNA after transcription. This injectable agent reduces LDL-C by up to 50%, and does so with a dosing scheme of only twice per year after a run-in period of two injections in three months [54, 55]. It has a favourable safety and tolerability profile. Inclisiran is currently being evaluated in clinical outcome trials. Multiple other agents are under investigation, including other monoclonal antibodies and anti-PCSK9 vaccines [24].

Approved in 2020, *Bempedoic acid* is the latest novel lipid-lowering agent currently on the market. Bempedoic acid inhibits ATP citrate lyase, thereby reducing LDL-C by about 20% as monotherapy [24]. When combined with ezetimibe, the LDL-C reduction was 48%. Bempedoic acid generally has a favourable safety and tolerability profile the

CLEAR Outcomes trial was designed to investigate the effect of bempedoic acid on the incidence of CVD and is expected to be completed in 2022. In the meantime, bempedoic acid has already been approved for clinical use [56].

There are more lipid-lowering strategies, which are used less frequently than the agents described above. The first we will discuss are the Bile acid sequestrants (BASs), which bind bile acids in the intestine and subsequently increase hepatic conversion of cholesterol into bile acids. The resulting decrease in hepatic cholesterol content results in increased hepatic LDL-R expression. *Colesevelam* is a novel BAS with a more favorable side-effect profile, as it is thought to bind with higher affinity compared to other BAS [57]. Although Colesevelam effectively lowered LDL-C levels, to date no data on clinical end points are available [48]. Moreover, it showed adverse effects similar to other BASs, including increased serum triglyceride levels and reduced intestinal uptake of several drugs, which means that these drugs should be taken more than 4 hours before Colesevelam [48].

CETP inhibitors: see CETP inhibitors under Genetic Causes for HDL-C Disorders.

Another novel approach to reducing LDL-C and TG is through inhibition of angiopoietin-like protein 3 (ANGPTL3). ANGPTL3 regulates lipid metabolism by inhibiting LPL and endothelial lipase [24]. Evinacumab is a novel monoclonal antibody that inhibits ANGPTL3. In HoFH patients, evinacumab reduced LDL-C and TG by 49% and 47%, respectively. Results from phase 3 clinical trials in other high-risk groups are expected in the near future. A second approach to inhibition of ANGPTL3 is through the N-Acetylgalactosamine (GalNAc)-modified antisense oligonucleotide (ASO) IONIS-ANGPTL3-Lrx, which is currently being evaluated in phase 2 trials [24].

Lomitapide is an oral small-molecule inhibitor of the microsomal triglyceride transfer protein (MTP), which facilitates the assembly of apo-B-containing lipoproteins. This leads to reductions in lipoprotein secretion and lowers LDL-C levels. After a single-arm, open-label, 78-week phase 3 trial including 29 patients, which showed promising results [58], Lomitapide was approved for treatment of HoFH. A larger registry (LOWER) was started in 2014 to evaluate the clinical long-term safety and effectiveness, including at least 300 patients for follow-up for at least 10 years [59]. A first report from this registry with 3-year data confirmed the risk-benefit profile that was described in the phase 3 trial [60].

Gene therapy is currently under investigation as a treatment option in HoFH. While the first trial in the early 1990s showed disappointing results, new advances paved the road to new trials. In gene therapy, patients are being treated with a recombinant adeno-associated virus (AAV) vector loaded with a functional transgene, for example, an LDL-R expressing transgene. The newest vector AAV8 is of interest because of its strong liver tropism and relatively low seroprevalence in Western populations, which is important because of immune responses. Clinical testing in mice showed promising results, with a total cholesterol of 227 versus 1032 mg/dL at day 56 post-vector administration. Metabolic effects were maintained for up to 20 weeks. Preliminary clinical trials of the AAV8.TBG.hLDLR compound in HoFH patients are currently ongoing [24]. Of note, an AAV1 vector expressing LPL was the first gene therapy agent approved in the Western world to treat LPL-deficient patients (reviewed below) [61].

Mipomersen is an ASO that in 2013 was approved by the FDA for use in patients with homozygous FH (HoFH), although it is not approved in Europe. It lowered LDL-C with 25% in patients already receiving lipid-lowering drugs, while also reducing Apo-B and Lp(a) and having no effect on HDL-C levels. Benefits in terms of clinical outcomes remain to be confirmed in clinical trials. Side effects, including flu-like symptoms and injection-site reactions, as well as adverse hepatic effects, could reduce compliance. Mipomersen is no longer marketed [62].

Extracorporal removal of lipids by apheresis is a last-resort option, indicated in a very small subset of patients with severely increased LDL-C (or triglycerides or Lp(a)) levels. This intervention is only indicated when established therapies do not suffice, and there are no RCTs conducted to evaluate the efficacy of this intervention [24]. It is plausible that research in novel therapies will further reduce the number of patients in who such an invasive intervention is warranted.

Finally, with respect to treatment of *children with FH*, several statin trials have been performed over the past decade [63], showing that statin treatment lowers LDL-C safely and effectively in children with FH [63, 64], In terms of clinical evidence, one study demonstrated reduced cIMT progression in FH adolescents on statin therapy [65], and a 20-year follow-up study of the same cohort showed that the cumulative incidence of CVD and death from cardiovascular causes in adulthood was much lower in these patients on statin therapy, compared to their parents at the same age [66]. On the basis of these studies, current guidelines in the United States and Europe recommend initial statin treatment in children with heterozygous FH at 6–10 years of age [45, 46]. Another international workforce published a consensus-based guideline applicable for most patients, which advocates for lifestyle modifications and consideration of the use of statin monotherapy starting from the age of 8 years and the eventual addition of ezetimibe or a BAS from the age of 10 years. For patients with homozygous FH, treatment with statins should start as early as possible [67]. In the United States, pravastatin is approved from the age of 8 years, and rosuvastatin from the age of 7 years for HoFH patients, while in Europe rosuvastatin is approved from the age of 6 years, although earlier treatment for severe FH phenotypes is allowed as well [68]. Ezetimibe is approved from the age of 10 years in both the United States and Europe. A recent study investigating the PCSK9 inhibitor alirocumab in children aged 8–17 years showed 45% reductions in LDL-C in the highest dose group, and an acceptable safety profile, paving the way for the use of PCSK9 antibodies to lower LDL-C in children with HeFH [69]. In the event of homozygous FH and rapidly progressive atherosclerosis, lomitapide and mipomersen could also be considered, although both drugs yet have to be tested in children, especially when apheresis is not an option [70].

In addition to pharmacological treatment of hypercholesterolemia, management should also comprise cascade screening of first-degree relatives. This is reviewed elsewhere [36].

Familial Defective Apolipoprotein B

Familial Defective Apolipoprotein B (*FDB*) is an autosomal dominant disorder, which resembles the clinical phenotype of FH. The mechanism underlying the hypercholesterolemia is the defective binding of apo-B100 of the LDL particle to the LDL receptor. The estimated prevalence is 1:1000 in US caucasians and Europeans [71]. Due to founder effects, prevalence up to 1:200 was observed in certain regions of Europe [72], while in Amish populations the prevalence sometimes even exceed the prevalence in founder populations for LDLR mutations in FH [71]. However, the exact prevalence remains unknown, since the phenotype overlaps with that of FH. Therefore, the prevalence of the phenotype of FH due to mutations in *LDLR, PCSK9, or Apo-B100* is around 1:250.

Genetics

FDB is caused by mutations in the *apo-B100* gene located on chromosome 2p23–24. So far, 11 functional mutations at the *apo-B* locus have been identified. The R3500Q mutation is the most frequent one, with a prevalence of 1:1000 in Caucasians [71].

Clinical Characteristics, Diagnosis, and Management

FDB is clinically indistinguishable from FH [73], although with slightly lower LDL-C levels [74]. FDB is diagnosed by genotyping or according to clinical diagnostic criteria for FH. Of note, the standard criteria for FH were found to underdiagnose r3500Q carriers [71]. Careful evaluation of all aspects of the patient suspected for FH is therefore warranted. Equal to FH, patients with FDB are treated with lipid-lowering medication combined with lifestyle modification.

Autosomal Recessive Hypercholesterolemia

ARH is the single known recessive disorder causing hypercholesterolemia. Only about 100 individuals with ARH have been identified worldwide [75], although the disease is not uncommon on the island of Sardinia with a frequency of 1:40.000 for homozygotes and compound heterozygotes and even 1:143 for heterozygotes [76]. In ARH, hepatic endocytosis of the LDL-R/LDL particle complex, mediated by the *LDL-R-adapting protein* (*LDLRAP*) is disrupted [30, 77].

Genetics

To date, 23 mutations in the *LDLRAP1* gene, located on chromosome 1p35–36.1, have been identified, the great majority being truncating mutations [75].

Clinical Characteristics

ARH is characterized by a phenotype, which resembles homozygous FH, consisting of severe hypercholesterolemia, large xanthomas, and premature CVD, although the phenotype in ARH is slightly milder, since patients tend to have higher HDL-C levels and are more responsive to lipid-lowering therapy and express a longer event-free survival when compared to homozygous FH patients [78]. The presence of residual LDL-R activity, as demonstrated in skin fibroblasts, might explain the favorable plasma cholesterol concentrations and the response to cholesterol-lowering medication in patients with ARH [79]. In general, no clinical symptoms before the age of 20 years are present in ARH. Heterozygous carriers of the *ARH* mutation usually have slightly elevated lipid levels within the normal range.

Diagnosis

ARH is diagnosed by genetic testing. Affected individuals meet clinical criteria for homozygous FH, as described in the section, "Clinical Characteristics"; however, based on the clinical evaluation of first-degree relatives, a lipid disorder of recessive origin, rather than homozygous FH, should be considered.

Management

Most patients currently described in the literature receive apheresis or a combination of apheresis and lipid-lowering therapy [80]. Patients with ARH are sensitive to treatment with statins and a cholesterol-lowering diet, and combinations with ezetimibe and lomitapide have also been described. Of note, the combination of any statin (with or without ezetimibe) and lomitapide led to the strongest reductions in LDL-C levels [80].

Familial Combined Hyperlipidemia

Familial combined hyperlipidemia (FCH) is a relatively common lipoprotein disorder, with a prevalence of 1:200. The disease is based on increased *VLDL synthesis,* due to an overproduction of apo-B100, sometimes combined with delayed hepatic clearance of VLDL [81].

Genetics

Initially, FCH was considered an autosomal dominant monogenetic disorder; however, the hereditary background might be *polygenetic*, as a handful of families display a convincingly autosomal dominant mode of inheritance, whereas, in others, a multifactorial basis is considered to be more likely. FCH might be best conceptualized as a phenotype with a common clinical presentation but with variable predisposing causes. Rare large-effect mutations are found in a fraction of patients, while multiple independently segregating small-effect mutations accumulate in a patient's genome, thereby raising LDL-C and triglycerides further [82].

Clinical Characteristics

FCH is phenotypically heterogeneous and, in most individuals, not manifest until adulthood. It is characterized by elevated LDL-C and/or triglyceride levels, a tendency to decreased HDL-C levels, and is often accompanied by central obesity, insulin resistance, and hypertension. In addition, there are no clinical stigmata such as in FH. Different phenotypes can be expressed within members of one affected family. In most cases, apo-B100 levels are elevated above 1.2 g/L and plasma triglycerides are mildly to moderately increased; however, cholesterol and triglyceride levels can vary over time within affected individuals. FCH patients have an increased risk of premature CVD [83].

Diagnosis

FCH is diagnosed based on a combination of plasma lipid abnormalities and a positive family history of dyslipidemia: either solitary elevated LDL-C, triglycerides, or both, with or without premature CVD in the index patient or family members. A nomogram has been developed to aid physicians in estimating the probability of FCH based on clinical criteria [84]. In short, a combination of apoB levels higher than 1.2 g/l and triglycerides higher than 1.5 mmol/l, both adjusted for age and sex, and present in 2 or more family members is regarded clinically suspicious for FCH [82].

Management

Untreated FCH patients are prone to premature CVD; therefore, aggressive lipid-lowering treatment equal to that for FH is required. Most FCH patients are treated with high-dose statins, with a target LDL-C of 2.5 or 1.8 mmol/L in subjects with CVD. In case triglyceride levels are elevated as well, patients can be treated with a *fibrate* on top of the statin, but not Gemfibrozil, since that combination increases the risk of rhabdomyolysis [85]. Novel therapeutic agents have yet to be evaluated in FCH patients. However, the expectation is that these agents will reduce CV risk with the same magnitude as in other hypercholesterolaemic patients. In addition, FCH patients should be treated with lifestyle modification, also in order to target the accompanying symptoms of obesity, insulin resistance, and hypertension. Finally, since FCH patients have functioning LDL receptors, the response to dietary interventions and pharmacological cholesterol lowering is generally better than observed in FH.

Sitosterolemia

Sitosterolemia is a rare autosomal recessive disorder characterized by premature atherosclerosis. Although hypercholesterolemia is not obligatory, elevations in LDL-C levels may be observed. The underlying defect in sitosterolemia is hyperabsorption of *plant sterols* and *sterols* and decreased biliary secretion of both cholesterol and plant sterols [86]. Plant sterols are structurally similar to cholesterol and are derived solely from the diet. Normally, plasma plant sterol levels in humans are extremely low due to active efflux, as achieved by the *ABCG5/G8 transporters.* In sitosterolemia, this mechanism is disrupted. Approximately 50 cases have been described worldwide and the global prevalence is estimated on one in 2.6 million for ABCG5 and one in 360.000 for ABCG8 [87].

Genetics

The *ABCG5* and *ABCG8* transporter genes are arranged in a head-to-head configuration on chromosome 2p21 [88]. Mutations in either the *ABCG5* or the *ABCG8* gene can cause sitosterolemia, either through homozygosity or compound heterozygosity [86, 89, 90]. All of the missense mutations in either *ABCG5* or *ABCG8* studied to date either prevent the formation of the obligate heterodimer or block the efficient trafficking of the heterodimer to the plasma membrane [19].

Clinical Characteristics

Sitosterolemia is characterized by xanthomas, arthralgias, anemia, and premature atherosclerosis [91]. Plasma cholesterol levels are not necessarily elevated; however, affected individuals are highly sensitive to dietary cholesterol and become markedly hypercholesterolemic when fed a high-cholesterol diet [92].

Diagnosis

The disease should be suspected in patients who develop xanthomas in early childhood, despite normal or only moderately elevated plasma cholesterol concentrations. Sitosterolemia can be diagnosed by genetic analysis or by plasma plant sterol levels exceeding 0.024 mM (1 mg/dL).

Management

Affected individuals should be restricted from a cholesterol- and plant sterol-rich diet, as well as from plant sterol-enriched food products. In addition, subjects benefit from treatment with ezetimibe, a cholesterol absorption inhibitor, which also inhibits intestinal absorption of plant sterols [93], alone or combined with a BAS [94]. Statins are not effective in lowering plant sterols, but are indicated when the patient also has elevated LDL-C levels.

Genetic Causes of HDL-C Disorders

Disorders of HDL-C identified in humans may result from interaction between genetic and environmental factors. Plasma HDL-C levels are under strong genetic influence, with heritability estimates ranging between 40% and 60% [95]. Several monogenetic defects in various proteins involved in HDL metabolism have been identified in humans to date. The genes encoding apolipoprotein-AI, ABCA1, and LCAT are essential for the de novo synthesis of HDL. A complete lack of any of these factors confers severe HDL deficiency, which is referred to as familial hypoalphalipoproteinemia. By contrast, CETP deficiency mostly induces accumulation of HDL in the circulation, the so-called hyperalphalipoproteinemia. However, the vast majority of cases with HDL-C deficiency, defined as an age- and sex-adjusted plasma HDL-C concentration below the tenth percentile, are polygenic and/or multifactorial in origin. Decreased HDL levels are often found in patients with genetically disturbed metabolic pathways such as hypertriglyceridemia, diabetes mellitus type 2, and obesity and metabolic syndrome [96]. In addition, multiple other factors have been identified to negatively influence HDL-C levels, such as smoking, physical inactivity, anabolic steroids, and certain medication or diseases such as rheumatoid arthritis and systemic lupus erythematosus [97].

The first step in the diagnostic workup of HDL deficiency consists of exclusion of these underlying conditions. Patients with a virtual absence of HDL must undergo a careful physical examination to unravel the clinical characteristics of certain HDL deficiency syndromes as described below. In addition, family studies should be initiated to show segregation of low HDL in the family. Definitive diagnosis requires specialized biochemical tests and the demonstration of a functionally relevant mutation in an HDL gene [96].

To date, no routinely used drug is able to increase HDL-C in patients with specific familial HDL deficiency syndromes. Moreover, the role of HDL as a therapeutic target has been the subject of debate for many years. Both Mendelian Randomization studies and clinical trials failed to show a causal relationship between HDL-C levels and CVD risk. However, basic research now suggests that HDL function could be considered as a therapeutic target [24]. These notions currently imply that the prevention of CVD in these patients must be focused on the avoidance and treatment of additional risk factors, at least until more evidence for HDL-C interventions becomes available. As such, current treatment guidelines do not recommend specific HDL treatment goals [45, 46]. For completeness, we will briefly discuss all HDL-C increasing interventions and therapeutic agents that have been investigated in recent years.

In general, several lifestyle and pharmacologic interventions have shown to modestly increase HDL, although the impact of these interventions on the functional quality of HDL is unclear. Lifestyle modifications such as weight reduction, exercise, and smoking cessation can increase HDL levels by approximately 10–15%. In addition, pharmacologic therapies with niacin, fibrates, and statins, alone or in combination, raise HDL. Niacin therapy is the most effective pharmacological agent currently available and results in significant HDL increases of 15–35%. Several mechanisms have been suggested, although it is not exactly clear how niacin raises HDL. The most common reason for treatment failure is the inability to tolerate cutaneous flushing. This can be reduced by prescribing the long-acting form, or by administering premedication with aspirin, or may diminish spontaneously after several days of therapy, as patients develop tolerance. Niacin used as monotherapy has shown benefit with regard to CHD risk reduction [98]. However, two recent clinical trials (AIM-HIGH, ([99]) HPS2 THRIVE [100]) in which niacin was added to statins in patients with established CVD and well-controlled LDL failed to confirm the clinical benefit in terms of CVD prevention, despite markedly increasing HDL levels. Fibric acid derivatives increase the synthesis of apo-A1, enhancing the formation of new HDL particles and raising HDL by 5–20%, with the largest increases seen in patients with hypertriglyceridemia. Triglycerides are reduced by 20–50%, but LDL is changed minimally, if at all, and are sometimes increased. To date, trial results are mixed, with two trials reporting a significant reduction in their primary outcome, while three others did not. Overall, patients with high triglyceride and low HDL cholesterol seem to benefit from fibrates, but it is debatable whether this is due to an increase in HDL concentration [101].

Promising new agents, which target both quantity and quality of HDL particles, are currently under development. These include CETP inhibitors, Apo-A1 and HDL mimetics, intravenous apo-A1 (Milano) infusion, and agonists of PPAR-alpha, LRH-1, and LXR [102]. CETP inhibitors, like torcetrapib, dalcetrapib (JTT- 705), evacetrapib, anacetrapib, and obicetrapib, are powerful HDL raisers and deserve special mentioning, since almost all CETP inhibitor clinical trials have failed or are discontinued by the manufacturer [103]. Still, it looks like there is a future for CETP inhibition: A phase III trial on anacetrapib initially showed a 9% reduction in major coronary events [104]. However, a post-trial follow-up study showed that the absolute reduction in major coronary events actually doubled at 6 years follow-up when compared to the end of the 4 year treatment period, without any safety concerns [101, 105]. Moreover, a recent Mendelian Randomization study suggested that the magnitude of cardiovascular benefit by CETP inhibitors is determined by the changes in ApoB-containing lipoproteins (for example, LDL-C), rather than changes in HDL-C [106]. This could explain the lack of efficacy for dalcetrapib and evacetrapib, since these agents had no effect on LDL-C levels and were neutral in CV benefit [24]. This Mendelian Randomization analysis also showed that the combination of CETP inhibition and HMGCR inhibition (the proxy for statins) leads to an attenuated reduction in ApoB particles and a proportionally attenuated reduction in risk for CVD [106]. This is thought to be the cause for the discordant findings in the clinical trials for anacetrapib, where the relatively large LDL-C reductions did not result in the anticipated reductions in CV risk. One last CETP inhibitor is still in development: Obicetrapib 10mg once daily monotherapy has shown to reduce LDL-C levels by 45.3 percent and ApoB levels by 33.7% [107]. Based on these potent reductions and the findings in the Mendelian Randomization study, obicetrapib was moved to phase III trials as an alternative to statin treatment.

Three products of Apo A-I infusion have recently been investigated in RCTs. For two compounds, there was no difference in the clinical endpoint of plaque volume as, measured by intravascular ultrasound imaging of the coronary arteries [24]. Both agents have been discontinued by their respective companies. In contrast, CSL-112 is currently being evaluated in 17,400 patients in a phase III outcome trial. CSL-112 is administered once weekly for four weeks, and the primary endpoint is a major cardiovascular event within 90 days [24]. The study is ongoing at the time of writing.

In this section, we will further focus on the established monogenetic disorders of HDL metabolism including Apo-A1, ABCA1, and LCAT. Also genetic disorders of CETP will be discussed.

Apolipoprotein AI Deficiency

Apo-A1 is the major protein component of HDL-C in plasma and plays a central role in cholesterol efflux from tissues to the liver for excretion. Apo-A1 deficiency is a rare autosomal recessive inherited disorder characterized by decreased HDL-C levels.

Genetics

The *apo-A1* gene is located on the long arm of chromosome 11, adjacent to the genes encoding the apolipoproteins C-III and IV. Of the approximately 70 reported distinctive mutations of this gene, mostly found in heterozygous state, some are functionally relevant, that is, are associated with reduced levels of apo-A1 and HDL-C [108].

Clinical Characteristics

Heterozygous carriers of a functionally relevant mutation usually present with half normal apo-A1 and HDL-C levels. Some mutations can even lead to more pronounced decreases. In most cases, heterozygous carriers of apo-A1 variants do not present with specific clinical symptoms. Important exceptions are some structural apo-A1 variants with amino acid substitutions in the N-terminus, which have been detected in patients with familial amyloidosis [109]. Surprisingly, susceptibility for premature coronary heart disease has been shown to differ markedly between apo-A1 variants. Low HDL-C levels due to heterozygosity for a specific apo-A1 mutation (p.L178P) were associated with vascular dysfunction, accelerated carotid arterial wall thickness, and an increased incidence of premature vascular events compared with their family controls [110]. By contrast, despite very low HDL levels, carriers of the *apo-A1* (p.R173C) Milano mutant did not differ from controls in terms of vascular function [111] and arterial wall thickness [112]. These differences are likely due to the profoundly different effects of the mutations at the protein level.

Table 23.2 Clinical hallmarks of familial HDL deficiency syndromes [96]

Apo-A1 deficiency		Tangier disease	Fish-eye disease	Familial LCAT deficiency
Affected gene	*APO-A1*	*ABCA1*	*LCAT*	*LCAT*
Enlarged tonsils	No	Occasionally	No	No
Hepato/splenomegaly	No	Occasionally	No	No
Neuropathy	No	Occasionally	No	No
Corneal opacities	+++	+	+++	+++
Xanthomas	Occasionally	No	No	Occasionally
Xanthelasma	Occasionally	No	No	No
Nephropathy	No	No	No	Yes
Hemolytic anemia	No	No	No	Yes

Patients with complete apo-A1 deficiency, due to homozygosity or compound heterozygosity, present with a virtually absent HDL-C. In adult patients, variable clinical manifestations have been described, such as abnormalities of the skin (xanthelasma and xanthomas) and/or eyes (corneal opacities) [96] (see Table 23.2). Remarkably, only 11 of the 25 reported cases with complete apo-A1 deficiency suffered from premature cardiovascular events. However, the remaining 14 cases were almost all below the age of 50 and may have been too young for clinical manifestations of atherosclerosis to occur. In addition, this small number of cases and differences in the type of apo-A1 gene defect makes conclusions on the susceptibility to premature coronary heart disease in these specific patients difficult [113]. Mendelian randomization studies suggest no relationship between HDL-C levels and CAD [114], but differences in HDL-C function might still explain some of the variation.

Diagnosis

The diagnosis of apo-A1 deficiency requires sequencing of the apo-A1 gene and the demonstration of a functionally relevant mutation.

Management

Since no routinely used drug is able to increase HDL-C levels in patients with familial low HDL cholesterol, the prevention of CVD in these patients must be focused on the avoidance and treatment of additional risk factors and the use of statins and additional lipid-lowering therapy, to obtain very low LDL-C levels [96].

ABCA1 Deficiency and Tangier Disease

ABCA1 mediates the efflux of cholesterol and phospholipids from peripheral tissues to lipid-poor apo-A1 in plasma and thereby plays a central role in forming HDL. Functionally relevant mutations in the *ABCA1* gene lead to cholesterol efflux defects, which subsequently cause low HDL-C and apo-A1 levels. Complete ABCA1 deficiency is the underlying cause of *Tangier disease*. The prevalence of Tangier disease worldwide is estimated at 1:640.000.

Genetics

The *ABCA1* gene resides on chromosome 9q31. To date, more than 90 mutations and several common and rare variants have been described in the *ABCA1* gene, with a wide range of biochemical and clinical phenotypes [115]. Several recent genome-wide association studies have identified common variants in *ABCA1* as a significant source of variation in plasma HDL cholesterol levels across multiple ethnic groups [116, 117] establishing *ABCA1* as a major gene influencing HDL levels in humans [118].

Clinical Characteristics

Heterozygote carriers of functionally relevant *ABCA1* mutations can present with a broad range of plasma HDL-C levels ranging from 30 to 83% of age- and sex-matched controls [118]. However, the majority of these mutations are associated with an approximately 50% reduction in serum HDL-C and apo-A1 levels and increased triglycerides. LDL levels are typically within the normal range.

Tangier disease, which is caused by complete ABCA1 deficiency due to homozygosity or compound heterozygosity, is characterized by profoundly decreased HDL-C plasma and apo-A1 levels. Frequently, serum levels of total and LDL cholesterol are also low, whereas serum levels of triglycerides are mildly elevated. The clinical presentation of Tangier disease varies considerably and if present clinical symptoms can be isolated or combined (see Table 23.2). It is likely that this phenotypic heterogeneity might at least in part be accounted for by the nature of the mutation and its effect on the protein [119]. Presenting features of Tangier disease include enlarged orange tonsils, hepatomegaly, and splenomegaly. Also, lymph nodes can have bright yellow streaks and morphologic characteristics as those present in the tonsils. A symptom with significant implications for quality of life is a peripheral neuropathy, which, however, has a highly variable expression. These clinical symptoms result from the accumulation of cholesterylesters in reticuloendothelial cells, that is, macrophages, Kupffer cells, or histiocytes, leading to the accumulation of these cells in various organs [96]. Despite the known role of ABCA1 in determining plasma HDL levels, the impact of ABCA1 on atherosclerosis remains controversial and incompletely understood [120]. Prior to the identification of *ABCA1* mutations as the genetic basis of Tangier disease in 1999, patients were identified based on their clinical phenotype, that is, extremely low HDL cholesterol in homozygotes, with the offspring and parents of homozygotes being obligate heterozygotes. Considering the wide variation in phenotype, misclassification of patients was likely and this complicated accurate CAD risk estimation.

Since the assignment of disease has been based on genotype, allowing a more unambiguous diagnosis, several studies have addressed the risk for CAD in these patients. Large family studies, studying several mutations, showed a more than threefold excess of CAD and increased carotid arterial wall thickness in affected family members when compared to unaffected members [121, 122]. In both studies, levels of cholesterol efflux correlated well with HDL-C levels and there was a strong correlation between levels of cholesterol efflux and CAD and/or carotid arterial wall thickness. However, these family studies potentially suffer from selection bias, as only families with the most severe phenotypes may have presented at clinics. Also, CAD risk estimates were based on few individuals and were not adjusted for age and other cardiovascular risk factors. Bypassing these problems, seven different *ABCA1* mutations were studied in two different population cohorts and a large case-control study, including a total of 109 heterozygotes, 6666 ischemic heart disease cases, and a total of 41,961 participants [123]. Four mutations were found to be associated with an average of 30% reduction in HDL-C and decreased cholesterol efflux. Carriers of these four mutations, however, did not display an increased risk of CVD. However, this conclusion should also be interpreted with caution as the variants studied were mild mutations, giving relatively small reductions in HDL cholesterol levels and cholesterol efflux [124]. The findings are also conflicting with several reports showing that common genetic variations of the ABCA1 gene influence the risk of CAD in the general population [123, 125, 126]. Interestingly, these associations with atherosclerosis are independent of effects on HDL levels. These findings, of an altered risk for CAD but without corresponding differences in lipid levels, suggest that although ABCA1 may be an important atherosclerosis susceptibility locus, the mechanism by which it exerts this effect is not necessarily by altering steady-state HDL-C levels. In conclusion, any specific *ABCA1* variant must be considered in relation to its impact on protein function, as different variants will have different effects on HDL and susceptibility to atherosclerosis [127].

Diagnosis

The findings of virtually absent HDL-C and low levels of apo-A1 are not sufficient to diagnose Tangier disease, which ultimately requires *ABCA1* gene sequence analysis. Cholesterol efflux defects can be demonstrated with the cholesterol efflux assay on cultivated skin fibroblasts. However, even in the absence of coding sequence mutations in *ABCA1*, cellular cholesterol efflux defects are a common feature in subjects with low HDL [128]. Foam cell formation, responsible for the clinical symptoms in Tangier disease, can be detected in the rectal mucosa by endoscopic examination as pale mucosa with studded 1–2-mm discrete orange-brown spots [96].

Management

To date, no specific treatment for Tangier disease exists. It is advised to identify and tightly regulate modifiable cardiovascular risk factors and possibly institute statin therapy as a means to drive LDL-C levels down even further.

Familial LCAT Deficiency and Fish-Eye Disease

Lecithin: cholesterol acyltransferase (*LCAT*) plays a key role in the maturation of small HDL by means of esterification of free cholesterol, primarily at the surface of the HDL particle (the so-called alpha-LCAT activity) but also on lipids transported by apo-B-containing lipoproteins (the so-called beta-LCAT activity). After esterification, the CE molecules migrate to the inner core of the lipoprotein, promoting further cholesterol efflux from peripheral tissues and leading to larger, cholesterylester-enriched HDL particles. Mutations in the *LCAT* gene causing LCAT deficiency represent another rare autosomal recessive disorder that underlies HDL deficiency. Low HDL-C values result from defective HDL maturation followed by rapid clearance of nascent HDL particles from the circulation. Depending on the mutation, patients with complete LCAT deficiency present with one of the two clinical phenotypes, *familial LCAT deficiency* (FLD) or *fish-eye disease* (FED).

Genetics

The gene encoding *LCAT* is located on chromosome 16, locus 16q22.1. Mutations in *LCAT* account for approximately 4% patients with low HDL-C [128]. Thus far, over 80 mutations in the *LCAT* gene have been described in reports that predominantly investigated single cases or small nuclear families [113].

Clinical Characteristics

Heterozygous carriers of *LCAT* mutations lack clinical symptoms, although they frequently present with up to 50% reduced HDL-C levels and mild hypertriglyceridemia [113]. Homozygous or compound heterozygous patients with mutations in the *LCAT* gene present with one of two clinical phenotypes, familial LCAT deficiency or fish-eye disease. In FLD, both alpha-LCAT, which is specific for HDL, and beta-LCAT, which is specific for VLDL and LDL, are deficient, that is, the deficient esterification is generalized. By contrast, patients with FED have a selective alpha-LCAT deficiency. Because LCAT is still partly active, these patients have, in general, a less severe phenotype. Both FLD and FED are characterized by corneal opacifications, which become apparent after the third decade (see Table 23.2). In addition, FLD is characterized by hemolytic anemia, and the deposition of foam cells in bone marrow, spleen, and particularly in kidneys. Progressive renal disease, with proteinuria and hematuria, which progresses to terminal renal insufficiency, has been described in a high percentage of these patients [81] (see Table 23.2). Biochemically, FLD and FED are both characterized by variable loss of LCAT activity and *HDL deficiency* (5–10% of normal HDL-C levels). Serum levels of apo-A1 are usually decreased but not as low as in patients with apo-A1 deficiency or Tangier disease. Additionally, hypertriglyceridemia is observed [113].

The association between *LCAT* gene mutations and atherosclerosis is still controversial, both because of the limited number of carriers and because of variable results in the studies performed. A 25-year follow-up of nine heterozygote family members [129], as well as a large family study, including 68 carriers of *LCAT* defects (of which 59 heterozygotes) and 74 family controls [113] which measured carotid arterial wall thickness indicated that heterozygous carriers of *LCAT* defects may have an increased risk of atherosclerotic vascular disease. Another study including 45 carriers of *LCAT* mutations reported an increase in aortic pulse wave velocity with both ultrasound and MRI, indicating increased arterial stiffness and carotid wall thickening [130]. However, a study including 540 LCAT mutation carriers from the IMPROVE study who underwent carotid echography showed no increase in intima wall thickening [131].

Diagnosis

The identification of LCAT deficiency needs either genetic testing or measurement of LCAT activity. Depending on the kind of mutation, immunoassays of LCAT detect either no, or slightly reduced concentrations of LCAT protein in plasma. Routine lipid and lipoprotein analyses do not help to distinguish patients with FLD and FED. However, patients with FLD show an increased proportion of unesterified cholesterol in plasma (80–100% instead of normal <30%). By contrast, the plasma of patients with FED has a normal or slightly elevated (up to 70%) unesterified cholesterol/cholesterol ester ratio [96].

Management

At this time, management of LCAT deficiency focuses on limiting the renal dysfunction. Because deposition of highly abnormal apo-B-containing lipoproteins in the kidneys of FLD patients has been implicated as the pathogenetic factor in the formation of renal disease, therapies that reduce the concentration of apo-B-containing lipoproteins (such as a fat-restricted diet and statins) are at least theoretically useful [96]. Recombinant LCAT therapy has been suggested as a possible acute treatment for acute coronary syndrome [132]. ACP-501 is a recombinant human LCAT, which has shown to transliently improve plasma lipids and HDL particle function. A phase 1 study including 16 patients showed dose-dependent HDL-C increases of up to 42%, as well as increases in HDL particle size [24].

Genetic Disorders of CETP

As a regulator of cholesterol flux through the RCT system, CETP may be viewed as potentially having both proatherogenic and antiatherogenic properties (see Fig. 23.1). By facilitating the exchange of cholesterylesters for triglycerides between HDL and Apo-B-containing lipoproteins (LDL and VLDL), CETP may decrease direct RCT via the HDL/hepatic SR-B1 route. In addition, pro-atherogenic effects of CETP activity may result from a reduction in overall HDL levels, potentially reducing cellular cholesterol efflux from the arterial wall, and from an increase in atherogenic LDL levels. However, the potentially pro-atherogenic activities of CETP may, to a large extent, be neutralized by an increase in indirect RCT via the LDL/hepatic LDL receptor route [133].

Genetics

CETP is encoded by a gene located on the long arm of chromosome 16. Several mutations of the *CETP* gene have been associated with altered CETP activity and HDL-c levels. Recent genome-wide association studies have reported that *CETP* genotypes are associated with HDL-C levels more strongly than any other locus across the genome [116, 117].

Clinical Characteristics

Significant differences between ethnic groups with regard to allele frequencies of *CETP* polymorphisms exist [134]. Particularly in Japan, *CETP* gene defects are common and there are appreciable numbers of individuals who are homozygous for mutations in the *CETP* gene. Not surprisingly, functional mutations of the *CETP* gene can produce significant changes in lipid and lipoprotein metabolism. Not all *CETP* gene mutations have an as-dramatic effect on CETP protein levels as the ones described above. Various single nucleotide polymorphisms of the *CETP* gene are associated with only small changes in plasma CETP levels and subsequently levels HDL-C levels [134]. Although sparse, there is evidence from clinical trials that elevated CETP levels, regardless of the cause, are associated with an increased risk of CVD [135–137]. However, studies on individuals with CETP protein deficiency, arising from different genetic mutations, have reported ambiguous findings on the relationship between CETP protein deficiency and CAD risk [138–140]. Overall cardiovascular risk is presumably dependent not only on the effect of CETP deficiency on overall levels of HDL-C but also on the effect on functionality of the HDL particles. Moreover, additional factors affecting the metabolic setting of the *CETP* gene mutation probably also play an important role. It was shown that high HDL-C resulting from simultaneous presence of *CETP*- and *LIPC* gene variants did not protect against CAD. By contrast, an increased risk for CAD was found in these patients [141]. In addition, high triglyceride levels have been suggested to enhance the effect of CETP concentration on CHD risk [137]. Also, potential joint effects of *CETP* genotypes with environmental determinants of HDL-C levels (e.g., exercise and alcohol) on the risk of coronary disease have been reported [142].

Genetic Causes of Elevated Triglycerides

Severely elevated *triglyceride* concentrations are a risk factor for developing *pancreatitis* and in the absence of other causes such as diabetes mellitus, alcohol abuse, chronic renal failure, or hypothyroidism, generally point to genetic disorders of triglyceride-rich lipoprotein-modulating enzymes or apolipoproteins. Mutations in several genes have been described, of which the *LPL, apo-CII,* and *Apo-E* genes are the most important ones. Very recently, the *GPIHBP1 gene* has been introduced as a contributor to *primary hypertriglyceridemia* [22, 143]. Two other new contributors described in a few families are the *APO-A5 gene* and the *LMF1 gene* [144]. On the other hand, loss-of-function mutations in apoC3 are associated with low levels of triglycerides and a reduced risk of CVD [12]. Next to the monogenic causes, polygenetic causes are also familial due to clustering of genetic mutations within families. Susceptibility then results from the accumulation of these mutations, because individual variants are insufficient to actually raise triglyceride levels significantly [144].

Regardless of its origin, the management of hypertriglyceridemia consists of therapeutic lifestyle changes aiming at dietary and weight control, as well as pharmacological treatment with fibrates, niacin, or high doses of fish oil, alone or in various combinations. In case triglyceride levels exceed 10 mmol/L (800 mg/dL), combinations of different drugs are usually required, in order to reduce the risk of pancreatitis [145]. The benefit of treating mild-to-moderate triglyceride elevations is less clear [146], although a causal association between triglycerides and the risk for CVD was found by Mendelian Randomization, and this study suggested that the CV risk reduction by lowering triglycerides was proportional to the absolute reduction in ApoB-containing lipoproteins [13]. Statins can lower triglyceride levels by 20–40% [147]. *Fibrates* lower triglyceride levels by approximately 40–60% and modestly raise HDL-C levels by approximately 15–25% [147]. A large clinical trial to investigate pemafibrate in diabetic patients is underway [148]. Patients who do not respond to *fibrates* can be treated with *niacin*, which lowers triglyceride levels by 30–50%, raises HDL-C levels by 20–30%, and lowers LDL-C levels by 5–25% [147, 149]. They are reviewed above. Fish oil with 2–4 g of *omega-3 fatty acids* daily can reduce triglyceride levels by 15–50%, depending on the dosage and different formulations [150]. Moreover, few adverse effects have been reported, mostly gastrointestinal. However, over-the-counter preparations usually contain far less than these required amounts, and an recent extensive cochrane review found little or no effect of omega-3 fatty acids on mortality or cardiovascular risk. [151, 152]. The new drug *lomitapide* (reviewed above) has also been shown to reduce triglyceride levels up to 40% [144]. Finally, Loss-of-function mutations of Apolipoprotein CIII (APOCIII) are associated with low levels of triglycerides and decreased incidence of CVD [12]. A new second-generation ASO inhibiting APOCIII, Volanesorsen, was found to reduce triglycerides by 77% in patients with reduced LPL activity [153]. Of note is the increased rate of thrombocytopenia in patients treated with Volanesorsen compared to placebo. The underlying mechanism is not clear. Volanesorsen saw its approval in 2019. Other ASO and siRNA compounds are still under investigation. Of note, in patients with *diabetes mellitus,* optimizing glycemic control might help to lower triglyceride levels without additional medication for hypertriglyceridemia.

Familial chylomicronemia syndrome: LPL Deficiency and Apo-CII Deficiency

Plasma LPL and its cofactor apo-CII are involved in the hydrolysis of triglyceride-rich particles such as chylomicrons and VLDL. Genetic *LPL deficiency* is a rare autosomal recessive disorder causing severe hypertriglyceridemia. Estimations of prevalence vary between 1:1,000,000 in the general population and 1:5000 in French Quebec [144]. The incidence of apo-CII deficiency is even lower than that of LPL deficiency.

Genetics

The *LPL* gene is located on chromosome 8p22 [154]. More than 114 mutations have been described and loss-of-function mutations in LPL account for more than 90% of the cases [144]. The *apo-CII* gene is located on chromosome 19, in which at least 13 mutations have been described [155]. In extremely rare occasions, mutations in *APOA5, LMF1*, and *GPIHBP1* have been described [22, 143, 144, 156–158].

Clinical Characteristics

Affected individuals have insufficient capacity to hydrolyze triglycerides, resulting in extremely high plasma triglyceride concentrations, often accompanied by recurrent episodes of *pancreatitis.* LPL deficiency typically manifests itself in early childhood with severe and repetitive colicky pain in the abdomen, acute pancreatitis, and failure to thrive. Eruptive xanthomas (Table. 23.1), lipemia retinalis, and hepatosplenomegaly can also be present. When one of the symptoms above is present, the diagnosis 'chylomicronaemia syndrome' can be made. Plasma is lipemic, reflecting increased plasma levels of both chylomicrons and VLDL. Loss-of-function mutations in *LPL* are associated with an increased risk of CVD, while gain-of-function mutations are protective [159–161]. However, the most serious manifestation of this syndrome remains pancreatitis, which has a 5–6% mortality rate [144].

Diagnosis

Fasting triglyceride levels above 10 mmol/l is suspect for chylomicronaemia. The first step is to rule out secondary causes, such as type 1 or 2 diabetes mellitus, diet, alcohol use, medication use, kidney disease or hypothyroidism [144]. Genetic *LPL* and *apo-CII deficiency* are diagnosed by genotyping, combined with the phenotype as described above. Apo-CII deficiency can also be diagnosed by a post-heparin LPL activity assay, in which the patient's post-heparin plasma is mixed with that of a nonaffected individual. In this experiment, triglyceride levels will decrease rapidly in an apo-CII-deficient patient, in contrast to subjects with LPL deficiency.

Treatment

Treatment consists of *dietary fat restriction.* Hypertriglyceridemia is treated as described above; however, in genetic *LPL* and *apo-CII* deficiency, most of these strategies do not result in a substantial reduction in triglyceride levels. Nevertheless, promising new compounds for the treatment of this patient group are under investigation, such as evinacumab (described above), agents targeting apolipoprotein C-II, apolipoprotein A-V and angiopoietin-like protein 4 [24, 162], and *antisense apo-CIII therapy* by volanesorsen [153]. *Alipogene tiparvovec* is an adeno-associated virus serotype 1-based gene therapy being the first gene therapy to be approved in the Western world. In clinical studies with 27 patients, it lowered plasma triglyceride levels for up to 26 weeks and after even 6 years of follow-up there were still clinically relevant reductions in the incidence of pancreatitis and acute abdominal pain events [163]. It is now approved for a small subset of patients with familial LPL deficiency suffering from recurrent severe pancreatitis under a fat-restricted diet. However, the drug is withdrawn from the market due to its costs.

Familial Dysbetalipoproteinemia (Apo E2/E2 Deficiency)

Familial dysbetalipoproteinemia (*FD*) is characterized by the defective clearance of VLDL- and *chylomicron-remnant particles* caused by homozygosity for apoE2, the type of apoE unable to bind to its receptor. There are three common apoE isoforms: apoE3, apoE2, and apoE4 [164]. Although approximately 0.5% of the population worldwide is homozygous for apoE2, only a small minority develops FD with an estimated prevalence of 1–2:10,000. This is due to the necessity of concomitant environmental, hormonal, and possibly genetic factors, inducing VLDL or chylomicron overproduction, such as a high caloric diet or alcohol abuse, diabetes mellitus, obesity, hypothyroidism, renal disease, or estrogen deficiency.

Genetics

Most people have an *apoE3/E3* genotype, with a ~ 55% prevalence; however, *apoE4* and *apoE2* also exist, with an estimated frequency of 0.5% for *apoE2/E2,* 15% for *apoE2/E3,* 25% for *apoE3/E4,* 1–2% for *apoE4/E4,* and 3–4% for *apoE2/E4*. *ApoE2* differs from *ApoE3* by a single substitution of cysteine for arginine at residue 158.

Less common, dominant-negative mutations may also cause the disorder. Over 25 dominant mutations have been described [165].

Clinical Characteristics

Clinically, apoE2/E2 patients present with *tubero-eruptive xanthomas* (see Fig. 23.4), palmar streaks, elevated TC, and triglyceride concentrations, and are at a high risk for premature CVD and peripheral vascular disease [166]. Tubero-

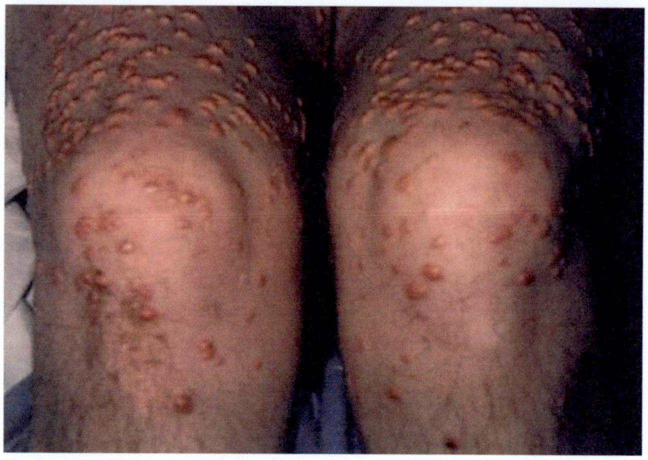

Fig. 23.4 Eruptive xanthomas

eruptive xanthomas begin as clusters of small papules on elbows, knees, or buttocks and can grow to the size of small grapes. Palmar xanthomas are orange-yellow discolorations of palm and wrist creases. Both are pathognomonic for FD, but their absence does not exclude the disorder, since many patients remain asymptomatic for a long time. Plasma TC concentrations usually exceed 8.0 mmol/L (300 mg/dL) and may approach 26.0 mmol/L (1000 mg/dL).

Triglyceride concentrations are within the same range. Dyslipidemia in FD rarely manifests before adulthood. The average age of clinically overt vascular disease is approximately 40 years in men and 59 in women.

Diagnosis

FD can be diagnosed by a combination of a lipid-phenotype and *apoE* genotyping. However, the absence of apoE2/E2 does not rule out the disease, as other genetic causes might also give rise to this trait. Phenotypically, either an ApoB/TC ratio of <0.15 g/mmol, or ApoB levels <1.2 g/L, TG >1.5 mmol/l, TG/ApoB <10 and TC/ApoB >6.2 are good differential determinants for the diagnosis of FD [167].

Management

Treatment of FD is aimed at reducing the overproduction of VLDL and/or chylomicrons, by means of dietary restrictions, including alcohol intake and weight reduction, combined with pharmacological treatment with statins, alone or combined with other compounds, as described above. Recently, a European cross-sectional study including 305 patients from seven academic hospitals in four European countries found that the majority of FD patients have non-HDL-C levels above the threshold of 3.3 mmol/L. However, less than half of these patients were adequately treated, increasing their cardiovascular risk [168]. PCSK9 antibodies could prove to be a treatment option [169], and A PCSK9 antibody trial in FD patients is currently underway.

Familial Combined Hyperlipidemia

FCH is discussed in the section, "Familial Combined Hyperlipidemia."

Familial Hypertriglyceridemia

Familial hypertriglyceridemia (*FHTG*) is a common disorder causing hypertriglyceridemia with the prevalence of 1:500. The genetic basis seems to be based on an accumulation of common and rare genetic mutations that increase susceptibility [170], and the onset of the disease depends on the presence of certain lifestyle factors. FHTG is discussed due to its high prevalence. The metabolic defect is a combination of hepatic VLDL overproduction and decreased catabolism of both VLDL and chylomicrons.

Clinical Characteristics

Typically, patients have moderately elevated plasma triglycerides, 3–10 mmol/L, often accompanied by low HDL-C levels. FHTG is associated with obesity, insulin resistance, hypertension, and hyperuricemia. The onset of hypertriglyceridemia is usually in adult age, when lifestyle factors, which increase triglyceride levels, such as obesity, become more prominent. When the hypertriglyceridemia becomes more severe, the clinical picture can resemble that of LPL deficiency. The association with CVD is weak, compared to the association of LDL-C with CVD [13].

Diagnosis

FHTG is diagnosed by exclusion of other causes of hypertriglyceridemia. A first-degree family member with the same disorder is useful for the diagnosis. FCH and FD should definitely be excluded, since these disorders are associated with a more pronounced CVD risk and therefore require a more stringent therapy.

Management

The first line of treatment is lifestyle modification, possibly combined with pharmacological treatment in case of more severe hypertriglyceridemia.

Summary

Disorders of lipoprotein metabolism are major contributors to CVD, a leading cause of mortality and morbidity worldwide. Dyslipidemia includes both elevated LDL-C levels, elevated triglycerides, and elevated remnant cholesterol, as well as decreased HDL-C levels.

LDL mediates cholesterol transport from the liver to peripheral tissues, including macrophages in the arterial wall, which, after uptake and accumulation of cholesterol, can transform into foam cells and atherosclerotic plaques. Conversely, HDL is thought to exert beneficial effects on the arterial wall through its role in the RCT, which involves the transport of cholesterol from peripheral tissues to the liver followed by biliary excretion and elimination via the feces.

The crucial role of increased plasma LDL-C levels in the pathogenesis of atherosclerosis has been firmly established, as well as the beneficial effects of LDL-C reduction accomplished by HMG-CoA reductase inhibitors or statins. In addition, decreased plasma HDL-C levels are an established independent predictor of CVD. However, pharmacological raising of plasma HDL levels has failed to reduce cardiovascular events thus far. It is therefore uncertain whether HDL plays a causative role in CVD protection or if it is merely an epiphenomenon or nonfunctional biomarker. Finally, the relationship between hypertriglyceridemia and CVD risk is weak but significant.

Most cases of CVD are multifactorial and/or polygenic in origin. However, when CVD occurs at a young age, a number of monogenetic disorders of lipoprotein are frequently seen. These monogenetic disorders of lipoproteins are the primary focus of this chapter.

Regarding LDL metabolism, mutations in four genes are currently identified to result in increased plasma LDL-C concentrations, namely the *LDLR* gene, *ApoB* gene, *LDLRAP1* gene, and most recently the *PCSK9 gene.* Clinical hallmarks of these disorders, of which familial hypercholesterolemia is the most frequent and well known, are elevated plasma LDL-C levels and, consequently, premature atherosclerosis.

To date, several rare monogenetic defects in various proteins involved in HDL metabolism have been identified in humans. The genes encoding apolipoprotein-AI, ABCA1, and LCAT, respectively, are essential for the de novo synthesis of HDL. A complete lack of any of these factors confers severe HDL deficiency, which is referred to as familial hypoalphalipoproteinemia. Although FHA patients display extremely low plasma HDL-C levels, the association of these genetic disorders with atherosclerosis is disputed. Since HDL is a heterogeneous class of lipoprotein particles, these different classes may have different associations with disease. Furthermore, the functionality of the HDL particles, rather than their abundance, may be an important determinant of their antiatherogenic effects.

Table 23.3 Steps in the diagnostic workup of dyslipidemias

1. Exclude underlying conditions
2. Suspected genetic cause? Profoundly decreased HDL-C levels? (<fifth percentile adjusted for age and sex), Profoundly increased LDL-C or TG levels. Presence of specific clinical hallmarks? (see text and Table 23.2) presence of familiar dyslipidemias/premature atherosclerosis?
3. Perform specialized biochemical tests and/or specific gene sequencing
4. Initiate family studies

Finally, severely elevated triglyceride concentrations can be induced by mutations in several genes, of which the *LPL*, *apo-CII,* and *Apo-E* genes are the most important ones. Next to the role of hypertriglyceridemia in athero-genesis, severely elevated triglyceride levels confer a health risk due to the increased risk of pancreatitis.

In general, the vast majority of dyslipidemia are polygenic and/or multifactorial in origin, which complicates the determination of the main cause, as well as quantification of the increased risk on CVD. Monogenic causes of lipid disorders result in a higher risk on CVD compared to polygenic causes and patients from the general population with similar lipid levels [15]. It is therefore extremely important to conduct a thorough diagnostic workup.

The first step in the diagnostic workup of dyslipidemias consists of the exclusion of underlying conditions through careful medical history taking, physical examination, and biochemical testing, which are reviewed in detail elsewhere. Suggestive for a genetic cause is the presence of specific clinical hallmarks (see text and Table 23.2) and/or the presence of familial dyslipidemias/premature atherosclerosis. When FH is suspected, multiple diagnostic criteria frameworks have been developed [171]. In cases where a genetic cause is suspected, specialized biochemical tests and/or the demonstration of a functionally relevant mutation in the involved genes should be performed to obtain a definitive diagnosis. In addition, family studies should be initiated to evaluate the inheritance pattern of the phenotype and to be able to timely diagnose family members and treat them accordingly (see Table 23.3).

Treatment consists of lifestyle modifications such as weight reduction, exercise, and smoking cessation to improve other atherogenic risk factors, possibly in combination with pharmacological agents. High-dose statins are currently the most effective pharmacological strategy to reduce CVD risk. Also in case of low HDL and hypertriglyceridemia, statin monotherapy, possibly in combination with other agents, reduces the risk of CVD. However, it should be noted that many new therapies are becoming available that could change current treatment guidelines in the years to come.

References

1. Yusuf S, Hawken S, Ôunpuu S, Dans T, Avezum A, Lanas F, et al. Effect of potentially modifiable risk factors associated with myocardial infarction in 52 countries (the INTERHEART study): case-control study. Lancet. 2004;364(9438):937–52. https://doi.org/10.1016/s0140-6736(04)17018-9.
2. Baigent C, Keech A, Kearney PM, Blackwell L, Buck G, Pollicino C, et al. Efficacy and safety of cholesterol-lowering treatment: prospective meta-analysis of data from 90,056 participants in 14 randomised trials of statins. Lancet. 2005;366(9493):1267–78. Available from: http://www.ncbi.nlm.nih.gov/pubmed/16214597
3. Genest JJ, Martin-Munley SS, McNamara JR, Ordovas JM, Jenner J, Myers RH, et al. Familial lipoprotein disorders in patients with premature coronary artery disease. Circulation. 1992;85(6):2025–33. https://doi.org/10.1161/01.cir.85.6.2025.
4. Briel M, Ferreira-Gonzalez I, You JJ, Karanicolas PJ, Akl EA, Wu P, et al. Association between change in high density lipoprotein cholesterol and cardiovascular disease morbidity and mortality: systematic review and meta-regression analysis. BMJ. 2009;338(1):b92. https://doi.org/10.1136/bmj.b92.
5. Ghali WA, Rodondi N. HDL cholesterol and cardiovascular risk. BMJ. 2009;338(1):a3065. https://doi.org/10.1136/bmj.a3065.
6. Hokanson JE, Austin MA. Plasma triglyceride level is a risk factor for cardiovascular disease independent of high-density lipoprotein cholesterol level: a meta-analysis of population-based prospective studies. J Cardiovasc Risk. 1996;3(2):213–9. https://doi.org/10.1097/00043798-199604000-00014.
7. Bansal S, Buring JE, Rifai N, Mora S, Sacks FM, Ridker PM. Fasting compared with nonfasting triglycerides and risk of cardiovascular events in women. JAMA. 2007;298(3):309. https://doi.org/10.1001/jama.298.3.309.
8. Nordestgaard BG, Benn M, Schnohr P, Tybjærg-Hansen A. Nonfasting triglycerides and risk of myocardial infarction, ischemic heart disease, and death in men and women. JAMA. 2007;298(3):299. https://doi.org/10.1001/jama.298.3.299.
9. Stauffer ME, Weisenfluh L, Morrison A. Association between triglycerides and cardiovascular events in primary populations: a meta-regression analysis and synthesis of evidence. Vasc Health Risk Manag. 2013;9(1):671–80.
10. Nordestgaard BG. Triglyceride-rich lipoproteins and atherosclerotic cardiovascular disease. Circ Res. 2016;118(4):547–63. Available from: http://circres.ahajournals.org/lookup/doi/10.1161/CIRCRESAHA.115.306249
11. Article O. Coding variation in *ANGPTL4, LPL,* and *SVEP1* and the risk of coronary disease. N Engl J Med. 2016;374(12):1134–44. https://doi.org/10.1056/NEJMoa1507652.
12. Jørgensen AB, Frikke-Schmidt R, Nordestgaard BG, Tybjærg-Hansen A. Loss-of-function mutations in APOC3 and risk of ischemic vascular disease. N Engl J Med. 2014;371(1):32–41. Available from: http://www.ncbi.nlm.nih.gov/pubmed/24941082
13. Ference BA, Kastelein JJP, Ray KK, Ginsberg HN, Chapman MJ, Packard CJ, Laufs U, Oliver-Williams C, Wood AM, Butterworth AS, Di Angelantonio E, Danesh J, Nicholls SJ, Bhatt DL, Sabatine MS, Catapano AL. Association of triglyceride-lowering variants and LDL-C–lowering variants with risk of coronary heart disease. JAMA. 2019;321(4):364.
14. Ference BA, Bhatt DL, Catapano AL, Packard CJ, Graham I, Kaptoge S, Ference TB, Guo Q, Laufs U, Ruff CT, Arjen C, Kees Hovingh G, Danesh J, Holmes MV, Smith GD, Ray KK, Nicholls SJ, Sabatine MS. Association of genetic variants related to combined exposure to lower low-density lipoproteins and lower systolic blood pressure with lifetime risk of cardiovascular disease. JAMA. 2019;322(14):1381.
15. Trinder M, Francis GA, Brunham LR. Association of monogenic vs polygenic hypercholesterolemia with risk of atherosclerotic cardiovascular disease. JAMA Cardiol. 2020;5(4):390.
16. Virani SS. Lipoprotein a and cardiovascular disease current state and future directions for an enigmatic lipoprotein. Front Biosci. 2018;23(3):1099–112.
17. Neeli I, Siddiqi SA, Siddiqi S, Mahan J, Lagakos WS, Binas B, et al. Liver fatty acid-binding protein initiates budding of prechylomicron transport vesicles from intestinal endoplasmic reticulum. J Biol Chem. 2007;282(25):17974–84. https://doi.org/10.1074/jbc.m610765200.
18. Davies JP, Levy B, Ioannou YA. Evidence for a Niemann–pick C (NPC) gene family: identification and characterization of NPC1L1. Genomics. 2000;65(2):137–45. https://doi.org/10.1006/geno.2000.6151.
19. Graf GA, Cohen JC, Hobbs HH. Missense mutations in ABCG5 and ABCG8 disrupt heterodimerization and trafficking. J Biol Chem. 2004;279(23):24881–8. https://doi.org/10.1074/jbc.m402634200.
20. Temel RE, Tang W, Ma Y, Rudel LL, Willingham MC, Ioannou YA, et al. Hepatic Niemann-pick C1–like 1 regulates biliary cholesterol concentration and is a target of ezetimibe. J Clin Invest. 2007;117(7):1968–78. https://doi.org/10.1172/jci30060.
21. Grundy SM. Absorption and metabolism of dietary cholesterol. Annu Rev Nutr. 1983;3(1):71–96. https://doi.org/10.1146/annurev.nu.03.070183.000443.
22. Beigneux AP, Davies BSJ, Gin P, Weinstein MM, Farber E, Qiao X, et al. Glycosylphosphatidylinositol-anchored high-density lipoprotein-binding protein 1 plays a critical role in the lipolytic processing of chylomicrons. Cell Metab. 2007;5(4):279–91. https://doi.org/10.1016/j.cmet.2007.02.002.
23. Lambert G, Sjouke B, Choque B, Kastelein JJP, Hovingh GK. The PCSK9 decade. J Lipid Res. 2012;53:2515–24.
24. Hegele RA, Tsimikas S. Lipid-lowering agents. Circ Res. 2019;124(3):386–404.
25. Lewis GF, Rader DJ. New insights into the regulation of HDL metabolism and reverse cholesterol transport. Circ Res. 2005;96(12):1221–32. https://doi.org/10.1161/01.res.0000170946.56981.5c.
26. Tall AR. Cholesterol efflux pathways and other potential mechanisms involved in the athero-protective effect of high density lipoproteins. J Intern Med. 2008;263(3):256–73. https://doi.org/10.1111/j.1365-2796.2007.01898.x.
27. van Tol A. Phospholipid transfer protein. Curr Opin Lipidol. 2002;13(2):135–9. https://doi.org/10.1097/00041433-200204000-00004.
28. Abifadel M, Varret M, Rabès J-P, Allard D, Ouguerram K, Devillers M, et al. Mutations in PCSK9 cause autosomal dominant hypercholesterolemia. Nat Genet. 2003;34(2):154–6. https://doi.org/10.1038/ng1161.
29. Quagliarini F, Vallvé J-C, Campagna F, Alvaro A, Fuentes-Jimenez FJ, Sirinian MI, et al. Autosomal recessive hypercholesterolemia in Spanish kindred due to a large deletion in the ARH gene. Mol Genet Metab. 2007;92(3):243–8. https://doi.org/10.1016/j.ymgme.2007.06.012.
30. Garcia CK, Willund K, Arca M, Zuliani G, Fellin R, Maioli M, et al. Autosomal recessive hypercholesterolemia caused by mutations in a putative LDL receptor adaptor protein. Science (80-). 2001;292(5520):1394–8. https://doi.org/10.1126/science.1060458.
31. Beheshti SO, Madsen CM, Varbo A, Nordestgaard BG. Worldwide Prevalence of Familial Hypercholesterolemia. J Am Coll Cardiol. 2020;75(20):2553–66.
32. Leitersdorf E, Tobin EJ, Davignon J, Hobbs HH. Common low-density lipoprotein receptor mutations in the French Canadian population. J Clin Invest. 1990;85(4):1014–23. https://doi.org/10.1172/jci114531.
33. Raal FJ, Sjouke B, Hovingh GK, Isaac BF. Phenotype diversity among patients with homozygous familial hypercholesterolemia: a cohort study. Atherosclerosis. 2016;248:238–44. https://doi.org/10.1016/j.atherosclerosis.2016.03.009.

34. Goldstein JL, Hobbs HH, Brown MS. Familial hypercholesterolemia. In: Scriver CR, Beaudet AL, Sly WS, Valle D, Childs B, et al., editors. The metabolic basis of inherited disease. 8th ed. New York: McGraw-Hill; 2001. p. 2863–913.
35. Leigh S, Futema M, Whittall R, Taylor-Beadling A, Williams M, den Dunnen JT, Humphries SE. The UCL low-density lipoprotein receptor gene variant database: pathogenicity update. J Med Genet. 2017;54(4):217–23.
36. Wiegman A, Gidding SS, Watts GF, Chapman MJ, Ginsberg HN, Cuchel M, et al. Familial hypercholesterolaemia in children and adolescents: gaining decades of life by optimizing detection and treatment. Eur Heart J. 2015;36:2425–37.
37. Slack J. Risks of ischæmic heart-disease in familial hyperlipoproteinæmic states. Lancet. 1969;294(7635):1380–2. https://doi.org/10.1016/s0140-6736(69)90930-1.
38. Souverein OW, Defesche JC, Zwinderman AH, Kastelein JJP, Tanck MWT. Influence of LDL-receptor mutation type on age at first cardiovascular event in patients with familial hypercholesterolaemia. Eur Heart J. 2007;28(3):299–304. https://doi.org/10.1093/eurheartj/ehl366.
39. Wiegman A, de Groot E, Hutten BA, Rodenburg J, Gort J, Bakker HD, et al. Arterial intima-media thickness in children heterozygous for familial hypercholesterolaemia. Lancet. 2004;363(9406):369–70. https://doi.org/10.1016/s0140-6736(04)15467-6.
40. Huijgen R, Vissers MN, Defesche JC, Lansberg PJ, Kastelein JJP, Hutten BA. Familial hypercholesterolemia: current treatment and advances in management. Expert Rev Cardiovasc Ther. 2008;6(4):567–81. https://doi.org/10.1586/14779072.6.4.567.
41. Besseling J, Reitsma JB, Gaudet D, Brisson D, Kastelein JJP, Hovingh GK, et al. Selection of individuals for genetic testing for familial hypercholesterolaemia: development and external validation of a prediction model for the presence of a mutation causing familial hypercholesterolaemia. Eur Heart J. 2016;38(8):565–73. Available from: http://www.ncbi.nlm.nih.gov/pubmed/27044878
42. Hovingh GK, Davidson MH, Kastelein JJP, O' Connor AM. Clinical update diagnosis and treatment of familial hypercholesterolaemia. Eur Heart J. 2013;34:962–71.
43. Prospective Studies Collaboration, Lewington S, Whitlock G, Clarke R, Sherliker P, Emberson J, et al. Blood cholesterol and vascular mortality by age, sex, and blood pressure: a meta-analysis of individual data from 61 prospective studies with 55,000 vascular deaths. Lancet. 2007;370(9602):1829–39. Available from: http://www.ncbi.nlm.nih.gov/pubmed/18061058
44. Besseling J, Sjouke B, Kastelein JJP. Screening and treatment of familial hypercholesterolemia e lessons from the past and opportunities for the future (based on the Anitschkow lecture 2014). Atherosclerosis. 2015;241(2):597–606. https://doi.org/10.1016/j.atherosclerosis.2015.06.011.
45. Mach F, Baigent C, Catapano AL, Koskinas KC, Casula M, Badimon L, Chapman MJ, De Backer GG, Delgado V, Ference BA, Graham IM, Halliday A, Landmesser U, Mihaylova B, Pedersen TR, Riccardi G, Richter DJ, Sabatine MS, Taskinen M-R, Tokgozoglu L, Wiklund O, Mueller C, Drexel H, Aboyans V, Corsini A, Doehner W, Farnier M, Gigante B, Kayikcioglu M, Krstacic G, Lambrinou E, Lewis BS, Masip J, Moulin P, Petersen S, Petronio AS, Piepoli MF, Pintó X, Räber L, Ray KK, Reiner Ž, Riesen WF, Roffi M, Schmid J-P, Shlyakhto E, Simpson IA, Stroes E, Sudano I, Tselepis AD, Viigimaa M, Vindis C, Vonbank A, Vrablik M, Vrsalovic M, Zamorano JL, Collet J-P, Koskinas KC, Casula M, Badimon L, Chapman MJ, De Backer GG, Delgado V, Ference BA, Graham IM, Halliday A, Landmesser U, Mihaylova B, Pedersen TR, Riccardi G, Richter DJ, Sabatine MS, Taskinen M-R, Tokgozoglu L, Wiklund O, Windecker S, Aboyans V, Baigent C, Collet J-P, Dean V, Delgado V, Fitzsimons D, Gale CP, Grobbee D, Halvorsen S, Hindricks G, Iung B, Jüni P, Katus HA, Landmesser U, Leclercq C, Lettino M, Lewis BS, Merkely B, Mueller C, Petersen S, Petronio AS, Richter DJ, Roffi M, Shlyakhto E, Simpson IA, Sousa-Uva M, Touyz RM, Nibouche D, Zelveian PH, Siostrzonek P, Najafov R, van de Borne P, Pojskic B, Postadzhiyan A, Kypris L, Špinar J, Larsen ML, Eldin HS, Viigimaa M, Strandberg TE, Ferrières J, Agladze R, Laufs U, Rallidis L, Bajnok L, Gudjónsson T, Maher V, Henkin Y, Gulizia MM, Mussagaliyeva A, Bajraktari G, Kerimkulova A, Latkovskis G, Hamoui O, Slapikas R, Visser L, Dingli P, Ivanov V, Boskovic A, Nazzi M, Visseren F, Mitevska I, Retterstøl K, Jankowski P, Fontes-Carvalho R, Gaita D, Ezhov M, Foscoli M, Giga V, Pella D, Fras Z, de Isla LP, Hagström E, Lehmann R, Abid L, Ozdogan O, Mitchenko O, Patel RS. 2019 ESC/EAS guidelines for the management of dyslipidaemias: lipid modification to reduce cardiovascular risk. Eur Heart J. 2020;41(1):111–88.
46. Grundy SM, Stone NJ, Bailey AL, Beam C, Birtcher KK, Blumenthal RS, Braun LT, de Ferranti S, Faiella-Tommasino J, Forman DE, Goldberg R, Heidenreich PA, Hlatky MA, Jones DW, Lloyd-Jones D, Lopez-Pajares N, Ndumele CE, Orringer CE, Peralta CA, Saseen JJ, Smith SC, Sperling L, Virani SS, Yeboah J. 2018 AHA/ACC/AACVPR/AAPA/ABC/ACPM/ADA/AGS/APhA/ASPC/NLA/PCNA guideline on the management of blood cholesterol. J Am Coll Cardiol. 2019;73(24):e285–350.
47. Cannon CP, Blazing MA, Giugliano RP, McCagg A, White JA, Theroux P, Darius H, Lewis BS, Ophuis TO, Wouter Jukema J, De Ferrari GM, Ruzyllo W, De Lucca P, Im KA, Bohula EA, Reist C, Wiviott SD, Tershakovec AM, Musliner TA, Braunwald E, Califf RM. Ezetimibe added to statin therapy after acute coronary syndromes. N Engl J Med. 2015;372(25):2387–97.
48. Reiner Ž. Management of patients with familial hypercholesterolaemia. Nat Publ Gr. 2015;12(10):565–75. https://doi.org/10.1038/nrcardio.2015.92.
49. Stoekenbroek RM, Kastelein JJP, Huijgen R. PCSK9 inhibition: the way forward in the treatment of dyslipidemia. BMC Med. 2015;13:1–6. https://doi.org/10.1186/s12916-015-0503-4.
50. Sabatine MS, Giugliano RP, Wiviott SD, Raal FJ, Blom DJ, Robinson J, et al. Efficacy and safety of evolocumab in reducing lipids and cardiovascular events. N Engl J Med. 2015;372(16):1500–9. Available from: http://www.ncbi.nlm.nih.gov/pubmed/25773607
51. Zhang X-L, Zhu Q-Q, Zhu L, Chen J-Z, Chen Q-H, Li G-N, et al. Safety and efficacy of anti-PCSK9 antibodies: a meta-analysis of 25 randomized, controlled trials. BMC Med. 2015;13(1):123. Available from: http://www.biomedcentral.com/1741-7015/13/123
52. Casula M, Olmastroni E, Boccalari MT, Tragni E, Pirillo A, Catapano AL. Cardiovascular events with PCSK9 inhibitors: an updated meta-analysis of randomised controlled trials. Pharmacol Res. 2019;143:143–50.
53. Nishikido T, Ray KK. Inclisiran for the treatment of dyslipidemia. Expert Opin Investig Drugs. 2018;27(3):287–94.
54. Raal FJ, Kallend D, Ray KK, Turner T, Wolfgang K, Scott Wright R, Wijngaard PLJ, Curcio D, Jaros MJ, Leiter LA, Kastelein JJP. Inclisiran for the treatment of heterozygous familial hypercholesterolemia. N Engl J Med. 2020;382(16):1520–30.
55. Ray KK, Scott Wright R, Kallend D, Koenig W, Leiter LA, Raal FJ, Bisch JA, Richardson T, Jaros M, Wijngaard PLJ, Kastelein JJP. Two phase 3 trials of inclisiran in patients with elevated LDL cholesterol. N Engl J Med. 2020;382(16):1507–19.
56. Markham A. Bempedoic acid: first approval. Drugs. 2020;80(7):747–53.
57. Florentin M, Liberopoulos EN, Mikhailidis DP, Elisaf MS. Colesevelam hydrochloride in clinical practice: a new approach in the treatment of hypercholesterolaemia. Curr Med Res Opin Informa Healthcare. 2008;24(4):995–1009. https://doi.org/10.1185/030079908x280446.
58. Averna M, Cefalù AB, Stefanutti C, Di Giacomo S, Sirtori CR, Vigna G. Nutrition, metabolism & cardiovascular diseases individual analysis of patients with HoFH participating in a

phase 3 trial with lomitapide: the Italian cohort. Nutr Metab Cardiovasc Dis. 2016;26(1):36–44. https://doi.org/10.1016/j.numecd.2015.11.001.

59. Blom DJ, Fayad ZA, Kastelein JJP, Larrey D, Makris L, Schwamlein C, et al. LOWER, a registry of lomitapide-treated patients with homozygous familial hypercholesterolemia: rationale and design. J Clin Lipidol. 2016;10(2):273–82. https://doi.org/10.1016/j.jacl.2015.11.011.
60. Underberg J, Cannon C, Larrey D, Makris L, Jurecka A, Blom D. Long-term safety and efficacy of lomitapide in patients with homozygous familial hypercholesterolemia: three-year data from the lomitapide observational worldwide evaluation registry (lower). J Am Coll Cardiol. 2018;71(11):A168.
61. Ajufo E, Cuchel M. Recent developments in gene therapy for homozygous familial hypercholesterolemia. Curr Atheroscler Rep. 2016;18(5):22. https://doi.org/10.1007/s11883-016-0579-0.
62. Fogacci F, Ferri N, Toth PP, Ruscica M, Corsini A, Cicero AFG. Efficacy and safety of mipomersen: a systematic review and meta-analysis of randomized clinical trials. Drugs. 2019;79(7):751–66.
63. Avis HJ, Vissers MN, Stein EA, Wijburg FA, Trip MD, Kastelein JJP, et al. A systematic review and meta-analysis of statin therapy in children with familial hypercholesterolemia. Arterioscler Thromb Vasc Biol. 2007;27(8):1803–10. https://doi.org/10.1161/atvbaha.107.145151.
64. Arambepola C, Farmer AJ, Perera R, Neil HAW. Statin treatment for children and adolescents with heterozygous familial hypercholesterolaemia: a systematic review and meta-analysis. Atherosclerosis. 2007;195(2):339–47. https://doi.org/10.1016/j.atherosclerosis.2006.09.030.
65. Rodenburg J, Vissers MN, Wiegman A, van Trotsenburg ASP, van der Graaf A, de Groot E, et al. Statin treatment in children with familial hypercholesterolemia: the younger, the better. Circulation. 2007;116(6):664–8. https://doi.org/10.1161/circulationaha.106.671016.
66. Luirink IK, Albert W, Meeike Kusters D, Hof MH, Groothoff JW, de Groot E, Kastelein JJP, Hutten BA. 20-year follow-up of statins in children with familial hypercholesterolemia. N Engl J Med. 2019;381(16):1547–56.
67. Reiner Ž. Impact of early evidence of atherosclerotic changes on early treatment in children with familial hypercholesterolemia. Circ Res. 2014;114(2):233–5.
68. P/229/2010: EMA decision of 23 November 2010 on the acceptance of a modification of an agreed paediatric investigation plan for rosuvastatin (calcium) (Crestor and associated names) (EMEA-000022-PIP01-07-M04). First published: 21/12/2010
69. Daniels S, Caprio S, Chaudhari U, Manvelian G, Baccara-Dinet MT, Brunet A, Scemama M, Loizeau V, Bruckert E. PCSK9 inhibition with alirocumab in pediatric patients with heterozygous familial hypercholesterolemia: The ODYSSEY KIDS study. J Clin Lipidol. 2020;14(3):322–330.e5.
70. Watts GF, Gidding S, Wierzbicki AS, Toth PP, Alonso R, Brown WV, et al. Integrated guidance on the care of familial hypercholesterolemia from the international FH foundation. J Clin Lipidol. 2014;8(2):148–72. https://doi.org/10.1016/j.jacl.2014.01.002.
71. Andersen LH, Miserez AR, Ahmad Z, Andersen RL. Familial defective apolipoprotein B-100: A review. J Clin Lipidol. 2016;10(6):1297–302.
72. Miserez AR, Muller PY. Familial defective apolipoprotein B-100: a mutation emerged in the Mesolithic ancestors of Celtic peoples? Atherosclerosis. 2000;148(2):433–6. https://doi.org/10.1016/s0021-9150(99)00470-0.
73. Defesche JC, Pricker KL, Hayden MR, van der Ende BE, Kastelein JJ. Familial defective apolipoprotein B-100 is clinically indistinguishable from familial hypercholesterolemia. Arch Intern Med. 1993;153(20):2349. https://doi.org/10.1001/archinte.1993.00410200071008.
74. Miserez AR, Keller U. Differences in the phenotypic characteristics of subjects with familial defective apolipoprotein B-100 and familial hypercholesterolemia. Arterioscler Thromb Vasc Biol. 1995;15(10):1719–29. https://doi.org/10.1161/01.atv.15.10.1719.
75. D'Erasmo L, Di Costanzo A, Arca M. Autosomal recessive hypercholesterolemia. Curr Opin Lipidol. 31(2):56–61.
76. Muntoni S, Pisciotta L, Muntoni S, Bertolini S. Pharmacological treatment of a Sardinian patient affected by autosomal recessive hypercholesterolemia (ARH). J Clin Lipidol. 2015;9(1):103–6. https://doi.org/10.1016/j.jacl.2014.08.009.
77. Eden ER, Sun X-M, Patel DD, Soutar AK. Adaptor protein Disabled-2 modulates low density lipoprotein receptor synthesis in fibroblasts from patients with autosomal recessive hypercholesterolaemia. Hum Mol Genet. 2007;16(22):2751–9. https://doi.org/10.1093/hmg/ddm232.
78. Cohen JC, Kimmel M, Polanski A, Hobbs HH. Molecular mechanisms of autosomal recessive hypercholesterolemia. Curr Opin Lipidol. 2003;14(2):121–7. https://doi.org/10.1097/00041433-200304000-00002.
79. Wilund KR, Campagna F, Arca M, Zuiliani G, Fellin R, Ho YK, et al. Molecular mechanisms of autosomal recessive hypercholesterolemia. Hum Mol Genet. 2002;11(24):3019–30. https://doi.org/10.1093/hmg/11.24.3019.
80. D'Erasmo L, Minicocci I, Nicolucci A, Pintus P, Roeters JE, Lennep V, Masana L, Mata P, Sánchez-Hernández RM, Prieto-Matos P, Real JT, Ascaso JF, Lafuente EE, Pocovi M, Fuentes FJ, Muntoni S, Bertolini S, Sirtori C, Calabresi L, Pavanello C, Averna M, Cefalu AB, Noto D, Pacifico AA, Pes GM, Harada-Shiba M, Manzato E, Zambon S, Zambon A, Vogt A, Scardapane M, Sjouke B, Fellin R, Arca M. Autosomal recessive hypercholesterolemia. J Am Coll Cardiol. 2018;71(3):279–88.
81. Wierzbicki A, Graham C, Young I, Nicholls D. Familial combined hyperlipidaemia: under – defined and under – diagnosed? Curr Vasc Pharmacol. 2008;6(1):13–22. https://doi.org/10.2174/157016108783331268.
82. Brahm AJ, Hegele RA. Combined hyperlipidemia: familial but not (usually) monogenic. Curr Opin Lipidol. 2016;27:131–40.
83. Schaefer EJ, Genest JJ, Ordovas JM, Salem DN, Wilson PWF. Familial lipoprotein disorders and premature coronary artery disease. Atherosclerosis. 1994;108:S41–54. https://doi.org/10.1016/0021-9150(94)90152-x.
84. Veerkamp MJ. Nomogram to diagnose familial combined hyperlipidemia on the basis of results of a 5-year follow-up study. Circulation. 2004;109(24):2980–5. https://doi.org/10.1161/01.cir.0000130646.93255.86.
85. Amend KL, Landon J, Thyagarajan V, Niemcryk S, McAfee A. Incidence of hospitalized rhabdomyolysis with statin and fibrate use in an insured US population. Ann Pharmacother. 2011;45(10):1230–9. Available from: http://www.ncbi.nlm.nih.gov/pubmed/21917557
86. Berge KE, Tian H, Graf GA, Yu L, Grishin NV, Schultz J, et al. Accumulation of dietary cholesterol in sitosterolemia caused by mutations in adjacent ABC transporters. Science. 2000;290(5497):1771–5. Available from: http://www.ncbi.nlm.nih.gov/pubmed/11099417
87. Hooper AJ, Bell DA, Hegele RA, Burnett JR. Clinical utility gene card for: Sitosterolaemia. Eur J Hum Genet. 2017;25(4):512.
88. Lu K, Lee M-H, Yu H, Zhou Y, Sandell SA, Salen G, et al. Molecular cloning, genomic organization, genetic variations, and characterization of murine sterolin genes Abcg5 and Abcg8. J Lipid Res. 2002;43(4):565–78. Available from: http://www.ncbi.nlm.nih.gov/pubmed/11907139
89. Hubacek JA, Berge KE, Cohen JC, Hobbs HH. Mutations in ATP-cassette binding proteins G5 (ABCG5) and G8 (ABCG8) causing sitosterolemia. Hum Mutat. 2001;18(4):359–60. https://doi.org/10.1002/humu.1206.

90. Reeskamp LF, Volta A, Zuurbier L, Defesche JC, Hovingh GK, Grefhorst A. ABCG5 and ABCG8 genetic variants in familial hypercholesterolemia. J Clin Lipidol. 2020;14(2):207–217.e7.
91. Bhattacharyya AK, Connor WE. β-Sitosterolemia and Xanthomatosis. J Clin Invest. 1974;53(4):1033–43. https://doi.org/10.1172/jci107640.
92. Salen G, Shefer S, Nguyen L, Ness GC, Tint GS, Shore V. Sitosterolemia. J Lipid Res. 1992;33(7):945–55. Available from: http://www.ncbi.nlm.nih.gov/pubmed/1431587
93. Salen G, von Bergmann K, Lütjohann D, Kwiterovich P, Kane J, Patel SB, et al. Ezetimibe effectively reduces plasma plant sterols in patients with sitosterolemia. Circulation. 2004;109(8):966–71. Available from: http://www.ncbi.nlm.nih.gov/pubmed/14769702
94. Salen G, Starc T, Sisk CM, Patel SB. Intestinal cholesterol absorption inhibitor ezetimibe added to cholestyramine for sitosterolemia and xanthomatosis. Gastroenterology. 2006;130(6):1853–7. https://doi.org/10.1053/j.gastro.2006.02.027.
95. Wang X, Paigen B. Genetics of variation in HDL cholesterol in humans and mice. Circ Res. 2005;96(1):27–42. Available from: http://www.ncbi.nlm.nih.gov/pubmed/15637305
96. von Eckardstein A. Differential diagnosis of familial high density lipoprotein deficiency syndromes. Atherosclerosis. 2006;186(2):231–9. https://doi.org/10.1016/j.atherosclerosis.2005.10.033.
97. Khovidhunkit W, Memon RA, Feingold KR, Grunfeld C. Infection and inflammation-induced proatherogenic changes of lipoproteins. J Infect Dis. 2000;181(s3):S462–72. https://doi.org/10.1086/315611.
98. Canner PL, Berge KG, Wenger NK, Stamler J, Friedman L, Prineas RJ, et al. Fifteen year mortality in coronary drug project patients: long-term benefit with niacin. J Am Coll Cardiol. 1986;8(6):1245–55. https://doi.org/10.1016/s0735-1097(86)80293-5.
99. Investigators AIM-HIGH, Boden WE, Probstfield JL. Anderson T, Chaitman BR, Desvignes-Nickens P, et al. niacin in patients with low HDL cholesterol levels receiving intensive statin therapy. N Engl J Med. 2011;365(24):2255–67. Available from: http://www.ncbi.nlm.nih.gov/pubmed/22085343
100. HPS2-THRIVE Collaborative Group, Landray MJ, Haynes R, Hopewell JC, Parish S, Aung T, et al. Effects of extended-release niacin with laropiprant in high-risk patients. N Engl J Med. 2014;371(3):203–12. Available from: http://www.ncbi.nlm.nih.gov/pubmed/25014686
101. Barter PJ, Rye K. Targeting high-density lipoproteins to reduce cardiovascular risk: what is the evidence ? Clin Ther Elsevier. 2015;37(12):2716–31. https://doi.org/10.1016/j.clinthera.2015.07.021.
102. Hausenloy DJ, Yellon DM. Targeting residual cardiovascular risk: raising high-density lipoprotein cholesterol levels. Heart. 2008;94(6):706–14. https://doi.org/10.1136/hrt.2007.125401.
103. Kosmas C, DeJesus E, Rosario D, Vittorio T. CETP inhibition: past failures and future hopes. Clin Med Insights Cardiol. 2016;10:37–42.
104. Bowman L, Hopewell JC, Chen F, Wallendszus K, Stevens W, Collins R, Wiviott SD, Cannon CP, Braunwald E, Sammons E, Landray MJ. Effects of Anacetrapib in Patients with Atherosclerotic Vascular Disease. N Engl J Med. 2017;377(13):1217–27.
105. Sammons E, on behalf of the REVEAL Study Collaborative Group (2019). The effects of anacetrapib on occlusive vascular events during post-trial follow-up of the REVEAL randomized trial. AHA Scientific Sessions.
106. Ference BA, Kastelein JJP, Ginsberg HN, Chapman MJ, Nicholls SJ, Ray KK, Packard CJ, Laufs U, Brook RD, Oliver-Williams C, Butterworth AS, Danesh J, Smith GD, Catapano AL, Sabatine MS. Association of Genetic Variants Related to CETP Inhibitors and Statins With Lipoprotein Levels and Cardiovascular Risk. JAMA. 2017;318(10):947.
107. Kees Hovingh G, Kastelein JJP, van Deventer SJH, Round P, Ford J, Saleheen D, Rader DJ, Brewer HB, Barter PJ. Cholesterol ester transfer protein inhibition by TA-8995 in patients with mild dyslipidaemia (TULIP): a randomised, double-blind, placebo-controlled phase 2 trial. Lancet. 2015;386(9992):452–60.
108. Pisciotta L, Fasano T, Calabresi L, Bellocchio A, Fresa R, Borrini C, et al. A novel mutation of the apolipoprotein A-I gene in a family with familial combined hyperlipidemia. Atherosclerosis. 2008;198(1):145–51. https://doi.org/10.1016/j.atherosclerosis.2007.09.017.
109. Joy T, Wang J, Hahn A, Hegele RA. Apoa1 related amyloidosis: a case report and literature review. Clin Biochem. 2003;36(8):641–5. https://doi.org/10.1016/s0009-9120(03)00110-3.
110. Hovingh GK, Brownlie A, Bisoendial RJ, Dube MP, Levels JHM, Petersen W, et al. A novel apoA-I mutation (L178P) leads to endothelial dysfunction, increased arterial wall thickness, and premature coronary artery disease. J Am Coll Cardiol. 2004;44(7):1429–35. https://doi.org/10.1016/j.jacc.2004.06.070.
111. Gomaraschi M, Baldassarre D, Amato M, Eligini S, Conca P, Sirtori CR, et al. Normal vascular function despite low levels of high-density lipoprotein cholesterol in carriers of the apolipoprotein A-IMilano mutant. Circulation. 2007;116(19):2165–72. https://doi.org/10.1161/circulationaha.107.705657.
112. Sirtori CR, Calabresi L, Franceschini G, Baldassarre D, Amato M, Johansson J, et al. Cardiovascular status of carriers of the apolipo- protein A-IMilano mutant: the Limone sul Garda study. Circulation. 2001;103(15):1949–54. https://doi.org/10.1161/01.cir.103.15.1949.
113. Hovingh GK, de Groot E, van der Steeg W, Boekholdt SM, Hutten BA, Kuivenhoven JA, et al. Inherited disorders of HDL metabolism and atherosclerosis. Curr Opin Lipidol. 2005;16(2):139–45. https://doi.org/10.1097/01.mol.0000162318.47172.ef.
114. Voight BF, Peloso GM, Orho-Melander M, Frikke-Schmidt R, Barbalic M, Jensen MK, et al. Plasma HDL cholesterol and risk of myocardial infarction: a mendelian randomisation study. Lancet. 2012;380(9841):572–80. Available from: http://www.ncbi.nlm.nih.gov/pubmed/22607825
115. Negi SI, Brautbar A, Virani SS, Anand A, Polisecki E, Asztalos BF, et al. Case study a novel mutation in the ABCA1 gene causing an atypical phenotype of Tangier disease. J Clin Lipidol. 2013;7(1):82–7. https://doi.org/10.1016/j.jacl.2012.09.004.
116. Kathiresan S, Melander O, Guiducci C, Surti A, Burtt NP, Rieder MJ, et al. Six new loci associated with blood low-density lipoprotein cholesterol, high-density lipoprotein cholesterol or triglycerides in humans. Nat Genet. 2008;40(2):189–97. https://doi.org/10.1038/ng.75.
117. Willer CJ, Sanna S, Jackson AU, Scuteri A, Bonnycastle LL, Clarke R, et al. Newly identified loci that influence lipid concentrations and risk of coronary artery disease. Nat Genet. 2008;40(2):161–9. https://doi.org/10.1038/ng.76.
118. Singaraja RR, Visscher H, James ER, Chroni A, Coutinho JM, Brunham LR, et al. Specific mutations in ABCA1 have discrete effects on ABCA1 function and lipid phenotypes both in vivo and in vitro. Circ Res. 2006;99(4):389–97. Available from: http://www.ncbi.nlm.nih.gov/pubmed/16873719
119. Singaraja RR, Brunham LR, Visscher H, Kastelein JJP, Hayden MR. Efflux and atherosclerosis: the clinical and biochemical impact of variations in the ABCA1 gene. Arterioscler Thromb Vasc Biol. 2003;23(8):1322–32. Available from: http://www.ncbi.nlm.nih.gov/pubmed/12763760
120. Rosenson RS, Jr Brewer HB, Ansell BJ, Barter P, Chapman MJ, Heinecke JW, et al. Dysfunctional HDL and atherosclerotic cardiovascular disease. Nat Publ Gr. 2015;13(01):48–60. https://doi.org/10.1038/nrcardio.2015.124.
121. Clee SM, Kastelein JJP, van Dam M, Marcil M, Roomp K, Zwarts KY, et al. Age and residual cholesterol efflux affect HDL choles-

terol levels and coronary artery disease in ABCA1 heterozygotes. J Clin Invest. 2000;106(10):1263–70. https://doi.org/10.1172/jci10727.
122. van Dam MJ, de Groot E, Clee SM, Hovingh GK, Roelants R, Brooks-Wilson A, et al. Association between increased arterial-wall thickness and impairment in ABCA1-driven cholesterol efflux: an observational study. Lancet. 2002;359(9300):37–41. https://doi.org/10.1016/s0140-6736(02)07277-x.
123. Frikke-Schmidt R, Nordestgaard BG, Stene MCA, Sethi AA, Remaley AT, Schnohr P, et al. Association of loss-of-function mutations in the ABCA1 gene with high-density lipoprotein cholesterol levels and risk of ischemic heart disease. JAMA. 2008;299(21):2524–32. Available from: http://www.ncbi.nlm.nih.gov/pubmed/18523221
124. Brunham LR, Singaraja RR, Duong M, Timmins JM, Fievet C, Bissada N, et al. Tissue-specific roles of ABCA1 influence susceptibility to atherosclerosis. Arterioscler Thromb Vasc Biol. 2009;29(4):548–54. https://doi.org/10.1161/atvbaha.108.182303.
125. Clee SM, Zwinderman AH, Engert JC, Zwarts KY, Molhuizen HOF, Roomp K, et al. Common genetic variation in ABCA1 is associated with altered lipoprotein levels and a modified risk for coronary artery disease. Circulation. 2001;103(9):1198–205. https://doi.org/10.1161/01.cir.103.9.1198.
126. Zwarts KY, Clee SM, Zwinderman AH, Engert JC, Singaraja R, Loubser O, et al. ABCA1 regulatory variants influence coronary artery disease independent of effects on plasma lipid levels. Clin Genet. 2002;61(2):115–25. https://doi.org/10.1034/j.1399-0004.2002.610206.x.
127. Brunham LR, Kastelein JJP, Hayden MR. ABCA1 gene mutations, HDL cholesterol levels, and risk of ischemic heart disease. JAMA. 2008;300(17):1997–8. Author reply 1998. Available from: http://www.ncbi.nlm.nih.gov/pubmed/18984885
128. Kiss RS, Kavaslar N, Okuhira K-I, Freeman MW, Walter S, Milne RW, et al. Genetic etiology of isolated low HDL syndrome: incidence and heterogeneity of efflux defects. Arterioscler Thromb Vasc Biol. 2007;27(5):1139–45. https://doi.org/10.1161/atvbaha.106.137646.
129. Ayyobi AF, McGladdery SH, Chan S, John Mancini GB, Hill JS, Frohlich JJ. Lecithin: cholesterol acyltransferase (LCAT) deficiency and risk of vascular disease: 25 year follow-up. Atherosclerosis. 2004;177(2):361–6. https://doi.org/10.1016/j.atherosclerosis.2004.07.018.
130. Van Den Bogaard B, Holleboom AG, Duivenvoorden R, Hutten BA, Kastelein JJP, Hovingh GK, et al. Patients with low HDL-cholesterol caused by mutations in LCAT have increased arterial stiffness. Atherosclerosis. 2012;225(2):481–5. https://doi.org/10.1016/j.atherosclerosis.2012.09.022.
131. Calabresi L, Baldassarre D, Simonelli S, Gomaraschi M, Amato M, Castelnuovo S, et al. Plasma lecithin: cholesterol acyltransferase and carotid intima-media thickness in European individuals at high cardiovascular risk. J Lipid Res. 2011;52:1569–74.
132. Saeedi R, Li M, Frohlich J. A review on lecithin: cholesterol acyltransferase de fi ciency. Clin Biochem. 2015;48:472–5.
133. Shah PK. Inhibition of CETP as a novel therapeutic strategy for reducing the risk of atherosclerotic disease. Eur Heart J. 2006;28(1):5–12. https://doi.org/10.1093/eurheartj/ehl392.
134. Tsai MY, Johnson C, Kao WHL, Sharrett AR, Arends VL, Kronmal R, et al. Cholesteryl ester transfer protein genetic polymorphisms, HDL cholesterol, and subclinical cardiovascular disease in the multi-ethnic study of atherosclerosis. Atherosclerosis. 2008;200(2):359–67. https://doi.org/10.1016/j.atherosclerosis.2007.12.038.
135. Klerkx AHEM, de Grooth GJ, Zwinderman AH, Jukema JW, Kuivenhoven JA, Kastelein JJP. Cholesteryl ester transfer protein concentration is associated with progression of atherosclerosis and response to pravastatin in men with coronary artery disease (REGRESS). Eur J Clin Investig. 2004;34(1):21–8. https://doi.org/10.1111/j.1365-2362.2004.01281.x.
136. Smilde TJ, van Wissen S, Awollersheim H, Trip MD, Kastelein JJP, Stalenhoef AFH. Effect of aggressive versus conventional lipid lowering on atherosclerosis progression in familial hypercholesterolemia (ASAP): a prospective, randomised, double-blind trial. Lancet. 2001;357(9256):577–81. https://doi.org/10.1016/s0140-6736(00)04053-8.
137. Boekholdt SM, Kuivenhoven J-A, Wareham NJ, Peters RJG, Jukema JW, Luben R, et al. Plasma levels of cholesteryl ester transfer protein and the risk of future coronary artery disease in apparently healthy men and women: the prospective EPIC (European prospective investigation into cancer and nutrition)-Norfolk population study. Circulation. 2004;110(11):1418–23. Available from: http://www.ncbi.nlm.nih.gov/pubmed/15337694
138. Agerholm-Larsen B, Tybjarg-Hansen A, Schnohr P, Steffensen R, Nordestgaard BG. Common cholesteryl ester transfer protein mutations, decreased HDL cholesterol, and possible decreased risk of ischemic heart disease: the Copenhagen City heart study. Circulation. 2000;102(18):2197–203. https://doi.org/10.1161/01.cir.102.18.2197.
139. Curb JD, Abbott RD, Rodriguez BL, Masaki K, Chen R, Sharp DS, et al. A prospective study of HDL-C and cholesteryl ester transfer protein gene mutations and the risk of coronary heart disease in the elderly. J Lipid Res. 2004;45(5):948–53. Available from: http://www.ncbi.nlm.nih.gov/pubmed/14967821
140. Moriyama Y, Okamura T, Inazu A, Doi M, Iso H, Mouri Y, et al. A low prevalence of coronary heart disease among subjects with increased high-density lipoprotein cholesterol levels, including those with plasma cholesteryl ester transfer protein deficiency. Prev Med (Baltim). 1998;27(5):659–67. https://doi.org/10.1006/pmed.1998.0340.
141. van Acker BAC, Botma G-J, Zwinderman AH, Kuivenhoven JA, Dallinga-Thie GM, Sijbrands EJG, et al. High HDL cholesterol does not protect against coronary artery disease when associated with combined cholesteryl ester transfer protein and hepatic lipase gene variants. Atherosclerosis. 2008;200(1):161–7. https://doi.org/10.1016/j.atherosclerosis.2007.11.019.
142. Mukherjee M, Shetty KR. Variations in high-density lipoprotein cholesterol in relation to physical activity and Taq 1B polymorphism of the cholesteryl ester transfer protein gene. Clin Genet. 2004;65(5):412–8. https://doi.org/10.1111/j.0009-9163.2004.0237.x.
143. Beigneux AP, Franssen R, Bensadoun A, Gin P, Melford K, Peter J, et al. Chylomicronemia with a mutant GPIHBP1 (Q115P) that cannot bind lipoprotein lipase. Arterioscler Thromb Vasc Biol. 2009;29(6):956–62. https://doi.org/10.1161/atvbaha.109.186577.
144. Brahm AJ, Hegele RA. Chylomicronaemia–current diagnosis and future therapies. Nat Publ Gr. 2015;11(6):352–62. https://doi.org/10.1038/nrendo.2015.26.
145. Brunzell JD. Hypertriglyceridemia. N Engl J Med. 2007;357(10):1009–17. https://doi.org/10.1056/nejmcp070061.
146. Birjmohun RS, Hutten BA, Kastelein JJP, Stroes ESG. Efficacy and safety of high-density lipoprotein cholesterol-increasing compounds: a meta-analysis of randomized controlled trials. J Am Coll Cardiol. 2005;45(2):185–97. Available from: http://www.ncbi.nlm.nih.gov/pubmed/15653014
147. Grundy SM, Cleeman JI, Merz CNB, Brewer HB, Clark LT, Hunninghake DB, et al. Implications of recent clinical trials for the National Cholesterol Education Program Adult Treatment Panel III guidelines. Circulation. 2004;110(2):227–39. Available from: http://www.ncbi.nlm.nih.gov/pubmed/15249516
148. Pradhan AD, Paynter NP, Everett BM, Glynn RJ, Amarenco P, Elam M, Ginsberg H, Hiatt WR, Ishibashi S, Koenig W, Nordestgaard BG, Fruchart J-C, Libby P, Ridker PM. Rationale and design of the pemafibrate to reduce cardiovascular outcomes

by reducing triglycerides in patients with diabetes (PROMINENT) study. Am Heart J. 2018;206:80–93.
149. McKenney J. New perspectives on the use of niacin in the treatment of lipid disorders. Arch Intern Med. 2004;164(7):697. https://doi.org/10.1001/archinte.164.7.697.
150. Pirillo A, Catapano AL. Update on the management of severe hypertriglyceridemia – focus on free fatty acid forms of omega-3. Drug Des Devel Ther. 2015;9:2129–37.
151. Hooper L, Ness A, Higgins JPT, Moore T, Ebrahim S. GISSI-Prevenzionetrial. Lancet. 1999;354(9189):1557. https://doi.org/10.1016/s0140-6736(05)76587-9.
152. Abdelhamid AS, Brown TJ, Brainard JS, Biswas P, Thorpe GC, Moore HJ, Deane KHO, AlAbdulghafoor FK, Summerbell CD, Worthington HV, Song F, Hooper L. Omega-3 fatty acids for the primary and secondary prevention of cardiovascular disease. Cochrane Database Syst Rev. 7(7):CD003177.
153. Witztum JL, Gaudet D, Freedman SD, Alexander VJ, Digenio A, Williams KR, Yang Q, Hughes SG, Geary RS, Arca M, Stroes ESG, Bergeron J, Soran H, Civeira F, Hemphill L, Tsimikas S, Blom DJ, O'Dea L, Bruckert E. Volanesorsen and triglyceride levels in familial chylomicronemia syndrome. N Engl J Med. 2019;381(6):531–42.
154. Merkel M, Eckel RH, Goldberg IJ. Lipoprotein lipase: genetics, lipid uptake, and regulation. J Lipid Res. 2002;43(12):1997–2006. Available from: http://www.ncbi.nlm.nih.gov/pubmed/12454259
155. Lam C-W, Yuen Y-P, Cheng W-F, Chan Y-W, Tong S-F. Missense mutation Leu72Pro located on the carboxyl terminal amphipathic helix of apolipoprotein C-II causes familial chylomicronemia syndrome. Clin Chim Acta. 2006;364(1–2):256–9. https://doi.org/10.1016/j.cca.2005.07.025.
156. Wang J, Hegele RA. Homozygous missense mutation (G56R) in glycosylphosphatidylinositol-anchored high-density lipoprotein-binding protein 1 (GPI-HBP1) in two siblings with fasting chylomicronemia (MIM 144650). Lipids Heal Dis. 2007;6(1):23. https://doi.org/10.1186/1476-511x-6-23.
157. Gin P, Beigneux AP, Davies B, Young MF, Ryan RO, Bensadoun A, et al. Normal binding of lipoprotein lipase, chylomicrons, and apo-AV to GPIHBP1 containing a G56R amino acid substitution. Biochim Biophys Acta Mol Cell Biol Lipids. 2007;1771(12):1464–8. https://doi.org/10.1016/j.bbalip.2007.10.005.
158. Péterfy M, Ben-Zeev O, Mao HZ, Weissglas-Volkov D, Aouizerat BE, Pullinger CR, et al. Mutations in LMF1 cause combined lipase deficiency and severe hypertriglyceridemia. Nat Genet. 2007;39(12):1483–7. https://doi.org/10.1038/ng.2007.24.
159. Benlian P, De Gennes JL, Foubert L, Zhang H, Gagné SE, Hayden M. Premature atherosclerosis in patients with familial chylomicronemia caused by mutations in the lipoprotein lipase gene. N Engl J Med. 1996;335(12):848–54. https://doi.org/10.1056/nejm199609193351203.
160. Saika Y, Sakai N, Takahashi M, Maruyama T, Kihara S, Ouchi N, et al. Novel LPL mutation (L303F) found in a patient associated with coronary artery disease and severe systemic atherosclerosis. Eur J Clin Investig. 2003;33(3):216–22. https://doi.org/10.1046/j.1365-2362.2003.01129.x.
161. Myocardial Infarction Genetics, CARDIoGRAM Exome Consortia Investigators. Coding variation in ANGPTL4, LPL, and SVEP1 and the risk of coronary disease. N Engl J Med. 2016;374(12):1134–44. Available from: http://www.ncbi.nlm.nih.gov/pubmed/26934567
162. Stroes ES, Nierman MC, Meulenberg JJ, Franssen R, Twisk J, Henny CP, et al. Intramuscular administration of AAV1-lipoprotein lipaseS447X lowers triglycerides in lipoprotein lipase-deficient patients. Arterioscler Thromb Vasc Biol. 2008;28(12):2303–4. https://doi.org/10.1161/atvbaha.108.175620.
163. Scott LJ. Alipogene tiparvovec: a review of its use in adults with familial lipoprotein lipase deficiency. Drugs. 2015;75:175–82.
164. Yuan G, Al-Shali KZ, Hegele RA. Hypertriglyceridemia: its etiology, effects and treatment. Can Med Assoc J. 2007;176(8):1113–20. https://doi.org/10.1503/cmaj.060963.
165. Charlotte Koopal A, Marais D, Westerink J, Visseren FLJ. Autosomal dominant familial dysbetalipoproteinemia: A pathophysiological framework and practical approach to diagnosis and therapy. J Clin Lipidol. 2017;11(1):12–23.e1.
166. Walden CC, Hegele RA. Apolipoprotein E in hyperlipidemia. Ann Intern Med. 1994;120(12):1026–36. Available from: http://www.ncbi.nlm.nih.gov/pubmed/8185134
167. Charlotte Koopal A, Marais D, Visseren FLJ. Familial dysbetalipoproteinemia. Curr Opin Endocrinol Diabetes Obes. 24(2):133–9.
168. Koopal C, Retterstøl K, Sjouke B, Hovingh GK, Ros E, De Graaf J, et al. Vascular risk factors, vascular disease, lipids and lipid targets in patients with familial dysbetalipoproteinemia: a European cross- sectional study. Atherosclerosis. 2015;240(1):90–7. https://doi.org/10.1016/j.atherosclerosis.2015.02.046.
169. Busygina K, Waldmann E, Parhofer K. The Effect of PCSK9 inhibition in familial dysbetalipoproteinemia (Type III hyperlipoproteinemia): 4 cases. J Am Coll Cardiol. 2018;71(11):A1759.
170. Lewis GF, Xiao C, Hegele RA. Hypertriglyceridemia in the genomic era: a new paradigm. Endocr Rev. 2015;36(1):131–47. Available from http://www.ncbi.nlm.nih.gov/pubmed/25554923
171. Haase A, Goldberg AC. Identification of people with heterozygous familial hypercholesterolemia. Curr Opin Lipidol. 23(4):282–9.

24 Genetics of (Premature) Coronary Artery Disease

Jeanette Erdmann and Heribert Schunkert

Introduction

Coronary artery disease (CAD) and its major complication, myocardial infarction (MI), remain the number one cause of death in industrialized society, causing approximately one in every six deaths in the United States in 2010 [1]. CAD is the clinical manifestation of a chronic pathomorphological process that occurs in the vascular wall [2]. Carl Müller (1886–1983) was the first to identify a link between high plasma cholesterol, xanthoma, and premature coronary heart disease in 1939, providing early evidence of a genetic component of CAD and its association with cholesterol [3]. Today, it is well established that CAD arises from the interaction of multiple genetic and environmental factors. Likewise, a multifactorial etiology applies to many of the underlying cardiovascular risk factors, including hypercholesterolemia, hypertension, diabetes mellitus, and smoking. Thus, endogenous (genetic) and exogenous (nutrition, physical activity, therapy, etc.) factors all contribute to the development of atherosclerotic lesions, directly in the arterial wall, indirectly via traditional risk factors, or interactively by augmentation or amelioration of other contributing processes [2]. On a cellular level, atherosclerosis is a complex process characterized by endothelial dysfunction, lipid and matrix accumulation, migration and local transformation of circulating cells, smooth muscle cell (SMC) proliferation, calcification, inflammation, and, finally, thrombus formation [2]. In this scenario, the potential influence of genetically modulated mechanisms may occur at multiple points during the development of the disease.

J. Erdmann (✉)
Institute for Cardiogenetics, University of Lübeck, Lübeck, Germany
e-mail: jeanette.erdmann@uni-luebeck.de

H. Schunkert
Deutsches Herzzentrum München, Klinik für Herz- und Kreislauferkrankungen, Technische Universität München, Munich, Germany
e-mail: schunkert@dhm.mhn.de

For years, evaluation of the family history served as a guide for assessing a patient's genetic risk for coronary events. While a positive family history exists in 20–30% of cases, modern molecular genetics revealed that genetic variants affecting the risk of CAD may be fairly common in our population. Indeed, the number of risk alleles identified since the year 2007 implies that basically all individuals share a variable number of genetic risk factors. For example, 75% of Western Europeans carry at least one variant of the chromosome 9p21.3 risk allele, which increases the probability of CAD by 25%, irrespective of family history [4].

Thus, genetic factors may play a variable role in nearly all cases of CAD, even when the family history is negative. Nevertheless, rare cases of families with multiple affected members have allowed for the identification of specific molecular gene defects that have become novel targets for risk prediction and enhanced our understanding of the pathophysiology of this disease [5].

Importance of Family History

Assessment of the family history is fundamental for understanding the genetic components of the complex disease processes leading to CAD. Familial predisposition is assumed when MI is diagnosed before 55 years in a male first-degree relative or before 65 years in a female first-degree relative. The Framingham Heart Study revealed that this type of positive family history for premature MI increases risk to slightly different extents depending on parental premature CAD (1.45-fold) or sibling CAD (1.99-fold) (Fig. 24.1).

Moreover, familial risk was found to increase with decreasing age of onset of disease in the affected relatives [6–8]. To a lesser degree, genetic factors affecting the risk of MI can be traced in affected second-degree relatives [9]. In families with several affected family members, traditional cardiovascular risk factors are often observed with increased frequency [10].

H. F. Baars et al. (eds.), *Clinical Cardiogenetics*, https://doi.org/10.1007/978-3-030-45457-9_24

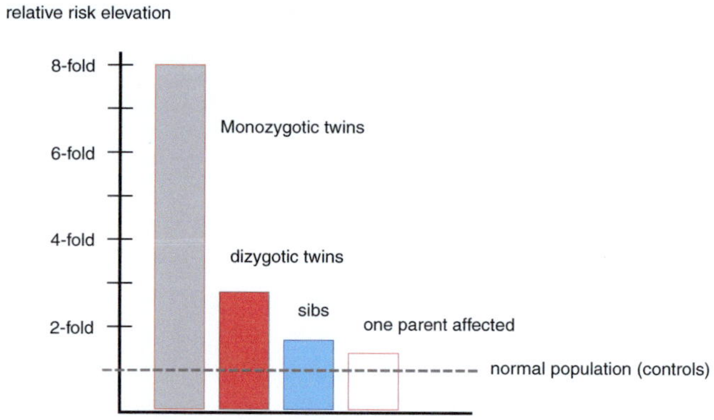

Fig. 24.1 The relative increase in the risk of MI/CAD is shown in relation to different familial backgrounds. The risk for monozygotic and dizygotic twins is based on the hypothesis that the partner twin died of MI at the age of 55 years

Furthermore, lifestyle habits associated with a raised incidence of MI (e.g., smoking) are more frequently shared in affected family members. Interestingly, both the Northwick Park Heart Study and the Reykjavik Cohort Study revealed that the increase in risk in terms of a positive family history remains highly significant (odds ratio 1.5–1.8) even after adjustment for traditional risk factors [11, 12]. Thus, the increased risk related to a positive family history is partially independent of traditional risk factors, suggesting that unrelated mechanisms may be causative in this respect [13].

Furthermore, a high rate of reoccurrence of MI was found in identical twins with MI. In these cases, a positive family history was related to an eightfold increased probability of death due to MI before the age of 55 years when the twin was affected at an early age as well [14]. The highest risk related to family history, however, is observed in families with a rare autosomal-dominant pattern of inheritance for MI [5, 15].

Familial Forms of Coronary Artery Disease

Some families present with an extremely high prevalence of CAD/MI. With the exception of two large families studied by Wang et al. [15] and Erdmann et al. [5] (see next section), most of these families could not be systematically analyzed genetically due to the high lethality of the disease. In the German MI Family Study, we specifically looked for MI in large families with at least four surviving affected individuals. Overall, these families represent less than 0.1% of cases of MI. Based on the analyses of 19 family pedigrees and statistical simulations, the presence of an autosomal-dominant inheritance pattern was plausible in all cases. These family pedigrees will hopefully extend the knowledge of genes involved in MI in the near future. However, as was shown for familial hypercholesterolemia, in a proportion of the extended families, complex oligogenic inheritance can masquerade as monogenic disease [16, 17].

MEF2A

Wang et al. reported a mutation in the gene of the transcription factor MEF2A in a family with an autosomal-dominant form of MI. This marked the first time that a familial genetic defect was shown to give rise to MI in humans [15]. A 21-bp deletion in the gene appeared to result in abnormal epithelium of the coronary walls, thus favoring plaque deposition that may ultimately lead to MI. Interestingly, the same pathway is crucial for preventing apoptosis in endothelial cells and death due to vascular obstruction in mice. However, at present, genetic studies do not support the significance of this gene with respect to CAD/MI morbidity in humans, as several reports showed no association between single nucleotide polymorphisms (SNPs) in the *MEF2A* gene and CAD/MI in other families in large case-control studies or GWA studies [18, 19].

GUCY1A1

Recently, the *GUCY1A1* gene (former designation was *GUCY1A3*), which encodes the α1-subunit of the soluble guanylyl cyclase (sGC) heterodimer consisting of the α1 and β1-subunits was linked to MI through a family study performed by our group [5]. The sGC complex acts as the receptor for nitric oxide (NO) and catalyzes the formation of the second messenger cGMP [20]. A loss-of-function (LOF) mutation was detected in *GUCY1A1* in an extended family with a history of MI upon exome sequencing of three affected family members. The mutation in *GUCY1A1* impairs its function by reducing the protein content of the α1-subunit, abolishing the activity of the sGC enzyme and reducing the production of cGMP [5]. Moreover, mice deficient in the α1-subunit displayed accelerated thrombus formation in the microcirculation upon local trauma. A contributory role of CCT7, which stabilizes the α1ß1 sGC dimer [21], was also established based on the identification of a second mutation found within the same family. Additionally, a number of rare variants in *GUCY1A1* with potential functional relevance were identified in MI patients (Fig. 24.2) [5].

Interestingly, in addition to these rare mutations, common variants in the *GUCY1A1* gene are significantly associated with CAD on a genome-wide basis (OR = 1.08; $p = 4.57 \times 10^{-23}$), as reported by a GWAS meta-analysis performed by the UK biobank and CARDIoGRAMplusC4D consortium (Fig. 24.3). The lead SNP rs7692387 is located in an intronic site that modulates *GUCY1A1* promoter activity. The transcription factor ZEB1 binds preferentially to the non-risk allele, leading to an increase in *GUCY1A1* expression,

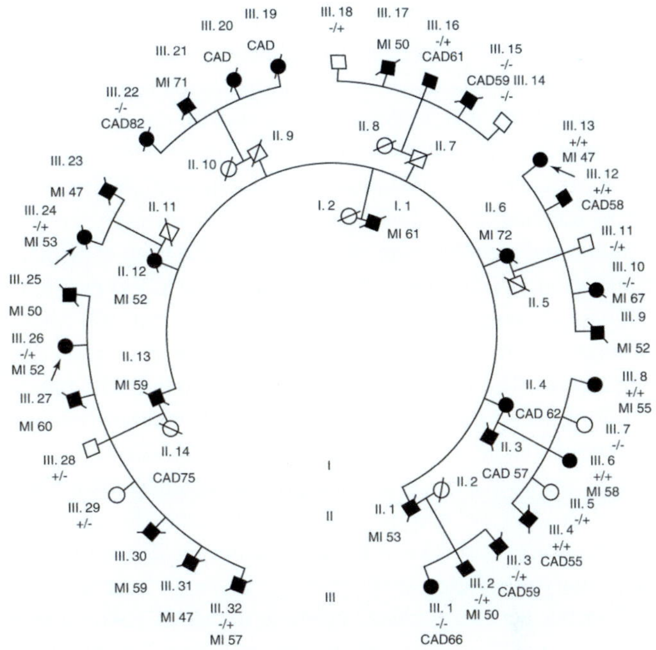

Fig. 24.2 Pedigree of the extended MI family with several individuals suffering from myocardial infarctions. White symbols denote healthy individuals, black symbols denote affected individuals; squares represent males, circles represent females. Crossed symbols represent deceased individuals. Age of onset is given next to the disease. *MI* myocardial infarction, *CAD* coronary artery disease. Persons III.13, III.24, and III.26 were exome-sequenced; 1/1 denotes double-mutation carriers (p. Leu163Phefs∗241/p.Ser525Leu2); 1/2 denotes probands carrying only the p.Leu163Phefs∗24 mutation in GUCY1A3; 2/1 denotes probands carrying only the p.Ser525Leu mutation in CCT7 [5]

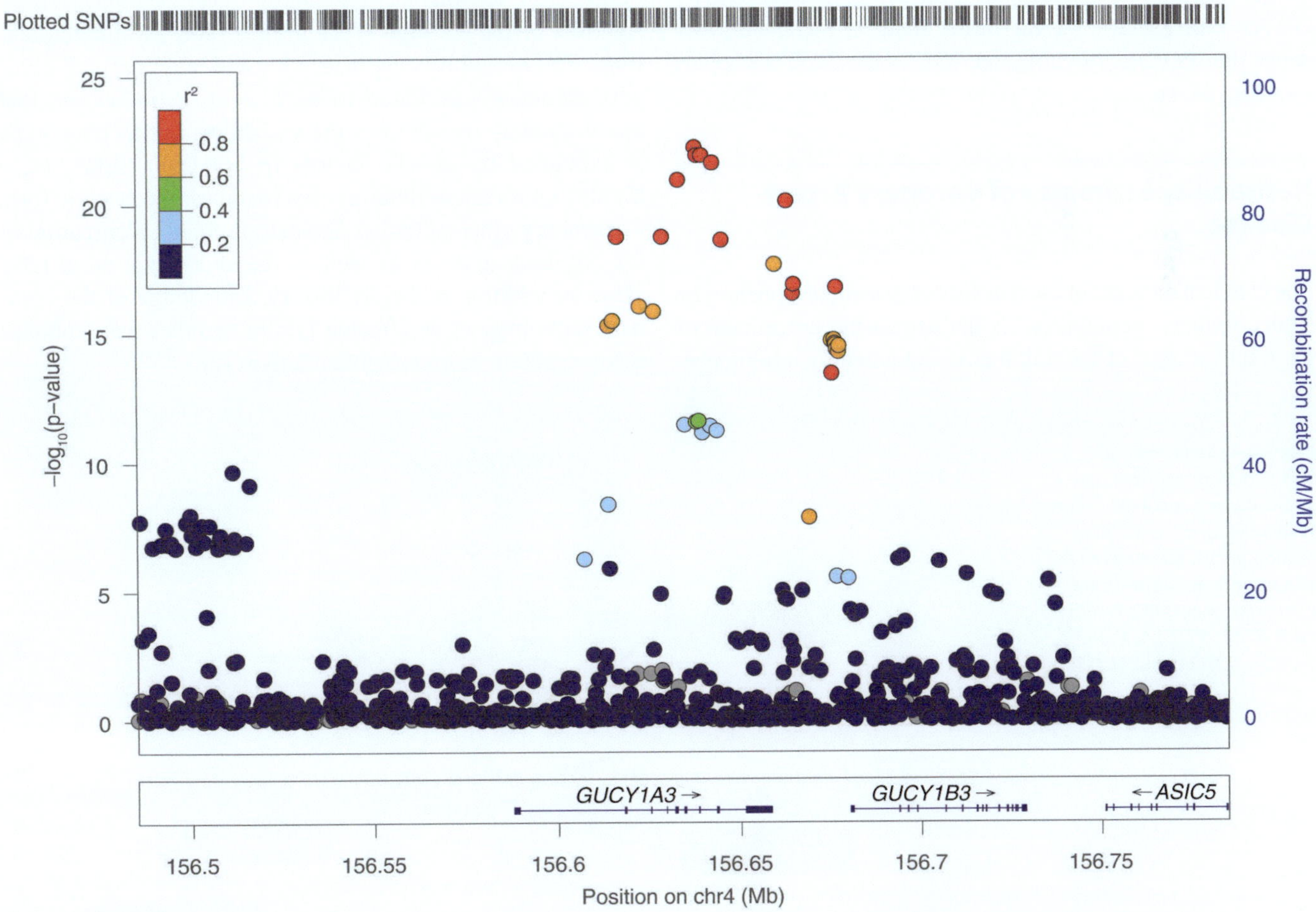

Fig. 24.3 Several common variants encompassing the *GUCY1A1* (formerly designated *GUCY1A3*) locus are genome-wide significant associated with CAD. This association plot is taken from the most recent GWAS meta-analysis comprising more than one million cases and controls

higher sGC levels, and higher sGC activity after stimulation [22]. Remarkably, Kessler et al. showed that homozygous *GUCY1A1* risk allele carriers are at increased risk of cardiovascular death or stent thrombosis within 30 days after coronary stenting, likely due to higher on-aspirin platelet reactivity. Whether *GUCY1A1* genotype helps to tailor antiplatelet treatment remains to be investigated [23]. Interestingly, in two randomized placebo-controlled trials in the setting of primary prevention, aspirin reduced the incidence of CVD events in individuals homozygous for the GUCY1A1 risk (G) allele, whereas heterozygote individuals had more events when taking aspirin. These findings present an example of the potential for genetics in precision medicine to differentiate between potential benefit and harm. Prospective, randomized, placebo-controlled trial studies of aspirin stratified by *GUCY1A1* genotype will be needed to further evaluate the extent to which aspirin may be useful for reducing incidence of CVD in primary prevention [24].

Further genetic evidence pointing to critical involvement of the NO-sGC-cGMP pathway in mediating CAD and MI risk has been shown by identifying the *NOS3* gene, encoding the endothelial NO synthase, as a further CAD risk gene by GWAS [20, 25, 26]. Furthermore, there is increasing evidence that *PDE1A*, *PDE3A*, and *PDE5A* are CAD risk genes too (Fig. 24.4).

Heritability Estimates of Coronary Artery Disease

The classical measure of the genetic component of a phenotype (trait), termed "heritability," is defined as the percentage of the total variance of the trait that is explained by inheritance. By examining the increased similarity of trait values in related individuals compared with unrelated or less-related individuals, one can estimate the heritability. The simplest conceptual study design in man is the comparison of monozygotic (MZ) and dizygotic (DZ) twins. MZ twins share 100% of their genes, whereas DZ twins share, on average, 50% of their genes. If a trait has a genetic component, MZ twins are more likely to resemble each other than DZ twins.

Because of the assumptions that are required to estimate heritability, the calculated numbers must be considered rough proxies. In particular, the high prevalence of risk alleles in apparently healthy subjects within a population may result in underestimation of the true role of the genetic factors involved.

Heritability of Coronary Anatomy and Pathology

We recently demonstrated that the heritability estimates of CAD depend in part on the pattern of coronary morphology. Particularly, left main disease and proximal coronary artery stenoses displayed high reoccurrence rates in affected siblings. The heritability estimate for ostial and proximal coronary stenoses was found to be $h^2 = 0.32$, indicating that approximately one-third of the variability in this phenotype is explained by genetic factors ($p = 0.008$). Likewise, a highly significant heritability was found for the ecstatic form of coronary atherosclerosis and extraluminal calcification of the coronary arteries, as well as the abdominal aorta [27]. Thus, in addition to family history, knowledge of the coronary pathology in an affected family member may enhance risk prediction in first-degree relatives [28].

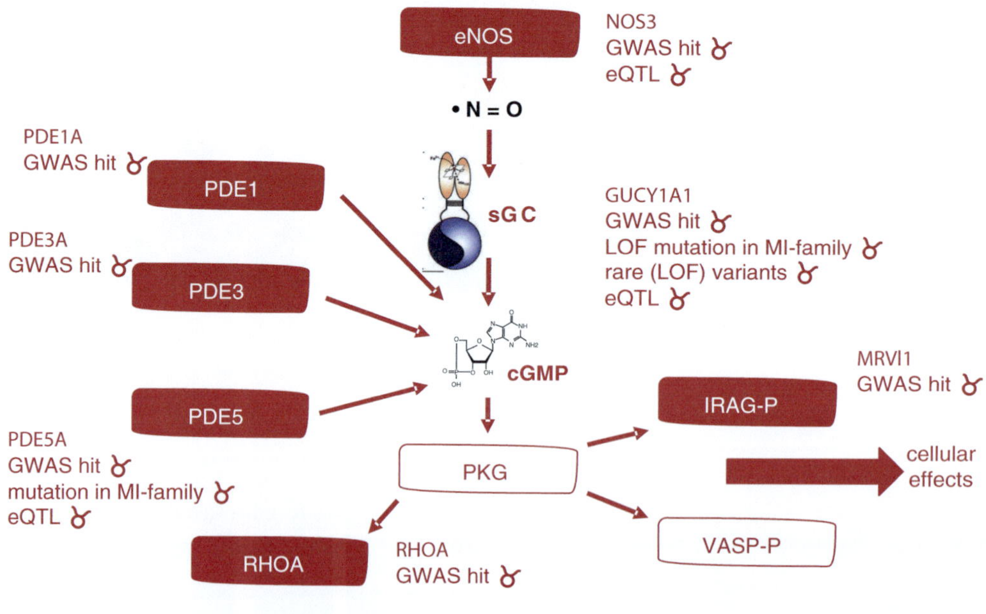

Fig. 24.4 Overview of NO-signaling pathway and genes that are involved. There is increasing evidence that several genes, all involved in this important pathway, are CAD risk genes, like *NOS3 GUCY1A1*, *PDE1A*, *PDE3A*, *PDE5A*, *RHOA*, and *MRVI1*

Genes Affecting Coronary Artery Disease

Over the past three decades, a great deal of research has focused on defining the genetic components of MI, CAD, and their risk factors. Initially, this research focused on candidate genes that hypothetically might affect known traits involved in the atherosclerotic process, including the renin-angiotensin system, lipoprotein metabolism, inflammation, or coagulation. However, the findings of many of these candidate gene studies were not replicated in consecutive studies. Consequently, at the beginning of the twenty-first century, novel strategies for gene identification were undertaken that allowed exploration of the entire genome. Without a priori hypothesis, genome-wide linkage analyses were performed that searched the entire genome for chromosomal regions shared by affected family members. While these studies resulted in the identification of several chromosomal loci harboring MI genes, these regions were too large for the elucidation of specific causative genes or molecular variants [29].

These efforts resulted in technological and methodological advances that initiated the advent of genome-wide association (GWA) studies in 2005 [30], and a new era of exploration of CAD and MI only 2 years later [31–34]. Within the last decade, these GWA studies have reproducibly identified thousands of gene variants associated with a broad spectrum of disorders such as coronary heart disease, high blood pressure, hypercholesterolemia, and diabetes mellitus. Surprisingly, most of the genes identified thus far were not expected to play a role in the development of atherosclerosis. Thus, an important task for the immediate future is to understand the fundamental pathophysiological mechanisms affected by these genes. Another difficulty in this research is that, unlike Mendelian traits, genetic studies on complex cardiovascular disorders are complicated by variable cosegregation of the risk allele and the disease. In fact, many genetic variants associated with these disorders were found to be relatively common in the overall population and therefore, albeit to variable degrees, prevalent in both healthy and affected individuals. Accordingly, functional information on these genetic factors and the related gene expression as well as protein expression patterns is crucial. Subsequently, genetic research may enhance diagnostic testing and identification of new treatment targets.

Genome-Wide Association Studies for CAD and MI: Novel Insights

Currently, commercially available DNA-arrays allow genotyping of up to 4,300,000 SNPs for statistical analysis [35]. To further increase the power of GWAS, an in-silico method called imputation can be used. This method, based on the overall haplotype structure of the human genome, allows for the inference of missing genotypes, harmonizes datasets for meta-analyses, and increases the overall number of markers available for association testing [36]. Based on the latest reference dataset from the 1000 Genomes Project [37], one can currently integrate more than 39 million variants for analysis [38]. Recently, the Haplotype Reference Consortium (HRC) [39] combined all whole-genome sequencing data sets into a single haplotype reference panel to facilitate genotype imputation. This technique significantly improves *p*-values, particularly for suggestive variants [40].

Over the past decade, GWAS for CAD/MI has seen much success, which was catapulted in 2007 with the discovery of 9p21, by independent research groups [31–34]. By 2009, 12 other genetic risk variants were discovered through GWAS to be associated with CAD [41]. Subsequently in 2013, with a larger sample size, the CARDIoGRAMplusC4D Consortium reported 46 loci associated with CAD, both confirming previously published and finding new variants [42]. This was followed by the identification of ten additional new loci in 2015. Currently, 2017 and 2018, CARDIoGRAMplusC4D data together with the UK Biobank data have proven to be a wealthy resource of genetic data reflected by the increase in new CAD associated loci to 164 by the beginning of 2018 (Fig. 24.5) [44].

In spite of these new CAD loci findings, less focus has been given to the X- and Y-chromosomes. It is common knowledge that there exists sexual dimorphism regarding the incidence, prevalence, morbidity, and mortality of CVD and/or MI with men having an increased risk compared to age-matched women. Much work remains for the inclusion of the sex-chromosomes in current GWAS efforts. Nevertheless, we can say that for the autosomal chromosomes there are currently a total number of 164 loci associated to CAD (Fig. 24.6).

Using the CAD/MI GWAS results thus far, we can conclude as following: (a) the majority of common variants found show modest CAD risk increase (odds ratio between 1.05 and 1.25); (b) most of the variants found are located outside protein-coding regions and might work through gene-regulation; (c) a large proportion of the variants show pleiotropy and (d) we have tremendously improved our understanding of CAD pathogenesis [44].

Annotation of CAD Loci and Druggability

In the last decade, GWAS have undoubtedly revolutionized the identification of genetic variants underlying an increased risk of complex diseases such as CAD. However, the functional interpretation of these loci has just begun [46]. The next step in unraveling the genetic causes of CAD is to analyze GWAS findings in detail, i.e., to map the genetic loci to genes and pathways. Getting from GWAS loci to the disturbed genetic

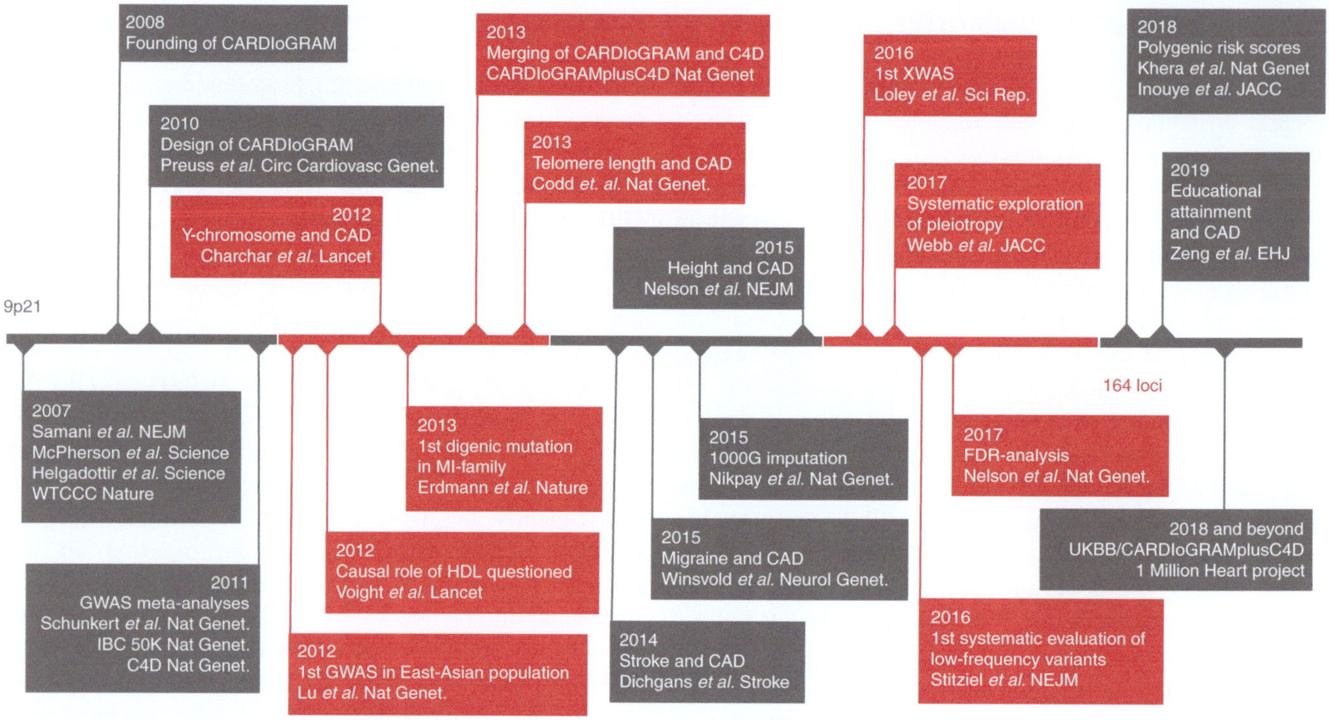

Fig. 24.5 Milestones in cardiovascular genetics from 2007 until 2018 and beyond [43]

mechanisms is, however, not straightforward, and cannot be accomplished solely using GWAS data. Indeed, identifying the underlying genetic cause is even more difficult, as most SNPs associated with complex disease lie in the noncoding regions of the genome and may have an effect on more than one gene including genes that are not necessarily close neighbors. Recent efforts to better understand the genetics underlying GWAS signals resulted in a detailed annotation of CAD loci by combining different datasets. More and more publicly available "omics" datasets, e.g., ENCODE data, have become available, facilitating in-depth loci characterization [47–49]. In a recent study performed by Brænne et al., all SNPs within known CAD loci (linkage disequilibrium, LD: $r^2 > 0.8$) were annotated with respect to their protein-coding sequence and influence on gene expression [50]. Influence on gene expression was estimated through quantitative trait loci, mi-RNA binding sites, or location within a promoter or other regulatory region. Based on the results of these in-silico studies, it is evident that most loci have an effect on regulatory gene function and do not act directly at the protein level. In addition, new genes have been functionally linked to known GWAS loci and a substantial number of genes, previously assigned to the loci (based on proximity), have not been validated [50]. Hence, systematic characterization of GWAS loci is necessary to better understand the disease pathways and develop new therapeutic treatment options [51]. A recent study by Lempiäinen et al., prioritized a number of genes as the most likely causal genes at genome-wide significant loci identified by GWAS of CAD and examined their regulatory roles in metabolic and vascular tissue gene–protein subnetworks ("modules"). These modules and genes within were then scored for CAD druggability potential. The scoring enriched for targets of cardiometabolic drugs currently in clinical use and in-depth analysis of the top-scoring modules validated established and revealed novel target tissues, biological processes, and druggable targets. This elegant study provides an unprecedented resource of tissue-defined gene–protein interactions directly affected by genetic variance in CAD risk loci [52].

To identify druggable CAD targets, Tragante et al. used publicly available GWAS results to predict relevant side effects, identified drug-gene interactions, and prioritized candidates for repurposing among existing drugs. Using such an approach of integration of genomic and pharmacological data proved beneficial for drug repurposing and development [53].

Chromosome 9p21.3

Each C-allele of SNP rs1333049 (G/C, MAF 0.46 in HapMap CEU), representing the CAD/MI locus on 9p21.3, is associated with a 25% increase in risk for CAD/MI (95% CI [1.16–1.35]). The high frequency of the risk allele (approximately 75% of all individuals in a Caucasian population carry at

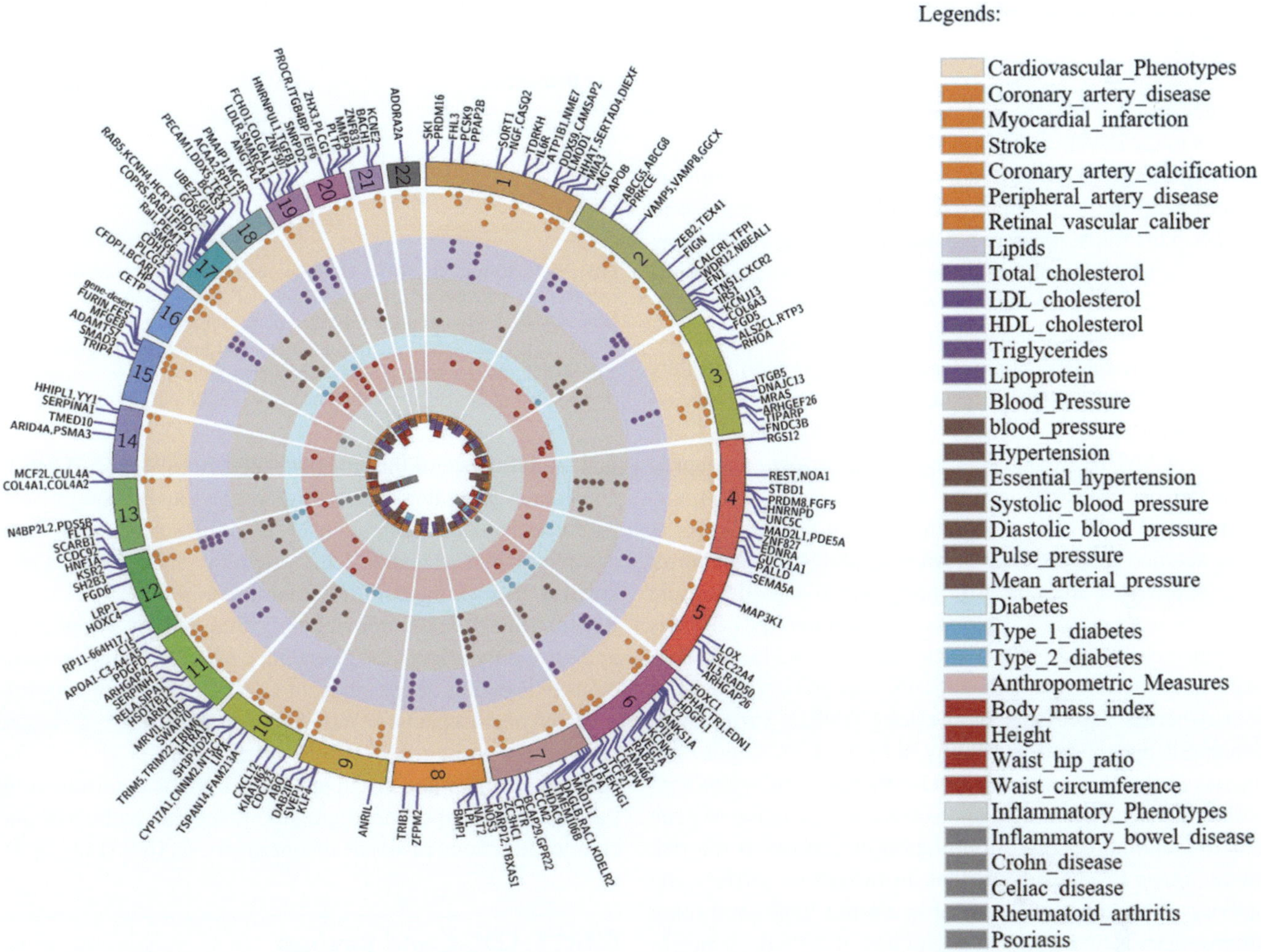

Fig. 24.6 CAD risk loci and level of pleiotropy. Shown are all known CAD risk loci (left) and their association with related traits (right). As can be seen a high proportion of the CAD risk loci are also associated with related traits at genome-wide significance. Data is taken from GWAS catalog [45]. Figure provided by Syed M. Ijlal Haider, Institute for Cardiogenetics

least one risk allele) explains why the proportion of CAD/MI risk that can be attributed to carrying the rs1333049 C-allele is fairly high (22%), even after adjustment for cardiovascular risk scores [31].

Pleiotropic Effects of Chromosome 9p21.3

Data show that this locus affects not only CAD/MI risk but also the risk of abdominal aortic aneurysm (AAA), intracranial aneurysm, peripheral arterial disease, and cardioembolic stroke in many populations [54]. In addition, Gschwendtner et al. (2009) reported that the 9p21.3 region represents a major risk locus for atherosclerotic stroke [55]. The effect of this locus on stroke appears to be independent of its relationship to CAD and other stroke risk factors and further supports a broad role for the 9p21 region in arterial disease. Recently, additional associations were reported between common variants located in 9p21.3 as well as a broad range of phenotypes not directly connected to atherosclerosis. The spectrum of these diseases ranges from periodontitis to various human cancers including glioma, basal cell carcinoma, and familial melanoma. Interestingly, the CDKN2A/2B tumor suppressor genes located in this region encode critical regulators of cell cycle and/or apoptosis. Of note, the CAD/MI risk haplotype does not appear to overlap completely with the cancer locus. While the associations of many of the phenotypes with 9p21.3 are only descriptive in nature, functional studies will help to unravel their relationship. For example, the same locus on chromosome 9p21.3 was also reported to be associated with type 2 diabetes mellitus (T2DM) in three out of five GWA studies. However, more detailed studies revealed that neighboring linkage disequilibrium (LD) blocks, but not the same SNPs, are responsible for T2DM (a risk factor for CAD) and CAD/MI [56].

Pathophysiology Behind Chromosome 9p21.3

The first insights into the pathophysiological mechanisms of 9p21.3 in CAD/MI came from Broadbent et al. (2008), who described lncRNA ANRIL, a long noncoding RNA that collocates with the CAD high-risk haplotype at chromosome 9p21.3. This transcript is expressed in tissues and cell types that are affected by atherosclerosis and is therefore a prime candidate for the chromosome 9p21.3 CAD/MI locus [57]. Liu et al. (2009) analyzed the expression of 9p21 transcripts in purified peripheral blood T-cells (PBTLs) from healthy probands [58]. They found significantly reduced expression of all INK4/ARF transcripts (p15(INK4b), p16(INK4a), ARF, and ANRIL) in subjects with CAD, stroke, and aortic aneurysm, while expression of methylthioadenosine phosphorylase (MTAP) was not influenced by the genotype. A more detailed analysis by Jarinova et al. (2009) using reporter gene expression analysis in primary aortic smooth muscle revealed that a conserved sequence within the 9p21.3 locus has enhancer activity [59]. Furthermore, whole blood RNA expression of short ANRIL variants was increased by 2.2-fold, whereas expression of the long ANRIL variant was decreased by 1.2-fold in healthy subjects homozygous for the risk allele. Moreover, relevant to atherosclerosis, genome-wide expression profiling demonstrated upregulation of gene sets modulating cellular proliferation in carriers of the risk allele. These results suggest that, in risk-allele carriers, the activity of an enhancer element is altered, thus promoting atherosclerosis by regulating expression of ANRIL, which in turn leads to altered expression of genes controlling cellular proliferation pathways. More insights into the pathogenetic mechanisms behind the chromosome 9p21.3 locus were reported by Visel et al. (2010), [60] who showed that deletion of the orthologous 70 kb noncoding CAD risk interval on mouse chromosome 4 affects the cardiac expression of neighboring genes, as well as the proliferation properties of vascular cells. Particularly, the cardiac expression levels of two genes near the noncoding interval, Cdkn2a and Cdkn2b, are severely reduced in chr4Δ70kb/Δ70kb mice, indicating that distant-acting gene regulators are located in the noncoding CAD risk interval. Primary cultures of chr4Δ70kb/Δ70kb aortic smooth muscle cells exhibited excessive proliferation and diminished senescence, a cellular phenotype consistent with accelerated CAD pathogenesis [60]. More recently, chromatin conformation capture analysis identified interactions between sequences at the 9p21.3 locus and sequences in the vicinity of the genes encoding CDKN2A and CDKN2B and MTAP in the short range, and between IFNW1 and interferon-α21 (IFNA21) in the long range, approximately one million base pairs upstream on chromosome 9 [61]. This finding is remarkable because it suggests that the influence of the enhancer sequences at 9p21.3 acts at considerably greater distances than previously thought. The pathomechanisms behind 9p21 is getting more and more complex if we add *ANRIL* into the play. *ANRIL* serves as a key risk effector molecule of atherogenesis at the 9p21 locus. Recent studies show convincingly that genetic variation at 9p21 not only affects the abundance of *ANRIL*, and in some cases expression of the adjacent *CDKN2A/B* tumor suppressors, but also impacts *ANRIL* splicing, such that 3′-5′-linked circular noncoding *ANRIL* RNA species are produced. The balance of linear and circular *ANRIL* RNA is determined by the 9p21 genotype and regulates molecular pathways and cellular functions involved in atherogenesis [62] (Fig. 24.7).

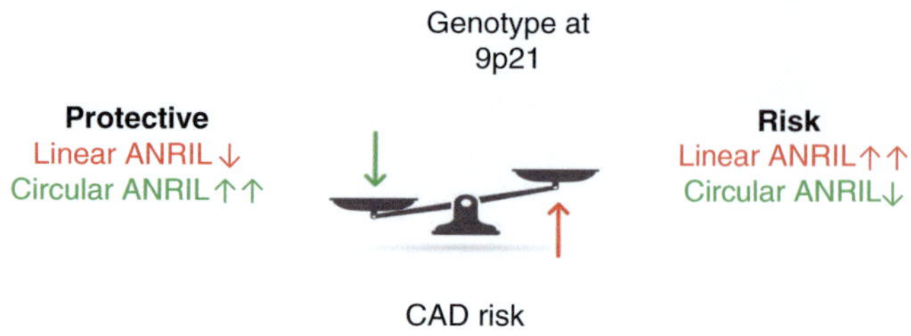

Fig. 24.7 Simplified model how the genotypes at chromosome 9p21 control the balance of linear and circular ANRIL RNA expression. Linear ANRIL upregulation regulates gene expression in trans and pro-adhesive, pro-proliferative, anti-apoptotic cell functions. High levels of circANRIL inhibit over-proliferation of vascular cells by controlling rRNA maturation. Figure is modified from Holdt and Teupser [62]

SORT1: LDL-C and Beyond

A locus on 1p13.3, represented by the SNP rs599839, was initially identified through a GWA study for CAD [31]. Interestingly, this locus has been linked with LDL-C in several other studies [63]. A minor allele in European populations (A/G, MAF 0.28 in HapMap CEU), SNP rs599839 is associated with a lower risk of CAD and lower levels of LDL-C. SNP rs599839 is responsible for approximately 1% of the variation in circulating LDL-cholesterol levels, equivalent to more established genes for LDL regulation, particularly APOE. SNP rs599839 lies in an approximately 97-kb large haplotype block on 1p13.3. This chromosomal region harbors four genes: proline/serine-rich coiled coil protein 1 (PSRC1), cadherin EGF LAG seven-pass G-type receptor 2 (CELSR2), myosin binding protein H-like (MYBPHL), and sortilin 1 (SORT1). The hepatic mRNA expression levels of PSRC1, CELSR2, and SORT1 were shown to correlate with LDL-C plasma levels in a mouse model of cardiovascular disease as well as in a human cohort. The CAD risk allele (A) was associated with lower levels of CELSR2 and SORT1 expression and with higher LDL-C levels. Both genes fall into the category of cell surface receptor-linked signal transduction [64]. SORT1 is a transmembrane receptor protein that binds to a variety of different ligands and is involved in the endocytosis and intracellular degradation of lipoprotein lipase (LPL) [65], a rate-limiting enzyme of triglyceride hydrolysis in lipoproteins. Recently, SORT1 was also linked to the endocytosis of APOA-V-containing chylomicrons [66]. Studies from our group confirmed association of the G allele of SNP rs599839 with higher sortilin mRNA levels in whole blood RNA [67]. Furthermore, we showed that overexpression of sortilin in transfected cells leads to increased uptake of LDL-particles into these cells. One possible explanation for association of the chromosome 1p13 variant with LDL-C and CAD might therefore be increased sortilin expression leading to enhanced LDL-uptake into tissues, which in turn results in lower LDL-C levels and subsequently lower risk of CAD [67]. Musunuru et al. reported that a common noncoding polymorphism at the 1p13 locus, rs12740374 (in high LD with rs599839), creates a C/EBP (CCAAT/enhancer binding protein) transcription factor binding site and alters hepatic expression of the SORT1 gene. Moreover, small interfering RNA (siRNA) knockdown and viral overexpression in mouse liver demonstrated that Sort1 alters plasma LDL-C and very low-density lipoprotein (VLDL) particle levels by modulating hepatic VLDL secretion. Thus, Musunuru et al. provided functional evidence of a novel regulatory pathway for lipoprotein metabolism and suggested that modulation of this pathway may alter risk for MI in humans [68]. However, sortilin also appears to be involved in the development of atherosclerosis by mechanisms not directly involving LDL-cholesterol, but possibly resulting from the attenuated secretion of proinflammatory cytokines, such as IL6 and TNFα, which accompanies sortilin deficiency in immune cells. In conclusion, the data indicate that sortilin plays an important role in the development of cardiovascular disease and functions beyond regulating LDL-cholesterol levels [69].

ADAMTS-7: Protective Role in Atherosclerosis

At the ADAMTS-7 locus, the major allele (A) of the most significant SNP identified, rs3825807, was associated with an 8% increase in the odds of developing CAD [70]. Interestingly, in subgroup analysis of MI and angiographic CAD phenotypes, this variant showed a greater association with atherosclerosis than MI (OR = 1.20 vs. 1.08) [70, 71]. Additional GWAS studies reported the association of ADAMTS-7 with human coronary calcification [72]. Variant rs3825807 is a nonsynonymous polymorphism, with an adenine (A) to guanine (G) change resulting in a serine (Ser) to proline (Pro) substitution in the pro-domain of ADAMTS-7. ADAMTS-7 is a disintegrin and metalloproteinase with thrombospondin motifs (ADAMTS) family member. Vascular smooth muscle cells (VSMCs) are key cells in migration and proliferation during the development of atherosclerosis, calcification, and restenosis. Previous studies sought to understand the underlying pathomechanisms involving ADAMTS-7 in VSMCs and their possible role in vascular disorders. Wang et al. reported previously the involvement of ADAMTS-7 in VSMC migration [73]. ADAMTS-7 was shown to promote neo-intima formation upon arterial injury through the degradation of cartilage oligomeric matrix protein (COMP). Furthermore, a recent study showed that rs3825807 has an effect on ADAMTS-7 maturation, thrombospondin-5 cleavage, and VSMC migration, as well as playing a potentially protective role against atherosclerosis and CAD [74]. Also, it was recently shown that ADAMTS-7 promotes VSMC and aortic calcification by altering the balance between the osteogenic protein BMP-2 and its natural inhibitor COMP [75]. Thus, based on these studies, there is increasing evidence linking ADAMTS-7 with VSMC function, which may explain, at least in part, its role in the development of atherosclerosis and vascular remodeling as well as calcification. However, the precise mechanisms linking ADAMTS-7 in vivo with vascular remodeling and atherosclerosis remain unclear. Very recently, a study conducted by our group employed ADAMTS-7 knockout (KO) mice to reveal the role of ADAMTS-7 in vascular remodeling. We demonstrated that Adamts-7-deficient mice are resistant to neo-intima formation after vascular injury. Thrombospondin-1 was identified as a potential substrate for ADAMTS-7 using liquid chromatography-tandem mass spectrometry secretome analysis. Furthermore, we demonstrated that the C terminus of ADAMTS-7 directly associates with and degrades thrombospondin-1 in vivo and in vitro [76]. Interestingly, at the same time, another group published findings on the protective effects of ADAMTS-7 inhibition on atherosclerosis in mice lacking Adamts-7 in an atherogenic background (Apoe-KO and/or LDL-KO) [77]. Thus, all findings reported thus far pinpoint a key role of ADAMTS-7 in VSMC function. ADAMTS-7 deficiency is beneficial for atherosclerosis and vascular remodeling, and its inhibition might represent a promising therapeutic target. Interestingly, the gnomAD data base (https://gnomad.broadinstitute.org/), a resource developed by an international coalition of investigators, with the goal of aggregating and harmonizing both exome and genome sequencing data from a wide variety of large-scale sequencing projects lists several probands carrying loss-of-function variants for *ADAMTS7*, including one male proband being homozygous for a loss-of-function variant (p.Trp1210CysfsTer88), leading to a human *ADAMTS7* knockout which is apparently healthy [78]. This data supports the notion that inhibiting ADAMTS7 is relatively safe and no harmful side-effects might be feared (Fig. 24.8).

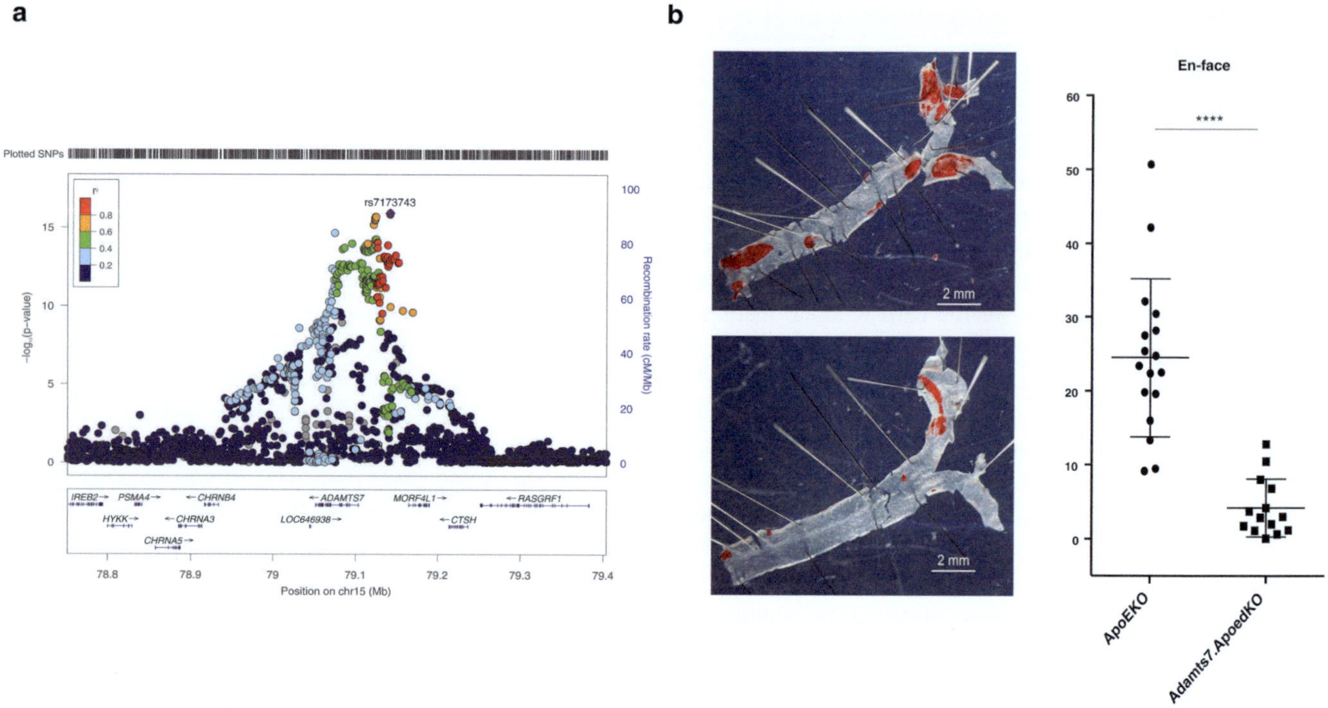

Fig. 24.8 A. Association plot for ADAMTS7 risk locus taken from the 1000G CARDIoGRAMplusC4D meta-analysis. B. ADAMTS7/APOE double knockout mice show significant decreased atherosclerosis, illustrated in en-face analysis of mice aorta

ZC3HC1: Single Nonsynonymous SNP Hit

This locus on chromosome 7 was reported in 2011 and contains only one genome-wide significant SNP, rs11556924 ($p = 2.22 \times 10^{-9}$, C to T), associated with CAD/MI [70]. rs11556924 lies within the coding region of the gene *ZC3HC1*, and there are no other SNPs in high LD. The wild-type allele, C, is associated with a higher risk of CAD/MI, and the minor allele, T, has a frequency of 15.58%. The SNP is nonsynonymous, causing substitution of arginine with histidine in the encoded protein at position 363. Although there is an eQTL-effect of the SNP rs11556924 on the neighboring gene *KLHDC10* [79], *ZC3HC1* is believed to be the better candidate gene for functional analyses, as the SNP leads to an amino acid exchange in the encoded protein [50].

ZC3HC1 encodes the protein NIPA (Nuclear interaction partner of ALK), which is involved in cell cycle control. It was first described in 2003 as a possible nuclear downstream target of the oncogenic tyrosine kinase nucleophosmin-anaplastic lymphoma kinase (NPM-ALK) [80]. Although NIPA directly binds NPM-ALK, it is not phosphorylated by this kinase. In subsequent studies, NIPA was found to be part of an SCF-type E3-ubiquitin ligase that interacts with cyclin B1 [81]. Cyclin B1 is a cell cycle regulating protein. During interphase, cyclin B1 is localized in the cytoplasm. Prior to mitosis, it is upregulated and transported to the nucleus. SCF-NIPA contributes to the regulation of cyclin B1 by targeting nuclear cyclin B1 and leading to its degradation [81]. Upon entry into M-phase, cyclin B1 enters the nucleus, whereupon NIPA is inactivated through phosphorylation. After inactivation of NIPA, cyclin B1 can carry out its function in promoting early events in mitosis [82].

Recent publications linked rs11556924 to hypertension in a Finnish population [83] and to a greater carotid intima-media thickness (cIMT) [84]. Another study in a Japanese population reported the SNP to be associated with atrial fibrillation, a common consequence of CAD/MI [85]. López-Mejías et al. found the homozygous nonrisk genotype to be associated with higher cIMT, an indicator of atherosclerosis. Yamase et al. also found the nonrisk allele to represent a risk factor for atrial fibrillation, whereas Kunnas et al. reported the homozygous risk genotype to be correlated with higher blood pressure. Although these publications appear to report contradictory results, they consolidate the link between the locus and CVD.

Chromosome 6q26–27: Haplotype Approach Links Risk SNPs to Lp(a)

Using a genome-wide haplotype approach, we were able to identify the SLC22A3-LPAL2-LPA gene cluster as a strong susceptibility locus for CAD [86]. Two haplotypes consisting of four SNPs (rs2048327 in the SLC22A3 gene, rs3127599 in the LPAL2 gene, and rs7767084 and rs10755578 in the LPA gene) were consistently associated with CAD/MI risk (CTTG haplotype, OR = 1.2 [95% CI,

1.13–1.28]; CCTC haplotype, OR = 1.82 [95% CI, 1.57–2.12]). Interestingly, this locus was not identified in previous genome-wide association (GWA) studies that focused on univariate analyses of SNPs. The proposed approach in the paper by Tregouet et al. may have wide utility for analyzing GWA data for other complex traits. The haplotype association analysis was performed using a sliding-windows approach. The locus partly overlaps the LPA gene, which encodes apolipoprotein(a), the main protein of lipoprotein(a) (Lp(a)), a well-known risk factor for CAD. Indeed, Tregouet et al. showed that the haplotypes associated with CAD were also associated with the highest Lp(a) levels, and, after adjustment for Lp(a) levels, were no longer associated with CAD, suggesting that their relation to risk is mediated by an effect on Lp(a) levels. Genetic variants, particularly a kringle repeat polymorphism, also affect the size of Lp(a) particles, and recent studies suggested that small Lp(a) particle size may be an independent risk marker. In light of these findings, Clarke et al. identified new risk variants (rs10455872 and rs3798220) with low allele frequency but strong effects on CAD (2.5-fold risk increase in individuals who carried at least two of these risk alleles) [87].

Genetic Architecture of (Premature) Coronary Artery Disease

Interestingly, the genetic components reflected by the multiple genetic variants identified in GWA studies cannot explain familial clustering of the disease as indicated by a positive family history. As mentioned, the variants identified in GWAS were characterized by a high allele frequency (i.e., each individual in a population is affected by multiple risk alleles to a greater or lesser degree) and a small effect size (i.e., only the cumulative effect of multiple variants may be of clinical relevance). A positive family history, on the other hand, appears to be mediated by rare deleterious mutations with a more profound effect [88, 89] or by specific interactions between more common genetic variants (epistasis) [90, 91]. Not surprisingly, the heritability of CAD and MI is only partially explained by currently known risk alleles.

Remarkably, there appears to be a marked overlap between the few genes that showed co segregation in family-based studies and those identified in GWAS. Indeed, almost all genes causing monogenic forms of CAD or MI also produce a signal in GWAS (i.e., *GUCY1A1*, *LDLR*, *PCSK9*, *APOB*, and *LPA*), giving rise to an allelic series ranging from rare, damaging alleles with profound effects to common alleles with mild effects. While monogenic forms are explained by rare damaging mutations in the coding sequence (Fig. 24.9: upper corner on the left side), GWAS signals most often arise from frequent variants with smaller effects in the very same genes or their regulatory regions (Fig. 24.9: lower corner of the right side) [5, 16, 42, 92].

Genetic Variants and Relevance for Therapeutic Development

Although over the last decades much research has focused on the identification of biological risk factors and developing medicines to modify them, actually only few medicines (e.g., aspirin, statins, and anti-hypertensive agents) have been proven to reduce the risk of CAD or MI. A novel promising

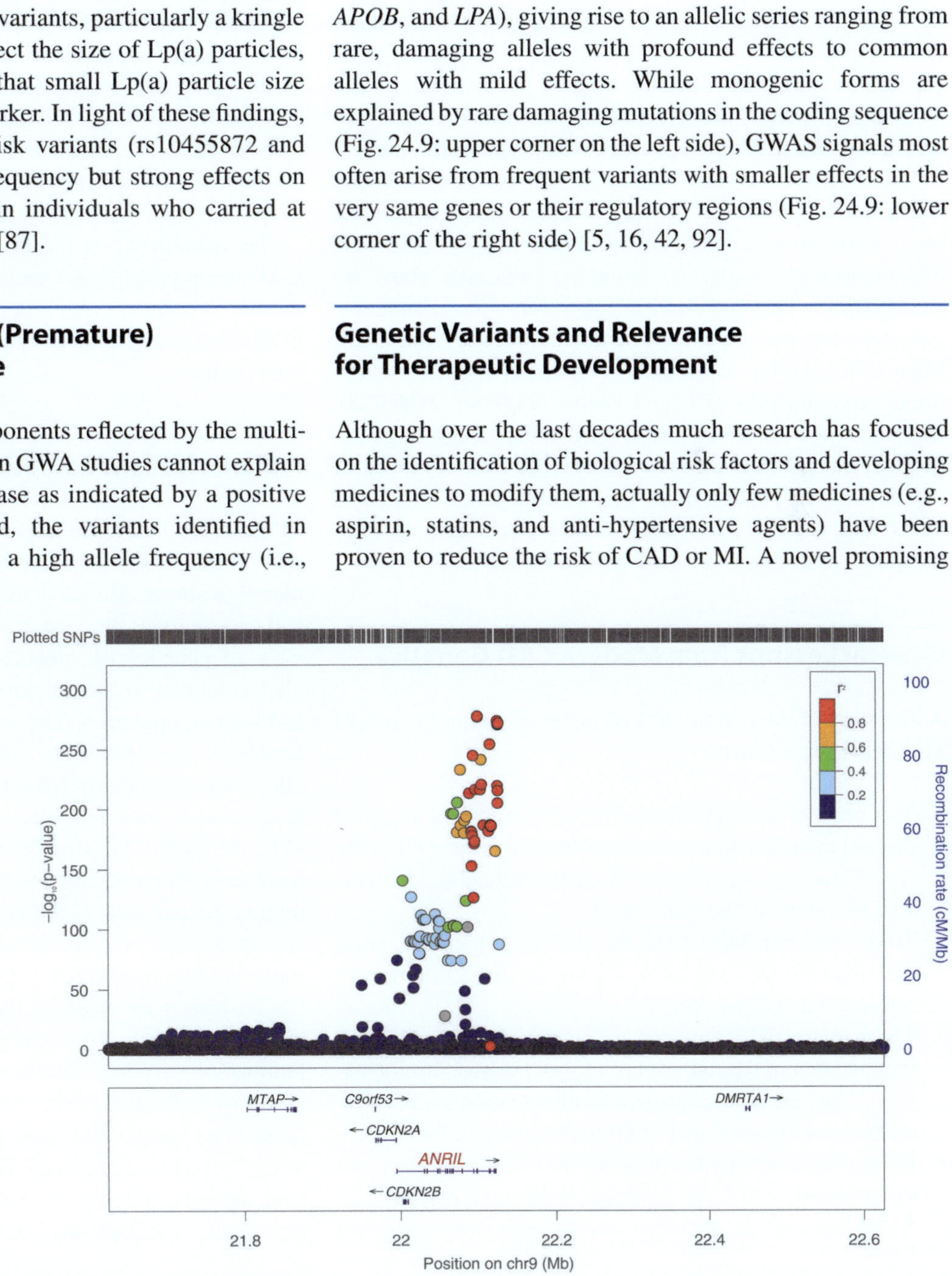

Fig. 24.9 Association plot presenting *ANRIL* and the *CAD* risk locus at chromosome 9p21. Data is obtained from the largest CAD GWAS meta-analysis performed so far including one million CAD cases and controls

Table 24.1 Examples of genes affecting CAD and MI risk identified by large-scale array-based and deep-sequencing projects with relevance for therapeutic development

Gene	PCSK9	NPC1L1	LPA	LPL	APOC3	ANGPTL4	ASGR1
Frequency	1 in 50 blacks	1 in 150	1 in 13	1 in 10	1 in 150	1 in 500	1 in 120
Phenotype	LDL	LDL	Lp(a)	TG	TG	TG	Non-HDL-C
Risk	80% lower risk	53% lower risk	14% higher risk	17% lower risk	40% lower risk	57% lower risk	34% lower risk
Therapy	Evolocumab Bococizumab Alirocumab Inclisiran	Ezetimibe	Antisense in develop-ment	?	Antisense in develop-ment	Mono-clonal antibodies in develop-ment	?
References	[97]	[98]	[87]	[93]	[99]	[93, 100]	[101]

TG triglycerides

approach for identifying potential therapeutically targets for drug development is through leveraging the human genome. Based on the presence of naturally occurring genetic variations that can be found in nearly every gene, including genes that are potential drug-specific targets. If these deoxyribonucleic acid (DNA) sequence variation modulate the function or expression of a gene, then the phenotypic consequences of this variation in the human population could predict whether a drug will safely reduce disease risk. Of significant interest are so-called human knockouts [96], people with biallelic loss-of-function mutations (as mentioned above for *ADAMTS7*). This innovative approach—the druggable genome—has now been applied to several drug-gene pairs. Some of these drugs are already in clinical use (such as ezetimibe, targeting *NPC1L1*, and statins, targeting *HMGCR*), and some are in development (including drugs targeting *APOC3* and just very recently *ASGR1*) (Table 24.1) [102]. A recent study by Nelson et al. showed that genes implicated by GWAS are twice as likely to succeed in clinical trials compared to targets without genetic support [103].

General Lessons from Modern CAD Genetics

A summary of the current data on genes affecting the risk of MI/CAD is as follows:

- The precise mechanisms linking chromosomal loci and disease manifestation are still unclear for almost all of the loci. However, it is foreseeable that mechanistic insights will be gained in the near future.
- Traditional risk factors mediate risk only partially, since the majority of loci (2/3) display no association with intermediate phenotypes.
- The genetic risk conferred by newly discovered loci is independent of the risk conferred by a positive family history. Thus, the molecular-genetic information for risk prediction goes beyond that of all traditional risk factors.
- Each of the currently known common risk alleles increases the probability of CAD by a relatively small margin, i.e., 5–30% per allele. In other words, individuals who are homozygous for the risk allele on chromosome 9p21.3 carry a 50% increased risk compared with the 25% of the European population who do not carry this allele.
- The high frequency of risk alleles, on the other hand, explains why the implications of the recently identified genetic factors at the population level are substantial, even though affected individuals carry only a relatively moderate risk increase.

This wealth of new information on the heritable aspects of CAD opens multiple avenues for scientific exploration. From a clinical point of view, the immediate needs concern risk prediction and (preventive) therapy for atherosclerosis (see next section).

Is Genetic Risk Prediction Feasible?

While CAD is a chronic process, its clinical manifestation may occur suddenly and fatally in the form of MI. Thus, there is a strong clinical demand for predicting disease onset and (preventive) therapy for atherosclerosis. A simplified view of genetic risk calculation could be a count of risk alleles, similar to the quantitative assessment of cholesterol levels in a population. The underlying assumption, that risk conferred by some alleles can be balanced by "protective" alleles at other loci, does not take into account that biological mechanisms, as well as effect sizes, at various loci are likely to be different. Thus, the development of genetic risk scores needs careful prospective testing. An open question for estimating genetic risk is the definition of a "control sample" free of genetic predisposition. The number of known chromosomal loci implicated in CAD is growing constantly, and the frequency of most of these alleles is high. Even in a "healthy" Western European population sample, the average number of currently known risk alleles is >50. Thus, if a group of individuals does not carry a specific risk allele, it cannot be expected that their genetic risk is "zero" but rather at the "population average." This population average is, however, heavily inflated by a multitude of perhaps untested genetically predisposing factors, minus the effect of the tested allele. Vice versa, the effect of a traditional risk factor, such as smoking, in a person who luckily does not carry any genetic predisposition, i.e., none of the CAD risk alleles, cannot be known. Is it outrageous to hypothesize that CAD could be eliminated altogether if the effects of susceptibility genes could be entirely neutralized? In this respect, it may be noteworthy that some mammalian species (mice) or vascular beds (internal mammary artery) do not develop atherosclerosis; in other words, even the presence of multiple established risk factors does not automatically result in the manifestation of CAD. Currently, only a relatively limited fraction (≈15%) of the overall genetic risk (heritability) of CAD is explained by the identified loci. This can be partly explained by the limited power of individual GWA studies to detect such loci. Global consortia (such as CARDIoGRAM and, later, CARDIoGRAMplusC4D) are in the process of analyzing genome-wide information from more than 80,000 cases of CAD and over 120,000 controls and have identified additional loci harboring even more common variants. Moreover, an increasing effort has been made to elucidate the role of rare variants, and this has been aided by the novel information on such variants coming out of the 1000 Genomes Project (https://www.1000genomes.org) and genotyping the exome array [93]. In parallel, statistical methods have been developed that make use of SNPs for risk prediction even when their statistical level of association with disease does not reach the conservative genome-wide significance threshold of $p < 5 \times 10^{-8}$. These algorithms take into account that analysis of all SNPs with association at significance levels of $p < 5 \times 10^{-6}$ or $p < 5 \times 10^{-5}$ will include multiple falsely associated SNPs. However, the predictive information derived from the large number of remaining truly associated SNPs may go far beyond the information derived from the relatively few "established" SNPs. Together, genetic susceptibility for MI, as well as for related risk factors, will soon become more transparent. In practical terms, the challenge is to utilize genomic information for the refinement of clinically utilized risk scores. These scores are largely dominated by the predictive information of age and gender and based on prediction of short-term risks. It is obvious that a man in his 70s has a higher risk than a young woman over the next 10 years, regardless of the genetic risk burden these two subjects may carry. The clinically relevant question is, what difference do genetic factors make in refining risk prediction in patients with similar characteristics (for example, two middle-aged men) to better target future preventive measures? Epidemiological studies with prospective DNA and data collection are ongoing to address these clinically important issues. The first promising results have been published already: a study of the placebo arms of four statin therapy trials demonstrated that genetic risk scores (GRS) adequately stratified CAD risk (HR for intermediate-risk vs. low-risk = 1.34; 95% CI, 1.22–1.47; HR for high-risk vs. low-risk = 1.72; 95% CI, 1.55–1.92). The analysis of the so-called ASCOT trial reported that individuals at high genetic risk for CHD derive greater benefit from statin therapy than those at low genetic risk. Indeed, the number needed to treat to prevent one event was 100 in those with low genetic risk, but 33 in those with high genetic risk [104]. Such prospective studies will help to understand the degree to which molecular-genetic prediction of CAD can improve personalized risk assessment beyond that approximated from family history or risk scores such as the Framingham or Euro Score.

The last few years the potential application of genomic research has widely been discussed in the literature. Especially, outcomes like the prediction of the risk of an individual for a complex disorder, such as CAD, and use of this information to encourage the adoption of preventive measures. Familial hypercholesterolemia (FH) is a condition characterized by monogenic mutations in the genes encoding *LDLR*, *PCSK9*, and *APOB*. Loss-of-function variants in these genes lead to increased cholesterol, and carriers have an up to fourfold elevated risk for CAD compared with non-carriers [105]. Early diagnosis, either on the basis of clinical criteria (including LDL cholesterol and family history) or DNA sequencing, can lead to timely treatment with lipid lowering medication and consequently lower the risk of cardiovascular disease to levels equivalent to those of the general population [106]. By contrast, the value of individual common variants is very limited for risk prediction. Polygenic risk scores (PRSs), derived by summing the number of risk variant alleles in each individual weighted by the impact of each allele on disease risk, perform better than individual variants; however, the predictive power remains limited [107].

Moreover, among participants at high genetic risk, adherence to a healthy lifestyle is associated with an almost 50% lower relative risk of CAD [108]. A novel approach, developed by Khera et al., which aggregated information from 6.6 million common variants to build a PRS [109], demonstrated convincingly that such a PRS can identify a fourfold increased risk for CAD in 2.5% of the population, comparable to FH mutation carriers (Fig. 24.10) [109].

On a cautionary note, the potential benefits of disclosing the genetic risk to patients must be weighed against possible unfavorable consequences, such as increased treatment costs, psychological distress or discrimination, and a sense of fatalism in high-risk individuals. However, a large Finnish study shows that giving personal genomic information to individuals can have a long-term beneficial effect on their lifestyles (Kardiokompassi.fi). Clearly, more work is needed to optimize the disclosure of genetic risk to patients and their healthcare providers, and to assess whether such disclosure can improve clinical outcomes.

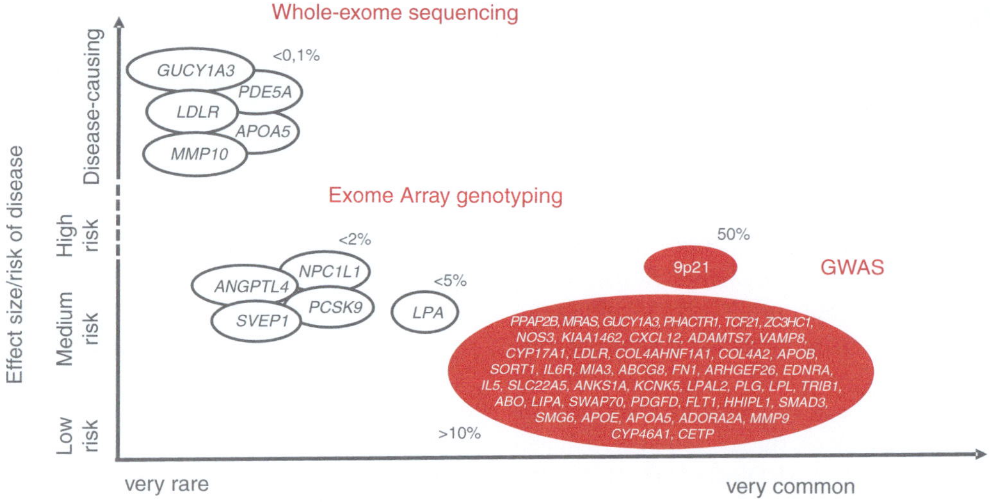

Fig. 24.10 Summary of the genetic architecture of CAD and MI. Rare, coding variants in *GUCY1A1*, *ADCY8*, *PDE5A*, *LDLR*, and *APOA5* have been identified by whole-exome sequencing (WES) in affected families. These variants confer large risk effects, displaying an almost monogenic inheritance pattern [5]. Low-frequency variants in *ANGPTL4*, *NPC1L1*, *PCSK9*, and *SVEP1* have been identified by WES or large-scale genotyping of the exome array [93]. Common variants in more than 160 genetic loci, conferring a low-risk effect, have been identified by GWAS [94]. Adapted from Manolio et al. [95]

Cardiovascular System Genetics

System genetics offer the potential to provide new insights into our understanding of the pathogenesis of CAD. The rationale for this approach is based on the hypothesis that an interacting network precipitates complex disease such as atherosclerosis. Players in this network modulate one another at multiple levels, including the genome, transcriptome (mRNA and miRNAs [110]), methylome/epigenome, proteome, and metabolome. The challenge is to comprehend the connections and interactions between individual constituents of this network. Specifically, it is of great interest to understand the communication between genetic (SNPs, CNVs), traditional, and environmental risk factors (SNPs, CNVs) at the level of the cell, tissue, and organ to ultimately describe the entire organism with respect to its predisposition to develop disease. The intention is to identify the biological networks that connect the different system elements, thereby defining the characteristics that describe the overall system. This information can then be used to derive mechanistic information on biological processes as well as identify potential target sites for therapeutic intervention (Figs. 24.11 and 24.12) [46, 111, 112].

Summary/Take Home Message

Molecular-genetic approaches applied to the study of CAD will continue to identify genes and pathways involved in predisposition to and pathophysiology of this life-threatening condition.

Moreover, future gene expression profiling studies will refine our understanding of the nature of atherosclerotic lesions within the vascular wall and promise discovery and validation of targets for therapeutic intervention.

Opportunities to translate genetic, genomic, proteomic, and metabolomic information into cardiovascular clinical practice have never been greater, but their implementation requires validation in large independent cohorts, which can be achieved only through collaborative efforts, such as CARDIoGRAM [43, 70] or CARDIoGRAMplusC4D [25]. Their continued success will depend on ongoing cooperation within the cardiovascular research community.

Advice for the Clinical Practice

Based on recent studies, risk prediction using PRS is feasible; however, the use of a PRS in clinical practice for risk reclassification in intermediate risk patients is not yet routine.

Genetic analysis (either specific SNPs or specific rare molecular gene defects) in patients with a strong family history of CAD after exclusion of familial hypercholesterolemia or in unaffected relatives is not yet recommended in a clinical setting, because individual findings are still difficult to interpret. However, in a research setting identification and analysis of patients with a strong family history are of utmost importance to further unravel the pathogenesis of the disease.

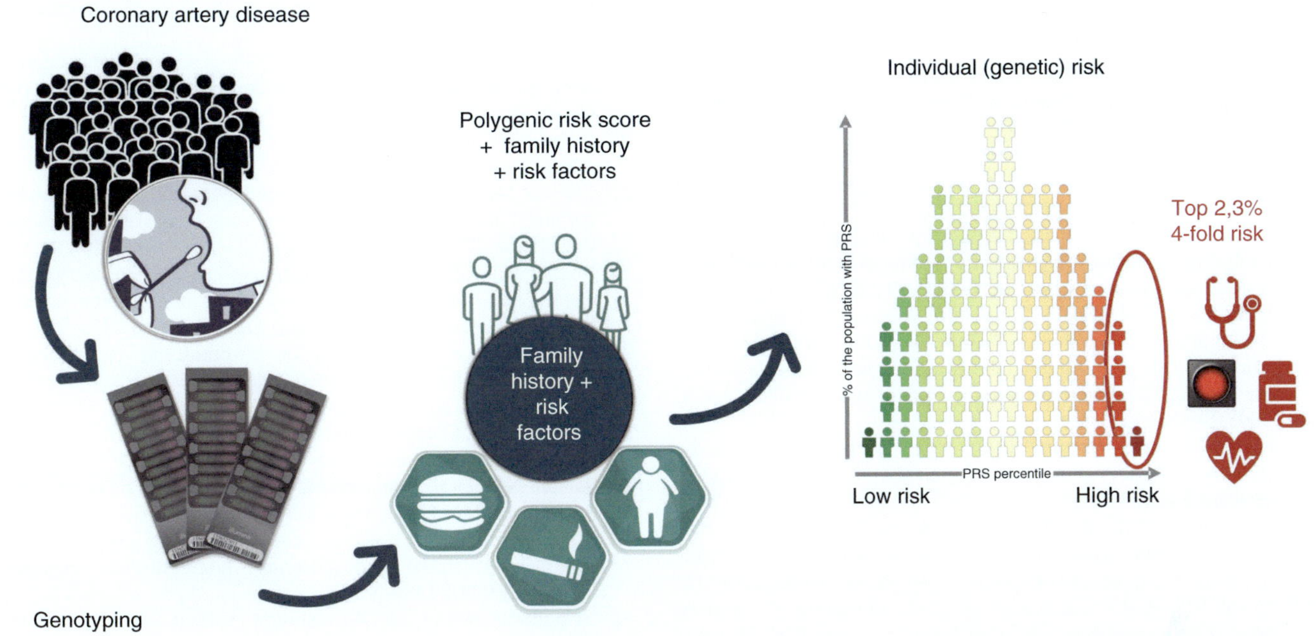

Fig. 24.11 A polygenic risk score can be calculated for every individual after genotyping a GWAS array. The polygenic risk score, in addition to family history and risk factors, can identify individuals at high risk for CAD. According to Khera et al. 2.3% of the population ("carriers") had inherited ≥4-fold increased risk for CAD and 0.5% ("carriers") had inherited ≥5-fold increased risk [109]

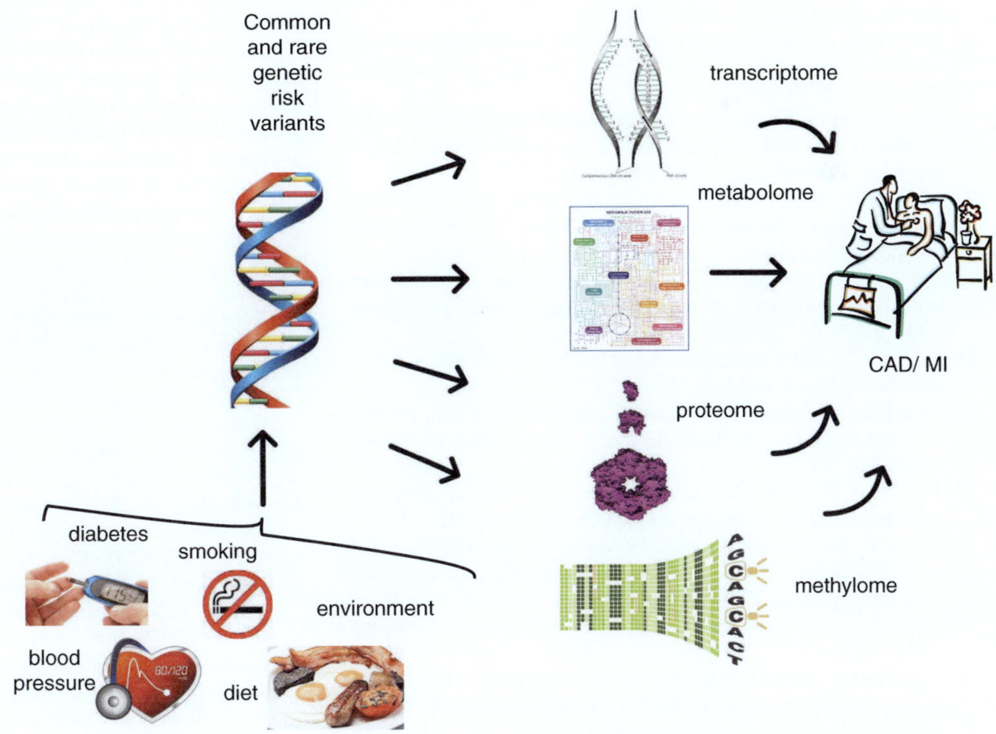

Fig. 24.12 Integrative view of genetic risk variants affecting gene expression or function in the context of traditional risk factors and hitherto unspecified environmental cofactors. Ultimately, biological networks may malfunction resulting in the precipitation of CAD and MI

References

1. Go AS, et al. Heart disease and stroke statistics—2014 update: a report from the American Heart Association. Circulation. 2014;129(3):e28–e292.
2. Lusis AJ. Atherosclerosis. Nature. 2000;407(6801):233–41.
3. Müller C. Angina pectoris in hereditary xanthomatosis. Arch Intern Med. 1939;64(4):675–700.
4. Schunkert H, et al. Repeated replication and a prospective meta-analysis of the association between chromosome 9p21.3 and coronary artery disease. Circulation. 2008;117(13):1675–84.
5. Erdmann J, et al. Dysfunctional nitric oxide signalling increases risk of myocardial infarction. Nature. 2013;504(7480):432–6.
6. Murabito JM, et al. Sibling cardiovascular disease as a risk factor for cardiovascular disease in middle-aged adults. JAMA. 2005;294(24):3117–23.
7. Myers RH, et al. Parental history is an independent risk factor for coronary artery disease: the Framingham Study. Am Heart J. 1990;120(4):963–9.
8. Lloyd-Jones DM, et al. Parental cardiovascular disease as a risk factor for cardiovascular disease in middle-aged adults: a prospective study of parents and offspring. JAMA. 2004;291(18):2204–11.
9. Horne BD, et al. Identification of excess clustering of coronary heart diseases among extended pedigrees in a genealogical population database. Am Heart J. 2006;152(2):305–11.
10. Hengstenberg C, et al. Siblings of myocardial infarction patients are overlooked in primary prevention of cardiovascular disease. Eur Heart J. 2001;22(11):926–33.
11. Andresdottir MB, et al. Fifteen percent of myocardial infarctions and coronary revascularizations explained by family history unrelated to conventional risk factors. The Reykjavik Cohort Study. Eur Heart J. 2002;23(21):1655–63.
12. Hawe E, et al. Family history is a coronary heart disease risk factor in the Second Northwick Park Heart Study. Ann Hum Genet. 2003;67(Pt 2):97–106.
13. Boer JM, et al. The joint impact of family history of myocardial infarction and other risk factors on 12-year coronary heart disease mortality. Epidemiology. 1999;10(6):767–70.
14. Marenberg ME, et al. Genetic susceptibility to death from coronary heart disease in a study of twins. N Engl J Med. 1994;330(15):1041–6.
15. Wang L, et al. Mutation of MEF2A in an inherited disorder with features of coronary artery disease. Science. 2003;302(5650):1578–81.
16. Stitziel NO, et al. Exome sequencing in suspected monogenic dyslipidemias. Circ Cardiovasc Genet. 2015;8(2):343–50.
17. Schunkert H, Bourier F. Deciphering unexplained familial dyslipidemias: do we have the tools? Circ Cardiovasc Genet. 2015;8(2):250–2.
18. Lieb W, et al. Lack of association between the MEF2A gene and myocardial infarction. Circulation. 2008;117(2):185–91.
19. Guella I, et al. Association and functional analyses of MEF2A as a susceptibility gene for premature myocardial infarction and coronary artery disease. Circ Cardiovasc Genet. 2009;2(2):165–72.
20. Wobst J, et al. Role of sGC-dependent NO signalling and myocardial infarction risk. J Mol Med (Berl). 2015;93(4):383–94.
21. Hanafy KA, Martin E, Murad F. CCTη, a novel soluble guanylyl cyclase-interacting protein. J Biol Chem. 2004;279(45):46946–53.
22. Kessler T, et al. Functional characterization of the GUCY1A3 coronary artery disease risk locus. Circulation. 2017;136(5):476–89.
23. Kessler T, et al. Association of the coronary artery disease risk gene GUCY1A3 with ischaemic events after coronary intervention. Cardiovasc Res. 2019;115(10):1512–8.
24. Hall KT, et al. Genetic variation at the coronary artery disease risk locus GUCY1A3 modifies cardiovascular disease prevention effects of aspirin. Eur Heart J. 2019:ehz384. https://doi.org/10.1093/eurheartj/ehz384.
25. Nikpay M, et al. A comprehensive 1,000 genomes-based genome-wide association meta-analysis of coronary artery disease. Nat Genet. 2015;47(10):1121–30.
26. Wobst J, et al. Molecular variants of soluble guanylyl cyclase affecting cardiovascular risk. Circ J. 2015;79(3):463–9.
27. Fischer M, et al. Distinct heritable patterns of angiographic coronary artery disease in families with myocardial infarction. Circulation. 2005;111(7):855–62.
28. Fischer M, et al. Familial aggregation of left main coronary artery disease and future risk of coronary events in asymptomatic siblings of affected patients. Eur Heart J. 2007;28(20):2432–7.
29. Broeckel U, et al. A locus on chromosome 10 influences C-reactive protein levels in two independent populations. Hum Genet. 2007;122(1):95–102.
30. Klein RJ, et al. Complement factor H polymorphism in age-related macular degeneration. Science. 2005;308(5720):385–9.
31. Samani NJS, et al. Genomewide association analysis of coronary artery disease. N Engl J Med. 2007;357(5):443–53.
32. McPherson R, et al. A common allele on chromosome 9 associated with coronary heart disease. Science. 2007;316(5830):1488–91.
33. Helgadottir A, et al. A common variant on chromosome 9p21 affects the risk of myocardial infarction. Science. 2007;316(5830):1491–3.
34. Wellcome Trust Case Control Consortium. Genome-wide association study of 14,000 cases of seven common diseases and 3,000 shared controls. Nature. 2007;447(7145):661–78.
35. Xing C, et al. Evaluation of power of the Illumina HumanOmni5M-4v1 BeadChip to detect risk variants for human complex diseases. Eur J Hum Genet. 2015;24(7):1029–34.
36. Marchini J, Howie B. Genotype imputation for genome-wide association studies. Nat Rev Genet. 2010;11(7):499–511.
37. The 1000 Genomes Project Consortium. A global reference for human genetic variation. Nature. 2015;526(7571):68–74.
38. Porcu E, et al. Genotype imputation in genome-wide association studies. Curr Protoc Hum Genet. 2013;Chapter 1:Unit 1.25
39. McCarthy S, et al. A reference panel of 64,976 haplotypes for genotype imputation. Nat Genet. 2016;48:1279–83.
40. Iglesias AI, et al. Haplotype reference consortium panel: practical implications of imputations with large reference panels. Hum Mutat. 2017;38(8):1025–32.
41. Roberts R. A genetic basis for coronary artery disease. Trends Cardiovasc Med. 2015;25(3):171–8.
42. CARDIoGRAMplusC4D Consortium. Large-scale association analysis identifies new risk loci for coronary artery disease. Nat Genet. 2013;45(1):25–33.
43. Schunkert H, Erdmann J, Samani NJS. CARDIoGRAM celebrates its 10th anniversary. Eur Heart J. 2019;40(21):1664–6.
44. Erdmann J, et al. A decade of genome-wide association studies for coronary artery disease: the challenges ahead. Cardiovasc Res. 2018;114(9):1241–57.
45. Buniello A, et al. The NHGRI-EBI GWAS catalog of published genome-wide association studies, targeted arrays and summary statistics 2019. Nucleic Acids Res. 2019;47(D1):D1005–12.
46. Bjorkegren JL, et al. Genome-wide significant loci: how important are they? Systems genetics to understand heritability of coronary artery disease and other common complex disorders. J Am Coll Cardiol. 2015;65(8):830–45.
47. Maurano MT, et al. Systematic localization of common disease-associated variation in regulatory DNA. Science. 2012;337(6099):1190–5.
48. Nicolae DL, et al. Trait-associated SNPs are more likely to be eQTLs: annotation to enhance discovery from GWAS. PLoS Genet. 2010;6(4):e1000888.

49. Schaub MA, et al. Linking disease associations with regulatory information in the human genome. Genome Res. 2012;22(9):1748–59.
50. Braenne I, et al. Prediction of causal candidate genes in coronary artery disease loci. Arterioscler Thromb Vasc Biol. 2015;35(10):2207–17.
51. Miller CL, Pjanic M, Quertermous T. From locus association to mechanism of gene causality: the devil is in the details. Arterioscler Thromb Vasc Biol. 2015;35(10):2079–80.
52. Lempiainen H, et al. Network analysis of coronary artery disease risk genes elucidates disease mechanisms and druggable targets. Sci Rep. 2018;8(1):3434.
53. Tragante V, et al. Druggability of coronary artery disease risk loci. Circ Genom Precis Med. 2018;11(8):e001977.
54. Helgadottir A, et al. The same sequence variant on 9p21 associates with myocardial infarction, abdominal aortic aneurysm and intracranial aneurysm. Nat Genet. 2008;40(2):217–24.
55. Gschwendtner A, et al. Sequence variants on chromosome 9p21.3 confer risk for atherosclerotic stroke. Ann Neurol. 2009;65(5):531–9.
56. Chen HH, et al. Functional genomics of the 9p21.3 locus for atherosclerosis: clarity or confusion? Curr Cardiol Rep. 2014;16(7):502.
57. Broadbent HM, et al. Susceptibility to coronary artery disease and diabetes is encoded by distinct, tightly linked SNPs in the ANRIL locus on chromosome 9p. Hum Mol Genet. 2008;17(6):806–14.
58. Liu Y, et al. INK4/ARF transcript expression is associated with chromosome 9p21 variants linked to atherosclerosis. PLoS One. 2009;4(4):e5027.
59. Jarinova O, et al. Functional analysis of the chromosome 9p21.3 coronary artery disease risk locus. Arterioscler Thromb Vasc Biol. 2009;29(10):1671–7.
60. Visel A, et al. Targeted deletion of the 9p21 non-coding coronary artery disease risk interval in mice. Nature. 2010;464(7287):409–12.
61. Harismendy O, et al. 9p21 DNA variants associated with coronary artery disease impair interferon-gamma signalling response. Nature. 2011;470(7333):264–8.
62. Holdt LM, Teupser D. Long noncoding RNA ANRIL: Lnc-ing genetic variation at the chromosome 9p21 locus to molecular mechanisms of atherosclerosis. Front Cardiovasc Med. 2018;5:145.
63. Samani NJS, et al. The novel genetic variant predisposing to coronary artery disease in the region of the PSRC1 and CELSR2 genes on chromosome 1 associates with serum cholesterol. J Mol Med (Berl). 2008;86(11):1233–41.
64. Schadt EE, et al. Mapping the genetic architecture of gene expression in human liver. PLoS Biol. 2008;6(5):e107.
65. Nielsen MS, et al. Sortilin/neurotensin receptor-3 binds and mediates degradation of lipoprotein lipase. J Biol Chem. 1999;274(13):8832–6.
66. Nilsson SK, et al. Endocytosis of apolipoprotein A-V by members of the low density lipoprotein receptor and the VPS10p domain receptor families. J Biol Chem. 2008;283(38):25920–7.
67. Linsel-Nitschke P, et al. Genetic variation at chromosome 1p13.3 affects sortilin mRNA expression, cellular LDL-uptake and serum LDL levels which translates to the risk of coronary artery disease. Atherosclerosis. 2010;208(1):183–9.
68. Musunuru K, et al. From noncoding variant to phenotype via SORT1 at the 1p13 cholesterol locus. Nature. 2010;466(7307):714–9.
69. Kjolby M, Nielsen MS, Petersen CM. Sortilin, encoded by the cardiovascular risk gene SORT1, and its suggested functions in cardiovascular disease. Curr Atheroscler Rep. 2015;17(4):496.
70. Schunkert H, et al. Large-scale association analysis identifies 13 new susceptibility loci for coronary artery disease. Nat Genet. 2011;43(4):333–8.
71. Reilly MP, et al. Identification of ADAMTS7 as a novel locus for coronary atherosclerosis and association of ABO with myocardial infarction in the presence of coronary atherosclerosis: two genome-wide association studies. Lancet. 2011;377(9763):383–92.
72. O'Donnell CJ, et al. Genome-wide association study for coronary artery calcification with follow-up in myocardial infarction. Circulation. 2011;124(25):2855–64.
73. Wang L, et al. ADAMTS-7 mediates vascular smooth muscle cell migration and neointima formation in balloon-injured rat arteries. Circ Res. 2009;104(5):688–98.
74. Pu X, et al. ADAMTS7 cleavage and vascular smooth muscle cell migration is affected by a coronary-artery-disease-associated variant. Am J Hum Genet. 2013;92(3):366–74.
75. Du Y, et al. Upregulation of a disintegrin and metalloproteinase with thrombospondin motifs-7 by miR-29 repression mediates vascular smooth muscle calcification. Arterioscler Thromb Vasc Biol. 2012;32(11):2580–8.
76. Kessler T, et al. ADAMTS-7 inhibits re-endothelialization of injured arteries and promotes vascular remodeling through cleavage of thrombospondin-1. Circulation. 2015;131(13):1191–201.
77. Bauer RC, et al. Knockout of Adamts7, a novel coronary artery disease locus in humans, reduces atherosclerosis in mice. Circulation. 2015;131(13):1202–13.
78. Lek M, et al. Analysis of protein-coding genetic variation in 60,706 humans. Nature. 2016;536(7616):285–91.
79. Erbilgin A, et al. Identification of CAD candidate genes in GWAS loci and their expression in vascular cells. J Lipid Res. 2013;54(7):1894–905.
80. Ouyang T, et al. Identification and characterization of a nuclear interacting partner of anaplastic lymphoma kinase (NIPA). J Biol Chem. 2003;278(32):30028–36.
81. Bassermann F, et al. NIPA defines an SCF-type mammalian E3 ligase that regulates mitotic entry. Cell. 2005;122(1):45–57.
82. Bassermann F, Peschel C, Duyster J. Mitotic entry: a matter of oscillating destruction. Cell Cycle. 2005;4(11):1515–7.
83. Kunnas T, Nikkari ST. Association of Zinc Finger, C3HC-type containing 1 (ZC3HC1) rs11556924 genetic variant with hypertension in a Finnish population, the TAMRISK Study. Medicine (Baltimore). 2015;94(32):e1221.
84. Lopez-Mejias R, et al. The ZC3HC1 rs11556924 polymorphism is associated with increased carotid intima-media thickness in patients with rheumatoid arthritis. Arthritis Res Ther. 2013;15(5):R152.
85. Yamase Y, et al. Association of genetic variants with atrial fibrillation. Biomed Rep. 2016;4(2):178–82.
86. Tregouet DA, et al. Genome-wide haplotype association study identifies the SLC22A3-LPAL2-LPA gene cluster as a risk locus for coronary artery disease. Nat Genet. 2009;41(3):283–5.
87. Clarke R, et al. Genetic variants associated with Lp(a) lipoprotein level and coronary disease. N Engl J Med. 2009;361(26):2518–28.
88. Braenne I, et al. Whole-exome sequencing in an extended family with myocardial infarction unmasks familial hypercholesterolemia. BMC Cardiovasc Disord. 2014;14:108.
89. Braenne I, et al. Systematic analysis of variants related to familial hypercholesterolemia in families with premature myocardial infarction. Eur J Hum Genet. 2016;24(2):191–7.
90. Lin C, et al. Gene-gene and gene-environment interactions in meta-analysis of genetic association studies. PLoS One. 2015;10(4):e0124967.
91. Mascheretti S, et al. An assessment of gene-by-gene interactions as a tool to unfold missing heritability in dyslexia. Hum Genet. 2015;134(7):749–60.
92. Do R, et al. Exome sequencing identifies rare LDLR and APOA5 alleles conferring risk for myocardial infarction. Nature. 2015;518(7537):102–6.

93. Myocardial Infarction Genetics and CARDIoGRAM Exome Consortia Investigators. Coding variation in ANGPTL4, LPL, and SVEP1 and the risk of coronary disease. N Engl J Med. 2016;374(12):1134–44.
94. Kessler T, Vilne B, Schunkert H. The impact of genome-wide association studies on the pathophysiology and therapy of cardiovascular disease. EMBO Mol Med. 2016;8(7):688–701.
95. Manolio TA, et al. Finding the missing heritability of complex diseases. Nature. 2009;461(7265):747–53.
96. Alkuraya FS. Human knockout research: new horizons and opportunities. Trends Genet. 2015;31(2):108–15.
97. Kathiresan S. A PCSK9 missense variant associated with a reduced risk of early-onset myocardial infarction. N Engl J Med. 2008;358(21):2299–300.
98. Myocardial Infarction Genetics Consortium Investigators. Inactivating mutations in NPC1L1 and protection from coronary heart disease. N Engl J Med. 2014;371(22):2072–82.
99. TG and HDL Working Group of the Exome Sequencing Project. National Heart, Lung, and Blood Institute, loss-of-function mutations in APOC3, triglycerides, and coronary disease. N Engl J Med. 2014;371(1):22–31.
100. Dewey FE, et al. Inactivating variants in ANGPTL4 and risk of coronary artery disease. N Engl J Med. 2016;374(12):1123–33.
101. Nioi P, et al. Variant ASGR1 associated with a reduced risk of coronary artery disease. N Engl J Med. 2016;374(22):2131–41.
102. Kathiresan S. Developing medicines that mimic the natural successes of the human genome: lessons from NPC1L1, HMGCR, PCSK9, APOC3, and CETP. J Am Coll Cardiol. 2015;65(15):1562–6.
103. Nelson MR, et al. The support of human genetic evidence for approved drug indications. Nat Genet. 2015;47(8):856–60.
104. Mega JL, et al. Genetic risk, coronary heart disease events, and the clinical benefit of statin therapy: an analysis of primary and secondary prevention trials. Lancet. 2015;385(9984):2264–71.
105. Benn M, et al. Mutations causative of familial hypercholesterolaemia: screening of 98 098 individuals from the Copenhagen General Population Study estimated a prevalence of 1 in 217. Eur Heart J. 2016;37(17):1384–94.
106. Louter L, Defesche J, van Lennep JR. Cascade screening for familial hypercholesterolemia: practical consequences. Atheroscler Suppl. 2017;30:77–85.
107. Hughes MF, et al. Genetic markers enhance coronary risk prediction in men: the MORGAM prospective cohorts. PLoS One. 2012;7(7):e40922.
108. Khera AV, et al. Genetic risk, adherence to a healthy lifestyle, and coronary disease. N Engl J Med. 2016;375:2349–58.
109. Khera AV, et al. Genome-wide polygenic scores for common diseases identify individuals with risk equivalent to monogenic mutations. Nat Genet. 2018;50(9):1219–24.
110. Nikpay M, et al. Genome-wide identification of circulating-miRNA expression quantitative trait loci reveals the role of several miRNAs in the regulation of cardiometabolic phenotypes. Cardiovasc Res. 2019;115(11):1629–45.
111. MacLellan WR, Wang Y, Lusis AJ. Systems-based approaches to cardiovascular disease. Nat Rev Cardiol. 2012;9(3):172–84.
112. Schadt EE, Bjorkegren JL. NEW: network-enabled wisdom in biology, medicine, and health care. Sci Transl Med. 2012;4(115):115rv1.

25 The Genetics of Mitral Valve Prolapse

Ana J. Pérez Matos, Toon Oomen, and J. Peter van Tintelen

Introduction

Mitral valve prolapse (MVP) is one of the most common forms of valvular heart disease.

It has long been recognized as an auscultatory phenomenon. It was not until 1966 that Barlow discovered the reason for the often-heard midsystolic click [1, 2]. Shortly afterwards, the introduction of echocardiography led to large numbers of patients diagnosed with MVP. Due to incorrect echocardiographic definitions and selection bias of studied populations, prevalences of up to 35% were reported in the 1970s and early 1980s [3]. A redefinition of echocardiographic criteria due to improved knowledge of mitral valve architecture provided a more accurate insight into the extent of the problem. Currently, the prevalence of MVP is known to range from about 0.5 to 3% in the general population [3–7]. It is equally distributed between men and women, yet patients with MVP tend to have a leaner stature [6].

Mitral valve prolapse (MVP) is defined as the billowing of one or both mitral valve leaflets across the plane of the mitral valve annulus into the left atrium during systole. By definition, the leaflets should reach more than 2 mm above the annular plane on the parasternal long axis view with echocardiography (Figs. 25.1 and 25.2).

The clinical presentation can be very diverse, ranging from an incidental finding within asymptomatic patients to dramatic cases with severe mitral regurgitation, heart failure, bacterial endocarditis, and in rare cases sudden cardiac death.

MVP may present as part of a systemic or syndromic disorder or as a solitary phenomenon. It may occur more frequently in connective tissue disorders such as Marfan syndrome, Loeys Dietz syndrome, and Ehlers Danlos syndrome. However, in most cases, it presents as a solitary entity; only a small minority, up to 1–2% of all patients with MVP have a connective tissue disorder or syndrome. This chapter focuses on the solitary forms that appear to be one of the most common Mendelian cardiovascular abnormalities in humans and it discusses the epidemiologic aspects of MVP, its pathophysiology, and the current status of genetic knowledge of this intriguing valvular disorder.

A. J. Pérez Matos · T. Oomen
Antonius Hospital Sneek, Department of Cardiology, Sneek, The Netherlands

J. P. van Tintelen (✉)
University Medical Center Utrecht, Department of Genetics, Sneek, The Netherlands
e-mail: j.p.vantintelen-3@umcutrecht.nl

Clinical Presentation, Diagnostics, Complications, and Pathophysiology of Mitral Valve Disease

The solitary forms of mitral valve disease are referred to as the classical prolapse, with the valve leaflet thickness exceeding 5 mm on echocardiography, and the nonclassical form, with leaflet thickness of less than 5 mm (both in the presence of a systolic upward displacement of 2 mm). Leaflet thickening or myxomatous degeneration is characterized by expansion of the spongiosa layer due to accumulation of proteoglycans. Also, structural alterations of collagen in all components of the valvular system and chordae can be found. It is thought that the mechanism underlying the expansion of the spongiosa layer is the result of a dysregulation of the balance between matrix protein synthesis and degradation [6]. From the pathologic anatomical point of view, accumulation of proteoglycans (myxomatous mitral valve) is the most common cause of MVP, leading to leaflet thickening and redundancy, chordeal elongation and interchordal hookings, and annular dilatation [7].

The clinical presentation of MVP is extremely heterogeneous, and to date hardly any specific set of predictors for disease progression has been identified (see Section "Ventricular Arrhythmias and Sudden Cardiac Death in MVP").

The diagnosis is in most cases made by physical examination. Typically, a midsystolic click is heard, often followed by a late systolic murmur [3]. The diagnosis is confirmed by two-dimensional echocardiography. MVP generally has a

H. F. Baars et al. (eds.), *Clinical Cardiogenetics*, https://doi.org/10.1007/978-3-030-45457-9_25

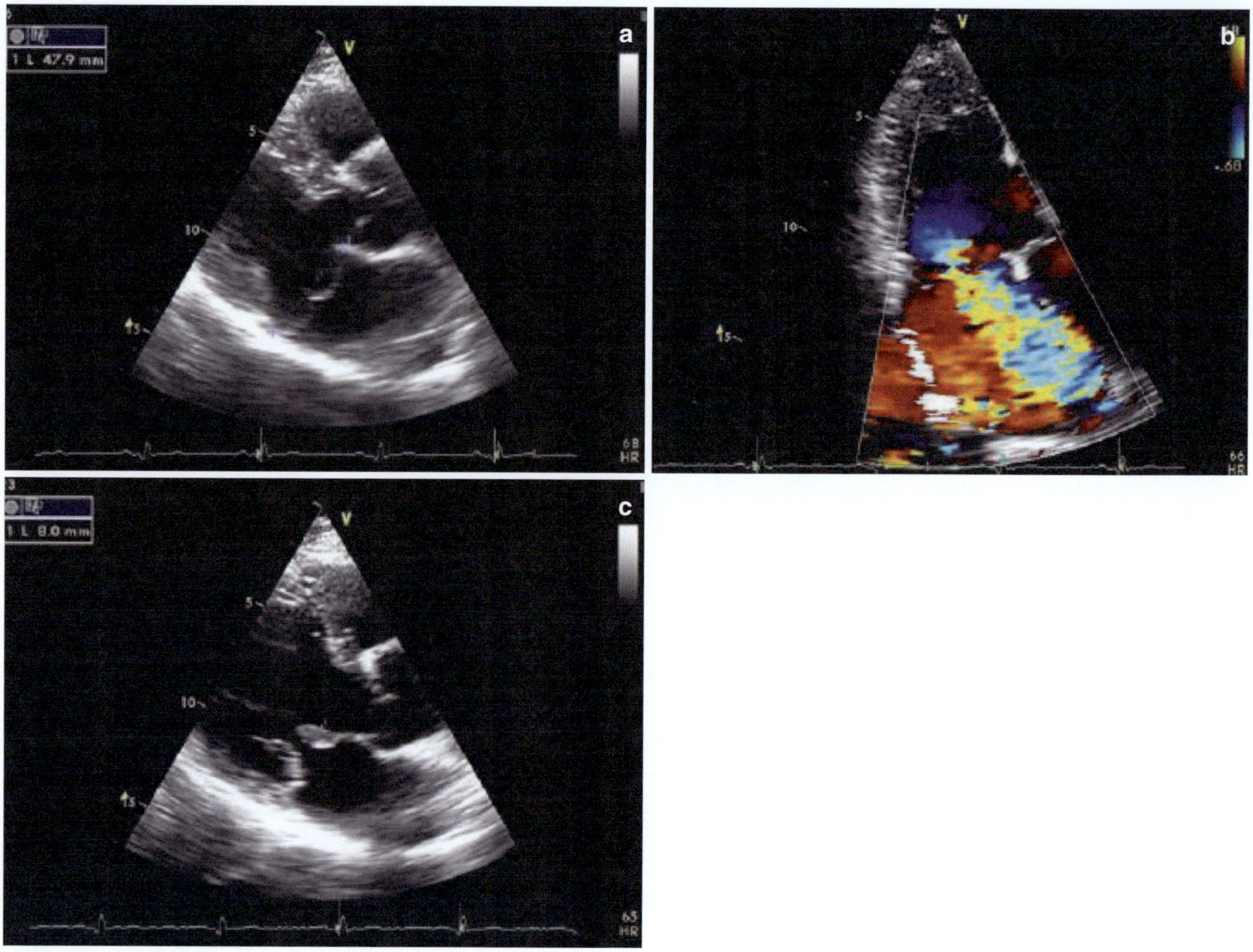

Fig. 25.1 (**a**) Parasternal long axis echocardiography showing classical mitral valve prolapse. Both posterior and anterior myxomatous mitral valve leaflets are billowing up to 6.5 mm in the left atrium during systole. (**b**) Apical three-chamber echocardiography with color Doppler flow measurement showing moderate to severe mitral regurgitation in the same patient. The left atrium is enlarged. (**c**) Parasternal long axis demonstrating myxomatous tips of both anterior and posterior mitral valves measuring 8 mm

good prognosis, however, in 25% of patients, MVP may progress to significant mitral regurgitation [9].

Complications such as severe mitral insufficiency, heart failure, thromboembolic complications, and sudden cardiac death are rare, especially in patients with nonclassical prolapse. Freed and coworkers, from the Framingham study group, found that these complications affected only 3% of all patients with MVP [6]. However, patients with classical prolapse carry a higher risk for complications [10]. It is not surprising that patients above 50 years who have a decreased left ventricular function, moderate to severe mitral regurgitation, and atrial fibrillation exhibit a high complication rate.

The risk for infective endocarditis was found to be raised; in a population study (Olmsted USA) where nearly 900 MVP patients were identified and followed up, the 15-year cohort risk of infectious endocarditis after MVP diagnosis was 1.1 ± 0.4% [11]. However, current guidelines for infectious endocarditis no longer advocate the use of prophylactic antibiotics in patients with MVP. Only patients who are known to have had endocarditis should receive infective endocarditis prophylaxis when appropriate [12].

Mitral regurgitation may, among other things, lead to atrial arrhythmias including atrial fibrillation and therefore to thromboembolic complications. Antithrombotic medication, on the other hand, should be given only if classical risk factors unrelated to MVP are present. Mitral valve reconstruction or replacement is advocated when severe mitral regurgitation leads to symptoms. In asymptomatic patients, when left ventricular (LV) abnormalities are present (LVEF $\leq$ 60% or LVESD $\geq$ 45 mm), surgery is indicated. Atrial fibrillation or pulmonary hypertension in asymptomatic patients with preserved LV function are reasons to consider surgery [13].

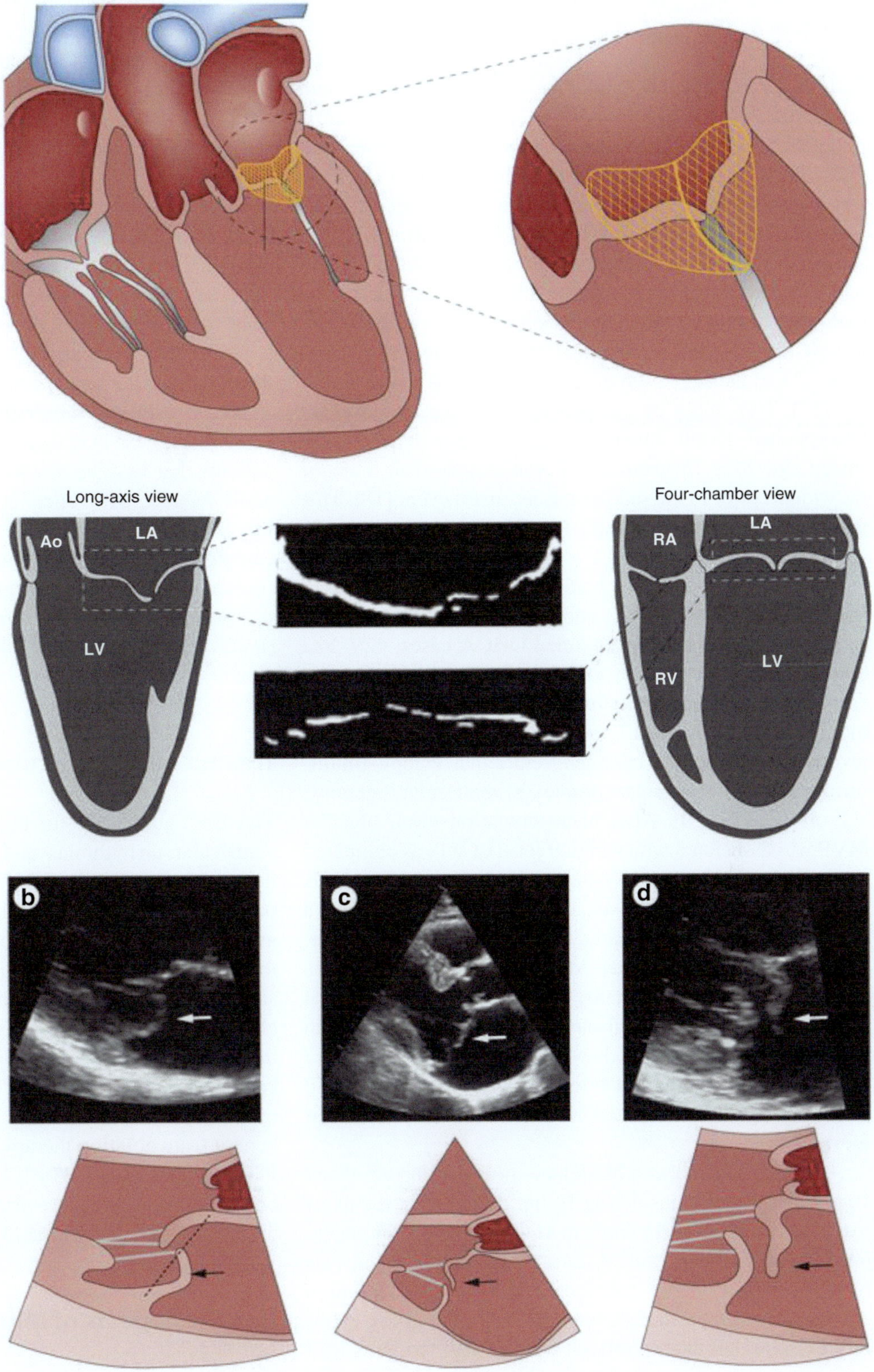

Fig. 25.2 Echocardiographic diagnosis of mitral valve prolapse. (**a**) Diagnosis of mitral valve prolapse must take into account the normal saddle shape of the valve and annulus, which produces opposite leaflet–annular relationships in perpendicular views. Mitral valve prolapse is most specifically diagnosed by leaflet displacement above the annular high points, imaged in long-axis views; and by leaflet misalignment at their point of coaptation. (**b**) Parasternal long-axis echocardiographic view of posterior leaflet prolapse (arrows) beyond the annular hinge points (dashed line). (**c**) Anterior leaflet prolapse and partial flail (partial eversion of the leaflet tip into the dilated LA; arrows) relative to the posterior leaflet, which is restricted, tethered by the dilated LV. These opposite leaflet displacements increase the regurgitant gap between the leaflets. (**d**) Patient with extensive leaflet thickening and anterior leaflet flail (arrows). *Ao* aorta, *LA* left atrium, *LV* left ventricle, *RA* right atrium, *RV* right ventricle. From Levine et al. [8]

Ventricular Arrhythmias and Sudden Cardiac Death in MVP

Sudden cardiac death occurs twice as often in patients with myxomatous valve disease/MVP as compared to the general population, with sudden death rates of 0.2–0.4% per year [10, 14]. SCD is found more often in patients with impaired left ventricular function, moderate to severe mitral regurgitation, and redundant chordae [15]. Interestingly, in a series of 200 victims of sudden cardiac death younger than 35 years, mitral valve prolapse was the only cardiac abnormality that could be found in as many as 10% of cases [16]. In a SCD series <40 years of age, recently studied by Basso et al., 7% of cases (13% females) had MVP as a sole anomaly [17]. This might be age dependent; in a recent Sudden Unexplained Death Syndrome general population study (mean age 70 ± 15 years) MVP was observed in 2.3% of individuals prior to the sudden cardiac arrest event [18]. This percentage is similar to, e.g., the Framingham Heart offspring study (2.4%) [6].

The involvement of two leaflets might also contribute to life-threatening arrhythmias and sudden cardiac death: in a series of 24 otherwise unexplained OHCA cases, 42% had bileaflet MVP. In addition to these abnormalities, patients with life-threatening arrhythmias were (mainly) females, more often demonstrated T wave abnormalities (biphasic, or inverted T-waves) and complex ventricular ectopy (multiform premature ventricular complexes, ventricular bigeminy, VT or VF) [19, 20]. Also, at a population level, bileaflet MVP was associated with a higher level of VTs as compared to single leaflet MVP and controls [19]. These individuals with bileaflet MVP, however, did not appear to portend a poor prognosis when compared to single leaflet MVP or controls. Interestingly, bileaflet MVP was associated with a lower rate of all-cause mortality [19]. These data suggest that bileaflet MVP may in a subset of cases be associated with structural changes that predispose to VT, but also reassure that, at least at the population level, incidentally noted MVP does not signal an elevated risk of fatal arrhythmias or mortality.

Although patients with MVP more often exhibit atrial and ventricular arrhythmias during Holter monitoring, the exact mechanism for pro-arrhythmia in MVP is not yet completely understood [21]. Mechanical stress on the papillary muscles resulting in fibrosis may contribute. On MRI late gadolinium enhancement suggesting fibrosis can be found in the papillary muscles and the inferobasal wall in MVP patients with complex ventricular arrhythmias [22]. These findings and additional pathological evidence of myocardial fibrosis in one or both papillary muscles and adjacent LV free wall and the inferobasal wall were recently described [17, 23].

Endocardial friction lesions from mechanical contact from the relapsing leaflets may also play a role; not only in inducing fibrosis but also in triggerring premature contractions resulting in ventricular arrhythmias [24]. So a combination of substrate-related fibrosis and mechanical effects may trigger premature contractions that subsequently may predispose to ventricular arrhythmias. In line with these observations, a common phenotype characterized by syncope, frequent, and repetitive premature ventricular contractions (PVCs) originating from the posterior papillary muscle was found in patients with “severe myxomatous MVP disease” (i.e. the combination of bileaflet prolapse, myxomatous mitral valve with thickened leaflet, and mitral annular disjunction) after aborted SCD [25].

These different observations and additional literature reviews suggest that there is a specific subgroup of MVP patients that may be at particular risk for SCD; i.e., young adult female, with bileaflet MVP, biphasic or inverted T waves in the inferior leads, and frequent complex ventricular ectopic activity with documented ventricular bigeminy or (polymorphic/RBBB morphology complex) ventricular tachycardia (VT) and premature ventricular contractions (PVCs) configurations of outflow tract alternating with fascicular or papillary muscle origin [17, 20, 26–28].

Treatment of Ventricular Arrhythmias in MVP

The ESC guidelines for the management of patients with ventricular arrhythmias and prevention of sudden cardiac death do not mention how to treat this specific group of patients. Assuming that the mechanism of ventricular arrhythmias is caused by a focus from the papillary muscles, then symptomatic patients with papillary muscle tachycardia should be treated with beta-blockade, Verapamil, or sodium channel blockers (class IC agents). If this treatment fails or the patient refuses using medication, catheter ablation should be considered [29]. A subset of patients with malignant ventricular arrhythmias like in bileaflet MVP syndrome may benefit from ablation therapy having less symptoms and less ICD shocks [20, 30]. An ICD is generally indicated as secondary prevention; however, data on the recurrence of cardiac arrest are still lacking [31].

Genetic Aspects of Mitral Valve Disease

Mitral valve prolapse has for many years been known to be familial in a subset of cases with an autosomal dominant mode of inheritance with reduced penetrance, influenced by age and sex [32–35]. Most patients with MVP present with a family history of valvular disease. MVP was found in 46% of first-degree relatives over 20 years, whereas only 16% of patients below that age were affected, suggesting progressive disease with age-dependent penetrance [36]. A recent population study showed that parental MVP is associated with an odds ratio of about 5 for MVP in offspring, also suggesting a genetic contribution to MVP.

Therefore, cardiac screening of first-degree family members may be considered in patients with MVP. When conducting family studies, echocardiography should be performed. Holter monitoring can be performed in the presence of complaints or a family history of sudden cardiac death.

Until today, three loci for genetic myxomatous autosomal dominant MVP have been identified, on chromosomes 16p11.2-p12.1, 11p15.4, and 13q31.3-q32.1 (MMVP1 [37], MMVP2 [38], and MMVP3 [39]). The genes underlying MMVP2 and MMVP3 have been identified so far. The gene in MMVP2, *DCHS1*, was identified in a large family and its role was confirmed in two smaller families [40]. a recent follow-up study showed that rare in silico predicted pathogenic variants in *DCHS1* can also be frequently identified in sporadic cases of MVP [41]. One has to be aware that the presence of a rare in silico predicted variant does not automatically implicate an explanation for the disease, as determining pathogenicity can be a challenge (see Chaps. 1 and 2). Extensive functional analysis has suggested a role for the DCHS1 protein in the development of cardiac valves [40].

The gene underlying MMVP3 was recently discovered in a single large family [42]. The gene, *DZIP1*, regulates the genesis of cilia protein and/or cilia signaling. Cilia are microtubule containing structures that are largely used to propel fluid or gametes, and also function to transduce mechanical, electrical, and chemical signals in a tissue-specific and time-dependent context. They relay information from the microenvironment to influence cell survival, differentiation, and tissue organization. The proportion of *DZIP1* in MVP cases still has to established, but this observation further opens the possibility that MVP may turn out to be a disease of valvular cilia defects [42].

The gene encoding Filamin A (*FLNA*) has been identified in X-linked myxomatous mitral valves in different unrelated families [43, 44]. Males carrying FLNA mutations exhibit a severe phenotype, often manifesting at young age (neonatally-40 years) with polyvalvular involvement, while females (heterozygotes) show milder manifestations of the disorder [45, 46]. The mitral valve degenerative lesions worsen over time, with a substantial lifetime risk (75%) of valve surgery in men [45]. Furthermore, a paradoxical restricted motion in diastole can be seen, which is unique in MVP diseases. Also, other structural cardiac abnormalities like atrial and ventricular septal defects and aortic root dilatation can be found in mutation carriers. Filamin A is an actin binding protein that plays a pivotal role in cell motility and membrane stability. Filamin A may contribute to the development of myxomatous changes of the cardiac valves by regulation of transforming growth factor-β (TGF-β) signaling through its interaction with Smads activated by TGF-β receptors [46, 47]. Defective signaling cascades that involve members of the TGF-β superfamily have been described in impaired remodeling of cardiac valves during development. A clear role for mutations in the *TGF-β* gene and its receptors in MVP has not yet been proven [44, 48].

The exact role of monogenic MVP still has to be elucidated: the larger pedigrees studied suggest that rare, highly penetrant genes may indeed underlie the disease phenotype, while familial clustering in the population may be due to either highly penetrant rare alleles with a strong effect size or (multiple common) variants with smaller effect sizes. GWAS studies have indicated risk loci for MVP in *LMCD1* (LIM and cysteine domain transcription factor) and *TNS1* (encoding the focal adhesion protein tensin 1) genes and a SNP in a metalloproteinase gene, *MMP2*, are associated with disease [49, 50].

Molecular Diagnostics

The role of molecular genetics in MVP is limited because only three genes have been identified so far. The selection for targeted screening of one of those genes can be based upon family history or the results of clinical evaluation of family members. These genes may also be included in larger panels that are generally designed to evaluate generalized connective tissue diseases like marfan and ehlers-danlos syndromes that may also be associated with MVP. The specific clinical features of these disorders can, however, in most cases, also be recognized by careful clinical evaluation. Clinical genetics centers often offer special clinics for diagnosing these patients.

Family Screening and Follow-Up in Relatives

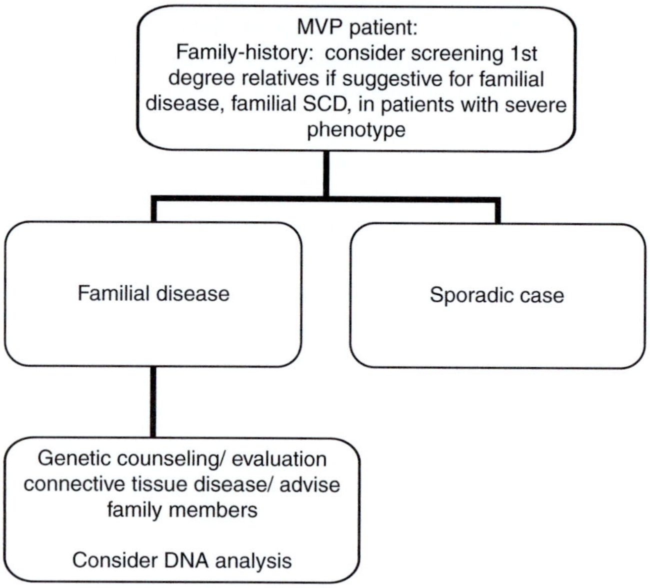

Summary

Mitral valve prolapse is the most common valvular disorder with a strong genetic contribution. The course of disease is benign in most cases, but serious complications such as heart failure, severe mitral regurgitation, bacterial endocarditis, ventricular arrhythmias, and sudden cardiac death occur, especially in patients with myxomatous degenerated valves. Bileaflet involvement, female sex, and substrate-related fibrosis and mechanical effects may trigger premature contractions that predispose to ventricular arrhythmias in a minority of patients. Until now, three chromosomal loci have been identified in autosomal dominant nonsyndromal MVP with *DCHS1* and *DZIP1* as the sole genes identified in dominant disease. Filamin A (*FLNA*) has been identified in X-linked myxomatous MVP, suggesting an underlying mechanism in the regulation of the valvular cytoskeleton. More genetic as well as clinical research is warranted to more precisely define patients at risk for this potentially lethal condition. First-degree relatives of patients with classical MVP and/or a history suggestive for familial disease (including signs of connective tissue disease such as aorta abnormalities) and/or SCD should undergo cardiac screening. In familial disease (MVP or connective tissue disease) or male patients with severe MVP or SCD, genetic screening should be considered.

Take Home Message

- MVP is a common, generally benign valvular disorder, with a familial character in a subset of cases
- Syndromal forms with MVP are rare and mainly consist of connective tissue disorders
- Sudden cardiac death rates are 0.2–0.4%/year
- Malignant arrhythmias infrequently occur: preliminary studies suggest that the substrate for arrhythmias seems related to fibrosis and mechanical effects that trigger premature contractions.
- Female patients with MVP, in particular those with bileaflet disease or posterior myxoid degeneration, repolarization abnormalities on ECG, and/or polymorphic/RBBB morphology complex ventricular arrhythmias may be at risk for SCD
- Cardiac screening should be considered in first-degree family members; particularly if a family history is positive for mitral valve disease, connective tissue disease, and/or sudden cardiac death
- Genetic screening/clinical genetic evaluation should be considered in males with severe (myxomatous) disease, X-linked pedigrees, or clear familial cases

References

1. Barlow JB, Bosman CK. Aneurysmal protrusion of the posterior leaflet of the mitral valve. An auscultatory-electrocardiographic syndrome. Am Heart J. 1966;71:166–78.
2. Cheng TO, John B. Barlow: the man and his syndrome. Int J Cardiol. 2014;177:311–6.
3. Weisse AB. Mitral valve prolapse: now you see it; now you don't: recalling the discovery, rise and decline of a diagnosis. Am J Cardiol. 2007;99:129–33.
4. Turker Y, Turker Y, Baltaci D, et al. The prevalence and clinical characteristics of mitral valve prolapse in a large population-based epidemiologic study: the MELEN study. Eur Rev Med Pharmacol Sci. 2015;19:2208–12.
5. Hepner AD, Ahmadi-Kashani M, Movahed MR. The prevalence of mitral valve prolapse in patients undergoing echocardiography for clinical reason. Int J Cardiol. 2007;123:55–7.
6. Freed LA, Levy D, Levine RA, et al. Prevalence and clinical outcome of mitral-valve prolapse. N Engl J Med. 1999;341:1–7.
7. Davies MJ, Moore BP, Braimbridge MV. The floppy mitral valve. Study of incidence, pathology, and complications in surgical, necropsy, and forensic material. Br Heart J. 1978;40:468–81.
8. Levine RA, Hagége AA, Judge DP, et al. Mitral valve disease—morphology and mechanisms. Nat Rev Cardiol. 2015;12:689–710.
9. Delling FN, Rong J, Larson MG, et al. Evolution of mitral valve prolapse: insights from the Framingham Heart Study. Circulation. 2016;133:1688–95.
10. Nishimura RA, McGoon MD, Shub C, et al. Echocardiographically documented mitral-valve prolapse. Long-term follow-up of 237 patients. N Engl J Med. 1985;313:1305–9.
11. Katan O, Michelena HI, Avierinos JF, et al. Incidence and predictors of infective endocarditis in mitral valve prolapse: a population-based study. Mayo Clin Proc. 2016;91:336–42.
12. Wilson W, Taubert KA, Gewitz M, et al. Prevention of infective endocarditis: guidelines from the American Heart Association: a guideline from the American Heart Association Rheumatic Fever, Endocarditis, and Kawasaki Disease Committee, Council on Cardiovascular Disease in the Young, and the Council on Clinical Cardiology, Council on Cardiovascular Surgery and Anesthesia, and the Quality of Care and Outcomes Research Interdisciplinary Working Group. Circulation. 2007;116:1736–54.

13. Falk V, Baumgartner H, Bax JJ, De Bonis M, Hamm C, Holm PJ, Iung B, Lancellotti P, Lansac E, Muñoz DR, Rosenhek R, Sjögren J, Tornos Mas P, Vahanian A, Walther T, Wendler O, Windecker S, Zamorano JL, ESC Scientific Document Group. 2017 ESC/EACTS Guidelines for the management of valvular heart disease. Eur J Cardiothorac Surg. 2017;52:616–64.
14. Düren DR, Becker AE, Dunning AJ. Long-term follow-up of idiopathic mitral valve prolapse in 300 patients: a prospective study. J Am Coll Cardiol. 1988;11:42–7.
15. Kligfield P, Levy D, Devereux RB, et al. Arrhythmias and sudden death in mitral valve prolapse. Am Heart J. 1987;113:1298–307.
16. Basso C, Corrado D, Thiene G. Cardiovascular causes of sudden death in young individuals including athletes. Cardiol Rev. 1999;7:127–35.
17. Basso C, Perazzolo Marra M, Rizzo S, et al. Arrhythmic mitral valve prolapse and sudden cardiac death. Circulation. 2015;132:556–66.
18. Narayanan K, Uy-Evanado A, Teodorescu C, et al. Mitral valve prolapse and sudden cardiac arrest in the community. Heart Rhythm. 2016;13:498–503.
19. Nordhues BD, Siontis KC, Scott CG, et al. Bileaflet mitral valve prolapse and risk of ventricular dysrhythmias and death. J Cardiovasc Electrophysiol. 2016;27:463–8.
20. Sriram CS, Syed FF, Ferguson ME, et al. Malignant bileaflet mitral valve prolapse syndrome in patients with otherwise idiopathic out-of-hospital cardiac arrest. J Am Coll Cardiol. 2013;62:222–30.
21. Hayek E, Gring CN, Griffin BP. Mitral valve prolapse. Lancet. 2005;365:507–18.
22. Han Y, Peters DC, Salton CJ, et al. Cardiovascular magnetic resonance characterization of mitral valve prolapse. JACC Cardiovasc Imaging. 2008;1:294–303.
23. Sheppard MN, Steriotis AK, Sharma S. Letter by Sheppard et al regarding article, "Arrhythmic mitral valve prolapse and sudden cardiac death". Circulation. 2016;133:e458.
24. Sniezek-Maciejewska M, Dubiel JP, et al. Ventricular arrhythmias and the autonomic tone in patients with mitral valve prolapse. Clin Cardiol. 1992;15:720–4.
25. Hourdain J, Clavel MA, Deharo JC, et al. Common phenotype in patients with mitral valve prolapse who experienced sudden cardiac death. Circulation. 2018;138:1067–9.
26. Spartalis M, Tzatzaki E, Spartalis E, et al. Mitral valve prolapse: an underestimated cause of sudden cardiac death-a current review of the literature. J Thorac Dis. 2017;9:5390–8.
27. Han HC, Ha FJ, Teh AW, et al. Mitral valve prolapse and sudden cardiac death: a systematic review. J Am Heart Assoc. 2018;7:e010584.
28. Nalliah CJ, Mahajan R, Elliott AD, et al. Mitral valve prolapse and sudden cardiac death: a systematic review and meta-analysis. Heart. 2019;105:144–51.
29. Priori SG, Blomström-Lundqvist C, Mazzanti A, et al. 2015 ESC Guidelines for the management of patients with ventricular arrhythmias and the prevention of sudden cardiac death: The Task Force for the management of patients with ventricular arrhythmias and the prevention of sudden cardiac death of the European Society of Cardiology (ESC). Eur Heart J. 2015;36:2793–867.
30. Syed FF, Ackerman MJ, McLeod CJ, et al. Sites of successful ventricular fibrillation ablation in bileaflet mitral valve prolapse syndrome. Circ Arrhythm Electrophysiol. 2016;9:e004005.
31. Basso C, Iliceto S, Thiene G, et al. Mitral valve prolapse, ventricular arrhythmias, and sudden death. Circulation. 2019;140:952–64.
32. Devereux RB, Brown WT, Kramer-Fox R, et al. Inheritance of mitral valve prolapse: effect of age and sex on gene expression. Ann Intern Med. 1982;97:826–32.
33. Strahan NV, Murphy EA, Fortuin NJ, et al. Inheritance of the mitral valve prolapse syndrome. Discussion of a three-dimensional penetrance model. Am J Med. 1983;74:967–72.
34. Weiss AN, Mimbs JW, Ludbrook PA, et al. Echocardiographic detection of mitral valve prolapse. Exclusion of false positive diagnosis and determination of inheritance. Circulation. 1975;52:1091–6.
35. Delling FN, Rong J, Larson MG, et al. Familial clustering of mitral valve prolapse in the community. Circulation. 2015;131:263–8.
36. Grau JB, Pirelli L, Yu PJ, et al. The genetics of mitral valve prolapse. Clin Genet. 2007;72:288–95.
37. Disse S, Abergel E, Berrebi A, et al. Mapping of a first locus for autosomal dominant myxomatous mitral-valve prolapse to chromosome 16p11.2-p12.1. Am J Hum Genet. 1999;65:1242–51.
38. Freed LA, Acierno JS Jr, Dai D, et al. A locus for autosomal dominant mitral valve prolapse on chromosome 11p15.4. Am J Hum Genet. 2003;72:1551–9.
39. Nesta F, Leyne M, Yosefy C, et al. New locus for autosomal dominant mitral valve prolapse on chromosome 13: clinical insights from genetic studies. Circulation. 2005;112:2022–30.
40. Durst R, Sauls K, Peal DS, et al. Mutations in DCHS1 cause mitral valve prolapse. Nature. 2015;525:109–13.
41. Clemenceau A, Bérubé JC, Bélanger P, et al. Deleterious variants in DCHS1 are prevalent in sporadic cases of mitral valve prolapse. Mol Genet Genomic Med. 2018;6:114–20.
42. Toomer KA, Yu M, Fulmer D, et al. Primary cilia defects causing mitral valve prolapse. Sci Transl Med. 2019;11:eaax0290.
43. Kyndt F, Gueffet JP, Probst V, et al. Mutations in the gene encoding filamin A as a cause for familial cardiac valvular dystrophy. Circulation. 2007;115:40–9.
44. Aalberts JJ, van Tintelen JP, Oomen T, et al. Screening of TGFBR1, TGFBR2, and FLNA in familial mitral valve prolapse. Am J Med Genet A. 2014;164A:113–9.
45. Le Tourneau T, Le Scouarnec S, Cueff C, et al. New insights into mitral valve dystrophy: a filamin-A genotype-phenotype and outcome study. Eur Heart J. 2018;39:1269–77.
46. Sasaki A, Masuda Y, Ohta Y, et al. Filamin associates with Smads and regulates transforming growth factor-beta signaling. J Biol Chem. 2001;276:17871–7.
47. Derynck R, Zhang YE. Smad-dependent and Smad-independent pathways in TGF-beta family signalling. Nature. 2003;425:577–84.
48. Disha K, Schulz S, Kuntze T, Girdauskas E. Transforming growth factor beta-2 mutations in Barlow's disease and aortic dilatation. Ann Thorac Surg. 2017;104:e19–21.
49. Dina C, Bouatia-Naji N, Tucker N, et al. Genetic association analyses highlight biological pathways underlying mitral valve prolapse. Nat Genet. 2015;47:1206–11.
50. Lima SM, Pitsis AA, Kelpis TG, et al. Matrix metalloproteinase polymorphisms in patients with floppy mitral valve/mitral valve prolapse (FMV/MVP) and FMV/MVP syndrome. Cardiology. 2017;138:179–85.

Induced Pluripotent Stem Cells

26

Alain van Mil, Klaus Neef, Geerthe M. Balk, Jan Willem Buikema, Joost P. G. Sluijter, and Pieter A. F. M. Doevendans

Introduction

In the past decade major advances in molecular biology and genomics have moved medicine toward a more causal and personalized approach, termed precision medicine. In cardiology, this approach is believed to be particularly favorable for patients with inherited cardiac disease [1]. Currently, for many inherited cardiac diseases, only symptomatic treatment is available and prognosis remains poor due to the lack of curative treatment strategies. The development of such curative treatments is severely hampered due to the fact that the underlying pathophysiological mechanism, by which genetic mutations result in disease, remains unknown for a large number of cardiac diseases. Additionally, patient-specific genetic variants are often of unknown significance, and only functional assessment of those DNA variants can ultimately prove or disprove pathogenicity. However, the limiting factor in studying the molecular mechanisms that trigger disease onset and progression has been the lack of a tractable, representative and predictive model system for the study of human heart disease. The main reason is that viable human myocardial cells, reflecting the disease phenotype, especially at the early stages, are extremely difficult to obtain and survive in culture for a very short time only. This unmet need for myocardial tissue and disease models has propelled advances in the stem cell field. With the discovery of induced pluripotent stem (iPS) cells [2] and the development of methods for their directed differentiation to cardiomyocytes (iPS-CM) [3], an exciting option for generating patient-specific cardiac cells to study inherited cardiac disease has emerged [4]. These iPS cells are generated by the transduction or transfection of adult cells with reprogramming factors, which results in epigenetic reprogramming of the adult cell genome into a pluripotent stem cell state [5–7]. The resulting iPS cells have the same genetic constitution as the person they were derived from and have the capacity to give rise to any cell type, including cardiac cells such as cardiomyocytes. With refined protocols for iPS cell generation and differentiation into iPS-CMs, a sustainable source of nontransgenic human cardiac cells has become available for in vitro disease modeling. Cardiomyocytes generated from iPS cells have several advantages over human embryonic stem cells (ESCs), to which they are molecularly and functionally equivalent [8]. IPS-CMs offer the unique possibility to functionally annotate patient-specific genetic variants, obtain a better understanding of the pathogenesis of inherited cardiac diseases, and eventually to develop and test strategies for treatment, including individualized patient therapy, before performing animal and first-in-man studies. Since the first study in 2010 [4], much progress has been made using patient-specific-iPS cell models to characterize cardiac diseases and study their molecular pathogenesis. Over 90 studies using iPS-CM models are now available. In the next paragraph, we have provided an overview of the current iPS-CM models of inherited cardiac disease.

iPS-CM Models of Inherited Cardiac Disease

The use of human iPS-CMs for cardiac disease modeling has progressed steeply since 2013, with over 25 new disease-specific mutations published each year (Table 26.1). iPS-CM models now exist for (1) several cardiomyopathies, including hypertrophic cardiomyopathy, dilated cardiomyopathy, arrhythmogenic cardiomyopathy, noncompaction cardiomyopathy, metabolic cardiomyopathy, cardiac amyloidosis, and mitochondrial cardiomyopathy, for (2) inherited arrhythmia syndromes, including long QT syndromes, catecholaminergic polymorphic ventricular tachycardia, and for (3)

A. van Mil (✉) · K. Neef · G. M. Balk · J. W. Buikema · J. P. G. Sluijter
Department of Cardiology, Division Heart and Lungs, University Medical Center Utrecht, Utrecht, Netherlands
e-mail: A.vanMil@umcutrecht.nl

P. A. F. M. Doevendans
Department of Cardiology, Division Heart and Lungs, University Medical Center Utrecht, Utrecht, Netherlands

Netherlands Heart Institute, Utrecht, Netherlands

H. F. Baars et al. (eds.), *Clinical Cardiogenetics*, https://doi.org/10.1007/978-3-030-45457-9_26

Table 26.1 Overview of mutations and genes studied using iPS-CMs

Disease	Mutation lines	References
HCM	MYH7 p.R663H	Lan, F. et al.
	MYH7 p.R663H	Liang, P. et al. (2013)
	MYH7 c.1324c>G, p.R422G	Han, L. et al.
	MYH7 E848G	Pioner, J. M. et al.
	TPM1 Arg91Cys (unknown if pathogenic)	Tanaka, A. et al.
	Unknown, no mutations in sarcomeric genes	Tanaka, A. et al.
	MYBPC3 Gly999-Gln1004del	Tanaka, A. et al.
	MYBPC3 c2373dupG [3 lines]	Dambrot, C. et al.
	MYBPC3 Gln1061X [2 lines]	Ojala, M. et al.
	TPM1 Asp175Asn [2 lines]	Ojala, M. et al.
	ALPK3 c.3792G>A, p.W1264X [2 lines]	Phelan, D. G. et al.
DCM	LMNA c.50insGCCA	Ho, J. C. Y. et al. & Siu, C. W. et al.
	LMNA R225X	Siu, C. W. et al.
	TNNT2 p.R173W [4 lines]	Sun, N. et al.
	DES c.940C>T, p.A285V	Tse, H. F. et al.
	TNNT2 R173W	Liang, P. et al. (2013)
	TNNT2 R173W	Wu, H. et al.
	PLN c.40_42del, p.R14del	Karakikes, I. et al.
	TTN W976R	Hinson, J. T. et al.
	TTN A22352fs	Hinson, J. T. et al.
	TTN P22582fs	Hinson, J. T. et al.
	TTN V6382fs (isogenic cell line, heterozygous mutation via Crispr-Cas)	Hinson, J. T. et al.
	TTN V6382fs (isogenic cell line, homozygous mutation via Crispr-Cas)	Hinson, J. T. et al.
	TTN N22577fs (isogenic cell line, heterozygous mutation via Crispr-Cas)	Hinson, J. T. et al.
	TTN N22577fs (isogenic cell line, homozygous mutation via Crispr-Cas)	Hinson, J. T. et al.
	TTN T33520fs (isogenic cell line, mutation via Crispr-Cas)	Hinson, J. T. et al.
	TTN p.Ser14450fsX4, c.43629insAT	Gramlich, M. et al.
	RBM20 c1906C>A, p.R636S	Wyles, S. P. et al.
	BAG3 exon 2 TALEN (loss of function heterozygous mutation)	Judge, L. M. et al.
	BAG3 exon 2 CRISPR/Cas9 (loss of function heterozygous mutation)	Judge, L. M. et al.
	BAG3 exon 2 TALEN (loss of function homozygous mutation)	Judge, L. M. et al.
	BAG3 exon 2 CRISPR/Cas9 (loss of function homozygous mutation)	Judge, L. M. et al.
	MYBPC3 mutant line TALEN	Judge, L. M. et al.
ARVC	PKP2 c.2484C>T	Kim, C. et al.
	PKP2 c.2013delC	Kim, C. et al.
	PKP2 c.1841t>C, L614P	Ma, D. et al.
	PKP2 c.9721InsT/N	Caspi, O. et al.
	PKP2 c.148_151delACAG/N	Caspi, O. et al.
	SCN5A p.R1898H, c.5693G>A	Te Riele, A. S. et al.
LVNC	TBX20 Y317* [6 lines—3 patients]	Kodo, K. et al.
	TBX20 Y317* [2 lines—1 patient]	Kodo, K. et al.
Pompe	GAA c.1935C>A, p. D645E	Huang, H. P. et al.
	GAA c.1935 C>A and c.2040+1G>T	Huang, H. P. et al.
	GAA exon18 del	Raval, K. K. et al.
	GAA 1336delT, 2233G>A	Raval, K. K. et al.
	GAA c.796C>T and c.1316T>A	Sato, Y. et al.
Fabry disease	GLA c.G485A, p.W162X	Itier, J. M. et al.
	GLA c.C658T, p.R220X	Itier, J. M. et al.
	GLA c.IVS4+919 G>A	Chien, Y. et al.
Danon disease	LAMP2 c.129-130insAT resulting in premature stop codon [2 lines]	Hashem, S. et al.
	LAMP2 female c.520C>T	Ng, K. M. et al.
	LAMP2 male c.520C>T	Ng, K. M. et al.
Metabolic CM	PRKAG2 N488I heterozygous patient	Hinson, J. T. et al.
	PRKAG2 N488I homozygous patient	Hinson, J. T. et al.
	PRKAG2 N488I heterozygous TALEN	Hinson, J. T. et al.
	PRKAG2 N488I homozygous TALEN	Hinson, J. T. et al.
Cardiac amyloidosis	TTR L55P	Leung, A. et al.
BTHS	TAZ c.517delG, p.Asp173Thrfs*12	Wang, G. et al.
	TAZ c.328T>C, p.Ser110Pro	Wang, G. et al.

Table 26.1 (continued)

Disease	Mutation lines	References
MERFF	MT-TK A8344G	Chou, S. J. et al.
LQTS1	KCNQ1 R190Q, c.569G>A	Moretti, A. P. D. et al.
	KCNQ1 1893delC, P631fs/33	Egashira, T. et al.
	KCNQ1 G279S	Liang, P. et al. (2013)
	KCNQ1 R190Q (safe harbour AAV integration in wt iPS line)	Wang, Y. et al.
	KCNQ1 G269S (safe harbour AAV integration in wt iPS line + 1 patient line [Liang, P. 2013])	Wang, Y. et al.
	KCNQ1 G345E (safe harbour AAV integration in wt iPS line)	Wang, Y. et al.
	KCNQ1 C.922~1,032 del, P.308~344del	Ma, D. et al.
	KCNQ1 G589D [2 lines]	Kiviaho, A. L. et al.
	KCNQ1 ivs7-2A>G [2 lines]	Kiviaho, A. L. et al.
JLNS	KCNQ1 c.478-2A>T	Zhang, M. et al.
	KCNQ1 c.1781G>A, p.R594Q	Zhang, M. et al.
	KCNQ1 c.1781A/A (gene-edited)	Zhang, M. et al.
LQTS2	KCNH2 A614V	Itzhaki, I. et al.
	KCNH2 Ala561Thr	Matsa, E. et al.
	KCNH2 R176W	Lahti, A. L. et al.
	KCNH2 c.A2987T, p.N996I	Bellin, M. et al.
	KCNH2 A561V	Mehta, A. et al.
	KCNH2 c.1264G>A, p.A442T	Spencer, C. I. et al.
	KCNH2 A614V (safe harbour AAV integration in wt iPS line + 1 patient line [Itzhaki, I. 2011])	Wang, Y. et al.
	KCNH2 A562P	Jouni, M. et al.
	KCNH2-IVS9-28A/G [2 lines]	Mura, M. et al.
LQTS3	SCN5A F1473C, KCNH2 K897T	Terrenoire, C. et al.
	SCN5A c.5287G>A, p.V1763M	Ma, D. et al.
	SCN5A c.716G>A, p.V240M	Fatima, A. et al.
	SCN5A c.1604G>A, p.R535Q	Fatima, A. et al.
	SCN5A c.1218C>A, p.N406K	Spencer, C. I. et al.
	SCN5A c.4931G>A, p.R1644 H	Malan, D. et al.
LQTS3-BrS mixed phenotype	SCN5A E1784K, c.5349G>A	Okata, S. et al.
Overlap syndrome of cardiac sodium channel disease	SCN5A c.5387_5389insTGA, p.1795insD	Davis, R. P. et al. & Portero, V. et al.
	SCN5A I230T, c.689T>C	Veerman, C. C. et al.
BrS	Unknown mutation [3 lines]	Veerman, C. C. et al.
	SCN5A R1638X	Kosmidis, G. et al.
	SCN5A W156X	Kosmidis, G. et al.
	SCN5A R620H and R811H [6 lines]	Liang, P. et al. (2016)
	SCN5A p.4189delT [2 lines]	Liang, P. et al. (2016)
ATS (LQTS7)	KCNJ2 R218W [2 lines]	Kuroda, Y. et al.
	KCNJ2 R67W [2 lines]	Kuroda, Y. et al.
	KCNJ2 R218Q [2 lines]	Kuroda, Y. et al.
TS (LQTS8)	CACNA1C p.G406R	Yazawa, M. et al.
LQTS14	CALM1 p.F142L [2 lines]	Rocchetti, M. et al.
LQTS15	CALM2 c.389A>G, p.D130G	Limpitikul, W. B. et al.
	CALM2 p.N98S, c.293A>G	Yamamoto, Y. et al.
CPVT	RYR2 p.F2483I, c.7447T>A	Fatima, A. et al. (2011) & Zhang, X.-H. et al.
	RYR2 p.P2328S	Kujala, K. et al. & Paavola, J. et al.
	RYR2 p.S406L, c.1217C>T	Jung, C. B. et al.
	RYR2 p.M4109R	Itzhaki, I. et al.
	CASQ2 p.D307H, c.1183G>C [2 lines]	Novak, A. et al. (2012)
	RYR2 c.6933G>C, p.Glu2311Asp	Di Pasquale, E. et al.
	RyR2 c.168-301 and c.273-722 del1228	Penttinen, K. et al.
	RyR2 c.7613C>G, p.T2538R	Penttinen, K. et al.
	RyR2 c.12343C>T, p.L4115F	Penttinen, K. et al.

(continued)

Table 26.1 (continued)

Disease	Mutation lines	References
	RyR2 c.1260A>G, p.Q4201R	Penttinen, K. et al.
	RyR2 c.13957G>T, p.V4653F	Penttinen, K. et al.
	RyR2 p.R420Q	Novak, A. et al. (2015)
	CASQ2 p.D307H [2 lines]	Novak, A. et al. (2015)
	TECRL c.331+1G>A heterozygous	Devalla, H. D. et al.
	TECRL c.331+1G>A homozygous	Devalla, H. D. et al.
	RyR2 L3741P, c.T11342C [2 lines]	Preininger, M. K. et al.
	RyR2 c.13759A>G, p.I4587V	Sasaki, K. et al.
	CASQ2 c.339-354, p.G112+5X [2 lines]	Lodola, F. et al.
	CASQ2 c.339-354, p.G112+5X [2 lines]	Lodola, F. et al.
	CASQ2 p.D307H	Maizels, L. et al.
CHD	GATA4 c.886G>A, p.G296S [4 lines]	Ang, Y. S. et al.
HLHS	Unknown mutation	Jiang, Y. et al.
	MYH6 R443P	Tomita-Mitchell, A. et al.
	MYH6 D588A	Tomita-Mitchell, A. et al.
	NOTCH4 exon1 c.17_28del and exon1:c.33_44del	Yang, C. et al.
	NOTCH2 exon25 c.C7075G	Yang, C. et al.
	NOTCH4 exon18 c.G2834A and exon25 c.C4028T	Yang, C. et al.
	NOTCH3 exon11 c.A1766C	Yang, C. et al.
CFCS	BRAF T599R	Josowitz, R. et al.
	BRAF Q257R A>G	Josowitz, R. et al.
NSML	PTPN11 p.T468M	Carvajal-vergara, X. et al.
FRDA	FXN GAA expansion (800/600)	Hick, A. et al.
	FXN GAA expansion (900/400)	Hick, A. et al.
	FXN GAA expansion	Lee, Y. K. et al. (2014, 2016)
	FXN GAA1/GAA2 1077/1077	Crombie, D. E. et al.
	FXN GAA1/GAA2 476/545	Crombie, D. E. et al.
	FXN GAA1/GAA2 733/943	Crombie, D. E. et al.
DMD	DYS del exon 45-52	Park, I.-H. et al. & Lin, B. et al.
	DYS Dp427m, del exon 4-43	Kazuki, Y. et al. & Zatti, S. et al.
	DYS del exon 48-50	Dick, E. et al.
	DYS del exon 47-50	Dick, E. et al.
	DYS c.3217G>T	Dick, E. et al.
	DYS del exon 45-52	Dick, E. et al.
	DYS c.10171C>T	Dick, E. et al.
	DYS c.4918-4919 delTG	Dick, E. et al.
	DYS c.7437G>A	Dick, E. et al.
	DYS del exon 50	Guan, X. et al. & Macadangdang, J. et al.
DM1	DM1 2829-3575 CTG repeats	Xia, G. et al. & Gao, Y. et al.
	DM1 1933-3152 CTG repeats	Xia, G. et al. & Gao, Y. et al.
Early-onset skeletal myopathy	HSPB5 343delT	Mitzelfelt, K. A. et al.
ALDH2	ALDH2*2 E487K [5 lines]	Ebert, A. et al.
ABL	MTTP c.C136G, p.R46G [2 lines]	Liu, Y. et al.

miscellaneous cardiac diseases, such as congenital heart defects, syndromes like cardiofaciocutaneous syndrome, Noonan syndrome with multiple lentigines, and Friedreich's ataxia, and for neuromuscular disorders, and other diseases with cardiac traits (Fig. 26.1). For most inherited cardiac diseases, multiple causative mutations have been investigated in iPS-CM models (Table 26.1).

Cardiomyopathies

Hypertrophic Cardiomyopathy

Hypertrophic cardiomyopathy (HCM) is associated with mutations in sarcomere protein-coding genes, causing left ventricular hypertrophy in the absence of a causative hemodynamic burden [9]. From 1400 different mutations known to cause HCM [10], to date, myosin heavy chain-β (*MYH7*), cardiac myosin binding protein C (*MYBPC3*) [11–13], and tropomyosin 1 (*TPM1*) [10, 14] are among the most frequent (Fig. 26.2).

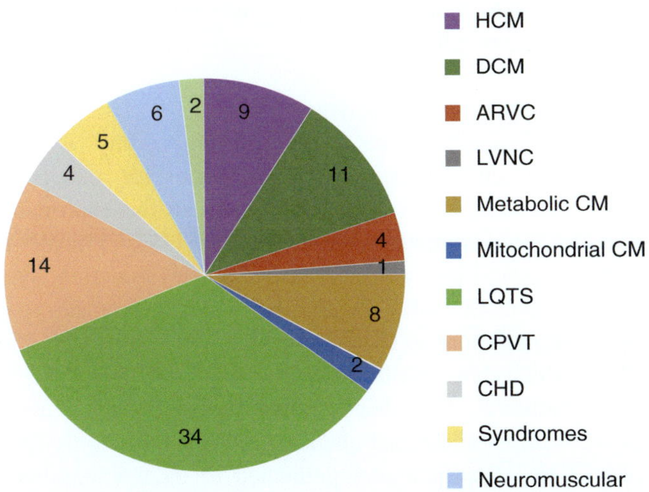

Fig. 26.1 The proportion of iPS cell lines generated per disease type

iPS-CM models have been used to study HCM-causing mutations in *MYH7*, *MYBPC3*, *TPM1*, and alpha kinase 3 (*ALPK3*) [10, 11, 13–19]. Disease phenotypes recapitulated by these models included irregularities in calcium handling, cardiomyocyte hypertrophy, sarcomere disarray, arrhythmias and hypercontractility [10, 16, 17, 19]. Downstream effects were reported in Endothelin-1 signaling [14], the canonical Wnt-pathway [17], and most prominently, calcineurin/NFATc4 signaling [14, 16, 17]. NFATc4 nuclear localization and disrupted calcium handling have been shown to be directly linked to the development of the pathognomonic cellular hypertrophic phenotype. However, ryanodine receptor 2 (RyR2) and sarco/endoplasmic reticulum Ca^{2+}-ATPase 2a (SERCA2a) expression levels in these models have been controversially reported as either increased [17] or decreased [10]. Furthermore, differences in the type of arrhythmogenic events were reported. Some mutations predominantly led to delayed afterdepolarization (DADs) [16], while others mainly led to early afterdepolarization (EADs) [10] or no DADs were seen at all [17]. These heterogeneities could presumably be due to the maturity of the iPS-CMs, since the duration of induced cardiac differentiation at the time point of measurement differed significantly between studies and maturation markers have not been specifically assessed.

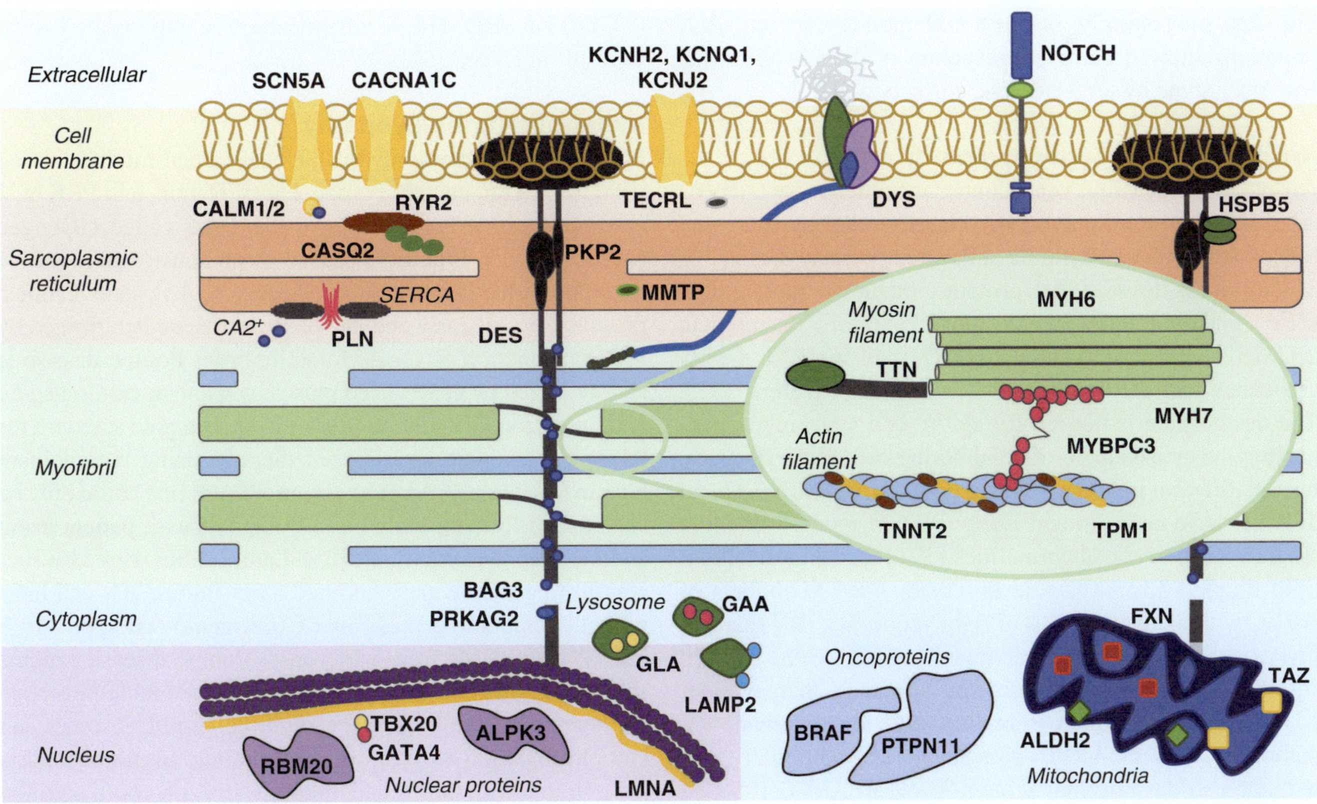

Fig. 26.2 The subcellular localization of disease-associated proteins studied using iPS-CM models

Dilated Cardiomyopathy

Dilated cardiomyopathy (DCM) is a common cardiomyopathy, characterized by left ventricular dilation and impaired systolic function, ultimately leading to heart failure. Mutations in more than 20 genes associated with the cytoskeleton, nuclear lamina, and sarcomeres have been shown to lead to the inherited form of DCM [20]. Mutations in the gene coding for lamin A/C (*LMNA*) lead to the most malignant subtypes, characterized by early-onset atrial fibrillation, conduction delay and sudden cardiac death [21]. Mutations in the desmin (*DES*) gene can cause DCM [22], and also HCM or ARVC [23]. Of all DCM cases, 30% arise due to mutations in the titin (*TTN*) gene [24].

Recent studies using iPS-CM disease models aimed at elucidating the molecular pathogenesis of mutations in *LMNA* [25], *DES* [26], *TTN* [27, 28], cardiac troponin T (*TNNT2*) [15, 29, 30], phospholamban (*PLN*) [31], RNA-binding motif protein 20 (*RBM20*) [32, 33], and chaperone regulator *BAG3* [34] (Fig. 26.2 and Table 26.1). A total of 13 mutations have been studied, in some cases both homozygous and heterozygous forms. iPS-CM models revealed disrupted sarcomeres, decreased contractile force and Ca^{2+} handling impairment, which is in agreement with observations in heart failure patients [35]. Accordingly, supplementing iPS-CM models of DCM with β-adrenergic blockers and calcium antagonists resulted in attenuation of sarcomeric disarray and apoptosis, as expected by clinical observations [30, 32]. Interestingly, two iPS-CM models carrying *PLN* mutations showed complete reversion of their in vitro disease phenotype by targeted gene correction [31, 36].

Arrhythmogenic Cardiomyopathy

Arrhythmogenic Right Ventricular Cardiomyopathy (ARVC) is an inherited cardiomyopathy characterized by increased risk of ventricular arrhythmia and sudden cardiac death [37]. Mutations in desmosomal proteins, including plakoglobin (*JUP*), plakophilin (*PKP2*), desmoplakin (*DSP*), desmoglein 2 (*DSG2*), and desmocollin 2 (*DSC2*) are most frequently associated with ARVC, present in 40–50% of patients [38]. The desmosome is needed for cell-to-cell attachment, connecting the cytoskeleton of neighboring cells (Fig. 26.2). So far, six different mutations in two different genes (*PKP2* and *SCN5A*) have been studied using iPS-CM models. In these studies, desmosome abnormalities [39–44] and intracellular lipid droplets [39, 40] were observed. iPS-CM models of ARVC with increased ratios of right ventricular (RV) cardiomyocytes, generated by enrichment for $Isl1^{+}$ cells, showed significantly more lipogenesis and apoptosis than without $Isl1^{+}$ enrichment, which is in line with the dominant RV pathology seen in ARVC patients [41]. Additionally, the reduction in desmosomal protein levels in ARVC iPS-CM models is in close agreement with histopathological data from ARVC patients [45]. Nonetheless, it remains questionable whether iPS-CMs cultured in the presence of various small-molecule compounds and hormones to switch metabolism and accelerate pathogenesis truly reflect the in vivo physiological environment [46]. Since the clinical ARVC phenotype may be provoked by exercise, possibly due to mechanical stress on the cardiomyocytes [47], it is specifically challenging to model all the external influences in vitro in this iPS-CM model, but is likely needed to elicit a more accurate disease phenotype.

Noncompaction Cardiomyopathy

Left Ventricular Noncompaction Cardiomyopathy (LVNC) is typically characterized by a prominent LV trabecular meshwork, deep intertrabecular recesses in the ventricular wall and a thin compacted epicardial layer [48]. Clinically it is characterized by systolic and diastolic dysfunction, systemic embolism, and arrhythmias. Many genes carrying causative mutations in LVNC are also involved in DCM and HCM, which show similar traits as LVNC [49]. Mutations in *MIB1*, however, have been shown to cause an exclusive LVNC without additional phenotypes [50]. In the only iPS-CM LVNC disease model published to date, it has been shown that a mutation in the cardiac transcription factor TBX20 led to reduced baseline proliferative capacity [51]. This recapitulates the cell cycle defects thought to play a role in LVNC pathogenesis. Furthermore, iPS-CMs showed dysregulated signaling of transforming growth factor beta (TGFβ) via PRDM16, in which certain mutations are known to result in LVNC [52].

Metabolic Cardiomyopathy

Four metabolic cardiomyopathies have been modeled using iPS-CMs so far, namely Pompe, Fabry, Danon, and PRKAG2 cardiomyopathy. Pompe disease [53], also called Glycogen Storage disease Type II, is caused by an autosomal recessive mutation in the acid alpha-glucosidase (*GAA*) gene. Clinical presentations of early and late onset forms are determined by residual function of GAA. Infantile-onset Pompe disease is characterized by generalized muscle weakness, cardiomegaly and hypertrophic cardiomyopathy [54]. The gold standard for therapy is enzyme replacement therapy, using recombinant human GAA (rhGAA). Initially, an iPS cell line could only be established from an early onset Pompe disease patient using an inducible *GAA* transgene [55]. Later studies were also successful to generate early and late onset Pompe iPS cell lines without temporal expression of transgenic wildtype GAA [56, 57]. iPS-CMs from early onset Pompe disease patients showed a typical cellular Pompe phenotype, including large glycogen-containing vacuoles, multiple large lysosomes and autophagosomes as well as deterioration of mitochondria [58]. In line with the clinical findings, rhGAA could partially reverse the pathological phenotype. Late onset Pompe iPS-CMs recapitulated part of the aforementioned findings and the cellular phenotype could be attenuated by lentiviral-mediated wildtype GAA expression [56]. Notably, protein hypoglycosylation was reported in early-onset Pompe iPS-CMs [57], associated with altered Ca^{2+} handling [59], which has been implicated with cardiac hypertrophy [16].

Fabry disease is caused by mutations in X-linked alpha-galactosidase A (*GLA*), leading to progressive accumulation of globotriaosylceramide (GL-3) in lysosomes. This can result in renal failure, left ventricular hypertrophy and increased risk of strokes [60], and is currently best treated with enzyme replacement therapy, similar to Pompe disease. Fabry iPS-CMs showed low GLA activity and accumulation of GL-3, causing abnormal sarcomere structure [61], consistent with clinical findings in endomyocardial biopsies [62]. Both glucosylceramide synthase inhibition and supplementation with recombinant GLA were shown to prevent and reverse the cellular phenotype. Other studies showed cellular hypertrophy, impaired contractile function, decreased metabolism [63], and increased IL-18 levels in iPS-CMs and sera of patient with LV hypertrophy progression [64]. Notably, neutralization of IL-18 reduced hypertrophy in vitro.

Danon disease (DD) is caused by mutations in the X-linked lysosomal-associated membrane protein type 2 (*LAMP2)* gene, leading to dysfunctional lysosomal and glycogen storage. DD patients suffer severe cardiac and skeletal muscle abnormalities resulting in HCM, heart failure and sudden cardiac death [65]. iPS-CMs from DD patients showed impaired autophagic flux, damaged mitochondria, and an increase in apoptosis [66]. Additionally, iPS-CMs were hypertrophic and displayed increased calcium decay times compared to healthy iPS-CMs, thus mimicking the ventricular hypertrophy and decrease in contractile function in DD patients. Early-onset fatal cardiomyopathy is observed predominantly in male DD patients, while female patients show a later onset and less-severe clinical phenotype. This has been attributed to random inactivation of the *LAMP2* gene on the X chromosome [67] and could be recapitulated in DD iPS-CMs recently [68].

PRKAG2 cardiomyopathy mimics some features of HCM, but with notable differences, such as a lack of myocardial fibrosis and the presence of ventricular pre-excitation (Wolff-Parkinson-White syndrome) and glycogen accumulation [69]. PRKAG2 is one of three regulatory subunits of the AMP-activated protein kinase (AMPK), and is highly expressed in the heart [70]. AMPK is a metabolic enzyme that can be activated by nutrient stress or genetic mutations, like missense mutations in PRKAG2. So far, one study has provided an iPS-CM disease model for PRKAG2 cardiomyopathy using both a patient line and a TALEN genome engineered line. Comparable to patients, this study showed an increase in AMPK activity and hypertrophy, glycogen accumulation, and inhibition of TGFβ2 production associated with cardiac fibrosis [71]. The attenuation of profibrotic signaling suggests therapeutic potential for molecules that provide tailored AMPK activation to target adverse cardiac remodeling. On the other hand, AMPK activation may incite cardiomyopathy, similar to *PRKAG2* mutations.

Cardiac Amyloidosis

A mutation in the transthyretin gene (*TTR*) leads to the hereditary autosomal-dominant form of amyloidosis (ATTR). ATTR patients suffer from multi-organ failure caused by expression and secretion of misfolded mutant TTR in hepatocytes, which aggregates and forms fibrils in affected organs, mainly the heart and peripheral nervous system. IPS cells derived from ATTR patients were differentiated into hepatic, neuronal, and cardiac lineages, thereby modeling the three major tissue types involved in this disease. Mutant TTR, secreted by iPS-hepatocytes decreased iPS-CM cell survival [72], emphasizing the potential of patient-specific iPS cells as models for studying disorders affecting multiple cell types and organs.

Mitochondrial Cardiomyopathy

Mitochondrial function is a key determinant of myocardial performance as the heart has an extremely high metabolic demand. Mutations in mitochondrial encoded genes or genes crucial for mitochondrial structure therefore often affect cardiac function. Barth syndrome (BTHS), for example, shows a multidimensional phenotype characterized by dilated cardiomyopathy, skeletal myopathy, neutropenia, growth retardation, and increased urinary excretion of 3-methylglutaconic acid in early childhood [73]. It is caused by a mutation in the tafazzin gene (*TAZ*), coding for the CoA-independent phospholipid acyltransferase, which is necessary for maturation of cardiolipin, a component of the inner mitochondrial membrane. An iPS-CM model of BTHS was used to show the functional link of TAZ mutations to the cellular phenotype [74]. Delivery of TAZ coding RNA and CRISPR/Cas9-based genome editing to correct the *TAZ* mutation could ameliorate cardiolipin levels, mitochondrial and ATP deficits, as well as the functional cellular phenotype, including sarcomere disarray and diminished contractility. Additionally, therapeutic treatment with linoleic acid, an essential unsaturated fatty acid precursor to cardiolipin, increased cellular cardiolipin levels, thereby improving sarcomere organization as well as twitch strength.

Myoclonic epilepsy with ragged-red fibers (MERRF) is an extremely rare mitochondrial disorder characterized by myoclonus, generalized epilepsy, cerebellar ataxia, myopathy, and ragged red fibers, resulting from mitochondrial aggregates, in muscle biopsies. In over 80% of cases, MERRF is caused by mutations in *MT-TK*, a mitochondrial gene encoding tRNA(Lys) [75]. An iPS-CM model of

MERRF, with the *MT-TK* A8344G mutation showed decreased mitochondrial respiration, increased ROS levels and upregulation of antioxidant gene expression. MERRF iPS-CMs contained numerous fragmented mitochondria, and increased expression of fission protein Drp1 [76]. Although the underlying mechanism remains unclear, the abnormal mitochondria with severe mitochondrial dysfunction show that the model is able to mimic pathophysiological features of MERRF disease.

Mitochondrial myopathy, encephalopathy, lactic acidosis, and stroke-like episodes (MELAS) syndrome is a more common and stereotypical example of a mitochondrial disorder leading to a cardiomyopathy. Cardiac dysfunction occurs in about a third of patients with MELAS syndrome, which shows an increase in abnormal mitochondria and mitochondrial inclusions, coupled with variable sarcomere thickening and a heterogeneous distribution of affected cardiomyocytes [77]. While the in vivo effects on cardiomyocytes are evident, MELAS syndrome has not been modeled using iPS-CMs, though MELAS iPS cells with a mutation in *MTTL1* have been established [78]. Similarly, Kearns-Sayre syndrome, a much rarer mitochondrial myopathy, is under investigation using iPS cells, but has not been published to date.

Inherited Arrhythmia Syndromes

Long QT Syndrome

The long QT syndrome (LQTS) is an autosomal dominant cardiac disease associated with over 500 different mutations in at least 15 genes [79] encoding ion channel (interacting) proteins. The characteristic prolonged repolarization phase (QT phase) on ECG measurements predisposes patients to potentially life-threatening ventricular arrhythmias, so-called *Torsades de pointes*, and sudden cardiac arrest. Patient-specific iPS-CM models have been predominantly used for LQTS1, LQTS2, and LQTS3, but recently also for Andersen-Tawil syndrome (LQTS7), Timothy syndrome (LQTS8), and calmodulinopathies (LQTS14/15).

Mutations in the genes *KCNQ1* and *KCNH2* are most prevalent and cause LQTS1 and LQTS2, respectively. The *KCNQ1* gene encodes for the α-subunit of the voltage-gated K^+ channel mediating the slow delayed rectifier current I_{Ks}. The KCNH2 or hERG channel is a K^+ channel needed for the rapid delayed rectifier current I_{Kr}. Nine different LQTS1 causing mutations in the *KCNQ1* gene have been studied using iPS-CM models [15, 80–88]. Multiple iPS-CM models showed a dominant *KCNQ1* mutation leading to a diminished I_{Ks} current due to a sarcolemmal deficiency of KCNQ1 channels [80, 81, 83]. In addition, electrophysiological abnormalities, including a prolonged corrected field potential duration were observed in LQTS1 iPS-CMs [81]. Interestingly, calcium antagonists could rescue the electrophysiological phenotype present in a LQTS1 iPS-CM model, indicating a functional link between *KCNQ1* mutations and calcium handling abnormalities [82]. Other studies reported protective effects of β-adrenergic antagonists [80] or the selective I_{Ks} activator ML277 [83].

Jervell and Lange-Nielsen syndrome (JLNS) is characterized by life-threatening ventricular tachycardia and bilateral deafness, and is caused by a homozygous or compound heterozygous mutation in *KCNQ1* or *KCNE1* [89], disrupting the function of the voltage-gated K^+ channel. Engineered and patient-derived JLNS iPS-CMs showed the electrophysiological JLNS phenotype, with increased action potential duration (APD) and sensitivity to proarrhythmic drugs [90].

LQTS2 iPS-CM models have been established from patients carrying eight different *KCNH2* mutations [82, 85, 91–99]. The LQTS2 clinical phenotype was reflected in iPS-CM models by decreased I_{Kr} currents, arrhythmia, and APD prolongation [92, 95]. Interestingly, iPS-CMs carrying the KCNH2 N996I mutation reported only a mild increase in APD without early afterdepolarizations (EADs) [97], agreeing well with the mild KCNH2 N996I clinical phenotype [100]. Furthermore, trafficking defects, affecting stability and localization of the gene product, were observed in some LQTS2 iPS-CM models [94, 99], presumably due to altered glycosylation of mutant KCNH2. Blocking Ca^{2+}-activated proteases (calpains) could rescue the electrophysiological phenotype [99]. LQTS2 iPS-CMs also showed calcium handling disturbances which could be rescued with calcium antagonists [93], similar to LQTS1 models. The dominant negative trait of LQTS2 could also be mimicked by RNAi-mediated knockdown of the mutant *KCNH2* allele, rescuing the electrophysiological phenotype [99].

LQTS3 and Brugada syndrome (BrS) are caused by *SCN5A* gene gain-of-function (increased activity) or loss-of-function (decreased activity) mutations, respectively [101]. SCN5A encodes the α-subunit of the main cardiac Na^+ voltage-gated channel ($Na_V1.5$), essential for the fast upstroke of the cardiac action potential.

LQTS3 is characterized by arrhythmic events generally occurring more frequently at rest and less likely to be triggered by adrenergic stress. In total, nine LQTS3-associated *SCN5A* mutations have been studied using iPS-CMs [93, 102–109], showing prolonged APD, either linked to slower inactivation [104] or faster recovery of $Na_V1.5$ from inactivation [102]. The sodium channel blocker mexiletine was reported to exert arrhythmogenic effects, and reverse elevated late sodium currents and prolonged APDs of LQTS3 iPS-CMs, in line with the therapeutic regime of LQTS3 patients [102, 105, 110].

BrS is characterized physiologically by an arrhythmogenic substrate, mostly located in the right ventricle outflow tract, and an increased risk of (supra)ventricular arrhythmias. So far, three publications report BrS iPS-CMs models [110–112], including iPS-CMs from patients who tested negative for mutations in the known BrS-associated genes, yet showing the characteristic disease phenotype. However, these iPS-CMs without identified mutations did not show any pathophysiological features mimicking the clinical phenotype [110]. Another study using BrS iPS-CMs with defined *SCN5A* mutations assessed reduced peak inward sodium density (I_{Na}) and maximal AP upstroke velocity, compared with the control cell line, thus relating a cellular electrophysiological phenotype to observed clinical features [111]. Furthermore, BrS iPS-CMs showed abnormal calcium transients and beating interval variations. Reversion of the underlying mutation by CRISPR/Cas9 genome editing resulted in reversal of the phenotype [112]. In an iPS-CM model of LQTS3/BrS overlap syndrome, electrophysiological abnormalities were found, including a significantly diminished I_{Na}, indicative of the BrS-specific loss-of-function mutation [106].

Andersen-Tawil Syndrome (ATS), also defined as LQTS7, is a rare autosomal dominant genetic disorder characterized, in addition to the symptoms of LQTS, by physical abnormalities typically affecting head, face, and limbs. Mutations in the *KCNJ2* gene account for approximately 70% of cases (ATS1), while the genetic cause of the remaining 30% (ATS2) is still unknown [113]. *KCNJ2* codes for the voltage-gated, inward-rectifying potassium channel protein Kir2.1 (Fig. 26.2), that contributes to the inward-rectifier potassium current (I_{K1}). So far iPS-CM models covering three KCNJ2 mutations have been established to elucidate ATS1 pathogenesis and find potential novel drug candidates [114]. ATS1 iPS-CMs mimicked the abnormal electrophysiological phenotype of ATS, showing strong arrhythmic events and irregular calcium release, which could be suppressed by the anti-arrhythmic agent flecainide through modulation of the Na^+/Ca^{2+} exchanger (NCX).

Timothy syndrome (TS) or LQTS8 is characterized by cardiac arrhythmias in combination with syndactyly and dysmorphic facial features. As of 2005, only 18 cases were reported [115]. TS is caused by a mutation in *CACNA1C*, a gene encoding for the sarcolemmal voltage-gated calcium channel, $Ca_V1.2$, the main cardiac L-type calcium channel (Fig. 26.2) [116]. To date, one TS iPS-CM model has been reported, showing DADs and a reduced beating rate in ventricular iPS-CMs, reflecting bradycardia often present in TS patients [117].

LQTS-associated calmodulinopathies (LQTS14 and LQTS15) result from mutations affecting calcium binding in at least one of three calmodulin genes (*CALM1*, *CALM2*, *CALM3*) [118]. Patients present with life-threatening arrhythmias that are often resistant to conventional therapies. LQTS14 iPS-CMs typically showed prolonged repolarization and failure to adapt to high pacing rates [119]. Strikingly, this study enhanced I_{K1} in iPS-CMs by dynamic-clamp to overcome the extremely low I_{K1} and thereby mimic a mature action potential profile. Consistent with clinical phenotypes [120], LQTS15 iPS-CMs exhibited significantly lower beating rates and prolonged APD compared to control cells, and showed a dominant negative effect of single heterozygous *CALM2* mutations on the suppression of L-type calcium channel (LTCC) inactivation [121, 122]. Interestingly, ablation of the mutant CALM2 allele could rescue the electrophysiological phenotype in iPS-CMs, opening up new perspectives for treatment [122].

Catecholaminergic Polymorphic Ventricular Tachycardia

Catecholaminergic Polymorphic Ventricular Tachycardia (CPVT) is characterized by ventricular arrhythmia related to physical or emotional stress, potentially leading to sudden cardiac death, even in young individuals [123]. The CPVT1 subtype is caused by mutations in the ryanodine receptor type 2 gene (*RYR2*), while CPVT2 is caused by a mutated calsquestrin-2 gene (*CASQ2*), both having essential roles in calcium handling. The RYR2 channel mediates calcium flow out of the sarcoplasmic reticulum (SR) during depolarization, while CASQ2 is a calcium-binding protein in the SR. Mutations in triadin (*TRDN*), *KCNJ2*, *TECRL*, and *CALM1/2* have also been described as causative for CPVT (Fig. 26.2 and Table 26.1). iPS-CM models have been established for 16 different CPVT-related mutations [124–139]. Arrhythmic events have been induced by adrenergic agonists, implicating an altered CaMKII signaling pathway [135], and pacing, inducing a negative inotropic effect as well as DADs in CPVT1 [124] and CPVT2 models [134]. Of note, a more immature phenotype of CPVT iPS-CMs was observed compared to control iPS-CMs [134, 138, 139], raising questions on the validity of the model. However, the response of CPVT iPS-CM to dantrolene, an inhibitor of sarcoplasmic calcium release, has been shown to be in line with clinical observations of CPVT patients [137].

Miscellaneous

Congenital Heart Defects

Congenital heart defects (CHD) are the most prevalent of all human developmental malformations [140]. Cardiac septal defects have been shown to be caused by mutations in the cardiac transcription factor *GATA4*, reducing affinity for its genomic target sequence and disrupting interaction with Tbx5 [141]. An iPS-CM model showed that this mutation leads to impaired contractility, calcium handling, and metabolic activity [142].

Next to GATA4 CHD, three iPS-CM models of hypoplastic left heart syndrome (HLHS) [143–145], characterized by a severely underdeveloped left heart, have been reported. HLHS iPS-CMs showed a more fetal-like gene expression profile and an immature cellular phenotype, consistent with observations in vivo [146]. Mutations in the *MYH6* gene [144] and the *NOTCH1* gene [145] could be correlated to HLHS defective heart development using iPS-CM models, as defective cardiomyogenesis was observed in *MYH6*-mutated iPS cell lines, and reactivation of NOTCH signaling was shown to partly rescue the in vitro disease phenotype.

Syndromic

Both Cardiofaciocutaneous syndrome (CFCS) and Noonan syndrome with multiple lentigines (NSML), formerly known as LEOPARD syndrome, have been modeled using iPS-CMs. Both syndromes are caused by mutations in genes involved in the RAS/MAP kinase pathway, and are therefore also referred to as "RASopathies." CFCS is characterized by the simultaneous occurrence of multiple congenital abnormalities and mental retardation. Most patients present with CHD like pulmonic stenosis or HCM [147]. To date, around 60 cases of CFCS have been published [148]. iPS-CM models carrying two BRAF mutations have been established, showing upregulation of a fetal gene program, including ANP, and incidence of arrhythmias [149, 150]. Furthermore, cocultured fibroblasts were shown to participate in developing the pathognomonic cardiomyocyte phenotype [149]. NSML is another very rare inherited syndromic disorder with cardiac traits, with approximately 85% of patients carrying a mutation in the *PTPN11* gene, encoding a member of the protein tyrosine phosphatase family. In addition to many other disease features, patients commonly develop HCM. The earliest iPS-CM model is the model for NSML, which showed that the HCM phenotype was indeed present in vitro, where preferential nuclear localization of NFATc4 and cardiomyocyte enlargement was shown [4].

Friedreich's ataxia (FRDA), yet another syndromic disease with cardiac traits, has been studied using iPS-CMs. It is caused by hyper-expansive GAA repeats in intron 1 of the frataxin (*FXN*) gene, leading to epigenetic silencing of the gene. *FXN* codes for frataxin, a small mitochondrially located protein involved in iron-sulfur cluster biosynthesis. FRDA usually presents with progressive ataxia between 10 and 15 years of age, causing dysarthria, muscle weakness and spasticity, and approximately two thirds of all FRDA patients suffer from hypertrophic cardiomyopathy [151]. In FRDA iPS-CMs, mitochondrial damage, fibrillary disarray, and calcium handling deficiency were present under standard culture conditions [152, 153], and challenging the iPS-CMs with increasing concentrations of iron also induced hypertrophy [154, 155]. Deferiprone, a drug counteracting iron overload in β-thalassemia, could relieve the stress-stimulation [155], consistent with clinical studies reporting a reduction in hypertrophy in FRDA patients [156]. Importantly, the extent of the GAA repeat was reported to change during the culture of FRDA iPS cells and stabilize during iPS-CM differentiation [152], which has to be taken into account when relating in vitro findings to the clinical phenotype as GAA length correlates with severity of FRDA symptoms including cardiac manifestations [157].

Neuromuscular

Duchenne muscular dystrophy (DMD) is a severe X-linked neuromuscular disorder, caused by mutations in the dystrophin (*DMD*) gene, which encodes a cytoplasmic protein anchoring the sarcomere to the extracellular matrix. DMD usually presents around the age of four with progressively worsening muscle weakness. Therapeutic improvements for DMD patients has led to a longer lifespan (up to 40 years), but resulted in cardiomyopathy becoming a prevalent cause of mortality [158]. The cardiac phenotype observed in DMD patients includes dilatation, arrhythmias, structural alterations and hemodynamic abnormalities. Nine different mutations in *DMD* have already been studied using iPS-CM models [159–163]. The differentiation to iPS-CMs was observed to be less efficient for the DMD iPS cell lines [160], and iPS-CMs showed increased cellular damage, apoptosis, altered calcium handling, and elevated cardiac injury markers [161, 162], which is in agreement with clinical data [164]. The use of 3D-engineered cardiac tissues, to create more mature and translationally relevant cardiomyocytes, was shown to be necessary to distinguish structural differences present in DMD myocytes, and has shed some light on the impaired response to external cues in DMD iPS-CMs, by showing a lower level of actin cytoskeleton turnover [163].

Myotonic Dystrophy type 1 (DM1) is a genetic multisystem disorder [165], with variable onset from birth to old age, and a broad spectrum of symptoms, including minor muscle pain to severe muscle weakness, myotonia, respiratory problems, and cardiac conduction defects. DM1 results from an unstable trinucleotide (CTG) repeat expansion in the dystrophia myotonica protein kinase (*DMPK*) gene [166]. A recent study aimed to develop a phenotype reversing gene therapy using DM1 iPS cells for use in autologous stem cell transplantations showed that removal of mutant transcripts by genome treatment led to reversal of the disease phenotype in the iPS-CMs [167].

Another gene related to multisystem disorders featuring cardiomyopathy and skeletal myopathy is *HSPB5*, which encodes a small heat shock protein [168]. In an iPS-CM model carrying the 343delT mutation, causing early-onset skeletal myopathy, aggregation of insoluble mutated protein and induction of a cellular stress response was observed [169]. In vitro refolding of 343delT mutated HSPB5 in the presence of wildtype rescued its solubility, which matches the recessive inheritance of the disease.

Other Diseases with Cardiac Traits

Abetalipoproteinemia (ABL), or Bassen-Kornzweig syndrome, is a rare autosomal recessive disorder of lipoprotein metabolism, resulting from mutations in the gene encoding the microsomal triglyceride transfer protein (*MTTP*), which is essential for creating beta-lipoproteins needed for normal absorption and transport of fat, cholesterol, and fat-soluble vitamins [170]. MTTP is expressed in the liver and intestine, and also in cardiomyocytes, which may be the reason why ABL patients can suffer from cardiac arrhythmias and heart failure [171]. Using iPS cells generated from an ABL patient with the homozygous missense mutation MTTPR46G, it was shown that both iPS-hepatocytes and iPS-CMs mimicked defects associated with ABL disease. ABL iPS-CMs failed to secrete apolipoprotein B (apoB) and showed intracellular lipid accumulation, and hypersensitivity to metabolic stress, increasing cell death [172]. These effects could be reversed by correction of the mutation via CRISPR/Cas9 gene editing.

Interestingly, iPS-CM disease models may also be useful to improve risk management of coronary artery disease (CAD), as shown by a study using iPS cells with an aldehyde dehydrogenase 2 (*ALDH2*) mutation (ALDH2∗2), as this mutation has been linked to an increased risk of CAD and more severe outcomes, and occurs in 8% of the human population [173, 174]. The model showed that the ALDH2∗2 mutation led to elevated ROS and toxic aldehydes, and induced cell cycle arrest and apoptosis, especially during ischemia, revealing new cues for therapeutic options.

Summary of the Cardiac Disease Models

Taken together, the current studies show that clinically relevant phenotypes are present in the inherited cardiac disease models, and that the use of these models can shed new light on the pathophysiological and molecular mechanisms, which is essential for the development of new therapies.

The predictive power of iPS-CM models and their potential to help establish patient-specific clinical regimens, and use as drug screening platforms has been especially clear in models of LQTS. For example, the pathological phenotype seen in a LQTS3 iPS-CM model could be mitigated by combining pacing and a pharmacological approach, which was analogous to the therapy used in these patients [102]. In another study, patients' susceptibility to develop a cardiotoxic response to sotalol, a QT-prolonging drug, could be reproduced with a panel of genetically diverse iPS-CMs [175]. Yet another striking example is the susceptibility to the serious cardiac arrhythmogenic side effects of cisapride seen in an iPS-CM model of LQTS. Previously, these side effects were seen in patients and led to the withdrawal of cisapride from the market [15].

Next to LQTS models, iPS-CM models of HCM, DCM, ARVC, and CPVT also agreed well with their in vivo characteristics, showing hypertrophy, calcium handling irregularities, sarcomeric disarray and arrhythmias (HCM), impaired calcium handling (DCM), and electrophysiological abnormalities (ARVC, CPVT). Since iPS-CM models reflect clinical phenotypes, the underlying pathological mechanisms leading to these phenotypes are present and can be studied using these models. This enabled researchers to gain new insights on the molecular pathogenesis of HCM, DCM, LVNC, LQTS, CHD, Pompe disease, NSML/LEOPARD, and Takotsubo cardiomyopathy, thereby providing new leads for individualized therapies [4, 14, 16, 17, 29, 57, 99, 142, 176, 177].

Advancing iPS-CM Disease Modeling

Before iPS-CM models of inherited cardiac disease will be able to fully recapitulate the disease in a dish, several hurdles need to be overcome. When looking at all the iPS-CM models discussed in this chapter, there are major differences in study design that will affect the quality of the disease model, the characteristics of the iPS-CMs and eventually the conclusions drawn. Important confounders that can potentially underlie the differences observed between a healthy control iPS-CM and the iPS-CM disease model are: the choice of control (matching for sex, ethnicity, family, or genome edited controls), cellular source (skin, blood, urine), induction of pluripotency (integrating vs. nonintegrating methods), adaptation to culturing conditions, and epigenetic status, which can, e.g., affect the capacity to differentiate to cardiomyocytes. So far, most studies have used healthy sex-matched control iPS-CMs, and an increasing number of studies has included (sex-matched) family members as controls, thereby reducing genetic differences by ~50% maximum. However, the effects of patient characteristics like ethnicity on the iPS-CM models have not been evaluated, while for example it has been established that ethnicity can influence the phenotypic expression of HCM [178]. The cell source used to generate the iPS cell line may also influence the iPS-CM model characteristics, as skin cells can contain UV-induced DNA damage, and the source cell type-specific epigenetic pattern has been shown to persist in iPS cell lines, affecting differentiation efficiency [179, 180]. More and more studies are shifting toward use of blood and urine cells for reprogramming, and the induction of pluripotency is moving from integrating vectors, e.g., retro- and lentiviruses, toward nonintegrating vectors, e.g., Sendai virus [181] or virus-free methods like episomal transfection [182], or mRNA delivery [183], avoiding insertional mutagenesis and potential transgene reactivation.

Fortunately, almost all of these confounders can now be eliminated by the use of isogenic control iPS cell lines, generated by genome editing techniques such as TALEN or CRISPR/Cas9. Isogenic controls are created by reversing the mutated, disease-inducing genes to the healthy wildtype, and are by far the best controls as they are matched for origin, epigenetic profile, culture conditions, and even differentiation capacity, providing a relevant and true "healthy control" [85, 97]. Several iPS-CM studies have already used isogenic controls to validate the pathogenicity of the specific mutation by showing complete reversal of the disease phenotype [28, 31, 36, 82, 167]. Moreover, these studies have laid the groundwork for developing targeted gene therapy for patients with inherited heart disease.

Other factors that may influence iPS-CM model characteristics are the differentiation protocol used (consistency, purity, CM subtypes), level of maturity, culture conditions, number of patient lines and clonal lines studied. When taking a detailed look at the currently published iPS-CM models, there are significant differences in the protocols used to differentiate iPS cells to cardiomyocytes. Differentiation is performed by either coculture with visceral endoderm-like cells [184], embryoid body formation in suspension [185], or monolayer culture with supplementation of specific differentiation factors [186]. The chemically defined monolayer protocol is increasingly used, most likely due to its high efficiency and ease of use [187, 188].

As a result of the use of different protocols, the percentage of cardiomyocytes obtained after differentiation varies greatly, as well as the time point of, e.g., first observed spontaneous beating, and the ratios of cardiomyocyte subtypes generated (ventricular, atrial, and nodal). Next to that, the level of cardiomyocyte maturity also greatly varies in the different studies, affecting the comparability of critical functional read-outs, like calcium handling and electrophysiological measurements. IPS-CMs have frequently been described to display a fetal-like phenotype, e.g., lacking mature sarcomere organization [46], showing low ratios of multinucleation [189], having underdeveloped t-tubule networks [190], and displaying altered calcium handling [191]. Cardiac maturation involves changes in cell size and morphology, cell–cell coupling, sarcomere density and organization, metabolism, mitochondrial content, and functional changes in calcium handling, contractility, and action potential characteristics [192]. Immature iPS-CMs might only partly recapitulate the disease phenotypes of several cardiac diseases, as many manifest exclusively in adulthood. However, only a limited number of studies thoroughly assessed features related to cardiomyocyte maturation, and electrophysiological assessments were mainly performed on spontaneously beating iPS-CMs, while preferably these cells should be paced in order to obtain robust data on potential arrhythmogenicity of the respective mutation. It is evident that both enhancing and proper assessment of iPS-CM maturation is important when establishing iPS-CM disease models. As a consequence, methods to enhance iPS-CM maturation are intensely studied, and have already led to numerous culture strategies to boost maturity like time in culture, substrate stiffness, electrical stimulation, 3D tissue formation, and growth substrate micropatterning [193–195]. The benefit of using 3D tissues for iPS-CM disease modeling was shown in an iPS-CM model of DCM linked to mutated titin, where small cardiac tissues composed of iPS-CMs, stromal cells, and a collagen type I/fibrinogen matrix showed the typical contractile-deficient phenotype associated with the disease, which was not present in the monolayer iPS-CM model [28]. Culture conditions may also be adapted to enhance disease models to be more comparable to the in vivo situation. Two good examples are the use of adrenergic agonist stimulation in CPVT iPS-CMs to attain the arrhythmic phenotype, and stimulation with adipogenic medium in ARVC iPS-CMs to enhance the disease-specific characteristics. Additionally, modeling ARVC might need an increase in model complexity, using multiple cell types, potentially generated by the same iPS cell line, to account for the crosstalk between different cell types and the fibro-fatty depositions present in these patients [39]. Even if protocols are fully optimized, standardized, and confounders are limited as much as possible, for example, by using isogenic controls, still not all confounding factors are eliminated. For instance, it has been shown that single nucleotide mutations occur spontaneously in different cell lines [196], including isogenic controls, indicating that lines can never be truly isogenic, thereby introducing a potential confounding factor. Additionally, expanding iPS lines for many passages results in selection pressure [197], thereby altering the cells with respect to, e.g., proliferation rate, and possibly capacity for differentiation. Finally, well-to-well variation in cell culture can induce phenotypic changes in the same iPS clonal line. Therefore, to increase rigidity and predictive power of cardiac disease modeling, not only several donors of cells to generate iPS lines but also multiple clonal lines derived from each reprogramming [198] and multiple samples per clonal line should be included to account for these possible confounders.

Naturally, standardization of these methodologies will be essential to enhance study reproducibility and intercomparability between labs. Finally, especially if standardization issues are tackled, as many cardiac disease-specific iPS cell lines as possible should be stored and made accessible through biobanks [199, 200]. Taken together these efforts will lead to advanced cardiac disease models with a better predictive power, enabling researchers to draw clinically relevant conclusions, without performing animal or first-in-man studies.

Take Home Message

Currently, over 150 human cardiac disease-specific iPS cell lines have been generated, differentiated, and studied. These patient-specific iPS-CM models have shown to be able to facilitate the study of many aspects of the disease phenotype and are particularly useful to elucidate the pathological molecular mechanisms associated with the specific cardiac disease. Importantly, iPS-CM models can predict the patient's response to existing and novel drugs, thereby facilitating personalized treatment. This clearly emphasizes the potential of using these models to advance our understanding and to develop targeted therapies for inherited cardiac diseases. However, to generate more robust and reproducible iPS-CM disease models, standardization of methodologies to minimize the confounding effects that can undermine study results is essential. In addition, the establishment of more predictive iPS-CM disease models that more closely mimic the disease are needed, as significant differences between the complex in vivo tissue architecture and pathophysiology, and simplified in vitro culture conditions can limit the capacity of the model to recapitulate disease-specific functional mechanisms.

References

1. MacRae CA, Vasan RS. The future of genetics and genomics. Circulation. 2016;133:2634–9.
2. Takahashi K, Yamanaka S. Induction of pluripotent stem cells from mouse embryonic and adult fibroblast cultures by defined factors. Cell. 2006;126:663–76.
3. Kattman SJ, et al. Stage-specific optimization of activin/nodal and BMP signaling promotes cardiac differentiation of mouse and human pluripotent stem cell lines. Cell Stem Cell. 2011;8:228–40.
4. Carvajal-vergara X, et al. Patient-specific induced pluripotent stem cell derived models of LEOPARD syndrome. Nature. 2010;465:808–12.
5. Aasen T, et al. Efficient and rapid generation of induced pluripotent stem cells from human keratinocytes. Nat Biotechnol. 2008;26:1276–84.
6. Seki T, Yuasa S, Fukuda K. Generation of induced pluripotent stem cells from a small amount of human peripheral blood using a combination of activated T cells and Sendai virus. Nat Protoc. 2012;7:718–28.
7. Zhou T, et al. Generation of induced pluripotent stem cells from urine. J Am Soc Nephrol. 2011;22:1221–8.
8. Choi J, et al. A comparison of genetically matched cell lines reveals the equivalence of human iPSCs and ESCs. Nat Biotechnol. 2015;33:1173–81.
9. Maron BJ, et al. Prevalence of hypertrophic cardiomyopathy in a general population of young adults. Circulation. 1995;92:785–9.
10. Ojala M, et al. Mutation-specific phenotypes in hiPSC-derived cardiomyocytes carrying either myosin-binding protein C or α-tropomyosin mutation for hypertrophic cardiomyopathy. Stem Cells Int. 2016;2016:Article ID1684792.
11. Dambrot C, et al. Serum supplemented culture medium masks hypertrophic phenotypes in human pluripotent stem cell derived cardiomyocytes. J Cell Mol Med. 2014;18:1509–18.
12. Richard P, et al. Hypertrophic cardiomyopathy: distribution of disease genes, spectrum of mutations, and implications for a molecular diagnosis strategy. Circulation. 2003;107:2227–32.
13. Birket MJ, et al. Contractile defect caused by mutation in MYBPC3 revealed under conditions optimized for human PSC-cardiomyocyte function. Cell Rep. 2015;13:733–45.
14. Tanaka A, et al. Endothelin-1 induces myofibrillar disarray and contractile vector variability in hypertrophic cardiomyopathy-induced pluripotent stem cell-derived cardiomyocytes. J Am Heart Assoc. 2014;3:1–26.
15. Liang P, et al. Drug screening using a library of human induced pluripotent stem cell-derived cardiomyocytes reveals disease-specific patterns of cardiotoxicity. Circulation. 2013;127:1677–91.
16. Lan F, et al. Abnormal calcium handling properties underlie familial hypertrophic cardiomyopathy pathology in patient-specific induced pluripotent stem cells. Cell Stem Cell. 2013;12:101–13.
17. Han L, et al. Study familial hypertrophic cardiomyopathy using patient-specific induced pluripotent stem cells. Cardiovasc Res. 2014;104:258–69.
18. Pioner JM, et al. Isolation and mechanical measurements of myofibrils from human induced pluripotent stem cell-derived cardiomyocytes. Stem Cell Rep. 2016;6:1–12.
19. Phelan DG, et al. ALPK3-deficient cardiomyocytes generated from patient-derived induced pluripotent stem cells and mutant human embryonic stem cells display abnormal calcium handling and establish that ALPK3 deficiency underlies familial cardiomyopathy. Eur Heart J. 2016;37:2586–90.
20. Burkett EL, Hershberger RE. Clinical and genetic issues in familial dilated cardiomyopathy. J Am Coll Cardiol. 2005;45:969–81.
21. Fatkin D, et al. Missense mutations in the rod domain of the lamin A/C gene as causes of dilated cardiomyopathy and conduction-system disease. N Engl J Med. 1999;341:1715–24.
22. Kostera-Pruszczyk A, Pruszczyk P, Kamińska A, Lee HS, Goldfarb LG. Diversity of cardiomyopathy phenotypes caused by mutations in desmin. Int J Cardiol. 2008;131:146–7.
23. Hedberg C, Melberg A, Kuhl A, Jenne D, Oldfors A. Autosomal dominant myofibrillar myopathy with arrhythmogenic right ventricular cardiomyopathy 7 is caused by a DES mutation. Eur J Hum Genet. 2012;20:984–5.
24. Herman DS, et al. Truncations of titin causing dilated cardiomyopathy. N Engl J Med. 2012;366:619–28.
25. Siu CW, et al. Modeling of lamin A/C mutation premature cardiac aging using patient-specific induced pluripotent stem cells. Aging. 2012;4:803–22.
26. Tse HF, et al. Patient-specific induced-pluripotent stem cells-derived cardiomyocytes recapitulate the pathogenic phenotypes of dilated cardiomyopathy due to a novel DES mutation identified by whole exome sequencing. Hum Mol Genet. 2013;22:1395–403.
27. Xiang X, et al. TREM2 deficiency reduces the efficacy of immunotherapeutic amyloid clearance. EMBO Mol Med. 2016;8:992–1004.
28. Hinson JT, et al. Titin mutations in iPS cells define sarcomere insufficiency as a cause of dilated cardiomyopathy. Science. 2015;349:982–6.
29. Wu H, et al. Epigenetic regulation of phosphodiesterases 2A and 3A underlies compromised β-adrenergic signaling in an iPSC model of dilated cardiomyopathy. Cell Stem Cell. 2015;17:89–100.
30. Sun N, et al. Patient-specific induced pluripotent stem cells as a model for familial dilated cardiomyopathy. Sci Transl Med. 2012;4:130ra47.
31. Karakikes I, et al. Correction of human phospholamban R14del mutation associated with cardiomyopathy using targeted nucleases and combination therapy. Nat Commun. 2015;6:6955.
32. Wyles SP, et al. Pharmacological modulation of calcium homeostasis in familial dilated cardiomyopathy: an in vitro analysis from an RBM20 patient-derived iPSC model. Clin Transl Sci. 2016;9:158–67.

33. Wyles SP, et al. Modeling structural and functional deficiencies of RBM20 familial dilated cardiomyopathy using human induced pluripotent stem cells. Hum Mol Genet. 2016;25:254–65.
34. Judge LM, et al. A BAG3 chaperone complex maintains cardiomyocyte function during proteotoxic stress. JCI Insight. 2017;2:1–17.
35. Yano M, Ikeda Y, Matsuzaki M. Altered intracellular Ca2+ handling in heart failure. J Clin Invest. 2005;115:556–64.
36. Stillitano F, et al. Genomic correction of familial cardiomyopathy in human engineered cardiac tissues. Eur Heart J. 2016;37:3282–4.
37. Norman MW, McKenna WJ. Arrhythmogenic right ventricular cardiomyopathy: perspectives on disease. Z Kardiol. 1999;88:550–4.
38. Finsterer J, Stoellberger C. Arrhythmogenic right ventricular dysplasia in neuromuscular disorders. Clin Med Insights Cardiol. 2016;10:173.
39. Ma D, et al. Generation of patient-specific induced pluripotent stem cell-derived cardiomyocytes as a cellular model of arrhythmogenic right ventricular cardiomyopathy. Eur Heart J. 2013;34:1122–33.
40. Caspi O, et al. Modeling of arrhythmogenic right ventricular cardiomyopathy with human induced pluripotent stem cells. Circ Cardiovasc Genet. 2013;6:557–68.
41. Kim C, et al. Studying arrhythmogenic right ventricular dysplasia with patient-specific iPSCs. Nature. 2013;494:105–10.
42. Cerrone M, et al. Missense mutations in plakophilin-2 cause sodium current deficit and associate with a brugada syndrome phenotype. Circulation. 2014;129:1092–103.
43. Te Riele ASJM, et al. Multilevel analyses of SCN5A mutations in arrhythmogenic right ventricular dysplasia/cardiomyopathy suggest non-canonical mechanisms for disease pathogenesis. Cardiovasc Res. 2017;113:102–11.
44. Akdis D, et al. Sex hormones affect outcome in arrhythmogenic right ventricular cardiomyopathy/dysplasia: from a stem cell derived cardiomyocyte-based model to clinical biomarkers of disease outcome. Eur Heart J. 2017;38:1498–508.
45. Asimaki A, et al. A new diagnostic test for arrhythmogenic right ventricular cardiomyopathy. N Engl J Med. 2009;360:1075–84.
46. Uosaki H, et al. Transcriptional landscape of cardiomyocyte maturation. Cell Rep. 2015;13:1705–16.
47. Kirchhof P, et al. Age- and training-dependent development of arrhythmogenic right ventricular cardiomyopathy in heterozygous plakoglobin-deficient mice. Circulation. 2006;114:1799–806.
48. Weiford BC, Subbarao VD, Mulhern KM. Noncompaction of the ventricular myocardium. Circulation. 2004;109:2965–71.
49. Arbustini E, Weidemann F, Hall JL. Left ventricular noncompaction: a distinct cardiomyopathy or a trait shared by different cardiac diseases? J Am Coll Cardiol. 2014;64:1840–50.
50. Luxán G, et al. Mutations in the NOTCH pathway regulator MIB1 cause left ventricular noncompaction cardiomyopathy. Nat Med. 2013;19:193–201.
51. Kodo K, et al. iPSC-derived cardiomyocytes reveal abnormal TGFβ signaling in left ventricular non-compaction cardiomyopathy. Nat Cell Biol. 2016;18:1031–42.
52. Arndt AK, et al. Fine mapping of the 1p36 deletion syndrome identifies mutation of PRDM16 as a cause of cardiomyopathy. Am J Hum Genet. 2013;93:67–77.
53. Journal A, Genetics M. Letter to the editor carrier frequency for glycogen storage disease type II in New York and estimates of affected individuals born with the disease. Am J Med Genet. 1998;72:69–72.
54. Nishigaki T. Glycogen storage disease type II. Ryoikibetsu Shokogun Shirizu. 1998;(19 Pt 2):349–52
55. Huang HP, et al. Human Pompe disease-induced pluripotent stem cells for pathogenesis modeling, drug testing and disease marker identification. Hum Mol Genet. 2011;20:4851–64.
56. Sato Y, et al. Disease modeling and lentiviral gene transfer in patient-specific induced pluripotent stem cells from late-onset Pompe disease patient. Mol Ther Methods Clin Dev. 2015;2:15023.
57. Raval KK, et al. Pompe disease results in a Golgi-based glycosylation deficit in human induced pluripotent stem cell-derived cardiomyocytes. J Biol Chem. 2015;290:3121–36.
58. Thurberg BL, et al. Characterization of pre-and post-treatment pathology after enzyme replacement therapy for pompe disease. Lab Investig. 2006;86:1208–20.
59. Fermini B, Nathan RD. Removal of sialic acid alters both T- and L-type calcium currents in cardiac myocytes. Am J Phys. 1991;260:H735–43.
60. Jakubowska E, Ryba M, Hruby Z. Fabry disease. Przegl Lek. 2006;63:218–9.
61. Itier JM, et al. Effective clearance of GL-3 in a human iPSC-derived cardiomyocyte model of Fabry disease. J Inherit Metab Dis. 2014;37:1013–22.
62. Chimenti C, et al. Myofilament degradation and dysfunction of human cardiomyocytes in Fabry disease. Am J Pathol. 2008;172:1482–90.
63. Chou S-J, et al. Energy utilization of induced pluripotent stem cell-derived cardiomyocyte in Fabry disease. Int J Cardiol. 2017;232:255–63.
64. Chien Y, et al. Interleukin-18 deteriorates Fabry cardiomyopathy and contributes to the development of left ventricular hypertrophy in Fabry patients with GLA IVS4+919 G>A mutation. Oncotarget. 2016;7:87161–79.
65. Nishino I, et al. Primary LAMP-2 deficiency causes X-linked vacuolar cardiomyopathy and myopathy (Danon disease). Nature. 2000;406:906–10.
66. Hashem S, et al. Brief report: oxidative stress mediates cardiomyocyte apoptosis in a human model of Danon disease and heart failure. Stem Cells. 2015;33:2343–50.
67. Majer F, et al. Danon disease: a focus on processing of the novel LAMP2 mutation and comments on the beneficial use of peripheral white blood cells in the diagnosis of LAMP2 deficiency. Gene. 2012;498:183–95.
68. Ng KM, et al. Amelioration of X-linked related autophagy failure in Danon disease with DNA methylation inhibitor. Circulation. 2016;134:1373–89.
69. Arad M, et al. Constitutively active AMP kinase mutations cause glycogen storage disease mimicking hypertrophic cardiomyopathy. J Clin Invest. 2002;109:357–62.
70. Lang T, et al. Molecular cloning, genomic organization, and mapping of PRKAG2, a heart abundant γ2 subunit of 5′-AMP-activated protein kinase, to human chromosome 7q36. Genomics. 2000;70:258–63.
71. Hinson JT, et al. Integrative analysis of PRKAG2 cardiomyopathy iPS and microtissue models identifies AMPK as a regulator of metabolism, survival, and fibrosis. Cell Rep. 2017;19:2410.
72. Leung A, et al. Induced pluripotent stem cell modeling of multisystemic, hereditary transthyretin amyloidosis. Stem Cell Rep. 2013;1:451–63.
73. Barth PG, et al. An X-linked mitochondrial disease affecting cardiac muscle, skeletal muscle and neutrophil leucocytes. J Neurol Sci. 1983;62:327–55.
74. Wang G, et al. Modeling the mitochondrial cardiomyopathy of Barth syndrome with induced pluripotent stem cell and heart-on-chip technologies. Nat Med. 2014;20:616–23.
75. Shoffner JM, et al. Myoclonic epilepsy and ragged-red fiber disease (MERRF) is associated with a mitochondrial DNA tRNALys mutation. Cell. 1990;61:931–7.
76. Chou SJ, et al. Impaired ROS scavenging system in human induced pluripotent stem cells generated from patients with MERRF syndrome. Sci Rep. 2016;6:23661.
77. Hsu YHR, et al. MELAS syndrome and cardiomyopathy: linking mitochondrial function to heart failure pathogenesis. Heart Fail Rev. 2016;21:103–16.

78. Kodaira M, et al. Impaired respiratory function in MELAS-induced pluripotent stem cells with high heteroplasmy levels. FEBS Open Bio. 2015;5:219–25.
79. Nakano Y, Shimizu W. Genetics of long-QT syndrome. J Hum Genet. 2016;61:51–5.
80. Moretti A, et al. Patient-specific induced pluripotent stem-cell models for long-QT syndrome. N Engl J Med. 2010;363:1397–409.
81. Egashira T, et al. Disease characterization using LQTS-specific induced pluripotent stem cells. Cardiovasc Res. 2012;95:419–29.
82. Wang Y, et al. Genome editing of isogenic human induced pluripotent stem cells recapitulates long QT phenotype for drug testing. J Am Coll Cardiol. 2014;64:451–9.
83. Ma D, et al. Characterization of a novel KCNQ1 mutation for type 1 long QT syndrome and assessment of the therapeutic potential of a novel IKs activator using patient-specific induced pluripotent stem cell-derived cardiomyocytes. Stem Cell Res Ther. 2015;6:39.
84. Kiviaho AL, et al. Distinct electrophysiological and mechanical beating phenotypes of long QT syndrome type 1-specific cardiomyocytes carrying different mutations. Int J Cardiol Heart Vasc. 2015;8:19–31.
85. Sala L, et al. A new hERG allosteric modulator rescues genetic and drug-induced long-QT syndrome phenotypes in cardiomyocytes from isogenic pairs of patient induced pluripotent stem cells. EMBO Mol Med. 2016;8:1065–81.
86. Kuusela J, et al. Effects of cardioactive drugs on human induced pluripotent stem cell derived long QT syndrome cardiomyocytes. Springerplus. 2016;5:234.
87. Kuusela J, Kim J, Räsänen E, Aalto-Setälä K. The effects of pharmacological compounds on beat rate variations in human long QT-syndrome cardiomyocytes. Stem Cell Rev Rep. 2016;12:698–707.
88. Kuusela J, Larsson K, Shah D, Prajapati C, Aalto-Setälä K. Low extracellular potassium prolongs repolarization and evokes early afterdepolarization in human induced pluripotent stem cell-derived cardiomyocytes. Biol Open. 2017;6:777–84.
89. Schwartz PJ, et al. The Jervell and Lange-Nielsen syndrome: natural history, molecular basis, and clinical outcome. Circulation. 2006;113:783–90.
90. Zhang M, et al. Recessive cardiac phenotypes in induced pluripotent stem cell models of Jervell and Lange-Nielsen syndrome: disease mechanisms and pharmacological rescue. Proc Natl Acad Sci USA. 2014;111:E5383–92.
91. Mura M, et al. The KCNH2-IVS9-28A/G mutation causes aberrant isoform expression and hERG trafficking defect in cardiomyocytes derived from patients affected by long QT syndrome type 2. Int J Cardiol. 2017;240:367–71.
92. Itzhaki I, et al. Modelling the long QT syndrome with induced pluripotent stem cells. Nature. 2011;471:225–9.
93. Spencer CI, et al. Calcium transients closely reflect prolonged action potentials in iPSC models of inherited cardiac arrhythmia. Stem Cell Rep. 2014;3:269–81.
94. Jouni M, et al. Toward personalized medicine: using cardiomyocytes differentiated from urine-derived pluripotent stem cells to recapitulate electrophysiological characteristics of type 2 long QT syndrome. J Am Heart Assoc. 2015;4:e002159.
95. Matsa E, et al. Drug evaluation in cardiomyocytes derived from human induced pluripotent stem cells carrying a long QT syndrome type 2 mutation. Eur Heart J. 2011;32:952–62.
96. Lahti AL, et al. Model for long QT syndrome type 2 using human iPS cells demonstrates arrhythmogenic characteristics in cell culture. Dis Model Mech. 2012;5:220–30.
97. Bellin M, et al. Isogenic human pluripotent stem cell pairs reveal the role of a KCNH2 mutation in long-QT syndrome. EMBO J. 2013;32:3161–75.
98. Matsa E, et al. Allele-specific RNA interference rescues the long-QT syndrome phenotype in human-induced pluripotency stem cell cardiomyocytes. Eur Heart J. 2014;35:1078–87.
99. Mehta A, et al. Re-trafficking of hERG reverses long QT syndrome 2 phenotype in human iPS-derived cardiomyocytes. Cardiovasc Res. 2014;102:497–506.
100. Moss AJ, et al. Increased risk of arrhythmic events in long-QT syndrome with mutations in the pore region of the human ether-a-go-go-related gene potassium channel. Circulation. 2002;105:794–9.
101. Wilde AAM, Amin AS. Clinical Spectrum of SCN5A mutations: long QT syndrome, Brugada syndrome, and cardiomyopathy. JACC Clin Electrophysiol. 2018;4:569–79.
102. Terrenoire C, et al. Induced pluripotent stem cells used to reveal drug actions in a long QT syndrome family with complex genetics. J Gen Physiol. 2013;141:61–72.
103. Ma D, et al. Modeling type 3 long QT syndrome with cardiomyocytes derived from patient-specific induced pluripotent stem cells. Int J Cardiol. 2013;168:5277–86.
104. Fatima A, et al. The disease-specific phenotype in cardiomyocytes derived from induced pluripotent stem cells of two long QT syndrome type 3 patients. PLoS One. 2013;8:e83005.
105. Malan D, et al. Human iPS cell model of type 3 long QT syndrome recapitulates drug-based phenotype correction. Basic Res Cardiol. 2016;111:1–11.
106. Davis RP, et al. Cardiomyocytes derived from pluripotent stem cells recapitulate electrophysiological characteristics of an overlap syndrome of cardiac sodium channel disease. Circulation. 2012;125:3079–91.
107. Veerman CC, et al. Switch from fetal to adult SCN5A isoform in human induced pluripotent stem cell–derived cardiomyocytes unmasks the cellular phenotype of a conduction disease–causing mutation. J Am Heart Assoc. 2017;6:e005135.
108. Okata S, et al. Embryonic type Na + channel β-subunit, SCN3B masks the disease phenotype of Brugada syndrome. Sci Rep. 2016;6:34198.
109. Portero V, et al. Anti-arrhythmic potential of the late sodium current inhibitor GS-458967 in murine Scn5a-1798insD+/− and human SCN5A-1795insD+/− iPSC-derived cardiomyocytes. Cardiovasc Res. 2017;113:829–38.
110. Veerman CC, et al. hiPSC-derived cardiomyocytes from Brugada Syndrome patients without identified mutations do not exhibit clear cellular electrophysiological abnormalities. Sci Rep. 2016;6:30967.
111. Kosmidis G, et al. Readthrough-promoting drugs gentamicin and PTC124 Fail to Rescue Na v 1.5 function of human-induced pluripotent stem cell-derived cardiomyocytes carrying nonsense mutations in the sodium channel gene SCN5A. Circ Arrhythm Electrophysiol. 2016;9:e004227.
112. Liang P, et al. Patient-specific and genome-edited induced pluripotent stem cell–derived cardiomyocytes elucidate single-cell phenotype of Brugada syndrome. J Am Coll Cardiol. 2016;68:2086–96.
113. Nguyen H-L, Pieper GH, Wilders R. Andersen–Tawil syndrome: clinical and molecular aspects. Int J Cardiol. 2013;170:1–16.
114. Kuroda Y, et al. Flecainide ameliorates arrhythmogenicity through NCX flux in Andersen-Tawil syndrome-iPS cell-derived cardiomyocytes. Biochem Biophys Rep. 2017;9:245–56.
115. Gillis J, et al. Long QT, syndactyly, joint contractures, stroke and novel CACNA1C mutation: expanding the spectrum of Timothy syndrome. Am J Med Genet Part A. 2012;158A:182–7.
116. Gez LS, Hagalili Y, Shainberg A, Atlas D. Voltage-driven Ca2+ binding at the L-type Ca2+ channel triggers cardiac excitation-contraction coupling prior to Ca 2+ influx. Biochemistry. 2012;51:9658–66.

117. Yazawa M, et al. Using iPS cells to investigate cardiac phenotypes in patients with Timothy syndrome. Nature. 2011;471:230–4.
118. Crotti L, et al. Calmodulin mutations associated with recurrent cardiac arrest in infants. Circulation. 2013;127:1009–17.
119. Rocchetti M, et al. Elucidating arrhythmogenic mechanisms of long-QT syndrome CALM1-F142L mutation in patient-specific induced pluripotent stem cell-derived cardiomyocytes. Cardiovasc Res. 2017;113:531–41.
120. Makita N, et al. Novel calmodulin mutations associated with congenital arrhythmia susceptibility. Circ Cardiovasc Genet. 2014;7:466–74.
121. Limpitikul WB, et al. A precision medicine approach to the rescue of function on malignant calmodulinopathic long-QT syndrome. Circ Res. 2017;120:39–48.
122. Yamamoto Y, et al. Allele-specific ablation rescues electrophysiological abnormalities in a human iPS cell model of long-QT syndrome with a CALM2 mutation. Hum Mol Genet. 2017;26:1670–7.
123. Leenhardt A, Denjoy I, Guicheney P. Catecholaminergic polymorphic ventricular tachycardia. Circ Arrhythm Electrophysiol. 2012;5:1044–52.
124. Fatima A, et al. In vitro modeling of ryanodine receptor 2 dysfunction using human induced pluripotent stem cells. Cell Physiol Biochem. 2011;28:579–92.
125. Kujala K, et al. Cell model of catecholaminergic polymorphic ventricular tachycardia reveals early and delayed afterdepolarizations. PLoS One. 2012;7:1–10.
126. Paavola J, et al. Slowed depolarization and irregular repolarization in catecholaminergic polymorphic ventricular tachycardia: a study from cellular Ca2+ transients and action potentials to clinical monophasic action potentials and electrocardiography. Europace. 2016;18:1599–607.
127. Preininger MK, et al. A human pluripotent stem cell model of catecholaminergic polymorphic ventricular tachycardia recapitulates patient-specific drug responses. Dis Model Mech. 2016;9:927–39.
128. Sasaki K, et al. Patient-specific human induced pluripotent stem cell model assessed with electrical pacing validates S107 as a potential therapeutic agent for catecholaminergic polymorphic ventricular tachycardia. PLoS One. 2016;11:e0164795.
129. Lodola F, et al. Adeno-associated virus-mediated CASQ2 delivery rescues phenotypic alterations in a patient-specific model of recessive catecholaminergic polymorphic ventricular tachycardia. Cell Death Dis. 2016;7:e2393.
130. Maizels L, et al. Patient-specific drug screening using a human induced pluripotent stem cell model of Catecholaminergic polymorphic ventricular tachycardia type 2. Circ Arrhythm Electrophysiol. 2017;10:1–15.
131. Devalla HD, et al. TECRL, a new life-threatening inherited arrhythmia gene associated with overlapping clinical features of both LQTS and CPVT. EMBO Mol Med. 2016;8:1390–408.
132. Jung CB, et al. Dantrolene rescues arrhythmogenic RYR2 defect in a patient-specific stem cell model of catecholaminergic polymorphic ventricular tachycardia. EMBO Mol Med. 2012;4:180–91.
133. Itzhaki I, et al. Modeling of catecholaminergic polymorphic ventricular tachycardia with patient-specific human-induced pluripotent stem cells. J Am Coll Cardiol. 2012;60:990–1000.
134. Novak A, et al. Cardiomyocytes generated from CPVT D307H patients are arrhythmogenic in response to β-adrenergic stimulation. J Cell Mol Med. 2012;16:468–82.
135. Di Pasquale E, et al. CaMKII inhibition rectifies arrhythmic phenotype in a patient-specific model of catecholaminergic polymorphic ventricular tachycardia. Cell Death Dis. 2013;4:e843.
136. Zhang X-H, Morad M. Calcium signaling in human stem cell-derived cardiomyocytes: evidence from normal subjects and CPVT afflicted patients. Cell Calcium. 2015;59:98–107.
137. Penttinen K, et al. Antiarrhythmic effects of dantrolene in patients with catecholaminergic polymorphic ventricular tachycardia and replication of the responses using iPSC models. PLoS One. 2015;10:1–17.
138. Novak A, et al. Functional abnormalities in iPSC-derived cardiomyocytes generated from CPVT1 and CPVT2 patients carrying ryanodine or calsequestrin mutations. J Cell Mol Med. 2015;19:2006–18.
139. Zhang X-H, et al. Ca2+ signaling in human induced pluripotent stem cell-derived cardiomyocytes (iPS-CM) from normal and catecholaminergic polymorphic ventricular tachycardia (CPVT)-afflicted subjects. Cell Calcium. 2013;54:57–70.
140. Hoffman JI, Kaplan S. The incidence of congenital heart disease. J Am Coll Cardiol. 2002;39:1890–900.
141. Garg V, et al. GATA4 mutations cause human congenital heart defects and reveal an interaction with TBX5. Nature. 2003;424:443–7.
142. Ang YS, et al. Disease model of GATA4 mutation reveals transcription factor cooperativity in human cardiogenesis. Cell. 2016;167:1734–49.e22.
143. Jiang Y, Habibollah S, Tilgner K, Collin J, Barta T, Al-Aama JY, Tesarov L, Hussain R, Trafford AW, Kirkwood G, Sernagor E, et al. Stem Cells Transl Med. 2014;3:416–23.
144. Tomita-Mitchell A, et al. The impact of MYH6 variants in hypoplastic left heart syndrome. Physiol Genomics. 2016;48:912–21.
145. Yang C, et al. Induced pluripotent stem cell modelling of HLHS underlines the contribution of dysfunctional NOTCH signalling to impaired cardiogenesis. Hum Mol Genet. 2017;26:3031–45.
146. Bohlmeyer TJ, et al. Hypoplastic left heart syndrome myocytes are differentiated but possess a unique phenotype. Cardiovasc Pathol. 2003;12:23–31.
147. Roberts A, et al. The cardiofaciocutaneous syndrome. J Med Genet. 2006;43:833–42.
148. Weiss G, Confino Y, Shemer A, Trau H. Cutaneous manifestations in the cardiofaciocutaneous syndrome, a variant of the classical Noonan syndrome. Report of a case and review of the literature. J Eur Acad Dermatol Venereol. 2004;18:324–7.
149. Josowitz R, et al. Autonomous and non-autonomous defects underlie hypertrophic cardiomyopathy in BRAF-mutant hiPSC-derived cardiomyocytes. Stem Cell Rep. 2016;7:355–69.
150. Cashman TJ, Josowitz R, Johnson BV, Gelb BD, Costa KD. Human engineered cardiac tissues created using induced pluripotent stem cells reveal functional characteristics of BRAF-mediated hypertrophic cardiomyopathy. PLoS One. 2016;11:1–17.
151. Bidichandani SI, Delatycki MB. Friedreich taxia. In: Adam MP, Ardinger HH, Pagon RA, editors. GeneReviews. Seattle, WA: University of Washington; 2011. p. 1–18.
152. Hick A, et al. Neurons and cardiomyocytes derived from induced pluripotent stem cells as a model for mitochondrial defects in Friedreich's ataxia. Dis Model Mech. 2013;6:608–21.
153. Crombie DE, et al. Friedreich's ataxia induced pluripotent stem cell-derived cardiomyocytes display electrophysiological abnormalities and calcium handling deficiency. Aging (Albany NY). 2017;9:1440–52.
154. Lee YK, et al. Modeling of Friedreich ataxia-related iron overloading cardiomyopathy using patient-specific-induced pluripotent stem cells. Pflugers Arch Eur J Physiol. 2014;466:1831–44.
155. Lee YK, et al. Efficient attenuation of Friedreich's ataxia (FRDA) cardiomyopathy by modulation of iron homeostasis-human induced pluripotent stem cell (hiPSC) as a drug screening platform for FRDA. Int J Cardiol. 2016;203:964–71.
156. Pandolfo M, Hausmann L. Deferiprone for the treatment of Friedreich's ataxia. J Neurochem. 2013;126:142–6.
157. Bit-Avragim N, et al. The GAA repeat expansion in intron 1 of the frataxin gene is related to the severity of cardiac manifestation in patients with Friedreich's ataxia. J Mol Med. 2000;78:626–32.

158. Spurney CF. Cardiomyopathy of Duchenne muscular dystrophy: current understanding and future directions. Muscle Nerve. 2011;44:8–19.
159. Dick E, et al. Exon skipping and gene transfer restore dystrophin expression in human induced pluripotent stem cells-cardiomyocytes harboring DMD mutations. Stem Cells Dev. 2013;22:2714–24.
160. Zatti S, et al. Complete restoration of multiple dystrophin isoforms in genetically corrected Duchenne muscular dystrophy patient-derived cardiomyocytes. Mol Ther Methods Clin Dev. 2014;1:1.
161. Guan X, et al. Dystrophin-deficient cardiomyocytes derived from human urine: new biologic reagents for drug discovery. Stem Cell Res. 2014;12:467–80.
162. Lin B, et al. Modeling and studying mechanism of dilated cardiomyopathy using induced pluripotent stem cells derived from Duchenne Muscular Dystrophy (DMD) patients. Dis Model Mech. 2015;8:457–66.
163. Macadangdang J, et al. Nanopatterned human iPSC-based model of a dystrophin-null cardiomyopathic phenotype. Cell Mol Bioeng. 2015;8:320–32.
164. Ramaciotti C, Iannaccone ST, Scott WA. Myocardial cell damage in Duchenne muscular dystrophy. Pediatr Cardiol. 2003;24:503–6.
165. Romeo V. Myotonic dystrophy type 1 or Steinert's disease. Adv Exp Med Biol. 2012;724:239–57.
166. Fu Y, et al. An unstable triplet repeat in a gene related to myotonic muscular dystrophy. Science. 1992;255:1256–8.
167. Gao Y, et al. Genome therapy of myotonic dystrophy type 1 iPS cells for development of autologous stem cell therapy. Mol Ther. 2016;24:1378–87.
168. Christians ES, Ishiwata T, Benjamin IJ. Small heat shock proteins in redox metabolism: implications for cardiovascular diseases. Int J Biochem Cell Biol. 2012;44:1632–45.
169. Mitzelfelt KA, et al. The human 343delT HSPB5 chaperone associated with early-onset skeletal myopathy causes defects in protein solubility. J Biol Chem. 2016;291:14939–53.
170. Wetterau JR, et al. Absence of microsomal triglyceride transfer protein in individuals with abetalipoproteinemia. Science. 1992;258:999–1001.
171. Zamel R, Khan R, Pollex RL, Hegele RA. Abetalipoproteinemia: two case reports and literature review. Orphanet J Rare Dis. 2008;3:19.
172. Liu Y, et al. Lack of MTTP activity in pluripotent stem cell-derived hepatocytes and cardiomyocytes abolishes apoB secretion and increases cell stress. Cell Rep. 2017;19:1456–66.
173. Ebert AD, et al. Characterization of the molecular mechanisms underlying increased ischemic damage in the aldehyde dehydrogenase 2 genetic polymorphism using a human induced pluripotent stem cell model system. Sci Transl Med. 2014;6:255ra130.
174. Zhang H, Gong DX, Zhang YJ, Li SJ, Hu S. Effect of mitochondrial aldehyde dehydrogenase-2 genotype on cardioprotection in patients with congenital heart disease. Eur Heart J. 2012;33:1606–14.
175. Stillitano F, et al. Modeling susceptibility to drug-induced long QT with a panel of subject-specific induced pluripotent stem cells. Elife. 2017;6:e19406.
176. Borchert T, et al. Catecholamine-dependent β-adrenergic signaling in a pluripotent stem cell model of takotsubo cardiomyopathy. J Am Coll Cardiol. 2017;70:975–91.
177. Caballero R, et al. Tbx20 controls the expression of the KCNH2 gene and of hERG channels. Proc Natl Acad Sci USA. 2017;114:E416–25.
178. Sheikh, N. et al. 170 Ethnic differences in phenotypic expression of hypertrophic cardiomyopathy. Heart. 2011;97:A95.
179. Kim K, et al. Donor cell type can influence the epigenome and differentiation potential of human induced pluripotent stem cells. Nat Biotechnol. 2011;29:1117–9.
180. Sanchez-Freire V, et al. Effect of human donor cell source on differentiation and function of cardiac induced pluripotent stem cells. J Am Coll Cardiol. 2014;64:436–48.
181. Fusaki N, Ban H, Nishiyama A, Saeki K, Hasegawa M. Efficient induction of transgene-free human pluripotent stem cells using a vector based on Sendai virus, an RNA virus that does not integrate into the host genome. Proc Jpn Acad Ser B Phys Biol Sci. 2009;85:348–62.
182. Yu J, et al. Induced pluripotent stem cell lines derived from human somatic cells. Science. 2007;318:1917–20.
183. Warren L, et al. Highly efficient reprogramming to pluripotency and directed differentiation of human cells with synthetic modified mRNA. Cell Stem Cell. 2010;7:618–30.
184. Mummery C, et al. Differentiation of human embryonic stem cells to cardiomyocytes: role of coculture with visceral endoderm-like cells. Circulation. 2003;107:2733–40.
185. Zhang J, et al. Functional cardiomyocytes derived from human induced pluripotent stem cells. Circ Res. 2009;104:e30–41.
186. Laflamme MA, et al. Cardiomyocytes derived from human embryonic stem cells in pro-survival factors enhance function of infarcted rat hearts. Nat Biotechnol. 2007;25:1015–24.
187. Burridge PW, Keller G, Gold JD, Wu JC. Production of de novo cardiomyocytes: human pluripotent stem cell differentiation and direct reprogramming. Cell Stem Cell. 2012;10:16–28.
188. Batalov I, Feinberg AW. Differentiation of cardiomyocytes from human pluripotent stem cells using monolayer culture. Biomark Insights. 2015;10:71–6.
189. Bergmann O, et al. Dynamics of cell generation and turnover in the human heart. Cell. 2015;161:1566–75.
190. Lieu DK, et al. Absence of transverse tubules contributes to non-uniform Ca 2+ wavefronts in mouse and human embryonic stem cell–derived cardiomyocytes. Stem Cells Dev. 2009;18:1493–500.
191. Hwang HS, et al. Comparable calcium handling of human iPSC-derived cardiomyocytes generated by multiple laboratories. J Mol Cell Cardiol. 2015;85:79–88.
192. Veerman CC, et al. Immaturity of human stem-cell-derived cardiomyocytes in culture: fatal flaw or soluble problem? Stem Cells Dev. 2015;24:1035–52.
193. Vunjak Novakovic G, Eschenhagen T, Mummery C. Myocardial tissue engineering: in vitro models. Cold Spring Harb Perspect Med. 2014;4:a014076.
194. Mills RJ, Voges HK, Porrello ER, Hudson JE. Disease modeling and functional screening using engineered heart tissue. Curr Opin Physiol. 2018;1:80–8.
195. Castilho M, et al. Melt electrowriting allows tailored microstructural and mechanical Design of Scaffolds to advance functional human myocardial tissue formation. Adv Funct Mater. 2018;28:1803151.
196. Smith C, et al. Whole-genome sequencing analysis reveals high specificity of CRISPR/Cas9 and TALEN-based genome editing in human iPSCs. Cell Stem Cell. 2014;15:12–3.
197. Brenière-Letuffe D, et al. Clonal dynamics studied in cultured induced pluripotent stem cells reveal major growth imbalances within a few weeks. Stem Cell Res Ther. 2018;9:1–11.
198. Vitale AM, et al. Variability in the generation of induced pluripotent stem cells: importance for disease modeling. Stem Cells Transl Med. 2012;1:641–50.
199. Stacey GN, Crook JM, Hei D, Ludwig T. Banking human induced pluripotent stem cells: lessons learned from embryonic stem cells? Cell Stem Cell. 2013;13:385–8.
200. De Sousa PA, et al. Rapid establishment of the European Bank for induced pluripotent stem cells (EBiSC)—the hot start experience. Stem Cell Res. 2017;20:105–14.

Prenatal Diagnosis and Preimplantation Genetic Testing for Inherited Cardiac Diseases

27

E. A. Nannenberg and Y. Arens

Introduction

As depicted in the previous chapters, most inherited cardiac diseases, i.e., cardiomyopathies and inherited arrhythmia syndromes, have an autosomal dominant pattern of inheritance and are characterized by incomplete penetrance and variable expression. Patients can be asymptomatic throughout life, but can also experience ventricular arrhythmias (SCD), heart failure, and embolic stroke as a result of the inherited cardiac disease. Cardiomyopathies and inherited arrhythmia syndromes can present in all age groups; from infancy to (late) adulthood [1, 2].

Treatment or preventive options are available for most of the inherited cardiac diseases. In case of genetic cardiomyopathies therapeutic options are available for treatment of the symptoms such as life style advices, antiarrhythmic drugs, heart failure medication, devices to treat life-threatening arrhythmias and, ultimately heart transplantation. These disorders cannot be cured nowadays. For most inherited arrhythmia syndromes preventive treatment options, such as life style advices (for instance alcohol and fever advices), betablockers, and ICDs, are available and have proven to substantially reduce the risk of SCD [3–6].

The discovery of genes known to be associated with cardiomyopathies and inherited arrhythmia syndromes has made genetic testing possible in many patients with one of these diseases [7]. When a disease-causing mutation is identified, predictive genetic testing of (asymptomatic) relatives can be performed to identify other individuals at risk, which then allows for timely treatment. For some inherited arrhythmia syndromes treatment can be offered before symptoms have developed. However, for inherited cardiomyopathies, the effect of treatment in a presymptomatic disease stage is still debated [6–9].

Predictive genetic testing is not only technically available after birth, but also during pregnancy by prenatal diagnosis. In addition there is the possibility of preimplantation genetic testing (PGT), previously called preimplantation genetic diagnostics (PGD). Consequently, mutation positive couples can be faced with difficult decisions regarding their reproductive options. In this chapter, we discuss the different techniques of prenatal diagnosis and preimplantation genetic testing, and provide an overview of prenatal diagnosis and preimplantation genetic testing for inherited cardiac diseases.

Prenatal Diagnosis (PND)

Prenatal diagnosis (PND) consist of a biopsy of placentary tissue (chorion villus sampling) through the abdominal wall or cervix performed between 10 and 13 weeks of gestation to obtain tissue for genetic analysis, or it consists of a puncture through the abdominal wall to obtain amniotic fluid (amniocentesis), performed from 15 weeks gestation (Fig. 27.1). Both procedures have an increased risk of miscarriage due to the invasiveness of the test. The estimated risk of a miscarriage associated with chorion villus sampling is 5 in 1000 (0.5%) and for amniocentesis it is estimated 3 in 1000 (0.3%) [10]. Subsequently, genetic analysis of the tissue can be performed to reveal the mutation status of the fetus. As previously mentioned, invasive prenatal procedures carry a risk of miscarriage and therefore are preferably performed only if the couple intends to terminate the pregnancy. Otherwise testing after birth could also be an option. Since PND may involve the termination of pregnancy of a fetus in case the fetus is mutation positive, emotional, religious, ethical, or moral considerations play an important role for many couples performing PND and should be thoroughly discussed with the involved couple.

E. A. Nannenberg
Department of Clinical Genetics, Amsterdam UMC, University of Amsterdam, AZ, Amsterdam, Netherlands
e-mail: e.a.nannenberg@amc.uva.nl

Y. Arens (✉)
Department of Clinical Genetics, Maastricht University Medical Center, Maastricht, Netherlands
e-mail: yvonne.arens@mumc.nl

H. F. Baars et al. (eds.), *Clinical Cardiogenetics*, https://doi.org/10.1007/978-3-030-45457-9_27

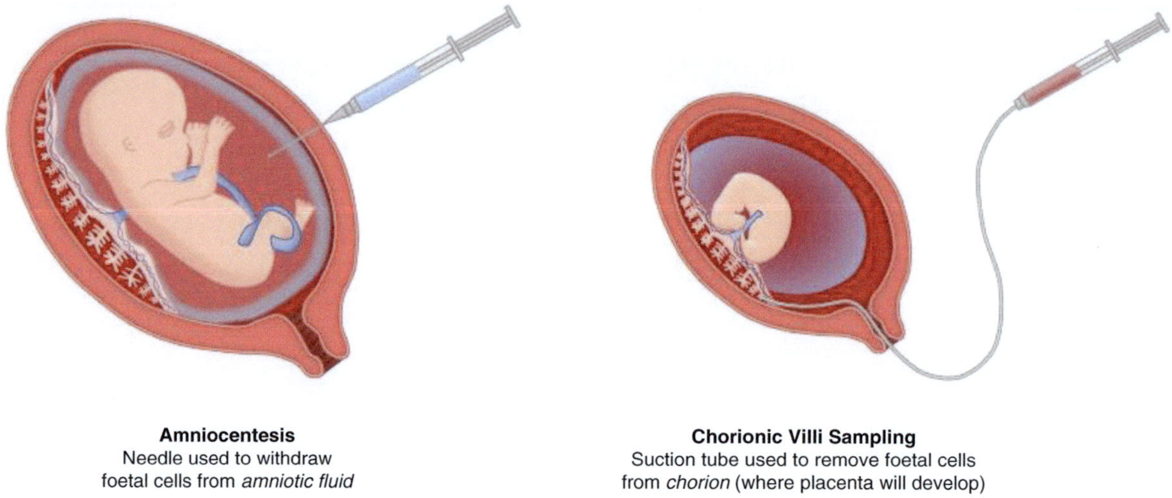

Fig. 27.1.

Preimplantation Genetic Testing (PGT)

Preimplantation genetic testing (PGT) is a reproductive option for mutation-positive patients of inherited diseases wishing to avoid transmission of the mutation to their offspring [11]. Since its introduction, preimplantation genetic testing (PGT) has been established as an alternative to PND to avoid pregnancy termination in couples who are at high risk of transmitting genetic disorders. PGT involves the use of in vitro fertilization (IVF) to create embryos that are biopsied and genetically tested Fig. 27.2. Only embryos without the mutation are transferred into the uterus [12, 13]. These couples are in general without fertility problems and only undergo an IVF treatment because of the embryo selection process. The IVF treatment involves risks as there is evidence that children born after IVF might have an increased risk of adverse perinatal outcome as prematurity and low and very low birth weight [14, 15].

For PGT of any genetic reason a specific test has to be developed, therefore there is a considerable timeframe involved, which might change by the development of new techniques in the future. In PGT only very small amounts of DNA are available, since PGT is performed on single embryonic cells or just a few embryonic cells. This implies a long process of fine-tuning the laboratory conditions to be able to get a reliable result. Linked markers are related to the disease causing mutation. For an efficient and accurate diagnosis in the embryo, participation of affected and non-affected family members is needed. This is often a time-consuming process [16–18].

PGT is an option for couples with a cardiogenetic disease who do not want to transmit the disease to the next generation. To be eligible and accepted for PGT in the Netherlands, patients have to meet specific criteria, described in Table 27.1.

Noninvasive Prenatal Diagnosis (NIPD)

In 1997, Lo et al. identified cell-free fetal DNA in the maternal circulation [19]. This scientific finding has paved the way to investigate the option of analyzing this fetal genetic material extracted from maternal blood for NIPD in monogenic disorders. Nowadays, there are a few reports of NIPD for a limited amount of single gene disorders (not for inherited cardiac diseases), but it is to be expected that NIPD for families at high risk of genetic conditions will become more widely available for monogenic disorders [20].

PND and PGT for Inherited Cardiac Diseases

In the literature, reports of PND and PGT for inherited cardiac diseases are scarce.

PND has been described in literature in a patient with hypertrophic cardiomyopathy (HCM) and a malignant family history of HCM caused by a pathogenic mutation in the *MYH7* gene [21]. In another report, 22 HCM patients were counseled for prenatal diagnosis, yet none of these couples eventually performed PND [22].

By contacting all clinical genetic departments in the Netherlands, we obtained the number of cases of PND for inherited cardiac diseases in the period 2001–2015. Between 2001 and 2015, PND has been performed 8 times for different inherited arrhythmia syndromes and cardiomyopathies in the Netherlands; 3 couples for HCM, 2 couples for dilated cardiomyopathy (DCM) and 1 for long QT syndrome (LQTS). This is approximately 0.3–0.7% of the total number of PNDs performed yearly and a fraction of the total number of patients counseled with a heart disease at the departments of clinical genetics (0.02–0.2%). In all families, a severe phenotype or a severe family history of sudden cardiac death was present [23].

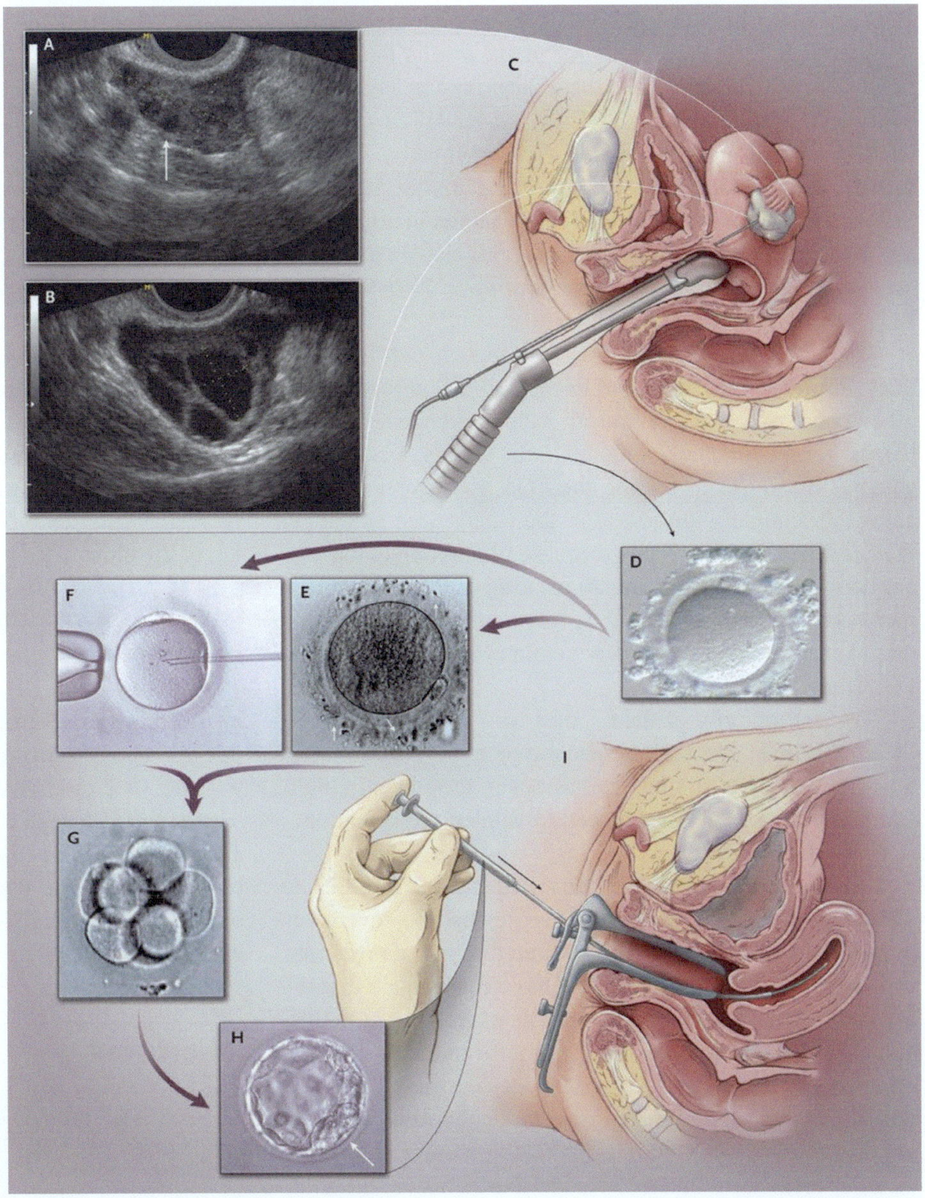

Fig. 27.2. (**a**, **b**) Hormonal stimulation; (**c**) oocyte retrieval; (**d**) oocyte; (**e**, **f**) IVF; (**g**, **h**) PGD; (**i**) embryo transfer

Table 27.1 PGT criteria in the Netherlands

PGT criteria	
Recurrence risk	High; >10%
Disease	Severe
Mutation	Known
Classification	Pathogenic or likely pathogenic
Technically	Possible
IVF	Semen analysis and hormonal evaluation normal
Age	<40 years female
BMI	35

Data on PGT performed for monogenetic diseases and the outcome of assisted reproductive techniques have been collected and published by the European Society for Human Reproduction and Embryology (ESHRE) from 1997 onwards. Until 2010, diagnoses were included in the reports. In 2006, the first cardiogenetic case, Brugada syndrome, was described.

Between 2006 and 2010, in total 24 PGT cycles have been performed in Europe for different inherited cardiac diseases (1 DCM, 7 HCM, 2 ARVC, 1 congenital cardiomyopathy, 4 LQTS, 7 BrS, and 2 CPVT) [24–26].

Furthermore, in literature, PGT has been described for DCM caused by a *LMNA* mutation, and for HCM caused by *MYBPC3* and *TNNI3* gene mutations. All patients had a severe phenotype and/or a family history with premature sudden death [27]. In the Netherlands, data of patients opting for PGT for inherited diseases is collected by the Dutch PGT consortium [28]. In total, 3280 couples were referred for PGT in the Netherlands between 1995 and 2017. Of these couples, 45 couples (~1%) with an inherited cardiac disease visited the PGT clinic for intake during this period. In 34 referred couples (76%) the indication was a cardiomyopathy. Couples came for PGT intake for HCM (n = 15), DCM (n = 16), noncompaction cardiomyopathy (NCCM) (n = 1), and arrhythmogenic cardiomyopathy-ACM (n = 2). Eleven couples were referred for a channelopathy (24%), i.e., Brugada syndrome (BrS) (n = 2), idiopathic VF (based on the dpp6 risk haplotype on chromosome 7) (n = 1), and LQTS (n = 3).

After intensive counselling, 11 couples (cardiomyopathies and idiopathic VF) continued the PGT procedure. All other couples decided to fulfill their child wish by other means, e.g., natural conception without testing, use of donor gametes or adoption. During the PGT procedure, the idiopathic VF couple withdrew after the customized single-cell PGT test had been designed, because of emotional and ethical considerations. Four mutation positive couples with an increased cardiomyopathy risk for their offspring became pregnant of a mutation negative child after PGT (data from PGDNederland) [28].

The vast majority of the couples who seek counseling at the PGT clinic have a severe phenotype or have experienced a family history of sudden cardiac death; teenagers dying of sudden cardiac death, or the need for a heart transplant or an ICD in young adults.

Although we know that in some patients and families the phenotype of inherited cardiac diseases can be severe, the number of patients, described in literature and reports, performing PND and PGT is small. One can speculate that due to incomplete penetrance and variable expression, it is difficult to predict to what extent the future mutation-carrying child will be at increased risk of (sudden) cardiac death. The possibilities to predict the expression of the mutation in an unborn child are very limited with the current (molecular genetic) techniques and knowledge. Furthermore, the availability of treatment options for some inherited cardiac diseases to reduce the risk of cardiac death, may also contribute to the low request for PND. The incomplete penetrance, variable expression, perceived burden of the disease, available preventive options, and lack of knowledge or information about reproductive options might play a role, but remains to be further elucidated in future research.

Case

A couple requested for PGT because of dilated cardiomyopathy (DCM). There was a family history of sudden death. A brother died at the age of 18 after a cardiac arrest. A core panel of 46 of the cardiac cardiomyopathy genes was performed and a Dutch *PLN* founder mutation was found (c.40_42del;p.Arg14del). The man turned out to have this heterozygous mutation. No signs of a cardiomyopathy were yet observed at cardiac evaluation. Counseling by a clinical geneticist and psychologist was performed. The PGT working group accepted the couple's request for PGT. A specific genetic test was set up, which took 9 months. During this period the couple was accepted for IVF by the gynecologist. The PGT treatment was planned 3 months later. The first attempt was without any suitable embryo, but after the second attempt an unaffected embryo could be transferred and the partner became pregnant. Prenatal testing was offered to the couple, because of the misdiagnosis risk of 2% due to the low amounts of DNA available in PGT. The couple declined. A healthy son was born 9 months later. DNA diagnostics can be performed after birth to confirm the mutation negative status of the child.

In Summary

PND and preimplantation genetic testing (PGT) are reproductive options for mutation carriers of inherited diseases wishing to avoid transmission of the predisposition to their offspring. Although inherited cardiac diseases can exhibit a severe phenotype or a severe family history of sudden cardiac death, the number of patients with inherited cardiac diseases opting for and continuing with PND and PGT is small.

References

1. Lieve KV, Wilde AA. Inherited ion channel diseases: a brief review. Europace. 2015;17(Suppl 2):ii1–6.
2. Kaski JP, Elliott P. Hypertrophic, dilated, and restrictive cardiomyopathies. In: Kumar D, Elliott P, editors. Principles and practice of clinical cardiovascular genetics. Oxford: Oxford University Press; 2010. p. 189–212.
3. Marian AJ, Braunwald E. Hypertrophic cardiomyopathy: genetics, pathogenesis, clinical manifestations, diagnosis, and therapy. Circ Res. 2017;121(7):749–70.
4. Weintraub RG, Semsarian C, Macdonald P. Dilated cardiomyopathy. Lancet. 2017;390(10092):400–14.
5. Authors/Task Force Members, et al. 2014 ESC Guidelines on diagnosis and management of hypertrophic cardiomyopathy: the Task Force for the Diagnosis and Management of Hypertrophic Cardiomyopathy of the European Society of Cardiology (ESC). Eur Heart J. 2014;35(39):2733–79.
6. Priori SG, Wilde AA, Horie M, et al. HRS/EHRA/APHRS expert consensus statement on the diagnosis and management of patients with inherited primary arrhythmia syndromes. Heart Rhythm. 2013;10:1932–63.
7. Wilde AAM, Behr ER. Genetic testing for inherited cardiac disease. Nat Rev Cardiol. 2013;10:571–83.

8. Wilde AAM, Amin A. Channelopathies, genetic testing and risk stratification. Int J Cardiol. 2017;237:53–5.
9. Aleksova N, Rutberg J, Green M, Haddad H. Genetic testing in cardiomyopathies: an update on indications and benefits. Curr Opin Cardiol. 2017;32(2):189–95.
10. Richtlijn NVOG Nota Prenatale Diagnostiek, 2017.
11. Derks-Smeets IA, Gietel-Habets JJ, Tibben A, Tjan-Heijnen VC, Meijer-Hoogeveen M, Geraedts JP, van Golde R, Gomez-Garcia E, van den Bogaart E, van Hooijdonk M, de Die-Smulders CE, van Osch LA. Decision-making on preimplantation genetic diagnosis and prenatal diagnosis: a challenge for couples with hereditary breast and ovarian cancer. Hum Reprod. 2014;29(5):1103–12.
12. Harton GL, De Rycke M, Fiorentino F, European Society for Human Reproduction and Embryology (ESHRE) PGD Consortium, et al. ESHRE PGD Consortium best practice guidelines for amplification-based PGD. Hum Reprod. 2011;26(1):33–40.
13. Harton GL, Harper JC, Coonen E, Pehlivan T, Vesela K, Wilton L, European Society for Human Reproduction and Embryology (ESHRE) PGD Consortium. ESHRE PGD Consortium best practice guidelines for fluorescence in situ hybridization-based PGD. Hum Reprod. 2011;26(1):25–32.
14. Hasson J, Limoni D, Malcov M, Frumkin T, Amir H, Shavit T, Bay B, Many A, Almog B. Obstetric and neonatal outcomes of pregnancies conceived after preimplantation genetic diagnosis: cohort study and meta-analysis. Reprod BioMed Online. 2017;35(2):208–18.
15. Liebaers I, Desmyttere S, Verpoest W, De Rycke M, Staessen C, Sermon K, Devroey P, Haentjens P, Bonduelle M. Report on a consecutive series of 581 children born after blastomere biopsy for preimplantation genetic diagnosis. Hum Reprod. 2010;25(1):275–82.
16. Feuer S, Rinaudo P. Preimplantation stress and development. Birth Defects Res C Embryo Today. 2012;96(4):299–314.
17. Zacchini F, Arena R, Abramik A, Ptak GE. Embryo biopsy and development: the known and the unknown. Reproduction. 2017;154(5):R143–8.
18. Ma H, et al. Correction of a pathogenic gene mutation in human embryos. Nature. 2017;548:413–9.
19. Lo YM, Corbetta N, Chamberlain PF, et al. Presence of fetal DNA in maternal plasma and serum. Lancet. 1997;350(9560):485–7.
20. Lench N, Barrett A, Fielding S, McKay F, Hill M, Jenkins L, White H, Chitty LS. The clinical implementation of non-invasive prenatal diagnosis for single-gene disorders: challenges and progress made. Prenat Diagn. 2013;33(6):555–62.
21. Charron P, Heron D, Gargiulo M, et al. Prenatal molecular diagnosis in hypertrophic cardiomyopathy: report of the first case. Prenat Diagn. 2004;24:701–3.
22. Charron P, Heron D, Gargiulo M, et al. Genetic testing and genetic counselling in hypertrophic cardiomyopathy: the French experience. J Med Genet. 2002;39:741–6.
23. Nannenberg EA. Mortality in inherited cardiac diseases. Thesis. 2014. https://pure.uva.nl/ws/files/2471991/153035_01_2_.pdf
24. Moutou C, Goossens V, Coonen E, et al. ESHRE PGD Consortium data collection XII: cycles from January to December 2009 with pregnancy follow-up to October 2010. Hum Reprod. 2014;29:880–903.
25. Goossens V, Traeger-Synodinos J, Coonen E, et al. ESHRE PGD Consortium data collection XI: cycles from January to December 2008 with pregnancy follow-up to October 2009. Hum Reprod. 2012;27:1887–911.
26. Harper JC, Coonen E, De Rycke M, et al. ESHRE PGD Consortium data collection X: cycles from January to December 2007 with pregnancy follow-up to October 2008. Hum Reprod. 2010;25:2685–707.
27. Kuliev A, Pomerantseva E, Polling D, et al. PGD for inherited cardiac diseases. Reprod BioMed Online. 2012;24:443–53.
28. https://www.pgdnederland.nl/jaarverslagen

MIX
Papier aus verantwortungsvollen Quellen
Paper from responsible sources
FSC® C105338

If you have any concerns about our products,
you can contact us on
ProductSafety@springernature.com

In case Publisher is established outside the EU,
the EU authorized representative is:
Springer Nature Customer Service Center GmbH
Europaplatz 3, 69115 Heidelberg, Germany

Printed by Libri Plureos GmbH
in Hamburg, Germany